# Medicine for Finals
# and Beyond

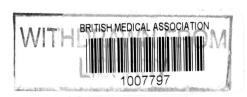

# Medicine for Finals and Beyond

## THIRD EDITION

Edited by

### John S. Axford
DSc MD FRCP FRCPCH
Emeritus Professor of Clinical Rheumatology
St George's Hospital
University of London
London UK

### Chris A. O'Callaghan
BM BCh MA DPhil DM FHEA FRCP
Professor of Medicine
Fellow of The Queen's College
Nuffield Department of Medicine
University of Oxford
Hon Consultant Physician and Nephrologist
Oxford University Hospitals
Oxford, UK

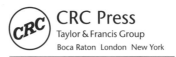

CRC Press
Taylor & Francis Group
Boca Raton  London  New York

CRC Press is an imprint of the
Taylor & Francis Group, an **informa** business

First edition published 2023
by CRC Press
2 Park Square, Milton Park, Abingdon, Oxon, OX14 4RN

and by CRC Press
6000 Broken Sound Parkway NW, Suite 300,

Boca Raton, FL 33487-2742

This title is a reworked and condensed version of *Medicine* published by Blackwell, 2004

CRC Press is an imprint of Informa UK Limited

*British Library Cataloguing-in-Publication Data*
A catalogue record for this book is available from the British Library

ISBN: 978-1-032-04526-9 (hbk)
ISBN: 978-0-367-15059-4 (pbk)
ISBN: 978-1-003-19361-6 (ebk)

DOI: 10.1201/9781003193616

Typeset in Palatino LT Std
by KnowledgeWorks Global Ltd.

Instructors can register to gain access to Figures Slides as PowerPoint or PDF. To register, they must request access at the following location: https://routledgetextbooks.com/textbooks/instructor_downloads/

Printed in Great Britain by Bell and Bain Ltd, Glasgow

# The editors

**John Axford** is a Consultant in Adult and Paediatric Rheumatology and Emeritus Professor of Clinical Rheumatology at St George's Hospital, University of London.

After training at University College Hospital he worked at The National Hospital for Neurology, The Hammersmith Hospital, The Royal Brompton Hospital, King's College Hospital and the New England Medical Center, Boston, Massachusetts, USA.

He has enjoyed teaching medicine throughout his career and pioneered video teaching to developing countries with the Royal Society of Medicine.

He is an author and editor of the textbook *UpToDate*.

**Chris O'Callaghan** is Professor of Medicine at the University of Oxford and a Consultant Physician (in Acute General Medicine) and Consultant Nephrologist in the Oxford University Hospitals.

He is Chief Examiner in Medicine for the University of Oxford, runs a research group, teaches medical students, and is a Fellow and former Dean of The Queens' College, Oxford.

After training and working in Oxford he worked at Guy's, St Thomas', Hammersmith, Brompton and Lewisham Hospitals in London, Royal Stoke University Hospital, the University of California, San Francisco, and the California Institute of Technology.

His other books include *The Kidney at a Glance* and *The MRCP Part I: a System Based Tutorial*.

# Contents

# Contributors

**Rachel L. Allen** BSc (Hons) DPhil
Professor & Director of the Institute of Medical and
    Biomedical Education
St George's, University of London
London, UK

**John S. Axford** DSc MD FRCP FRCPCH
Emeritus Professor of Clinical Rheumatology
St George's Hospital
University of London
London, UK

**Kevin C.R. Baynes** BA (Oxon) MBBS PhD FRCP
Consultant in Diabetes & Endocrinology
London North West University Healthcare NHS Trust
London, UK

**Gary Bell** BA MB BS FRCPsych
Consultant Psychiatrist
Cognacity
London, UK

**Christopher J. Black** MB BS(Hons) PhD MRCP
Consultant Gastroenterologist
Leeds Teaching Hospitals NHS Trust
Leeds, UK

**Jim Bolton** MB BS BSc(Hons) FRCPsych
Consultant Psychiatrist
Department of Liaison Psychiatry
St Helier Hospital
London, UK

**Pierre-Marc Bouloux** BSc MB BS (Hons) MD FRCP
Director and Consultant Endocrinologist
Centre for Endocrinology
Royal Free Campus
UCL
London, UK

**Christopher B. Bunker** MA MD FRCP
Consultant Dermatologist
and Honorary Professor of Dermatology
UCL and Chelsea & Westminster Hospitals,
and
University College and Imperial College
London, UK

**Ruth Corrigan** BM BCh PhD
Academic Clinical Lecturer in Microbiology and Infectious
    Diseases
Nuffield Department of Clinical Laboratory Sciences
University of Oxford
Oxford, UK

**Paul I. Dargan** MB BS FRCP FEAPCCT FAACT
Professor of Clinical Toxicology
Guy's & St Thomas' NHS Foundation Trust
and King's College Hospital
London, UK

**Gareth R. Davies** BSc (Hons) MD FRCP
Consultant Physician and Gastroenterologist
Harrogate District Hospital
Harrogate, UK

**Maria Dudareva** BM BCh PhD MRCP
NIHR Doctoral Research Fellow
Bone Infection Unit
Oxford University Hospitals NHS Trust
Oxford, UK

**Susanna Dunachie** BM ChB PhD FRCP FRCPath
Professor of Infectious Diseases
University of Oxford
Oxford, UK

**Hanif Esmail** MA MBBS MRCP PhD FRCPath
Associate Professor and Honorary Consultant in Infectious
    Diseases
University College London and Hospital for Tropical
    Diseases
University College London Hospitals
London, UK

**Keeley Fairbrass** BSc(Hons) MBChB(Hons) MRCP
Gastroenterology Registrar and Clinical Research Fellow
Leeds Teaching Hospitals NHS Trust
Leeds, UK

**Thomas A. Fox** BSc MB ChB MSc MRCP FRCPath
Department of Haematology
University College Hospital
London, UK

**Faye Gishen MB BS BSc FRCP EdD PFHEA**
Professor of Medical Education & Palliative Medicine
UCL Medical School
London, UK

**Harrison Howarth BSc (Hons) MB BS MRCPsych**
Core Psychiatry Trainee
Camden and Islington NHS Foundation Trust
London, UK

**Jeffrey Lee MB BS (Hons) FRCP**
Consultant Rheumatologist
Royal Free Hospital
London, UK

**Alexander Lyon MA BM BCh PhD FRCP FHFA**
Senior Lecturer and Honorary Consultant Cardiologist
Imperial College London and Royal Brompton Hospital
London, UK

**Malcolm R. Macleod BSc(Hons) MB ChB PhD FRCP FRSB**
Professor of Neurology and Translational Neurosciences
    (University of Edinburgh)
and Honorary Consultant Neurologist (NHS Forth Valley)
Edinburgh, UK

**Alison J. Maycock MB BChir (Cantab) MA MRCGP**
General Practitioner Partner, Trainer and Appraiser
Hollow Way Medical Centre
Oxford, UK

**Emma C. Morris BA MA MB BChir PhD FRCP FRCPath FMedSci**
Professor of Clinical Cell & Gene Therapy
UCL Division of Infection and Immunity
Hon Consultant Haematologist
University College London Hospitals NHS Foundation Trust
and Royal Free London Hospitals NHS Foundation Trust
London, UK

**James Neuberger DM FRCP**
Hon Consultant Physician
The Liver and Hepatobiliary Unit
Queen Elizabeth Hospital
Birmingham, UK

**Chris A. O'Callaghan BM BCh MA DPhil DM FHEA FRCP**
Professor of Medicine
Fellow of The Queen's College
Nuffield Department of Medicine
University of Oxford
Hon Consultant Physician and Nephrologist
Oxford University Hospitals
Oxford, UK

**Ian Pavord MA MBBS DM FRCP FERS FMedSci**
Professor of Respiratory Medicine
Respiratory Medicine Unit and Oxford Respiratory NIHR BRC
Nuffield Department of Clinical Medicine
University of Oxford
and John Radcliffe Hospital
Oxford, UK

**Nayia Petousi MA MB BChir MRCP DPhil**
Consultant Respiratory Physician
Oxford University Hospitals NHS Foundation Trust
Oxford, UK

**Nick Talbot BM BCh MA DPhil MRCP**
Departmental Lecturer
Department of Physiology, Anatomy and Genetics
University of Oxford
Consultant in Respiratory Medicine
Oxford University Hospitals NHS Foundation Trust
Oxford, UK

**Adrian Tookman MB BS FRCP**
Consultant Palliative Medicine
Former Medical Director Marie Curie Hospice
London, UK

**Richard E. Watchorn MB BCh BAO MD FRCP**
Consultant Dermatologist
Beaumont Hospital, Dublin
and Honorary Consultant Dermatologist
University College London Hospitals NHS Foundation Trust
Honorary Clinical Senior Lecturer
Royal College of Surgeons of Ireland
and Imperial College London
London, UK

# Acknowledgements

All those who contributed to editions of this book's predecessor, Medicine—this new book builds on their work especially: Stephen H. Gillespie (Chapter 3), Chris Sonnex (Chapter 3), Christopher Carne (Chapter 3), Emma M. Clark (Chapter 5), Jon Tobias (Chapter 5), M.J. Walshaw (Chapter 6), Charles Hind (Chapter 6), C.W. Pumphrey (Chapter 6), J.C. Kingswood (Chapter 8), D.K. Packham (Chapter 8), D.S. Rampton (Chapter 10), D.J. Betteridge (Chapter 11), Felicity Kaplan (Chapter 12), Gerard S. Conway (Chapter 12), C.J. Mumford (Chapter 13), D.H. Bevan (Chapter 15), A.C. Kurowska (Chapter 16), A.K. Fletcher (Chapter 17) and F.P. Morris (Chapter 17). Peter Saugman was a key supporter from the start.

Jo Koster and Jordan Wearing for superb editorial support with this edition. Nora Naughton for her outstanding and incredibly efficient project management of the production of this book. Becky Freeman and Susan Smyth for their tireless efforts copy-editing and proof-reading respectively.

M. Ali Abbasi, Christine Heron and Andrew Hine for radiology advice. Julia Steed for keeping the text under control.

The following doctors for reviewing the text and providing helpful feedback: Nina Agarwal, Pat Woo Mark Cassar, Vijay Hadela, Marcus Hughes, Simon Lambracos, Brian Lunn, Mike Mendall, Muthana Al Obaidi, Sanjeev Patel, Johnathan Rogers, Malcolm Rustin, Paddy Stone and Malcolm Walker.

Our excellent colleagues for their valued expertise and discussions of medicine.

# Introduction

**Our focus in this condensed third edition is on helping you to pass your final assessments and examinations with ease and confidence.**

*Medicine for Finals and Beyond* contains all the information that you need to qualify as a doctor. The contributing authors are experts in their respective fields, as well as experienced writers and teachers. The book has been strongly influenced by input from many students and colleagues. Much has changed since the second edition was published and some chapters needed further refinement as the pandemic unfolded.

## DESIGNED FOR LEARNING

To pass examinations and to practise medicine well, it is important to understand the basics. There are many textbooks of medicine, but we believe that they are generally not well designed for learning. Some have grown thicker with each edition and include detail that is beyond the needs of students and, indeed, of many qualified doctors. This can make it difficult to see the 'wood for the trees' and slows and complicates learning.

*Medicine for Finals and Beyond* has been carefully crafted to avoid the overwhelming. Each system is presented in an integrated chapter, with sections on the basic structure, function and biology of the system, on clinical presentations, on the approach to the patient and on the diseases affecting that system. There is a clear focus on evidence-based medicine as well as consideration of the social, caring and communicative aspects of practice and the impact of disease and treatment on the lives of patients.

The material in this edition has been arranged to aid learning and recall. The amount of information on each topic has been carefully regulated. Important topics are readily identifiable and deliberately presented in detail if they are very common or are often examined. Illustrations have been used extensively to aid learning.

The book is written for students but will also be of use to doctors and other healthcare workers who are trying to understand or revise medicine, so it will remain useful as you advance beyond your student years.

## HOW TO USE THIS BOOK

Chapter 1 provides an overview of the human dimension to clinical medicine and Chapter 2 reviews the basic science. Together, these help you to understand what underpins modern medical practice. The chapters which follow cover systems. Navigation is aided by the coloured page end-tabs that label each chapter. Drugs are referred to by their Recommended International Non-proprietary Name (rINN) although, in a few cases, older names are also provided if they are still in use.

## CHAPTER LAYOUT

The system chapters cover structure and function, approach to the patient and diseases and their management. Aids to learning within each chapter highlight important material:

- **At a Glance boxes** summarize core topics for rapid revision.
- **History and Examination boxes** outline key features to elicit from the patient.
- **Emergency boxes** summarize essential information about emergencies.
- **Must-know checklists** highlight key points.

The editors and authors have enjoyed creating this third edition and are confident that students will find it a useful and enjoyable book as they learn medicine and particularly in the pressured run-up to final exams. The editors suggest that you remember:

'the patient is always right…'

and therefore……….

'if in doubt, ask the patient.'

Enjoy your career and REMEMBER to have fun outside medicine too.

**John Axford and Chris O' Callaghan**

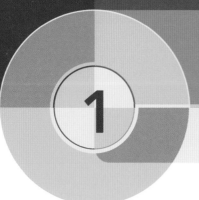

# The Human Aspects of Medicine

## CHRIS O'CALLAGHAN & ALISON MAYCOCK

## INTRODUCTION

This chapter considers the context in which the clinical facts and details discussed in the other chapters are gathered and deployed. It is intended to help the student or clinician reflect on how to make the most effective use of the information contained in the other chapters.

The effectiveness of doctors rests not just on their *knowledge of clinical facts* but also on *good communication, clear clinical reasoning* and *reflective practice*. The General Medical Council (GMC), which regulates medical practice in the UK, captures these elements in its guidance 'Good medical practice'. This is divided into different domains and specifies how doctors should act.

- Knowledge, skills and performance
  - o Have patient-centred care as their first concern.
  - o Be competent and up to date.
  - o Recognize and work within their competence.
- Safety and quality
  - o Act promptly if patient safety, dignity or comfort is at risk.
  - o Protect and promote the health of patients and the public.
- Communication partnership and teamwork
  - o Treat patients politely and considerately.
  - o Respect patients' confidentiality.
  - o Listen to patients and respond to their concerns and preferences.
  - o Give patients the information they want or need in a form they can understand.
  - o Respect patients' right to contribute to decisions about their management.
  - o Support patients in their self-care.
  - o Work effectively with colleagues in the patients' interest.
- Maintaining trust
  - o Be honest and open and act with integrity.
  - o Never discriminate unfairly against patients or colleagues.
  - o Never abuse patient trust or public trust in the profession of medicine.

These elements form the basis of doctors' mandatory annual appraisal and the 5-yearly revalidation of their licence to practise in the UK.

A key element of medical practice is communication and the clinician is involved in a complex communication network (**Figure 1.1**).

## COMMUNICATION WITH PATIENTS

Being a *skilled listener* is fundamental to the process of understanding the problems that patients present and their significance for the patient across all aspects of their life. Consultations are usually face-to-face, but increasingly occur via telephone, video, email or even social media, and each medium presents different challenges.

*Patient-centredness* and *shared decision-making* should be the defining features of the consultation. The patient's values and goals should be established by the clinician and incorporated into a negotiated plan of action. Agreeing a plan is important, as the patient has to live with its consequences. A negotiated and agreed plan is much more likely

DOI: 10.1201/9781003193616-1

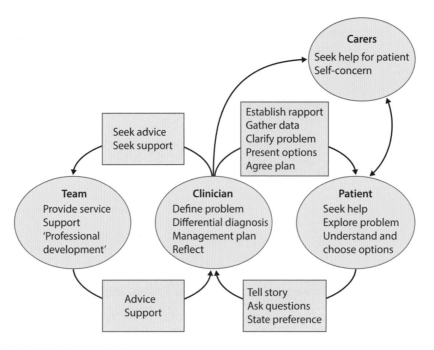

**Figure 1.1** The network of clinical communication.

to be effective than an instruction given by the doctor to the patient. We all engage more fully in plans we have helped devise.

Consider the *structure of a consultation*, its main phases and tasks (**Figure 1.2**).

During these processes, the clinician *provides a structure to the consultation for the patient* to understand, tackles their problem and also *builds a relationship* with the patient. Let us look in more detail at some of these elements.

## OPENING THE CONSULTATION

### Preparation

- Gather any data already available (e.g. test results, letters from other clinicians).
- Manage your own feelings and needs (e.g. hunger, tiredness, anxiety or stress).
- Be clear about your own agenda (e.g. you may wish to achieve an audit target or reduce your clinic numbers).
- Choose a comfortable setting.

### Establishing rapport

- Make eye contact and smile.
- Identify yourself by name and role.
- Confirm that the patient is ready to talk.
- Ensure the patent is comfortable, appropriately covered and positioned.
- Ensure any other people in the room are appropriate and the patient consents to their presence.
- Put the patient at their ease with a kind and gentle manner.

- Explain any use of computers or other technology as needed.
- Involve the patient and ask questions in a friendly manner. Use non-verbal gestures such as smiling, nodding and allowing silence.
- Acknowledge and respond to each point made by the patient.
- Notice how the patient looks and behaves and draw this into the consultation, if appropriate.

## GATHERING INFORMATION

People generally consult doctors because they think that they have a medical problem that should be diagnosed and treated, or because something is adversely affecting them and their coping mechanisms are failing.

Start by asking open and wide questions to capture all the important information from your perspective and the patient's, such as:
- Why have you come to see me today?
- What outcome are you hoping we will achieve?
- What is it about this problem that worries you?
- What do you think the problem is?
- What next steps do you have in mind?
- Is there anything else that has been bothering you?

Follow each of these by an open prompt, such as:
- Can you tell me a bit more about that?

Clarify with open specific questions, such as:
- Do you have a cough?

Pin down your diagnosis by asking increasingly specific closed questions, such as:
- Does anything bring the cough on?
- Does exercise bring the cough on?

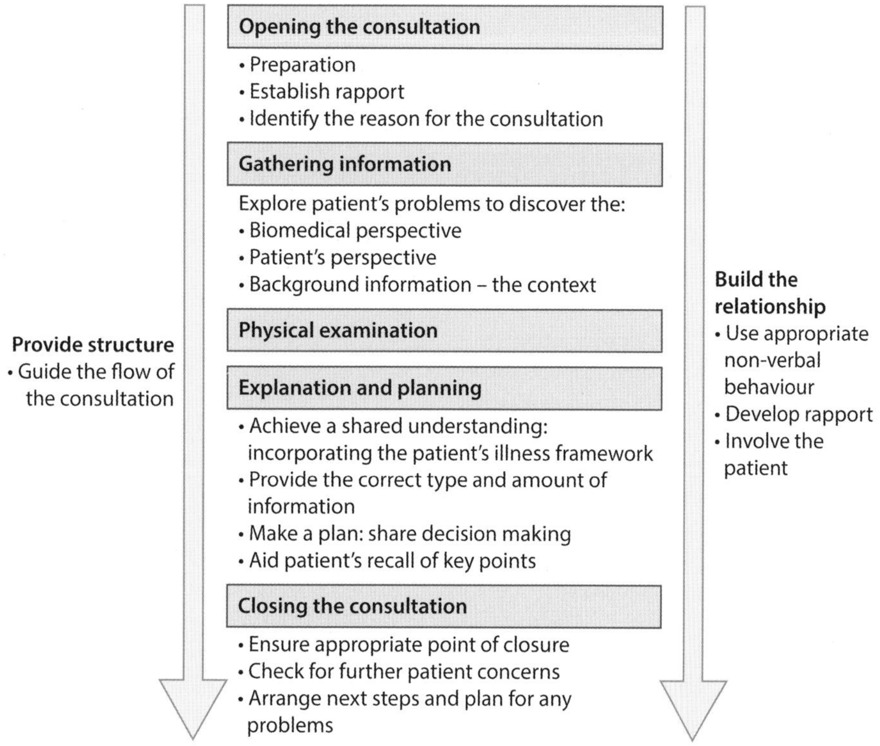

**Figure 1.2** The tasks and processes of the consultation.

Avoid negative leading questions, such as:

- You do not have the cough at night then?
- You don't get any side effects from these medications?

## PHYSICAL EXAMINATION

Tailor your examination according to the history and your differential diagnosis.

## EXPLANATION AND PLANNING

### Achieve a shared understanding of the problem

- Clarify and summarize what has been said.
- Establish in your own mind your differential diagnosis.
- Use non-specialist language to explain your conclusions.
- Ask for the patient's opinions, suggestions and preferences.
- Relate explanations to the patient's own terms or concepts.
- Explicitly check the patient's understanding.

### Provide the correct type and amount of information

- Deliver information in small chunks.
- Provide written material, such as patient information leaflets or web links.

### Make a plan

- Agree the forward plan with the patient.
- Empower the patient to manage their own illness and self-care.
- Document key points carefully.

## CLOSING THE CONSULTATION

- Check for any outstanding patient concerns.
- Advise whom the patient may contact with further questions.
- Advise what to do in situations that need action and especially those which are a threat to patient safety.

## COMMUNICATION WITH RELATIVES AND CARERS

It is important to bear in mind the following, when talking to relatives and/or carers.

- Obtain appropriate consent from the patient for the discussion.
- Establish the identity and role of the carer or relative.
- Be sensitive to the impact of the patient's illness on the individual carer or relative.
- Establish what they already know and what more they wish to know.

- Use the skills of the patient consultation, such as active listening, breaking information into small chunks and providing written material, as appropriate.

## COMMUNICATION WITH COLLEAGUES

Most doctors work in teams and this can be challenging, rewarding and enjoyable. Good team working requires showing respect and consideration for others. This includes listening to the concerns and points of view of other people and acknowledging and valuing their contributions. Effective communication is needed to optimize efficiency and patient safety.

- Keep accurate and concise records, which are signed and dated or appropriately validated electronically.
- Formulate requests for help as clearly as possible, to obtain the most useful response.
- Be sensitive to the roles and competencies of colleagues.
- Promote a fair and supportive work environment.
- Be willing to help colleagues but realistic about what can be done.
- Obtain patient consent for discussion with outside teams or agencies.

## COMMUNICATION IN CHALLENGING CIRCUMSTANCES

Communication with patients or relatives or carers can be especially challenging in certain situations, such as the following:

- The patient and clinician do not speak the same *language*. An interpreter should be used.
- The patient has *impaired hearing*. A hearing aid or signing interpreter should be used as appropriate.
- The patient has impaired cognitive skills or *lacks capacity*. The clinician must establish the level of understanding and the capacity of the patient for each specific decision. Mental capacity is always assumed and is demonstrated for a specific decision when a patient can:
  o Understand the information given and the decision required
  o Retain the information
  o Weigh up the information to make a decision
  o Communicate that decision
- The patient displays *strong emotions*. The clinician should remain calm, speak quietly, acknowledge the emotion displayed and show a willingness to listen further.
- The clinician must *break bad news*. The clinician should choose a quiet, comfortable place, ask if the patient wants someone else to be present and check what

they already know. It can be helpful to offer a warning along the lines of 'I am sorry, but I have some difficult information for you…'.

- The clinician is communicating a complex concept such as *risk*. Advise the patient of absolute risk (not relative). Give numbers not percentages. Use visual decision-making aids if possible (e.g. **Figure 1.3**, a patient decision-aid chart). Discuss the likelihood of a problem both occuring and not occuring. For example, in the hypothetical situation illustrated in **Figure 1.3**, if discussing the option of taking a statin with a patient who has a 10-year cardiovascular disease (CVD) risk of 30%, you might say:

  'If there were 100 people like you in the room, over the next 10 years, on average it is likely that 30 of them would have heart pain, a heart attack or stroke and 70 of them would not. If they all take this medicine every day for the next 10 years, then 20 of them would be likely to have a problem and 80 would not. Therefore, 10 people would be likely to avoid the problem.'

- There is *uncertainty* of diagnosis, prognosis or benefits of intervention options. The doctor should be honest with patients about the limitations of medical certainty and predictability, but should offer reassurance regarding what is known and can be done.
- There are *medically unexplained symptoms*. Medically unexplained symptoms can be frustrating for both the doctor and patient. The doctor should be explicit about the limitations of current medicine to explain every symptom. It is important to acknowledge that even when no organic illness can be diagnosed, a patient may be significantly affected by their symptoms and

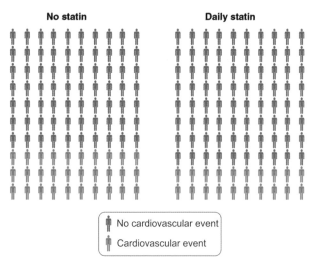

**Figure 1.3** Patient decision aid to communicate the benefit of a statin on cardiovascular risk. This hypothetical decision aid could be used to demonstrate how taking a statin might reduce the likely number of cardiovascular events over a 10-year period from 30 to 20 per 100 people.

the doctor can still offer to support the patient in managing their problem.

- The patient is making *a complaint*. Clinicians have a statutory duty of candour in the UK. This means they must tell patients about any medical errors. Complaints should be handled according to local complaints procedures, which usually involve providing the complainant with:
  - A clear written description of what happened
  - A clear description of how it was investigated
  - An apology for any errors and acknowledgement of the impact on the patient
  - An indication of how future problems will be avoided
  - An invitation to meet to discuss the matter
- Obtaining *informed consent*. When obtaining consent for a procedure, the emphasis is now on providing the information which a reasonable patient can be expected to want to know. This includes side effects or consequences which are common and those which are uncommon or rare but which are serious. In the UK, this follows the High Court findings in the case of *Montgomery v Lanarkshire*. In this situation, a mother sued the hospital trust for not informing her of the risks of a vaginal delivery to her unborn baby. The mother was small and the baby was large. The baby suffered injury during delivery and the court ruled that she should have been informed of this small but important risk.
- The patient has *strong cultural or personal values* and beliefs which may affect the medical process. This may be refusing certain treatments, such as blood products in the case of some Jehovah's Witnesses, or gelatin-containing capsules for some Muslims. Clinicians must be sensitive to diversity and avoid making assumptions. They must be alert for cues indicating embarrassment regarding being examined or talking about intimate issues.
- The clinician is working *outside their area of competence*. In this case, the doctor should explain to the patient that this is so and further advice should be sought from a colleague with appropriate expertise.

## COMMUNICATION AND CONFIDENTIALITY

Patients' trust in doctors is, in part, founded on confidentiality. The clinician should not disclose identifiable patient details without consent. Implied consent can be assumed for aspects of direct patient care and local audit as specified in GMC guidance in the UK. All other disclosure requires explicit consent except in the following circumstances:

- Disclosure is in the public interest if it is required to prevent serious crime or communicable disease. For example, clinicians have a duty to inform the

sexual contact of a patient who has HIV infection if the patient is not prepared to prevent the risk of transmitting the infection. A doctor also has a duty in the UK to inform the police or Driver and Vehicle Licensing Agency (DVLA) if a patient is not fit to drive and is continuing to do so.
- The patient lacks capacity and disclosure is in the best interest of the patient.
- A court orders disclosure of information.

In any case of disclosure without consent, the clinician must carefully document the efforts they made to obtain consent and inform the patient of their plans before disclosure or, if this is not possible, as soon as possible thereafter.

Patient confidentiality must be safeguarded when patient information is shared electronically, and any such communication must use systems which are compliant with the appropriate security standards. In the UK, nhs.net accounts currently fulfil these requirements. Outside this facility, clinicians should check the security of the system they are using or remove all patient-identifying data from the communication. When emailing patients, the clinician should make them aware of the potential limitations for security and document the patient's consent for this type of communication.

In the UK, the British Association of Dermatologists has published GMC-approved guidance on how to take clinical images and email these images for direct patient care. This guidance states that securely configured devices and NHS email or secure data transfer apps must be used. The images must then be deleted immediately after transfer. In any other circumstance, patient data must be completely anonymized.

## CLINICAL REASONING OR JUDGEMENT

Clinicians make sense of the information they gather by a process of clinical reasoning, which aims at making a working or differential diagnosis and management plan. Clinical reasoning has several stages which may be reiterated until a best course of action is identified. We have already identified some of the key components of this and a framework for understanding clinical reasoning is summarized in **Figure 1.4**.

## MAINTAINING PATIENT TRUST

Patients often put enormous trust in the medical profession. When interacting with doctors, patients may feel, and be, very vulnerable. Their health and well-being may be under serious threat. It is unlikely that they are familiar with the concepts and information which form the basis for the decisions they are being asked to make. There is therefore a duty on clinicians to respect and safeguard patient trust by acting honourably and in the patient's best interests at all times. These requirements are identified by the GMC

**Gather information**
Review the clinical records. Use questions to clarify the presentation. Start with open, wide questions to capture the maximum relevant information. Increasingly focus questions to pin down detail. Try to rule in or out important diagnoses.

↓

**Establish a differential diagnosis**
Use patterns identified from study and experience together with formal and informal diagnostic algorithms. Be aware of the limitations of these tools in any particular case; illnesses vary in their presentation and people vary in what they remember and say

↓

**Examination and investigation**
Design investigations to refine the list of differential diagnoses – making some options more likely and some less likely

↓

**Revise the list of working diagnoses**
As the clinical situation unfolds, more information emerges which may or may not reinforce the working diagnosis and so this must always remain open to revision

↓

**Balance competing demands**
Weigh the burden of investigation on patients against the likelihood of gaining information that will improve care. It is best to share with the patient the decision on how to balance and prioritize goals

↓

**Decide on a course of action**
In agreement with the patient, make a plan that is likely to be effective and minimize risk

↓

**Plan ahead**
Anticipate likely outcomes of the interventions chosen and identify situations that might need action – especially those related to patient safety. Acknowledge any uncertainty of diagnosis and outcome

**Figure 1.4** Stages in clinical reasoning.

as outlined earlier. They contribute to what we think of as professionalism.

## REFLECTIVE PRACTICE

In the UK, the ongoing professional development of doctors has been formalized in statutory annual appraisal and a 5-yearly revalidation process. The GMC has recently drawn attention to the *key role played by reflection in enabling individuals to develop professionally*. In essence, reflection involves taking time to step back and think about a particular event and consider what went well, what could have gone better and how

best to address the learning or other need required to enable better practice in future. The final step is to identify what will confirm that practice has improved.

The professional development of doctors also involves looking after ourselves and building resilience to withstand the demands of the job. We need to have enough time and energy to pursue our interests, both medical and non-medical. We need to nurture ourselves as individuals as well as professionals in order to deal with stress and to avoid burnout. Time for reflection and planning is part of this self-care, as is sharing worries or dilemmas with peers or seniors, forming small peer-support groups or finding a mentor or coach. It is important to remember that doctors are normal people and may, like their patients, need help at times.

## PROVIDING LEADERSHIP

As doctors gain in experience and become more senior, they take on more leadership activities, although any doctor may be required to show leadership at any stage. For example, any junior doctor may be asked to organize how the team divides up the tasks they need to do. Being a leader means taking responsibility for the functioning of the team as a whole. Again, the basic skills of communication are key: achieving rapport, listening, clarifying issues and sharing decisions as far as is practical. However, it is the leader of a team who has to take the final decision and, with that, the final responsibility for the actions taken.

## LIFE AS A CLINICIAN

The role of the clinician makes enormously varied demands on the individual. These include demands on memory and knowledge, experience, logical reasoning, emotional intelligence, social skills, self-reflection and self-management. Demands are also made on the imagination and creativity of the doctor, as they must help generate a plan with the patient in every circumstance they encounter. It is, however, a role that can reward the individual with a marvellously varied professional life.

**MUST-KNOW CHECKLIST**
- Effective communication is an essential aspect of clinical medicine.
- If time permits, prepare and plan each consultation.
- Always listen to patients.
- Patient confidentiality is of the utmost importance.

**Questions and answers** to test your understanding of Chapter 1 can be found by clicking 'Support Material' at the following link: https://www.routledge.com/Medicine-for-Finals-and-Beyond/Axford-OCallaghan/p/book/9780367150594

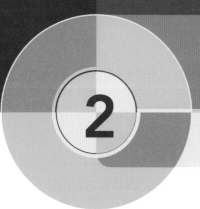

# The Scientific Basis of Medicine

**2**

CHRIS O'CALLAGHAN & RACHEL ALLEN

In this chapter, we outline some of the scientific foundations of modern medicine, highlighting how scientific advances have opened up the potential for new therapies and diagnostic tests.

## BIOLOGICAL MACROMOLECULES

### NUCLEIC ACIDS

Genetic information is stored and transferred in the form of the nucleic acids *deoxyribonucleic acid (DNA)* and *ribonucleic acid (RNA)*. These molecules provide the necessary information for protein production. Like many biological molecules, nucleic acids are multimers of smaller units; which in this case are known as nucleotides. A set of four nucleotide components is used to generate DNA or RNA. *Adenine (A)*, *guanine (G)* and *cytosine (C)* are common to both DNA and RNA. *Thymine (T)* is found in DNA but absent from RNA, with *uracil (U)* present in its place.

DNA strands consist of nucleotides joined by *phosphodiester bonds* linking the sugar of one nucleotide to the phosphate group of the next. DNA coils into a *double helix* of two antiparallel strands (**Figure 2.1**). *Complementary base pairing* of adenine with thymine and guanine with cytosine ensures the fidelity of DNA transcription and replication. When DNA is copied, each parental strand acts as a template for replication: incoming nucleotides form hydrogen bonds with an appropriate base on the template strand. Base mispairing, induced by damage or mutation, introduces structural alterations which can be detected and/or removed by DNA repair proteins.

RNA differs from DNA in its sugar content and usually exists as a single strand. RNA is a versatile molecule that is fundamental to protein synthesis; information from a DNA strand is copied (transcribed) into a new strand of RNA, which acts as a template for protein production. Some viruses use RNA as their hereditary material; retroviruses such as human immunodeficiency virus (HIV) encode their genome on a single strand of RNA, which is reverse transcribed into DNA upon infection of a host cell.

### PROTEINS

*Proteins* are long chains of *amino acids* held together by peptide bonds. Each amino acid is composed of an amino group, a carboxyl group and the particular side chain that defines their chemical nature. Individual proteins are constructed from a library of 20 amino acids, which may be subgrouped according to the acidic, basic, uncharged polar or non-polar character of their side chains (**Figure 2.2**). Like all large molecules, proteins adopt a conformation that confers the most stability. Protein modifications can result from the addition of other substances, such as metal ions (e.g. iron in haemoglobin), lipids (lipoproteins) or carbohydrates (glycoproteins).

### CARBOHYDRATES

Carbohydrates are composed of carbon, hydrogen and oxygen with a general formula $C_x(H_2O)_y$. They range from simple *monosaccharides* of three to six carbons to large complex *polysaccharides* (**Figure 2.3**). Glycoproteins are usually generated by covalent attachment of carbohydrate groups to the amino acids asparagine, threonine or serine. Some diseases, such as cancers and arthritis, may have characteristic glycosylation patterns, which can be useful for diagnosis and for predicting prognosis.

Long-term complications associated with diabetes can result from hyperglycaemia. In a non-enzymatic process, glucose attaches to the amino group of proteins such as collagen (e.g. in blood cell walls). Consequent chemical

DOI: 10.1201/9781003193616-2

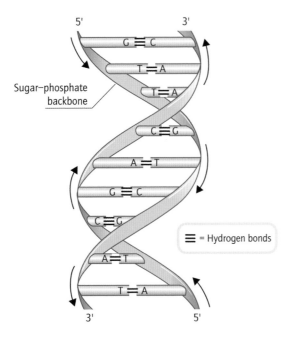

Figure 2.1 The DNA double helix.

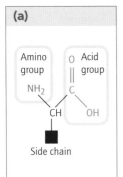

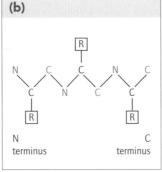

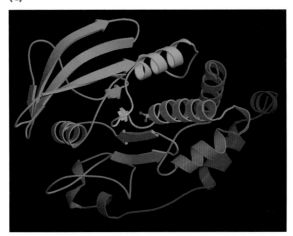

**Figure 2.2** **(a)** Amino acid side chains (designated by a black box) may be acidic, basic or hydrophobic in nature. **(b)** Amino acids join to form a polypeptide chain. **(c)** Protein secondary structure is composed of α-helices and β-sheets, both of which can be seen in the structure of human tyrosine phosphatase 1B. An example of an α-helix is shown in red and an example of a β-sheet is shown in green.

rearrangements irreversibly generate *advanced glycosylation end products (AGE)*. AGE have a range of pathological effects including peptide cross-linking.

## LIPIDS

The structural units of lipids are fatty acids, containing long chains of 4–24 carbon atoms joined to a carboxylic acid group (**Figure 2.4**). Fatty acids may be *saturated* or *non-saturated* depending on the presence of double bonds within their hydrocarbon tail. *Polyunsaturated* fatty acids contain multiple double bonds. One of the most important *in vivo* functions performed by lipids is the formation of cellular membranes. *Phospholipids* contain a hydrophilic phosphate group, linked by glycerol to a hydrophobic fatty acid tail. The amphipathic nature of phospholipids allows them to form a sealed membrane bilayer in aqueous solution. Another physiologically important group of lipids are the cholesterol derivatives (steroids). These molecules contain four hydrocarbon rings, one of which carries a hydroxyl group which gives the molecule an amphipathic nature.

## CELL BIOLOGY

### CELL STRUCTURE

Cells are the basic structural unit of all living organisms. Each cell has the means to maintain itself within the organism and interact with other cells and body systems. Subcellular organelles compartmentalize processes such as respiration or digestion (**Figure 2.5**).

The fluid nature of the outer phospholipid membrane that surrounds the cell allows proteins to move around its surface. The *cytosol* is the site of many cellular reactions and contains all the necessary machinery for protein synthesis. A *cytoskeleton* of microfilaments, intermediate filaments and microtubules provides physical support for the various organelles and forms transport routes between them.

The membrane-bound *nucleus* acts as a store for genetic information. Nuclear pores facilitate exchange of protein and RNA between the nucleus and the rest of the cell. Newly formed proteins destined for transport to lysosomes or the cell surface are inserted into the *endoplasmic reticulum (ER)*, a system of folded membranes. Initial *protein glycosylation* may also occur within the ER. From the ER, proteins progress through a related system of compartments known as the *Golgi complex*, where further modifications take place. The Golgi complex sorts macromolecules for onward transport and, on leaving it, proteins progress through a system of vesicles until they reach their ultimate location.

Endocytosed proteins and other materials are degraded within membrane-bound *lysosomes*, which store the hydrolytic enzymes required for such degradation. Deficiency of a lysosomal enzyme causes the neurological condition *Tay–Sachs disease* in which gangliosides accumulate in the brain causing neural degeneration and early death.

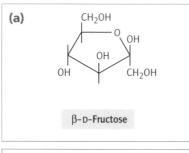

**Figure 2.3** Carbohydrate structures. Most common monosaccharides adopt a ring conformation in aqueous solution. **(a)** Fructose and **(b)** glucose are examples of 5-carbon (pentose) and 6-carbon (hexose) monosaccharides, respectively. **(c)** Lactose is a disaccharide formed from galactose and glucose subunits. **(d)** Heparin is a polysaccharide.

*Mitochondria* are the powerhouses of the cell. These maternally inherited organelles carry their own small genome encoding various components of the respiratory process.

## CELL DIVISION

### Mitosis

In order to divide successfully, a cell must copy its DNA so that each daughter cell receives its full set of chromosomes. This is achieved by a tightly regulated mitosis following the cell cycle pathway (**Figure 2.6**). Passage through the cell cycle is controlled by *cyclin* proteins, in a cascade of phosphorylation events. Each cyclin acts as a catalytic subunit in partnership with a *cyclin-dependent kinase (CDK)*. Upon cyclin binding, CDKs phosphorylate target proteins that are required for cell-cycle progression. *CDK-specific inhibitors (CDKIs)* bind cyclin–CDK complexes to regulate their activity and can themselves be regulated by other proteins. During mitosis, one member of each chromosome pair becomes attached to a centriole. Centrioles move to opposite ends of the cell, taking the chromosomes with them. In order to prevent inappropriate proliferation of cells, mitosis is tightly controlled, with various checkpoints to ensure

that every part of the mitotic process is completed correctly before the next stage begins. Because uncontrolled proliferation is a hallmark of cancer, the cell cycle provides an obvious target for therapy. CDKIs often act as tumour suppressors and are potentially useful anticancer agents.

### Meiosis

A more specialized form of cell division generates gametes bearing a single set of chromosomes. *Meiosis* requires two rounds of cell division, with DNA replication occurring during the first round of division. The second division results in each daughter cell inheriting a single set of chromosomes.

## APOPTOSIS

An effective mechanism is required to remove cells that are damaged or no longer necessary. This programmed cell death is generally known as *apoptosis* (**Figure 2.7**), and follows a carefully controlled series of events allowing the cell to condense its cytoskeleton and fragment its DNA. Apoptosis is driven by members of the caspase protein family. Bcl proteins regulate caspase activity. Programmed cell

**Figure 2.4** Lipids. **(a)** Saturated and **(b)** unsaturated fatty acids are termed according to the presence of double bonds within their hydrocarbon tail. **(c)** Steroid molecules such as cholesterol are based on a skeleton of four carbon rings. **(d)** Phospholipids are amphipathic molecules with two hydrophobic (green) hydrocarbon tails attached to a hydrophilic polar head group (blue). **(e)** In aqueous solution, phospholipids form a bilayer with a hydrophobic interior. This arrangement forms the basis for eukaryotic cellular membranes.

death can be triggered in response to stimuli such as cell surface signals or mitochondrial stress. Following ligand binding, cell-surface death receptors such as Fas recruit adaptor proteins to trigger procaspase activation, and thus elicit apoptosis. Mitochondria can initiate an alternative apoptotic pathway in response to DNA damage or intracellular oxidative stress. A dying cell will show membrane blebbing, cell shrinkage and protein fragmentation as it collapses in upon itself. Within the nucleus, chromatin condensation and DNA degradation occur. Finally, the cell is flagged for uptake by phagocytic cells.

## CELLULAR HOMOEOSTASIS AND COMMUNICATION

The human body maintains a stable environment for its cells and tissues through a combination of physiological and biochemical processes. Cell membranes form a barrier to large molecules, allowing the cell to maintain a constant internal environment. Specific transport mechanisms are therefore required to transfer material in and out of the cell. Membranes contain many different proteins that actively or passively facilitate the movement of ions or molecules across

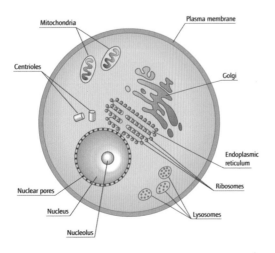

**Figure 2.5** Cell structure.

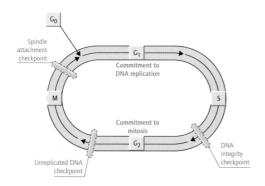

**Figure 2.6** The cell cycle. Cells resting between divisions are held indefinitely in the quiescent ($G_0$) phase. Upon appropriate stimulation (e.g. exposure to growth factors) cells enter 'gap 1' ($G_1$), the first stage of the cell cycle, during which various RNAs and proteins are synthesized. The cell then enters a period of DNA synthesis termed the 'S-phase'. Once each chromosome has been replicated, a second 'gap' phase, $G_2$ takes place. When the cell is ready to divide, mitosis begins (M phase). During mitosis, chromosomes condense and the nuclear envelope breaks down, allowing paired chromosomes to attach to centrioles by a microtubule spindle. Chromosome pairs separate and are moved to opposite ends of the cell preceding cytoplasmic division (cytokinesis). Positive and negative control points operate throughout the cell cycle. Various commitment points and regulatory checkpoints are marked in red and green, respectively. Cell cycle control proteins include p21, p53 and Rb (the retinoblastoma protein).

membranes. Three major classes of transport protein are membrane channels, pumps and transporters.

Cells can use extracellular molecules to communicate with one another. Signal transduction pathways translate these stimuli into an appropriate cellular response, usually through a series of phosphorylation reactions leading to novel gene transcription in the nucleus. Signalling pathways play a role in the development of many cancers.

## MOLECULAR BIOLOGY

### CHROMOSOMES

The human *genome* organises our entire genetic information into a set of 46 *chromosomes*, which segregate our DNA for storage or transcription. Humans have 23 pairs of chromosomes, with one set inherited from each parent. These include 22 pairs of standard chromosomes and one pair of sex chromosomes (XX in females, XY in males). In the absence of transcription or replication, DNA is packed into chromosomes as *chromatin* with DNA wrapped tightly around very many *nucleosome* cores. The most densely packed form, *heterochromatin*, has a closed structure to maintain genes in a transcriptionally inactive state. In

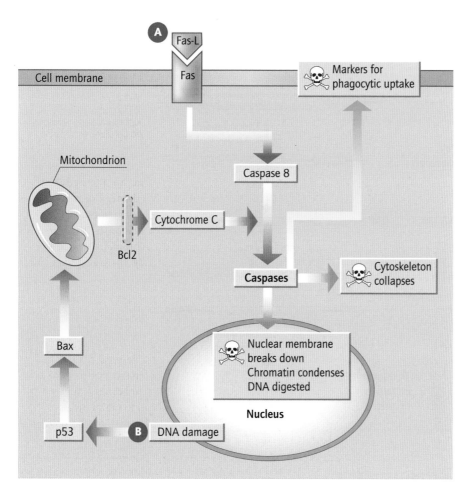

**Figure 2.7** Apoptosis. There are two major pathways of apoptosis. (A) Death signals from cell surface receptors such as Fas (CD95) trigger activation of caspase 8 to initiate a signalling cascade through downstream enzymes. Mitochondria host a range of pro-apoptotic factors including cytochrome C, which is necessary for downstream caspase activation. A second apoptotic pathway (B) operates through these organelles. Triggers such as DNA damage (signalled through p53 and Bax) initiate the release of pro-apoptotic factors from mitochondria. Bcl2 acts as an anti-apoptotic regulator of this process.

contrast, genes that are being expressed in order to produce protein are located within open *euchromatin*, to allow access for the necessary transcriptional machinery.

To neutralize the tendency of chromosomes to shorten with each round of DNA replication, the telomerase enzyme elongates the ends of each chromosome to form a blocked *telomere* structure. Telomerase is usually active in stem cells and germ cells or during oncogenesis, but is not found in healthy somatic tissues. Modulation of telomerase enzyme has therefore become a subject of interest for anti-ageing and anticancer research.

## GENE STRUCTURE

Every protein is encoded by a DNA sequence within a *gene* at a defined *locus* on a chromosome. *Codons* of three sequential nucleotides encode a single amino acid or a stop signal. Regulatory regions containing target sites for various DNA-binding proteins flank the coding sequence and control gene expression. These regions form a vital part of the gene and their loss can have profound effects on protein expression. Mutations in control regions can cause disease, as evidenced by some of the haemoglobin gene mutations that cause thalassaemia. An upstream *promoter* provides binding sites for RNA polymerase and transcription factors. Functionally related *enhancer* sequences are located further afield and recruit various DNA-binding proteins that can regulate the efficiency of gene transcription. The transcriptional unit

contains *exons* of coding DNA separated by *introns*, which play no part in the finished protein. A large portion of our genome is composed of *repetitive DNA* of unclear function.

## FROM GENE TO PROTEIN – TRANSCRIPTION AND TRANSLATION

When a gene is active, the chromatin structure loosens to allow access for RNA polymerase to generate an RNA molecule (**Figure 2.8**). This messenger RNA (mRNA) precursor is then processed for translation into an amino acid sequence. Gene splicing removes introns from the coding sequences to leave a continuous series of exons for translation. Once within the cytosol, mRNA attaches to large ribonucleoprotein particles known as ribosomes. Ribosomes read along mRNA, generating proteins by polymerizing amino acids donated by transfer RNA (tRNA) molecules bearing an appropriate anticodon.

## GENE EXPRESSION PATTERNS

Every somatic cell carries an identical set of genes. *Housekeeping genes* are required for basic cellular functions and are constitutively expressed. Additional subsets of expressed genes determine the phenotype and differentiation state of the cell. Access of transcriptional proteins to the gene promoter will be restricted if it is tightly packed within heterochromatin. *CpG islands* are stretches of cytosine

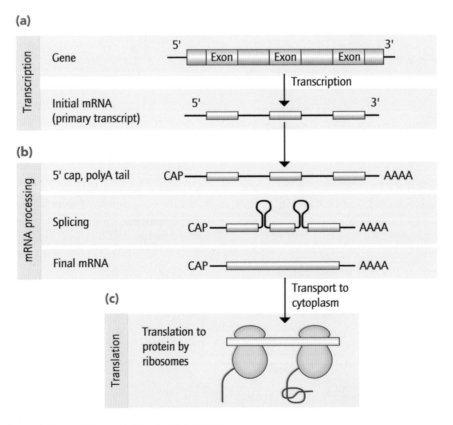

**Figure 2.8** Gene transcription, mRNA processing and translation.

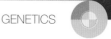
and guanine found at the 5′ end of genes. Methylation of cytosine (C) within CpG islands can prevent a gene from becoming expressed. An extreme form of methylation control is exercised on one of the X chromosome pair in every somatic female cell. This process results in hypermethylation of the inactive chromosome to prevent gene transcription. The field of epigenetics studies how processes such as DNA methylation or the modification of histone proteins in nucleosomes are regulated, how they control gene expression and their influence in health and disease. Epigenetic modification of cell cycle control genes is commonly observed in cancer.

Gene activation can occur in response to various internal or external stimuli through the action of receptor proteins and signalling pathways. The end point of these pathways is usually the expression or activation of one or more DNA-binding proteins that, in turn, stimulates gene expression. In addition to the regulation of transcription, factors such as mRNA stability, transcriptional regulation and differential splicing may influence protein expression.

Developmental regulation of gene expression has clinical significance in a number of areas. For example, different haemoglobin genes are activated in the fetus compared to those expressed by adults. One therapeutic approach for thalassaemia is to reactivate fetal haemoglobin genes to compensate for abnormalities in their adult counterparts.

## PHARMACOLOGY

At their site of action, drugs interact with molecules termed drug 'receptors' or 'targets'. These are often actual biological receptors, such as hormone receptors, but they may also be any other type of molecule, such as an enzyme or membrane channel. The *affinity* of a drug-receptor interaction is a measure of how tightly the two molecules bind. An *agonist* is a substance that has an effect on a specific drug receptor, causing activation of the function of the receptor molecule. A *partial agonist* has the same type of effect on the function of the receptor molecule, but even at the maximal effect of the drug, the function of the receptor molecule is not activated to its maximal level. An *antagonist* is a drug that binds, to but opposes, the natural activity of the receptor molecule. *Competitive antagonists* compete with agonists for the same receptor, but they do not exert an agonist effect themselves and so reduce the effect of any agonist present. In these circumstances, the overall effect will depend on the relative concentrations of agonist and antagonist. A *non-competitive antagonist* does not compete for the same site but opposes the effect of the agonist by another mechanism. Finally, an *irreversible antagonist* is an antagonist that inactivates the receptor molecule permanently once it has bound. This effect cannot be reversed, even at high concentration of agonist. Many drug receptors are bound by naturally occurring agonists and antagonists, including hormones and neurotransmitters.

*Pharmacodynamics* describe the distribution of a drug through various body compartments as a function of time. In contrast, *pharmacokinetic* studies follow the actions and effects of drugs on living tissue. *Dose–response curves* relate the biological effect of a drug to its administered dose. Sometimes, this effect is directly proportional to the dose, so that doubling the dose will double the effect. However, this is often not the case and it may, for example, take a 10-fold increase in dose to achieve a doubling of effect. Drug dosage is affected by many factors including the absorption, distribution, metabolism and excretion of the drug. Although these effects are complex, clinically useful decisions about drug dosage can be made if the drug half-life is known. The *half-life* of a drug is the time taken for plasma levels of the drug to fall to half of their original value. Drugs are usually administered orally, intravenously (IV), subcutaneously (subcut) or intramuscularly (IM). Before distribution to its site of action, a drug must first be absorbed from its administration site (e.g. gut, skin or muscle) unless it is injected IV. The most rapid effects are obtained by IV administration, which immediately delivers the drug into the blood for direct transport to the tissues. When a drug has been absorbed, it equilibrates throughout its *volume of distribution*, which may not include all tissues. Most orally administered drugs are absorbed in the small bowel and must pass through the liver before they can reach the systemic arterial circulation. This means that they may be altered by metabolism in the liver, a process known as 'first pass metabolism'. Once any drug has been administered, it may be inactivated by metabolism (especially in the lungs) or excreted by the kidney in urine or, less commonly, by the liver in bile. Metabolism frequently alters drug activity. *Phase 1 reactions* cause oxidation, reduction or hydrolysis of the drug and involve cytochrome p450 mixed-function oxidases. *Phase 2 reactions* add groups such as glucuronides or sulphates to the drugs, increasing their water solubility and making them suitable for excretion by the liver in bile or by the kidney in urine. Within the kidney, anion and cation transporters are capable of transporting drugs into the renal tubules for excretion in the urine.

Many drugs are bound by *plasma proteins*; acidic drugs bind albumin and basic drugs bind to α1 acid glycoproteins. If a drug is strongly bound by a plasma protein, it will tend to remain within the circulation. If a drug is poorly bound by plasma proteins, its distribution will depend upon its *lipid-solubility*. Water-soluble drugs tend to remain within extracellular fluids, whereas lipid-soluble drugs cross cell membranes to enter cells and may even become concentrated in adipose tissue.

## GENETICS

### MUTATIONS

There is genetic variation between individuals and polymorphic genetic variants (known as alleles) are distributed throughout populations. These genetic variations may influence disease susceptibility. Defects in a single gene may be responsible for a particular disease such as cystic fibrosis, but within a given gene, mutations may occur at multiple sites. These mutations may vary in their penetration – the most common mutation seen for cystic fibrosis is a deletion in the CFTR protein that results in misfolded protein, which is then retained inside the cell leading to a severe disease phenotype. Other mutations allow the CFTR protein to reach the cell surface, but reduce its activity and cause less severe forms of disease.

Point mutations are the simplest form of DNA alteration (**Figure 2.9**). In this case, a single nucleotide of the DNA sequence is affected. If a mutation affects the protein-coding sequence of a gene, it is termed *silent* if it does not alter the encoded amino acid. A *missense* mutation occurs when DNA alterations encode a different amino acid. Sometimes, the effects are more drastic; a mutation which introduces an early stop codon (*nonsense* mutation) will terminate protein translation and full-length protein will not be produced.

Similarly, gain or loss of one or two nucleotides will alter the subsequent reading frame of the protein and the remainder of the correct sequence will be lost. Pathogenic mutations may also occur outside a protein-coding sequence; alterations to promoter regions or splice sites can have profound effects on gene expression.

Background levels of mutation arise from normal cellular and environmental interactions. Mutation rates also reflect the fidelity of DNA replication and its proofreading and/or correction potential. Trinucleotide repeats are known to be particularly unstable and are associated with a range of genetic diseases including Huntington's chorea, myotonic dystrophy and fragile X syndrome. Disease severity is usually proportional to the increase in repeat length.

## MONOGENIC AND POLYGENIC DISORDERS

*Monogenic* diseases are the simplest genetic disorders to study as they tend to follow Mendelian genetics. Dominant and recessive diseases have characteristic patterns of

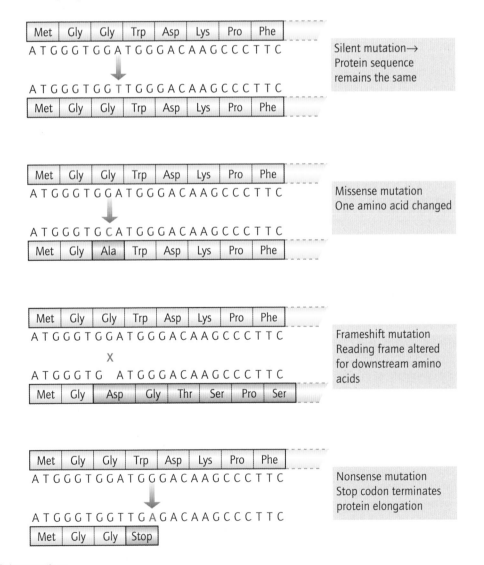

**Figure 2.9** Point mutations.

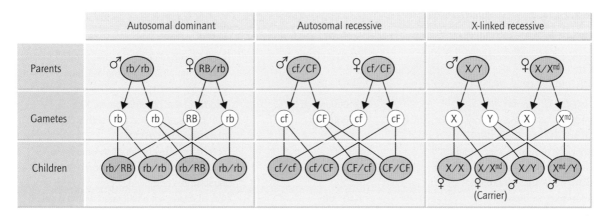

**Figure 2.10** Inheritance patterns. Diseased phenotypes are indicated in pink, dominant alleles in capitals and recessive alleles in lower case. For autosomal dominant disorders such as retinoblastoma, children have a 50% chance of inheriting the disease allele (RB) from an affected parent. In the case of autosomal recessive disorders including cystic fibrosis, children of two carrier parents have a 25% chance of inheriting two copies of the disease allele (cf). Ratios are altered for X-linked recessive disorders such as muscular dystrophy where daughters have a 50% chance of inheriting the disease allele ($X^{md}$) from their mother to become carriers themselves. Sons have a 50% chance of inheriting the disease allele from their mother; as there is no compensatory allele on the Y chromosome these sons are affected with the disease.

inheritance (**Figure 2.10**). *Dominant* traits require only one defective copy to generate a disease phenotype. In contrast, *recessive* disorders are only visible when both copies of a gene are mutated. Recessive disorders often result from a loss in biological activity for the relevant protein. Sex linkage alters Mendelian genetics, as males carry only one copy of the X chromosome; recessive mutations carried on this chromosome behave as if dominant in men, while heterozygous females act as asymptomatic 'carriers'. *Polygenic disorders* have a known genetic component (such as type 1 diabetes) but involve many genes and often environmental factors too (**Table 2.1**). In such cases, disease results from a combination of multiple polymorphisms, acting in concert with external factors. The risk of disease conveyed by each individual genetic variant in a polygenic disorder is relatively low and much lower than that conveyed by a genetic mutation in a monogenic disorder.

## CHROMOSOMAL ABNORMALITIES

A range of clinical syndromes can be caused by chromosomal abnormalities such as abnormal chromosome numbers or structural alterations (**Table 2.2**). Normal individuals carry two complete sets of chromosomes (*diploid*). An abnormal number of chromosomes (*aneuploidy*) can result in physical abnormality or prenatal death. Aneuploidy follows a failure of chromosomes to segregate correctly, usually during meiotic cell division. Thus, one of the two daughter cells inherits an extra copy of the relevant chromosome (*trisomy*), while the other lacks a copy (*monosomy*). Inheritance of extra sets of chromosomes (*polyploidy*) arises from a diploid gamete, fertilization by two spermatozoa or failure to complete cell division. Polyploid zygotes are non-viable.

The main cause of chromosomal structural abnormality is double-stranded DNA breakage. DNA breakage occurs

**Table 2.1** Common or important genetic diseases

| Disease | Approximate frequency | Nature |
|---|---|---|
| Rheumatoid arthritis | 1/100 | Polygenic |
| Haemochromatosis | 1/400 | Monogenic; autosomal recessive, mutations in *HFE* gene |
| Type 1 diabetes mellitus | 1/500 | Polygenic |
| Familial hypercholesterolaemia | 1/500 | Monogenic; autosomal dominant, various mutations in LDL receptor gene |
| Von Willebrand's disease | 1/1000 | Monogenic; autosomal, usually dominant, mutations in *VWF* gene |
| Polycystic kidney disease | 1/1000 | Monogenic; autosomal dominant |
| Fragile X syndrome | 1/1250 males | Monogenic; X-linked recessive, mutations in *FMR1* gene |
| Ulcerative colitis | 1/1500 | Polygenic |
| Cystic fibrosis | 1/2000 | Monogenic; autosomal recessive, mutations in *CFTR* gene |
| Huntington's disease | 1/2000 | Monogenic; autosomal dominant, repeat length mutation in Huntingtin (*HT*) gene |
| Haemophilia A | 1/5000 males | Monogenic; X-linked recessive, mutations in factor VIII gene |

**Table 2.2** Chromosomal abnormalities

| Disease | Approximate frequency | Genetic nature |
|---|---|---|
| Trisomy 21 (Down syndrome) | 1/700 (at birth) | Three copies of chromosome 21 (4% of cases result from a balanced translocation involving chromosome 21) |
| Klinefelter syndrome | 1/1000 males | Trisomy of sex chromosomes: XXY |
| Hereditary motor and sensory neuropathy type 1 (Charcot–Marie–Tooth disease) | 1/2600 | Most cases are associated with a duplication of chromosome 17p11.2 |
| Trisomy 18 (Edwards syndrome) | 1/3000 | Three complete copies of chromosome 18 |
| Turner syndrome | 1/5000 females | Monosomy of the X chromosome (XO) |
| Trisomy 13 (Patau syndrome) | 1/5000 | Usually three complete copies of chromosome 13 |
| Prader–Willi syndrome | 1/10 000 | 75% of cases are associated with a deletion from chromosome 15 |

as a natural feature of meiosis, but can also be triggered by ionizing radiation. Broken ends of DNA are rapidly repaired by specific enzymes. Abnormal repair generates structural abnormalities including translocations, deletions, duplications and inversions of DNA segments. *Translocations* represent a transfer of DNA between two chromosomes. This exchange does not necessarily result in loss of DNA, so an individual carrier may remain healthy. However, chromosome translocations can interfere with meiosis such that offspring cells may receive a partial trisomy or monosomy. *Deletions* result in a loss of genetic material, often spanning many genes. Their effects can be severe, resulting in congenital malformation. *Duplications* of a DNA stretch are generally less harmful than deletions. Introduction of two separate double-stranded breaks can generate an *inversion* if the chromosomal fragment is reinserted in a back-to-front orientation. Although no DNA is lost or gained in this process, inversions can obstruct chromosome pairing during meiosis.

## CANCER GENETICS

Cancers result from an accumulation of genetic abnormalities within somatic cells. The majority of these defects arise spontaneously (often as a result of exposure to mutagens) as *somatic mutations* that are not in the germline, although some can be inherited (e.g. mutations in the cancer-causing *BRCA* genes). An inherited predisposition to cancer is often characterized by disease onset at an early age and increased disease incidence in other family members. Cell proliferation is central to tumour formation, as cancers arise from a single cell. Thus, mutations in genes that promote or inhibit cell proliferation, control apoptosis or regulate DNA repair (often known as oncogenes) can have profound effects.

*Tumour suppressor genes* restrict cell proliferation and induce repair or apoptosis in response to DNA damage. *p53* is the classic example of a tumour suppressor gene, and is the most commonly mutated gene in tumours (**Figure 2.11**). *DNA repair genes* remove the damage induced by mutagenesis. Point mutations, translocations and gene amplification

can all play a part in tumorigenesis. Chromosomal translocations can generate hybrid oncogenes, as seen with the Philadelphia chromosome in chronic myeloid leukaemia (see Chapter 15, Haematological disease).

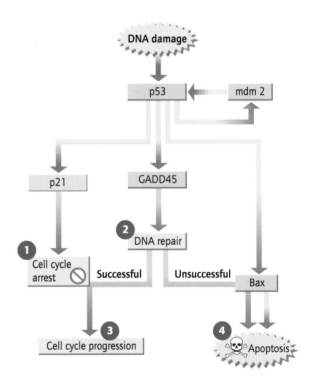

**Figure 2.11** The tumour suppressor protein p53 acts to maintain genetic stability by controlling cell cycle and apoptosis pathways. The wide-ranging influence of p53 reflects its status as the most commonly mutated protein in cancer (p53 is implicated in 50% of colon cancers, 50% of lung cancers and over 50% of breast cancers). p53 is usually localized to the nucleus where it acts as a transcription factor, thus the majority of pathogenic p53 mutations affect its DNA-binding domain. In response to DNA damage, p53 triggers the expression of various proteins including p21, which arrests the cell cycle (1) by inhibiting CDKs, and GADD45, a DNA repair protein (2). Cell cycle block is lifted following successful DNA repair (3). If DNA repair is unsuccessful, however, pro-apoptotic factors such as bax (also induced by p53) trigger cell death (4). p53 also stimulates expression of its own negative regulator, mdm2.

## PERSONALIZED MEDICINE

Advances in technologies that can be applied to study the human genome, along with measurement of specific mRNA and protein levels, continue to develop at a rapid pace. These 'omic' technologies include whole genome sequencing, exome sequencing of protein-coding regions, transcriptome analysis of transcribed mRNA and proteomic profiling of expressed proteins. Whole genome sequencing can be used for the diagnosis of rare childhood conditions and to better inform their treatment where this is possible. Characterizing disease phenotypes at the molecular level within individual patients allows the development of tailored treatments and molecular diagnostic tools. This approach is most advanced in the field of cancer medicine where, for phenotypically similar cancers, analysis of somatic mutations in the cancer cells and the levels of mRNA or protein expression proteins can indicate whether individual patients will benefit from particular drug therapies. Breast cancers which express high levels of the HER2 protein, a growth factor receptor, can be treated effectively using trastuzumab, which binds to this receptor. Combining pharmacology with genomics (pharmacogenomics) may be used to determine the most effective medication for individual patients and avoid adverse drug reactions. For example, the liver enzyme CYP2D6 is involved in metabolizing up to 25% of currently available drugs. Genetic variations in CYP2D6 can have profound effects on the speed of drug metabolism, with implications for the effectiveness of drugs between individuals. As personalized medicine continues to develop, we will be better able to inform prescribing and reduce the potential for side effects.

## HUMAN GENE THERAPY

Advances in molecular biology techniques have enabled the development of *gene therapy* approaches for a number of conditions. Gene therapies receiving approval to date have been applied to somatic cells, whose DNA cannot be inherited by the patient's descendants. To date, the majority of these are applied *ex vivo*, for example taking haematopoietic stem cells out of the body, modifying them and then re-infusing them into patients to generate anti-cancer immune responses. The potential use of gene editing (e.g. using clustered regularly interspaced short palindromic repeats (CRISPR) technology) to modify heritable DNA in sperm, eggs or embryos remains controversial and has considerable ethical implications.

## IMMUNOLOGY AND INFLAMMATION

The human immune system has evolved complex strategies to detect and destroy anything it regards as non-self or altered-self. This requires it to manage a delicate balance between providing a vigorous response to foreign or altered self, but maintaining tolerance to healthy self-antigens in order to prevent autoimmunity.

The *innate* immune response provides an immediate and relatively non-specific response to challenge. In contrast, the *adaptive* immune system, involving T cells and antibodies secreted by B cells, requires an initial priming stage followed by cell proliferation when it encounters a target for the first time. Adaptive immunity is highly specific for individual antigens and, following an initial encounter, can persist to provide a memory response.

Key cells of the innate immune system include phagocytes, such as macrophages and dendritic cells, which destroy exogenous particles by phagocytosis and can process ingested proteins for presentation to T cells. Through this process, dendritic cells are able to prime naive T cells. Recognition of microbial components or damage-associated molecular patterns by innate immune receptors on phagocytes can elicit the production of cytokines, which in turn trigger inflammation and inform the responses of other immune cells.

B and T lymphocytes equip the adaptive immune response with its specificity, diversity and memory. The initial activation of naive T cells requires recognition of antigen by the *T-cell receptor (TCR)* and sufficient co-stimulatory signalling and appropriate cytokines. Co-stimulation is regulated by proteins which serve as immune checkpoints to restrain the activation of adaptive immunity. Successful activation of naive T cells leads to the proliferation of a population of effector cells which, in the case of *helper T cells ($T_H$ cells)*, support the functions of B cells and *cytotoxic T cells (CTLs)*.

B-cell specificity is conferred by the *B-cell receptor (BCR)* (**Figure 2.12**), which can be expressed as a membrane-bound receptor or in a soluble form as an *antibody (Ab)* or *immunoglobulin (Ig)*. The human immune system can produce a highly diverse repertoire of B-cell receptors and antibodies through *combinatorial rearrangements* of multiple gene segments and *somatic mutation*. Each antibody clone can bind a specific target epitope, exerting immune functions by blocking or neutralising the target antigen, or flagging it for destruction by other immune cells.

There are various types of T cells. CTLs are responsible for killing infected cells and tumour cells. $T_H$ cells perform a range of functions mediated through the action of secreted cytokines. *Regulatory T cells (Treg)* play a role in inhibiting immune responses and inadequate Treg function may be a factor in autoimmune diseases. T-cell specificity is determined by the TCR (**Figure 2.12**), which like antibodies, uses combinatorial gene rearrangement to achieve the necessary diversity of receptors. T-cell receptors recognize short peptide fragments presented on the surface of target cells by *major histocompatibility complex (MHC)* proteins, which are also referred to as *human leukocyte antigens (HLAs)*.

HLA proteins are highly diverse, and the combination of MHC alleles expressed by an individual is referred to as

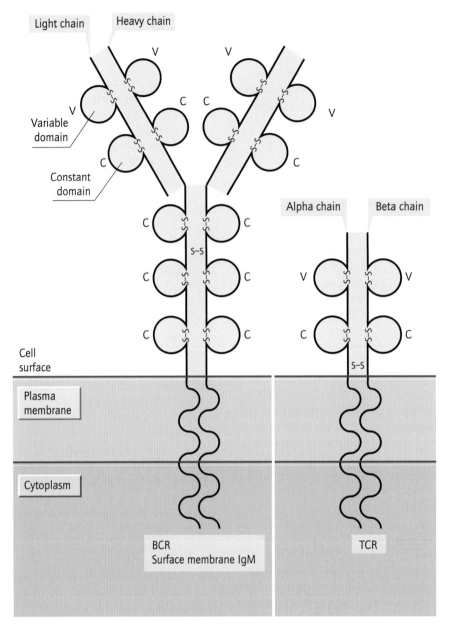

**Figure 2.12** Schematic diagram of BCR and TCR. Both comprise variable (V) and constant (C) immunoglobulin-like domains. The structure of the BCR is a typical immunoglobulin molecule anchored within the membrane of the B cell. B cells and plasma cells produce immunoglobulins with the same specificity but with different heavy chain constant regions which allow them to be secreted from the cell as soluble antibody molecules.

their HLA *haplotype*. Certain HLA alleles and haplotypes are associated with disease (**Table 2.3**). In addition to disease association, HLA typing has direct relevance to tissue transplantation and haematopoietic stem cell transfer.

Cytokines are soluble immune mediators that behave in a similar manner to hormones: they can act locally on the cell that secreted them, on nearby cells or at a distance and their expression is tightly regulated. Cytokines have been systematically subgrouped in several ways, and may be categorized according to their structure, origin or effects. Chemokines (*chemo*tactic cyto*kines*) are involved in leucocyte activation and migration. Particular cytokine profiles,

particularly of those that act as inflammatory mediators, are often observed in disease situations. This has therapeutic relevance as regulation of cytokine activity could be used to enhance or inhibit immune reactions.

## IMMUNE-BASED THERAPEUTICS

The high specificity of monoclonal antibodies for antigens has led to their development as precision therapeutics to block protein interactions, prevent receptor signalling, or label their targets for destruction. Antibody-based therapies are now the dominant class of biopharmaceuticals and

**Table 2.3** MHC disease associations

| Disease | HLA association | Relative risk |
|---|---|---|
| Rheumatoid arthritis | HLA-DR4 | 2–6 |
| Systemic lupus erythematosus | HLA-DR3 (white people) | 2–5 |
| | HLA-DR2 (Japanese) | 2 |
| Ankylosing spondylitis | HLA-B27 | 90 |
| Type 1 diabetes mellitus | HLA-DR3 | 3–6 |
| | HLA-DR4 | 2–7 |
| | DR3/DR4 combined | 14 |
| Multiple sclerosis | HLA-DR2 | 2–4 |
| Myasthenia gravis | HLA-DR3 | 2–3 |

HLA, human leucocyte antigen.

are used to treat a variety of diseases. When new therapeutic targets are identified, antibodies can provide a rapid route to modifying their functions. Monoclonal antibody treatments have proved particularly effective in the treatment of rheumatoid arthritis, where the inflammatory cytokines TNF-alpha and IL-6 are important mediators of disease pathogenesis. Biologic disease-modifying antirheumatic drugs include monoclonal antibodies specific for TNF-alpha, IL-6 and the receptor for IL-6 (see Chapter 4, Rheumatic disease). Recombinant proteins can also be used as therapeutics. For example, the drug anakinra is a modified form of the IL-1 receptor antagonist used for the treatment of rheumatoid arthritis. Disadvantages of such therapies include their high cost and potential to increase susceptibility to infections such as tuberculosis.

## CANCER IMMUNOLOGY

Although cancers are 'self' in origin, the molecular changes that result in tumorigenesis can result in the production of tumour-specific antigens and tumour-associated antigens which are recognized by the immune system as altered self. Cancer cells can employ a number of mechanisms to reduce their immunogenicity, including the upregulation of immune checkpoint proteins to inhibit the immune responses against the tumour and so prevent the killing of tumour cells. Checkpoint inhibitor therapies use monoclonal antibodies that specifically bind checkpoint proteins such

as PD-L1 and CTLA4 and so block their ability to inhibit T cells. Checkpoint inhibitors are effective in a number of cancers, such as melanoma, but the immune activation that they cause increases the risk of autoimmune disease, such as colitis or diabetes (see Chapter 4, Rheumatic disease). Combination of checkpoint therapies is likely to increase the power of their effects, while further research is required to enhance our knowledge of immune checkpoint pathways and reduce the potential of the autoimmune related adverse events that can result from their use.

### MUST-KNOW CHECKLIST

- Females have two X chromosomes; males have one X and one Y chromosome.
- Germline gene mutations can cause genetic disease or alter disease risk.
- Somatic mutations can cause cancer.
- The half-life of a drug is the time for the plasma level to fall to half its original level.

**Questions and answers** to test your understanding of Chapter 2 can be found by clicking 'Support Material' at the following link: https://www.routledge.com/Medicine-for-Finals-and-Beyond/Axford-OCallaghan/p/book/9780367150594

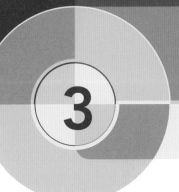

# Infectious Disease

SUSANNA J. DUNACHIE, HANIF ESMAIL,
RUTH CORRIGAN & MARIA DUDAREVA

## INTRODUCTION

Three hundred years ago most people in the world died from infection, and the average life expectancy was estimated to have been 30–40 years. Nowadays, non-communicable diseases such as ischaemic heart disease and chronic respiratory illnesses are the biggest global killers. In high-income settings, infectious diseases are lower down the list of causes of death, and even in low- and middle-income countries, where there remains a large burden of infectious disease, the pattern of disease is changing. The devastating impact of the outbreak of the SARS-CoV-2 coronavirus causing COVID-19 in December 2019 on global mortality and the social and economic lives of billions demonstrates the importance of infectious diseases.

Infectious diseases remain an important cause of illness and death worldwide. In some countries, many children still die before their fifth birthday; acute respiratory infection, gastroenteritis, measles and malaria are among the biggest killers. Infection is also the biggest cause of hospital admission in the UK.

The dramatic reduction in the burden of infectious diseases in high-income countries since the 19th century has occurred through a combination of factors, including:

- Better living conditions
- Improved nutrition
- Sanitation (safe water and drainage)
- Immunization
- Effective drug therapy
- Improved diagnosis and management of contagious people

Infectious diseases remain important due to:

- The discovery of newly recognized diseases, e.g. severe acute respiratory syndrome (SARS), SARS-CoV-2 causing COVID-19, and Middle East respiratory syndrome (MERS)
- The emergence and re-emergence of outbreak pathogens capable of causing pandemics, e.g. Ebola, Zika and swine influenza virus
- The failure to control existing global infections including human immunodeficiency virus (HIV), tuberculosis (TB) and malaria
- Rapidly increasing antimicrobial resistance (AMR) leading to multidrug-resistant TB, extended spectrum beta-lactamase (ESBL) Gram-negative bacteria and methicillin-resistant *Staphylococcus aureus* (MRSA) among other drug-resistant infections

DOI: 10.1201/9781003193616-3

- Rising concern around hospital-acquired infections caused by pathogens such as *Clostridium difficile*, Norovirus and drug-resistant bacteria
- The increased risk of hospital-acquired infection following invasive procedures and complex treatments in frail and elderly people
- Widespread international travel leading to new exposures to tropical diseases, and global spread of diseases such as dengue, influenza and ESBL *Escherichia coli*
- Growing interest in the role of the gut microbiome in health and disease
- Increasing recognition of the role of infectious agents in triggering other diseases such as cancer, inflammatory bowel disease and arthritis

Infectious diseases affect all branches of medicine. This chapter is a summary of the main infectious diseases. Diseases are discussed in groups according to their main presentation (e.g. fever with a rash), or by system (e.g. infections of the respiratory tract). **Table 3.1** shows the definitions of key terms used in infectious diseases.

There is increasing interest in the human microbiome (**Figure 3.1**), which is all the microbes (bacteria, viruses, fungi and protozoa) that live on or inside the human body, including the gut, respiratory tract, genitourinary system and skin. The microbiome is a key contributor to human health, with gut bacteria helping to digest food, regulate the immune system and produce vitamins. People with chronic conditions such as obesity, diabetes and autoimmune disease are known to have an altered microbiome.

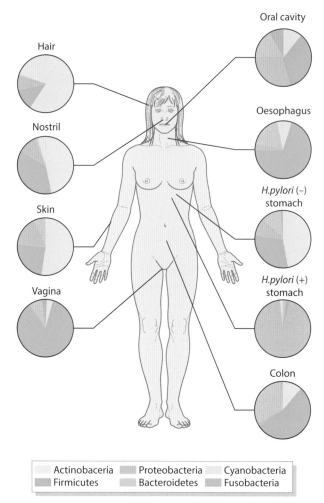

Figure legend:
- Actinobaceria
- Firmicutes
- Proteobacteria
- Bacteroidetes
- Cyanobacteria
- Fusobacteria

**Figure 3.1** The human microbiome by anatomical site. Reproduced from Cho I & Blaser MJ. The human microbiome: at the interface of health and disease (2012) *Nat Rev Genet* 13, 260–70. https://doi.org/10.1038/nrg3182, with permission from Springer Nature.

## SOURCES OF INFECTION AND ROUTES OF TRANSMISSION

There are four sources for microorganisms that give rise to disease.
- *The host's normal flora* (**Figure 3.2**): e.g. poor dental hygiene leading to oral bacteria such as *Streptococcus sanguis* being deposited on heart valves, causing endocarditis; perforation of the large bowel allowing

**Table 3.1** Definitions of terms

| Term | Definition |
|---|---|
| Pathogen | A microorganism capable of establishing itself in the human body where it causes disease |
| Commensal | A microorganism capable of establishing itself in the human body without causing disease |
| Pathogenicity | The ability of a microorganism to invade the host |
| Virulence | The ability of an organism to cause serious disease |

intestinal contents to escape into the peritoneum, resulting in peritonitis
- *Other humans:* e.g. the spread of measles by transmission of airborne virus from an infected person's respiratory exhalations; sexual transmission of HIV
- *Animals:* e.g. *Salmonella* food poisoning from eating infected chicken; rabies from the bite of an infected dog
- *The environment:* e.g. *Legionella* infection arising from a contaminated air-conditioning system; *Clostridium tetani* entering a wound from contaminated soil to cause tetanus

Routes of transmission include:
- *Respiratory droplets:* Pathogens are projected short distances in droplets by coughing, sneezing or exhaling, e.g. *Streptococcus pneumonia*, SARS-CoV-2 and influenza.
- *Airborne:* Aerosolized pathogens travel across rooms, e.g. measles, chickenpox and TB.

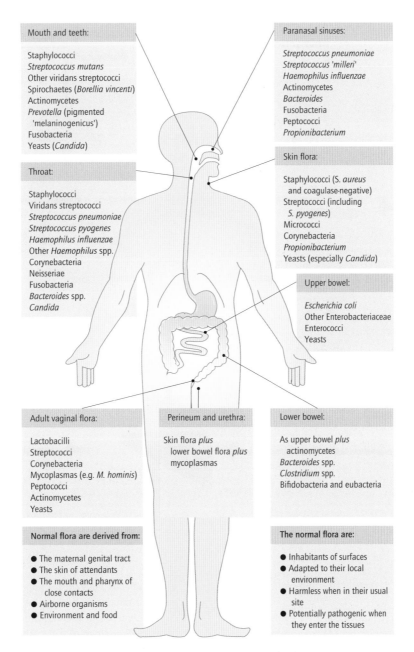

**Figure 3.2** Normal human flora. Reproduced from Bannister B, Begg N & Gillespie S, *Infectious Disease*, 2000, 2nd edn (Wiley-Blackwell, Oxford) with permission.

- *Ingestion (faecal–oral route):* Organisms are transmitted by contaminated food or water, e.g. *Salmonella* Typhi and tapeworms.
- *Direct contact:* Pathogens are spread by direct contact with people or contaminated objects (fomites), e.g. *Clostridium difficile* and scabies.
- *Parenteral:* Transmission may be via blood transfusions, non-sterile injections, tattooing or intravenous (IV) drug misuse: e.g. hepatitis C and HIV.
- *Sexual:* The pathogen is typically fragile and does not survive long outside the body, e.g. *Neisseria gonorrhoeae* and HIV.

## DISEASE MECHANISMS IN INFECTIOUS DISEASES

Microorganisms have evolved an armoury of weapons to enhance survival, transmission, immune evasion and spread.

- *Enhanced survival in the environment:* e.g. spore formation by *Clostridium difficile*
- *Attachment to host surfaces:* e.g. attachment of *Neisseria gonorrhoeae* to genital mucosa by specialized organelles called fimbriae or pili, or attachment of *Plasmodium falciparum* (malaria)-infected red blood cells to host brain capillaries via a parasite-encoded protein

23

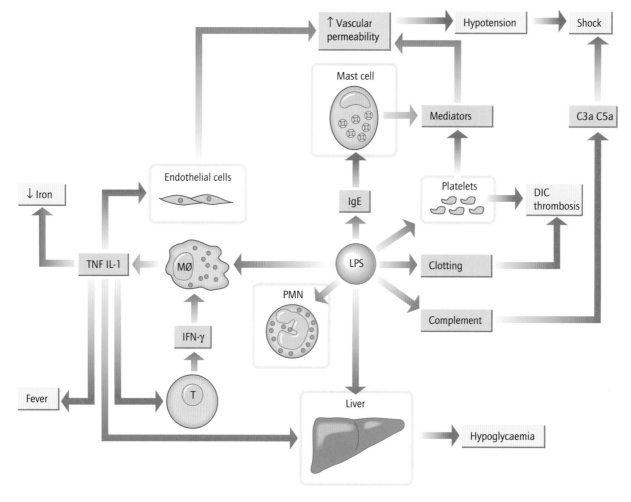

**Figure 3.3** Action of bacterial LPS. Bacterial LPS (endotoxin) activates nearly all immune mechanisms and the clotting pathway, thus making LPS one of the most powerful immune stimuli recognized. DIC, disseminated intravascular coagulation.

- *Motility:* e.g. *Vibrio cholerae* is able to move using its flagellum
- *Immune evasion* where pathogens have evolved counter-mechanisms to bypass human immune defence: includes avoiding destruction by host phagocytes due to a polysaccharide capsule (e.g. *Streptococcus pneumoniae*), mechanisms to survive inside host macrophages (e.g. prevention of fusion of the phagosome with the digestive lysosome by *Mycobacterium tuberculosis*), and antigenic variation (e.g. influenza and *Plasmodium falciparum*)
- *Endotoxins,* which are part of the structure of bacteria that are released when bacteria cells die or during normal bacterial cell turnover, and induce an innate immune response: e.g. Gram-negative bacteria express a lipopolysaccharide (LPS) on their outer membrane that causes disease by activating host macrophages to produce interleukin 1 (IL-1) and tumour necrosis factor (TNF) (**Figure 3.3**)
- *Exotoxins,* which are toxins released by bacteria to harm the host and help bacterial spread: e.g.

*Streptococcus pyogenes* releases a hyaluronidase into the tissues to break down connective tissue; *Vibrio cholera* releases cholera toxin that binds to the cell surface of gut cells and increases the concentration of cyclic adenosine monophosphate (cAMP) within the cell, resulting in secretion of fluid

## CLASSIFICATION OF INFECTIOUS DISEASES

A pathogen causes an infectious disease which presents as a clinical syndrome. There is a 'many-to-many' relationship between pathogens and diseases, whereby one microorganism can cause many different clinical syndromes, and one clinical syndrome can have several microorganisms as the aetiological agent. **Tables 3.2–3.11** give a classification of infectious organisms with their associated diseases.

**Table 3.2** Some medically important Gram-positive cocci and associated diseases

| Genus and species | Associated diseases |
|---|---|
| **Staphylococcus (aerobic, facultatively anaerobic, arranged in clusters)** | |
| Staph. aureus (coagulase-positive) | Skin infection, septicaemia, osteomyelitis, pneumonia (especially post-influenza), food poisoning (enterotoxin-producing strains), toxic shock syndrome (TSS toxin-producing strains) |
| | Endocarditis (especially in IV drug users) |
| Staph. epidermidis and other 'coagulase-negative' staphylococci | Rarely pathogenic, but septicaemia in immunocompromised, and infection of prostheses and cannulas |
| **Streptococcus (aerobic, facultatively anaerobic, arranged in pairs or chains, classified by α or β haemolysis, and by Lancefield grouping)** | |
| Group A β haemolytic Strep. pyogenes ('Group A Strep.', GAS') | Pharyngitis, scarlet fever, septicaemia |
| | Erysipelas, cellulitis, pyoderma |
| | Rheumatic fever (post-infective complication) |
| | Acute glomerulonephritis (post-infective complication) |
| Group B Strep. agalactiae ('Group B Strep') | Neonatal meningitis, pneumonia and septicaemia |
| Group C Strep. equi, Strep. dysgalactiae | Pharyngitis, endocarditis |
| Group D Strep. bovis | Endocarditis |
| | Bacteraemia associated with colonic carcinoma |
| **Viridans α haemolytic streptococci** | |
| Strep. mitis | Endocarditis |
| Strep. sanguis | Endocarditis |
| Strep. anginosis, Strep. constellatus, Strep. intermedius | Deep-seated abscesses (e.g. liver abscess, empyema) |
| Strep. pneumoniae | Pneumonia, bacteraemia, otitis media, osteomyelitis |
| | Meningitis |
| **Enterococcus** | |
| E. faecalis | Urinary and abdominal infections |
| E. faecium | Endocarditis |
| | Bacteraemia in intensive care |

**3**

**Table 3.3** Some medically important Gram-positive rods and associated diseases

| Genus and species | Associated disease |
|---|---|
| **Bacillus (spore-bearing aerobes)** | |
| B. cereus | Food poisoning |
| B. anthracis | Anthrax |
| **Listeria monocytogenes** | Neonatal meningitis |
| | Meningitis and septicaemia in pregnancy and immunocompromised |
| **Corynebacterium** | |
| C. diphtheriae | Diphtheria |
| C. pyogenes | Skin infection |
| **Clostridium (spore-forming anaerobes)** | |
| Cl. tetani | Tetanus |
| Cl. botulinum | Botulism |
| Cl. perfringens | Food poisoning, wound infection, gas gangrene |
| Cl. difficile | Antibiotic-associated colitis |

**Table 3.4** Some medically important Gram-negative cocci, coccobacilli and associated diseases

| Genus and species | Associated disease |
|---|---|
| **Neisseria** | |
| N. gonorrhoeae | Gonorrhoea, pelvic inflammatory disease |
| N. meningitidis | Meningitis, septicaemia |
| **Moraxella catarrhalis** | Bronchitis, pneumonia, sinusitis, otitis media |
| **Acinetobacter baumannii** | Ventilator-associated pneumoniae, bacteraemia |
| **Haemophilus** | |
| H. influenzae | Meningitis, epiglottitis, lower respiratory tract infection |
| H. ducreyi | Chancroid |
| **Bordatella pertussis** | Whooping cough |
| **Brucella abortus** | Brucellosis |
| **Pasteurella multocida** | Sepsis after an animal bite |

**Table 3.5** Some medically important Gram-negative rods and associated diseases

| Genus and species | Associated disease |
|---|---|
| **Enterobacteriaceae** | |
| ***Klebsiella, Serratia, Enterobacter, Citrobacter, Proteus*** | Urinary tract infection, hospital-acquired sepsis (e.g. peritonitis, pneumonia, septicaemia) and neonatal sepsis |
| ***Escherichia*** | |
| *E. coli* | Urinary tract infection, hospital-acquired sepsis and neonatal sepsis, traveller's diarrhoea |
| ETEC | Traveller's diarrhoea |
| EIEC | Dysentery |
| EHEC or VTEC (often serotype 0157) | Haemolytic–uraemic syndrome |
| ***Yersinia pestis*** | Plague |
| ***Salmonella*** | |
| *S. Typhi, S. Paratyphi A, B* | Enteric fever |
| Non-typhoid *Salmonella* | Enteritis |
| ***Shigella*** | |
| *S. flexneri, S. boydii, S. dysenteriae, S. sonnei* | Dysentery |
| ***Vibrio cholerae*** | Cholera |
| ***Pseudomonas aeruginosa*** | Urinary tract infection, hospital-acquired sepsis (e.g. peritonitis, pneumonia, septicaemia), otitis externa (especially in diabetes) |
| ***Burkholderia*** | |
| *B. pseudomallei* | Melioidosis |
| *B. cepacia* | Chronic destructive chest infection in cystic fibrosis |
| ***Legionella pneumophila*** | Legionnaires' disease |
| ***Bartonella henselae*** | Cat scratch fever |
| ***Bacteroides fragilis*** | Surgical sepsis |

EHEC, enterohaemorrhagic *E. coli*; EIEC, enteroinvasive *E. coli*; ETEC, enterotoxigenic *E. coli*; VTEC, verotoxin-producing *E. coli*.

## BACTERIA

Bacteria are identified or speciated by using a series of physical characteristics (see **Figure 3.8**). Some of these are listed below.

- *Gram reaction* to staining with crystal violet: Gram-positive bacteria stain purple due to their thick layer of peptidoglycan in the cell wall retaining the dye, while Gram-negative bacteria stain red, because their thinner peptidoglycan wall does not retain the crystal violet dye during the decolouring process. Gram-positive and Gram-negative bacteria respond differently to antibiotics.

**Table 3.6** Medically important spiral organisms and associated diseases

| Genus and species | Associated disease |
|---|---|
| **Treponema** | |
| *T. pallidum* | Syphilis |
| *T. endemicum* | Endemic non-venereal syphilis |
| *T. pertenue* | Yaws |
| *T. carateum* | Pinta |
| **Borrelia burgdorferi** | Lyme disease |
| **Leptospira interrogans** | Leptospirosis (Weil's disease), aseptic meningitis |
| **Campylobacter jejuni** | Enteritis |
| **Helicobacter pylori** | Gastritis, peptic ulcer disease |

**Table 3.7** *Rickettsia*, *Chlamydia*, *Mycoplasma* and associated diseases

| Genus and species | Associated disease |
|---|---|
| ***Rickettsia*** | |
| *R. prowazekii* (louse-borne) | Epidemic typhus |
| *R. typhi* (flea-borne) | Murine typhus |
| *R. rickettsii* (tick-borne) | Rocky Mountain spotted fever |
| *R. conorii* (tick-borne) | Boutonneuse fever, African tick fever |
| *R. akari* (mite-borne) | Rickettsial pox |
| ***Orientia tsutsugamushi*** (mite-borne) | Scrub typhus |
| ***Coxiella burnetti*** | Q fever |
| ***Chlamydia*** | |
| *C. trachomatis* | Genital tract infection, trachoma, lymphogranuloma venerum |
| *C. psittaci* | Psittacosis |
| *C. pneumoniae* | Pneumonia |
| ***Mycoplasma*** | |
| *M. pneumoniae* | Upper respiratory tract infection, pneumonia, otitis media |
| *M. hominis* | Genital tract infection |
| ***Ureaplasma urealyticum*** | Genital tract infection |

**Table 3.8** Some medically important mycobacteria

| Genus and species | Associated disease |
|---|---|
| **Mycobacterium** | |
| M. tuberculosis | TB |
| M. bovis | TB |
| M. avium-intracellulare | Bacteraemia and pulmonary infection in immunocompromised patients including advanced HIV Lymphadenopathy in children |
| M. kansasii, M. xenopi | TB-like syndrome in those with chronic chest disease |
| M. leprae | Leprosy |

*Note:* non-tuberculosis mycobacteria are often called 'atypical mycobacteria'

- *Cell shape:* Bacteria can be cocci, bacilli or spirals.
- *Atmospheric preference:* Organisms are aerobic, requiring oxygen, or anaerobic, requiring an atmosphere with very little or no oxygen. Organisms that grow in either atmosphere are known as facultative anaerobes.
- *Requirement for special media or intracellular growth.*

More detailed biochemical, antigenic and molecular tests are performed to identify organisms to species level. Many laboratories use automated processes such as MALDI-TOF (matrix-assisted laser desorption/ionization time-of-flight mass spectrometry) or VITEK-2®.

Medically important bacteria are shown in **Tables 3.2–3.8**. Mycobacteria (**Table 3.8**) include *Mycobacterium tuberculosis* and *M. leprae* (the cause of leprosy) as well as other environmental mycobacteria that chiefly cause opportunistic infections in people with impaired immune systems such as in advanced HIV infection.

## VIRUSES

Viruses are classified according to their nucleic acid genetic material, as shown in **Figure 3.4**.

- DNA viruses (**Table 3.9**) are either double-stranded (dsDNA, e.g. herpes simplex virus (HSV)) or single-stranded (ssDNA, parvovirus).
- RNA viruses (**Table 3.10**) possess a single strand of RNA and are further classified by how the RNA is translated into protein.
  - Positive-sense RNA viruses (+ssRNA) such as polio virus in the Picornaviridae family serve directly as messenger RNA (mRNA) for translation into proteins in the host cell.
  - Negative-sense RNA viruses (-ss) such as rabies in the Rhabdoviridae family have RNA that is complementary to mRNA and needs to be converted to positive RNA by RNA polymerase before translation.

**Table 3.9** DNA viruses

| Family and virus | Associated disease |
|---|---|
| **Papovaviridae** | |
| Human wart viruses | Warts |
| **Polyomaviridae** | |
| JC virus | Progressive multifocal leucoencephalopathy |
| BK virus | Haemorrhagic cystitis in the immunosuppressed |
| **Adenoviridae** | |
| Adenovirus A–F | Upper respiratory tract infection, coryza, conjunctivitis, gastroenteritis, sepsis in the immunocompromised |
| **Herpesviridae** | |
| Herpes simplex Types 1 and 2 | Primary stomatitis, orogenital herpes, encephalitis, keratitis, neonatal sepsis |
| Cytomegalovirus (CMV) | Congenital infection, infection in the immunocompromised |
| Epstein–Barr virus (EBV) | Infectious mononucleosis, Burkitt lymphoma, nasopharyngeal carcinoma |
| Varicella-zoster virus (VZV) | |
| Primary | Chickenpox |
| Recurrent | Shingles |
| Human herpesvirus 6 | Roseola infantum |
| **Poxviridae** | |
| Variola virus | Smallpox |
| Molluscum contagiosum virus | Molluscum contagiosum (benign epidermal tumours) |
| Orf | Orf |
| **Parvoviridae** | |
| Parvovirus (B19) | Erythema infectiosum, aplastic crisis |
| **Hepadnaviridae** | |
| Hepatitis B | Acute, fulminant and chronic hepatitis, hepatocellular carcinoma |

**Table 3.10** RNA viruses

| Family | Virus | Associated disease |
|---|---|---|
| **Picornoviridae** | | |
| Enteroviruses | Polioviruses 1–3 | Polio |
| | Echoviruses | Aseptic meningitis |
| | Coxsackie viruses | Aseptic meningitis, hand foot & mouth disease, myocarditis, endocarditis |
| | Hepatitis A virus | Acute hepatitis |
| Rhinoviruses | | Coryza ('common cold') |
| Caliciviruses | Norovirus (Norwalk agent) | Gastroenteritis |
| Astroviruses | | Gastroenteritis |
| Togavirus | | |
| Alphaviruses | Chikungunya | Fever with bone pain |
| (all arboviruses) | O'nyong-nyong, Ross River | Fever with bone pain |
| Flaviviruses | Dengue 1–4 | Fever with bone pain, haemorrhagic fever |
| (all arboviruses) | Yellow fever | Haemorrhagic fever and hepatitis |
| | Japanese encephalitis | Encephalitis |
| | St Louis encephalitis | Encephalitis |
| | Tick-borne encephalitis (TBE) | Encephalitis |
| Rubiviruses | Rubella virus | Rubella |
| Orthomyxoviruses | Influenza viruses A, B, C | Influenza |
| Paramyxoviruses | Parainfluenza viruses 1–4 | Acute respiratory infections |
| | Mumps virus | Mumps |
| | Measles virus | Measles |
| | Respiratory syncytial virus | Bronchiolitis in infants, acute respiratory infections |
| Coronaviruses | SARS-CoV | Severe acute respiratory illness (especially in older/ immunocompromised people) |
| | SARS-CoV-2 | COVID-19 |
| | MERS-CoV | MERS |
| | Various human coronaviruses | Coryza ('common cold') |
| Arenaviruses | Lassa virus | Lassa fever |
| Bunyaviruses | Congo–Crimea haemorrhagic fever | Haemorrhagic fever |
| (all arboviruses) | Rift valley fever | Haemorrhagic fever |
| Retroviruses | HTLV I | T-cell leukaemia and lymphoma |
| | HIV | HIV / AIDS |
| Rhabdoviruses | Rabies virus | Rabies |
| Filoviruses | Marburg virus | Haemorrhagic fever |
| | Ebola virus | Haemorrhagic fever |
| Reoviruses | Rotavirus | Gastroenteritis |
| Unclassified RNA viruses | Norwalk-like viruses (SRSVs) | Gastroenteritis |
| | Hepatitis C virus | Chronic hepatitis, hepatocellular carcinoma |
| | Hepatitis D virus | Acute and chronic hepatitis in the presence of coexistent (delta agent) hepatitis B virus infection |
| | Hepatitis E virus | Epidemic and sporadic faeco-oral acute and fulminant hepatitis |

HTLV, human T-cell leukaemia/lymphoma virus; SRSV, small round-structured virus.

○ Retroviruses (+ss RNAr) such as HIV possess single-stranded positive (-sense) RNA that cannot act as mRNA. It is transcribed into DNA by reverse transcriptase. The DNA is incorporated into host DNA. The subsequent transcription is under the control of host transcriptase enzymes to make mRNA and viral genomic RNA.

## PROTOZOA

Protozoa are unicellular organisms, some of which are important pathogens of humans. They include *Plasmodium*, the causative organism of malaria, which is responsible for around one million deaths each year worldwide. Some protozoa have a complex life cycle that includes a vector, whereas

Possible structural components

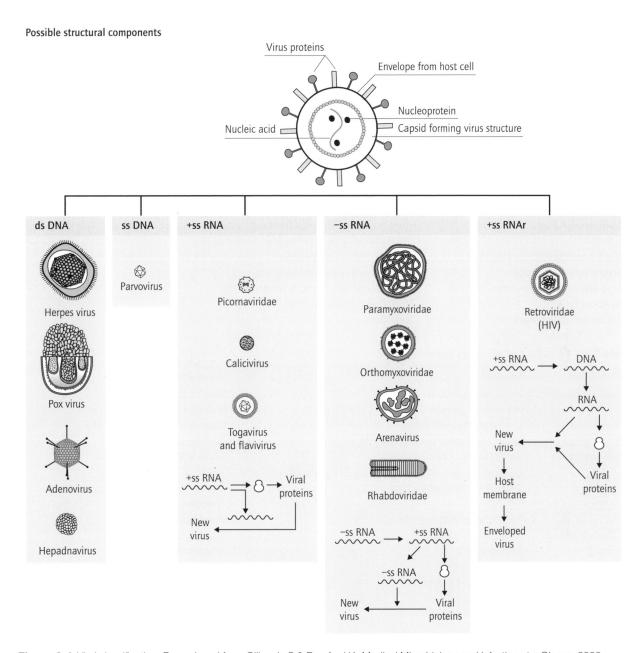

**Figure 3.4** Viral classification. Reproduced from Gillespie S & Bamford K, *Medical Microbiology and Infection at a Glance*, 2000 (Wiley-Blackwell, Oxford) with permission.

others spread from person to person by the faecal–oral route. Many protozoa such as *Leishmania* and *Trypanosoma* are adapted to an intracellular environment (**Table 3.11**).

## HELMINTHS

Parasitic worms (helminths) are complex infectious agents (**Table 3.12**) that have co-evolved over millions of years in parallel with their hosts, producing low-grade chronic infections. Most helminths do not complete their life cycle within one host individual, and typically a human host harbours one or more stages of the parasite but the complete life cycle includes a period outside the host, often involving

another host species. Parasitic worms are classified into roundworms (nematodes), tapeworms (cestodes) and flukes (trematodes).

## FUNGI

Fungi are widely distributed in the environment and only rarely cause human disease. They may have a yeast-like morphology such as *Candida* and *Cryptococcus* or be filamentous such as *Aspergillus*. A wide variety of diseases can arise when invasion occurs, ranging from cutaneous dermatophyte infections to systemic *Candida* or *Aspergillus* infection in the severely immunocompromised patient (**Table 3.13**).

**Table 3.11** Protozoa and associated diseases

| Genus and protozoan | Associated disease |
|---|---|
| *Plasmodium* | |
| *P. vivax, P. ovale, P. malariae, P. falciparum* | Malaria |
| *Trypanosoma* | |
| *T. brucei gambiense, T. brucei rhodesiense* | African trypanosomiasis |
| *T. cruzi* | South American trypanosomiasis |
| *Leishmania* | |
| *L. donovani, L. infantum* | Visceral leishmaniasis |
| *L. tropica, L. major, L. aethiopica* | Old World cutaneous leishmaniasis |
| *L. braziliensis, L. mexicana* | New World cutaneous leishmaniasis, mucocutaneous leishmaniasis |
| *Giardia lamblia* | Diarrhoea |
| *Toxoplasma gondii* | Congenital abnormalities, fever with lymphadenopathy, retinitis and brain abscess (in immunosuppression such as advanced HIV) |
| *Acanthamoeba* (various species) | Amoebic meningitis, keratitis |
| *Entamoeba histolytica* | Amoebic colitis, amoebic liver abscess |
| *Cryptosporidium parvum* | Acute diarrhoea (chronic in advanced HIV) |
| *Isospora belli* | Diarrhoea in advanced HIV |
| *Trichomonas vaginalis* | Vaginitis |

**Table 3.12** Helminths and associated infections

| Classification | Species | Associated disease |
|---|---|---|
| Filarial nematodes | *Wuchereria bancrofti* | Elephantiasis |
| | *Onchocerca volvulus* | River blindness |
| | *Loa loa* (African eye worm) | Calabar swelling |
| | *Dracunculus medinensis* (guinea worm) | Chronic leg ulcer |
| Gut nematodes | *Ascaris lumbricoides* (roundworm) | Minor abdominal symptoms |
| | *Ancylostoma duodenale* and *Necator americanus* (hookworm) | Anaemia |
| | *Trichuris trichiura* (whipworm) | Minor abdominal symptoms, nutritional deficiency |
| | *Enterobius vermicularis* (threadworm) | Pruritus ani |
| Other nematodes | *Strongyloides stercoralis* | Larva currens |
| | *Toxocara canis* | Visceral larva migrans |
| | *Trichinella spiralis* | Fever, muscle pain |
| Trematodes | *Schistosoma mansoni* | Colitis, portal hypertension, pulmonary hypertension |
| | *Schistosoma haematobium* | Haematuria, hydronephrosis, carcinoma of the bladder |
| | *Clonorchis sinensis* and *Opisthorchis* spp. ('liver flukes') | Cholangitis, cholangiocarcinoma |
| | *Fasciola hepatica* | Fever, painful hepatomegaly |
| | *Paragonamus* spp. | Chronic cavitating lung disease |
| Cestodes (tapeworm) | *Taenia saginata* (beef tapeworm) | Minor abdominal symptoms |
| | *Taenia solium* (pork tapeworm) | Cysticercosis, epilepsy |
| | *Echinococcus granulosus* | Hydatid cysts |

## APPROACH TO THE PATIENT

### HISTORY

Infection results from a complex interaction between an individual, an organism and the environment. A detailed history (HISTORY & EXAMINATION 3.1, HISTORY 3.2) should include enquiry about:

- Age, sex and race
- Occupation (e.g. farmer – brucellosis, Q fever) and hobbies (e.g. triathlete – leptospirosis from contaminated water exposure)
- Travel history (**Table 3.14**)
- Sexual history
- Past medical history
  - Skin conditions with a break in the protective surface predisposing to infection

**Table 3.13** Fungi and associated diseases

| Organism | Associated disease | Principal target organs | Geographical distribution |
|---|---|---|---|
| *Microsporum* sp. | Ringworm | Skin | Worldwide |
| *Trichophyton* sp. | Ringworm, athlete's foot | Skin, nails | Worldwide |
| *Malassezia furfur* | Tinea versicolor | Skin | More common in hot climates |
| *Sporothrix shenkii* | Sporotrichosis | Subcutaneous | Tropics/subtropics |
| *Madurella* sp. and others | Madura foot, mycetoma | Subcutaneous, bone | Tropics |
| *Cryptococcus neoformans* | Cryptococcosis | Lung, meninges (often opportunistic) | Worldwide |
| *Histoplasma capsulatum* | Histoplasmosis | Lung/disseminated (opportunistic) | North America and many tropical areas |
| *Histoplasma duboisii* | African histoplasmosis | Skin, bones, disseminated | Africa |
| *Blastomyces dermatitidis* | Blastomycosis | Skin, lung, bone | North America and Africa |
| *Coccidiodes immitis* | Coccidiodomycosis | Lung, bone, skin, disseminated | South-western USA, Mexico, Argentina, Paraguay |
| *Paracoccidiodes braziliensis* | Paracoccidiodomycosis | Lung, lymph nodes, disseminated | South America |
| *Candida albicans* | Candidiasis | Mucous membranes, commonly | Worldwide opportunistic, rarely disseminated |
| *Pneumocystis carinii* | Opportunistic infection | Lungs | Worldwide |
| *Aspergillus fumigatus* | Aspergillosis | Opportunistic (especially lungs) | Worldwide |
| *A. flavus, A. niger* | | Also, allergic bronchopulmonary aspergillosis | |

---

**HISTORY & EXAMINATION 3.1**

**Questions to be addressed by the history and examination of a patient with an infectious disease**

What is the site of the infection?
What is the probable infecting organism?
Is there any associated tissue damage and/or organ failure?
Is there an underlying disease predisposing the patient to infection?
Are there any other predisposing factors (e.g. lifestyle, travel)

---

**HISTORY 3.2**

**Important questions to ask a patient with an infection**

**About the patient**
Where have you been recently?
Have you been abroad? If so, where and for how long?
What is your occupation?
Have you been exposed to animals or insect bites?

**Symptoms**
When were you last well?
Do you have any localized features?
Does the fever have a pattern?
Do you have any symptoms other than fever (e.g. headache, joint aches, rash, diarrhoea, stomach upset, nausea)?
Have you lost any weight?
Do you have sweats during the night?

**Drug history**
Have you taken any antibiotics?
Have you taken any medicines to bring down your fever?
Are you taking any other medicines or tonics, either prescribed or obtained from other sources including health food shops?

**Past medical history**
What infections have you had in the past?
What immunizations have you had?
Have you had any transfusions?

**Family history**
Is anyone in your family immunosuppressed?
Has anyone in your family had an unusual infection?
Does anyone in your family have a skin condition?

**Sexual history**
See HISTORY & EXAMINATION 3.1

---

**Table 3.14** Some causes of fever and infection in a traveller

| Area visited | Infection |
|---|---|
| Tropics and subtropics | Malaria, typhoid, TB, hepatitis A, dengue, Zika, chikungunya |
| Africa (rural) | Filariasis (West Africa), typhus, viral haemorrhagic fever (e.g. Ebola), yellow fever (West Africa) |
| Middle East | Brucellosis, MERS |
| Asia | Japanese encephalitis |
| South America | Viral haemorrhagic fever, Oroya fever |
| Oceania | Malaria, filariasis |
| North America | Rocky Mountain spotted fever, Lyme disease |
| Worldwide | Sexually transmitted diseases, HIV |

- o Immunocompromise due to a range of causes including genetic, infection (e.g. HIV), drug therapy (e.g. steroids, chemotherapy)
- o Sickle cell anaemia resulting in a functional splenectomy
- History of exposure to infection (e.g. measles or TB)
- Blood transfusions and IV drug use (risk of blood-borne viruses such as HIV, hepatitis B and hepatitis C)
- Animal contact (e.g. birds – psittacosis, extrinsic allergic alveolitis; dogs – toxocariasis, rabies; cats – toxoplasmosis, cat-scratch disease)
- Time-course of symptoms

## SYMPTOMS

Infectious diseases can present with a wide range of symptoms including:
- Fever
- Headache
- Malaise and fatigue
- Gastrointestinal (GI) disturbance including anorexia, nausea, vomiting, diarrhoea or constipation
- Myalgia and arthralgia
- Rash
- Focal symptoms for localized infection (e.g. dysuria for urinary tract infection, joint pain for septic arthritis)

## EXAMINATION

A thorough examination should be undertaken (EXAMINATION 3.3), paying careful attention to the following:
- Vital signs including temperature (fever >37.5 °C), pulse, blood pressure and respiratory rate
- Level of consciousness and signs of meningism
- Hydration status
- Presence of a rash, blistering (**Figure 3.5**) or an eschar from a tick bite (**Figure 3.6**)
- Detection of jaundice
- Needle marks from IV drug use
- Full lymph node examination including axillae and groin
- Presence of an enlarged liver or spleen

## GENERAL PRINCIPLES OF MANAGEMENT

- Prior to patient contact, a risk assessment should be made to exclude the possibility of a highly contagious high-risk pathogen (e.g. Ebola) and to evaluate whether additional infectious control measures are required to minimize the risk of spread (e.g. diarrhoea, known AMR, varicella).
- If there are signs of sepsis, prompt resuscitation and empirical antibiotic therapy following cultures is essential.

### EXAMINATION 3.3

**Examination of a patient with an infection**

**Look**

*Inspect the skin*
Look for rashes, eschars, petechiae, ulceration, scars from previous shingles and needle marks.
*Examine the eyes/fundi*
Look for petechiae, keratitis and retinal lesions (e.g. CMV).
*Inspect the mouth*
Look for evidence of oral thrush, state of dentition.
*Inspect the ears*
Look for evidence of otitis media.

**Feel**

*Palpate the lymph nodes (cervical, axillary and inguinal)*
Note any enlargement.
*Palpate the liver and spleen*
Hepatosplenomegaly may suggest a non-infective infiltrative cause of a fever (e.g. lymphoma).
Hepatomegaly may occur with a liver abscess.
Splenomegaly is a feature of glandular fever, malaria and visceral leishmaniasis.
*Palpate the abdomen for tenderness and masses*
*Feel the nerves*
Note any thickening if considering leprosy.
*Palpate the sinuses*
Note any tenderness suggesting sinusitis.
*Feel for skin nodules*
Skin nodules can be felt in cysticercosis.

**Move**

*Move the joints*
Look for septic arthritis.
*Move the neck*
Look for meningeal irritation.

**Percuss**

*Percuss the chest*
Look for evidence of an effusion (TB) or consolidation (pneumonia).

**Listen**

Note the whoop of pertussis (whooping cough).
Listen to the heart for the murmurs of subacute bacterial endocarditis.
Listen to the lungs for signs of pneumonia.

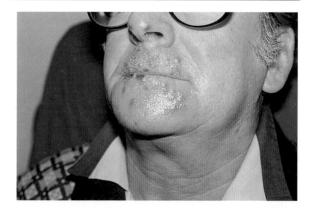

**Figure 3.5** Herpes simplex reactivation lesion (cold sore). Reproduced from Bannister B *et al.*, *Infectious Disease*, 1996 (Wiley-Blackwell, Oxford) with the permission of the authors.

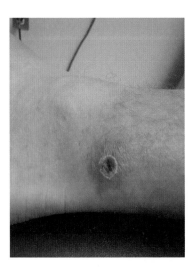

**Figure 3.6** Tick typhus: a black eschar at the site of the infecting tick bite.

- Early evaluation by the intensive care team should be considered if there are warning signs of severe illness such as tachycardia, hypotension, reduced level of consciousness or a petechial rash.
- Diagnostic samples for microbiological culture should be drawn prior to initiating antimicrobial treatment, unless this will delay life-saving treatment.
- Symptomatic treatment includes analgesia, oral or IV hydration, and antiemetics if required.
- Empirical antimicrobial therapy can be commenced if appropriate, using local antimicrobial guidelines, and stopped or fine-tuned later according the results of diagnostic tests.
- For many patients, especially those with suspected viral infections, reassurance and observation is the most appropriate management.
- Where a collection such as an abscess is present, surgical drainage is the mainstay of treatment rather than antibiotics.

## DIAGNOSIS OF INFECTIOUS DISEASES

Diagnostic tests will be driven by the history and examination, but may include:
- Full blood count, renal and liver profile
- C-reactive protein (CRP)
- Blood culture if history of fever or suspected systemic infection
- Serology (e.g. EBV, CMV, HIV, hepatitis B, hepatitis C)
- A 'serum save', which can be requested from the laboratory, in order to add on specific serological tests later as further information becomes available
- The threshold for HIV testing should be low, explaining to the patient that you are screening the

function of their immune system; with HIV it is now much better to know if you are positive than not know, as highly effective treatments are available, allowing a near-normal life expectancy
- Blood for molecular testing (e.g. *N. meningitidis* by polymerase chain reaction [PCR])
- Nasopharyngeal swab for respiratory viruses (e.g. SARS CoV-2, influenza)
- Urine dipstick and culture
- Stool culture (including a request for microscopy for ova, cysts and parasites if a gut parasite infection is suspected)
- Sputum for microscopy and culture to detect mycobacteria if TB is suspected (sputum culture in non-mycobacterial respiratory infections has low diagnostic value due to the high rate of commensal organisms detected)
- Cerebrospinal fluid (CSF) microscopy and culture if signs of meningism and/or suspected central nervous system (CNS) disease
- Bone marrow microscopy culture is indicated in some cases (e.g. suspected visceral leishmaniasis or miliary TB)
- Radiology (e.g. chest radiograph, abdominal ultrasound, CT scan)
- Biopsy (e.g. of enlarged lymph node for histopathology and culture)

An overview of investigation for a pyrexia of unknown origin (PUO) is shown in **Figure 3.8**.

## LABORATORY DIAGNOSIS OF PATHOGENS

- Blood culture bottles arriving in the laboratory are placed in an incubator. If bacterial growth occurs, the resulting increase in $CO_2$ production will change the colour of a $CO_2$-sensitive disc on the base of the blood culture bottle. Automated incubator systems such as BACTEC® machines detect the colour change and sound an alarm. 'Positive' blood cultures can then be examined under the microscope with Gram stain (**Figure 3.8a,b**), and plated out on agar plates.
- Different types of agar plates select different pathogens. Blood agar is the commonest agar media and supports the growth of most bacteria. MacConkey agar is selective for Gram-negative gut pathogens (**Figure 3.9**). Sabouraud agar selects fungi such as *Aspergillus*.
- When bacteria grow on agar plates, the species can then be identified using biochemical tests. Biochemical kits such as the 'API' system can be used, but many laboratories now use automated systems. MALDI-TOF uses mass spectrometry to identify bacteria, while the VITEK system is an automated platform for bacterial diagnosis by biochemical testing followed by automated antimicrobial susceptibility testing (AST).

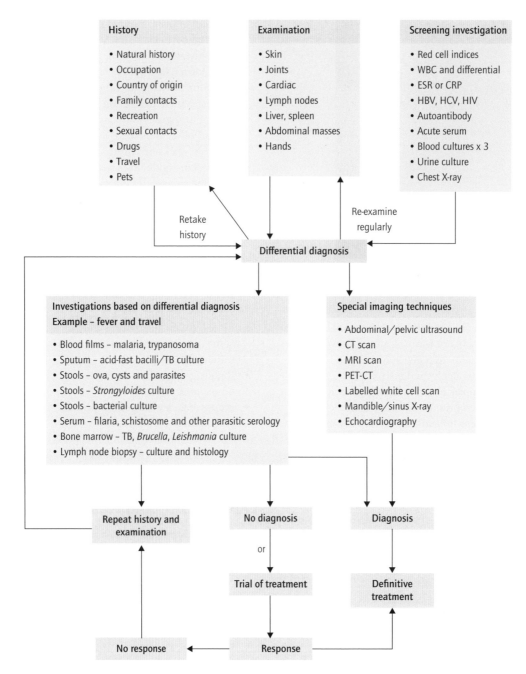

**History**

- Natural history
- Occupation
- Country of origin
- Family contacts
- Recreation
- Sexual contacts
- Drugs
- Travel
- Pets

**Examination**

- Skin
- Joints
- Cardiac
- Lymph nodes
- Liver, spleen
- Abdominal masses
- Hands

**Screening investigation**

- Red cell indices
- WBC and differential
- ESR or CRP
- HBV, HCV, HIV
- Autoantibody
- Acute serum
- Blood cultures x 3
- Urine culture
- Chest X-ray

Retake history

Re-examine regularly

**Differential diagnosis**

**Investigations based on differential diagnosis**
**Example – fever and travel**

- Blood films – malaria, trypanosoma
- Sputum – acid-fast bacilli/TB culture
- Stools – ova, cysts and parasites
- Stools – *Strongyloides* culture
- Stools – bacterial culture
- Serum – filaria, schistosome and other parasitic serology
- Bone marrow – TB, *Brucella*, *Leishmania* culture
- Lymph node biopsy – culture and histology

**Special imaging techniques**

- Abdominal/pelvic ultrasound
- CT scan
- MRI scan
- PET-CT
- Labelled white cell scan
- Mandible/sinus X-ray
- Echocardiography

**Repeat history and examination**

**No diagnosis**

**Diagnosis**

or

**Trial of treatment**

**Definitive treatment**

**No response**

**Response**

**Figure 3.7** Pyrexia of unknown origin. Adapted from Gillespie S & Bamford K, *Medical Microbiology and Infection at a Glance*, 2003 (Wiley-Blackwell, Oxford) with permission.

- The sensitivity of bacteria to antimicrobials is tested in the laboratory by AST, according to guidelines such as EUCAST or CLSI.
- For the Kirby-Bauer disc diffusion method of AST, a suspension of bacteria is spread on an agar plate and then discs containing antibiotics are added (**Figure 3.10**). Following incubation, the ability of each antibiotic to inhibit bacterial growth is determined by measuring the zone of inhibition. Sensitivity or resistance is determined by comparing the inhibition zone size against standard criteria in the guidelines.

- For the E-test method, a strip containing graduated amounts of one antimicrobial is placed on the agar plate following spread of bacteria.
- Diagnosing fungi, parasites and helminths in the laboratory requires expert knowledge of their microscopic appearance.
- Although historically viruses were identified by viral culture and electron microscopy, this is now rare, and serology or molecular approaches are generally used.
- Multiplex PCR panels for specific syndromes can be used to test for several aetiological agents at once

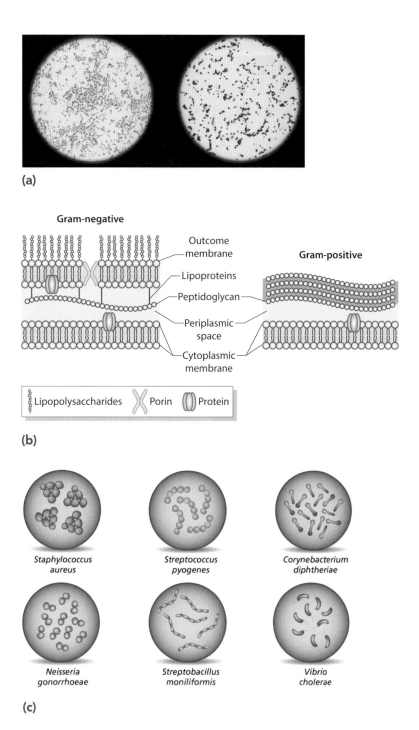

**Figure 3.8** Gram staining of bacteria. **(a)** Appearance under light microscope of Gram-negative (left) and Gram-positive (right) bacteria. With permission of Shutterstock/Schira. **(b)** Structural difference between Gram-negative bacteria (thin peptidoglycan layer surrounding cell) and Gram-positive bacteria (thick peptidoglycan cell wall). **(c)** Shapes of bacteria.

(e.g. a CSF multiplex panel might test for enterovirus, herpes simplex, varicella virus among others).

- TB can be diagnosed by Ziehl–Neelsen staining of sputum to detect acid-fast bacilli (**Figure 3.11**). Xpert MTB/RIF is a cartridge-based nucleic acid amplification technique (NAAT) that detects *Mycobacterium tuberculosis* directly from clinical samples such as sputum by detection of DNA, with simultaneous identification of rifampicin resistance by detection of the *rpo* gene. This platform has been successfully deployed in many low-income settings and allows rapid diagnosis and control of TB.

- Histopathology of biopsy specimens is also important for the diagnosis of many infections including CMV, *Leishmania* and TB, but it does not allow AST.

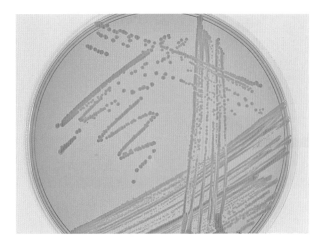

**Figure 3.9** *E. coli* isolated on MacConkey agar.

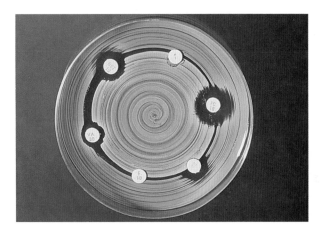

**Figure 3.10** Disc sensitivity testing: antibiogram of an isolate of *Staphylococcus epidermidis* from the blood of a patient in intensive care. Reproduced from Bannister B *et al.*, *Infectious Disease*, 1996 (Wiley-Blackwell, Oxford) with permission of the authors.

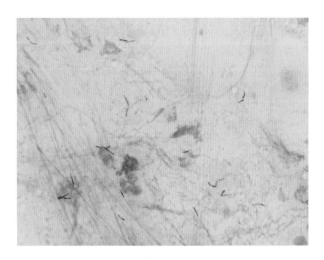

**Figure 3.11** Ziehl–Neelsen-stained smear of sputum, showing acid-fast bacilli. With permission of Shutterstock/Sudarma.

- Quality control is essential in microbiology laboratories. The use of internal controls (reference strains of bacteria with known characteristics), participation in external quality assurance schemes (EQA) and laboratory accreditation are important.

## ANTIMICROBIAL THERAPY

Antimicrobial agents have their effect because of selective toxicity. They interfere with microbial metabolism or functions but have minimal effect on the host. A number of different strategies have been used in their design. Key mechanisms of action of antibiotics are shown in **Figure 3.12**.

Knowledge of the pharmacology of antimicrobial agents is required to ensure that adequate concentrations of free antibiotic can penetrate to sites of infection, and to avoid toxicity. Body weight, renal function, liver function, and the use of other medicines (especially cytochrome P450 inducers such as phenytoin or inhibitors such as metronidazole) influence bioavailability of drugs. Some antimicrobials require IV administration due to poor oral absorption, reduced oral tolerance, or the patient having vomiting and diarrhoea.

There are two important concepts in understanding antibacterial chemotherapy:

- *Minimum inhibitory concentration (MIC):* The lowest concentration at which the growth of the organism is inhibited. The concentration of antimicrobials at the site of the infection should exceed the MIC.
- *Minimum bactericidal concentration (MBC):* The lowest concentration at which the organism is killed. Some antimicrobials are not bactericidal (kill bacteria) but are only bacteriostatic (prevent growth of bacteria but do not kill).

Toxic effects caused by antimicrobials include renal toxicity (e.g. by aminoglycosides such as gentamicin), liver toxicity (e.g. by anti-TB drugs such as rifampicin), bone marrow toxicity (e.g. by high-dose co-trimoxazole) and Stevens–Johnson syndrome (severe oropharyngeal blistering, e.g. by co-trimoxazole).

## ANTIBIOTIC CLASSES

### Penicillins

- Penicillins are beta-lactam antibiotics that work by inhibiting cross-linking of bacterial peptidoglycans.
- Bacteria become penicillin-resistant by producing a beta-lactamase or penicillin-binding proteins.
- Penicillin has good activity against *Streptococcus* unless resistance is present.
- Flucloxacillin, a modified penicillin, has excellent activity against *Staph. aureus* (but not MRSA).
- Co-amoxiclav is amoxicillin combined with the beta-lactamase inhibitor clavulanic acid. It has a spectrum

## Common antibiotic mechanisms

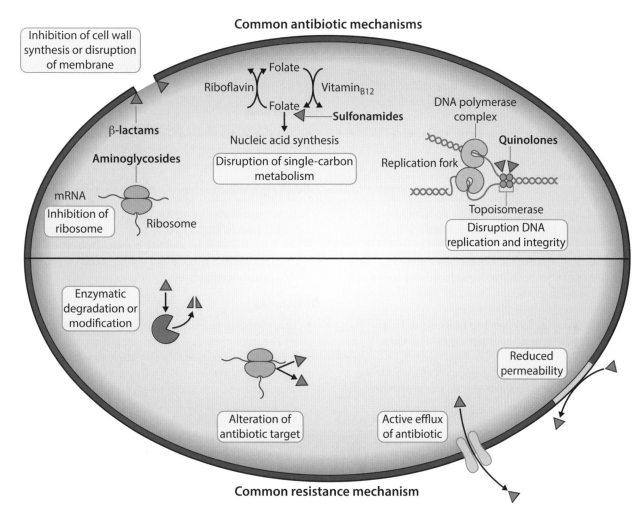

**Figure 3.12** Common mechanisms of action and resistance for antibiotics.

of activity including many Gram-positive and Gram-negative bacteria.

- Piperacillin is a penicillin given in combination with the beta-lactamase tazobactam, giving broad-spectrum activity including against *Pseudomonas*.

### Cephalosporins

- Cephalosporins are beta-lactam antibiotics related to penicillin.
- 1st generation cephalosporins (e.g. cefalexin) have mainly a Gram-positive spectrum of activity.
- 2nd generation (e.g. cefuroxime) have slightly more Gram-negative coverage than 1st generation.
- 3rd generation have broader activity still; ceftriaxone has excellent CNS penetration and is used for meningitis among other indications, while ceftazidime includes cover against *Pseudomonas*.
- 4th generation (e.g. cefepime) have greater resistance to beta-lactamases.
- 5th generation are reserved for resistant infections (e.g. ceftaroline covers MRSA).

- Cephalosporins are a group of antibiotics associated with increased risk of *C. difficile* diarrhoea

### Aminoglycosides

- Aminoglycosides work by inhibiting protein synthesis.
- They need to be given IV.
- They can cause ototoxicity and renal toxicity.
- Gentamicin is commonly used to treat Gram-negative infections such as pyelonephritis and has good activity against *Staph. aureus* including most MRSA strains.
- Several aminoglycosides including streptomycin have activity against TB but are now uncommonly used.

### Monobactams

- A monobactam is a beta-lactam antibiotic with a broad Gram-negative activity but no Gram-positive activity.
- Aztreonam is an example.

### Carbapenems

- Carbapenems are an important beta-lactam antibiotic class with a broad spectrum of activity;

they should be reserved for severe multidrug resistant infections.

- Examples include meropenem, imipenem and ertapenem.
- Carbapenem-resistant Enterobacteriaceae (CRE) have acquired resistance by one of several mechanisms such as developing carbapenemases that cleave the beta-lactam ring, or developing efflux pumps to actively transport the drug out of cells.

## Glycopeptides

- Vancomycin and teicoplanin are glycopeptides that work by disruption of cell walls via inhibition of formation of peptidoglycan polymers.
- They are active against Gram-positive bacteria only.
- They form the mainstay of therapy for MRSA.
- Glycopeptides are not absorbed orally, although oral vancomycin can be used to treat *C. difficile* diarrhoea by working within the gut lumen.
- If vancomycin is given too quickly, 'red man syndrome' can occur due to mass histamine release.
- Vancomycin-resistant enterococci (VRE) evade the antibiotic's actions by alterations in the peptidoglycan synthesis pathway.

## Oxazolidinones

- Linezolid is an oxazolidinone antibiotic that inhibits the initiation of bacterial protein synthesis.
- It is active against all Gram-positive bacteria including MRSA and VRE.
- *It also has activity against TB and is a core component of drug-resistant TB therapy.*
- Linezolid requires close monitoring because bone marrow suppression can occur.
- Resistance is currently rare.

## Lipopeptides

- Daptomycin is a lipopeptide antibiotic that disrupts bacterial cell membrane function.
- It shows activity against Gram-positive bacteria only and is reserved for severe infections such as endocarditis or bone infection where resistance or allergy rules out first-line options.
- It needs to be given IV.
- Resistance is currently rare.

## Macrolides

- Macrolides act by interfering with protein synthesis.
- Erythromycin has activity against a broad range of Gram-positive and Gram-negative bacteria, some anaerobes, *Mycoplasma* and *Chlamydia*.
- Erythromycin can also be used as a gut motility agent (e.g. in ITU patients).
- Clindamycin has excellent oral availability and good tissue penetration and covers Gram-positive bacteria

and anaerobes, but it may be associated with more risk of *C. difficile* diarrhoea than other choices.
- Azithromycin has good coverage of enteric pathogens such as *Salmonella* and *Campylobacter* but resistance is growing.

## Tetracyclines

- Tetracyclines act by interfering with protein synthesis.
- Activity is against a broad range of Gram-positive and Gram-negative bacteria.
- Tetracyclines are often used in the treatment of acne.
- Doxycycline is also active against leptospirosis, rickettsiae, *Borrelia burgdorferi* (Lyme disease), malaria and *E. Histolytica*.
- This group should be avoided in pregnant women and children under 8 years of age due to effects on skeletal and dental development.

## Quinolones

- Quinolones impair bacterial DNA synthesis by DNA gyrase inhibition.
- Ciprofloxacin has good Gram-negative activity including against *Pseudomonas* and excellent oral bioavailability. It used to be first choice for severe diarrhoea caused by enteric pathogens such as *Salmonella* and *Shigella* but resistance is now widespread.
- Moxifloxacin has better Gram-positive cover, including against *Streptococcus pneumoniae*, but narrower Gram-negative activity and does not cover *Pseudomonas. It also has activity against TB and is a core component of treatment for drug-resistant TB.*

## Chloramphenicol

- Chloramphenicol inhibits protein synthesis in the ribosome.
- It is a cheap, broad-spectrum antibiotic still used in low-income countries, but due to concerns about bone marrow suppression, it is used infrequently by the oral or IV route in high-income countries.
- Chloramphenicol is still used worldwide as a highly effective topical treatment in eye ointments for the treatment of bacterial conjunctivitis.

## Nitroimidazoles

- Metronidazole treats anaerobic bacterial infections and some protozoa such as *Giardia*.
- Metronidazole is very well absorbed orally and should never be prescribed IV unless the patient cannot eat and drink.
- Alcohol should not be consumed with metronidazole or else a very unpleasant vomiting reaction occurs.

## Sulphonamides

- Sulphonamides inhibit bacterial folic acid synthesis.
- Trimethoprim is useful for treating urinary tract infections, although resistance is now common.

- Co-trimoxazole is a very useful drug for treating a range of infections including *Staphylococcus aureus* skin infections and *Pneumocystis* pneumonia (PCP), as well as being used to prevent infections in people with low CD4+ counts due to advanced HIV.
- Co-trimoxazole can cause rashes and, rarely, Stevens–Johnson syndrome.

## Rifampicin

- Rifampicin inhibits DNA-dependent RNA polymerase activity by forming a stable complex with the enzyme, which prevents initiation of RNA synthesis.
- Rifampicin is bactericidal against both intracellular and extracellular organisms and is used in combination therapy for the treatment of TB and non-tuberculous mycobacteria.
- It is sometimes used in the treatment of a range of other infections including MRSA, *Borrelia burgdorferi* (Lyme disease) and *Neisseria gonorrhoeae* (particularly as prophylaxis).

## ANTIVIRALS

The intracellular location of viruses and their use of host cell systems make it difficult to develop antiviral therapy. Despite this, there are a growing number available. Some of the more important are listed below.

### Amantadine and rimantadine

- Amantadine prevents viral uncoating and release of viral RNA within the infected cell.
- It has some action against influenza A if given prophylactically or early in the infection, but its use is usually restricted to individuals at high risk of severe illness.

### Neuraminidase inhibitors

- Neuraminidase (NA) inhibitors such as zanamivir (Relenza®) and oseltamivir (Tamiflu®) prevent viral release from infected cells.
- Resistance occurs by mutations in coding for the haemagglutinin (HA) binding site or by alteration of the sequence in the active site of the gene encoding NA.
- Zanamivir must be given by nasal drops, spray, nebulized mist or dry powder aerosol.
- Oseltamivir has good oral bioavailability.
- Zanamivir and oseltamivir bring a modest reduction in the duration of influenza symptoms among patients treated within 48 hours of the onset of symptoms.
- NA inhibitors can prevent influenza in immunocompromised patients when the drug is given for 14 days during an influenza epidemic.

### Nucleoside analogues

- Nucleoside analogues inhibit herpesvirus DNA polymerase.
- Acyclovir is active against HSV and VZV, and it is also used for prophylaxis against herpes infections in the immunocompromised.
- Valaciclovir is the prodrug for acyclovir and has better absorption.
- Ganciclovir and its prodrug valganciclovir are active against HSV and CMV and are indicated in the treatment of life- or sight-threatening CMV infections in immunocompromised individuals.
- Ribavirin has activity against RSV, influenza A and B, parainfluenza virus, Lassa fever and other arenaviruses. It is most commonly used by aerosol for treatment of severe RSV infection in infants.

## ANTIRETROVIRAL COMPOUNDS

The introduction of highly active antiretroviral therapy (HAART) has transformed the clinical landscape of HIV care. For patients, this therapy has brought about improvement in the CD4 count and a fall in the HIV viral load.

- 'Treatment as prevention' means that successful suppression of HIV viral load by HAART makes the risk of transmission of HIV from an infected person to their uninfected partner negligible.
- Some HAART regimens are now available as combined single-tablet, once a day treatment.
- Anti-HIV drugs are used as post-exposure prophylaxis (PEP), e.g. for a healthcare worker who receives a needlestick injury from someone with known uncontrolled HIV, or after high-risk sexual intercourse (PEPSI).
- It has recently been established that prescribing antiretrovirals to people at high risk of acquiring HIV through their sexual lifestyle is effective in lowering transmission (pre-exposure prophylaxis, PrEP).

### Nucleoside reverse transcriptase inhibitors or nucleoside analogues

- Nucleoside reverse transcriptase inhibitors (NRTIs) are nucleoside analogues that inhibit the action of reverse transcriptase, the viral enzyme that converts viral RNA into a DNA copy.
- NRTIs include the longest established antiretroviral drug zidovudine (AZT), lamivudine, tenofovir, abacavir, entecavir and emtricitabine. They are the mainstay of retroviral therapy and are used in combination in initial therapy.
- Tenofovir and lamivudine are also effective against hepatitis B.

### Protease inhibitors

- Protease inhibitors inhibit HIV protease and are central to HAART.
- Examples include indinavir, ritonavir, lopinavir, atazanavir and darunavir.
- Ritonavir is also used in low dose as a booster drug.

### Non-nucleoside reverse transcriptase inhibitors

- Non-nucleoside reverse transcriptase inhibitors (NNRTIs) inhibit reverse transcriptase by an alternative mechanism to NRTIs.
- Examples include efavirenz, etravirine and nevirapine.
- Because of their potential for resistance after a single mutation event, they should only be used in regimens designed to be maximally suppressive.

### Integrase inhibitors

- Integrase inhibitors block the action of integrase, a viral enzyme that inserts the viral genome into the DNA of the host cell.
- Examples are dolutegravir and raltegravir.

### Chemokine receptor 5 inhibitors

- Chemokine receptor 5 (CCR5) inhibitors stop HIV binding to the CCR5, preventing infection of CD4+ T cells.
- Maraviroc was the first licenced CCR5 antagonist.

## TREATMENT OF HEPATITIS C

Recent years have seen a revolution in the treatment of chronic hepatitis C, with the addition of effective, well-tolerated oral therapies (directly active antiviral (DAA) therapies) to the older treatments of PEG-interferon-$\alpha$ and ribavirin.

- Pegylated-interferon-$\alpha$ augments human natural antiviral immune responses to increase viral clearance, but it has marked side effects of flu-like symptoms.
- DAA are taken for 8–12 weeks and clear hepatitis C (cure) in over 90% of patients.
- DAA include the protease inhibitor simeprevir and the non-nucleoside polymerase (NSSA) inhibitors sofosbuvir and ledipasvir. DAA are used alone or in combination, depending on patient characteristics and their hepatitis C strain type.

## ANTIFUNGAL AGENTS

- Azoles such as fluconazole and itraconazole block cytochrome P450 and sterol 14$\alpha$-demethylase in the fungal membrane. Fluconazole is used to treat yeasts such as *Candida* and *Cryptococcus*, while itraconazole can also treat filamentous fungi such as *Aspergillus* and the dermatophytes that cause ringworm, etc.

- Echinocandins such as caspofungin and micafungin inhibit the synthesis of $\beta$-glucan in the fungal cell wall. They are used to treat certain fungal infections such as some *Candida* species and *Aspergillus*. They are also used as prophylaxis and empirical therapy in transplant patients.
- Amphotericin B is used for severe fungal infections where other agents are not effective and is also used to treat leishmaniasis. The liposomal formulation is mostly used due to lower side effects, but it is expensive.
- Other antifungals in clinical use include nystatin, flucytosine and terbinafine.

## ANTIPARASITIC AGENTS

- Quinine is the oldest specific anti-infective agent known and comes from the bark of the *Cinchona* tree. It remains effective treatment for malaria, although it can have toxic side effects such as cardiotoxicity (especially QT interval prolongation), hypoglycaemia and ringing in the ears.
- Chloroquine and mefloquine are synthetic derivatives of quinine that are used to prevent and treat malaria, but resistance has emerged to both, especially chloroquine.
- Artemisinin comes from the plant *Artemisia annua* or qinghaosu, which has a long history of use in traditional Chinese medicine for the treatment of malaria. This drug is now first-line treatment for malaria worldwide, but worrying signs of resistance are now reported in South East Asia.
- Atovaquone is combined with proguanil for use as an effective prophylactic agent against malaria (Malarone®).
- Antihelminth drugs include ivermectin, albendazole and praziquantel.

## ALLERGY

- Allergies to antibiotics are very common, and can include rash or more severe Type 1 reactions such as angio-oedema or anaphylaxis.
- Those with significant penicillin should not be prescribed other $\beta$-lactam antibiotics as cross-reaction can occur in up to 10%.
- A careful history should be taken if allergy is reported, sometimes including checking with other sources such as the patient's registered GP surgery (primary care provider), because drug intolerances while ill (e.g. vomiting after oral penicillin, or a rash when amoxicillin is given during EBV infection) can be recorded permanently as allergy, leading to unnecessary restrictions in the patient's management.

## ANTIMICROBIAL SENSITIVITY AND RESISTANCE

Antimicrobial agents have a limited spectrum of activity: only some bacteria are susceptible to their action. This is usually because the metabolic process with which they interfere occurs in only some bacteria. For example, vancomycin interferes with peptidoglycan synthesis but can only do this in Gram-positive organisms; all Gram-negative organisms are therefore naturally resistant.

AMR is growing rapidly and is now a global concern. The Global Burden of Disease Study estimated that there were 1.27 million deaths directly attributable to AMR worldwide in 2019. Some mechanisms of resistance are shown in **Figure 3.12**. There is evidence that inappropriate use of antimicrobials in humans is a major driving force for AMR, with contributions from poverty, globalization, poor sanitation and hygiene practices, and use of antimicrobials in farming and agriculture. Antimicrobial stewardship is essential to limit the spread of AMR.

Some examples of medically important AMR bacteria:
- MRSA
- ESBL Gram-negative infections
- *Streptococcus pneumoniae* resistance to penicillin
- CRE
- VRE
- Gut pathogens including *Salmonella* species, *Shigella* and *Campylobacter* that are resistant to fluoroquinolones such as ciprofloxacin
- Drug-resistant *Mycobacterial tuberculosis* including multidrug resistant (MDR-TB) and extremely resistant (XDR-TB) tuberculosis
- *Neisseria gonorrhoeae* resistant to fluoroquinolones such as ciprofloxacin and azithromycin

AMR is also a problem for antiviral agents. HIV rapidly develops resistance to antiretrovirals if monotherapy or poor compliance occurs. Resistance is also a major problem in the control of malaria, with widespread global resistance to chloroquine, established resistance to mefloquine and resistance to artemisinin now reported in South East Asia. AMR can also occur for other antiparasite agents, and for antifungal agents such as fluconazole (used in the treatment of *Candida* infections).

## INFECTION PREVENTION AND CONTROL

Infection prevention and control (IPC) is now an essential, integrated component of the delivery of healthcare, whether in the community or the hospital setting. It is the responsibility of all healthcare professionals. Principles include:

- Antimicrobial stewardship (see below)
- Excellent hand hygiene at every opportunity before and after patient contact
- Minimizing the use of invasive foreign material such as IV catheters, urinary catheters and drains, and applying best practice guidelines to the insertion, monitoring, care and removal of lines
- Excellence in wound care
- Physiotherapy and early mobilization to reduce healthcare associated pneumonia
- Maintenance of standards for cleaning of clinical areas, bathrooms and medical equipment, waste disposal management and the preparation and serving of food
- Identification and isolation or cohorting of patients with contagious pathogens such as norovirus, varicella and MRSA
- Use of personal protective equipment (PPE) to reduce transmission by staff
- Coordination of response to outbreaks of infectious disease
- Maintenance and surveillance systems to prevent the transmission of environmental pathogens such as *Legionella* or *Pseudomonas* via air-conditioning systems, plumbing, etc.
- Measures to minimize hospital stay and use of invasive procedures
- Occupational health screening and annual administration of influenza vaccine
- High-profile leadership within organizations and teams to support best practices around IPC
- Public health campaigns

## ANTIMICROBIAL STEWARDSHIP

Antimicrobial stewardship is the oversight of use of antimicrobial drugs in a healthcare system and in the wider community. Principles include:

- Restrictions in the availability of antibiotics without prescription to the public
- Use of guidelines for empirical antibiotic therapy for clinical syndromes, driven by local knowledge of aetiological and resistance patterns, using the narrowest spectrum agents possible to treat the likely causative agent(s)
- Reduction in indication for using antimicrobials
- Reduction in duration of courses of antimicrobials
- Availability of expert advice from microbiologists, infectious disease specialists and pharmacists to manage complex cases
- Screening for the presence of AMR in selected patients (e.g. those transferred from another facility with a high prevalence of AMR)
- Oversight of prescribing practice by pharmacists
- Regular audit and feedback of practice against guidelines

## PREVENTION AND CONTROL OF INFECTION IN THE COMMUNITY

Alongside antimicrobial stewardship, IPC in the community is driven by public health bodies and includes:

- Enforcement of regulations in the food, livestock, agriculture and leisure (e.g. petting farms) industries
- Control of waste disposal, vectors and vermin
- Maintenance of Health and Safety standards for housing, sanitation and workplace provision
- Health education
- Immunization programmes
- Monitoring of notifiable disease trends for early outbreak detection and management, with testing and contact tracing when available

# INFECTIONS AND THEIR MANAGEMENT

## SYSTEMIC INFECTIONS

### SEPSIS

Sepsis is a life-threatening clinical syndrome caused by a dysregulated inflammatory response to infection that can lead to multi-organ failure and death.

#### Epidemiology

The global burden of sepsis is difficult to measure, but there are an estimated 30 million cases of sepsis per year worldwide and 6 million deaths. In the UK, the number of cases per year is approximately 123 000, with 37 000 deaths.

#### Disease mechanisms

- A wide range of infections can cause sepsis. Gram-positive bacteria, such as *S. aureus* and Group A *Streptococcus*, and Gram-negative bacteria, such as *E. coli* and *Klebsiella pneumoniae*, are the commonest causes but a sepsis syndrome can also be the result of fungal infections (e.g. *Candida* spp.), viruses (e.g. influenza, SARS-CoV-2, Ebola) and parasites (e.g. *P. falciparum* malaria).
- In around half of cases, the cause is never identified.
- Sepsis is characterized by an uncontrolled intravascular inflammatory response to the pathogen, with dysfunction in endothelium, coagulation and perfusion.
- Pro-inflammatory cytokines including L-1, IL-6, TNF, and interferon gamma (IFN-γ) stimulate activation of polymorphonuclear leukocytes (PMNs), macrophages and lymphocytes, leading to organ dysfunction.

### Clinical features

- Clinical features include fever, rigors, altered consciousness and localizing symptoms and signs of infection (e.g. cough and chest signs for pneumonia, dysuria and loin pain for pyelonephritis).
- Use of alert systems in hospitals to identify unwell patients at risk of sepsis from vital signs such as heart rate, blood pressure and oxygen saturation is important.
- The underlying infection can affect any organ including skin, bone and joint or CNS.
- The qSOFA score is used to evaluate people with suspected or known infection, where up to 3 points are given for the presence of a respiratory rate ≥22 breaths/minute, altered level of consciousness, and systemic blood pressure ≤100 mmHg.
- Severe sepsis is sepsis with organ dysfunction.
- Septic shock is when severe circulatory, cellular and metabolic abnormalities are present and there is a high mortality.

### Differential diagnosis

Differential diagnosis of sepsis is wide and includes non-infectious conditions that can cause the syndrome that overlaps with sepsis called systemic inflammatory response syndrome (SIRS), including heart failure, alcohol withdrawal, acute pancreatitis, burns, pulmonary embolism, thyrotoxicosis, anaphylaxis and adrenal insufficiency.

### Investigation

- Full blood count, kidney and liver function, and inflammatory markers such as CRP and procalcitonin (if available)
- Microbiological culture of blood, urine and other relevant clinical samples according to presentation
- Arterial blood gases, with focus on $PaO_2$, pH and lactate
- Chest X-ray and further imaging (e.g. CT chest/abdo/pelvis) depending on presentation

### Management

- IV fluid
- Empirical antibiotics according to local antimicrobial stewardship guidelines to cover the most likely bacteria (e.g. co-amoxiclav and gentamicin for community-acquired sepsis), with fine tuning once further information is available from imaging and culture results
- The 'door-to-needle time' of administering antibiotics as fast as possible (within 1 hour) following presentation to a healthcare provider with sepsis is crucial, but pressures to restrict antibiotic use due to antimicrobial stewardship and concerns about AMR means skilled triage is required to identify sepsis patients rapidly
- Supportive care and monitoring of end-organ function, including ICU if required, to maintain organ

perfusion and respiration, such as vasopressor therapy and ventilation

- Source control (e.g. radiologically guided aspiration or surgery for a pus collection)

## Prognosis

- The case fatality rate from sepsis is high, and estimated to be 10– 52% for hospitalized patients, depending on setting.
- The qSOFA score can help predict mortality, including in low- and middle-income settings, but the site of infection, aetiological agent and underlying host factors all contribute to the risk of mortality.
- Patients who survive sepsis to hospital discharge have increased risk of mortality and readmission to hospital.

## PYREXIA (OR FEVER) OF UNKNOWN ORIGIN

PUO is defined as several episodes of fever ≥38.3 °C during a period of illness of at least 3 weeks, without a diagnosis despite reasonable attempts at investigation in a secondary care setting.

## Epidemiology

- PUO affects fewer than 3% of patients admitted to hospital.
- As diagnostic tests including radiologically guided biopsy, cross-sectional and radionuclide imaging are more readily accessible, a smaller proportion of patients investigated for febrile illness will fulfil this definition.
- Inflammatory and neoplastic causes of PUO are now more common than infections.
- Despite investigation, up to one in five patients presenting with PUO do not have a definitive cause for fever identified.

## Disease mechanisms

- PUO represents distinct clinical syndromes that are context-specific: classical PUO, PUO associated with immune compromise, and nosocomial (healthcare-associated) PUO.
- These syndromes may arise from a broad range of underlying diseases (**Table 3.15**).

**Table 3.15** Underlying diseases responsible for classical pyrexia of unknown origin

| Type of disorder | Disease |
|---|---|
| Connective tissue disorders, inflammatory and autoimmune diseases | Rheumatoid arthritis |
| | Still's disease, juvenile idiopathic arthritis |
| | Systemic lupus erythematosus |
| | Sarcoidosis |
| | Granulomatous vasculitides (ANCA+) |
| | Giant cell arteritis in older patients |
| | Polymyalgia rheumatica in older patients |
| | Aortitis and retroperitoneal fibrosis |
| | Inflammatory bowel disorders |
| Haematological disorders | Autoimmune haemolytic anaemia |
| | Thrombotic thrombocytopaenic purpura |
| | Cyclical neutropaenia |
| | Lymphoma and chronic lymphocytic leukaemia |
| | Castleman disease |
| | Histiocytosis disorders |
| Malignancies | Haematological malignancies (see above) |
| | Renal cell carcinoma |
| | Hepatocellular carcinoma |
| | Colorectal carcinoma |
| | CNS neoplasms |
| | Atrial myxoma |
| Infections | Infection in an unexpected site, e.g. liver abscess, pancreatitis, culture-negative endocarditis, pericarditis, discitis, prostatic abscess |
| | Systemic infection, e.g. HIV, malaria, leishmaniasis, TB, brucellosis, relapsing fever, Q fever, bartonellosis, Whipple disease, HCV |
| Other | Deep vein thrombosis, pulmonary embolism, resorbing haematoma |
| | Drugs: drug fever, serum sickness-like reactions, drug reaction with eosinophilia and systemic symptoms (DRESS) syndrome, alcoholic hepatitis |
| | Hereditary conditions: Fabry disease, familial Mediterranean fever |
| | Endocrine disorders: Addison's disease, thyrotoxicosis, pheochromocytoma |

3

- Fever appears to be mediated through elevated levels of pro-inflammatory cytokines including IL-6, IL-1 and TNF.

## Clinical features

To identify the underlying cause of PUO, a thorough history is essential. This should include:
- Specific details of recent and previous travel
- Unwell contacts
- Exposure to animals, insects, guano and urine
- Medications, alcohol and drugs
- Vaccination
- Family history
- History of cardiac valve abnormalities and systemic infections

## Examination

This should include:
- Fundoscopy
- Oropharyngeal examination
- Temporal artery palpation in older patients
- Abdomen, including spleen
- Lymph node palpation (cervical, axillary, inguinal)
- Joints and spine
- Skin (with particular attention for rashes), nails and hair
- Genitalia, rectum and prostate
- Lower limbs for deep vein thrombosis and rash

## Investigation

- Investigations should be directed towards possible aetiologies identified on history and examination in the first instance.
- Blood cultures, HIV serology, blood film and abdominal ultrasound should be undertaken if not previously performed.
- Echocardiography, CT, MRI imaging, and $^{18}$F-fluorodeoxyglucose positron emission topography CT (FDG-PET/CT scan) should be considered.
- Biopsies guided by imaging may yield the diagnosis.
- Bone marrow biopsy may be helpful if there are abnormal cell counts, anaemia or thrombocytopaenia.
- In cases where investigation is uninformative, a fever diary or period of observation may be fruitful.
- The drug chart needs careful review

## Management

Management of PUO should be targeted towards identifying life-threatening and treatable causes, and supportive care, pending diagnosis.

## INFLUENZA

Influenza ('flu') is a common viral illness caused by an RNA virus in the Orthomyxoviridae family.

## Epidemiology

- Influenza A and B cause seasonal outbreaks of flu.
- Influenza A viruses are classified into subtypes according to the combination of the HA and the NA proteins, which are viral envelope glycoproteins.
- Outbreaks occur in winter months in temperate zones but can occur throughout the year in tropical zones.
- The attack rate is typically 10–20% but can be higher in closed communities (such as nursing homes, prisons and cruise ships) and during pandemics.
- In 2017, the World Health Organization (WHO) estimated that 290 000–650 000 deaths are associated with respiratory diseases from seasonal influenza each year.
- Avian flu (e.g. H5N1) mainly affects birds but can rarely affect humans in close proximity to birds, and it has a high case fatality rate.

## Disease mechanisms

- Influenza is transmitted by droplet spread through coughing and sneezing, and by contaminated hands and surfaces.
- Influenza HA binds to sialic acid on respiratory epithelial cells to enable infection of host cells. After viral replication, NA cleaves the binding of new virions to host cells to enable spread of virions.
- After an outbreak of flu in a community, recovered people have acquired immunity to HA and NA to prevent reinfection with the same viral strain. However, major changes in the structure of HA and NA by genome reassortment, known as antigenic shift, and minor changes by point mutations, known as antigenic drift, mean that the population is not immune to new flu strains.
- Antigenic shifts are associated with global epidemics and pandemics of influenza A (as occurred in 1918 – H1N1 ('Spanish flu'), 1957 – H2N2 ('Asian flu'), 1968 – H3N2 ('Hong Kong flu') and 2009 – H1N1, known to the public as 'swine flu'), while antigenic drifts are associated with local outbreaks.

## Clinical features

- Clinical features of flu include fever, dry cough, headache, muscle and joint pains, sore throat and coryza.
- The incubation period is 1–4 days, and serological surveys have shown a wide spectrum of disease from asymptomatic to severe.
- Complications include primary influenza pneumonia, secondary bacterial pneumonia with *Streptococcus pneumoniae*, *Staphylococcus aureus* and other species, Guillain–Barré syndrome, and heart problems including myocardial infarction and myocarditis.
- People at increased risk of severe infection and death include the elderly, pregnant women and those with chronic conditions such as cancer, heart disease, diabetes and renal disease or immunosuppression.

### Investigation

- A clinical diagnosis may be sufficient for most cases of flu in the community, but formal diagnosis reduces investigation for other aetiologies, reduces use of antibiotics, can inform infection control and direct use of antiviral medicines.
- Rapid diagnostic tests (RDTs) for influenza detect antigen and can be useful in both community and hospital settings.
- Molecular tests such as rapid molecular tests and multiplex reverse transcription-polymerase chain reaction (RT-PCR) assays have higher sensitivity but are not always available or cost-effective.

### Management

- Most cases of flu can be managed symptomatically at home, with rest, fluids and paracetamol.
- Patients at high risk of complications of flu probably benefit from antiviral treatment with an NA inhibitor such as zanamivir or oseltamivir.
- Severe cases require supportive care in hospital.
- Hand hygiene is an important infection control measure to reduce the spread of flu.
- Each year the WHO predicts which strains of the virus are most likely to be circulating in the next year, and this knowledge is used to make the annual seasonal flu vaccine.
- Flu vaccine is offered to those at increased risk of severe infection, young children (who are probably responsible for a lot of transmission) and healthcare workers. Healthcare workers can be a significant cause of transmission, and staff absences due to sickness create service risks during flu outbreaks. It is therefore essential that all healthcare workers receive an annual flu vaccine to help protect their patients.

### Prognosis

The vast majority of people with flu make a full recovery, but fatalities can occur, especially in those with underlying diseases. At an epidemiological level, a large proportion of excess mortality in winter months is attributed to flu and its complications such as secondary bacterial pneumonia.

## COVID-19

COVID-19 is a viral infection caused by the novel coronavirus SARS-CoV-2, that can lead to severe respiratory illness – especially in older adults and people with underlying health conditions.

### Epidemiology

- COVID-19 emerged as a severe pneumonia in Wuhan, China, at the end of 2019.
- During the first few months of 2020, the virus spread to 210 countries and territories across the world and was declared a pandemic by the WHO.
- Viral spread is likely to be influenced by international travel, population density, population demographics and the timing and extent of control measures including vaccination, wearing of face coverings, social distancing and good ventilation.
- Variants of concern have emerged, including the Omicron variant where mutations in the spike protein led to loss of vaccine-induced neutralizing antibody function and a resurgence of high case numbers but lower mortality.

### Disease mechanisms

- Coronaviruses are enveloped, single-stranded RNA viruses.
- SARS-CoV-2 is thought to be chiefly by person-to-person spread via respiratory droplets released when an infectious person talks, coughs or sneezes, but a significant role of airborne transmission is increasingly acknowledged..
- The virus has been detected in blood, stool and semen but the role of these routes for transmission is unclear.
- SARS-CoV-2 can be transmitted by asymptomatic people and in the pre-symptomatic period (before a person develops symptoms).
- The viral spike protein binds to ACE2 receptors on lung epithelial cells and other cell types to enter cells.
- In patients with severe disease, increased pro-inflammatory cytokines including IL-6, IL-1ß and TNF can result in cytokine dysregulation leading to increased vascular permeability, thrombosis and multi-organ failure.

### Clinical features

- Incubation period is around 5 days (range 2–14).
- Cardinal symptoms include fever, dry cough and alteration in smell/taste.
- A range of other symptoms and presentations are known, including shortness of breath, myalgia, malaise, fatigue, diarrhoea and rash. Sore throat and coryza can also occur in COVID-19 but are more typical of 'common cold' upper respiratory tract infections.
- A wide spectrum of disease is seen, ranging from asymptomatic through to severe and fatal pneumonia often associated with hyperinflammation and hypercoagulability.
- Risk factors include increasing age, obesity and underlying health conditions including diabetes, heart disease, chronic respiratory disease and immunocompromise.
- The degree of hypoxia may be disproportionate to the patient's symptoms and signs on chest examination.

### Investigation

- PCR testing of nasopharyngeal swab using an adequate swabbing technique is used for diagnosis, but a negative swab does not exclude COVID-19.
- Lymphopenia is typically seen.
- Other laboratory abnormalities include elevations in aminotransaminase, lactate dehydrogenase (LDH),

CRP, troponin, and d-dimers, alongside acute kidney injury.
- Arterial blood gases to quantify hypoxia and exclude Type II respiratory failure are useful.
- Chest X-ray may show consolidation and ground glass opacities, which are typically peripheral, bilateral, and more in the lower lung zones. Radiographs may be normal in early or mild disease. CT chest adds sensitivity, and a low threshold for low resolution CT pulmonary angiogram should be used to detect embolus where the hypoxia is out of proportion to imaging findings.

### Management

- The mainstay of management is supportive care with oxygen if required to maintain saturations above 92%, and monitoring of end-organ function.
- Clinical trials continue to reveal beneficial adjuvant therapies for COVID-19, including dexamethasone, antivirals (remdesevir, molnupiravir and Paxlovid), IL-6 blockade (tocilizumab) and monoclonal antibodies (Ronapreve and Sotrovimab). Local up-to-date management guidelines should be consulted.
- Prophylaxis against venous thromboembolic disease should be given.
- Consider antibiotics for community-acquired pneumonia according to local antibiotic stewardship guidelines if bacterial infection is a significant alternative or additional diagnosis.
- Individualized 'ceilings of care' decisions should be considered early and discussed openly and compassionately with patients and their families.
- Patients who are not responding to oxygen should be considered for continuous positive airway pressure (CPAP) and intubation on ICU.
- Strict infection control with hand hygiene, PPE, enhanced cleaning and isolation/cohorting of confirmed patients is essential.
- In the community, social distancing and wearing face coverings are used as control measures around the world.
- Licenced vaccines include those targeting the viral spike protein - mRNA vaccines (Pfizer-BioNTech and Moderna), viral vectors (Oxford-AstraZeneca and Jaassen/Johnson & Johnson), protein subunit (Novavax), as well as whole killed vaccines (Sinopharm, Sinovac and Bharat-Biotech).
- Vaccination to reduce probability of infection and prevent severe disease is the most important control strategy, but vaccine inequality is vast with only 1 in 10 people living in low-income countries having received a single vaccine dose in early 2022.
- Licenced vaccines include those targeting the viral spike protein - mRNA vaccines (Pfizer-BioNTech and Moderna), viral vectors (Oxford-AstraZeneca and Jaassen/Johnson & Johnson), protein subunit (Novavax), as well as whole killed vaccines (Sinopharm, Sinovac and Bharat-Biotech).

- Vaccination to reduce probability of infection and prevent severe disease is the most important control strategy, but vaccine inequality is vast with only 1 in 10 people living in low-income countries having received a single vaccine dose in early 2022.

### Prognosis

- The case fatality ratio varies by amount of testing performed and clinical context, but the infectivity mortality ratio (the proportion of people dying who were infected even if asymptomatic) prior to the vaccination era was estimated to be around 0.5–1%, with mortality rising steeply with age and higher in men.
- Vaccination and past infection have transformed rates of hospitalisation, ICU admission and death per diagnosed case, but unvaccinated people and those with immunocompromise continue to be vulnerable.
- The long-term health consequences of the pandemic are yet to be known, with harms including Long COVID, mental health impacts, and disruption of healthcare for other conditions.

## INFECTIOUS MONONUCLEOSIS AND EPSTEIN–BARR VIRUS INFECTION

Infectious mononucleosis (IM), also known as 'glandular fever' (UK) or 'mono' (USA), is caused by the Epstein–Barr virus, a member of the herpes family.

### Epidemiology

- There are two peaks of infection in high-income countries: early childhood (birth to 6 years), and in adolescence or early adulthood.
- 90% of adult populations are seropositive.
- In low-income settings with poorer sanitation, 90% of children are seropositive by 2 years of age.
- EBV infections are usually subclinical in young children, but around 50% of young people acquiring EBV infection have IM.
- Outbreaks occur when young people join close communities for the first time (e.g. university starters and military recruits).

### Disease mechanisms

- EBV is mainly transmitted by the oral route (e.g. via kissing or poor hygiene.)
- The virus establishes an infection in the phalangeal epithelium followed by proliferation of B cells.
- During IM, the peripheral blood is dominated by atypical mononuclear cells.
- Primary infection is followed by lifelong latency.
- Seropositive people shed the virus in their saliva.

### Clinical features

- Symptoms are sore throat, fever, cervical lymphadenopathy and fatigue, lasting 2–6 weeks.

- Examination may show palatal petechiae, generalized lymphadenopathy, splenic enlargement (up to 50%) and jaundice (around 5%).
- Two rashes can occur: a transient morbilliform rash early in the disease course; or a maculopapular rash occurs in almost 100% of IM patients given amoxicillin.
- Complications include splenic rupture, pharyngeal obstruction, CNS disease (meningitis, encephalitis and the Guillain–Barré syndrome) and haematological complications (e.g. haemolytic and aplastic anaemia, haemophagocytic syndrome).
- EBV is associated with a number of cancers including Burkitt lymphoma, nasopharyngeal carcinoma and lymphomas in the immunosuppressed and is also associated with haemophagocytic lymphohistiocytosis (HLH), a rare immune activation syndrome with poor prognosis.

### Differential diagnosis

Differential diagnosis includes other viral infections (e.g. influenza, rhinovirus, coronavirus, CMV, HIV seroconversion illness), streptococcal throat infection (Group A *Streptococcus*) and acute toxoplasmosis.

### Investigation

- Diagnosis is by the detection of heterophile antibodies (weak antibodies with non-specific binding), also known as the monospot test.
- Blood film shows lymphocytosis with atypical mononuclear cells.
- A positive EBV viral capsid antigen IgM confirms the diagnosis.
- Liver function tests are deranged in most cases of IM.
- Ultrasound may confirm an enlarged spleen but does not usually change the management.

### Management

- Symptomatic management with rest, fluids and analgesia is the mainstay of treatment.
- Steroids are sometimes given for severe pharyngitis although the evidence of benefit unless started within 12 hours of illness onset is not strong.
- There is no evidence that antivirals such as acyclovir improve clinical symptoms in IM.
- Antibiotics should be avoided; if given because Strep throat is strongly suspected in the differential, penicillin V should be used.
- Patients with an enlarged spleen should avoid contact sports for 3 weeks to reduce rupture risk.
- There is no current vaccine.

### Prognosis

- Uncomplicated IM is a self-limiting illness, although a prolonged period of post-viral fatigue is well described.
- Deranged liver function including hepatitis typically settles.

- Disease in immunocompromised people such as those with advanced HIV or organ transplantation may be chronic and require specialist care.

## CYTOMEGALOVIRUS

- CMV is an acute infection caused by the herpes virus cytomegalovirus.
- In the immunocompetent, infection with CMV is usually asymptomatic but can cause a glandular fever-like illness with lymphadenopathy, which is usually self-limiting in healthy people.
- Transmission occurs by multiple routes including close contact, sexual transmission, congenital and via organ transplantation.
- Between 40% and 100% of adults have antibodies to CMV, with seropositivity seen at an earlier age in low- and middle-income countries.
- Reactivation of latent CMV or reinfection with a novel strain can occur.
- In immunosuppressed people such as transplant patients or advanced HIV, CMV infection may cause a progressive illness with severe organ involvement including severe colitis, mucosal ulceration, retinitis (especially in advanced HIV), interstitial pneumonitis and/or hepatitis.
- Features of congenital CMV include petechial rash, jaundice, microencephaly and sensorineural hearing loss.
- Diagnosis is by detection of DNA in blood by RT-PCR. Histology of tissue biopsy may reveal a characteristic appearance with 'owl's eye' inclusion bodies. Seroconversion can support a diagnosis of infection.
- Treatment is with ganciclovir or foscarnet, ideally alongside reversal/reduction (of immunosuppression, e.g. lowering immunosuppression in transplant recipients where possible, or commencing antiretrovirals in advanced HIV).

## TOXOPLASMOSIS

- Toxoplasmosis is an infection caused by the protozoan parasite *Toxoplasma gondii*, whose definitive host is the cat.
- Humans are usually infected by eating undercooked meat, but contact with cats may be relevant.
- Seroprevalence varies from country to country depending on the culinary habits but, in general, the rate of seropositivity rises with age.
- Infection in healthy hosts is usually asymptomatic; if symptomatic, it may cause fever, lymphadenopathy (which may persist for several months) and rash. Most then develop an ongoing latent infection which can reactivate if the person later becomes immunocompromised.
- Toxoplasmosis can be spread from mother to infant *in utero*, which can lead to severe outcomes for the fetus

including intracranial calcification, hydrocephalus and echogenic bowel.

- Eye disease and brain abscess occur in immunocompromise such as advanced HIV due to reactivation of a latent infection.
- Diagnosis is supported by positive IgM antibodies and seroconversion on follow-up from negative to positive IgG antibodies
- Treatment is in consultation with an infectious diseases specialist; a number of treatment regimens are available including trimethoprim-sulfamethoxazole.

## VIRAL FEVERS OF CHILDHOOD WITH RASH

A group of viral rash illnesses (see varicella, and **Table 3.16**) are traditionally thought of as diseases of children but, with routine immunization against them, their incidence in children is falling. These viruses are now increasingly seen in adults, where people missed immunization and did not meet the disease during childhood, while others have developed only poor immunity in response to immunization. Vaccine hesitancy leading to lower rates of vaccination against measles, mumps and rubella (MMR) can lead to loss of herd immunity and outbreaks of disease. In adults, the presentation of these diseases can be atypical and the course modified.

## VARICELLA – CHICKENPOX AND ZOSTER

Chickenpox is a highly contagious viral illness caused by primary infection with VZV. Like all herpes viruses, the infection then usually persists. Zoster, or shingles, is a painful, blistering illness resulting from reactivation of latent VZV.

### Epidemiology
#### Chickenpox

- Chickenpox is common in childhood in countries such as UK that do not offer routine immunization against VZV.
- Incidence peaks in winter and early spring.
- The household attack rate from a chickenpox case to a non-immune person is around 90%.
- In the UK, 90% of adults show seropositivity to VZV.
- Countries with routine vaccination such as USA have lower incidence rates but outbreaks occur.
- In tropical countries, less of the population is immune, and a higher proportion of chickenpox cases are in adults.

#### Zoster

- Zoster is common in older adults and immunocompromised people but can occur in children and young adults.
- Age-related decline in cell-mediated immunity leads to increased incidence and severity of zoster with age.

Older adults are vaccinated to boost immunity and prevent reactivation.

- Re-exposure to chickenpox cases is also protective against zoster, believed to be by boosting VZV-specific cell-mediated immunity.

### Disease mechanisms

- Chickenpox is highly contagious and is transmitted chiefly by droplet spread from respiratory secretions.
- VZV can also be transmitted by direct contact with the blisters of chickenpox and zoster.
- In the primary infection, VZV invades the oropharyngeal mucosa to infect T cells.
- VZV replication in the skin results in the characteristic vesicles.
- After the primary chickenpox infection, VZV becomes latent in neuronal cell bodies in the ganglia.
- Latent VZV becomes reactivated at times of stress or immunosuppression, leading to zoster.

### Clinical features
#### Chickenpox

- Chickenpox has a characteristic blistering itchy rash (**Figure 3.13**), which appears in crops, first on the trunk and face.
- The rash starts as a pruritic rash which forms vesicles, then pustules, then crusts over.
- Prior to the onset of the rash children may have a fever and be non-specifically unwell.
- Chickenpox is contagious from 1–2 days before the onset of the rash until all lesions have crusted over.
- The incubation period is 10–21 days.
- Disease is more severe in adolescents and adults.
- Immunocompromised children and adults may have severe disseminated VZV.
- Complications include secondary bacterial skin infections and sepsis including Group A *Streptococcus*, VZV pneumonitis, encephalitis and cerebellar ataxia, and haemorrhage.

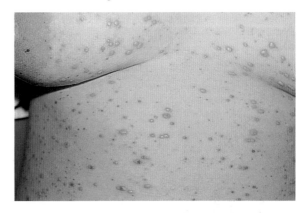

**Figure 3.13** Chickenpox: typical rash showing non-coalescing lesions at all stages of development. Reproduced from Bannister B *et al.*, *Infectious Disease*, 1996 (Wiley-Blackwell, Oxford) with permission of the authors.

**Table 3.16** Common childhood exanthema compared

| | Measles | Chickenpox | Rubella (German measles) | Erythema infectiosum | Mumps |
|---|---|---|---|---|---|
| **Causative virus** | Paramyxovirus (RNA) | Herpesvirus (DNA) | Togavirus (RNA) | Parvovirus (DNA) | Paramyxovirus (RNA) |
| **Spread** | Droplet | Droplet, fomite | Droplet | Droplet | Droplet |
| **Incubation period** | 8–14 days | 14–21 days | 14–21 days | | 4–18 days |
| **Infectious period** | 2–3 days before rash | Until crusts dry | | | 15 days before to 4 days after parotitis |
| **Prodrome** | Conjunctival suffusion, cough, fever, Koplik's spots on the palate | Fever, malaise of a few hours or no prodrome | Malaise or no prodrome | Malaise, arthralgia | Sore throat, fever, pain at angle of jaw |
| **Rash** | Blotchy macular rash becoming confluent appears about day 4, beginning on the forehead, spreading onto trunk and limbs over 3–4 days. Clears after 4–5 days, often with fine desquamation and brown discoloration | Pink macules, mainly central (trunk, face) – rapidly evolve into papules and vesiculate, dry and crust over. Different stages present at the same time | Fine macular rash develops over face and upper arms and spreads down. Fades after 3 days | 'Slapped cheek' appearance, and a lacy rash on thighs | None |
| **Other clinical features** | | Mild conjunctivitis, sore throat and cervical adenopathy, especially post-cervical, occipital and postauricular Forchheimer spots may be seen | Fever and generalized arthralgia | | Meningitis |
| **Complications** | Mainly respiratory – secondary viral pneumonia and rarely giant cell pneumonia, bronchitis and otitis media. Myocarditis, encephalitis, hepatitis and SSPE are rare complications | Secondary bacterial pneumonia, chickenpox pneumonitis, bacterial infection of spots, disseminated chickenpox (especially in the immunosuppressed), cerebellar ataxia (may precede or follow the rash), haemorrhagic chickenpox | Asymmetrical large joint arthropathy, teratogenicity | Persisting arthralgia, aplastic crisis in those with haemolytic disease | Swollen parotid, submandibular gland, pancreatitis, orchitis, mastitis, sterility (controversial – it has proved difficult to show that sterility following orchitis is a consequence of the orchitis and sterility is not inevitable), meningitis |

- Chickenpox in pregnancy can cause severe congenital abnormalities.
- *Differential diagnosis* includes hand, foot and mouth disease (Coxsackie virus), enterovirus, impetigo, syphilis, pemphigus and bullous pemphigoid.

### Zoster

- Zoster usually affects one dermatome corresponding to the dorsal root ganglion that is the site of infection, but multiple dermatome or disseminated presentations can occur in immunocompromised patients (e.g. with HIV).
- A prodrome of pain, itching or tingling at the dermatome site often precedes the characteristic vesicular rash, and there may be systemic illness with fever, myalgia and malaise.
- The pain may be severe prior to rash eruption, and depending on site can mimic acute myocardial infarction, acute cholecystitis or renal colic.
- Thoracic dermatomes are commonly affected, and the rash should not affect the midline.
- Ophthalmic zoster is infection of the first division of the trigeminal nerve root and can have sight-threatening ocular involvement.
- In Ramsay Hunt syndrome (peripheral facial weakness, zoster rash and pain inside the ear, and loss of taste in the anterior part of the tongue), the VII and VIII cranial nerve roots are affected.
- As for chickenpox, the rash is contagious until crusted over.
- Complications include severe chronic pain (post-herpetic neuralgia), meningoencephalitis, cranial nerve palsies, keratitis, retinopathy, pancreatitis and hepatitis.
- *Differential diagnosis* includes HSV, contact dermatitis, insect bites, folliculitis, impetigo and scabies.

### Investigation

- Diagnosis of both chickenpox and zoster is usually made on clinical grounds.
- PCR of vesicle fluid for VZV can confirm diagnosis of chickenpox or zoster if required.
- VZV IgG antibodies performed to check for immunity in immunocompromised people or pregnant women following a history of exposure.
- Chest radiograph should be performed for adults with chickenpox to check for pneumonitis.
- PCR of CSF for VZV if CNS disease is suspected.

### Management

### Chickenpox

- Treatment of children with chickenpox in the community is mainly symptomatic, with fluids, paracetamol, chlorpheniramine and topical calamine cream.
- Aspirin should be avoided in children with chickenpox due to the risk of Reye's syndrome.

- NSAIDs should be avoided due to a possible association with necrotizing soft-tissue infections and invasive Group A *Streptococcus*.
- Adolescents >13 years, adults and immunocompromised children should be treated with acyclovir or valacyclovir (the latter has better oral absorption).
- Immunocompromised people with chickenpox should be admitted to hospital, and admission should be considered for adults with chickenpox.

### Zoster

- Acyclovir/valacyclovir should be offered to >50 year-olds with zoster.
- Steroids may reduce pain and duration of zoster, but there is no evidence they reduce the risk of post-herpetic neuralgia.
- Analgesia options for zoster include topical lidocaine, paracetamol, NSAIDs, oxycodone and amitriptyline.
- Ophthalmic zoster cases should be reviewed by an ophthalmologist.

### Infection prevention and control

- Children with chickenpox should be kept at home where possible and avoid nurseries, schools, public transport and crowded places until all the lesions have crusted over.
- Zoster is not contagious if the lesions are covered.
- If hospitalized with chickenpox or zoster in an exposed area (e.g. ophthalmic), the patient should be in a side room.
- Immunoglobulin (VZIG) can be given if available to non-immune vulnerable people (immunocompromised and pregnant) following exposure.

### Vaccination

- The varicella vaccine is a live attenuated vaccine.
- Vaccine efficacy against chickenpox is >90% for the two-dose regimen, with breakthrough infections typically mild.
- The chickenpox vaccine is used routinely in children in many countries around the world.
- The UK does not yet have chickenpox vaccination in the routine immunization schedule due to concerns about its cost-effectiveness and prioritizing improving immunization uptake rates for existing vaccines in a society with a degree of vaccine scepticism. The chickenpox vaccine is given for non-immune healthcare workers and non-immune contacts of immunocompromised people, and it is also available on private prescription.
- The zoster vaccine is a higher dose of the chickenpox vaccine and is given to older adults to give reduced risk of zoster and milder disease.

### Prognosis

- Chickenpox is usually a mild self-limiting illness, however there is a hospitalization rate of around 5 in 1000 cases and a case fatality rate of 2–3/100 000.
- Zoster can result in post-herpetic neuralgia, with the risk increasing with age (30% of >80-year-olds).
- Zoster recurs in up to 6% of people.

## MEASLES

Measles is a highly contagious systemic infection, caused by the measles virus.

### Epidemiology

- Measles occurs worldwide, with WHO estimates of around 6.7 million cases and 110 000 deaths globally in 2017.
- In high-income countries with effective vaccination schemes, measles is rare, although outbreaks occur in settings with reduced vaccination uptake.
- In low- and middle-income countries, measles remains a common cause of mortality in children less than 5 years old.

### Disease mechanisms

- Measles is caused by an RNA paramyxovirus and is highly infectious, with an attack rate of around 90% when a non-immune person has exposure to the virus.
- Transmission of measles is by direct person-to-person spread and airborne spread of droplets from the respiratory secretions of an infected person.
- Natural infection confers life-long immunity.

### Clinical features

- Incubation is 6–21 days.
- Fever, coryza, cough, conjunctivitis and characteristic morbilliform rash occur (**Figure 3.14a,b**), associated with pathognomonic white Koplik's spots (**Figure 3.14c**) in the mouth.

- Measles may be complicated by primary or secondary pneumonia or encephalitis.
- Diarrhoea is common in the tropics and is often severe. Myocarditis and laryngitis are reported.
- Neurological complications include encephalitis (1 in 1000 measles cases), acute disseminated encephalomyelitis (ADEM), and the late complication of subacute sclerosing panencephalitis (SSPE). SSPE is a rare, fatal, demyelinating encephalopathy caused by the measles virus remaining latent within the CNS producing this rare encephalitis many years later.

### Investigation

- Diagnosis of measles has traditionally been made on clinical grounds, but it needs confirmation for public health and control purposes.
- Measles is confirmed by positive serum measles IgM antibodies, a significant rise in measles IgG antibodies between acute and convalescent titres, isolation of measles virus in culture, or detection of measles virus RNA by RT-PCR.

### Management

- Treatment of measles is mainly supportive.
- Vitamin A should be given to all children with measles because deficiency is associated with poorer outcomes even in high-income countries.
- Ribavirin is used for severe cases and immunocompromise, although further trials are needed.
- People with measles should be kept in isolation until 4 days after the rash appears, or for the duration of illness in immunocompromised people.
- The MMR vaccine is a highly effective live vaccine. Two doses are required.
- Claims in 1998 that the MMR vaccine is linked to autism have been comprehensively discredited. Vaccine hesitancy for MMR remains an ongoing worldwide issue, requiring further understanding and action.

**3**

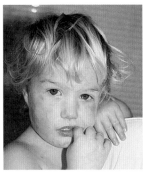
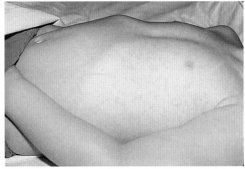
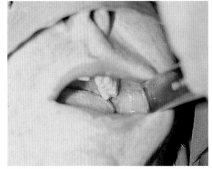

(a)  (b)  (c)

**Figure 3.14** Measles. **(a)** Facies on the development of the rash. **(b)** Evolution of the maculopapular rash. Second day, the rash has reached the hips. **(c)** Koplik's spots. All figures reproduced from Bannister B *et al.*, *Infectious Disease*, 1996 (Wiley-Blackwell, Oxford) with permission of the authors.

### Prognosis

- The prognosis of uncomplicated measles is good.
- Morbidity is usually caused by secondary bacterial infection and is much higher in low- and middle-income countries, especially in children <12 months and where malnutrition is present.

## CHRONIC FATIGUE SYNDROME

Chronic fatigue syndrome (CFS) is a diagnosis provided to those with a predominant symptom of extreme tiredness that is not explained by an identifiable medical or psychiatric condition, i.e. of unknown pathophysiology. The term myalgic encephalopathy (ME) is sometimes used, although pathological evidence of encephalopathy has not been clearly demonstrated. CFS is often referred to infectious diseases specialists, as patients frequently report that symptoms are triggered by an infection.

### Epidemiology

- The true frequency of CFS in a population is difficult to know due to case heterology and differences between studies in CFS definitions and study methodology.
- The UK prevalence of CFS has been estimated to be 0.11–2.6%.
- Women are twice to three times more likely to be affected than men.
- Two peaks in age for incidence are seen: adolescence and between 30 and 50 years.

### Disease mechanisms

- The aetiology of CFS is unknown.
- CFS cases are heterologous, but some may have an inflammatory component.
- Research has sought to identify initiating triggers for CFS, and a range of factors have been investigated including infection (e.g. EBV, *Mycoplasma pneumonia*, *Giardia*), immunological disorders (e.g. IgG deficiencies), neuroendocrine, GI and psychological factors, but no clear common cause has been found.
- Twin studies support a genetic contribution.
- Current research is examining the role of mitochondrial dysfunction and metabolic disturbances in disease pathogenesis and maintenance.
- CFS may represent a common clinical manifestation of multiple diseases with discrete aetiologies.

### Clinical features

- Chronic and disabling fatigue (otherwise unexplained) of at least 6 months' duration, accompanied by several other symptoms including pain, sleep disturbance, neurological and cognitive changes, motor impairment, and altered immune and autonomic responses.
- Post-exertional malaise and memory or concentration problems are commonly reported.

### Investigation

- Screening to exclude infectious, endocrine or rheumatological causes includes full blood count (FBC), renal, liver and thyroid function tests, C-reactive protein, serology (EBV, CMV, HIV, HBV, HCV), erythrocyte sedimentation rate (ESR).
- Further laboratory or radiological investigations are of limited yield in the absence of specific findings in the history and examination.

### Management

- CFS is a real and incapacitating disease, and a supportive relationship between the patient and doctor is essential.
- Therapeutic goals should be agreed which could include accomplishing activities of daily living, maintaining hobbies and a social life, and returning to work (if applicable).
- Any accompanying medical conditions, including depression, should be treated.
- Cognitive behavioural therapy (CBT) and exercise therapy are helpful for some patients.

### Prognosis

- 20–50% of adults with CFS improve in the medium term (1–4 years), but only 6% return to their previous level of functioning.
- Children with CFS have better outcomes than adults.

## INFECTIONS OF THE NERVOUS SYSTEM

## BACTERIAL MENINGITIS

Meningeal inflammation is caused by a bacterial pathogen.

### Epidemiology

- UK incidence in adults is approximately 1.5/100 000/ year.
- The region of sub-Saharan Africa known as the meningitis belt can have incidence >100/100 000/ year.

### Disease mechanisms

- Neonates are colonized with potential pathogens in the birth canal. In adults and children, potential pathogens are transmitted via droplet spread with initial colonization of nasopharynx.
- Meningeal infection occurs either via bacteraemic spread or direct infection through anatomical defect.
- Causative bacteria vary with age.

o *Common*:
- Streptococcus pneumoniae (adult/children)
- *Neisseria meningitidis* (adult/children)
- *Escherichia coli* (neonates)
- Group B *Streptococcus* (neonates)
o *Less common:*
- *Listeria monocytogenes* (elderly, pregnancy, neonates, immunocompromised)
- *Haemophilus influenzae* (rare following widespread Hib vaccination)

### Clinical features

Acute presentation is of fever, headache, neck stiffness, vomiting and sepsis (reduced conscious level if delayed treatment).

### Differential diagnosis

Differential diagnosis includes viral meningitis, TB meningitis, systemic sepsis, general viral infection, and other causes of headache (see Chapter 13, Neurological disease).

### Investigation

- *CSF microscopy:* neutrophil predominance, elevated protein concentrations, Gram stain may be helpful (low sensitivity but important when positive)
- *CSF biochemistry:* glucose reduced (<50% in comparison to serum); lactate elevated; protein elevated
- *CSF culture:* gold standard to identify pathogen and antimicrobial susceptibility
- *CSF PCR:* bacterial DNA can be amplified by PCR; multiplex reactions can cover a whole panel of potential pathogens

### Management

- Lumbar puncture with CSF analysis is a crucial investigation and does not need to be delayed for CT head unless there are features that may be associated with increased risk of a space-occupying lesions such as: a reduction in conscious level, immunosuppression, focal neurology, seizure activity or other clinical signs of raised intercranial pressure (such as papilloedema).
- Administer antibiotics promptly
  o Empirical treatment in adults is ceftriaxone 2 g BD IV.
  o If there are risk factors for listeria (pregnancy, immunosuppression, >55 years old), amoxycillin 2 g QDS IV should be added.
- If pneumococcal disease is suspected or confirmed, dexamethasone 10 mg QDS IV can be added.
- Patients should be managed in a side room with standard PPE.
- The disease is notifiable in the UK.
- Close contacts of meningococcal disease require preventive therapy with rifampicin or ciprofloxacin.
- A vaccine is available for *S. pneumoniae*, HiB and *N. meningitidis*.

### Prognosis

- If untreated, bacterial meningitis has a very high mortality, hence the need for prompt treatment.
- Complications of pyogenic meningitis are caused by inflammation and cerebral oedema and include: cranial nerve palsy, deafness, hydrocephalus, mental retardation and epilepsy.

## VIRAL MENINGITIS

In viral meningitis, the meningeal inflammation is caused by viral infection, which is usually less serious than bacterial meningitis.

### Epidemiology

- UK incidence is approximately 3/100 000/year.
- Disease caused by enterovirus is more common in the summer months and is spread faeco-orally with occasional outbreaks reported.
- Only a minority of viral infections result in clinical signs of meningitis.

### Disease mechanisms
*Common*

- Non-polio enteroviruses (i.e. echovirus, Coxsackie virus)
- HSV-2 > HSV-1 (recurrent HSV-2 meningitis – Mollaret syndrome)
- VZV

*Rare*

- Other herpesviruses (CMV/EBV)
- HIV (as part of seroconversion illness)
- Measles (uncommon with vaccination)
- Mumps (uncommon with vaccination)
- Lymphocytic choriomeningitis virus (LCMV) (rare – excreted in rodent urine)

### Clinical features

Symptoms are headache, fever, neck stiffness with no signs of encephalitis (see below), which develop acutely over 1–2 days.

### Differential diagnosis

Differential diagnosis includes bacterial meningitis, TB meningitis, general viral infection, and other causes of headache (see Chapter 13, Neurological disease).

### Investigation

- *CSF microscopy:* this is typically lymphocytic.
- *CSF biochemistry:* protein concentrations may be slightly raised, glucose and lactate are usually normal.
- *CSF PCR:* viral nucleic acid can be amplified by PCR. Multiplex reactions can cover a whole panel of potential pathogens.
- Frequently, the causative pathogen is not isolated.

3

## Management

There is no specific treatment for the viruses responsible for aseptic meningitis so patients should be treated symptomatically.

## Prognosis

Viral meningitis is usually a self-limiting condition with complete recovery within a few days.

# VIRAL ENCEPHALITIS

Viral encephalitis is inflammation of the brain caused by a virus.

## Epidemiology

- Viral encephalitis is a rare disease. Incidence is approximately 1/100 000/year in the UK with HSV and VZV being the most frequently isolated organisms.
- Incidence of arbovirus encephalitis varies globally, and is a very rare presentation in the UK.
- Cases of TBE and West Nile virus encephalitis are seen in Europe in the summer months.
- Japanese encephalitis is the most common arbovirus encephalitis globally with 30 000–50 000 cases/year mainly in Asia.

## Disease mechanisms

### Commonest causes in high-income countries

- HSV with HSV1 > HSV2
- VZV

### Other global causes

- Other herpes viruses (HHV-6 in severely immunocompromised)
- Arthropod-borne (arbo) flaviviruses: West Nile, Japanese encephalitis, St Louis encephalitis, Murray Valley encephalitis, TBE, Louping ill virus
- Arthropod-borne (arbo) alpha virus: Eastern equine encephalitis, Western equine encephalitis, Venezuelan equine encephalitis

## Clinical features

Symptoms are headache, fever, reduced conscious level, confusion, irritability, bizarre behaviour, seizures, which develop acutely over 1–2 days.

## Differential diagnosis

Differential diagnosis includes ADEM, autoimmune encephalitis and acute confusional state (see Chapter 13, Neurological disease).

## Investigation

- *CSF microscopy:* typically, lymphocytic protein concentrations may be slightly raised, glucose are usually normal. However, concentrations can be normal.
- *CSF PCR:* viral RNA can be amplified by RT-PCR. Multiplex reactions can cover a whole panel of potential pathogens. Diagnostics for rare viral causes may only be available at reference laboratories.
- *MRI scan* may show bilateral asymmetrical involvement of the limbic system, medial temporal lobes.
- *EEG* may show focal abnormalities such as spike and slow- or periodic sharp-wave patterns over the involved temporal lobes in HSV encephalitis, or diffuse slowing.
- *Brain biopsy* is rarely indicated.
- *Autoantibodies:* include N-methyl-D-aspartate (NMDA) and Voltage Gated Potassium Channel (VGKC) to exclude non-infective, autoimmune causes (see Chapter 13, Neurological disease).

## Management

- Treat for HSV encephalitis with IV acyclovir continued for 14–21 days if confirmed.
- There are no specific infection control issues.

## Prognosis

- Prognosis is poor compared to viral meningitis.
- Mortality for HSV encephalitis is 10–15% and there is a high frequency of neurological sequelae in surviving patients.

# CENTRAL NERVOUS SYSTEM TUBERCULOSIS

This disease of the CNS is caused by *Mycobacterium tuberculosis*. The two main manifestations are tuberculous meningitis (TBM) and tuberculomas (space-occupying lesions within the brain parenchyma or spinal cord).

CNS TB can occur as isolated manifestation of extrapulmonary disease or associated with disseminated or miliary disease especially in advanced HIV and children <2 years.

## Epidemiology

- CNS TB represents only 1% of the total number of TB cases.
- It results in death or severe disability in 50% globally. Even in high-resource settings, such as the UK, mortality is approximately 10%.

## Disease mechanisms

- During the initial dissemination of bacilli, small tuberculous granuloma may emerge within the CNS, termed 'Rich foci'. Rich foci that subsequently progress may extend into the subarachnoid space or ventricles resulting in meningitis or, if located more deeply, may develop into tuberculoma or abscesses.
- The inflammatory exudate accompanying meningeal involvement, typically over the basal surface of the brain, may obstruct the CSF flow resulting in hydrocephalus or can cause a vasculitis. These complications increase morbidity and mortality.

## Clinical features

- TBM in adults usually presents subacutely, with symptoms typically developing over >5 days.
- Symptoms include low-grade fever, headache and neck stiffness. Confusion or a reduced Glasgow coma score is present in 30–60%. Cranial nerve palsies occur in 30–50%. Tuberculoma may present with focal neurology or seizures.
- Metabolic complications are common, with hyponatraemia occurring in 50% of cases.

## Differential diagnosis

Differential diagnosis includes other causes of subacute lymphocytic meningitis (e.g. *Cryptococcus*, viral infection, Lyme disease, syphilis, partially treated bacterial meningitis and brucella).

## Investigation

- *CSF examination:* a large volume sample is needed (8–10 mL).
  - Cell count: white cell count is usually elevated (lymphocyte predominance). Protein and lactate concentration can be markedly raised and the CSF : serum glucose is usually <50%.
  - Culture: rarely positive prior to 10 days incubation. Sensitivity is only 80% against a clinical diagnosis of TBM.
  - Ziehl–Neelsen stain: this generally has a poor sensitivity (10–20%), which can be improved by concentration of a large volume, microscopist expertise and time spent looking at the slide.
  - Xpert MTB/RIF assay: rapid, automated, NAAT, in comparison to CSF culture sensitivity is 80% and specificity is 99%.
- *Diagnostic imaging*
  - Gadolinium-enhanced MRI brain has greater sensitivity for abnormalities over contrast CT; however, 15% of those in early stages of TBM will still have normal MRI.
  - Common findings on brain imaging are basal meningeal enhancement, hydrocephalus, infarction and space-occupying lesions.
  - Chest radiographs of all patients with suspected TBM should be undertaken to assess for evidence of pulmonary or miliary disease.

## Management

- Drugs for treating drug-sensitive CNS TB are the same as for other forms of TB except the recommended duration is rifampicin and isoniazid for 12 months supplemented by ethambutol and pyrazinamide for the first 2 months.
- There is a strong evidence base to support that adjunctive steroid tapered over 6–8 weeks reduces mortality and severe disability in patients with TBM.

## Prognosis

Overall prognosis and risk of death relate to the conscious level and extent of neurological impairment at presentation, which largely reflects the presence of hydrocephalus or cerebral vasculitis.

# PYOGENIC BRAIN ABSCESS

This is an abscess in the brain tissue, caused by bacteria.

## Epidemiology

- Incidence is estimated to be 0.3–0.9/100 000 in high-income countries.
- The median age at presentation is 30–40 years.

## Disease mechanisms

- Infection can arise from contiguous spread (40–50%) from ear, sinus, mastoid infection or in relation to skull fracture, penetrating injury or neurosurgical intervention.
- Haematogenous spread accounts for 30–40% of brain abscesses, where bacteria spread in the bloodstream from a distant pyogenic infection at another site (e.g. dental or pulmonary infection) or from septic embolism from an intravascular source of infection (e.g. endocarditis).
- In 10–20%, the source of infection is unclear.
- Causative organisms reflect aetiology; however, brain abscesses are frequently polymicrobial (in about 25%),
- *Strep. anginosus–constellatus* group organisms (previously *Strep. milleri*), *Staph. aureus*, Enterobacteriaceae and anaerobes are common pathogens.

## Clinical features

The classic triad is fever, headache and focal neurology or seizures. However, only 20% have all three of these features and presentation can be atypical or subacute.

## Differential diagnosis

Differential diagnosis includes brain tumour (primary or metastasis), other infective mass lesions (tuberculoma, neurocysticercosis, toxoplasmosis, nocardia) and stroke.

## Investigation

- *Contrast CT:* peripheral rim-enhanced lesion surrounded by a vasogenic oedema. Brain abscesses on CT appear as a single abscess in about 80%, and are most commonly located in frontal or temporal lobes.
- *MRI:* this has better resolution than CT and is more discriminating between tumour and infection.
- *Aspiration:* brain abscess should be referred to a neurosurgeon for consideration of stereotactic aspiration/biopsy, typically undertaken if the lesion is

>1 cm. Samples should be sent for microscopy, culture (including TB and fungal) and histology.

## Management

- Empirical therapy in adults is typically ceftriaxone 2 g BD IV + metronidazole 400 mg PO TDS, with a total treatment duration of 4–6 weeks.
- Therapy is often kept broad even if results are available as polymicrobial infection is common.

## Prognosis

- Outcome of brain abscess in high-income settings has improved with improvements in imaging and neurosurgical technique.
- Typically, case fatality is around 10% with approximately 70% making a good recovery.

## OTHER IMPORTANT CNS INFECTIONS

### Tetanus

- Tetanus results from a cutaneous infection with the anaerobic bacteria *Clostridium tetani*. *C. tetani* spores are commonly present in soil globally. Following a local infection, typically from a soil-contaminated wound, the organism secretes a potent neurotoxin that can cause severe muscle spasms and rigidity, compromising respiration.
- The disease can be prevented by pre-exposure vaccination, which is part of the childhood vaccination programme, hence disease is uncommon in high-resource settings. However, there are more than 500 000 cases worldwide annually.
- Post-exposure management of contaminated wounds is important in disease prevention. Heavily contaminated wounds require cleaning and debridement. Passive immunization with IV anti-tetanus toxin immunoglobulin can be used to eliminate unbound toxin.
- In those who develop neurological symptoms, management is largely supportive. However, removal of the organism and toxin with surgical debridement, immunoglobulin and antibiotics therapy with penicillin and or metronidazole is also important.
- With supportive care such as sedation and intubation on ICU for as long as it takes for recovery, most patients in high-income settings survive. However, in resource-limited settings, the case fatality rate is estimated to be between 8% and 50%, and higher for neonatal tetanus.

### Botulism

- Botulism is a rare neurological condition caused by toxins from the anaerobic bacteria *Clostridium botulinum*.
- The illness typically presents with signs of bulbar palsy, often double vision or palatal paralysis.

Paralysis can be progressive until respiration is compromised. Treatment is supportive and often involves intensive care support unless mild, but mortality may be more than 25%.

- Acquisition can occur through three routes:
  - *Food-borne botulism:* In the right conditions, spores of *C. botulinum* can germinate within food (e.g. preserved meat and vegetables) and produce a neurotoxin which is then ingested.
  - *Wound-related botulism:* This can occur following intramuscular injection with contaminated batches of heroin where injection of spores of *C. botulinum* can lead to a local infection local resulting in toxin production.
  - *Infant botulism:* Children under 1 year old can be susceptible to infection with *C. botulinum* following ingestion of the spores which may be present in honey.

### Leprosy

- This is a chronic granulomatous disease caused by *Mycobacterium leprae* and spread by nasal secretions. It can affect many tissues, especially skin and nerves, and it develops slowly. Nerve damage causes motor and sensory loss, which lead to traumatic damage to tissues.
- Disease manifests as a spectrum influenced by the host's cell-mediated immune response. Lepromatous leprosy occurs with poor cellular immunity and high pathogen numbers, resulting in tissue thickening and damage. Tuberculoid leprosy occurs with substantial cellular immunity and is usually localized within an area of hypopigmented anaesthetic skin supplied by a thickened nerve.
- Treatment is usually with a combination of rifampicin, dapsone and clofazimine.

### Rabies

- Rabies is zoonotic infection caused by a bullet-shaped RNA virus. It spreads to humans following the bite of an infected animal to cause a viral encephalitis, which is fatal once symptoms develop. The virus can infect a wide and diverse range of mammals. The most important reservoir for human transmission is wild and domestic canines and bats.
- The killed rabies vaccine is effective and safe. It can be given before exposure to those at particular risk or as PEP after a possibly infected bite. Additionally, immunoglobulin may also be given following high-risk exposure. Present regimens prevent the onset of rabies in the great majority of cases. However, it is essential that prophylaxis is started as soon as possible after any skin abrasion caused by any mammal in an endemic area.

## Poliomyelitis (polio)

- Polio is an enteroviral infection that destroys anterior horn cells, leading to severe paralysis.
- It is spread by either the faeco-oral or respiratory routes. The disease is now rare and may soon be eliminated following the efforts of an international vaccination programme.
- Patients usually present with a febrile paralysis. Pain or hyperaesthesia often herald the onset of paralysis, which characteristically manifests as an asymmetrical flaccid weakness and can evolve rapidly over a few hours or progressing more gradually over a week or more. Respiratory or bulbar paralysis may be prominent

features. The asymmetry and complete absence of any sensory defect differentiates polio from Guillain–Barré syndrome and peripheral neuropathies.

## INFECTIONS OF THE GASTROINTESTINAL SYSTEM

Infections of the GI tract are common and include diarrhoeal diseases, dental infections and hepatitis. Blood-borne viruses including hepatitis B and hepatitis C will be discussed in Chapter 9, Liver, biliary tract and pancreatic disease. The common infections of the GI system are listed in **Table 3.17**.

**Table 3.17** GI infections

| Location | Syndrome | Organism |
|---|---|---|
| Mouth | Dental caries | *Streptococcus mutans* |
| | Gingivitis | Anaerobes |
| | 'Cold sore' (herpes labialis) | Herpes simplex type 1 |
| | Candidiasis (thrush) | *Candida* |
| | Vincent's angina | *Fusobacterium fusiformis* |
| | | *Borrelia vincenti* |
| Stomach | Gastritis, ulcer | *Helicobacter pylori* |
| Small intestine | Malabsorption/chronic diarrhoea | Bacterial overgrowth |
| | | Traveller's diarrhoea |
| | | TB |
| | | *Yersinia enterocolitica* |
| | | (Tropical sprue) |
| | Enterotoxin | *Staphylococcus aureus* |
| | | *Bacillus cereus* |
| | | *Vibrio parahaemolyticus* |
| | | *Vibrio cholerae* |
| | | Enterotoxigenic *E. coli* |
| | Renal dysfunction | *Giardia* |
| | Invasive | *Salmonella* |
| | | *Campylobacter* |
| | | Rotavirus |
| | | *Cryptosporidium* |
| Large intestine | Dysentery | *Shigella* |
| | | Amoebae |
| | | *Campylobacter* |
| | | Enteroinvasive *E. coli* |
| Liver | Acute hepatitis | Hepatitis A–E |
| | | EBV |
| | | CMV |
| | | Arboviruses (yellow fever) |
| | | Leptospirosis |
| | | Septicaemia |
| | | *Legionella* |
| | | *Chlamydia* |
| | Chronic hepatitis | Hepatitis B |
| | | Hepatitis C |
| | | Hepatitis D |

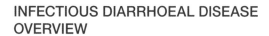

## INFECTIOUS DIARRHOEAL DISEASE OVERVIEW

Diarrhoea is defined by the WHO as the passage of three or more loose or liquid stools per day (or more frequent passage than is normal for the individual). Infections are a common cause worldwide, but there are many other causes of diarrhoea, as discussed in Chapter 10, Gastrointestinal disease.

### Epidemiology

- Worldwide there are over 6 billion episodes of diarrhoeal illness each year, and around 1.6 million annual deaths from diarrhoea predominantly in infants and young children due to dehydration.
- The majority of GI infections are in low- and middle-income countries, and are transmitted by the faeco-oral route, through ingestion of contaminated food or contact with infected people.
- Diarrhoeal disease is more likely in insanitary conditions and when services are disrupted by war or natural disaster.
- Outbreaks can occur clustered around restaurants, hospitals or institutions, especially with norovirus and *Salmonella*.

### Disease mechanisms

- Common causes are Gram-negative bacteria, viruses or intestinal parasites, as outlined below.
- Diarrhoea results from dysregulation of the normal bidirectional process of absorption and secretion of water and electrolytes in the lumen of the GI tract.
- Diarrhoea can be osmotic, due to osmotically active contents in the gut lumen, secondary due to toxins or enterocyte abnormalities, or due to excess motility.

### Clinical features

Diarrhoea is the prominent symptom for GI infections trans-mitted by this route, which may be accompanied by abdomi-nal pain, vomiting, fever and other systemic symptoms.

### Differential diagnosis

There are many non-infectious causes of diarrhoea, as dis-cussed in Chapter 10, Gastrointestinal disease. They include irritable bowel syndrome, diet, inflammatory (e.g. Crohn's, ulcerative colitis), endocrine (e.g. hyperthyroidism), malig-nancy (e.g. carcinoid, colon cancer), drug-related (e.g. anti-biotics, chemotherapy) and malabsorption (e.g. coeliac disease).

### Investigation

- The majority of diarrhoeal episodes are short-lived and do not merit formal tests.
- Investigation of persistent or severe cases should include FBC (a neutrophilia is common in bacterial GI infections), urea and electrolytes, and stool culture +/- molecular tests, microscopy for ova, cysts and parasites, serology, plus sigmoidoscopy for non-resolving diarrhoea.

### Management

- Many cases of diarrhoea are self-limiting and are managed symptomatically with oral rehydration therapy (ORT).
- Antimotility agents such as loperamide have a role in some cases.
- Antibiotics may prolong diarrhoea and resistance is widespread, so these should be reserved for severe culture-confirmed cases where sensitivities are available.
- Prevention includes public health measures to raise and maintain sanitation standards, adequate cooking of food, avoidance of contaminated water and excellent hand hygiene.
- Vaccines are available for some aetiological agents such as rotavirus and *Salmonella* Typhi, but they are not efficacious in all people.

### Prognosis

- While the majority of cases of infectious diarrhoea resolve, diarrhoea remains one of the leading causes of death in small children in the world's poorest regions.
- Following resolution of self-limiting diarrhoea, post-infectious lactate intolerance and irritable bowel symptoms can occur.
- Non-infectious sequelae of infectious diarrhoea can occur such as Guillain–Barré disease and reactive arthritis.

## *ESCHERICHIA COLI* INFECTIONS

- *E. coli* is a normal commensal of the intestinal tract present worldwide, but it may cause diarrhoea in humans, especially in travellers.
- Transmission is by the faeco-oral route.
- Several medically important strains of *E. coli* occur, including enterotoxigenic *E. coli* (ETEC), which is a common cause of traveller's diarrhoea, and enterohaemorrhagic *E. coli* (EHEC), which can cause severe and haemorrhagic diarrhoea, with the rare complication of haemolytic–uraemic syndrome.
- Treatment involves ORT and, in severe cases, antibiotics (e.g. co-trimoxazole, ciprofloxacin).
- Prognosis is usually excellent with recovery within days, although haemolytic–uraemic syndrome in ETEC is associated with a significant mortality.

## SHIGELLOSIS

- Shigellosis is an acute intestinal infection by *Shigella* spp., associated with superficial haemorrhagic disease in the colon.

- *Shigella* is spread by the faeco-oral route and the infective dose is very low.
- Shigellosis is common throughout the world and infection is most likely in children between the ages of 6 and 10 years, although all age groups are at risk.
- Intestinal infection is caused by one of four species: *Shigella dysenteriae*, *S. flexneri*, *S. boydii* and *S. sonnei*.
- Infection is usually self-limiting but severe disease with blood-stained mucus, fever, rigors, headache and abdominal pain can occur. Death may result from dehydration, endotoxic shock, bowel necrosis and perforation, or haemolytic–uraemic syndrome.
- Prompt diagnosis and treatment of serious cases leads to full recovery.

## SALMONELLOSIS

- *Salmonella* is a common cause of intestinal infection that may spread beyond the gut to cause septicaemia.
- There are two species: *Salmonella enterica* and *Salmonella bongori*.
- *S. enterica* comprises six subspecies and is further divided into serovars based on serological tests in the laboratory to O, H and Vi antigens. For simplicity, strains are often referred to by the genus name (*Salmonella*) followed by the serovar name with a capital letter and no italics, e.g. *Salmonella* Typhi.
- *S.* Typhi and *S.* Paratyphi cause a systemic infection known as enteric fever; other *Salmonella* are referred to as non-*Salmonella* Typhi (NTS).
- Clinical syndromes include:
  o Enteric fever (see below)
  o Enterocolitis and gastroenteritis
  o Carrier state: *Salmonella* may remain in the gallbladder and be excreted from the bowel for over a year, causing outbreaks when food handlers are affected
  o Localized infection (e.g. osteomyelitis, meningitis and arthritis)
- Antibiotics should be reserved for severe cases. Resistance to ciprofloxacin is now common and azithromycin resistance is increasing, and so ceftriaxone while awaiting culture and susceptibility testing may be used.
- Three vaccines are currently available for typhoid: killed whole-cell vaccine; subcellular vaccine containing the Vi antigen; and the oral live attenuated *Salmonella* Ty21A.

## ENTERIC FEVER

- Also known as typhoid fever, enteric fever is caused by *S.* Typhi and *S.* Paratyphi.
- Enteric fever starts gradually with a headache, cough, sore throat, initial constipation and gradually increasing remittent fever.

- Physical signs in the first week are a systemic upset, relative bradycardia, a transient erythematous maculopapular rash on the abdomen ('rose spots' – very rare!), mild splenomegaly and abdominal tenderness.
- Diarrhoea may occur after the first week.
- The third week may be complicated by intestinal perforation and haemorrhage, and more rarely, osteomyelitis, acute cholecystitis, lobar pneumonia, haemolytic anaemia, meningitis, peripheral neuropathy and urinary tract infection.

## CAMPYLOBACTER JEJUNI

- *Campylobacter jejuni* can cause diarrhoea, fever and cramping abdominal pains.
- It is the most common type of infective diarrhoea in many developed countries, usually caused by eating either undercooked meat, such as chicken which was infected with *Campylobacter*, or salad contaminated during preparation by chopping boards used for raw meat.
- Guillain–Barré syndrome is associated with *Campylobacter* infection.
- Most cases are self-limiting, but erythromycin or ciprofloxacin can be used for severe cases, guided by culture and sensitivity testing if available.

## CLOSTRIDIUM DIFFICILE DIARRHOEA

- *Clostridium difficile* can cause a toxin-mediated diarrhoeal disease.
- Prior antibiotic use disrupts the gut microbiome and causes a disturbance in the gut flora, allowing *C. difficile* to flourish.
- *C. difficile* is typically a healthcare-associated infection and person-to-person spread occurs.
- Clinical features include diarrhoea, fever, abdominal pain and a raised white cell count.
- Severe cases have dilation of the colon with colonic wall thickening on imaging, which can lead to perforation.
- Sigmoidoscopy in severe cases shows pseudomembranes: small white-yellow plaques situated on the mucosal surface of the rectum and sigmoid colon (pseudomembranous colitis).
- Hospitalized patients with diarrhoea (e.g. passing more than three stools per day) should have stool tested for *C. difficile* toxin (CDT) by ELISA, have antibiotics stopped or narrowed where possible, and be commenced on empirical treatment for *C. difficile* pending clearance by a negative CDT result.
- Treatment for *C. difficile* should follow local guidelines, but options include oral vancomycin (which is not absorbed), metronidazole or fidaxamicin.
- Infection control measures include isolation or cohorting of suspected cases, barrier nursing with

**3**

gown and gloves, and hand washing with soap and water as alcohol gels do not adequately destroy *Clostridium* spores.

## CHOLERA

- Cholera is a secretory diarrhoeal disease caused by *Vibrio cholerae.*
- There is profuse watery diarrhoea, up to 20 L/day, leading to fluid depletion and renal failure, with a high case fatality rate if untreated.
- The organism is spread rapidly in water or contaminated food.
- Cholera bacilli produce an enterotoxin with A and B subunits. The B subunit irreversibly binds to enterocytes by specific GM1 ganglioside receptors; the A subunit activates intracellular adenyl cyclase, leading to massive secretion of water and electrolytes into the gut lumen.
- Cholera outbreaks occur where socioeconomic conditions are poor, or during war, famine and other disasters.
- Cholera may remain endemic in a community.
- The disease is capable of spreading rapidly across the world (a phenomenon known as a pandemic).
- The El Tor biotype has replaced the classical strain as the major cause of cholera.
- The mainstay of treatment is rehydration with ORT or IV fluids, and tetracycline or doxycycline shorten the duration of the illness.

## VIRAL DIARRHOEA

- Rotavirus is a well-established cause of self-limiting, often severe diarrhoea in young children. Most people acquire immunity early in life but, because this wanes with increasing age, the elderly are again vulnerable.
- Norovirus (winter vomiting disease) occurs in epidemics of mild and short-lived gastroenteritis, often associated with upper respiratory tract symptoms and sometimes with a fever, and it is extremely common in temperate climates.
- Astroviruses, caliciviruses and fastidious adenoviruses have all been implicated as causes of transient diarrhoea. These organisms can cause outbreaks in the hospital environment.

## DIARRHOEA CAUSED BY PARASITES
## AMOEBIASIS

- Amoebiasis is an intestinal infection caused by the protozoan *Entamoeba histolytica.*
- The incubation period is variable, ranging from a few days to several months.
- Amoebic colitis may start gradually, first with an intermittent diarrhoea, which later becomes bloody

and mucopurulent. There may also be headache, nausea and anorexia.
- Fulminant amoebic dysentery like that of shigellosis can occur.
- Complications include amoebic liver abscess, toxic megacolon with perforation and peritonitis, and colonic stricture.
- Treatment involves metronidazole, followed by an agent to eradicate the cyst stage and prevent relapse and late complications, such as paromomycin.

## GIARDIASIS

- This is an intestinal infection caused by the flagellate protozoan *Giardia duodenalis* (previously *Giardia lamblia*).
- It is common in tropical countries, and can occur in temperate zones including high-income countries.
- Giardia cysts are resistant to killing by standard methods of chlorination.
- Giardia causes acute watery diarrhoea and can lead to chronic milder diarrhoea or an asymptomatic carrier state.
- Some chronic infections are associated with partial villous atrophy and malabsorption.
- Metronidazole and tinidazole are first-line therapies. AMR is increasingly reported, and second-line options include albendazole and other antiparasitic drugs.
- Mucosal immunity is important in controlling the infection – individuals with IgA deficiency are particularly prone to chronic or recurrent giardiasis.

## CRYPTOSPORIDIOSIS

- This is an intestinal infection with the protozoan *Cryptosporidium parvum.*
- Human infection occurs either as a sporadic zoonosis or in water-borne outbreaks, including in swimming pools with faulty filtration systems.
- The infection generally causes a mild and self-limiting watery diarrhoeal illness.
- Infection can be persistent and progressive in patients with immunodeficiency, including AIDS, where the cornerstone of management is improving the host immune system (with antiretrovirals in HIV).

## INFECTIONS OF THE RESPIRATORY TRACT

The common infections of the respiratory tract are listed in **Table 3.18**. Many of these are treated by respiratory physicians.

**Table 3.18** Respiratory infections

| Location | Syndrome | Organism |
|---|---|---|
| Upper respiratory tract | Acute tonsillitis | Group A streptococci |
| | Diphtheria | *Corynebacterium diphtheriae* |
| | Pharyngitis | *Haemophilus influenzae* |
| | | *Mycoplasma* |
| | | *Mycobacterium tuberculosis* |
| | Coryza | Rhinovirus |
| | Whooping cough | *Bacillus pertussis* |
| Lower respiratory tract | Lobar pneumonia | *Streptococcus pneumoniae* |
| | Atypical pneumonia | *Mycoplasma* |
| | | *Legionella* |
| | | *Chlamydia* |
| | | *Staphylococcus aureus* |
| | | Viral |
| | | Gram-negative bacteria |
| | Lung abscess | *Staph. aureus* |
| | | Gram-negative bacteria |
| | | Anaerobes |
| | Empyema | *Strep. pneumoniae* |
| | | *M. tuberculosis* |
| | Mycobacterial infection | *M. tuberculosis* |
| | | Non-tuberculous mycobacteria (NTM) |
| | Mycotic infection | Bronchopulmonary aspergillosis |
| | | Phycomycosis |
| | | Histoplasmosis |

## INFECTIONS OF THE CARDIOVASCULAR SYSTEM

The common infections of the cardiovascular system are listed in **Table 3.19**. Many of these are treated by cardiologists.

## TROPICAL INFECTIONS

Tropical infections are diseases that occur solely or predominantly in hot and humid regions and are often associated with poverty. The cause of tropical infections may be bacterial, viral, fungal or parasitic, and transmission may be via airborne spread, contaminated food and water, sexual contact or via the bites of insects or animals. The intersection between tropical infections and malnutrition, pollution and non-communicable diseases such as diabetes is increasingly recognized as important in pathogenesis.

## MALARIA

Malaria is one of the world's biggest infectious killers and is caused by protozoa in the *Plasmodium* genus.

### Epidemiology

- 1.1 billion people in 91 countries and territories worldwide are at high risk of malaria infection, throughout most of the world's tropics.

- The WHO estimates that there were 212 million cases of symptomatic malaria in 2016 with 429 000 deaths.
- The global incidence of malaria reduced by 37% between 2000 and 2015.

**Table 3.19** Infections of the cardiovascular system

| Syndrome | Organism |
|---|---|
| Infective endocarditis | |
|   Native valves | *Streptococcus viridans* |
| | Other streptococci (*S. sanguis*, *S. mitis*, *S. anginosus*, etc.) |
| | Enterococci |
| | *Staphylococcus aureus* |
| | *Coxiella burnetti* (Q fever) |
|   Prosthetic valves | The above plus *Staphylococcus epidermidis* |
| Myocarditis | Coxsackie and echovirus |
| | Influenza, mumps, EBV, CMV |
| | *Mycoplasma pneumoniae* |
| | *Leptospira* spp. |
| | Pyogenic organisms |
| | Trypanosomiasis (Chagas' disease) |
| | Coxiella (Q fever) |
| Acute pericarditis | Coxsackie and influenza viruses |
| | *Mycoplasma pneumoniae* |
| | *Streptococcus pneumoniae* |
| | *Mycobacterium tuberculosis* |

CMV, cytomegalovirus; EBV, Epstein–Barr virus.

- Malaria is caused by one of six human infective species of *Plasmodium*. *P. falciparum* causes the largest burden of disease and predominates in sub-Saharan Africa, Papua New Guinea, Haiti and the Dominican Republic.
- *P. vivax* is more common in the Americas and Western Pacific.
- The prevalence of *P. falciparum* and *P. vivax* is similar in the Indian subcontinent, South East Asia and Oceania. *P. malariae* and *P. ovale* are much less common.
- The significance of human infections with the primate parasites *P. knowlesi* and *P. simian* is still not fully understood.

## Disease mechanisms

- *Plasmodia* are transmitted by the female *Anopheles* mosquito (**Figure 3.15**).
- Very rarely, malaria can be acquired congenitally or via contaminated blood products or needles.
- Severity of infection depends on parasite and human factors:
  - Parasite virulence factors include variable surface antigens such as PfEMP-1 that mediate sequestration of infected red cells to capillary endothelium.
  - Host factors include absence of Duffy antigens, which are involved in erythrocyte invasion by *P. vivax*, and HbS heterozygosity, which results in reduced parasite growth and increased clearance of infected sickle cells.
- Malarial immunity is thought to be exposure-dependent and therefore children, travellers and those returning to endemic countries after significant periods away are most at risk, as are pregnant woman due to pregnancy-related changes to the immune system.

## Clinical features

- Malaria should be suspected in all travellers returning from an endemic area with fever.
- Symptoms can be non-specific such as malaise, myalgia and fatigue. Other symptoms may include headache, cough, nausea, abdominal pain and diarrhoea, and these may be associated with tachycardia, tachypnoea and hepatosplenomegaly.
- The classic relapsing tertian or quartan fevers are rare.
- Severe malaria is more likely to occur in *P. falciparum* infection. Markers of severe malaria include impaired consciousness, generalized weakness (prostration), convulsions, acidosis, hypoglycaemia, anaemia, renal impairment, jaundice, pulmonary oedema, significant bleeding, shock and hyperparasitaemia (parasitaemia >2%).
- Blackwater fever is characterized by haemoglobinuria causing 'Coca-Cola'-coloured urine resulting from haemolysis. The free haemoglobin damages the glomeruli, leading to renal failure.
- Cerebral malaria results from parasitized red cells obstructing the cerebral capillaries. It is associated with impaired consciousness, coma, fits and psychosis. Focal signs are uncommon.
- Pulmonary oedema is a complication of malaria, and fluid balance needs attention to prevent fluid overload.

## Differential diagnosis

Differential diagnosis of malaria is broad and includes:

- Dengue fever
- Chikungunya virus
- Typhoid fever
- Leptospirosis
- Bacterial or viral meningitis
- Bacterial pneumonia
- Viral haemorrhagic fever

## Investigation

- Malaria is diagnosed by demonstrating *Plasmodium* parasites in the peripheral blood by one of the following methods:
  - Rapid antigen tests detect conserved parasite proteins in 15–20 minutes.
  - Light microscopy, although labour-intensive, allows speciation (**Figure 3.16**) and an estimation of parasitaemia.
  - PCR.
- Three negative blood films across 3 consecutive days are required to exclude malaria.
- Patients with malaria typically have a low platelet count, and anaemia can occur alongside renal impairment and derangement of liver function.
- Patients presenting with suspected malaria should also have blood and urine culture performed to check for an alternative diagnosis or co-infection.

## Management

### Treatment

- Malaria is treated on the assumption that it is *P. falciparum* (until the species is known).
- Oral treatment is with quinine, atovaquone with proguanil hydrochloride (Malarone™) or artemeter with lumefantrine (Riamet™).
- If the patient is unable to take tablets or has features of severe infection (including parasitaemia >2%), treatment with IV quinine or artesunate (from a specialist centre) should be commenced.
- If the patient has been taking malaria prophylaxis, a different agent from the one used for prophylaxis should be used for treatment.
- Non-falciparum malaria is treated with Riamet™ or chloroquine, alongside primaquine to eliminate the

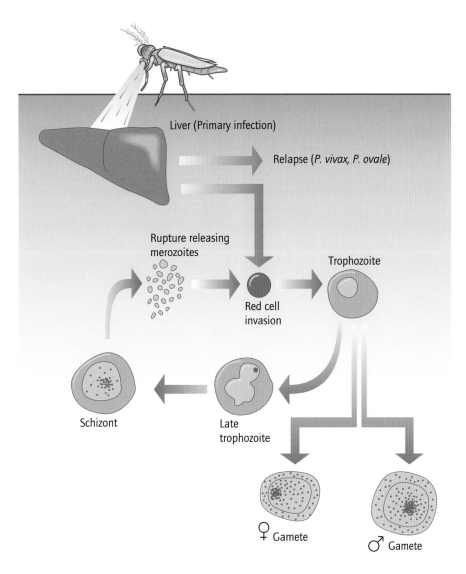

**Figure 3.15** Malaria life cycle.

3

hypnozoites of *P. vivax* and *P. ovale*. Before starting primaquine, patients should be tested for glucose-6-phosphate dehydrogenase (G6PD) deficiency because the drug can cause haemolysis in G6PD-deficient patients.

- In the UK, malaria is a notifiable disease.

*Prevention and control*
Globally, strategies to disrupt malaria transmission include adequate distribution and uptake of antimalarial drugs, mass drug administration, personal protection from mosquito bites including bed nets, vector control efforts and vaccine development.

- Malaria prophylaxis is recommended when travelling to countries with high malaria transmission. The medication offered depends upon local resistance patterns and patient preference. Vaporized insecticides such as diethyltoluamide (DEET) and the wearing of long sleeves and trousers at dawn and dusk are also recommended.

- The use of insecticide-impregnated bed nets has been shown to reduce malaria-attributable mortality by up to 30%. There is however, growing resistance of mosquitoes to pyrethroid insecticides (including permethrin).

- Vector control efforts including insecticide spraying with DDT have historically been very popular. However, concerns regarding mosquito resistance and the environmental and health effects mean that insecticides are now only recommended by the WHO as part of an indoor residual spraying strategy, whereby insecticides are sprayed on the inside walls of dwellings in endemic areas.

- The pursuit of an effective malaria vaccine is ongoing. RTS,S is a recombinant vaccine based upon the circumsporozoite protein, which is an antigen from the parasite's pre-erythrocyte stage. It was approved for use by the WHO in 2015 and shows moderate effectiveness in clinical trials in Africa.

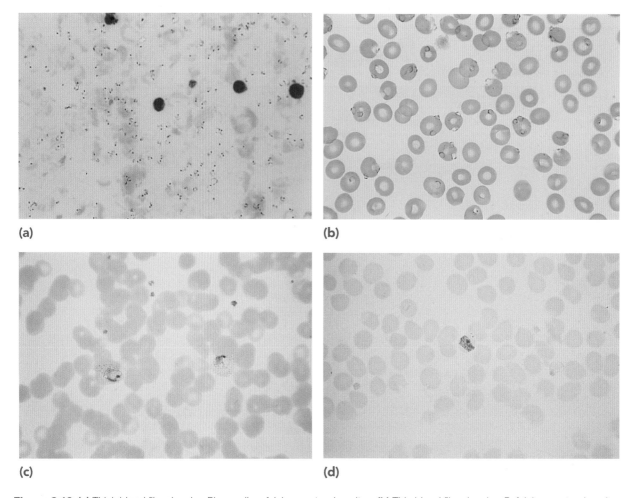

**Figure 3.16** **(a)** Thick blood film showing *Plasmodium falciparum* trophozoites. **(b)** Thin blood film showing *P. falciparum* trophozoites. **(c)** Thin blood film showing *P. vivax* trophozoites. **(d)** Thin blood film showing *P. malariae* trophozoites. Images **(c)** and **(d)** reproduced from Gillespie S, *Medical Microbiology Illustrated*, 1994 (Butterworth–Heinemann, Oxford) with permission of the author and publisher.

- Several other approaches to a malaria vaccine are in development, including targeting the *P. falciparum* reticulocyte-binding protein homologue 5 (PfRH5), a conserved protein involved in erythrocyte invasion.
- Due to only partial vaccine efficacy of current vaccines under research, it is likely that vaccines will be used as part of a combined strategy with vector control, targeted and mass drug administration and other control measures rather than vaccines offering a single solution in the prevention of malaria.

### Prognosis

*P. vivax*, *P. ovale* and *P. malariae* infections are benign, with fatal infections rare in immunologically competent patients. *P. falciparum* infection can have a rapidly progressive course and high mortality in those with no immunity such as children and travellers.

## DENGUE

Dengue is a febrile viral infection that is spread by mosquitoes.

### Epidemiology

- Dengue is endemic in more than 100 tropical and subtropical countries and is transmitted by *Aedes aegypti* or *Aedes albopictus* mosquitoes.
- There are an estimated 390 million infections each year, of which approximately 96 million are clinically apparent.

### Disease mechanisms

- Dengue is caused by one of four virus serotypes (DEN-1, DEN-2, DEN-3, DEN-4), which are types of flavivirus (a single-stranded RNA virus).
- Severe infection is more common when individuals are infected for a second time with a different serotype from the first infection.

### Clinical features

- Clinical manifestations of dengue infection are varied, from asymptomatic to a mild febrile illness to a life-threatening toxic shock syndrome.
- Mild symptoms include fever, nausea and vomiting, rash, headache, eye pain, and muscle or joint pain.

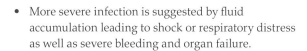

- More severe infection is suggested by fluid accumulation leading to shock or respiratory distress as well as severe bleeding and organ failure.

## Differential diagnosis

Differential diagnosis of dengue includes:
- Other viral haemorrhagic fevers
- Chikungunya
- Zika
- Malaria
- Typhoid fever
- Leptospirosis
- Acute HIV infection
- Viral hepatitis
- Rickettsial infection
- Sepsis due to bacteraemia

## Investigation

- Diagnosis of dengue in the acute phase is based on clinical suspicion, supported by leukopaenia and increased haematocrit with a rapid reduction in platelet count.
- A positive tourniquet test (the appearance of more than 10–20 petechiae per square inch, after application of an inflated tourniquet to the midpoint of systolic and diastolic pressure for 5 minutes) is also suggestive of a diagnosis of dengue.
- A rapid test for dengue, the NAT test, detects dengue IgM antibodies and is widely used in endemic areas.
- Diagnosis can be confirmed by positive serology and PCR-based amplification methods of viral RNA.

## Management

- The incubation period of infection with dengue virus ranges from 3 to 14 days.
- The disease has three phases: a febrile phase, a critical (plasma leakage) phase and a convalescent (reabsorption) phase.
- Treatment of acute infection is supportive, paying particular attention to fluid balance and bleeding.
- Infection control measures largely depend upon mosquito control methods, such as insecticides and removal of standing water.
- There is a dengue vaccine (CYD-TDV (Dengvaxia)) which is protective against development of severe dengue in people with serological evidence of prior dengue infection.

## Prognosis

- The majority of dengue infections are self-limiting, and some may be asymptomatic.
- Warning signs of severe dengue necessitating hospital admission are intense abdominal pain, lethargy, persistent vomiting, hepatomegaly (>2 cm), postural hypotension, mucosal bleeding and a progressive increase in haematocrit.

- Untreated, mortality from severe dengue can be greater than 20%, but with early recognition and supportive care mortality is <1%.

## EBOLA

Ebola virus disease (previously known as Ebola haemorrhagic fever) is a severe and often fatal disease of humans caused by the Ebola virus, a single-stranded RNA virus. There are five strains of Ebola virus.

### Epidemiology

- The Ebola virus was first discovered in 1976 near the Ebola River in the Democratic Republic of Congo (DRC).
- The largest outbreak occurred in 2014–16 in West Africa. It was caused by the Zaire strain of the virus. There were 28 616 reported cases with a case fatality rate of 39%.
- Fruit bats are considered the natural host of Ebola virus.
- Human-to-human transmission occurs via direct contact with blood or body fluids of infected people, and via surfaces contaminated with these fluids.

### Disease mechanisms

- The pathogenesis of Ebola virus is not fully understood.
- The Ebola virus can enter almost any human cell type using a variety of entry mechanisms.
- It can induce immune dysregulation via cytokine production, cell modulation and cell death resulting in organ failure, capillary leakage and haemorrhage.

### Clinical features

Symptoms typically occur within 2–21 days of exposure, with an average of 5–7 days, and include:
- Fever and chills
- Headache
- Myalgia
- Nausea and vomiting
- Diarrhoea
- Unexplained haemorrhage (bleeding or bruising)

### Differential diagnosis

- Malaria
- Typhoid fever
- Marburg virus
- Lassa fever
- Crimean–Congo haemorrhagic fever
- Bacterial sepsis

### Investigation

- Diagnosis is made by PCR.
- Laboratory findings include lymphopaenia, thrombocytopaenia, elevated liver enzymes, abnormal coagulation, abnormal renal function and electrolytes.
- The haematocrit may be raised as fluid leaves the capillaries.

3

## Management

- Management primarily involves supportive care.
- Recent evidence from a clinical trial conducted during the 2018–19 outbreak in DRC suggests that treatment of patients with monoclonal antibodies against Ebola can improve survival.
- Clinical trials for a vaccine are also underway.
- Patients should be isolated with strict procedures for use of PPE and waste disposal for clinical and laboratory staff, as transmission to these staff has frequently occurred during outbreaks.
- Management algorithms for suspected cases of viral haemorrhagic fever are available (e.g. Public Health England).

## Prognosis

- Prognosis is poor.
- Case fatality rate is dependent on the virus strain but can be up to 90%.
- Survivors may experience post-infection sequelae such as tiredness, muscle aches and pains, and eye problems.
- Stigma associated with survival is not uncommon in affected communities.

## ZIKA

Zika is a tropical viral infection spread by the bites of *Aedes* mosquitoes of importance due to concern about infection during pregnancy affecting CNS development of the foetus.

### Epidemiology

- Zika was first identified in Uganda in monkeys in 1947, with the first human case in 1952.
- Outbreaks of Zika virus have occurred in Africa, South East Asia, the Pacific Islands, Central and South America and the Caribbean.
- The first major outbreak occurred in Micronesia in 2007, followed by large outbreaks in French Polynesia (2013) and Brazil (2015).
- In 2018, Zika virus was reported to the WHO in 86 countries and territories.

### Disease mechanisms

- Zika infection is caused by Zika virus, a flavivirus related to yellow fever and dengue.
- It is transmitted primarily by bites from *Aedes aegypti* and *Aedes albopictus* mosquitoes, but it can also be transmitted congenitally, sexually and via blood products.

### Clinical features

Symptoms occur within 3–14 days of transmission and include:

- Rash: typically, sudden onset maculopapular rash which is itchy and may start on the head and move to the trunk, arms and legs, as well as affecting the palms and soles
- Low-grade fever (<38.5 °C)
- Non-purulent conjunctivitis, arthralgia and joint swelling as well as other non-specific symptoms such as headache, myalgia, nausea and vomiting

### Differential diagnosis

- Dengue
- Chikungunya
- Parvovirus
- Rubella
- Measles
- Leptospirosis
- Malaria
- Rickettsial infection

### Investigation

- Infection with Zika virus should be suspected in all individuals with recent travel to an endemic area and suggestive symptoms.
- Diagnosis is confirmed by positive serology or detection of viral antigens or viral RNA by PCR in body fluids.

### Management

- Management of acute infection is symptomatic.
- Infection prevention methods involve reducing risk of mosquito bites during travel to an endemic area as well as, upon return to a non-endemic area, reducing the risk of transmission to others.
- Due to the risks of congenital infection (see below), pregnant women are advised not to travel to Zika endemic areas, and men and women are advised to avoid conception for a period of time on return.
- Vaccine development is underway.

### Prognosis

- Acute infection is usually mild and symptoms resolve after approximately 1 week.
- Zika virus infection has been associated with Guillain–Barré syndrome. This complication has a higher mortality and likelihood of ITU admission than uncomplicated Zika infection.
- Congenital infection with Zika virus is associated with miscarriage as well as CNS and joint problems in the new born. Most severely, this can manifest as microcephaly and even anencephaly, as well as severe deformities of the hands and feet.

## LEISHMANIASIS

Leishmaniasis is a tropical infection with three clinical types: visceral (kala-azar, VL), cutaneous (CL) and mucocutaneous.

## Epidemiology

An estimated 50 000–90 000 cases of VL occur each year, predominantly in East Africa, South East Asia and Brazil. CL is common in the Middle East, Central Asia, Central and South America and the Mediterranean, with a global annual incidence of up to one million cases. The mucocutaneous form is rarer and occurs mostly in South America. In addition to humans, a wide variety of animal species can be infected. This extensive animal reservoir hampers efforts to control disease.

## Disease mechanisms

- Leishmaniasis is caused by parasites in the protozoan *Leishmania* genus and is transmitted by the bite of infected female phlebotomine sandflies.
- There are more than 20 species of *Leishmania* that cause disease, including:
  o *Leishmania donovani* and *L. infantum* – VL
  o *L. braziliensis* and *L. mexicana* – 'New World' (American) CL
  o *L. tropica* and *L. major* ('Old World' CL)
- The incubation period following an infected bite can be several months.

## Clinical features

- Patients with VL present with anorexia, malaise and weight loss, and they may complain of abdominal discomfort resulting from splenic enlargement. Signs include anaemia and cachexia, and the liver and spleen are enlarged.
- CL starts as a small itchy papule that forms a chronic ulcer, with regional lymphadenopathy.
- Mucocutaneous leishmaniasis features destructive lesions of the nose, mouth and throat which can be disfiguring and disabling.

## Investigation

- Patients with VL have a normocytic normochromic anaemia, thrombocytopaenia and leucopoenia.
- Biopsy of bone marrow, tissue or splenic aspirate should be studied for the presence of *Leishmania* by histopathology (**Figure 3.17**), PCR and culture.
- Serology shows anti-*Leishmania* antibodies but may represent past exposure, and sensitivity is reduced in immunocompromised people.

## Management

- First-line treatment of VL is liposomal amphotericin B.
- Other therapeutic options include miltefosine and pentavalent antimonial therapy.
- For CL, treatment options include local therapies (cryotherapy, topical ointments/creams with paromomycin and other ingredients, intralesional injections of pentavalent antimonial drugs and laser treatment), systemic treatments as for VL, or careful observation in selected low-risk cases.

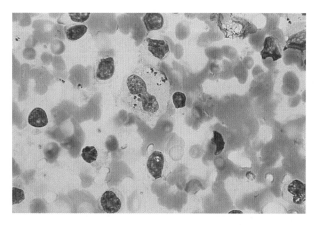

**Figure 3.17** Amastigotes of *Leishmania donovani*. Reproduced from Gillespie S, *Medical Microbiology Illustrated*, 1994 (Butterworth–Heinemann, Oxford) with permission of the publisher and author.

- Prevention of disease is by avoiding sandfly bites; there is no current vaccine.
- Early diagnosis and treatment of infected people helps to control the spread of disease.

## Prognosis

- Without treatment, VL is fatal in 95% of cases.
- CL heals in uncomplicated cases to leave a depressed white or brown scar.

## OTHER GLOBALLY IMPORTANT BACTERIAL INFECTIONS

A number of diseases occur worldwide transmitted by exposure to vectors, animals and the environment. A *zoonosis* is a disease that is transmitted from animals to humans. Many of these diseases are treatable with doxycycline. Prevention measures include rodent control, insect bite prevention, avoidance of stagnant water and animal farm water runoff, and protection of food from animal contamination.

## RICKETTSIAL DISEASE

- Rickettsial infections are caused by intracellular bacteria that, like *Chlamydia* and viruses, are only capable of replication within another cell.
- A range of genera cause disease around the world. A selection of some of the key Rickettsial infections are shown in **Table 3.20**.
- They are transmitted between their mammalian hosts by a vector such as a louse, tick, flea or mite.
- Typically, the natural mammalian host is a rodent, with humans acquiring the infection as a zoonosis. Only epidemic typhus is primarily a disease of humans.
- Clinical features include fever, rash, lymphadenopathy and an eschar – a dry, dark scab that looks like a

**Table 3.20** Key rickettsial diseases

| Disease (cause) | Geographical distribution | Vector | Animal reservoir |
| --- | --- | --- | --- |
| Rocky Mountain spotted fever (*Rickettsia rickettsii*) | The Americas (North, Central and South) | Tick | Rodents |
| Mediterranean spotted fever (*Rickettsia conorii*) | Southern Europe, Africa, Southern and Western Asia | Tick | Rodents, dogs |
| Rickettsialpox (*Rickettsia akari*) | Former Soviet Union countries, Balkans, Turkey, South Africa, Korea, North and South America | Mite | Rodents |
| Japanese spotted fever (*Rickettsia japonica*) | Japan | Tick | Rodents |
| African tick bite fever (*Rickettsia africae*) | Sub-Saharan Africa, Caribbean | Tick | Ruminants |
| Epidemic typhus (*Rickettsia prowazekii*) | Central Africa, Asia, the America (North, Central and South) | Human body louse | Humans, flying squirrels |
| Murine typhus (*Rickettsia typhi*) | Temperate, subtropical and tropical regions worldwide | Flea | Rodents |
| Scrub typhus (*Orientia tsutsugamushi*) | Asia-Pacific region, Africa, Chile | Larva mite (chigger) | Rodents |

cigarette burn and forms at the site of the insect bite (see **Figure 3.6**).

- Diagnosis is often clinical (e.g. fever with an eschar, or when other causes of fever have been excluded) but can be confirmed by rising antibody titres from paired serum samples 4 weeks apart. PCR is also available in some settings although lacks sensitivity.
- Treatment is with doxycycline.

## MELIOIDOSIS

- Melioidosis is a Gram-negative sepsis caused by the soil-dwelling bacterium *Burkholderia pseudomallei*.
- Transmission is via inhalation, skin inoculation or ingestion of contaminated drinking water.
- The disease is best recognized in South East Asia and Northern Australia, but it is now known to occur in tropical regions across the globe, with an estimated 165 000 cases per year and 89 000 deaths.
- Most melioidosis patients have a risk factor such as diabetes, chronic kidney disease, alcohol excess or older age. People with diabetes have a 12-fold increased risk.
- A wide range of clinical presentations occur, including sepsis, pneumonia, abscess formation in any organ and skin disease. Subacute and chronic disease may mimic TB.
- Diagnosis requires culture, with the bacterium growing easily but often misidentified as an environmental *Pseudomonas* of low pathogenicity.
- *B. pseudomallei* is intrinsically resistant to first-line antibiotics including penicillins, quinolones and aminoglycosides. Treatment requires at least 2 weeks of IV ceftazidime or a carbapenem, with follow-on

therapy for 3 months with oral trimethoprim-sulfamethoxazole to avoid relapse.

## Q FEVER

- Q fever is a zoonosis caused by *Coxiella burnetti*, a small intracellular bacterium related to the *Rickettsia*.
- Q fever occurs worldwide, including in the UK, and the most common animal reservoirs are cattle, sheep and goats. Transmission is most often by aerosol to farm and abattoir workers, or occasionally via infected milk.
- The acute illness presents as a fever and atypical pneumonia, sometimes accompanied by granulomatous hepatitis.
- *Coxiella burnetti* is also an important cause of culture-negative endocarditis and a cause of PUO.
- Diagnosis relies on serology, and treatment is with doxycycline.

## LEPTOSPIROSIS

- Leptospirosis is a zoonosis caused chiefly by *Leptospira interrogans*.
- Leptospirosis is found throughout the world and is spread from rats and other animals to humans directly or through contact with their urine. Humans become infected through occupational exposure (e.g. agricultural, abattoir and sewage workers) or while participating in outdoor pursuits such as triathlons. Cases are usually sporadic but outbreaks can occur.
- Clinical features include headache, myalgia, conjunctival suffusion and fever. Disease can be subclinical or mild, but in severe cases renal disease, hepatitis, meningitis, vasculitis and myocarditis can

occur. The combination of jaundice and acute renal failure is also known as Weil's disease.

- Diagnosis is clinical supported by serology; confirmation by PCR is available in some settings.
- Treatment is with doxycycline or ceftriaxone, plus supportive care (such as renal dialysis) in severe cases

## BRUCELLOSIS

- Brucellosis is a zoonosis caused by Gram-negative coccobacilli from the genus *Brucella* with three species usually implicated in human disease: *B. melitensis* in goats, *B. abortus* in cattle and *B. suis* in pigs.
- Disease is transmitted to humans from livestock, either directly or via food. It no longer occurs within the UK.
- Clinical features include fever, malaise, night sweats and arthralgia. Complications include endocarditis and bone and joint disease. It is also a cause of PUO.
- Diagnosis is difficult and depends on rising antibody titres, although the bacteria sometimes can be isolated with prolonged culture. Molecular diagnosis is now possible using 16S rRNA gene sequencing on diseased tissue such as heart valves or bone biopsy.
- Treatment consists of a prolonged course of doxycycline combined with another agent such as rifampicin.

## PLAGUE

- Plague is caused by *Yersinia pestis* and is a disease of rodents transmitted to humans by flea bites.
- Human-to-human transmission of pneumonic plague occurs by respiratory transmission.
- Recent DNA testing confirmed *Y. pestis* as the cause of the Black Death in medieval Europe.
- Plague is now limited to a small number of endemic foci where the disease continues in Western USA, South America, Central Africa and the Far East, with a large outbreak in Madagascar in 2017 causing 2348 confirmed or suspected cases.
- Three clinical syndromes are well described: bubonic plague (fever, headache and swollen, painful lymph nodes known as 'buboes'), septicaemic plague (fever, shock and haemorrhage), and pneumonic plague (fever, respiratory failure and shock).
- Diagnosis is by microbiological culture and serology, and a rapid antigen detection test is now available for field use.
- A number of antibiotics are active against *Y. pestis*, including gentamicin, doxycycline, quinolones and trimethoprim-sulfamethoxazole.

## LYME DISEASE

- Lyme disease is caused chiefly by the bacterium *Borrelia burgdorferi*.
- The disease is transmitted to humans by the bite of infected black-legged ticks and is the most common tick-borne infection in the USA (predominantly North-eastern states) and Europe. It has also been reported in Russia, Japan and China.
- Clinical features of acute Lyme disease are fever, headache, fatigue and a typical rash called *erythema migrans*. Complications of untreated infection include neurological disease such as meningitis, peripheral nerve neuropathies and encephalopathy, heart disease such as conduction disorders and cardiomyopathy, ocular disease, arthritis and skin disease.
- Diagnosis may be clinical, based on a history of possible exposure to tick bites and the characteristic rash, confirmed by serology.
- Treatment options include doxycycline, amoxicillin, azithromycin, or ceftriaxone for disseminated disease.

## NEGLECTED TROPICAL DISEASES

- Neglected tropical diseases (NTDs) are a group of communicable diseases that occur in resource-limited countries and are estimated to collectively affect over a billion people.
- Most of the global burden of NTDs is borne by people living in poverty, in conditions of poor sanitation, and in close contact with animals and vectors such as mosquitoes.
- The WHO maintains a list of NTDs (as shown in **Table 3.21**).
- Six of the NTDs on the WHO list can be controlled and/or potentially eliminated by mass drug administration of safe and effective medicines, which can be delivered in combinations to target several diseases at once.
- Improving access to safe drinking water, sanitation and hygiene (WASH) is vital to prevent and treat NTDs.
- Tackling NTDs requires expert knowledge of local epidemiology, and coordination of political, health, logistical and sociological frameworks.
- There are also many 'forgotten diseases' which cause much morbidity and mortality worldwide but have not made it onto the WHO's NTD list for reasons including lack of advocacy and/or absence of effective tools for prevention and control. Examples include leptospirosis, loa loa and melioidosis.

3

**Table 3.21** The WHO neglected tropical diseases list (2017)

| Name | Cause | Transmission |
| --- | --- | --- |
| Buruli ulcer | *Mycobacterium ulcerans* | Chronic bacterial skin infection, route of transmission unknown |
| Chagas disease | *Trypanosoma cruzi* | Protozoan parasite, spread by the triatomine bug ('kissing bug'). |
| Dengue and chikungunya | Viruses in the *Flavivirus* (dengue) and *Alphavirus* genera (chikungunya) | Viral infection spread by mosquitoes (chiefly *Aedes aegypti*) |
| Dracunculiasis (guinea-worm disease) | *Dracunculus medinensis* | Chronic parasitic worm infection of the skin, transmitted by ingestion of larvae-infected water |
| Echinococcosis | *Echinococcus granulosus* and *Echinococcus multilocularis* | Parasitic tapeworms acquired by ingestion of contaminated soil, water or food |
| Food-borne trematodiases | *Clonorchis, Fasciola, Opisthorchis* and *Paragonimus* | Parasitic flatworms known as flukes, transmitted by ingestion of infected fish (*Clonorchis* and *Opisthorchis*), salad (*Fasciola*) or crustaceans (*Paragonimus*) |
| Human African trypanosomiasis (sleeping sickness) | *Trypanosoma brucei gambiense* and *Trypanosoma brucei rhodesiense* | Protozoan parasite transmitted by the tsetse fly |
| Leishmaniasis | *Leishmania* species | Protozoan parasite transmitted by the sandfly |
| Leprosy | *Mycobacterium leprae* | Chronic bacterial infection with presumed person-to-person spread (via skin or respiratory route) |
| Lymphatic filariasis (elephantitis) | *Wuchereria bancrofti, Brugia malayi* and *Brugia timori* | Parasitic worms known as filariae, transmitted by several mosquito species |
| Mycetoma, chromoblastomycosis and other deep mycoses | >20 species of fungi and bacteria including *Nocardia* and *Actinomyces* | Fungal or bacterial infection transmitted from contaminated soil through skin inoculation |
| Onchocerciasis (river blindness) | *Onchocerca volvulus* | Parasitic worms known as filariae, spread by black flies |
| Rabies | Rabies virus | Viral infection transmitted by bite or scratch from infected animal |
| Scabies and other ectoparasites | *Sarcoptes scabiei* var. *hominis* | Parasitic mite infection, spread by direct person-to-person contact |
| Schistosomiasis | *Schistosoma* genus including *S. haematobium* and *S. mansoni* (Figure 3.18) | Parasitic flatworms known as flukes, transmitted by skin penetration after exposure to contaminated freshwater |
| Geohelminths | Several including *Ascaris lumbricoides, Trichuris trichiura, Ancylostoma duodenale, Strongyloides stercoralis* | Parasitic worms transmitted by faeco-oral route or through the skin following contact with soil |
| Snakebite envenoming | Around 250 species of medical importance including black mamba, Indian cobra and Russell's viper | Injection of toxins from bite of venomous snake |
| Taeniasis/Cysticercosis | *Taenia solium* | Ingestion of tapeworm larvae from undercooked pork |
| Trachoma | *Chlamydia trachomatis* | Bacterial infection spread by personal contact or flies |
| Yaws (endemic treponematoses) | *Treponema pallidum* subsp. *pertenue* | Bacterial infection transmitted person-to-person by direct skin contact |

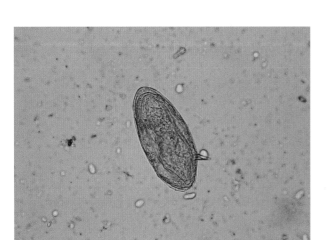

**Figure 3.18** Egg of *Schistosoma mansoni* in the stool. The lateral spine is characteristic of this species. *S. haematobium* has a terminal spine and *S. japonicum* is more rounded with a small spine. Reproduced from Gillespie S, *Medical Microbiology Illustrated*, 1994 (Butterworth–Heinemann, Oxford) with permission of the publisher and author.

## SEXUALLY TRANSMITTED INFECTIONS

### APPROACH TO THE PATIENT

- People commonly present to a genitourinary medicine (GUM) clinic because they have genital symptoms or because they suspect that they may have contracted an infection. As patients are often embarrassed and anxious, it is essential to have a sensitive and non-judgemental approach and also to employ measures to ensure strict confidentiality.
- In addition to routine medical history, all those attending a GUM clinic should be asked the questions relating to sexual history and preferences, recent sexual contacts and time interval since last sexual contact, risk factors for HIV, hepatitis B, hepatitis C and syphilis acquisition, use of contraception, recreational drug use, symptoms relating to the genitourinary system in particular, urethral/vaginal/anal discharge, anogenital ulceration, pain, bleeding and discomfort.
- Examination should be guided by symptoms and include:
  o General: palpation for inguinal lymphadenopathy, visual inspection of external anogenital region for warts, lice, ulceration, rash, local inflammation and discharge
  o Men: testicular examination (for tenderness/lumps), examination for urethral discharge
  o Women: bimanual per vaginal (PV) examination for adnexal/cervical tenderness and masses, vaginal speculum examination for vaginitis, cervicitis and discharge

- Investigations (see specific diseases for details):
  o Men: first-catch urine (FCU), urethral swab for microscopy, Gram stain, culture and NAAT; >4 polymorphonuclear cells (PMN) per high-power field suggests urethritis
  o Women: FCU, high vaginal swab for microscopy, Gram stain, culture, wet mount, pH and potassium hydroxide (KOH) test, endocervical swab for microscopy, Gram stain, culture and NAAT; >30 PMN per high-power field suggests cervicitis
- Once a sexually transmitted infection (STI) has been diagnosed, patients must be advised:
  o That sexual contacts should attend a GUM clinic for investigation
  o To abstain from sexual contact until both they and their partner are cured, either after a course of the treatment completes or in some instances after a test of cure has been performed
  o That serological tests for syphilis and HIV may need to be repeated after a window period to ensure that they are not infected
  o How to avoid contracting infections in the future (e.g. use of condoms, etc.)
- All patients attending a GUM clinic should receive treatment directly from the clinic free of charge to encourage patients with STIs to attend and comply with treatment.

### CHLAMYDIA

Chlamydia is an STI caused by serovars D–K of the intracellular bacteria *Chlamydia trachomatis*. The L1, L2 and L3 serovars of *C. trachomatis* are associated with the presentation of lymphogranuloma venerum (LGV), resulting in more severe inflammatory pathology and lymph node involvement.

#### Epidemiology

- Chlamydia is the most common bacterial STI in the UK and USA.
- Prevalence is highest in the 15–24 years age group.
- Transmission to sexual partners is common, with 75% concordance rate.
- 3–15% of cases have co-infection with *Mycoplasma genitalium*.
- The LGV presentation is more common in tropical regions among heterosexuals, but it occurs in outbreaks in men who have sex with men (MSM) in high-resource settings.

#### Disease mechanisms

Transmission of *C. trachomatis* occurs via direct inoculation of mucosal membranes with infected secretions during sexual activity.

**3**

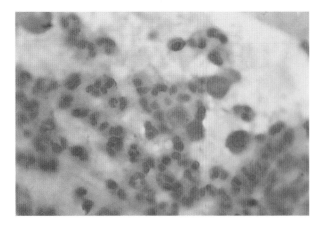

**Figure 3.19** Gram stain appearance of urethral discharge showing polymorphs. NB *Chlamydia* cannot be seen on routine microscopy.

## Clinical features

- The incubation period is 1–3 weeks.
- Genital infection with *C. trachomatis* is asymptomatic in 85% of women and >50% of men, which facilitates transmission.
- When symptomatic, men most commonly experience a mucopurulent urethral discharge and women an endocervical discharge (**Figure 3.19**). Rarely epididymo-orchitis may complicate infection in men and pelvic inflammatory disease (see below) in women.
- Reactive arthritis (Reiter's syndrome) complicates <1% of cases.
- Rectal infection is usually asymptomatic in both sexes but can present with anal discharge. LGV proctitis often presents with bloody anorectal discharge, pain, tenesmus and change in bowel habit.
- Neonatal infection presents with conjunctival discharge and chemosis and swelling of eyelids within 1–3 weeks of birth.

## Investigation

- Chlamydia cannot be routinely cultured or visualized by microscopy.
- NAATs are gold standard.
  - ○ In women: vulvovaginal sampling has higher sensitivity than endocervical sampling and sensitivity of FCU is variable.
  - ○ In men: FCU sample is as sensitive as urethral sampling.
- Rectal swabs have variable sensitivity of anorectal disease.
- Chlamydia DNA may be detectable for 3–5 weeks following successful treatment.

## Management

- Doxycycline 100 mg BD for 7 days is the treatment of choice for all presentations of chlamydia.

- Test of cure is not recommended for uncomplicated chlamydia other than rectal disease.

## Prognosis

- Untreated, 50% would clear the infection within 12 months.
- Treatment failure is more common in rectal disease.

## GONORRHOEA

Gonorrhoea is an STI caused by the Gram-negative diplococcus *Neisseria gonorrhoea*.

### Epidemiology

- Gonorrhoea is the second most common bacterial STI in the UK and USA, with incidence rising.
- AMR is an increasing problem with concern about reduced susceptibility to cephalosporins and azithromycin.

### Disease mechanisms

- Transmission of *N. gonorrhoea* occurs via direct inoculation of mucosal membranes with infected secretions during sexual activity. While the urethra and endocervix are most frequently involved, the rectum and pharynx can also be infected.
- The conjunctiva of neonates can be infected during birth.

### Clinical features

- The incubation period is 2–5 days.
- Genital infection with *N. gonorrhoea* is more frequently asymptomatic in women (50%) than in men (10%). Men most commonly experience a mucopurulent urethral discharge. Symptomatic women usually have endocervical discharge at presentation. Symptomatic rectal infection typically presents with anal discharge or pain. Pharyngeal infection is usually asymptomatic in both sexes though may present with discomfort.
- Rarely, epididymo-orchitis may complicate infection in men and pelvic inflammatory disease (PID) (see below) may complicate infection in women.
- Neonatal infection presents with conjunctival discharge and chemosis and swelling of eyelids within 5 days of birth.

### Investigation

- *Microscopy*: Gram stain of infected secretions allows for rapid visualization. Although sensitivity is high for urethral discharge in symptomatic men (95%), it is generally poor for endocervical secretions in women (<50%) and for pharyngeal infection.
- *NAATs*: these have high sensitivity in urine and urethral samples in men and endocervical and vaginal

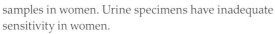

samples in women. Urine specimens have inadequate sensitivity in women.

- *Culture:* this allows confirmatory identification and AST.

## Management

- Treatment is indicated for all those with positive microscopy, NAAT or culture. Epidemiological treatment of sexual partners may be indicated.
- For treatment of cases of uncomplicated anogenital or pharyngeal gonorrhoea and their partners, treatment with a single dose of ceftriaxone 1G IM is recommended.
- Patients should be advised to return for test of cure and abstain from unprotected sex until 7 days after they and their partners complete treatment.

## Prognosis

AMR is making treatment failure and relapse more common.

## ANOGENITAL HERPES

Anogenital herpes is a common STI caused by the viruses herpes simplex virus-1 (HSV-1) and herpes simplex virus-2 (HSV-2), resulting in genital ulceration and pain.

### Epidemiology

- Seroprevalence of HSV-2 in US and UK adults is approximately 23%.
- HSV-1, more typically associated with orolabial herpes, is now the commonest cause of anogenital herpes, particularly in the 15–24 years age group.

### Clinical features

- Symptoms develop in about one-third following primary infection. Painful blistering and ulceration are typical, which may cause dysuria depending on location of lesion. This may also be associated with systemic symptoms of fever and myalgia. Lymphadenitis is common in primary infection.
- Rarely, infection can be complicated by aseptic meningitis, myeloradiculitis and urinary retention.
- Symptoms of recurrent episodes of herpes are generally milder.

### Disease mechanisms

- Virus begins to be shed prior to the appearance of ulcers and is spread by direct contact with lesions or infected secretions.
- Incubation period is typically 2–12 days.
- Following primary infection, the virus remains latent in local sensory ganglia, reactivating periodically, which may or may not be associated with symptoms. Subclinical reactivation and viral shedding are common.
- Barrier contraception use and suppressive antivirals can reduce risk of transmission.

### Investigation

- *NAAT:* direct detection of HSV from lesions using nucleic acid amplification tests is the gold standard investigation. Viral culture is less sensitive and more laborious.
- *Serology:* HSV-1 and HSV-2 antibodies can be detected in serum. HSV-1 antibodies do not distinguish between orolabial and genital herpes, though HSV-2 antibodies are suggestive of genital herpes. Seroconversion on paired samples a few weeks apart supports recent infection.

### Management

- *Supportive therapy:* Pain and discomfort can be reduced by use of simple analgesia, saline bathing and topical lignocaine ointment
- *Primary infection:* 5 days of oral acyclovir 400 mg TDS, valaciclovir 500 mg BD or famciclovir 250 mg TDS commenced within 5 days of lesion appearance can reduce severity and duration of initial episode however will not alter likelihood of recurrence.
- Recurrence can be managed by supportive therapy, episodic oral therapy or continuous suppressive therapy depending on severity and frequency of recurrence.

### Prognosis

Following primary infection, approximately 80% of those with HSV-2 and 50% with HSV-1 will experience at least one recurrence. Recurrence rates are typically higher for HSV-2 (approximately four times a year) than HSV-1 (approximately once a year).

## SYPHILIS

Syphilis is an STI caused by the spirochete (spiral-shaped) bacterium *Treponema pallidum* subspecies *pallidum*.

### Epidemiology

- Syphilis was common in Europe until the development of antibiotics and widespread use of barrier contraception.
- Antenatal seroprevalence is now less than 0.1% in the UK but as high as 6% in some countries in sub-Saharan Africa. In MSM, rates of syphilis have been increasing over the last 15 years, reflecting falling condom use and changes in sexual behaviour in this population.

### Clinical features

- *Primary:* This is marked by the appearance of a painless chancre (ulcer, **Figure 3.20**) at the site of entry around the genitalia/anus after an incubation period of approximately 2–4 weeks. Few other symptoms are present and the chancre will heal after 3–6 weeks with or without treatment.

**3**

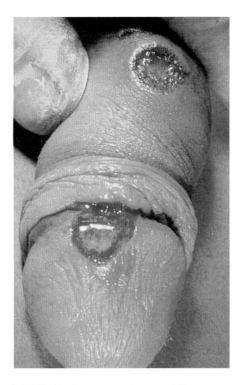

**Figure 3.20** Penile chancres – primary syphilis.

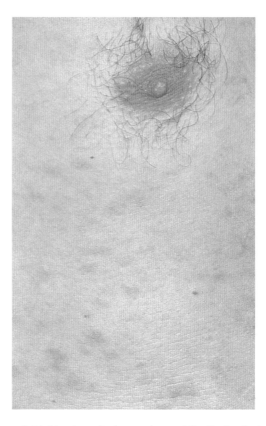

**Figure 3.21** Macular rash of secondary syphilis affecting the trunk.

- *Secondary:* If untreated, the individual may progress to the secondary stage approximately 2–4 months after the initial infection. This is characterized by a non-pruritic maculopapular (**Figure 3.21**) or pustular rash which often involves palms and soles (**Figure 3.22**). Wart-like lesions, known as condyloma latum, may appear around mucous membranes. The rash may be accompanied by fever and lymphadenopathy and other constitutional symptoms. Untreated, these symptoms will resolve but a latent infection will persist.
- *Tertiary:* In a proportion of those who remain untreated, tertiary syphilis can develop 3–30 years after initial infection, affecting multiple organ systems with a wide variety of presentations. Gummatous syphilis (soft tumours of skin and bone), neurosyphilis (meningitis, dementia, peripheral neuropathy), cardiovascular syphilis (aortitis/aneurysm). Untreated, tertiary syphilis can result in death.
- *Congenital syphilis:* This is now a rare condition due to vertical transmission *in utero*. It may result in miscarriage though is frequently asymptomatic. Symptomatic presentation may result in hepatosplenomegaly, dental and skeletal abnormalities.
- *Neurosyphilis:* Syphilis of the CNS can occur at any stage of the disease. Lymphocytic meningitis is the most common presentation in early syphilis, occurring more frequently in those who are HIV co-infected. In tertiary syphilis, meningovascular disease can cause ischaemia or parenchymal disease, resulting in variety

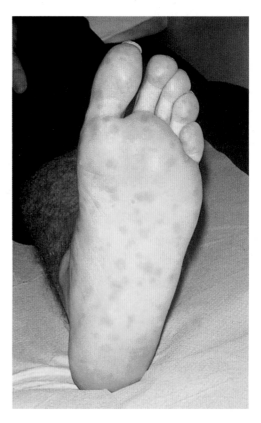

**Figure 3.22** Macular rash of secondary syphilis affecting the soles of the feet.

of abnormalities, degenerative myelopathy (tabes dorsalis), Argyll Roberson pupils (accommodate but do not react to light) and dementia (generalized paresis).

### Disease mechanisms

- Chancres contain numerous organisms that can pass though mucosal membranes or breaks in skin. The bacteria cannot survive outside the human host.
- Transmission occurs sexually through direct contact with the lesion or vertically.

### Investigation

- *Dark field microscopy: Treponema* can be directly visualized.
- *NAAT:* The organism can be detected from biopsy or lesion sampling.
- *Serology:* Typically classified into treponemal antibody (ab) tests and non-treponemal ab tests, diagnosis is made by performing a screening test using one class followed by a confirmatory test with another class.
  - Treponemal ab tests (IgM and IgG) are specific for *Treponema pallidum* but cannot distinguish the different subspecies that cause syphilis from bejel and yaws. They can be used as screening or confirmatory tests but are not used to stage disease or monitor treatment.
  - Non-treponemal ab tests (such as RPR and VDRL) target lipid antigens released from the treponema. They can be used as screening or confirmatory tests, are quantitative and are helpful in staging disease and monitoring treatment response. However, they can be non-specific, cross-reacting with other ab and giving false positives.
- *CSF examination:* Used for investigation of neurosyphilis. Those with symptomatic neurosyphilis will typically have abnormal CSF WCC (>5 cells (lymphocytes)/mm). CSF ab testing can be helpful (if not bloody tap), VDRL being more sensitive than RPR, but false negatives and positives are not uncommon.

### Management

- *Early syphilis (primary, secondary, early latent (<2 years)):* benzathine penicillin G 2.4 MU IM single dose
- *Late syphilis (late latent (> 2years), tertiary (not neurological)):* benzathine penicillin 2.4 MU IM weekly for 3 weeks (three doses)
- *Neurosyphilis:* benzylpenicillin IV for 14 days

### Prognosis

Outcome is very good with treatment of early disease. Left untreated, however, it can be fatal.

## HUMAN PAPILLOMA VIRUS

Human papilloma virus (HPV) is a non-enveloped, double-stranded (ds) DNA virus. There are over 150 HPV types, 40 of which are transmitted sexually, some of which are associated with anogenital warts and cancer of the cervix, throat, anus and external genitalia.

HPV types 16 and 18 are highest risk for cervical cancer (involved in >70%) and HPV-types 6 and 11 are highest risk for anogenital warts (involved in >90%). These four HPV-types are included in recombinant form in the quadrivalent HPV vaccine.

### Epidemiology

- Seroprevalence of HPV rapidly rises in women from age of 14. In the UK, prevalence of HPV infection at cervical smear was 40% in women in their early twenties prior to vaccination.
- Anogenital warts are the most commonly diagnosed viral STI.
- HPV-associated cancers make up over 5% of total cancers worldwide (greater in low- and middle-income countries). Smoking and HIV infection are important cofactors.

### Disease mechanisms

- HPV infects and proliferates within the basal keratinocytes of stratified epithelium, exposed through microabrasions to epithelial surface.
- HPV integrates into the host DNA. Expression of viral oncoproteins E6 and E7 inactivated tumour suppressor protein modifies the cell cycle, promoting viral assembly and increasing the risk of malignant transformation.

### Clinical features

- The incubation period for presentation of warts is 3 weeks to 8 months. For cancer, presentation is usually years after initial infection.
- The majority of infections are asymptomatic and 90% clear HPV within 2 years.
- Warts present as lumps of varying size in the anogenital region. They are usually rough and hard on dry, keratinized skin but soft on moist, non-keratinized skin. Growths can be multiple.
- They can cause irritation and bleeding and distress due to appearance.

### Investigation

- Warts are usually diagnosed clinically on visual inspection. Biopsy is rarely required.

### Management

- Warts will clear spontaneously in one-third but can be treated with topical therapy (e.g. with podophyllotoxin) or physical ablation (e.g. excision, cryotherapy, electrosurgery) if needed, dependent on location and preference.
- Condom use can reduce transmission of HPV.

3

- The quadrivalent vaccine (HPV-6, 11, 16 and 18) is offered to girls and boys aged 12–13 years in UK to prevent acquisition of HPV.
- Most high-income countries have screening programmes for cervical cancer. In the UK, women aged 25–65 years are invited for periodic cervical smear tests, evaluated cytologically for abnormal cells and microbiologically for HPV.

### Prognosis

Relapse of anogenital warts following treatment is common, particularly in immunosuppressed patients.

## PELVIC INFLAMMATORY DISEASE

- PID usually results from ascending infection from the female lower genital tract to the upper genital tract, which can result in endometritis, parametritis, salpingitis, oophoritis or pelvic abscess formation. Rarely, infection spreads beyond the pelvis to organs within the abdomen (e.g. causing a perihepatitis called Fitz-Hugh–Curtis syndrome).
- PID is most commonly a complication of *Chlamydia trachomatis* and *N. gonorrhoeae* infection. *Mycoplasma genitalium* may also be a causative agent. Other possible causes include *Gardnerella vaginalis* and other anaerobic species.
- Intrauterine contraceptive device insertion is a risk factor for PID.
- Symptoms of PID include lower abdominal or pelvic discomfort/pain, abnormal vaginal discharge, intermenstrual or post-coital bleeding and deep dyspareunia. Systemic signs of infection may also be present and occasionally patients may develop sepsis. On vaginal examination, pain on cervical movement (cervical excitation) and adnexal tenderness may be present. However, PID can also be asymptomatic.
- Treatment must include an agent that is active against *C. trachomatis* and *N. gonorrhoeae*. First-line outpatient therapy is ceftriaxone 1G IM + doxycycline 100 mg BD for 14 days + metronidazole 400 mg TDS for 14 days.
- PID carries a risk of significant long-term complications. Even after a single episode, 10–20% of women are infertile as a result of tubal damage, 20% of women experience chronic pelvic pain and the risk of ectopic pregnancy is increased sevenfold.

## OTHER COMMON GU PRESENTATIONS

### *Trichomonas vaginalis*

- *Trichomonas vaginalis* is a flagellated protozoan parasite transmitted sexually, infecting the urethra and or vagina.
- Asymptomatic carriage is common, although common symptoms include vaginal or penile discharge and dysuria.

- Diagnostic investigations: Microscopy of wet preparation of high vaginal or penile swab (sensitivity <50%, higher in women than men), culture or NAAT (gold standard).
- Treatment (including sexual partners) is with nitroimidazoles (either metronidazole or tinidazole 2 g stat or metronidazole 400 mg TDS for 5–7 days).

### Bacterial vaginosis

- Bacterial vaginosis (BV) is the commonest cause of abnormal vaginal discharge.
- It is caused by an imbalance of vaginal microbiome with increases in anaerobe species and reduction in lactobacilli and is associated with a raised vaginal pH >4.5.
- Risk factors include vaginal douching, smoking, antibiotic use, new sexual partner and IUD contraceptives.
- The main symptom is an offensive-smelling, thin vaginal discharge. BV is not usually associated with signs of inflammation.
- Diagnosis can be aided by use of:
  o Amstel criteria: three out of four of the following present:
    – Thin, white/yellow, homogenous discharge
    – Clue cells on microscopy
    – pH of vaginal fluid >4.5
    – Release of fishy odour on adding 10% potassium hydroxide (KOH)
  o Hay/Ison criteria for Gram stain of vaginal fluid:
    – Grade 1 (normal): *Lactobacillus* morphotype predominates
    – Grade 2 (intermediate): mixed flora with some lactobacilli present but *Gardnerella* or *Mobiluncus* morphotypes also present
    – Grade 3 (BV): predominantly *Gardnerella* and/or *Mobiluncus* morphotypes with few or absent lactobacilli
- Management: Patients should be instructed to avoid vaginal douching and may benefit from treatment with nitroimidazoles (either metronidazole or tinidazole 2 g stat or metronidazole 400 mg TDS for 5–7 days).

### Vaginal candidiasis

- Vaginal candidiasis is a common inflammatory vulvitis/vaginitis (**Figure 3.23**) caused by mucosal invasion by commensal *Candida* species (yeast).
- Risk factors include antibiotic use, diabetes, pregnancy, hormonal contraceptive use, steroid use, HIV infection.
- Symptoms are vulval itch/discomfort, vaginal discharge typically curdy and non-offensive, superficial dyspareunia.
- Diagnosis is by microscopy and culture.
- Management:
  o Avoid tight-fitting synthetic clothing and irritants (e.g. perfumed products).

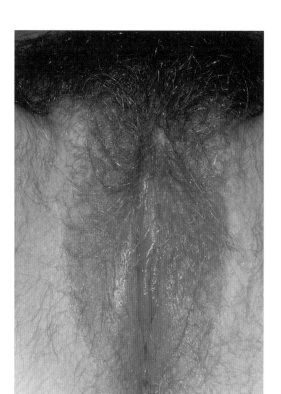

**Figure 3.23** Vulvitis caused by candidiasis.

o Treatment is with topical azoles (e.g. clotrimazole pessary/cream or oral azoles (e.g. fluconazole 150 mg stat).

# HUMAN IMMUNODEFICIENCY VIRUS 1 AND 2

HIV is a viral infection that causes immunocompromise; untreated, it leads to acquired immunodeficiency syndrome (AIDS).

## Epidemiology

- Around 37 million people worldwide live with HIV, and 25% do not know they are infected.
- Two-thirds of people living with HIV are in the WHO Africa region.
- HIV is responsible for 1.2 million deaths per year worldwide.
- In the UK, around 100 000 people live with HIV (1.9/1000 prevalence).
- The risk of HIV infection is highest in key groups worldwide: MSM, sex workers, transgender people, people who inject drugs and prisoners.
- HIV testing is recommended yearly for people in high-risk groups and their partners, and routine testing should be offered for anyone seeking healthcare in a high-incidence area.
- Most HIV in the world is caused by HIV-1, but globally 1–2 million people have HIV-2 infection, predominantly in West Africa. Dual infection with HIV-1 and HIV-2 is possible. HIV-2 is characterized by lower transmissibility, a longer asymptomatic stage and less rapid decline of CD4+ T cells.
- 1 in 4 people with HIV in the world do not know their status.

## Disease mechanisms

- The HIV virion has a viral envelope and a core (capsid). The envelope has the glycoproteins gp120 and gp41, which bind to and enter the host cell. The capsid contains two copies of the (positive sense) ssRNA genome, the enzymes reverse transcriptase, integrase and protease, the major core protein and some minor proteins (**Figure 3.24**).
- HIV attaches to the CCR5 or CXCR4 co-receptor and CD4 receptor on CD4 T lymphocytes using gp120, transcribes the RNA genome to DNA in the cell cytoplasm using error-prone viral reverse transcriptase following fusion and uncoating, and

3

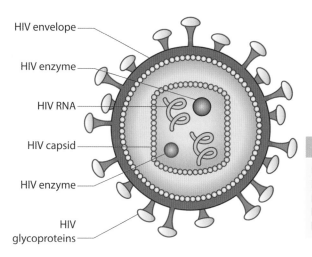

HIV envelope

HIV enzyme

HIV RNA

HIV capsid

HIV enzyme

HIV glycoproteins

**Figure 3.24** Structure of the HIV virion.

**Key to terms**

**HIV capsid:** HIV's core that contains HIV RNA
**HIV envelope:** Outer surface of HIV
**HIV enzymes:** Proteins that carry out steps in the HIV life cycle
**HIV glycoproteins:** Protein 'spikes' embedded in the HIV envelope
**HIV RNA:** HIV's genetic material

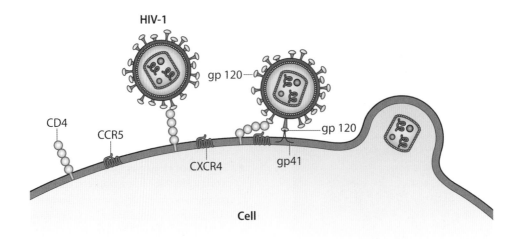

**Figure 3.25** Entry of HIV into the CD4 T cell.

integrates the DNA copy into the cell genome using integrase (**Figure 3.25**).

- Infected CD4 T cells may transcribe integrated viral DNA to RNA, producing billions of virions, or remain quiescent as a reservoir for virus integrated within the cell genome (**Figure 3.26**). Inaccurate viral copying leads to genetic diversity within an infected individual, hindering the immune response.
- Activation and CD8 cytotoxic T-cell attack depletes CD4 T cells over time, resulting in cardiovascular disease from persistent immune activation, immune senescence and susceptibility to opportunistic infection.

### Clinical features

- Primary HIV infection can be asymptomatic or a seroconversion illness of various severity: flu-like illness often with maculopapular rash, lymphadenopathy, aseptic meningitis.
- Persistent generalized lymphadenopathy may follow primary infection.
- There is an asymptomatic latent phase but typically, without treatment, the CD4 count will fall and the RNA viral load will rise over the years (**Figure 3.27**).
- Patients may eventually present with a range of symptoms including weight loss, chronic diarrhoea, skin complaints or dementia.
- AIDS involves complications of immune deficiency (infection or malignancy).

### Differential diagnosis

- Primary infection has similarities with IM (EBV, CMV) and lymphoma.
- HIV should be considered in any patient presenting with AIDS-defining opportunistic infections (**Table 3.22**), HIV-associated malignancies and other indicator conditions (**Table 3.23**).

### Investigation

- HIV serology testing combines enzyme-linked immunosorbent assays for antibodies against HIV-1, HIV-2, and viral p24 antigen. This is highly sensitive and specific, with a false negative 'window period' of around 10 days in primary HIV infection.
- A positive result requires confirmation with a second assay.

**Table 3.22** Opportunistic infections in AIDS

| Class of infection | Infection |
| --- | --- |
| Bacterial | *Mycobacterium tuberculosis* |
| | *M. avium* complex (MAC) |
| | *M. kansasii* |
| | Pneumonia (≥2 episodes in 12 months) |
| | *Salmonella* |
| | Recurrent septicaemia |
| Viral | CMV, retinitis, visceral infection |
| | Herpes simplex chronic ulcers, bronchitis or pneumonitis |
| | Progressive multifocal leukoencephalopathy (PMLE, caused by JC virus) |
| Fungal | PCP caused by *Pneumocystic jiroveci* (**Figure 3.28a**) |
| | Candidiasis, oesophageal or invasive |
| | Cryptococcosis, extrapulmonary (especially meningitis) |
| | Systemic histoplasmosis, coccidioidomycosis and talaromycosis |
| Parasitic | Cerebral toxoplasmosis (**Figure 3.28b**) |
| | *Cryptosporidium* chronic diarrhoea |
| | *Isospora* chronic diarrhoea |
| | Atypical disseminated leishmaniasis |
| | Reactivation of American trypanosomiasis |

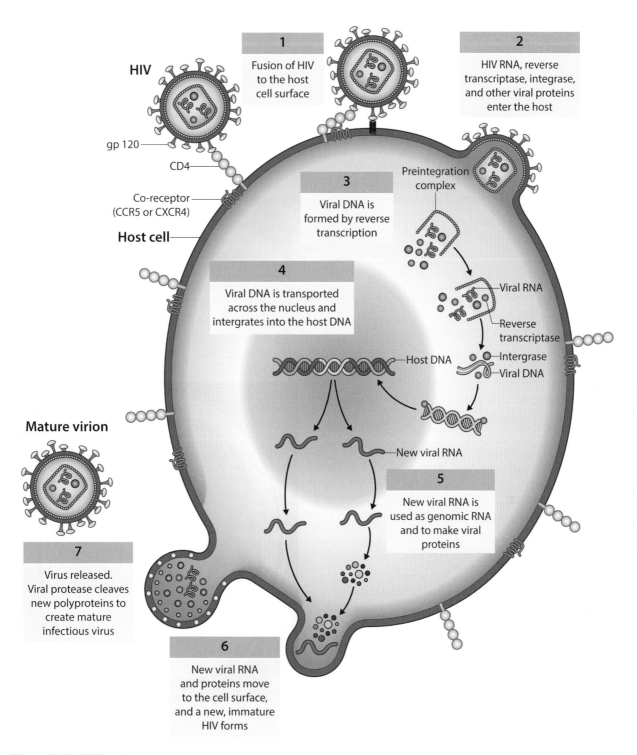

**HIV**

gp 120

CD4

Co-receptor
(CCR5 or CXCR4)

**Host cell**

**Mature virion**

**1** Fusion of HIV to the host cell surface

**2** HIV RNA, reverse transcriptase, integrase, and other viral proteins enter the host

Preintegration complex

**3** Viral DNA is formed by reverse transcription

**4** Viral DNA is transported across the nucleus and intergrates into the host DNA

Viral RNA

Reverse transcriptase

Host DNA

Intergrase

Viral DNA

New viral RNA

**5** New viral RNA is used as genomic RNA and to make viral proteins

**7** Virus released. Viral protease cleaves new polyproteins to create mature infectious virus

**6** New viral RNA and proteins move to the cell surface, and a new, immature HIV forms

**Figure 3.26** HIV life cycle.

- Self-testing using validated immunoassays should be confirmed with serology.
- The threshold for testing for HIV needs to be low as it is much better to diagnose and manage early before life-threatening infections occur. It is important to emphasize to patients when testing for HIV and delivering positive results that HIV is a highly treatable disease with a near-normal life expectancy in high-income settings if compliant with treatment.
- Recommended laboratory investigations following a new diagnosis of HIV, for baseline monitoring and screening, are shown in **Table 3.24**.

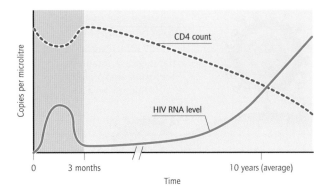

**Figure 3.27** HIV RNA and CD4 counts over time.

## Management

### Prevention

- HIV is an STI, and most transmission occurs through heterosexual intercourse.
- Close social or household contact does not pose a risk.

**Table 3.23** HIV-associated malignancies and indicator conditions for which testing for HIV is indicated

| Category | Conditions |
|---|---|
| HIV-associated malignancies | Cervical cancer |
| | Non-Hodgkin lymphoma |
| | Kaposi's sarcoma (**Figure 3.29**) |
| HIV indicator conditions | TB and other systemic mycobacterial infections |
| | Cerebral space-occupying lesions |
| | Disseminated fungal infections |
| | Severe parasitic infections |
| | Chronic diarrhoea |
| | STIs |
| | Hepatitis B or C |
| | Mononucleosis-like illness (glandular fever) |
| | Community-acquired pneumonia |
| | Invasive pneumococcal disease |
| | Shingles |
| | Invasive *Candida* infection |
| | Ocular, pulmonary or GI CMV disease |
| | Chronic parotitis |
| | Lymphoma |
| | Cervical and anal cancer or dysplasia |
| | Lung cancer |
| | Oral hairy leucoplakia |
| | Persistent lymphadenopathy |
| | Seborrhoeic dermatitis |
| | Subcortical dementia |
| | Persistent leukocytopaenia or thrombocytopaenia |
| | Unexplained chronic diarrhoea, chronic renal impairment, fever or weight loss, or neurological disease |

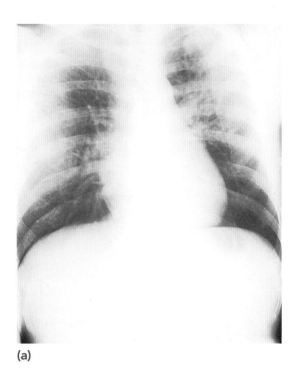

**(a)**

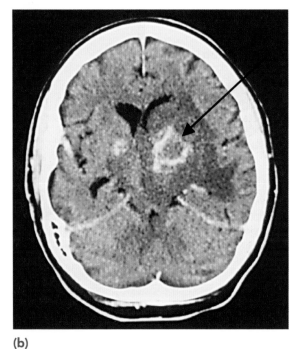

**(b)**

**Figure 3.28 (a)** Chest X-ray showing lung shadowing consistent with *Pneumocystis* pneumonia. **(b)** Ring enhancement in toxoplasmosis. Reproduced from Leach RM, *Critical Care Medicine at a Glance*, 2014 (Wiley-Blackwell, Oxford) with permission.

- Condoms, PrEP with antiretrovirals and PEP are effective at reducing transmission.
- Infectivity is related to viral load, so effective treatment reduces the risk of onward transmission.
- Routine screening in pregnancy, initiation of antiretroviral therapy (ART) before 24 weeks'

**Table 3.24** Investigations following new diagnosis of HIV

| Investigation | Reason |
|---|---|
| HIV plasma viral load | Related to infectivity and treatment monitoring |
| CD4 count and percentage | Prognosis |
| Antiretroviral drug resistance testing | |
| STI screen | |
| Cervical cytology in women | |
| FBC | |
| Urea and electrolytes | HIV-associated nephropathy, tenofovir use |
| Liver function test | Drug monitoring |
| Serology for CMV, VZV, toxoplasma, HBV, HCV and syphilis | |
| Urine dip | Protein in HIV-associated nephropathy |
| QRISK-2 cardiovascular risk assessment including glucose and lipid profile | Complication of HIV, abacavir use |
| HLA-B57*01 | Abacavir use contraindicated if positive |
| TB interferon gamma release assay | |

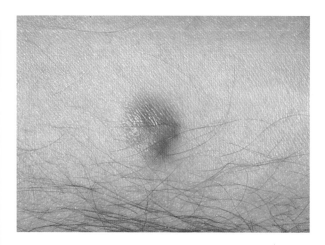

**Figure 3.29** Lesion of Kaposi's sarcoma.

gestation, Caesarean section, avoidance of breastfeeding, and post-partum treatment of the newborn prevent mother-to-child transmission.
- In healthcare settings, universal precautions (gloves for body fluid contact, single use and safe disposal of sharps, screening of blood products) must be used to prevent transmission between patients and to healthcare staff.
- Despite intensive research, an effective vaccine to prevent HIV remains elusive.

*Treatment*

- Combination ART, usually with three drugs, is recommended from the time of diagnosis to render the viral load undetectable (**Table 3.25**), as this hugely reduces opportunistic infection and mortality as well as infectivity – 'undetectable = untransmissible' according to the latest research.
- If the CD4 T-cell counts fall below 200 cells/microlitre, primary preventative treatment with co-trimoxazole to prevent *Pneumocystis jirovecii* pneumonia is recommended.
- If the CD4 count <200 at diagnosis, formal ophthalmology review to exclude CMV retinitis is recommended.
- Aggressive management of cardiovascular risk factors (including stopping smoking and encouraging exercise) is important due to increased IHD in HIV.
- Encourage participation in cancer screening programmes due to increased risk of malignancy.

**3**

**Table 3.25** Antiretroviral drugs

| Class of antiretroviral drug | Examples | Action |
|---|---|---|
| Nucleo(s/t)ide reverse transcriptase | Tenofovir | Two drugs of this class form the backbone of ART for most patients |
| | Abacavir | |
| | Lamivudine | Inhibit initial transcription of viral RNA to DNA |
| | Emtricitabine | |
| Integrase inhibitors | Dolutegravir | Prevent HIV DNA integrating into the CD4 T-cell genome |
| | Raltegravir | |
| Protease inhibitors | Darunavir | Inhibit the maturation of virions |
| | Atazanavir | Ritonavir is a potent enzyme inhibitor and is used to prolong the action of other antiretroviral drugs |
| | Ritonavir | |
| NNRTIs | Efavirenz | Are not effective against HIV-2 |
| | Nevirapine | Viral resistance in HIV-1 is becoming more common |
| CCR5 antagonists | Maraviroc | Inhibit viral entry to the cell |

- If presenting with TB and HIV and a low CD4 count, ART should be delayed to 2–8 weeks after commencing anti-TB therapy, or else administered with prednisolone, to decrease the risk of immune reconstitution inflammatory syndrome (IRIS).
- Counselling and social support may be needed.

## PROGNOSIS

- Early diagnosis and effective treatment to suppress the infection can provide near-normal life expectancy for people living with HIV.

- Diagnosis and treatment when opportunistic infection or malignancy is present (AIDS) leads to reduced life expectancy; untreated, people with AIDS have a median life expectancy of around 3 years.

### MUST-KNOW CHECKLIST

- How to take a history and examine patients with infections
- How presentation of infection can vary in different age groups
- The routes of transmission of infective agents and how to prevent their spread in the hospital and the community
- The main bacterial, viral, fungal and parasitic infections in humans
- The spectrum, mechanisms of action and key resistance mechanisms for the main anti-infective agents
- The importance of antimicrobial stewardship and the challenge of AMR
- The ways in which the laboratory can be used to make a diagnosis of infectious diseases and how laboratory can help understand transmission dynamics (e.g. the role of whole genome sequencing)
- How to recognize and treat sepsis
- How to approach investigation and management of PUO
- Maintain up-to-date knowledge of SARS-CoV-2 and other emerging outbreak pathogens
- Recognize the main causes and management of viral rash illness in children
- Have an informed and up-to-date approach to the management of CFS
- The common presentations, aetiologies, investigation and management of neurological infections including meningitis and intracranial TB
- The key infectious causes of diarrhoea
- Be familiar with major tropical infections including malaria, dengue, Ebola, Zika and leishmaniasis
- Appreciate that sexual history-taking requires an understanding, non-judgemental approach
- The common causes of genital ulceration, genital lumps and pathological vaginal discharge
- The clinical presentation and control of chlamydia and gonorrhoea
- The epidemiology and diagnosis of HIV, alongside knowledge of opportunistic infections and malignancy in HIV
- A firm understanding that HIV is now a very treatable condition

**Questions and answers** to test your understanding of Chapter 3 can be found by clicking 'Support Material' at the following link: https://www.routledge.com/Medicine-for-Finals-and-Beyond/Axford-OCallaghan/p/book/9780367150594

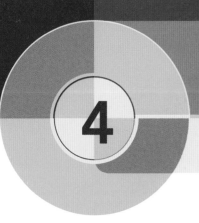

# Rheumatic Disease

## 4

JOHN AXFORD

## INTRODUCTION

Rheumatic diseases are common, and osteoarthritis (OA) is one of the most frequent causes of disease. They form a significant part of a doctor's workload and lead to large annual health bills for doctors, drugs and hospital care. Approximately 15% of patients on an average GP's list have an arthritis-related condition and take up approximately 27% of consulting time. Many working days are lost each year because of arthritis and related conditions.

Rheumatic diseases affect people of all ages and both sexes, but some are more common in certain age groups and races, and in males or females.

Joint pain is a feature of most rheumatic diseases, but these disorders may present in different guises with other symptoms to a variety of specialist clinics ranging from dermatology to genitourinary medicine. The last two decades have seen a revolution with the discovery and application of monoclonal antibodies. All patients with inflammatory arthritis can now expect that treatment will put their disease into remission.

## STRUCTURE AND FUNCTION

Arthritis is the most common factor linking the rheumatic diseases, and a knowledge of joint structure is required to understand the disease processes. Extra-articular manifestations involve skin, lung and kidney, for example, and an understanding of the structure of such organs is also necessary.

### JOINTS

In the context of musculoskeletal disease, joints may be either *fibrocartilaginous* (allowing moderate movement) or *synovial* (allowing considerable mobility).

#### Fibrocartilaginous joints

Fibrocartilaginous joints include the pubic symphysis, the sacroiliac joint and the intervertebral discs.

#### Synovial joints

A typical synovial joint consists of articulating bone surfaces, *articular cartilage, synovium, synovial fluid, capsule and tendons* inserting into the capsule (see below) together with

DOI: 10.1201/9781003193616-4

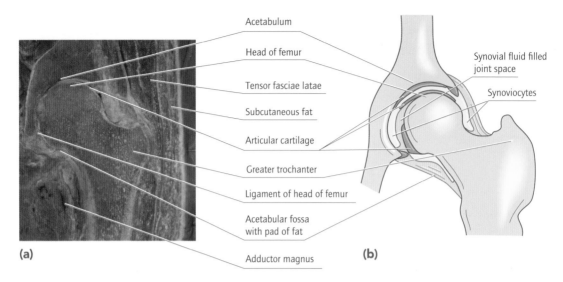

Labels:
Acetabulum
Head of femur
Tensor fasciae latae
Subcutaneous fat
Articular cartilage
Greater trochanter
Ligament of head of femur
Acetabular fossa with pad of fat
Adductor magnus
Synovial fluid filled joint space
Synoviocytes

**(a)**

**(b)**

**Figure 4.1** The hip joint is a synovial joint. **(a)** Cross-section. **(b)** Diagram of a cross-section.

nerve and blood supply. It may contain fibrocartilage (e.g. knee menisci), and be surrounded by tendons, ligaments and bursae (**Figure 4.1**).

Joint stability depends on the shape of the joint, its associated tendons, ligaments and muscles, and the presence of synovial fluid, which seals the joint surfaces together.

## APPROACH TO THE PATIENT

### HISTORY

Most rheumatological diagnoses can be made clinically, although some diseases may resemble each other at first and evolve over time (e.g. autoimmune rheumatic diseases).

It is important to obtain a good history and to examine a patient thoroughly. Your aims should be to define:

- Symptoms and their location and effect
- Differential diagnosis
- Useful investigations
- Appropriate treatment

If the patient is managed over many years, a well-recorded presenting history and examination will prove valuable for charting disease progression.

### ABOUT THE PATIENT

Age, sex, race and occupation are associated with certain rheumatic diseases:

- Sexually acquired reactive arthritis (SARA) and systemic lupus erythematosis (SLE) or lupus are more common in a younger age group (25–35 years) than OA and polymyalgia rheumatica (PMR), which are more common in those over 50 years of age.
- Gout and ankylosing spondylitis (AS) are more common in men, but RA is more common in women.
- White people are more prone to PMR, while Afro-Caribbeans are more susceptible to SLE.

- Musicians, dancers, keyboard operators and labourers may repetitively traumatize certain joints or surrounding structures, and exposure to toxic agents (e.g. polyvinyl chloride) is associated with a scleroderma-like disease.

## RHEUMATIC SYMPTOMS

Some symptoms are common in rheumatic diseases so pain, stiffness and joint swelling should be explored in depth. The important questions to ask a patient are listed in HISTORY & EXAMINATION 4.1.

Joint pain may arise from the joint itself, or from adjacent bone or surrounding soft tissue, or be referred from other systems (e.g. cardiac pain may be referred to the arm). Joint swelling always indicates disease.

### First symptoms

First symptoms may provide clues to the diagnosis:

- Patients with AS often have peripheral arthritis early in the disease.
- Infection and gout are typified by an acute onset.
- OA has chronic characteristics.

### Pattern of joint involvement

- *Monoarthritis* (involvement of one joint) may indicate infection; *oligoarthritis* (two to four joints) occurs in psoriatic arthritis (PsA); and *polyarthritis* (at least five joints) is common in RA.
- Any joint may be involved in any disease but some joints are commonly associated with certain diseases.
- OA involves interphalangeal (IP) hand joints, cervical and lumbar spine, hips and knees.
- RA involves metacarpophalangeal (MCP) joints, wrists, cervical spine, knees, ankles and metatarsophalangeal joints.

## HISTORY & EXAMINATION 4.1

### Important questions to ask a patient with rheumatic disease

#### About the patient

How old are you?

What is your occupation?

#### Joint symptoms

*Stiffness*

How severe is it?

*Joint swelling*

Is it persistent, intermittent or progressive?

#### Pattern of disease

*Onset and progression*

What were your first symptoms?

Over what period of time did they develop?

How many joints were affected (is it a mono-, oligo- or polyarthritis)?

Which joints were affected (symmetrical or asymmetrical)?

How many joints are affected now?

Which joints are affected now?

When are your symptoms most severe?

Does the overall severity of your symptoms change?

How have your symptoms responded to different treatments?

*Associated features*

Have you lost weight?

Do you have a fever?

Have you noticed any changes in your skin (indicating vasculitis, psoriasis or inflammation)?

Have you lost any hair and/or noticed any changes in your nails (suggesting SLE or psoriasis)?

Do you get eye pain and/or irritation (features of keratoconjunctivitis sicca and AS)?

Has your bowel habit changed (suggesting systemic sclerosis [SSc] or inflammatory bowel disease [IBD])?

(Men only) Do you have a urethral discharge (indicating SARA)?

Do you have any unusual sensations or loss of sensation in your arms and/or your legs (a feature of vasculitis and some compression syndromes)?

#### Disease impact

*Work*

Has there been any change in ability to perform certain types of work?

Has early retirement been necessary?

Has hospitalization affected career plans?

*Home*

Can household jobs be carried out?

Is assistance needed for personal care?

Are household aids necessary?

*Social*

Have social and sporting activities changed?

Is transport now necessary?

#### Drug history

What medication are you taking?

For how long has any treatment been prescribed?

Have there been any favourable or adverse reactions?

Have any drugs been discontinued and if so, why?

Do you take your medication as prescribed?

#### Past medical history

Have you ever had a miscarriage?

Have you ever had a peptic ulcer?

#### Family history

Does anyone in your family have:
- A rheumatic condition?
- An autoimmune condition?
- A skin condition?
- IBD?

---

- RA can usually be distinguished from spondyloarthropathies because of its symmetrical joint involvement.
- RA and seronegative spondyloarthritis (SpA) are characterized by exacerbations and remissions.
- Gout is episodic.
- RA is associated with early morning joint stiffness.
- OA is characterized by an increase in symptoms during the day.

### Other symptoms

Do not disregard associated features that do not seem to be relevant. Many rheumatic diseases are accompanied by non-rheumatic manifestations.

## PATTERN OF DISEASE

The pathophysiological processes of some rheumatic diseases give rise to recognizable disease patterns in terms of first symptoms, progression and associated features. Certain events (e.g. trauma, drugs, illness) may trigger the disease.

### Disease progression

The number, location and pattern (symmetrical or asymmetrical) of the joints affected, the severity of the joint symptoms and the presence of associated symptoms may reveal milestones or stages of disease progression.

## DISEASE IMPACT

Chronic rheumatic diseases may not only alter a patient's way of life at home and work and socially but can also test personal relationships and strain financial resources. It is therefore important to find out whether there has been any functional change in the patient in these settings.

Try to understand the patient's views of their disease and expectations of treatment.

## DRUG HISTORY

A detailed summary of past and present medication and physical therapy is essential. Some drugs can trigger rheumatic disease: thiazide diuretics can induce gout; minocycline can cause lupus syndrome; and corticosteroids can cause avascular necrosis of bone.

## PAST MEDICAL HISTORY

Consider whether previous illnesses are:
- Related to the presenting complaint (e.g. spontaneous miscarriage and lupus)
- Affected by the current condition (e.g. subacute bacterial endocarditis and septic arthritis)
- Relevant to drug management (e.g. peptic ulcer and non-steroidal anti-inflammatory drug [NSAID] therapy)

## FAMILY HISTORY

Ask whether there is any family history of rheumatic disease or diseases that may have an arthritic component, such as psoriasis, Crohn's disease or haemochromatosis.

## EXAMINATION

Examination of a rheumatological patient should not differ from that for other patients, except in its increased emphasis on the musculoskeletal system. All other systems should be examined in detail, especially those commonly involved in rheumatic disease, such as the skin, respiratory system and neurological system. In particular, look for the extra-articular manifestations listed in RHEUMATIC DISEASE: CLINICAL FEATURES AT A GLANCE.

To avoid missing the unexpected, a methodical approach to rheumatological examination is advised. Examination is best conducted with the patient standing, then sitting, supine and prone (in that order). First look, then feel and then move the area under examination as appropriate (**Figure 4.2**).

Compare affected joints or muscles with their counterparts. Passive movement is a reliable measure of range of movement. Muscle tenderness may indicate an inflammatory disorder and should be investigated. Tell the patient what is happening, particularly if it may hurt.

Neurological features of rheumatological disease include:
- Spastic paraparesis caused by cervical cord compression resulting from OA or RA involvement of the cervical spine
- Signs of root and nerve entrapment in disease of the lumbosacral spine and carpal tunnel syndrome
- Sensory motor neuropathy in vasculitis

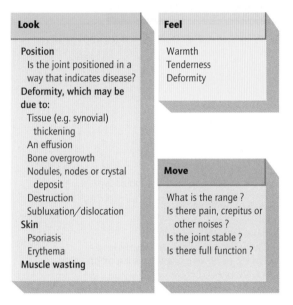

**Figure 4.2** How to examine a joint.

## INVESTIGATION

Investigations should be interpreted in the context of a careful history and physical examination.

## HAEMATOLOGY

### Full blood count

#### Haemoglobin
- *Anaemia:* This is common in rheumatic disease. It may be:
  - *Microcytic* (e.g. blood loss resulting from treatment with analgesics or NSAIDs)
  - *Normocytic* (e.g. a manifestation of chronic disease)
  - *Macrocytic* (e.g. folate deficiency, as may occur in RA)
- *White cell count:* This may be increased or decreased:
  - *Neutrophilia:* may accompany septic arthritis
  - *Eosinophilia:* may occur in polyarteritis nodosa (PAN)
  - *Neutropenia:* a feature of Felty's syndrome and drug sensitivity
  - *Leucopenia:* a manifestation of lupus and treatment with cytotoxic drugs (e.g. azathioprine)
- *Platelets:* These may be increased (e.g. in RA), or reduced, as in lupus and as a side effect of treatment with cytotoxic agents.

### Acute phase proteins and erythrocyte sedimentation rate

Erythrocyte sedimentation rate (ESR) and C-reactive protein (CRP), an acute phase protein, are both non-specific guides to inflammatory activity, as seen for example in RA

## RHEUMATIC DISEASE: CLINICAL FEATURES AT A GLANCE

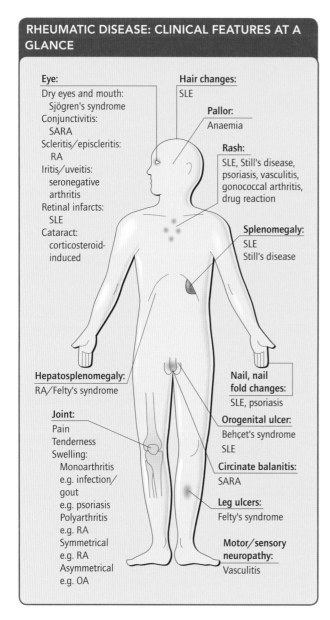

**Eye:**
Dry eyes and mouth:
  Sjögren's syndrome
Conjunctivitis:
  SARA
Scleritis/episcleritis:
  RA
Iritis/uveitis:
  seronegative
  arthritis
Retinal infarcts:
  SLE
Cataract:
  corticosteroid-
  induced

**Hair changes:**
SLE

**Pallor:**
Anaemia

**Rash:**
SLE, Still's disease,
psoriasis, vasculitis,
gonococcal arthritis,
drug reaction

**Splenomegaly:**
SLE
Still's disease

**Hepatosplenomegaly:**
RA/Felty's syndrome

**Joint:**
Pain
Tenderness
Swelling:
  Monoarthritis
  e.g. infection/
  gout
  e.g. psoriasis
Polyarthritis
  e.g. RA
Symmetrical
  e.g. RA
Asymmetrical
  e.g. OA

**Nail, nail fold changes:**
SLE, psoriasis

**Orogenital ulcer:**
Behçet's syndrome
SLE

**Circinate balanitis:**
SARA

**Leg ulcers:**
Felty's syndrome

**Motor/sensory neuropathy:**
Vasculitis

## EXAMINATION 4.2

### Musculoskeletal examination

#### Useful screening questions

*To detect significant musculoskeletal abnormalities*

Do you suffer from any pain or stiffness in your arms or legs, neck or back?

Do you have any difficulty with washing and dressing or with stairs and steps?

#### Useful screening examination

*To detect significant musculoskeletal abnormalities*

Check for joint swelling and deformity, plus pain and difficulty with movements (see **Figure 4.2**).

**Four components of the musculoskeletal system need to be assessed (in any order): gait, arms, legs, spine (GALS)**

*Gait*
Observe the patient walking

*Arms* (sitting)
* Hold out hands
* Turn the hands over
* Make a fist
* Pinch the tip of the index and middle finger to the thumb
* Flex and extend the elbows
* Put hands behind the head

*Legs* (lying)
* Inspect the feet
* Flex each knee
* Internally rotate the hip
* Extend each knee
* Palpate the knee

*Spine (sitting and standing)*
* Bend the neck from side to side
* Inspect the whole spine
* Bend forward and touch the toes
* Palpate lumbar vertebrae

Record the outcome of the examination in the notes (e.g. GALS) as simply as possible.

---

and lupus. Normally, ESR is less than 20 mm/hour and CRP is less than 10 mg/L.

A normal ESR generally excludes active inflammation. A falsely low ESR can occur in sickle cell disease, anisocytosis, spherocytosis, polycythaemia and heart failure. A falsely raised ESR can result from prolonged blood storage or a measurement error. ESR and CRP levels may be inappropriately low in some patients (e.g. seronegative arthritis and LE respectively) and are not infallible markers of inflammation.

## BIOCHEMISTRY

* *Uric acid:* may be raised in gout
* *Urea and creatinine levels:* may increase with renal involvement
* *Alkaline phosphatase and other tests of liver function:* may be altered as a result of drug therapy (e.g. with methotrexate) or with bone disease

## IMMUNOLOGY

A number of markers of immune system function (e.g. antibodies, complement) that may be associated with specific diseases or disease groups can be measured. Autoantibodies and complement tests are discussed here because they are reliable and are commonly carried out.

### Autoantibodies

Autoantibodies bind to a wide spectrum of antigens (**Table 4.1**), but their pathogenic relationship to disease has not been determined in most cases. The presence of autoantibodies may, however, be used clinically to:

* *Confirm a diagnosis:* anti-cyclic citrullinated peptide antibodies (ACPAs) and RA
* *Indicate an exacerbation of disease:* anti-DNA and lupus

**4**

**Table 4.1** Antigen binding and disease associations of commonly measured autoantibodies

| Bound antigen | Disease |
|---|---|
| IgG-Fc (rheumatoid factor) | RA (associated with severity) |
| ACPAs | RA |
| DNA (double-stranded) | Lupus (correlates with disease activity) |
| **Extractable nuclear antigens** | |
| SS-A/Ro | Sjögren's syndrome |
| | Lupus; fetal heart block |
| SS-B/La | Sjögren's syndrome |
| | Lupus |
| SM/RNP | Lupus (highly specific) |
| U1 RNP | Overlap syndromes |
| Jo-1 (t-RNA synthetase) | Myositis |
| SCL70 (topoisomerase) | SSc |
| Centromere | SSc |
| Phospholipids (anticardiolipin, lupus anticoagulant) | Lupus; associated with thrombotic events, thrombocytopenia, fetal loss |
| Neutrophil cytoplasmic | Vasculitis |
| Proteinase III (PR3-ANCA) | Granulomatosis with polyangiitis (GPA) |
| Myeloperoxidase (MPO-ANCA) | Microscopic polyangiitis |
| | PAN |
| | Eosinophilic GPA (EGPA) |

*ANCA, antineutrophil cytoplasmic antibody; c-, cytoplasmic; GN; glomerulonephritis; p-, peripheral; RNA, ribonucleic acid; RNP, ribonuclear protein.*

- *Suggest early treatment:* coexistence of rheumatoid factor (RF) and reduced immunoglobulin G (IgG) galactosylation in RA is associated with severe disease later

### Complement

Total haemolytic complement, C3 and C4, are the factors usually measured to assess complement levels.

The main indication for these measurements is to diagnose lupus where immune complex activation of the classical pathway is thought to cause a reduction in these components. A genetic deficiency of the protein C2 is associated with lupus.

Complement proteins may show a rise in inflammatory rheumatic diseases (e.g. RA).

### HLA typing

*HLA-B27* (class I) may be useful in diagnosing axial spondyloarthritis (axSpA) (see **Table 4.2**).

## SYNOVIAL FLUID

Arthrocentesis or joint aspiration is safe and easy to perform.

**Table 4.2** Differential diagnosis of arthritis

| Type of arthritis | Causes |
|---|---|
| Monoarthritis/ oligoarthritis | OA, infectious arthritis (bacterial, viral, fungal) |
| | Crystal arthritis |
| | Trauma |
| | Haemarthrosis |
| | Juvenile idiopathic arthritis (JIA) (pauciarticular) |
| | Lyme disease |
| | Neuropathic joint (e.g. diabetes mellitus) |
| | Sarcoidosis |
| | Malignancy (osteogenic sarcoma, lymphoma, leukaemia) |
| | AxSpA |
| Polyarthritis | OA |
| | RA |
| | Other autoimmune rheumatic diseases |
| | JIA |
| | Haemochromatosis |

Synovial fluid is commonly examined for:
- *Infection:* Gram stain acid-fast methods and culture for bacteria
- *Crystal identification:* to detect urate (needle-shaped negatively birefringent crystals) and calcium pyrophosphate (rectangular-shaped positively birefringent crystals)

## DIAGNOSTIC IMAGING

Diagnostic imaging is often necessary to allow an accurate diagnosis in rheumatology, and some techniques are more appropriate than others for certain disorders.

### Plain radiography

Radiography (**Figure 4.3a**) can demonstrate changes occurring in all components of the joint, and characteristic changes are seen, for example, in OA, RA and AS. Serial radiography can be useful to document disease progression.

### Ultrasonography

Ultrasound is a useful non-invasive technique that can define changes to normal anatomy and with colour Doppler can determine whether inflammation is present (**Figure 4.3c**).

### Computed tomography

Computed tomography (CT) is an imaging technique that has revolutionized medical imaging. It is widely available, fast, and provides a detailed view of the internal organs and structures (**Figure 4.3b**).

CT is especially useful for:
- Visualizing lungs and coronary arteries
- Assessing for bone fractures
- Evaluating metastatic lesions

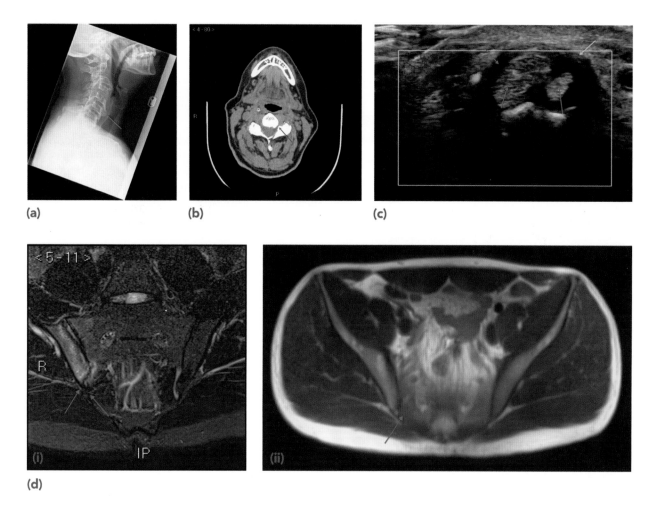

**Figure 4.3** **(a)** Lateral radiograph of a patient with OA of the cervical spine. Note the large osteophytes (red arrow) arising from the C3- C5 vertebral endplates. **(b)** Axial CT image of the cervical spine. The left neural foramen is stenosed (red arrow) due to a prominent complex of osteophyte and disc. This will result in compression of the ipsilateral exiting cervical nerve. **(c)** DQTS ultrasound. These are the two tendons in the first extensor compartment of the wrist otherwise known as the De Quervain's tendons which consist of the abductor pollicis longus (red arrow) and the extensor pollicis brevis (blue arrow). Both tendons appear dark/charcoal in colour indicating tendinosis. Note the thickened tendon sheath (green arrow) and the hyperaemia within the sheath (yellow arrow) indicating that there is tenosynovitis. **(d)(i)** MRI. Coronal oblique STIR image of the sacroiliac joints. The red arrow demonstrates oedema in the right sacroiliac join on both the sacral and iliac side. It also shows erosive changes (blue arrow). **(d)(ii)** Axial image of fused PET-MRI of pelvis. The red arrow demonstrates tracer uptake in the right sacroiliac joint on both the sacral and iliac side indicating inflammation.

4

### Magnetic resonance imaging

Magnetic resonance imaging (MRI) is an imaging technology using non-ionizing radiofrequency radiation inside a strong magnetic field.

MRI is useful in evaluation of non-calcified body tissues including menisci, articular cartilage, cruciate ligaments, tendons and joint fluid (**Figure 4.3d**).

### Nuclear medicine imaging

There are a number of nuclear imaging examinations available including bone scan labelled leucocyte scintigraphy, gallium scan and positron emission tomography. Single proton and positron emission tomography (PET) are more sensitive techniques in defining inflammation, especially when combined with CT.

## ARTHROSCOPY

Arthroscopy is useful both diagnostically and therapeutically. Unlike needle biopsy, it allows a direct view of the joint and synovial fluid, and biopsy samples can be taken from multiple sites within the joint. The joint most commonly examined by arthroscopy is the knee. The technique is often used to investigate trauma (e.g. sport injury).

## HISTOPATHOLOGY

It may sometimes be necessary to take a tissue biopsy to help make a diagnosis:

- *Synovial membrane and bone biopsy*: in suspected infection
- *Kidney biopsy*: in suspected lupus

- *Liver biopsy:* in suspected iatrogenic and autoimmune liver disease
- *Lung biopsy:* in suspected granulomatosis with polyangiitis (GPA)

## DIFFERENTIAL DIAGNOSIS

The differential diagnoses of arthritis are shown in **Table 4.2**.

## GENERAL PRINCIPLES OF MANAGEMENT

The management of rheumatic diseases is summarized in **Table 4.3**.

### SUPPORTIVE TREATMENT

#### The multidisciplinary team

Patients with rheumatic disease may require medical supervision for many years, perhaps a lifetime. This can best be provided by a multidisciplinary team of specialists who educate, treat and support the patient. Such a team will include:

- Doctors
- Specialist nurses
- Physiotherapists
- Podiatrists
- Dietitians
- Occupational therapists
- Physicians + Physician assistants
- Social workers
- Psychiatrists/psychologists
- Orthopaedic surgeons

Rheumatic disorders such as RA can bring social, financial, emotional and physical disadvantage, and as the disease fluctuates so does the patient's ability to cope with it.

Anxiety and depression are common and occur in up to 20% in RA. Psychological support is very important.

#### Patient education

The patient and their family need to understand how the disease will affect them and what the probable outcome will be. They should also understand their role in the treatment programme. Reassure the patient that disease progression can usually be slowed and sometimes halted with few sequelae.

This information can be built up and reinforced over successive visits to the rheumatology team. Free literature describing the disease and its treatment is helpful.

Smoking cessation advice is mandatory. Smoking is associated with increased incidence and severity of arthritis, increased risk of atherosclerosis and coronary heart disease, and it may diminish the efficacy of drugs (e.g. hydroxychloroquine).

### SPECIFIC TREATMENT

#### Drug treatment

This is aimed at:
- *Alleviating pain:* analgesics (**Table 4.4**)
- *Modifying the inflammation once it has been triggered:* NSAIDs
- *Modifying the immunological events leading to inflammation:* drugs that suppress the disease process (**Table 4.5**)

Patients should be provided with written information detailing the drugs they should be taking, especially if they are taking corticosteroids.

#### *Analgesics*

Analgesics commonly used in rheumatic disease are summarized in **Table 4.4**.

#### *Non-steroidal anti-inflammatory drugs*

Analgesic and anti-inflammatory activities to varying degrees as a result of decreasing the synthesis of prostaglandins, prostacyclin and thromboxane by the inhibition of cyclo-oxygenase (COX-1, COX-2). The use of NSAIDs has been limited by their adverse effects (e.g. upper GI toxicity, nephrotoxicity). COX-1 enzymes are expressed constitutively in gastric mucosa, kidneys and other organs and are not thought to be inducible. COX-2 enzymes are not constitutively expressed in tissues but can be induced by certain molecules (e.g. cytokines at sites of inflammation). Selective COX-2 inhibitors have minimal effects on the COX-1 enzyme and have less upper GI toxicity. NSAIDs are indicated for pain associated with inflammation and generally not indicated for pain secondary to joint destruction (e.g. OA), where simple analgesics are more appropriate. It may be necessary to try several before finding one that suits an individual patient.

#### *Corticosteroids*

Corticosteroid has been demonstrated to retard the development of radiological bony erosions. Corticosteroids:
- Inhibit leucocyte chemotaxis
- Prevent circulating polymorphs, monocytes and lymphocytes from reaching sites of inflammation
- Reduce vascular permeability
- Inhibit the production of cytokines and arachadonic acid metabolites such as prostaglandins and leukotrienes

However, corticosteroids may:
- Affect bone metabolism resulting in osteoporosis
- Interfere with glucose metabolism and be diabetogenic
- Cause salt and water retention and precipitate or exacerbate hypertension
- Interfere with ocular lens metabolism resulting in cataract formation
- Be immunosuppressive and increase susceptibility to bacterial and opportunistic infections (e.g. herpes zoster virus and fungal infections)

**Table 4.3** Management of rheumatic diseases

An integrated approach to treatment between hospital and community is essential. Regular patient follow-up is useful to reinforce treatment.

**Support**

*Education*

Patients should be fully aware of the diagnosis and treatment and the part they should play to maximize therapy.

Encourage walking, swimming and jogging if joint inflammation is controlled. Joining support groups can be useful in chronic disease. Advise to dress warmly, stop smoking, and avoid drugs causing vasoconstriction in Raynaud's disease.

Dietary advice is useful in most rheumatic disorders.

*Physiotherapy*

To maintain joint function and increase mobility

*Occupational therapy*

To maintain activities in daily life

Advice on work environment may be useful

*Podiatry*

Improves foot and toe posture and function

Foot care advice may be useful (e.g. to prevent local infection)

**General treatment**

Sunscreens to help prevent lupus skin involvement

Ointments and creams and attention to ulcers for cutaneous manifestations in SSc

Artificial tears, saline nasal sprays and mouthwashes in Sjögren's syndrome

**Drugs**

Analgesics: e.g. paracetamol, codeine phosphate

Tricyclic antidepressants: e.g. amitriptyline, for pain control

NSAIDs: ibuprofen, diclofenac, naproxen, celecoxib, etoricoxib

Corticosteroids: oral and injection; are powerful anti-inflammatory agents

*Immunization*

Immunization should be considered for children and adults.

Immunization status, particularly with regard to chickenpox, should be checked before starting corticosteroids and immunosuppressant drugs.

Immunization with live vaccines is usually contraindicated if immunosuppressant drugs are being taken.

*Chemical disease-modifying drugs*

Methotrexate, sulfasalazine, leflunomide

*Biological disease modifying drugs*

Anticytokine: inhibition of TNF, IL-1, IL-6, IL-17, IL-12/23

Costimulation blockade:

- abatacept: B-cell depletion and inhibition
- rituximab (anti CD20)

Kinase inhibition: tofacitinib

*Immunosuppressive drugs*

Azathioprine, cyclophosphamide

**Complementary therapies**

Complementary therapies are popular. You should be aware of what is available and what your patient may be receiving.

**Surgery**

Joint replacement – hip, knee, elbow, shoulder

Joint removal – metatarsal head

Joint reconstruction – hands

**Ophthalmology**

Eye examination may be necessary as the following can occur:

- Scleritis – RA
- Uveitis – AS, JIA, especially antinuclear antibody-positive pauciarticular disease
- Retinitis – lupus

**4**

**Table 4.4** Analgesics commonly used in rheumatic disease

| | |
|---|---|
| **Aspirin** | Side effects (rare): rash, blood dyscrasias, acute pancreatitis, hepatic and renal damage after overdose |
| Aspirin has both analgesic and anti-inflammatory actions. | Contraindications: hepatic and renal impairment, alcohol dependence |
| Indications: pain relief and as an anti-inflammatory and antipyretic | Aspirin and paracetamol may be usefully combined with certain opiate analgesics (e.g. codeine phosphate and dihydrocodeine) |
| Side effects (mild and infrequent): gastrointestinal (GI) irritation, increased bleeding time, bronchospasm, skin reactions, rash, blood dyscrasis, acute pancreatitis, hepatic and renal damage after overdose | **Opiate analgesics** |
| Contraindications: children under 12 years of age, breastfeeding women, GI ulceration, haemophilia, gout, asthma, hepatic and renal impairment, alcohol dependence | Codeine phosphate<br>• Co-codamol (combination with paracetamol)<br>Tramadol<br>Buprenorphine (patches and oral) |
| **Paracetamol** | |
| Indications: non-narcotic analgesia | |

**Table 4.5** Drugs that suppress the rheumatic disease process. These drugs are usually used in the treatment of autoimmune rheumatic diseases and SpA and are called disease-modifying antirheumatic drugs (DMARDs)

| | |
|---|---|
| **Pharmacological action** | *IL-17 inhibition:* |
| DMARDs are thought to affect the disease process. | • Secukinumab |
| They do not produce an immediate therapeutic effect – it may take up to 4–6 months of treatment to obtain a full response. The treatment should be discontinued at 6 months if no objective benefit has been achieved. | • Ixekizumab<br><br>*IL-12/23 blockade:*<br>• Ustekinumab<br>• Guselkumab |
| **Indications** | *TNF inhibition:* |
| Start early in rheumatic disease before joints start to become destroyed because joint components, principally articular cartilage, have little regenerative potential. | • Soluble receptor antagonists:<br>  ○ Etanercept:<br>    – Fusion proteins comprising the p75 TNF<br>    – Receptor linked to the Fc portion of the human IgG1 |
| Use in children requires early referral to a specialist and expert advice. | • Monoclonal antibodies:<br>  ○ Infliximab<br>  ○ Adalimumab |
| **Chemical DMARDs** | ○ Golimumab (HuIgG1kappamAb) |
| *Methotrexate* | ○ Humanized Fab fragment + polyethylene glycol |
| A folic acid analogue interfering with thymidylate synthesis, which explains its antiproliferative effects | *Co-stimulation blockade:* |
| Inhibits purine nucleotide synthesis and causes errors in DNA transcription | • Abatacept (CTLA-4 – Ig)<br>• Soluble fusion protein comprising CTLA–4 and the Fc portion of IgG inhibitory signal |
| Can be given orally or subcutaneously for better efficacy | *B cell depletion and inhibition:* |
| *Sulfasalazine* | • Rituximab (anti-CD20) |
| An acid azo compound of 5-aminosalicylic acid and sulfapyridine | • Belimumab (anti-B lymphocyte stimulator) |
| *Leflunomide* | *Kinase inhibition:* |
| Similar in efficacy to sulfasalazine and methotrexate, leflunomide is an isoxazole derivative which inhibits pyrimidine synthesis. It is structurally unrelated to other DMARDs and has a distinct mechanism of action | • Tofacitinib<br>• Baricitinib |
| *Hydroxychloroquine* | *Azathioprine* |
| An antimalarial drug | Inhibits purine nucleotide synthesis and causes errors in DNA transcription |
| **Biological DMARDs** | |
| *IL-1 inhibition:* | *Cyclophosphamide* |
| • Anakinra (rhIL-1Ra)<br>• Canakinumab<br>• Rilonacept | Alkylating agents substitute alkyl radicals into other molecules and interfere with their function |
| *IL-6 inhibition:* | |
| • Tocilizumab<br>• Sarilumab | |

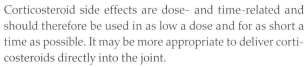

Corticosteroid side effects are dose- and time-related and should therefore be used in as low a dose and for as short a time as possible. It may be more appropriate to deliver corticosteroids directly into the joint.

In patients receiving prolonged periods of treatment, it is important to protect against the development of osteoporosis. Dietary advice should therefore be provided and drugs such as vitamin D and bisphosphonates may be used (see Chapter 5, Metabolic bone disease).

### Biological therapies

As the fundamental mechanisms of the immune response are becoming clearer, novel approaches to therapy are being developed for the treatment of RA and other systemic inflammatory diseases associated with autoimmunity. The major biological therapeutics in clinical use include protein molecules, such as monoclonal antibodies, and small molecule kinase inhibitors. Biological therapeutics have been developed that can:

- Interfere with cytokine function, signal transduction or production
- Inhibit the 'second signal' required for T-cell activation
- Deplete B cells

An overview of biological agents currently used can be found in **Table 4.5**.

## DISEASES AND THEIR MANAGEMENT

### AUTOIMMUNE RHEUMATIC DISEASE

Autoimmune rheumatic diseases include:

- Rheumatoid arthritis
- Sjögren's syndrome
- Systemic lupus erythematosus (lupus)
- Vasculitis syndromes
- Inflammatory myopathies
- SSc

## RHEUMATOID ARTHRITIS

RA is a multisystem disorder in which immunological abnormalities characteristically result in symmetrical joint inflammation, articular erosions and extra-articular complications. It is the most common and disabling autoimmune arthritis, and genetic susceptibility is well defined.

### Epidemiology

- RA affects approximately 1–3% of the UK population. There is increased incidence in certain racial groups (e.g. Pima Indians, Afro-Caribbeans and Asians).
- Prevalence increases with age but peaks between 30 and 55 years.

- Premenopausal women are two to three times more susceptible than men. There is no apparent sex difference in the elderly.
- There are associations with the major histocompatibility complex (MHC) as well as an increased prevalence in first-degree relatives and monozygotic twins. In RA, immunoglobulins have reduced galactose in their sugar component and it is thought that this is also associated with inflammatory mechanisms.

### Clinical features

#### Systemic

Systemic manifestations can arise weeks or months before the arthritis and affect approximately 70% of patients. There may be significant weight loss.

#### Musculoskeletal

Joint involvement in RA is characteristically symmetrical, affecting any synovial joint. Symptoms and signs include:

- *Stiffness:* common and most severe on waking, the joints becoming more mobile as the day progresses
- *Pain*
- *Warmth:* resulting from joint inflammation
- *Joint swelling:* usually results from an effusion or synovial hypertrophy (rings feel tight)
- *Deformity:* may develop insidiously

#### Specific joint and tendon involvement

*Hand and foot changes* In RA, there are characteristic changes in the hands and feet. Distal interphalangeal (DIP) joints are not usually involved, in contrast to their frequent involvement in OA and PsA.

Some RA clinical signs are now fortunately historical with the advent of a better understanding of the disease mechanism and how to intervene, especially with biological therapies.

Some characteristic, but now rare, RA clinical features are:

*Finger deformities*

- Ulnar deviation of the fingers (**Figure 4.4**)
- *Swan-neck deformity* (**Figure 4.5**)
- *Boutonnière deformity:* flexion at the proximal interphalangeal (PIP) joint and hyperextension at the DIP joint
- *Z-shaped deformity:* palmar subluxation of the proximal phalanges and flexion at the MCP joint, making it difficult to pinch the thumb

*Other changes*

- The upper cervical spine is often involved, and subluxation of the vertebrae is a serious but now rare complication. The earliest and most common symptom of cervical subluxation is pain radiating up into the occiput.
- Fixed flexion deformity at the elbow can be an early manifestation.

4

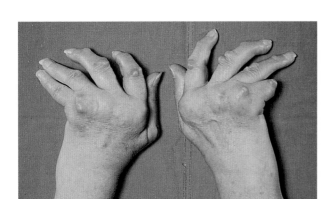

**Figure 4.4** MCP destruction causing ulnar deviation of the digits. There is relative sparing of the DIP and PIP joints and multiple rheumatoid nodules are present.

- Popliteal (Baker's) cysts may accompany knee involvement, and rupture into the popliteal fossa can occur, which may clinically resemble deep-vein thrombosis.
- Tendon sheaths of the fingers and wrists may be involved, especially early in the disease.
- Synovitis at the wrist and of the wrist flexor tendons may result in carpal tunnel syndrome, which is often bilateral and a useful clinical sign.

### Muscle and bone involvement

- Muscle weakness may result from the disease process itself or from disuse muscular atrophy.
- Osteoporosis may be associated with active disease or complicate corticosteroid treatment. It may cause spontaneous fractures.

### Dermatological involvement

- *Rheumatoid nodules:* These are firm, round, non-tender and often multiple cutaneous lesions that are now

uncommon. They are found at pressure points in association with friction, particularly extensor surfaces of forearms.
- *Rheumatoid vasculitis:* Although now uncommon with improved treatment, this may present with palmar erythema, dermal (especially nailfold) infarcts, peripheral sensory neuropathy, and mononeuritis multiplex (may cause foot drop).

### Ocular involvement

Painful eyes are:

- Usually caused by Sjögren's syndrome, which occurs in 15–20% of patients with RA
- Characterized by dryness and grittiness (together with a dry mouth), or episcleritis and scleritis, which cause red inflamed eyes (**Figure 4.6**).

Corticosteroid-induced cataracts may occur.

### Disease pattern in RA

Clinical progression in RA is variable. The onset may be rapid or insidious, and there may be single or multiple but usually symmetrical joint involvement, with exacerbations and remissions. Patients are now presenting earlier and hence the diagnosis may not be confirmed at first presentation.

### Investigation

Investigations are carried out to:

- Support the diagnosis
- Assess disease activity and response to treatment
- Assess internal organ involvement
- Identify drug toxicity

### Haematology

- *Full blood count (FBC):* Anaemia is common in RA, resulting from many factors, and is normally normochromic and normocytic but may be hypochromic and microcytic, reflecting a failure of iron utilization. Thrombocytosis is common in active RA.
- *ESR:* This is often raised in active RA.

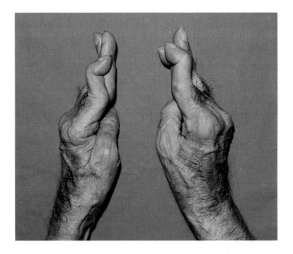

**Figure 4.5** Swan-neck deformity of the forefingers caused by hyperextension at the PIP joint with flexion at the DIP joint.

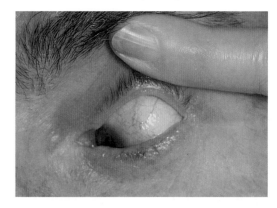

**Figure 4.6** Scleritis is common in RA and causes painful red eyes.

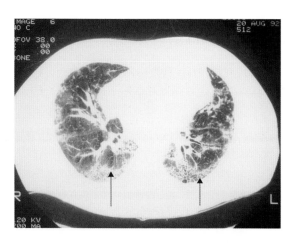

**Figure 4.7** High-resolution CT. Lung fibrosis in RA. Interstitial changes are present predominantly in the periphery (arrows).

### Biochemistry

*Liver function tests (LFTs):* Active disease is associated with a slight increase in alkaline phosphatase and transaminase. CRP (an acute phase reactant) can be used to monitor disease activity.

### Immunology

Rheumatoid factors (RFs) are autoantibodies directed against the Fc portion of immunoglobulin G. High-titre IgM RF is relatively specific for the diagnosis of RA. Anti-citrullinated protein antibodies (ACPA) are also useful in the diagnostic evaluation of patients for RA. Sensitivity varies between 50% and 75% and specificity is usually over 90%. Measurement of ACPA is useful in the differential diagnosis of early polyarthritis.

### Diagnostic imaging

See **Figure 4.7**, and **Figure B** in RHEUMATOID ARTHRITIS AT A GLANCE

- *Ultrasound and MRI:* are useful in demonstrating joint and tendon synovitis and help demonstrate efficacy of treatment
- *Joint radiography:* reveals the extent of joint destruction, which is now uncommon

## Diagnosis

A disease pattern may not be evident in early disease; clinical suspicion may be all there is.

There is no diagnostic test for RA and a diagnosis is based upon symptoms (e.g. significant early morning joint stiffness) and clinical signs (e.g. symmetrical arthritis and rheumatoid nodules), together with investigations, such as the presence of serum RFs and anti-CCP antibodies and characteristic imaging changes.

## Management

Non-drug and preventative treatments are key to successful management (see **Table 4.3**). They include:
- Patient education + counselling

- Physical therapy
- Occupational therapy
- Nutrition + dietary therapy
- Bone protection
- Modifying risk factors for atherosclerosis
- Vaccinations

The multidisciplinary team is central to efficient and effective treatment of the patient with RA.

Drug treatment in RA is outlined in 'Specific treatment' (above). Current management theory is that disabling joint damage begins early in disease. The longer active disease persists, the less response there is to therapy. DMARDs should be commenced within 3 months of onset and tight control of disease activity is important, leading to improved radiographic and functional outcomes. Most patients will require a combination of drug therapies at some stage in the disease process. Immunomodulatory drugs have been shown to be of significant benefit to those patients unresponsive to other drug therapies. Surgery is carried out mainly for pain relief, but large joint replacement (hip, knee or shoulder) can increase functional ability in a selected population.

## Prognosis

The introduction of methotrexate in the 1980s was the turning point to successful management of RA. The development of targeted biological therapy in the 1990s has further improved management such that disease remission should be expected. Poor prognostic factors remain:
- Functional limitation at diagnosis
- Extra-articular disease
- RF-positive or presence of ACPAs
- Bony erosions documented radiographically

## SJÖGREN'S SYNDROME

Sjögren's syndrome is a chronic autoimmune disorder characterized by the progressive destruction of exocrine glands, which leads to mucosal and conjunctival dryness (xerostomia and keratoconjunctivitis sicca respectively) and polyarthritis.

The syndrome may occur in isolation (primary Sjögren's syndrome) or be accompanied by a variety of other autoimmune rheumatic diseases (secondary Sjögren's syndrome). Secondary Sjögren's syndrome is evident in 15–20% of patients with lupus, 10–15% of patients with RA and 1–5% of patients with SSc.

### Epidemiology

- Primary Sjögren's syndrome commonly presents between 30 and 50 years of age.
- 90% of patients are female.
- Primary Sjögren's is associated with *HLA-B8* and *HLA-DR3* in white people.

**4**

# RHEUMATOID ARTHRITIS AT A GLANCE

## Clinical features

*Constitutional*
- Fatigue
- Anorexia
- Weight loss
- Mild pyrexia

*Joints*
- Symmetrical joint involvement causing:
- Pain
- Swelling
- Stiffness
- Deformity
- RA has a predilection for the MCP and PIP joints of the hands, wrists, shoulders, cervical spine, knees and feet, although any synovial joint may be affected.

*Immunological*
- Lymphadenopathy

*Haematological*
- Anaemia

*Skin*
- Rheumatoid nodules
- Vasculitis

*Bones and muscles*
- Muscle weakness
- Osteoporosis

*Eyes*
- Sjögren's syndrome: keratoconjunctivitis
- Scleritis

*Nervous system*
- Carpal tunnel syndrome and cord compression

*Heart*
- Pericarditis and effusion

*Lungs*
- Pleuritis and effusion
- Fibrosing alveolitis

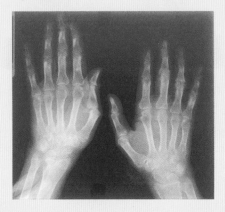

**Figure B** Radiography of the hands of a patient with RA demonstrates erosive changes in the PIP joints of the right hand, the IP joints of the thumbs, the MCP joint of the left thumb, several of the carpal bones and the wrist and distal radio-ulnar joint of the left hand. In addition, there is characteristic juxta-articular osteopaenia.

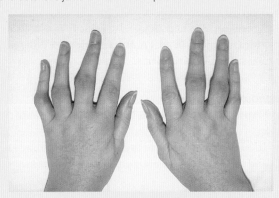

**Figure C** MCP joint and IP joint synovitis and deformity in a patient with 5-year history of RA.

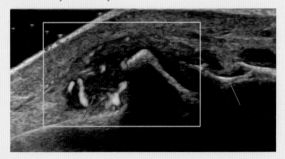

**Figure D** Ultrasound longitudinal image of a PIP joint with Doppler in a patient with RA. Note the severe synovial hypertrophy (red arrow) with the increased vascularity (hyperaemia) on Doppler suggestive of synovitis. Note also the erosion in head of the proximal phalanx (blue arrow).

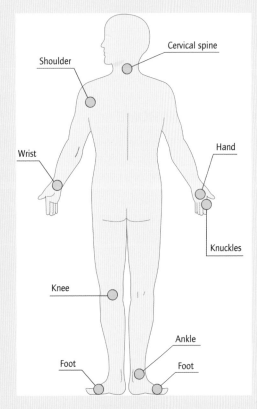

Cervical spine

Shoulder

Wrist

Hand

Knuckles

Knee

Ankle

Foot

Foot

**Figure A** Pattern of joint involvement in RA.

## Disease mechanisms

- Sjögren's syndrome is characterized by salivary gland involvement and autoantibody production, although other organs may also be affected.
- Associated autoantibodies are IgM RF, SSA (anti-**Ro**bair) and SSB (anti-**La**timer), which are present in at least 90%, 70% and 48%, respectively, of patients with primary Sjögren's syndrome (see **Table 4.1**).
- The lymphocyte infiltration may become progressive and is termed pseudolymphoma when gland enlargement occurs; rarely, a malignant B-cell lymphoma may develop.

## Clinical features

The clinical features of primary Sjögren's syndrome result from:

- *Exocrine gland involvement:* affects the eyes, mouth, respiratory system, GI system, kidneys and skin
- *Extraglandular involvement:* affects the musculoskeletal system, thyroid, nervous system and blood vessels

### Salivary glands

Salivary gland involvement results in reduced pooling of saliva in the floor of the mouth. When severe, there may be lip cracking or ulceration, angular stomatitis, oral soreness, fissuring and ulceration of the tongue, atrophy of the oral mucosa, secondary candidiasis and dental caries.

### Eyes

Keratoconjunctivitis sicca causes various ocular symptoms, including the sensation of a foreign body, burning, tiredness, dryness, redness, blurred vision, itchiness, soreness, pain, photosensitivity and excessive secretion.

### Skin

A common symptom is skin dryness (xeroderma) – vaginal dryness causes a burning sensation and dyspareunia.

### Musculoskeletal

Myalgia and arthralgia. Some patients develop a mild relapsing non-erosive polyarthritis that usually affects the large joints.

### Lung

Recurrent bronchitis and pneumonitis are common.

### Gastrointestinal

- Mild dysphagia or chronic gastritis resulting from GI involvement
- Acute or chronic pancreatitis, enlargement of the liver and spleen (Sjögren's syndrome is associated with primary biliary cirrhosis and other autoimmune liver diseases)

### Renal

Renal involvement may cause nephrogenic diabetes insipidus, renal tubular acidosis, interstitial nephritis or glomerulonephritis.

### Neurology

Peripheral sensory, sensorimotor and cranial (especially trigeminal) neuropathy, and other manifestations of CNS involvement (e.g. seizures, movement disorders) may be seen.

### Vessels

Vasculitis of small and medium-sized vessels may lead to skin and neurological features.

### Pregnancy

The presence of anti-Ro/La antibodies is associated with the development of complete heart block and heart failure in neonates.

## Diagnosis

Diagnosis of Sjögren's syndrome can generally be made from the combination of eye and mouth symptoms, and the presence of serum autoantibodies (see below). An opthalmological examination should be carried out to evaluate eye dryness.

## Management

Sjögren's syndrome is initially treated symptomatically. Additional management is similar to that for other rheumatic disorders (see **Table 4.3**). The management of autoimmune liver disease is discussed in Chapter 9, Liver, biliary tract and pancreatic disease.

## Prognosis

- Primary Sjögren's syndrome is rarely life-shortening, but there may be reduced quality of life.
- Severe exocrine gland disease is associated with increased risk of lymphoma.
- The prognosis of secondary Sjögren's syndrome relates to the severity of the underlying disease.

## SYSTEMIC LUPUS ERYTHEMATOSUS

Systemic lupus erythematosus (SLE), or lupus, is a multisystem disease in which autoantibodies and immune complexes may cause cellular and tissue damage. This results in a wide spectrum of clinical manifestations, which have a tendency towards exacerbation and remission. There may be significant overlap with other autoimmune rheumatic disorders such as RA and SSc.

## Epidemiology

- In the USA, there are 20–150 cases per 100 000. In women, the prevalence is 164 (white) to 406 (African-American) per 100 000.

- Presentation is usually at 25–35 years old.
- 90% of patients are women (99% in child-bearing years).
- Afro-Caribbean females are affected more commonly than white females.
- Genetic susceptibility is present (see below).

## Disease mechanisms

The aetiology of lupus is probably multifactorial and, as with other autoimmune rheumatic disease, involves environmental factors and genetic susceptibility.

The monozygotic twin concordances are between 24% and 60% and dizygotic 5%. Complement deficiencies are associated with lupus. Lupus is more common in women.

The basic abnormalities in lupus are thought to be the production of autoantibodies and immune complexes, and the inability of the immune system to suppress them. In lupus, antibodies are directed mainly against the cell nucleus (antinuclear and cytoplasmic proteins). These nuclear and cytoplasmic molecules may have important cellular functions that include storage of genetic materials (e.g. histone) and gene transcription (e.g. smRNA). A detailed list of lupus-associated antibodies is given in **Table 4.1**. For a summary of lupus, see LUPUS AT A GLANCE.

## Clinical features

The multisystem involvement of lupus gives rise to a spectrum of clinical features that vary in severity. Systemic manifestations are common. Fatigue is common and may reflect a flare of the disease. Other causes may be associated with depression and cardiovascular disease.

### Skin

A 'butterfly' rash, acute cutaneous lupus erythema over the cheeks and the bridge of the nose, exacerbated by ultraviolet light, is characteristic of lupus. Livedo reticularis may be present. Raynaud's phenomenon will occur in approximately 50% of patients at presentation. This describes the colour changes of the hands that occur as a result of digital vasospasm, usually associated with cold weather. Typically, the fingers turn white (ischaemia), blue–purple (deoxygenation of the blood) and then red (reperfusion hyperaemia).

Discoid lupus may occur in isolation. Patchy alopecia can be permanent but usually rapid hair loss is associated with active disease and regrowth will occur when the disease remits. Other cutaneous manifestations are oral and vaginal mucosal ulceration, periungual erythema, angio-oedema and cutaneous vasculitis.

### Musculoskeletal

Musculoskeletal involvement is manifest as arthralgia and a symmetrical non-erosive arthritis (Jaccoud's) affecting mainly the PIP and MCP joints, wrists and knees. Deformity is unusual. Myalgia caused by muscle involvement is common, but myositis is uncommon.

### Kidneys

Renal disease (lupus nephritis) develops in 50% of patients with lupus at some time. There is a broad spectrum of severity; it is often asymptomatic but may result in hypertension or renal failure.

### Central nervous system

CNS involvement is an important cause of morbidity (**Figure 4.8**). Neuropsychiatric symptoms may range from cognitive impairment through seizures to strokes. Migraine is more common in patients with lupus than in the general population, particularly those with antiphospholipid antibodies. Neuropsychiatric features may also be a result of drug treatment (e.g. corticosteroids), infection, hypertension, renal failure (e.g. uraemia) or increased coagulation (e.g. antiphospholipid syndrome [APS]). Depression may also be a feature associated with any chronic disorder.

### Blood

Haematological abnormalities include haemolytic anaemia and lymphopenia and occur in 10% of patients.

### Heart and lungs

Heart and lung involvement can result in:

- *Pericarditis:* may be associated with a pericardial effusion
- *Myocarditis:* can cause arrhythmia and cardiac failure
- *Libman–Sacks endocarditis:* rarely, gives rise to emboli and aortic and mitral regurgitation
- *Peripheral vasoconstriction:* causes Raynaud's phenomenon in 50% of patients
- *Pleural effusion*
- *Pneumonitis:* may cause fever, dyspnoea and cough, and, rarely, leads to fibrosis
- *Loss of lung volume:* resulting in elevation of both hemidiaphragms and restricted lung fields (**Figure 4.9**)
- *Adult respiratory distress syndrome and intra-alveolar haemorrhage:* rare
- *Pulmonary embolism:* as a result of increased coagulation in APS

### Eyes

Conjunctivitis, episcleritis and optic neuritis are features of lupus, and retinal vasculitis can cause infarcts (cystoid bodies). Approximately 15–20% of patients have Sjögren's syndrome.

### Osteoporosis

This is a common complication of lupus.

## Investigations

### Haematology

Haematological abnormalities are common and all three blood cell lines can be affected:

- Anaemia of chronic disease
- Leucopenia and mild thrombocytopenia: 50% of patients
- *Coagulation tests:* abnormalities may be detected predisposing to thrombosis (see Chapter 15, Haematological disease)
- *ESR:* may correlate with disease activity

## LUPUS AT A GLANCE

### Clinical features

*Constitutional*

- Malaise
- Fever

*Skin*

- Mucocutaneous
- Alopecia
- Malar 'butterfly' rash
- Discoid lupus
- Mucosal ulcers
- Vasculitic rash
- Raynaud's phenomenon
- Nailfold/pulp infarcts

*Joints*

- Arthralgia
- Symmetrical arthritis (Jaccoud's)

*Muscles*

- Myalgia
- Myositis

*Kidneys*

- Hypertension
- Lupus nephritis

*Neuropsychiatric*

- Psychomotor changes
- Epilepsy
- Stroke

*Blood*

- Anaemia: thrombocytopenia
- Lymphopenia
- Coagulation abnormalities

*Heart and circulation*

- Raynaud's phenomenon
- Accelerated atherosclerosis
- Pericarditis
- Myocarditis (Libman–Sacks)

*Lungs*

- Pleural effusion
- Loss of lung volume
- Pulmonary embolism

*Eyes*

- Sjögren's syndrome: episcleritis
- Retinal infarcts
- Optic neuritis

*Abdomen*

- Hepatosplenomegaly

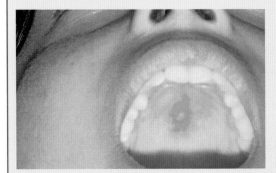

**Figure A** Mucosal ulceration of the roof of the mouth.

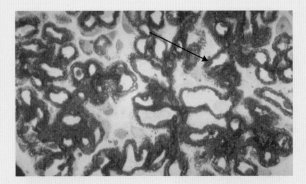

**Figure B** Membranous glomerulonephritis. The peripheral capillary loops of the glomerulus exhibit spikes (arrow), some of which show cross-linking (arrows) (Jones silver stain: high power).

**4**

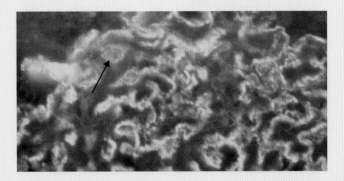

**Figure C** Membranous glomerulonephritis–IgG. The peripheral capillary loops exhibit granular ('lumpy-bumpy') deposition of IgG (arrow).

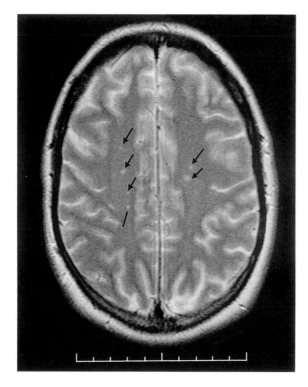

**Figure 4.8** MRI T2-weighted axial image through the brain, demonstrating small foci of high signal intensity within the deep white matter (arrowed). These magnetic resonance appearances are non-specific but, in the correct clinical context, are in keeping with small vessel ischaemia.

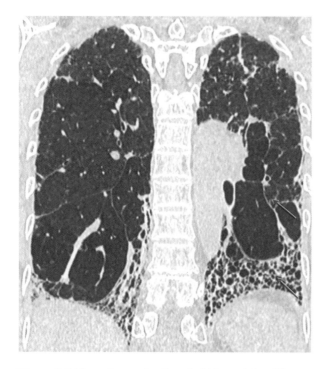

**Figure 4.9** Coronal reconstruction of a high-resolution CT demonstrates exuberant honeycombing with a sharp delineation of the fibrotic lung in the craniocaudal plane (the 'straight-edge' sign), both recognized signs of autoimmune rheumatic disease-associated fibrotic interstitial lung disease. Courtesy of Dr Arjun Nair, Consultant Radiologist, UCL Hospital, London, UK.

### Biochemistry
- *Renal function:* This can be assessed initially by serum creatinine estimation. Urinalysis by dipstick testing and microscopy of the urine will indicate renal abnormality (see Chapter 8, Renal disease).
- *CRP:* This is usually normal and, when increased, may be an indication of infection.

### Immunology
- *Autoantibodies:* Autoantibodies to nuclear and cytoplasmic antigens may be present (see **Table 4.1**). The antinuclear antibody (ANA) test is the best screening test for lupus as it is usually positive. Anti-dsDNA antibodies are specific for lupus and may reflect disease activity, while RF is found in 30–50% of patients. Anti-**Sm**ith RNA antibodies are also virtually confined to individuals with lupus but are present in less than 20% of such patients.
- *Antiphospholipid antibodies:* These may be associated with a thrombotic tendency (see below).
- *Complement:* Low levels of total C3 and total C4 may reflect disease activity.

### Diagnostic imaging
- *MRI and spectroscopy*
- *CT scanning of the brain:* useful in the diagnosis of neuropsychiatric lupus and may reflect electroencephalogram (EEG) abnormalities (see **Figure 4.8**)

### Histopathology
- *Renal biopsy:* may be indicated to diagnose glomerulonephritis
- *Skin biopsy:* may be useful

### Diagnosis

Diagnosis of lupus rests on recognizing a constellation of clinical and laboratory findings. Because it may be drug-induced, a detailed drug history is essential.

Disease activity indices have been developed and are generally used for research purposes. They may have general applicability to clinical practice if simplified. Examples include the SLE Disease Activity Index 2000 (SLEDAI-2K) and British Isles Lupus Assessment Group 2004 (BILAG-2004).

### Management

Patients with lupus need assiduous care so that any increase in disease activity can be treated immediately and appropriately (for a general summary of management, see **Table 4.3**). Systemic corticosteroids and cytotoxic agents are required for severe life-threatening events (e.g. lupus nephritis).

There is no evidence that treatment during remission alters progression of the disease. It is safe and useful to immunize patients with influenza, tetanus and pneumococcal vaccine to prevent infection and the likelihood of a possible disease flare.

## Prognosis

Complete remission is rare but, with optimal diagnostic awareness and management, the overall 10-year survival of lupus is 90% and most patients live a normal lifespan and die from non-lupus causes. Infection is the main cause of death now that renal support and transplantation are so successful. The complications of corticosteroid therapy can cause considerable morbidity.

## ANTIPHOSPHOLIPID SYNDROME

APS can occur as a primary condition or in association with lupus and other autoimmune rheumatic diseases.

### Clinical features

APS is characterized by vascular thrombosis, thrombocytopenia and recurrent spontaneous miscarriage, and there are associated antibodies reactive with phospholipid.

### Investigation

Phospholipid antibodies are specific markers for APS. There are a wide range (e.g. cardiolipin, phosphatidylserine, phosphatidylethanolamine and phosphatidylinositol). Antibodies in APS are directed mainly to phospholipid-binding plasma proteins and in particular $\beta_2$-glycoprotein-1. The functional activity of phospholipid antibodies (lupus anticoagulants) is detected using coagulation assays. Both types of assay should be used in evaluating a patient for APS.

### Lupus and pregnancy

- Pregnancy is not contraindicated in a patient in remission with good renal function.
- Fertility rate is normal, but there is a high spontaneous miscarriage rate (30–50%), especially if antiphospholipid antibodies are present.
- Adverse fetal outcomes include miscarriage, prematurity and stillbirth, and a disease flare may occur, usually in the first trimester or postpartum.
- Treatment with prednisolone is safe during pregnancy. In aPL-positive patients with pre-eclampsia or HELLP syndrome (haemolysis elevated liver enzymes and low platelet count in association with pregnancy), the possibility of the evolving catastrophic APS must be considered.
- Neonatal lupus is rare. Clinically, there may be a transient rash or permanent congenital heart block, which is related to SS-A (Ro), SS-B (La) antibody in maternal serum. The neonate may have a transient positive ANA test and thrombocytopenia resulting from maternal antiplatelet antibodies, haemolytic anaemia and leucopaenia.

**Table 4.6** Drugs in pregnancy and breastfeeding

| Relatively safe |
|---|
| NSAIDs (NB Avoid conception, 1st and 3rd trimester) |
| Glucocorticoids |
| Azathioprine |
| Sulfasalazine |
| Hydroxychloroquine |
| Intravenous immunoglobulin |
| TNF-alpha blockers (NB Infants: avoid live vaccines in first 6/12) |
| **Contraindicated** |
| Methotrexate |
| Mycophenolate mofetil |
| Leflunomide |

## Management

This is aimed at preventing thrombotic complications using aspirin, intravenous immunoglobulin and heparin. Pregnancy outcome in APS-positive mothers with recurrent fetal loss is also improved with regular fetal and maternal monitoring, and anticoagulation in some cases.

Drugs safe and contraindicated for use during pregnancy and when breastfeeding are listed in **Table 4.6**.

## VASCULITIS SYNDROMES

The primary vasculitis syndromes are a heterogeneous group of autoimmune diseases characterized by inflammation and damage to blood vessels. The resulting disease depends on the type, size and location of involved blood vessels (**Table 4.7**). Secondary vasculitis may be associated

**Table 4.7** Common vasculitides

| Vessel | Disease |
|---|---|
| Large-vessel vasculitis | GCA |
| | Takayasu's arteritis |
| Medium-vessel vasculitis | PAN |
| | Kawasaki's disease |
| | EGPA |
| Small-vessel vasculitis | ANCA-associated vasculitis: |
| | • Microscopic polyangiitis |
| | • GPA |
| | • EGPA |
| | Immune complex small-vessel vasculitis: |
| | • Antiglomerular basement membrane disease |
| | • IgA vasculitis (Henoch–Schönlein) |
| Vasculitis associated with systemic disease | Lupus vasculitis |
| | Rheumatoid vasculitis |
| | Sarcoid vasculitis |
| | Behcet's syndrome |

ANCA, anti-neutrophil cytoplasm antibody.

## VASCULITIS AT A GLANCE

A heterogeneous group of autoimmune diseases characterized by inflammation and damage to blood vessels

**Aetiology**

Antigen trigger:

- *Exogenous:* drug, microbe, immunization
- *Endogenous:* immunoglobulin, DNA, tumour antigen

**Clinical features**

Constitutional: fever, weight loss

*Heart and lungs*

- Cough
- Chest pain

*Joints*

- Arthralgia
- Arthritis

*Eyes*

- Conjunctivitis
- Scleritis

*Skin*

- Purpura
- Macules
- Ulcers

*Neurology*

- Cerebral vasculitis
- Sensory motor impairment

*Kidneys*

- Renal failure

*Gastrointestinal*

- Mouth ulcers
- Abdominal pain
- Other diseases associated (e.g. lupus, malignancy)

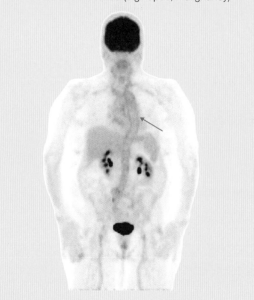

**Figure A** Maximum intensity projection image from PET study. This is showing increased tracer uptake due to vasculitis of the aorta (red arrow) and large vessels. Courtesy of Dr Simon Wan, Institute of Nuclear Medicine, University College Hospital, London, UK.

---

with other autoimmune diseases such as RA and lupus, infection such as hepatitis B and HIV and drugs such as sulphonomides, penicillins and thiazide diuretics (for a summary, see VASCULITIS AT A GLANCE).

Vasculitis may be the main component of a disease or a secondary component, as in RA, and may involve single or multiple organs.

### Common clinical features

See VASCULITIS AT A GLANCE, **Figure 4.10** and **Figure 4.11**.

### Investigation

- Investigations utilize blood and tissues (e.g. skin and kidney) to define inflammation, immunopathology and organ involvement.
- Imaging further aids the diagnosis of specific organ involvement (e.g. vessels, lung, brain and kidney).

### Immunology

Serum antibodies are increased. In Henoch–Schönlein purpura (HSP), IgA is the antibody class commonly involved in the immune complexes. Antibodies to both cytoplasmic (c-) serine proteinase 3 (PR3) and peripheral (p-) myeloperoxidase (MPO) associated neutrophil cytoplasmic antigens (ANCA) may be detected. Disease association with these antibodies may overlap, although 90% of GPA patients are PR-3 ANCA-positive.

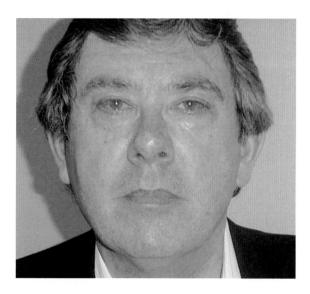

**Figure 4.10** Episcleritis in GPA.

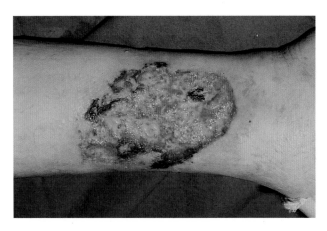

**Figure 4.11** Vasculitis can cause skin infarction and ulcer formation. These ulcers may take many weeks to heal and are a significant cause of morbidity.

### Diagnostic imaging

- *Echocardiography:* to detect heart involvement
- *Arteriography* (MRI can be used): may show characteristic aneurysms in the small and medium-sized renal and visceral arteries (**Figure 4.12**)

### Histopathology (biopsy)

- *Vessel:* Temporal artery biopsy should be carried out if giant cell arteritis (GCA) is suspected and may show a panarteritis. This should be performed before corticosteroids are commenced if possible. The biopsy may be normal if there is segmental involvement.
- *Skin:* This shows vasculitis, IgA deposits in HSP.
- *Nasal:* Biopsy to show granulomas in GPA.
- *Renal:* This provides a histological diagnosis of glomerulonephritis.

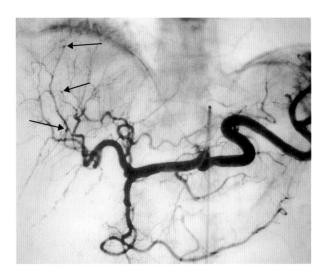

**Figure 4.12** Digital subtraction angiography of the coeliac axis in PAN. Microaneurysm formation can be seen affecting branches of the hepatic artery (arrows).

### Urinalysis

Haematuria and proteinuria may be present.

### Management

Treatment depends on the size of vessel and organ involvement, and small vessel vasculitis such as HSP may require no therapy. However, there is a wide spectrum of treatments available:

- High doses of corticosteroids (e.g. 40–60 mg prednisolone), which may be required in systemic necrotizing vasculitis
- Cytotoxic drugs (cyclophosphamide, azathioprine, methotrexate)
- Plasmapheresis in patients with pulmonary haemorrhage and severe renal disease
- Intravenous immunoglobulin in Kawasaki's disease
- Co-trimoxazole for limited GPA (without renal involvement)

## PRIMARY VASCULITIC DISEASES

## GIANT CELL ARTERITIS AND POLYMYALGIA RHEUMATICA

### Epidemiology

- GCA is relatively common in Europe and the USA with a prevalence of 2 in 1000. Polymyalgia rheumatica (PMR) has a prevalence of approximately 5 in 1000 population.
- Patients are usually over 55 years of age.
- GCA and PMR are more common in women.
- They are rare in Afro-Caribbeans.

### Pathology

- GCA is a systemic disease involving medium- and large-sized arteries.
- GCA is characterized histologically by a panarteritis with inflammatory mononuclear cell infiltrates and giant cell formation. Inflammatory changes may not affect the entire length of the artery and 'skip' lesions are common.
- IL-6 is important in disease pathogenesis.

### Clinical features

#### GCA

- Non-specific systemic symptoms include malaise and weight loss, and 50% of patients will have symptoms of PMR.
- If the temporal artery is involved, it may be nodular and tender to touch (**Figure 4.13**). Pulsation may be absent or reduced.
- There may be associated scalp pain, noticed on hair brushing, and pain on chewing, resulting from jaw claudication.

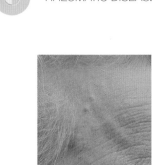
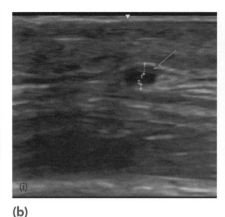
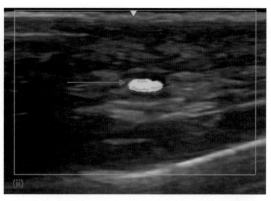

**(a)**     **(b)**

**Figure 4.13 (a)** GCA. The temporal artery may be visible and tender to the touch. **(b)** Ultrasound. Intima media thickening in the mid portion of the right frontal branch of the superficial temporal artery, indicated by blue arrow in **(i)**, with halo sign on colour Doppler, indicated by red arrow in **(ii)**, and persistence of a visible Bessel wall on compression of the lumen with the US probe. A positive 'compression sign' test (blue arrow in **(i)**) indicates intima media oedema/thickening **(b)** Courtesy of Dr. Rizwan Rajak, Croydon University Hospital, Croydon, UK.

- Ischaemic optic neuritis may lead to severe visual impairment (amaurosis fugax) and sudden blindness, and may occur within weeks or months of the systemic symptoms.

### PMR

- Bilateral muscle stiffness and ache, and pain in the neck, shoulders, lower back, hip and thigh are characteristic. These symptoms will be greater in the morning and may cause sleep disturbance due to pain. There may be functional limitations such as dressing and mobility disturbance.
- There may be systemic signs and symptoms such as malaise, fatigue, depression, anorexia and weight loss with low-grade fever.
- There may be peripheral arthritis.
- Approximately 15% of patients will have GCA.

### Diagnosis

- The diagnosis may be difficult and is often delayed. It is based on clinical and laboratory findings, and is aided by temporal artery biopsy and ultrasound.
- ESR is normal in 25% of patients with PMR.

### Management

#### GCA

- High-dose prednisolone (60 mg/day) at first; gradually decrease to maintenance regimen (7.5–10 mg/day). Length of treatment may extend from one to unlimited years.
- Methotrexate and tocilizumab (anti-IL-6) may additionally be required in more severe cases.

#### PMR

- Treat with low-dose corticosteroid (prednisolone starting at 15 mg/day), gradually reducing each month.

- Close follow-up is required to detect symptoms of GCA. The ESR is used to monitor disease activity.

### Prognosis

- GCA and PMR both have a good prognosis if treatment is started promptly because corticosteroids prevent blindness and other vascular complications.
- PMR usually remits after 6 months to 2 years.
- Relapses may occur upon lowering prednisolone.

### Takayasu's arteritis

Takayasu's arteritis (aortic arch syndrome) has a predilection for the aortic arch and its branches. It may result in loss of pulses, claudication – especially affecting the upper limbs – as well as arterial bruits.

### Polyarteritis nodosa

#### Pathology

PAN is caused by necrotizing vasculitis. It characteristically affects bifurcations and branches of the renal and visceral arteries. There is an acute neutrophil infiltration of all layers of the vessel wall and perivascular areas, resulting in intimal proliferation, degeneration, fibrinoid necrosis, immune vessel narrowing, infarction of the tissues supplied by the vessel and, sometimes, haemorrhage.

Aneurysmal dilatation (up to 1 cm) is characteristic along involved arteries. Glomerulonephritis occurs in 30% of patients (see LUPUS AT A GLANCE).

#### Clinical features

- The disease may have an abrupt onset, and 50% of patients experience fever, weight loss and malaise.
- Specific features reflect the location and degree of involvement of affected vessels. For example, a patient with PAN may present with nephritis and hypertension, an acute abdomen, mononeuritis multiplex or polyarthritis.

- Cutaneous lesions are often present and include palpable purpura, digital infarcts, livedo reticularis and mucocutaneous ulceration.
- Approximately 70% of patients have renal involvement, and proteinuria is common.

### Management
Long-term remission can be obtained using corticosteroids and cytotoxic drugs (e.g. cyclophosphamide).

### Prognosis
The 5-year survival rate for untreated PAN is 13%. Death is usually brought about by renal failure and intestinal and cardiovascular complications, which may be compounded by hypertension.

### Kawasaki's disease (mucocutaneous lymph node syndrome)

- This is one of the most common vasculitides of childhood. The majority are children under 5 years of age, with greater prevalence in Japanese children. It is a self-limiting condition with an average duration of 12 days without therapy.
- Rash occurs involving lips, oral cavity, limbs, trunk, palms and soles of feet. There may be skin desquamation. In addition, conjunctivitis and other manifestations of inflammation including fever and lymphadenopathy are common.
- Cardiovascular findings are present in up to 30% of patients at diagnosis (e.g. coronary artery dilatation).
- Treatment with anti-inflammatory and immunomodulation, principally with intravenous immunoglobulin, may be necessary (**Figure 4.14**).

### Granulomatosis with polyangiitis
GPA is a vasculitis affecting the upper (bloody nasal discharge and saddle nose deformity) and lower respiratory tracts (**Figure 4.15**). An association with renal impairment resulting from glomerulonephritis is seen is some patients.

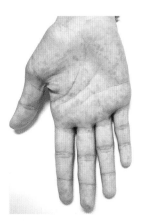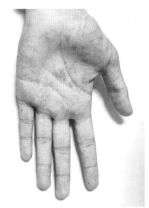

**Figure 4.14** Erythematous macular rash on both palms, as seen in Kawasaki disease. With permission from Charlie Chulapornsiri/Shutterstock.

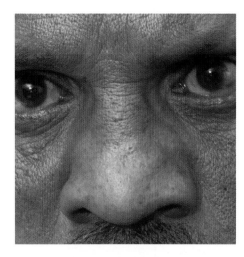

**Figure 4.15** Saddle-nose deformity in GPA.

### Eosinophilic granulomatosis with polyangiitis
Patients with EGPA may specifically present with atopy (late-onset asthma), lung infiltrates, rash and arthritis. This may occur several years before the start of systemic disease. There may be associated cardiac and neurological involvement.

### IgA vasculitis (Henoch–Schönlein purpura)
#### Disease mechanisms
Usually, IgA vasculitis occurs without a known antecedent event, but antigens implicated as triggers include viruses and bacteria (especially *Streptococcus*), drugs, foods, insect bites and immunizations.

#### Clinical features
Clinically, the disorder is characterized by an abrupt onset with malaise. Flu-like symptoms are common. Other features include:
- *Palpable purpura:* usually distributed over the buttocks and lower limbs (**Figure 4.16**)
- *Transient non-migratory polyarthritis:* a common symptom
- *Intestinal symptoms:* including colicky pain, nausea and vomiting, diarrhoea, constipation and the passage of blood and mucus rectally
- *Haematuria, moderate proteinuria and casts:* indicating glomerulonephritis, occurs in 50% of patients

#### Management
- In children, the condition is generally self-limiting and treated symptomatically, although corticosteroids may be required for severe renal disease, but benefit is unproven.
- In adults, IgA can be associated with increased morbidity.

#### Prognosis
The symptoms may recur over weeks or months, and there is a 40% recurrence rate in adults.

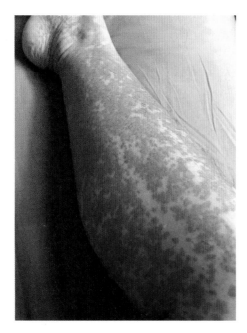

**Figure 4.16** HSP. Palpable purpuric plaques occur on the lower legs. There may also be multifocal areas of haemorrhage or necrosis.

## Immunoglobulin G4-related disease

Immunoglobulin G4-related diseases (IgG4-RD) are immune-mediated fibroinflammatory conditions that share similar pathological serological and clinical features. There are four main clinical phenotypes:

- Pancreatohepatobiliary disease
- Retroperitoneal fibrosis and/or aortitis
- Head and neck limited disease
- Classic Mikulicz syndrome – enlarged lacrimal, parotic and submandibular glands with systemic involvement

The pathogenesis of IgG4-RD is not completely understood. The evidence is that it is a T-cell mediated autoimmune disease in which the IgG4 antibodies are not themselves pathogenic. The diagnosis, if possible, is confirmed with biopsy and, before treatment is initiated, the extent of the disease needs to be evaluated. Treatment is with immunosuppression and relapses are common following discontinuation of therapy. Significant organ dysfunction may arise from uncontrolled and progressive inflammatory and fibrotic changes in affected tissues.

## INFLAMMATORY MYOPATHIES

The inflammatory myopathies are a group of disorders sharing the common feature of immune-mediated muscle injury.

The idiopathic inflammatory myopathies (IIMs) encompass eight categories:

- Dermatomyositis (DM) in adults
- Juvenile dermatomyositis
- Amyopathic DM
- Cancer-associated DM
- Polymyositis (PM)

- Immune-mediated necrotizing myopathy
- Inclusion body myositis
- Overlap myositis

### Polymyositis

The onset of PM is insidious and progressive, usually over weeks or months; it is rarely acute. It may occur at any age and the female to male ratio is 2 : 1.

Symptoms include:

- *Systemic features:* e.g. fever, weight loss, fatigue and malaise
- *Raynaud's phenomenon:* may occur in approximately 20–30% of patients
- *Symmetrical muscle weakness:* of the proximal limb muscles (especially hips and thighs), pharyngeal and upper oesophageal muscle (causing dysphagia) and the diaphragm (causing respiratory impairment)
- *Muscle pain and tenderness:* causing aching in the buttocks, thighs and calves
- *Cardiac abnormalities:* causing ECG changes, arrhythmias, myocarditis and heart failure
- *Lung involvement:* as a result of interstitial lung disease (30–40%), muscle weakness and, in severe disease, as a consequence of aspiration pneumonia

### Dermatomyositis

Skin changes may precede or follow muscle involvement and include:

- Classic lilac-coloured (heliotrope) rash and oedema on the upper eyelids (**Figure 4.17a**)
- Scaly violaceous eruption over the extensor surfaces of joints, commonly the knuckles, elbows and knees (Gottron's papules) (**Figure 4.17b**)
- Subcutaneous calcification and ulceration
- Facial erythema: mimicking acute cutaneous lupus erythema
- Photodistributed poikiloderma (hyper- and hypopigmented skin) classically involving the upper back (shawl sign), and on the lateral aspects of the thighs (holster sign)
- Generalized erythroderma
- Periungual abnormalities: abnormal capillary nail bed loops
- Ragged cuticles
- Psoriasiform changes in the scalp

### Antisynthetase syndrome

- Patients with DM/PM may have a constellation of clinical findings termed the antisynthetase syndrome. These findings include acute disease onset, constitutional symptoms, myositis, Raynaud's phenomenon, mechanic's hands, non-erosive arthritis and interstitial lung disease.
- Affected patients have antibodies to aminoacyl transfer ribonucleic acid (tRNA) synthetase enzymes.

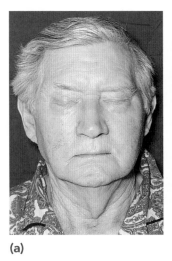
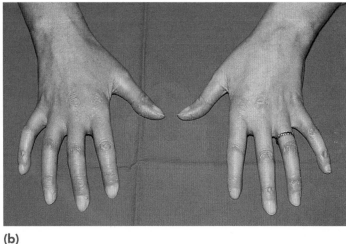

**(a)**            **(b)**

**Figure 4.17** PM. **(a)** Primary DM. This patient has the classic lilac-coloured (heliotrope) rash on the eyelids, together with periorbital oedema. **(b)** Primary DM causes a characteristic rash over the knuckles, sometimes referred to as Gottron's papules or collodian patches.

### Childhood-onset DM

- Childhood-onset DM is not associated with malignancy, and its characteristic manifestations are:
  - Inflammatory myopathy, with atrophy and contractures
  - Subcutaneous calcification
  - Vasculitis affecting the skin, muscle and gut
- Peak incidence is between 5 and 10 yearss.

### Diagnosis

Diagnosis of PM is based on a typical clinical picture accompanied by characteristic electromyograph (EMG) changes, an elevated serum creatinine kinase and a characteristic muscle biopsy. The muscle biopsy may be normal in 10% of patients with myositis because of the patchy nature of the disease.

### Investigation

#### Haematology

ESR is raised in active disease.

#### Biochemistry

- *Muscle enzymes:* Serum skeletal muscle enzymes creatine kinase, aldolase, asparate-amino transferase, lactate dehydrogenase and alanine-amino transferase are elevated.
- *Urine myoglobin:* Myoglobinuria may be detected if there is acute muscle destruction.

#### Immunology

Antinuclear antibodies may be present in up to 80% of patients with DM/PM. Autoantibodies divide into two classifications: myositis-specific antibodies (MSAs), which are almost exclusively present in IIM, and myositis-associated antibodies (MAAs), which are present in other systemic autoimmune disease. MSAs are closely associated with distinct clinical phenotypes and can help predict potential complications. MSAs include aminoacyl transfer (tRNA) synthetase antibodies and MAAs include Ro and La antibodies.

#### Diagnostic imaging

- *Chest radiography:* to look for diaphragmatic involvement and suspected malignancy
- *MRI:* of muscles involved (e.g. thigh) may aid diagnosis and assist biopsy

#### Histopathology

- Muscle biopsy serial sections should be examined. Changes include necrosis, muscle fibre regeneration and lymphocyte infiltration.
- Skin biopsy shows characteristic findings including perivascular lymphocytic infiltration in the dermis.

#### Other investigations

- *EMG abnormalities:* These are present in 90% of patients. Characteristic changes are low-amplitude polyphasic action potentials, pseudomyotonic high-frequency pattern and spontaneous fibrillation with positive sharp waves in resting muscle.
- *ECG abnormalities:* These are present in 5–10% of patients.
- *Respiratory function tests:* These should be carried out if lung involvement is suspected.

### Management

- In the future, MSA testing will play an increasingly important role in the selection of treatment for DM/PM and in the assessment of prognosis.

**4**

- Current treatment is with high-dose corticosteroids for several months, and long-term maintenance therapy may be required.
- Regular muscle strength and serum creatine kinase level tests are necessary to detect any relapse, together with tests of respiratory function, as diaphragmatic involvement is common.
- Immunosuppressive and cytotoxic drugs may be required if the disease is severe, fails to respond to corticosteroids or relapses (see **Table 4.5**).

### Prognosis

- Death is usually brought about by malignancy, infection and pulmonary complications.
- Early treatment improves the prognosis.
- The 5-year survival rate is 68–80%. Within 5 years, 25% make a full recovery and discontinue therapy, 50% have inactive disease but residual weakness and 25% have active disease.

## AUTOINFLAMMATORY DISEASES

This is a family of disorders characterized by aberrant activation of inflammatory pathways in the absence of antigen-directed autoimmunity. Many of these diseases present with recurrent fevers and are termed the periodic fever syndromes (**Table 4.8**).

### Clinical features

- Recurrent episodes of inflammation over months or years, unexplained by another cause
- First disease manifestations in childhood
- Fever, rash, serositis (pleuritic/peritonitis), arthritis, meningitis, uveitis

### Diagnosis

Once a clinical pattern is determined to be consistent with one of the major autoinflammatory disorders, genetic testing is then typically employed to confirm a clinically suspected entity.

### Differential diagnosis

Differential diagnosis includes relapsing fever, malignancy, cyclic neutropenia, systemic JIA, adult-onset Still's disease.

**Table 4.8** Autoinflammatory diseases

| |
|---|
| Familial Mediterranean fever (FMF) |
| Tumour necrosis factor receptor 1-associated periodic fever (TRAPS) |
| Hyperimmunoglobulin D syndrome (HIDS) |
| Cryopyrin-associated periodic fever syndrome (CAPS) |
| Muckle–Wells syndrome (MWS) |
| Neonatal-onset multisystem inflammatory disorder (NOMID) |
| Periodic fever with aphthous stomatitis, pharyngitis and adenitis (PFAPA) |

## CHECKPOINT INHIBITOR IMMUNOTHERAPY

A wide range of rheumatological disorders have been observed with these treatments, including inflammatory arthritis, myositis and salivary gland dysfunction (sicca syndrome).

T-lymphocyte associated antigen 4 (CTLA4) and programmed cell death receptor 1 (PD-1) are targets for immunological checkpoint inhibition. These treatments have a dramatic impact on the care of patients with advanced melanoma and are rapidly being used for other malignancies. Treatment is associated with immune-related adverse events that may involve the skin, bowel, liver and endocrine system.

## FIBROMYALGIA/CHRONIC FATIGUE SYNDROME

This is a condition characterized by muscle pain with tender points, fatigue and sleep disturbance. It occurs most frequently in the 30–60-year age group and women predominate. Synonyms include postviral syndrome and myalgic encephalopathy.

All investigations, including those of inflammation and immunopathology, are normal. If any tests are abnormal, then other causes of fatigue and muscle pain must be sought.

The aetiology of the disorder is multifactorial and poorly understood. In some cases, there is a significant psychological component. Severity may vary and FMS/CFS may coexist with other rheumatological disorders. Treatment is therefore patient-specific and usually responds to a graded exercise programme in association with tricyclic antidepressants. Patients require significant support. It is estimated that 60% of patients still have moderate symptoms 3 years after diagnosis.

## SYSTEMIC SCLEROSIS SYNDROMES

SSc is a multisystem syndrome causing inflammation, fibrosis and vascular damage to the skin and internal organs; the GI tract, lungs, heart and kidneys are predominantly involved. A wide spectrum of disease may result and need not be progressive. Scleroderma is a descriptive word for the skin involvement and means 'hard skin'.

### Epidemiology

- SSc is seen at any age but is most common in 30–50 year-olds.
- Approximately 80% of patients are female.
- There are regional differences in incidence (e.g. higher rates are seen in USA/Australia than in Japan or Europe and in Black people than White).

### Clinical features

SSc may develop rapidly or insidiously (see SYSTEMIC SCLEROSIS SYNDROMES AT A GLANCE).

- *Raynaud's phenomenon:* This characteristically affects the fingers, but may involve the toes, nose and ears (**Figure E** in SYSTEMIC SCLEROSIS SYNDROMES AT A GLANCE)

## SYSTEMIC SCLEROSIS SYNDROMES AT A GLANCE

**Clinical features**

*Skin*

- Raynaud's phenomenon
- Sclerodactyly
- Fixed flexion contractures
- Ulceration
- Increased pigmentation
- Vitiligo
- Telangiectasia
- Disorganization of the nailfold capillary bed
- Subcutaneous and periarticular calcium deposits

*Kidney*

- Hypertension
- Progressive renal failure

*Gastrointestinal*

- Gastro-oesophageal regurgitation
- Malabsorption
- Constipation
- Diarrhoea

*Musculoskeletal*

- Arthralgia
- Asymmetrical polyarthritis (25%)
- Carpal tunnel syndrome
- Acute myositis (15%)

*Central nervous system*

- Headaches
- Seizures
- Strokes
- Radiculopathy and myelopathy

*Lung*

- Pulmonary fibrosis
- Pulmonary hypertension

*Cardiovascular*

- Cardiac failure
- Arrhythmias
- Cardiomyopathy
- Pericarditis
- Venous thromboembolism

*Genitourinary*

- Erectile dysfunction
- Dispareunia

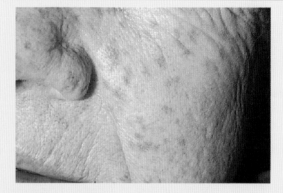

**Figure B** Telangiectasia in a patient with SSc.

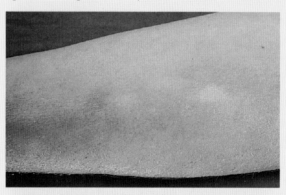

**Figure C** Morphoea. This is a localized patch of skin thickening.

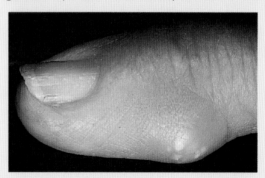

**Figure D** Subcutaneous and periarticular calcium deposits may occur and can be extemely painful.

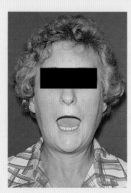

**Figure A** Scleroderma may cause thickening of the skin around the mouth and an inability to open the jaw fully.

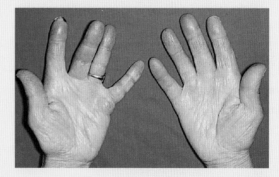

**Figure E** Raynaud's disease. Cyanosis of the fingers occurs because of arterial vasoconstriction, which in this patient has resulted in an area of infarction of the left forefinger.

4

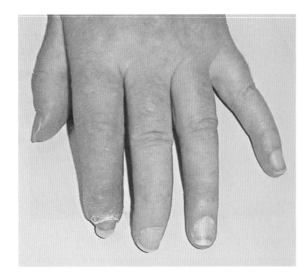

**Figure 4.18** Scleroderma of the fingers and irreversible ischaemia.

and in 90% of patients is the first sign of SSc. It is episodic and there are clearly demarcated colour changes from white (ischaemia) then blue (stasis) then red (reactive hyperaemia). Usually these changes are in response to cold, but they may occur in response to stress.

- *Skin:* Skin is firm, thick (morphea), dry and leathery, tightly bound to subcutaneous tissue with associated hair loss; this is called sclerodactyly when involving fingers (**Figure 4.18**). Ulceration of the skin may occur and the fingertip is the most common site. There may be limited and diffuse cutaneous SSc (dcSSc), and prognosis depends upon extent of skin involvement. If digital ulceration and ischaemia are severe, irreversible tissue damage may occur and may be associated with gangrene. Calcitosis cutis describes calcium hydroxyapatite-containing nodules that appear on the digits, extensor surface of the forearms, elbows and knees. Telangiectasia typically occurs in association with the limited form on the fingers initially.
- *CREST syndrome:* Patients with limited cutaneous systemic sclerosis (LCSSC) may have manifestations of **C**alcinosis cutis, **R**aynaud's phenomenon, **E**sophageal dysmotility, **S**clerodactyly and **T**elangectasia.

### Investigation

#### Immunology
Autoantibodies are present. Those commonly found are:
- *ANA:* 95%
- *Anticentromere antibody:* associated with limited cutaneous scleroedema (5%)
- *Antitopoisomerase-1 (Anti-Scl-70 antibody):* associated with dcSSc and severe interstitial lung disease

- *Anti-RNA polymerase 3 antibody:* associated with dcSSc and rapidly progressive skin involvement

#### Diagnostic imaging
- *Radiography of the hand:* may show resorption of the tuft of the distal phalanx
- *High-resolution CT scanning and chest X-ray:* to check for lung involvement
- *Doppler echocardiography:* initial assessment for pulmonary arterial hypertension
- *Barium meal:* typically shows dilatation, and delayed gastric emptying

#### Histopathology
- *Renal biopsy:* may show changes of arterial intimal proliferation as well as fibrinoid necrosis caused by hypertension
- *Skin biopsy:* is rarely required

#### Other investigations
Pulmonary function tests reveal low diffusion capacity and $P_{O_2}$ on exercise.

### Management
- The principles of management of SSc are organ-based. Specific therapy for SSc pathology may involve DMARDs, corticosteroid, and cytotoxic drugs (e.g. cyclophosphamide).
- In hypertensive renal crisis, renin-angiotensin blocking drugs (e.g. captopril, enalapril) are useful.

### Prognosis
The prognosis of systemic sclerosis depends on the extent of heart, lung and kidney involvement. Pulmonary hypertension is a major cause of morbidity and mortality.

## SPONDYLOARTHRITIS

SpA is characterized by inflammation of the axial skeleton and peripheral joints.
- SpA with axial involvement is designated axial SpA (axSpA). This comprises:
  - AS with radiographic sacroiliitis on plain radiography
  - Non-radiographic axSpA (nr-axSpA) without plain radiographic changes, but MRI changes, of sacroiliitis
- SpA with peripheral involvement is designated (pSpA) which comprises:
  - Peripheral arthritis
  - Peripheral enthesitis
  - Dactylitis

## Epidemiology

- SpA affects 0.1–0.5% of the population.
- Those affected are commonly 20–30 years old.
- AxSpA is more common in men, but this is probably because it is more severe in men than women and more easily diagnosed.
- It is rare in Japanese people and Black Africans.
- It is associated with the *HLA-B27* gene, which is equally distributed between males and females.

## Disease mechanisms

- *HLA-B27* seems to be a major susceptibility gene. Approximately 80% of White people with AS have the *HLA-B27* gene compared to 8% of White people without AS.
- Children of an *HLA-B27* individual have a 50% chance of carrying the gene, and the risk of a child of an *HLA-B27* AS patient developing AS is approximately 17%. Randomly selected *HLA-B27* individuals have a 2–10% risk of developing AS.
- Twin concordance is 75% for monozygotes. Thus, a positive test for *HLA-B27* alone is not diagnostic for axSpA and a negative test for *HLA-B27* does not exclude the diagnosis of axSpA.

## Pathology

- Involvement is common in:
  - *Synovial joints:* apophyseal, costovertebral, sacroiliac, hip, shoulder and peripheral joints
  - *Cartilaginous joints:* intervertebral discs, the manubriosternal joint and symphysis pubis
  - *Entheses:* where ligaments, tendons and the joint capsule attach to bone
- Sites commonly involved are the annulus fibrosus (leading to syndesmophyte formation and the radiographical appearance of bamboo spine), iliac crests, ischial tuberosities, greater trochanters, calcaneae and patellae.

## Clinical features

See ANKYLOSING SPONDYLITIS AT A GLANCE.

### Bones and joints

- *Back pain and stiffness:* These symptoms are most severe in the early morning and after prolonged rest, and may be relieved by activity. Pain in the hips, buttocks and shoulders may be a feature. Advanced disease results in the classic bamboo spine and marked thoracic kyphosis ('question mark' posture). Symptoms may be persistent or intermittent, with deformities evolving over 10 or more years without treatment.
- *Asymmetrical peripheral arthritis:* Approximately 20% of patients have asymmetrical peripheral arthritis at the same time as the back symptoms, although it may precede back symptoms in 10–20% of patients, particularly teenagers. 30% of those under 20 years of age have hip disease.

---

## ANKYLOSING SPONDYLITIS AT A GLANCE

**Clinical features**

*Constitutional*
- Fatigue
- Fever
- Weight loss

*Joints*
- Low back pain and stiffness
- Pain in hips, buttocks and shoulders
- Asymmetrical peripheral arthritis

*Muscles*
- Costosternal and vertebral muscle enthesitis

*Haematological*
- Anaemia

*Eyes*
- Acute anterior uveitis (4–5%)

*Heart*
- Aortic valve incompetence
- Cardiac conduction defects

*Lungs*
- Bilateral upper lobe fibrosis

*Neurological manifestations*
- Spinal cord injury
- Atlantoaxial subluxation
- Corda equina syndrome

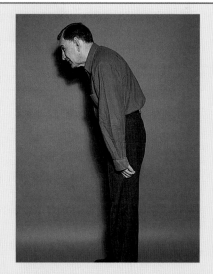

**Figure A** Spine. AS can cause a marked thoracic kyphosis with increased wall–tragus measurement.

4

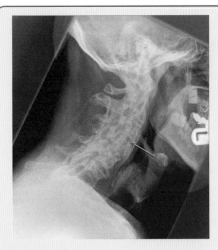

**Figure B** Lateral radiograph of the cervical spine of an adult patient with chronic AS demonstrating 'bamboo spine'. Note the fusion of vertebral bodies due to ossification of the spinal ligaments ('syndesmophytes'; blue arrow).

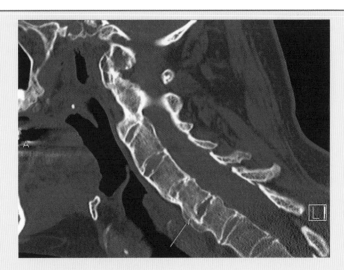

**Figure C** CT sagittal reconstruction image of the cervical spine of an adult patient with chronic AS demonstrating 'bamboo spine'. Note the fusion of vertebral bodies due to ossification of the spinal ligaments ('syndesmophytes'; red arrow).

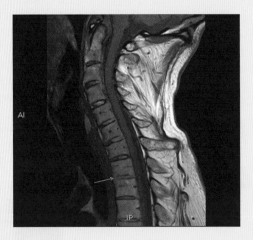

**Figure D** Sagittal T1-weighted MR image of the cervical spine of an adult patient with chronic AS demonstrating 'bamboo spine'. Note the fusion of vertebral bodies due to ossification of the spinal ligaments ('syndesmophytes'; blue arrow).

- *Dactylitis (sausage digits):* There may be diffuse swelling of toes and fingers (6%).
- *Enthesitis:* This is inflammation at a ligamentous bone junction (e.g. Achilles tendon or plantar fascia). Pleuritic chest pain can occur on deep breathing as a result of inflammation at the costosternal and vertebral muscle insertions.

### Diagnosis

Diagnosis is usually delayed and it is not unusual for a decade to pass before definitive treatment is commenced.

### Investigation

#### Haematology

- *FBC:* Chronic anaemia is a feature.
- *ESR:* This may be raised but does not reflect disease activity.

#### Diagnostic imaging

- *Radiography:* There may be no radiographical changes early in the disease, but changes that may be seen as the disease progresses are described in **Table 4.9**. Chest X-ray is necessary if interstitial lung disease is suspected.
- *MR scanning:* MRI can detect areas of active inflammation, as well as enthesitis, before there are radiographical changes.
- *Ultrasound:* This is useful in detecting enthesitis and evidence for peripheral arthritis.

### Management

- The aims of management are to prevent or minimize spinal deformities and to maximize skeletal mobility. (For a general summary of management, see **Table 4.3**.)

**Table 4.9** Radiographical changes in AS

| Location | Radiographical change |
|---|---|
| Vertebral bodies | Early squaring; later bony bridging and fusion of adjacent vertebrae (syndesmophytes) leads to a bamboo spine appearance; erosion and sclerosis at vertebral body margins (Romanus sign) |
| Sacroiliac joint (anteroposterior view) (may involve lower third on one side early in disease) | Blurring of the joint margins, irregular subchondral erosions and patchy sclerosis, at first. Later, sclerosis becomes marked, joint space is lost and osteoporosis becomes evident |
| Ligamentous bony junctions (most commonly the pelvis, greater trochanters, plantar fascia and Achilles tendons) | Inflammation (enthesitis) and secondary ossification lead to proliferative bone margins, spicules and spurs |
| Atlantoaxial joint | Subluxation |

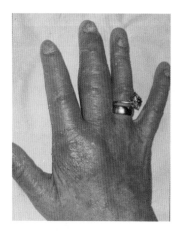

**Figure 4.19** Right hand showing middle finger dactylitis, rash and nail dystrophy.

- Treatment includes non-pharmacological interventions and initial drug therapy with NSAIDs. Biological therapies have significant efficacy in putting the disease into remission.

### Prognosis

Without treatment, approximately 10% of patients with axSpA develop progressive crippling disease. With physiotherapy, anti-inflammatory drugs and biological disease-modifying drugs, however, most patients should lead a normal life and have a normal life expectancy.

## PSORIATIC ARTHRITIS

PsA is an inflammatory arthritis associated with psoriasis. It is distinct from RA.

### Epidemiology

- PsA affects approximately 10% of patients with psoriasis (0.1–0.2% of the population).
- Those affected are usually 30–40 years old.
- Approximately 50% of those with PsA, but not peripheral arthritis, have the *HLA-B27* gene.

### Clinical features

Generally, PsA is mild and intermittent and affects few joints. Spontaneous remission may occur.

For 15% of patients, arthritis precedes the rash (**Figure 4.19**), but these manifestations often begin together. A search for psoriasis should include the scalp,

natal, cleft and feet, and lesions may also affect the genitalia and tongue. There is no correlation between the extent of skin involvement or nail onychodystrophy and severity of the arthritis (**Figure 4.20**). Peripheral joints may be warm, swollen and tender, and flexion contractures and ankylosis may occur. The characteristic patterns of joint involvement are detailed in **Table 4.10**. Ocular disease (conjunctivitis, iridocyclitis, episcleritis) is rare. Some patients may present with more than one pattern and many change the pattern of their arthritis during follow up. PsA usually presents in association with peripheral joint involvement.

### Investigation

As for axSpA, diagnostic imaging can reveal joint destruction (**Figure 4.21**).

### Management

See **Table 4.3**.

The risk of cardiovascular disease is increased in patients with PsA.

### Prognosis

Approximately 5% of patients develop a severe disabling and deforming arthritis.

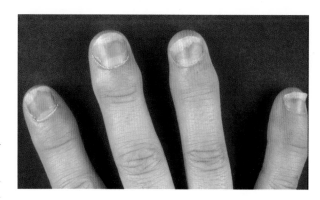

**Figure 4.20** Nail dystrophy with adjacent DIP joint arthritis.

**Table 4.10** Characteristic patterns of joint involvement in PsA

| Pattern | Percentage of patients (%) | Features |
|---|---|---|
| Asymmetrical oligoarthritis | 70 | Commonly involves proximal joints of hands and feet. Finger dactylitis, similar to those in SARA (**Figure 4.19**) |
| AxSpA | 25 | May occur alone or with the other forms of arthritis |
| Symmetrical polyarthritis | 10 | Similar to RA with systemic symptoms |
| DIP joint involvement | 10 | Nail changes are usual, and associated with dactylitis (**Figure 4.19**) |
| Arthritis mutilans | 5 | Destructive and deforming polyarthritis, ankylosis, dissolution of bone and telescoping of fingers, and spinal ankylosis may occur (**Figure 4.21, Figure 4.22**) |

DIP, distal interphalangea.

# SEXUALLY ACQUIRED REACTIVE ARTHRITIS

SARA is characterized by the reactive arthritis triad of sero-negative oligoarticular asymmetrical arthritis, urethritis and/or cervicitis and conjunctivitis.

## Epidemiology

- SARA is uncommon. Approximately 1% of people with urethritis develop SARA.
- Those affected are usually 16–35 years of age.
- Approximately 95% of patients are male.
- The *HLA-B27* gene is present in 60–90% of patients.

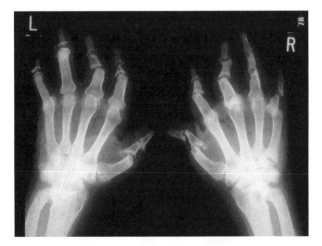

**Figure 4.21** Radiograph of hands showing joint destruction resulting from arthritis mutilans.

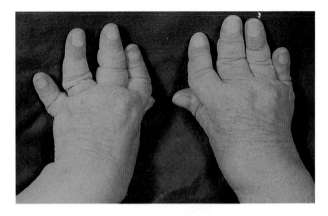

**Figure 4.22** Arthritis mutilans. Joint destruction has caused dissolution of bone and telescoping of fingers. Remarkably, some function may be preserved.

## Disease mechanisms

- SARA is probably triggered by an infectious agent in the urogenital system interacting with a predisposing genetic background. The organisms thought to be responsible are *Chlamydia trachomatis* and *Ureaplasma urealyticum*.
- The arthritis is 'reactive' because it is not caused by a direct infection of the joint.
- Disseminated gonococcal infection (*Neisseria gonorrhoeae*) can cause tenosynovitis dermatitis and polyarthralgia.

## Clinical features

There may be mild systemic symptoms, malaise and fever at first in both sexes and an associated intermittent muco-purulent penile discharge in men. It may be difficult to diagnose in women at this stage, but urethral ulcers may be present.

### Musculoskeletal involvement

- Rheumatic features arise later and include arthritis, Achilles tenosynovitis, enthesitis and plantar fasciitis and axSpA (**Figure 4.23**).
- The characteristic sausage-shaped digits (dactylitis) are caused by enthesitis and arthritis.
- The arthritis is usually acute, asymmetrical and oligoarticular, and it affects mainly the knees, ankles, metatarsophalangeal joints and IP joints of the feet.

### Skin involvement

- Keratoderma blenorrhagica is common and indistinguishable from pustular psoriasis; the papules are commonly on the palms, soles and glans penis.
- Painless mucocutaneous lesions in the mouth and on the glans penis (circinate balanitis) are also common.

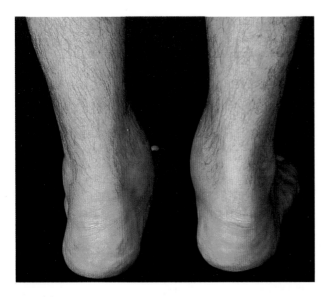

**Figure 4.23** Sexually acquired reactive arthritis (SARA). Achilles tendinitis (on the left side in this patient) is sometimes a feature of SARA.

- Subungual cornification can accumulate and lift the nail plate, but there is no pitting.

### Eye involvement

Conjunctivitis, uveitis, keratitis and optic neuritis are rare.

### Differential diagnosis

- The main differential diagnosis is gonococcal arthritis, for which there is a greater female incidence, no family history and usually a response to penicillin.
- There is no association with *HLA-B27*.
- The arthritis is usually acute and non-recurrent.

### Investigation

The investigations and their results are the same as those for axSpA.

### Management

Ensure that the predisposing infection has been adequately treated in the patient and their partner. (For a general summary of management, see **Table 4.3**).

### Prognosis

Most patients recover from the initial symptoms within several months, but 33% have recurrent or sustained disease and 15–25% of these develop permanent disability.

## ARTHRITIS ASSOCIATED WITH GASTROINTESTINAL DISEASE

GI diseases associated with arthritis (enteric reactive arthritis) include:

- Dysentery, causing postdysenteric reactive arthritis
- IBD, Crohn's disease and ulcerative colitis (UC)

### Epidemiology

- The prevalence of post-dysenteric reactive arthritis is up to 27 in 100 000. The two patterns of IBD-associated arthritis are peripheral arthritis, which affects 12% of patients with UC and 20% of patients with Crohn's disease, and axSpA, which affects 6% of patients in each group.
- IBD-associated peripheral arthritis most commonly presents at 25–45 years of age.
- IBD-associated axSpA is associated with the presence of *HLA-B27* in approximately 50% of patients.
- Post-dysenteric reactive arthritis is more common in mainland Europe than in the UK.

### Disease mechanisms

The organisms thought to be responsible for post dysenteric reactive arthritis are *Shigella dysenteriae*, *Shigella flexneri*, *Salmonella typhimurium*, *Yersinia enterocolitica*, *Clostridium difficile* and *Campylobacter jejuni*.

### Clinical features

- The peripheral arthritis usually follows IBD by 6 months to several years and there is a close temporal relationship between exacerbations of IBD and the arthritis.
- The spondylitis is indistinguishable from axSpA.
- Sacroiliac joint involvement is evident in 5–15% of patients, but will not usually become symptomatic or progress.
- The clinical features of post-dysenteric reactive arthritis are similar to those of SARA.

### Investigation

- Investigations and their results are as for axSpA.
- If IBD is suspected, specific investigations are required (see Chapter 10, Gastrointestinal disease).

### Management

- IBD-associated arthritis is managed by controlling the IBD; topical corticosteroids may help.
- Bowel resection may prevent acute attacks of peripheral disease associated with UC but not those associated with Crohn's disease. Otherwise, the treatment for enteric reactive arthritis is similar to that for axSpA.

### Prognosis

- Peripheral joint destruction in IBD-associated arthritis is rare. An attack of peripheral arthritis subsides within weeks and resolves without damage. The axial type of arthritis usually progresses without treatment despite any remission of IBD or colectomy.
- The prognosis for post-dysenteric reactive arthritis is similar to that for SARA.

**4**

## RHEUMATIC DISEASE IN CHILDREN

Children may present with a wide variety of musculoskeletal complaints, most of which are benign. Most conditions are unique to childhood, but may overlap with adult disease, even though their presentation may be similar to those in adults (e.g. gait disturbance or joint pain stiffness and swelling). This uniqueness may be as a result of congenital anomalies (e.g. scoliosis) or developmental anomalies (e.g. slipped femoral capital epithesis). This section highlights the variety of conditions that may occur.

## JUVENILE IDIOPATHIC ARTHRITIS

There are a variety of different causes of childhood arthritis as listed in **Table 4.11**. JIA is the principal form of chronic idiopathic synovitis.

There are different patterns of JIA (**Table 4.12**), which have different characteristics and prognoses and are probably distinct diseases. Remember that children will not

**Table 4.11**  Causes of childhood arthritis

**Trauma**
- Sports injury
- Non-accidental injury (NAI)

**Mechanical**
- Slipped capital femoral epiphysis

**Viral infection**
- Rubella
- Mumps
- Chickenpox
- Parvovirus

**Bacterial (infective)**
- *Haemophilus influenzae* (especially neonates)
- *Staphylococcus aureus*
- *Mycobacterium tuberculosis*

**Bacterial (reactive)**
- β-haemolytic *Streptococcus* (rheumatic fever)
- *Borrelia burgdorferi* (Lyme arthritis)
- SARA

**Idiopathic**
- JIA
- Autoimmune rheumatic disease
- HSP
- DM
- Lupus
- Malignancy
- Leukaemia
- Lymphoma
- Haemophilia
- Haemarthoses

**Table 4.12**  Subtypes of JIA

**Oligoarthritis** (four joints or fewer, 50% of patients)
- 70% are female, who are usually ANA-positive.
- Extended oligoarthritis may develop (more than four-joint involvement) after the first 6 months of disease.
- See JUVENILE IDIOPATHIC ARTHRITIS AT A GLANCE **Figure A**.

*Oligoarthritis subtypes*
- Oligoarthritis (persistent and extended): majority are girls under 5 years, likely to be ANA-positive with associated chronic uveitis
- Enthesitis-related arthritis: commonly adolescent boys with arthritis of the hips, knees and sacroiliac joints, enthesopathy and acute iritis. Often ANA-negative and 70% are *HLA-B27*-positive
- PsA

**Polyarticular onset** (five joints or more; 40% of patients)
- 25% are RF-positive.
- 75% are RF-negative.
- See JUVENILE IDIOPATHIC ARTHRITIS AT A GLANCE **Figure B**.
- Those affected are predominantly females.
- Age of presentation has two peaks: the first between the ages of 2 and 5 years, and the second between 10 and 14 years.

**Systemic onset or Still's disease** (10% of patients)
- This can occur at any age, has no sex predisposition and is characterized by systemic symptoms, a rash and arthritis.
- See JUVENILE IDIOPATHIC ARTHRITIS AT A GLANCE **Figure C**.
- Macrophage activation syndrome is a severe complication of systemic JIA and may be life-threatening.

describe their symptoms as adults may; for example, a parent may describe inability to walk or participate in games, but children with arthritis may avoid sporting activity. The criteria for diagnosis are arthritis for at least 6 weeks in a patient of 16 years of age or less. See **Figure A** in JUVENILE IDIOPATHIC ARTHRITIS AT A GLANCE.

Arthritis may appear after weeks or months and there are three disease course patterns:
- Monophasic, where the disease becomes quiescent after 4–6 months
- Polycyclic, with inactive periods ranging from a few months to years
- Persistent, the most common course with systemic manifestations and/or arthritis

A similar presentation may occur in adults. It is rare, with similar laboratory features and may become intermittent or chronic. Treatment is similar.

### Diagnosis

The criteria for the diagnosis of JIA are:
- Persistent arthritis of one or more joints for at least 6 weeks
- Exclusion of other causes of arthritis (see **Table 4.2**)

## JUVENILE IDIOPATHIC ARTHRITIS AT A GLANCE

JIA is arthritis for at least 6 weeks in a patient of 16 years of age or less.

There are three different patterns of JIA:

- Pauciarticular (50%)
- Polyarticular (40%)
- Systemic (10%)

### Clinical features

*Arthritis*

*Skin*

- Köbner's phenomenon
- Pale pink macular (Still's) evanescent rash

*Systemic*

- Temperature chart: spiking temperature
- Malaise and lymphadenopathy

*Eyes*

- Chronic uveitis
- ANA is strongly associated with occurrence of uveitis. This is a cause of childhood blindness

*Heart and lungs*

- Pericarditis
- Pleural effusion
- Patients may be of small stature and have limb growth discrepancy because of inflammation and corticosteroid treatment if treatment is delayed

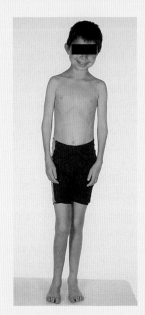

**Figure A** Pauciarticular JIA. This child has a monoarthritis affecting the right knee.

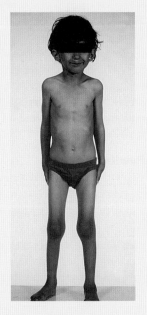

**Figure B** Polyarticular JIA. This child has arthritis principally affecting the knees, hips, wrists, elbows, cervical spine and temporomandibular joints.

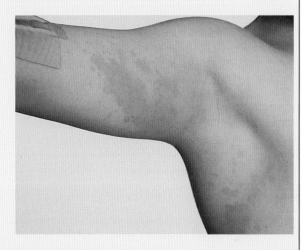

**Figure C** Systemic JIA. The pale pink evanescent macular rash is found in the child's axilla.

## Investigation

### Haematology

- *FBC:* usually reveals anaemia, a raised white cell count and thrombocytosis
- *ESR:* is raised in polyarthritis and systemic JIA

### Immunology

- *Autoantibodies:* ANAs and RFs may be present
- *Viral antibodies:* rarely useful, but should be requested if a specific infection is suspected (e.g. parvovirus B19)
- *Antistreptolysin O titre:* raised in β-haemolytic streptococcal infection

### Diagnostic imaging

Ultrasound and MRI of affected joints help to confirm a diagnosis of arthritis.

- *Radiography:* may show changes similar to those of RA and AS
- *Abdominal ultrasound and echocardiography:* may be necessary to detect hepatosplenomegaly and pericarditis

## Management

- Oligoarticular JIA is usually responsive to NSAIDs and intra-articular corticosteroids.
- Methotrexate and other immunosuppressive drugs are recommended for children with disease that extends to involve five of more joints or require repeat injections. Alternatives are sulfasalazine and leflunomide.
- Biological agents are typically used in patients with uveitis and in patients with extended oligoarticular

**4**

and polyarticular JIA; typically, tumour necrosis factor inhibitor, adalimumab, etanercept or infliximab.

- Treatment is most successful when there is prompt and long-term attention to maintaining joint mobility and avoiding or controlling complications.
- Corticosteroid use in the treatment of systemic JIA can now be reduced with the use of biological therapies such as tocilizumab (anti-IL-6), canakinumab (anti-IL-1) and anakinra (IL-1 receptor antagonist), and hence prognosis has dramatically improved (see **Table 4.5**).
- Great emphasis is placed on support for the child's family. Liaison between GP, and educational services is paramount.
- Physiotherapy is aimed at preventing joint deformity and maintaining function.
- Regular eye examinations are necessary, especially for those with ANA-positive pauciarticular-onset JIA. Up to 50% of children with uveitis are asymptomatic and, if untreated, disease may lead to blindness.

*Immunizations*

Routine childhood vaccines should be administered to all children with JIA, regardless of disease activity. In general, live vaccines should not be given to children who are receiving systemic immunosuppression.

### Prognosis

- The overall prognosis of JIA is variable, however, there are now multiple treatment options and the goal is for disease remission.
- Mortality is usually caused by infection or pericarditis.
- Morbidity is substantial and may be psychological, educational, social and medical. Medical morbidity is associated with chronic anterior uveitis, which may lead to visual impairment, growth disturbance as a result of localized inflammation or corticosteroid treatment and joint failure. Osteoporosis is now less common. Temporomandibular joint involvement can result in micrognathia.
- Poor prognostic indicators are polyarticular RF-positive disease associated with joint erosion. Poor drug compliance is also a significant prognostic factor.
- Joint replacement is now uncommon.

## NON-INFLAMMATORY MUSCULOSKELETAL DISORDERS

### Hypermobility syndrome

Joint hypermobility syndrome in children is a common clinical finding and does not usually cause symptoms (**Figure 4.24**). The criteria for diagnosis are given in **Table 4.13**.

Hypermobility syndrome is estimated to affect 7–12% of schoolchildren.

It is probable that up to 40% of children with hypermobility have recurrent joint pain. This typically affects

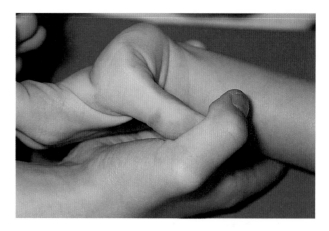

**Figure 4.24** Hypermobility. This patient has a hypermobile thumb!

the knees, but it may also affect the ankles, hips, back and upper limbs to a lesser extent. The condition is relatively benign, but there may be an increased risk of OA in later life. If treatment is necessary, exercises to increase muscle bulk may be helpful and orthoses may be useful to correct joint deformity.

### Paediatric pain

Evaluation of paediatric pain includes determining the underlying type of pain (nociceptive versus neuropathic pain), source and location of pain, and the severity of pain. If the child is able to understand and report their pain severity, self-reporting can be used with the visual analogue scales and faces scale. If the child is unable to perform self-reporting, behavioural observational scales can be used e.g. revised face/legs/activity/cry/consolability (r-FLACC) tool.

### *Growing pains*

Growing pains are defined as pain waking a child at night who is otherwise without any manifestation of musculoskeletal problems. Growing pains are a common musculoskeletal condition (15% of children). The aetiology is unknown.

There are, however, certain common clinical features:
- They occur commonly in pre-school and school-age children.
- They primarily affect the lower extremities.

**Table 4.13** Criteria for the diagnosis of joint hypermobility

The ability to perform three or more of the following:
- Passive hyperextension of the fingers, with extension of the wrist until the fingers are parallel to the forearm
- Passive opposition of the thumb to touch the forearm with the wrist flexed
- Hyperextension of the elbow greater than 10°
- Hyperextension of the knees greater than 10°
- Flexion of the trunk and hips with the knees extended until the palms of the hands touch the floor

- There may be symptom-free periods lasting days/weeks/months.
- Nocturnal pain usually resolves by morning.
- Pain is relieved by massage/heat/analgesics (e.g. ibuprofen).
- Normal activity is maintained.
- Physical examination is normal.
- Associated complaints of recurrent abdominal pain and/or headache occur in approximately one-third of patients.
- Family history of growing pains or rheumatic complaint is common.

### Management

- Treatment usually involves the resources of the rheumatology team and is aimed at educating both patients and their parents about the benign nature of these disorders.
- Physiotherapy and a graded exercise programme have been shown to be beneficial.
- Psychological support and coping strategies, and drug treatment with analgesia and NSAIDs, may be helpful.
- Patients and parents need reassurance that the condition will improve spontaneously.

### Congenital dislocation of the hip

Congenital dislocation of the hip is one of the most common causes of hip disability in children and of OA in later life.

### Epidemiology
- More common in girls
- Occurs in 1 in 15 000 births

### Clinical features
The left hip is more often involved. Congenital dislocation of the hip should be recognized at birth by detection of an abnormal click as the infant's hip is abducted and adducted. Later, abnormalities of hip movement, femoral shortening and pain may become evident.

### Investigation
Radiography shows that the acetabulum is oblique (increased angle from the horizontal), shallow and directed anterolaterally (**Figure 4.25**). It is insufficient to cover the femoral head, which is usually anteverted relative to the femoral shaft and is small and often deformed.

### Management
Treatment is splinting in abduction.

### Prognosis
- Prognosis for full restoration to normal anatomy is excellent.
- Late diagnosis requires more complex treatment and is accompanied by an increased risk of OA in later life.

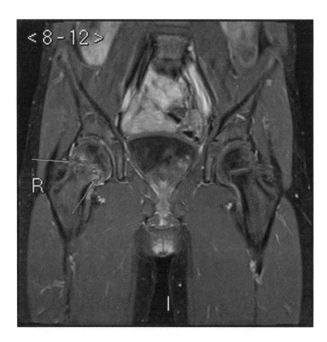

**Figure 4.25** Slipped femoral capital epiphysis. Coronal fat-saturated MR image of the pelvis of a paediatric patient. This demonstrates oedema of the right capital femoral epiphysis (blue arrow) and mild medial subluxation of the femoral physis (red arrow).

### Slipped femoral capital epiphysis

### Epidemiology
This is common in 10- to 17-year-old boys.

### Disease mechanisms
Slipped femoral capital epiphysis may result from acute trauma to the hip. However, before closure of the proximal femoral epiphysis, the femoral head can slip, displacing medially and posteriorly in relation to the shaft of the femur. There may be associated endocrine abnormalities.

### Clinical features
- The disorder produces an abduction, lateral rotation and extension deformity and there may be shortening of the leg and associated pain (**Figure 4.25**).
- The child is frequently hypogonadal and obese.
- Avascular necrosis of the femoral head may occur.

### Investigation
Lateral hip radiography is usually diagnostic.

### Management
Surgical correction is often necessary.

### Prognosis
The prognosis is usually good.

## ISCHAEMIC BONE DISEASE

Ischaemic bone disease in childhood or osteochondrosis are conditions that refer to non-traumatic ischaemic necrosis, which typically affects a growth or ossification centre.

### Osgood–Schlatter disease

#### Disease mechanisms
Osgood–Schlatter disease is idiopathic osteochondrosis of the tibial tubercle and may represent a partial avulsion of the tibial tubercle.

#### Clinical features
This disorder is most common in boys aged 10–16 years, who may present with pain, prominence and tenderness over the patellar tendon insertion into the distal extension of the proximal tibial epiphysis.

#### Investigation
Radiography may show soft-tissue swelling, as well as irregular ossification of the anterior portion of the epiphysis. Small fragments of bone may also be noted in the tendon.

#### Management
- Pain usually disappears when the ossicle fuses to the underlying tibia.
- Athletic activity should be discontinued or reduced until pain resolves.
- Analgesics and NSAIDs may be useful (see **Table 4.4**).

#### Prognosis
Osgood–Schlatter disease is self-limiting and resolution usually occurs 1–2 years after epiphyseal closure.

### Perthes' disease

See **Figure 4.26**.

#### Disease mechanisms
Perthes' disease is idiopathic osteonecrosis of the proximal femoral capital epiphysis. Its aetiology is unknown.

#### Clinical features
Clinically the patient (most commonly a boy 3–12 years of age) presents with a limp, which may be painful and associated with limited abduction and internal rotation, and a fixed flexion deformity. It is bilateral in 15% of patients and may be associated with a modest degree of delayed skeletal maturation.

#### Investigation
Radiography shows disease progression through four phases: death of the bone, fragmentation, gradual revascularization and restoration of structure.

#### Management
Restoration of normal bone structure may result in a large, flat femoral head with a wide, short neck (coxa magna et plana). Treatment is based on the extent of the lesion. Surgical realignment may be necessary.

#### Prognosis
Therapy is most beneficial if started early in young children. Otherwise, the prognosis is relatively poor and many patients will develop painful hips in adult life.

## CRYSTAL ARTHRITIS

Three types of crystals may be deposited in joints and cause arthritis:
- *Monosodium urate deposition:* causes gout and commonly affects the first toe
- *Calcium pyrophosphate dihydrate (CPPD) deposition:* causes pseudogout and commonly affects the knee
- *Basic calcium phosphate (apatite) deposition:* commonly affects the knee and shoulder

## GOUT

Gout is a heterogeneous group of diseases, which are manifest by increased serum urate concentration, recurrent arthritis, aggregated urate deposits (tophi), renal disease and nephrolithiasis.

Gout is one of the most painful rheumatological conditions. There is a rapid onset (within hours) of joint pain, swelling and inflammation. It is associated with hypercholesterolaemia and hypertension, and hence with cardiovascular disease.

### Epidemiology
- Prevalence of hyperuricaemia and gout is approximately 3% of adults and has been increasing since the 1970s.
- Prevalence increases with increasing age.
- 90% of people with primary gout are male. Normal urate levels increase at puberty and the menopause, and are higher in men. Gout is extremely unusual in premenopausal women who are not taking diuretics.
- Studies suggest a multifactorial inheritance, and a family history may be obtained from 6–18% of patients with gout.

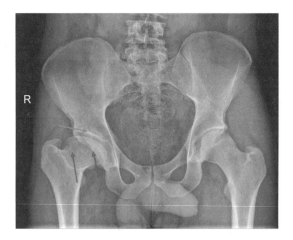

**Figure 4.26** Anteroposterior radiograph of an adult patient with features of chronic Perthes' disease. Note the enlarged and deformed femoral neck 'coxa magna' (red arrow) and the flattened and widened femoral head 'coxa plana' (blue arrow), with secondary changes in the acetabulum (green arrow).

## Disease mechanisms

Hyperuricaemia may be a primary or secondary manifestation, occurring as part of another disease or as an effect of drug treatment (**Table 4.14**).

Uric acid is formed from the oxidation of purine bases and approximately 70% is excreted in the urine; the rest is excreted into the GI tract.

The mean serum urate level in healthy individuals is approximately 300 μmol/L in males and 240 μmol/L in females, while the saturation value of serum urate is approximately 400 μmol/L. The risk of gouty arthritis and/or renal stones increases with increasing serum urate level and with duration of hyperuricaemia.

## Clinical features

The natural history of gout can be considered in four stages:

1  Asymptomatic hyperuricaemia
2  Acute gouty arthritis
3  Intercritical gout
4  Chronic tophaceous gout

There may also be renal manifestations (see GOUT AND PSEUDOGOUT AT A GLANCE).

**Table 4.14** Causes of hyperuricaemia and gout

| |
|---|
| **Primary** |
| *Reduced uric acid clearance (90%)* |
| Undefined abnormality in otherwise normal kidneys |
| *Overproduction of uric acid (10%)* |
| Specific X-linked enzyme defects (increased PRPP synthetase activity, partial deficiency of HGPR transferase) |
| **Secondary** |
| *Reduced uric acid clearance* |
| Renal failure (permanent or reversible) |
| Lead poisoning |
| Drugs (e.g. diuretics, which enhance reabsorption and decrease filtration of uric acid, low-dose aspirin, pyrazinamide, nicotinic acid, ethambutol, alcohol, ciclosporin) |
| *Competitive inhibition of uric acid excretion* |
| Starvation, alcoholic ketosis, diabetic ketoacidosis, lactic acidosis |
| Overproduction of uric acid |
| Increased purine biosynthesis |
| Deficiency or absence of glucose-6-phosphatase (e.g. autosomal recessive glycogen storage disease type I or Von Gierke's disease) |
| X-linked HGPR transferase deficiency (Lesch–Nyhan syndrome in which the major clinical manifestations are unrelated to hyperuricaemia) |
| Increased nucleic acid turnover |
| Myeloproliferative and lymphoproliferative disorders, carcinoma |
| Severe psoriasis |
| High alcohol consumption |
| Obesity |

HGPR, hypoxanthine guanine phosphoryl; PRPP, phosphoryl pyrophosphate.

## Differential diagnosis

The most important differential diagnosis of gout is infective arthritis. Others include soft-tissue infection, inflamed bunions, local trauma, RA, OA with acute inflammation, acute sarcoidosis, PsA, pseudogout, acute calcific tendonitis, SARA and xanthomatosis.

## Investigation

### Haematology
- *ESR and CRP:* may be raised
- *Neutrophilic leucocytosis:* may develop

### Biochemistry
- *Serum uric acid:* elevated in 90% of patients with gout, but may be normal during an acute attack
- *Serum creatinine and urea:* elevated in renal failure

### Microbiology
Gram stain and culture of synovial fluid should be performed to exclude infection.

### Diagnostic imaging
Plain radiography, MRI and US are useful for showing soft-tissue swelling at first, but later tophi and peri-articular erosions are seen. Rheumatoid erosions are articular.

### Other investigations
Synovial fluid monosodium urate crystals are slender needle-shaped and negatively birefringent (bright yellow when parallel to the axis of slow vibration) under compensated polarized light microscopy. Crystals remain detectable after weeks or months of storage.

## Management

Treatment of gout is aimed at relieving the acute synovitis with anti-inflammatory medication and preventing further crystal formation. Dietary advice for patients with hyperuricaemia is listed in **Table 4.15**.

### Asymptomatic hyperuricaemia
There is no evidence that chronic renal disease or joint deformity will develop if it is not treated. Diuretic substitution

**Table 4.15** Advice for patients with hyperuricaemia to prevent gout and nephrolithiasis

| |
|---|
| Dietary: |
| • Lose weight (if indicated) |
| • Avoid foods containing large amounts of purine (e.g. sardines, bacon, liver, kidneys) |
| • Supplement diet with foods containing small amounts of purines (e.g. cereals, cheese, vegetables) |
| • Avoid excess alcohol |
| • Drink plenty of fluid |
| Avoid aspirin and diuretics |
| Make sure that shoes fit and are comfortable |

**4**

## GOUT AND PSEUDOGOUT AT A GLANCE

### Gout

Increased serum urate concentration (**Figure 4.27b**), recurrent arthritis, aggregated urate deposits: tophi, renal disease and neph-rolithiasis. Associated with hypercholesterolaemia, hypertension and cardiovascular disease. Differentiation from infective arthritis is important.

### Pseudogout

CPPD (**Figure 4.27a**) deposition disease. May be secondary to another disease, e.g. haemochromatosis, hypomagnesaemia, hypo-phosphatasia, hypercalcaemia, hyperparathyroidism, gout, ochronosis, Wilson's disease.

### Clinical features

*Gout*

- *Asymptomatic hyperuricaemia:* 5% of hyperuricaemics develop gout. The first attack of gouty arthritis comes after many years of hyperuricaemia.
- *Acute gouty arthritis:* This first affects the big toe in 50% of patients (**Figure 4.27a**).
- *Intercritical gout:* An asymptomatic period after the first attack may last up to 10 years. 60% of patients have a further attack within the first year.
- *Chronic tophaceous gout:* If gout is not treated, crystals of monosodium urate (tophi) will deposit in cartilage (e.g. in the helix of the ear) (**Figure 4.27b,c**), in synovial membranes (e.g. in the olecranon bursa), in tendons (e.g. in the Achilles tendon) and in soft tissues (e.g. of the ulnar surface of the forearm). A polyarticular pattern may develop late in the course of untreated gout.
- *Renal manifestations:* Gouty patients also have an increased incidence of calcium-containing renal stones.

*Pseudogout*

- *Acute* (pseudogout): symptoms peak within 36 hours and may last for 1–4 weeks
- *Subacute* (pseudorheumatoid): may develop over weeks to months in 5% of patients
- *Chronic* (pseudo-osteoarthritis): progressive symmetrical polyarthritis with acute attacks
- *Asymptomatic:* a coincidental finding of chondrocalcinosis

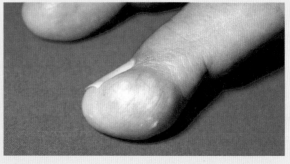

**Figure B** Gouty tophus with uric acid crystals exuding from the fingertip.

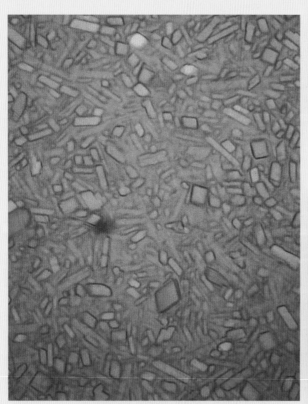

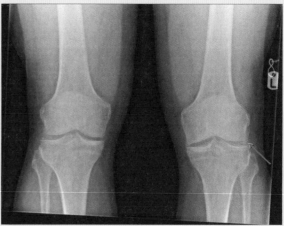

**Figure A** Calcium pyrophosphate dihydrate (CPPD) crystals (extracted from synovial fluid). These are pleomorphic, rectangular and weakly positively birefringent. The axis of slow vibration is from bottom left to top right.

**Figure C** Anteroposterior radiograph of both knees. Extensive calcification of the lateral menisci bilaterally (blue arrow) typical of chondrocalcinosis.

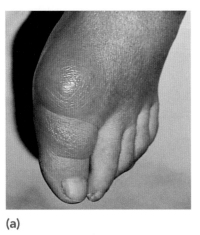 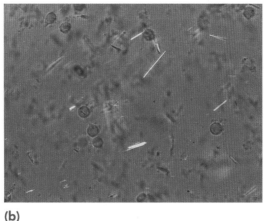 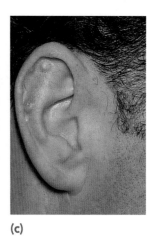

(a) (b) (c)

**Figure 4.27** Gout. **(a)** Acute gouty arthritis affecting the big toe. This is exquisitely painful. **(b)** Synovial fluid microscopy under compensated polarized light showing the slender needle-shaped and negatively birefringent urate crystals. The axis of slow vibration is from bottom left to top right. **(c)** Urate crystal deposition in the cartilage of the ear.

and dietary change are advisable, but the only indications for hypouricaemic drug treatment are:

- Family history of renal stones with a similar degree of hyperuricaemia
- Clear-cut uric acid overproduction (over 1100 mg/day urinary excretion on a controlled diet or resulting from chemotherapy for haematological malignancies)
- Repeated uric acid levels above 775 µmol/L in males and 550 µmol/L in females

### Acute gout

Acute gout is treated with an NSAID. If an NSAID is contra-indicated (e.g. because of asthma, congestive cardiac failure or duodenal ulceration) or if it is ineffective, colchicine can be used instead, until the attack subsides. If oral therapy is not effective, the attack can usually be terminated by oral or intramuscular corticosteroid injection or, if possible (knee involvement), joint aspiration and an intra-articular cortico-steroid injection. Biological treatment with anakinra (IL-1 antagonist), and canakinumab (monoclonal antibody against IL-1beta) are emerging as treatments for acute gout and prevention of gouty flares.

Treatment is not indicated for intercritical gout unless there is a history of renal calculi or uric acid excretion and/or uric acid levels are raised (see above).

If there are repeated attacks of gout and the disease is likely to become chronic, a xanthine oxidate inhibitor such as allopurinol is used to reduce serum uric acid levels and prevent further attacks (**Table 4.16**). The aim is to keep serum uric acid levels below 360 µmol/L (<6 mg/dL) and 300 µmol/L (<5 mg/dL) in tophaceous gout.

**Table 4.16** Urate-lowering therapies

- Xanthine oxidate inhibitors: allopurinol, febuxostat
- Uricosuric agents: probenecid, benzbromarone, lesinurad
- Uricase: pegloticase, rasburicase

When using allopurinol:

- Allopurinol should not be started during an acute attack because its use will lead to a worsening of the inflammation.
- It should be given with an NSAID or colchicine for 1 month after the hyperuricaemia has been corrected.
- It need not be stopped if an acute attack occurs during treatment.
- Allopurinol is associated with a variety of rashes, which can be severe.

Dietary advice aimed mainly at decreasing purine intake together with measures to prevent gout and nephrolithiasis are listed in **Table 4.15**.

## CALCIUM PYROPHOSPHATE DIHYDRATE DEPOSITION DISEASE OR PSEUDOGOUT

CPPD deposition disease is the most common cause of acute monoarthritis in middle-aged and elderly adults.

### Epidemiology

- Prevalence is estimated to be 1 in 1000 population.
- There is increasing prevalence with increasing age.

### Disease mechanisms

CPPD deposition disease may be primary. If present in a person under 55 years of age, CPPD deposition disease may arise secondary to other diseases such as haemochromato-sis, hypomagnesaemia, hypophosphatasia, hypercalcaemia (caused by primary hyperparathyroidism), hypothyroidism, gout, ochronosis and Wilson's disease.

The pathogenesis of pseudogout is unknown.

### Clinical features

#### Acute attacks (pseudogout)

- Acute attacks (pseudogout) are characterized by rapidly developing arthritis, which peaks within

123

36 hours and lasts for 1–4 weeks. An attack may be provoked by trauma, surgery or illness.

- A single joint (commonly the knee) is usually affected, and becomes erythematous, warm and painful. There may be associated fever. Other joints may be affected, including the MTP joint of the great toe.
- Radiography may show chondrocalcinosis.

### Subacute attacks (pseudorheumatoid)

- 5% of patients present with subacute attacks.
- Many joints (commonly knees, wrists and elbows) become involved over weeks to months, and there may be morning stiffness, pain, deformity and fatigue.

### Chronic calcium pyrophosphate dihydrate deposition disease (pseudo-osteoarthritis)

Chronic CPPD deposition disease affects mainly middle-aged women and causes progressive symmetrical multiple joint (knees, wrists, MCP joints, hips, shoulders, elbows and ankles) degeneration associated with acute attacks.

### Asymptomatic calcium pyrophosphate dihydrate deposition disease

Asymptomatic CPPD deposition disease is detected by coincidental finding of chondrocalcinosis.

## Diagnosis

Diagnosis of CPPD deposition disease is based on the pattern of clinical features, the presence of chondrocalcinosis and CPPD crystal identification.

## Differential diagnosis

The differential diagnosis is mainly between gout and infective arthritis – but pseudogout, gout, OA and sepsis may occur together.

## Investigation

### Biochemistry, immunology and microbiology

These tests are as for gout.

### Diagnostic imaging

Joint radiography shows chondrocalcinosis in the articular hyaline cartilage, fibrocartilage and tendons in 75% of patients. In the articular cartilage, fine linear densities are seen parallel to and separated from the underlying bone, while fibrocartilage contains thick irregular densities within the central portion of the joint cavity. Commonly involved fibrocartilage includes the menisci of the knee, the triangular cartilage of the wrist, the symphysis pubis and the annulus fibrosus of the intervertebral discs.

### Other investigations

- *Synovial fluid:* CPPD crystals are pleomorphic, rectangular and weakly positively birefringent (yellow when at right angles to the axis of slow vibration). There is a marked decline in CPPD crystals if the fluid is stored for more than 1 day.

- *Look for an underlying cause* (e.g. haemochromatosis): In patients with early-onset disease (those who are under 55 years of age), there may be an underlying cause.

## Management

Specific treatment may be required for protracted recurrent cases (see **Table 4.3**).

## Prognosis

CPPD disease is usually self-limiting and resolves within 1–3 weeks.

# BASIC CALCIUM PHOSPHATE (APATITE) DISEASE

Basic calcium phosphate crystals are deposited mainly in the knee and shoulder (Milwaukee shoulder) and may also cause calcific periarthritis, tendonitis and bursitis.

The crystals are too small to be seen with light microscopy but are visible with electron micrography, and joint radiographs are similar to those of CPPD deposition disease. NSAIDs and intra-articular corticosteroids are the treatment of choice.

## REGIONAL MUSCULOSKELETAL DISORDERS

Regional musculoskeletal disease refers to localized rheumatic disorders that cause pain. They may be associated with systemic disease (e.g. diabetes mellitus, malignancy, other rheumatic disorders such as RA and SARA) but for most the cause is non-specific and multifactorial.

Diabetes mellitus has a close association with musculoskeletal conditions. The prevalence of hand and shoulder disorders is higher in patients with diabetes than in controls and correlates with the duration but not the type of diabetes. Hand abnormalities are common and are associated with vascular connective tissue and peripheral nerve pathology. Common conditions include carpal tunnel syndrome, Dupuytren's contracture, tenosynovitis of flexor tendons of the finger, and frozen shoulder.

These disorders are sometimes referred to as 'soft-tissue' disorders because they describe the extra-articular structures that are often involved.

## Management

- Treatment is with analgesics, NSAIDs, ultrasound and local ice application.
- Local injections of corticosteroid and lignocaine (lidocaine) can be useful when the pain is acute and well localized. Hydrocortisone is the corticosteroid of choice for injection because it is less commonly

associated with complications such as subcutaneous fat necrosis and scarring than the long-acting corticosteroids. Specific treatment is discussed for specific conditions.

## HAND AND WRIST DISORDERS

Common disorders in the hand and wrist are trigger finger, ganglions, Dupuytren's contracture, de Quervain's tenosynovitis and carpal tunnel syndrome.

Patients may express considerable anxiety with regard to hand pain, especially if there is occupation involvement (e.g. musicians and keyboard operators).

### Trigger finger

- Trigger finger is caused by stenosing tenosynovitis and most commonly affects the flexor tendons of the third and fourth fingers.
- It is often associated with repeated manual trauma and results from a nodular enlargement of the tendons.

### Ganglions

Ganglions may be painful and are firm dorsal swellings that contain synovial and mucinous material and are connected to joints or tendon sheaths, usually around the wrist and in the hand.

### Dupuytren's contracture

- This is associated with diabetes mellitus, alcoholism, trauma and HIV infection.
- The contracture is a painless thickening of the palmar aponeurosis that produces gradual flexion, initially of the little and ring fingers.

### De Quervain's tenosynovitis

- De Quervain's tenosynovitis is a form of wrist tenosynovitis involving the tendons of extensor pollicis brevis and abductor pollicis longus in the most lateral compartment of the wrist adjacent to the radial styloid.
- Pain is located in the anatomical snuff box, and can be elicited by forced ulnar deviation, placing the patient's thumb in the palm (Finkelstein's test).

### Carpal tunnel syndrome

#### Disease mechanisms

Carpal tunnel syndrome is the most common entrapment neuropathy and results from compression of the median nerve in the carpal tunnel of the wrist (**Figure 4.28**). The median nerve supplies the sensory branches to the thumb, index and middle fingers, and half of the ring finger, together with motor branches to all anterior forearm muscles except flexor carpi ulnaris and flexor digitorum profundus to the ring and little fingers. It may be occupational

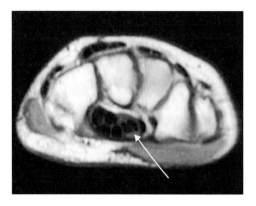

**Figure 4.28** MRI of the wrist demonstrating the carpal tunnel. The median nerve and flexor tendons pass through the carpal tunnel, which is bound dorsally and laterally by the carpal bones, and on the anterior aspect by the transverse carpal ligament.

because of repeated deviation of the wrist from neutral position, and may be associated with RA, gout, myxoedema, acromegaly, diabetes mellitus, and pregnancy where it may be bilateral.

#### Clinical features

- Early symptoms are painful tingling in the wrist and hands at night that mainly affects the thumb and index and middle fingers, but which may extend up the arm. The patient may also complain of numbness in the median nerve supply, as well as thenar weakness and atrophy.
- Examination may reveal a positive Tinel's sign (percussion of the wrist causing finger paraesthesiae) and reproduction of the pain and paraesthesiae with the Phalen manoeuvre (flexing the patient's hand at the wrist).
- To determine motor loss, test the thenar muscles: abductor pollicis brevis (with the thumb adducted towards the fifth finger, ask the patient to abduct the thumb against resistance); opponens pollicis (ask the patient to oppose the tip of the thumb with the tip of the fifth finger and try to break the pinch).
- Inspection of the hand may reveal atrophy of the thenar muscles.

#### Investigation

Nerve conduction testing will show a prolonged distal median nerve motor latency, as well as delayed sensory latency across the wrist.

#### Management

- Initial treatment includes wrist splinting, analgesia and local corticosteroid injection.
- If the symptoms are not relieved, especially if weakness is present, hand surgery is recommended.

**4**

# ELBOW DISORDERS

Common disorders at the elbow are humeral epicondylitis and olecranon bursitis.

## Humeral epicondylitis

- Lateral or medial humeral epicondylitis is usually caused by mechanical overload on the tendons.
- Lateral involvement (tennis elbow) causes localized tenderness that is exacerbated by resisted wrist extension and supination. Grip strength may be reduced. Medial involvement (golfer's elbow) causes localized tenderness induced by resisted flexion of the wrist and pronation.
- Ultrasound and MRI may be useful to define tendon damage.
- Treatment is conservative at first with rest, but local corticosteroid injection is often required. Muscle strengthening exercises are necessary when the pain subsides. If the cause is sport- or occupation-related, preventive advice should be given. Elbow splints may be useful.

## Olecranon bursitis

- Olecranon bursitis is commonly caused by acute trauma, gout, RA or infection.
- There is pain, swelling and inflammation over the olecranon.
- Treatment is by aspiration (to check for gout and infection) and corticosteroid injection.

# SHOULDER DISORDERS

The shoulder consists of three joints (the acromioclavicular, sternoclavicular and glenohumeral joints), all of which can be involved by inflammation.

Arm elevation is facilitated by the rotator cuff of muscles consisting of supraspinatus, infraspinatus, terres minor and subscapularis. These muscles act together to depress the humoral head to allow the deltoid muscle to elevate the arm. They are also involved in assisting internal and external rotation of the shoulder.

Causes of shoulder pain are listed in **Table 4.17**.

**Table 4.17** Causes of shoulder pain

| |
|---|
| Referred pain from the cervical spine: cervical spondylosis |
| Tendinitis: rotator cuff tendinitis (commonly affects the supraspinatus insertion into the humeral head), biceps tendinitis or associated with mild trauma or impingement of the rotator cuff under the acromion; partial or complete tears may result (**Figure 4.29**) |
| Bursitis: subacromial bursa may become inflamed with a coexistent rotator cuff tendinitis |
| Joint disease: adhesive capsulitis can result from tendinitis, glenohumeral arthritis and polymyalgia rheumatic; pain present on palpation |

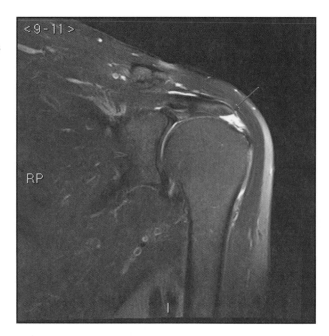

**Figure 4.29** Coronal fat-saturated MR image of the shoulder. Retracted tendon of the anterior supraspinatus tendon (blue arrow).

# COMPLEX REGIONAL PAIN SYNDROME

Complex regional pain syndrome (CRPS) is characterized by pain in a distal extremity and often accompanied by sensory-motor, autonomic and trophic signs. The most common inciting events are: fractures, blunt traumatic injuries (e.g. sprains) and surgery. A temperature difference between affected and unaffected side may be present (warm or cold CRPS).

Two subtypes of CRPS are recognized.
- Type 1: (formerly known as reflex sympathetic dystrophy) in which there is no evidence of peripheral nerve injury; 90%
- Type 2: (formerly known as causalgia) in which peripheral nerve injury is present; 10%.

## Clinical features

- Pain is the most prominent and debilitating symptom, and there may be a burning/stinging/tearing sensation deep inside the limb. It may be distal in the limb, sometimes in stocking/glove distribution, and can be worse at night.
- Sensory: There may be hyperalgesia, allodynia or hypaesthesia.
- Motor (65%): Functional motor impairment is related to pain.
- Autonomic: There may be differences in skin temperature, skin colour, sweat or oedema. Fifty percent of patients may have an absolute difference in skin temperature ≥1 °C. Oedema may occur as a result of inflammation or autonomic dysfunction.

- Trophic: There may be increased hair growth, increased/decreased nail growth, contraction and fibrosis of joints and fascia, and skin atrophy.

### Diagnosis

Diagnosis is based upon clinical features, history and physical examination. There is no test or method for confirming the diagnosis.

### Management

A multidisciplinary team approach is essential.
Treatment involves:
- Patient education
- Physical therapy and occupational therapy
- Psychosocial and behavioural management
- Pain control:
  o NSAIDs
  o Amitriptyline
  o Gabapentin/pregabalin
  o Bisphosphonate
  o Topical lignocaine/capsaicin

## HIP AND KNEE DISORDERS

Hip and knee disorders include trochanteric bursitis, chondromalacia patellae, patella tendinitis, prepatellar tendinitis, popliteal cyst, meniscal tears and ligament injuries.

### Trochanteric bursitis

The trochanteric bursa lies over the lateral aspect of the greater trochanter and under the fascia lata.

Bursitis causes acute pain over the lateral side of the hip and proximal thigh that usually radiates distally and may cause swelling. The pain is often worsened by sitting. Trochanteric bursitis may be one of the presenting features of PMR.

### Chondromalacia patellae

Chondromalacia patellae results from fibrillation of the patellar articular surface.

### Clinical features

- There may be a localized dull ache which is aggravated by sitting and walking up and down stairs, and which may be relieved by extending the knees. This may be accompanied by clicking and crepitus and a sensation of the knees giving way or locking.
- Destruction of the patella cartilage may cause swelling and stiffness.
- Pain may be elicited by compressing the patella in knee extension, and crepitus may be detected on knee movement.

### Investigation
MRI is diagnostic.

### Management
Treatment involves rest and avoidance of activities that precipitate the pain. NSAIDs are used if necessary. Rehabilitation is aimed at strengthening the quadriceps.

### Prepatellar bursitis (housemaid's knee)

- Prepatella bursitis can result from repetitive local trauma and gout.
- There is stiffness and limited movement and pain on kneeling.
- Synovial fluid should be removed for examination.
- Knee protection with a foam cushion may be necessary if recurrence is likely.

### Popliteal cyst (Baker's cyst)

- A popliteal cyst usually arises from a posterior rupture of the knee joint. It may be an incidental finding or may cause pain because of its size.
- When large, it may rupture into the calf, causing severe pain and may mimic an acute deep-vein thrombosis (**Figure 4.30**).
- Treatment is aimed at the knee abnormality.

### Meniscal tears

- Menisci are torn by compressive, rotational and shearing forces in the knee.
- Pain from medial and lateral tears is common, particularly after twisting injuries.
- Examination will reveal specific joint line tenderness. There may be swelling and a reduced range of movement.

**Popliteal cyst**

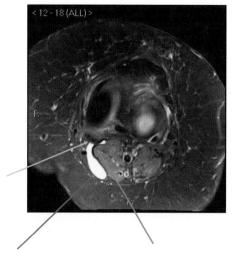

**Figure 4.30** Fat saturated axial MR of the knee. Fluid filled popliteal or Baker's cyst arising from the posteromedial aspect of the knee joint. The cyst extends between the medial head of gastrocnemius (green arrow) and the semimembranosus (yellow arrow) which is a characteristic location, hence also known as a semimembranosus bursa.

4

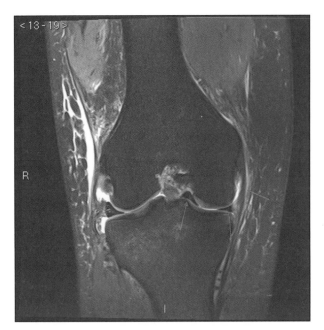

**Figure 4.31** Coronal fat-saturated MR image of the knee showing a meniscal terar. The blue arrow shows the residual medial meniscus. The red arrow shows the flipped fragment of the medical meniscus which now lies in the intercondylar notch. The green arrow shows a grade 2 sprain of the medial collateral ligament.

- MRI is diagnostic (**Figure 4.31**).
- Treatment is conservative, with rest and pain relief. If a full range of movement is not possible and pain does not subside, partial or total meniscectomy or repair may be necessary.

*Ligament injuries*

- Four major ligaments provide knee stability: the anterior and posterior cruciate, and the lateral and medial collateral ligaments. Injury to the knee may involve these ligaments, the joint capsule and other joint structures.
- Pain, swelling and a reduced range of movement can result.

# LOWER LEG DISORDERS

Common problems of the soft tissues of the lower leg, ankle and foot include ligament injuries, Achilles tendinitis, plantar fasciitis and hallux valgus.

## Ligament injuries

- The common mechanisms of injury to the major ankle ligaments are plantar flexion and inversion, dorsiflexion and eversion. The lateral ankle ligaments are most commonly injured.
- There may be swelling because of haemarthrosis and local swelling over the site of the ligament damage.
- The area of maximal tenderness is defined by palpation, and the entire length of the fibula should be palpated as there may be associated proximal fibular fractures.

## Achilles tendinitis

- Achilles tendinitis is associated with gout and SpA.
- The peroneus longus and posterior tibial tendons commonly become inflamed.
- The pain of Achilles tendinitis is usually in the region of the tendon insertion (enthesis) into the calcaneal tuberosity.

## Plantar fasciitis

- Plantar fasciitis is usually idiopathic but may be associated with a SpA. It causes tenderness on weight-bearing along the plantar surface of the metatarsal heads at the inferomedial surface of the calcaneus at the site of attachment of the plantar fascia.
- Radiographs may show a plantar spur caused by calcification at the fascial attachment (**Figure 4.32**).
- A metatarsal head support and a foam doughnut over the painful area may provide relief. If not, a local corticosteroid injection around the attachment of the plantar fascia to the calcaneus is usually beneficial.

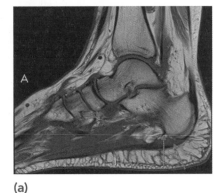

(a)

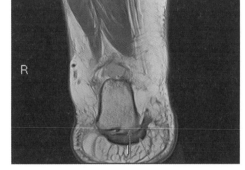

(b)

**Figure 4.32** Plantar fasciitis. **(a)** Sagittal and **(b)** coronal T1-weighted MR images of the ankle. Severe plantar fasciitis with thickening and heterogeneity of the plantar fascia (red arrows) and a calcaneal spur (blue arrows).

### Hallux valgus (bunion)

- Hallux valgus causes bursal inflammation because of prolonged pressure over the bony prominence.
- It commonly results in valgus deformity that may require surgical correction of the hallux.

## LOW BACK PAIN

Low back is defined as the area of the back and spine below the thoracolumbar junction (T12/L1) and the costophrenic angles. Movement in the spine occurs at the synovial apophyseal joints, and at the intervertebral discs. In the lumbar region, there is little rotation and maximum flexion is approximately 45°.

### Epidemiology

- Low back pain is a serious cause of morbidity in the population and results in considerable time off work. It is also an expensive occupational health problem, accounting for many work-related injuries and subsequent litigation.
- It is common and accounts for approximately 4% of GP consultations and 33% of all rheumatological symptoms.
- Prevalence increases with age.

### Disease mechanisms

Low back pain can be caused by:
- *Any component of the thoracolumbosacral area:* vertebrae, intervertebral discs, apophyseal joints, ligaments and paraspinal and abdominal muscles
- *Associated structures:* may be retroperitoneal (kidneys, uterus and associated structures), genitourinary (bladder, prostate) or vascular (aortic aneurysm)
- *Systemic disease:* sickle cell disease, infection

Specific causes are listed in LOW BACK PAIN AT A GLANCE. Common causes of low back pain in children are osteochondrosis (Scheuermann's disease) and scoliosis. Abnormal posture is also a common cause of back pain. This may be associated with seating that may not offer sufficient back support or wearing high-heeled shoes, which may cause an exaggeration of lumbar lordosis. Additionally, unequal leg length may be present.

Associated risk factors include occupation (e.g. heavy manual work), anxiety, depression and pregnancy.

Lumbar disc disease usually causes root syndromes, because the spinal cord ends at L2. The lumbar nerve root exits high in its foramen and is usually above a prolapsing disc, which compresses the nerve root passing to the interspace immediately below (**Figure 4.33**).

### Clinical features

Clinical features that may help in the diagnosis of back pain are:
- *History of previous trauma*
- *Characteristics of the pain*: acute pain suggests bone or soft-tissue injury; radiating pain, nerve root compression; early morning stiffness, inflammatory arthritis; and neurogenic claudication, characterized by pain on exertion – especially walking – and relieved by rest and stooping forward, suggests spinal stenosis
- *Symptoms of malignancy or systemic infection*
- *Peripheral arthritis*: the spondyloarthropathies
- *Metabolic bone disorders* (e.g. Paget's disease; see Chapter 5, Metabolic bone disease)
- *Aggravating and relieving factors*: coughing and sneezing aggravates compression on nerve roots, whereas bed rest may be beneficial, and anti-inflammatory drugs may relieve inflammatory arthritis

**4**

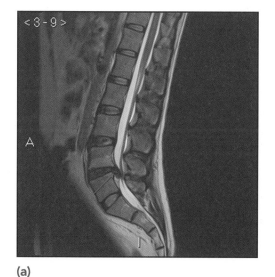

(a)

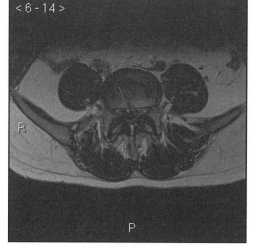

(b)

**Figure 4.33** Prolapsed intervertebral disc. **(a)** Sagittal and **(b)** axial T2-weighted MR images of the lumbar spine in an adult patient. Severe canal stenosis from large prolapsed disc (red arrows) causing compression of the cauda equina roots (blue arrow).

**Table 4.18** Clinical features of inflammatory and mechanical back pain

| Clinical feature | Inflammatory back pain | Mechanical back pain |
|---|---|---|
| Nature | Constant | Precipitated by movement, etc. |
| Onset | Gradual | Sudden |
| Worst pain | On rest or in the morning | Evening |
| Location | Bilateral | Unilateral leg and buttock |
| Morning stiffness | Present | Absent |
| Effect of exercise | Relieves pain | Aggravates pain |
| Relieving factors | Exercise | Rest |

- *Other neurological symptoms*: paraesthesiae indicate nerve route compression and may indicate the level of involvement, while weakness, numbness and bowel or bladder dysfunction suggest significant nerve root or corda equina compression

The contrasting nature, onset, location and characteristics of inflammatory and mechanical back pain are shown in **Table 4.18**.

On examination, spinal alignment, tenderness and movement should be noted. Straight leg raising is useful for eliciting sciatic nerve irritation (L4, L5 and S1 roots). Restriction to 45° or less indicates significant root irritation. The level of the lesion will be revealed by the sensory motor and reflex findings of a neurological examination (**Table 4.19**; see Chapter 13, Neurological Disease).

A prolapsed intervertebral disc is unlikely if:

- There is no evidence of nerve root compression.
- More than one root is involved.
- There is bilateral nerve involvement.
- There is diffuse pain and tenderness.
- Pain is worse on resting.

*Corda equina compression* may result from a central protrusion and causes saddle-shaped sacral anaesthesia, flaccid paralysis of the legs and sphincter involvement. *This is a surgical emergency* (see EMERGENCY PRESENTATION 4.1).

**Table 4.19** Neurological features of lumbar disc prolapse

| Disc (nerve root) | Sensory features (pain and dysthaesia) | Motor signs (weakness and wasting) | Decreased reflexes |
|---|---|---|---|
| L3–4 (L4 root) | Anterior leg, medial foot | Ankle dorsiflexion (tibialis anterior) | Knee |
| L4–5 (L5 root) | Lateral leg and thigh, central foot | Extension of great toe, extensor hallucis longus | Non-specific |
| L5–S1 (S1 root) | Posterior leg, lateral foot | Eversion of foot (peroneals) | Ankle |

## LOW BACK PAIN AT A GLANCE

**Mechanical**
- Prolapsed intervertebral disc
- Vertebral body and apophyseal OA
- Spinal stenosis
- Spondylolisthesis
- Fracture
- Non-specific abnormal posture

**Neoplastic**
- Bone primary or secondary (bone metastases commonly originate from carcinoma of the breast, bronchus, kidney, thyroid and prostate)
- Myeloma
- Spinal cord and coverings

**Inflammation**
- AxSpA and other SpA

**Infection**
- *Mycobacterium tuberculosis*
- *Salmonella*
- *Brucella*

**Metabolic**
- Osteoporosis
- Osteomalacia
- Haemochromatosis
- Ochronosis
- Wilson's disease
- Paget's disease

**Referred pain**
- Pelvic pathology
- GI tract (e.g. pancreatitis)
- Vasculature (e.g. aortic aneurysm)

## Investigation

### Haematology

- *FBC:* may reveal malignancy (e.g. lymphoproliferative disorder such as myeloma) or chronic anaemia (e.g. spondylitis)
- *ESR:* may be increased in infection, an inflammatory arthritis or malignancy

## EMERGENCY PRESENTATION 4.1

**Red flags for possible serious spinal pathology**

Age of presentation > older

Violent trauma

Constant progressive non-mechanical pain

Thoracic pain

Previous history of carcinoma

Systemic steroids

Drug abuse/HIV infection

Systemically unwell

Weight loss

Persisting severe restriction of lumbar flexion

Widespread neurological signs and symptoms

Structural deformity

## Biochemistry

Calcium, phosphate, alkaline phosphatase may reveal evidence of metabolic disease (e.g. osteomalacia, Paget's disease).

## Microbiology and histopathology

Aspiration or biopsy is usually necessary for culture or cytology to identify a source of infection.

## Diagnostic imaging

- *Radiography:* Plain radiographs are rarely helpful, particularly if taken early in the course of an episode of back pain. Plain radiographs may show the degenerative and regenerative changes of OA; osteoporosis, spondylitis, scoliosis or kyphosis; vertebral anomalies (hemivertebrae, spina bifida occulta); vertebral body or pedicle destruction (caused by neoplasia or infection); pathological fracture; or spondylolisthesis (forward subluxation of the body of one vertebra onto the one below, usually at L5/S1.
- *CT scan:* This may be used to visualize the spinal canal.
- *MRI:* This may be used for detecting disc lesions (see **Figure 4.33**).
- *Nuclear medicine imaging:* Although this is useful for detecting infection, it will also appear abnormal in degenerative disease.

## Management

- When there is no evidence of serious underlying disease, a reduction in daily activities may be advised, but total bed rest should be avoided if at all possible (see **Table 4.3**).
- Physiotherapy, particularly to correct posture, and a progressive exercise programme with weight reduction may be useful when acute symptoms have resolved.
- Drug treatment includes diazepam for muscle relaxation, and simple analgesics for pain relief (see **Table 4.4**). NSAIDs and low-dose antidepressants (e.g. amitriptyline) may be useful.
- Transcutaneous nerve stimulation may be used to inhibit the sensation of pain.
- Further medical or surgical treatment may be indicated according to the diagnosis.

## Prognosis

The symptoms of mechanical back pain usually resolve with treatment and at least 92% of acute back pain symptoms will settle within 6 weeks. A few patients develop chronic pain, which is associated with considerable morbidity.

## NECK PAIN

Neck pain is common and probably has a similar prevalence to low back pain.

**Table 4.20** Neurological features of cervical disc prolapse

| Disc | Nerve root | Sensory features | Motor loss | Decreased reflexes |
|------|------------|------------------|------------|--------------------|
| C4–5 | 5 | Neck to outer shoulder and arm | Deltoid | Biceps/ supinator |
| C5–6 | 6 | Outer arm to thumb and index finger | Biceps and brachioradialis | Biceps/ supinator |
| C6–7 | 7 | Posterior forearm to dorsum middle finger | Triceps and forearm extensors | Triceps |
| C7–T1 | 8 | Inner arm to fourth and fifth fingers | Thumb and finger extensors | None |

## Disease mechanisms

The causes of neck pain are similar to those of low back pain and may be summarized as in LOW BACK PAIN AT A GLANCE, except that mechanical pain is limited to OA or prolapsed cervical disc or is non-specific in nature (e.g. posture) and referred pain commonly relates to visceral or cardiovascular disease (e.g. cardiac ischaemia).

## Clinical features

These may be similar to those described for low back pain (see LOW BACK PAIN AT A GLANCE) apart from those features specific to the lumbar spine and pelvis. The cervical spine is specifically involved in RA and AS, and in these conditions, there is a consequent increase in the incidence of atlantoaxial subluxation. The features of cervical disc prolapse may be difficult to diagnose because of the referred nature of pain away from the neck, which is summarized in **Table 4.20**.

## Investigation and management

These are the same as for low back pain.

## DISORDERS OF BONE, CARTILAGE AND CONNECTIVE TISSUE

Bone, cartilage and connective tissue can be involved in a wide variety of pathological conditions, from infection to genetic abnormalities (**Table 4.21**). Examples of the more common conditions are covered in this section, while bone metabolism and metabolic bone disorders are discussed in Chapter 5, Metabolic bone disease.

## OSTEOARTHRITIS

OA is a multifactorial disease and can affect all joints, particularly those that are weight-bearing and frequently used.

**Table 4.21** Disorders of bone, cartilage and connective tissue

OA

Metabolic bone diseases (see Chapter 5, Metabolic bone disease):
- Osteomalacia
- Osteoporosis
- Hyperparathyroidism
- Hypocalcaemia disorders
- Renal bone disease

Bone and joint infection

Paget's disease of bone

Primary tumours of bone and synovium

Ischaemic bone disease:
- Osteonecrosis

Dysplastic bone disease:
- Fibrous dysplasia
- Osteopetrosis
- Achondroplasia
- Hypertrophic osteoarthropathy

Inheritable disorders of connective tissue

Disorders of fibrous elements:
- Osteogenesis imperfecta
- Ehlers–Danlos syndrome
- Marfan's syndrome
- Pseudoxanthoma elasticum

Disorders of proteoglycan metabolism:
- Mucopolysaccharidoses

Inborn errors of metabolism:
- Ochronosis
- Homocystinuria

**Table 4.22** Causes of secondary OA

| Cause | Disorders | |
|---|---|---|
| Mechanical | Congenital and developmental | Hip dysplasia |
| | | Slipped femoral capital epiphysis |
| | | Hypermobility disorders |
| | Trauma | Major trauma |
| | | Repetitive occupational trauma |
| | | Surgery |
| | Bone disease | Paget's disease |
| | | Osteonecrosis (Perthes' disease) |
| | Neuropathic joints | Diabetes mellitus |
| | | Syphilis |
| | | Syringomyelia |
| | Endocrinopathies | Acromegaly |
| | | Cushing's syndrome |
| | Metabolic | CPPD disease |
| | | Gout |
| | | Ochronosis |
| | | Wilson's disease |
| | | Haemochromatosis |
| | Inflammatory arthritis | RA |
| | | Infection |
| Drugs | Intra-articular corticosteroid | |
| Haematological | Haemophilia | |
| | Sickle cell disease | |

*CPPD, calcium pyrophosphate dihydrate.*

## Epidemiology

- Approximately 50% of the population will have clinical symptoms by 60 years of age.
- Prevalence increases with age.
- Under 45 years of age the prevalence is higher in men than in women, between 55 and 75 years it is higher in women, and over 75 years the sex distribution is equal. Women experience more severe hand and knee involvement and greater symptoms.

## Disease mechanisms

OA has a multifactorial aetiology and may result from a primary abnormality, or be secondary to a predisposing factor. Aetiological factors include biochemical abnormalities of cartilage (probably as a result of gene defects), genetic predisposition, obesity and mechanical abnormalities. Causes of secondary OA are listed in **Table 4.22**.

OA involves all joint structures, but characteristic changes affect the cartilage, subchondral bone and synovium:
- Loss of cartilage
- Increased bone and cartilage remodelling
- Patchy synovial inflammation

In view of the proliferative changes described above, OA can be best described as a metabolically active regenerative disease.

Specific changes may occur in the spine where OA affects the two principal joints (the synovial posterior apophyseal joints and the cartilaginous intervertebral discs). Secondary OA may result from mechanical or biochemical abnormalities (**Table 4.22**). It may involve joints not usually affected in primary disease.

## Clinical features

OA results in painful stiff joints with limited movement but, unlike RA, there is no systemic involvement. The pain develops gradually on use and weight-bearing, and is usually limited to only one or a few joints. Stiffness increases with inactivity (gelling), may occur at night, be aggravated by cold or damp and lasts no longer than 30 minutes. Deformity can result from swelling, osteophytes, subluxation and node formation around the IP joints, and is not usually associated with pain. An effusion may also develop.

Primary OA may be:
- *Localized:* consisting only of Heberden's nodes with no other joint involvement

- *Generalized:* involving three or more joints
- *Erosive:* involving the DIP and PIP joints of the hands, with osteophyte and erosive changes on radiography

OA has a characteristic pattern of hand, hip, knee and spine involvement, and this is discussed below and summarized in OSTEOARTHRITIS AT A GLANCE.

### Hand involvement
- Causes flexion and lateral deviation of the DIP joints, and enlargement of the first carpometacarpal (thumb) joint with radial subluxation, giving the hand a square appearance
- Bony swellings: over the DIP joints (Heberden's nodes) and PIP joints (Bouchard's nodes)

### Hip involvement
- Equally common in men and women and often unilateral
- Causes pain in the groin over the greater trochanter, in the buttock or down the inner or anterior thigh
- Standing may be difficult and the patient may limp
- Contralateral disease often develops later

### Knee involvement
- Associated with obesity
- Causes pain on kneeling, climbing stairs and getting in and out of cars
- Medial compartment disease results in a genu varus deformity and instability; patellofemoral disease causes loss of side-to-side patellar mobility and anterior knee pain
- An effusion with inflammation may be associated with a popliteal (Baker's) cyst if intra-articular pressure is raised

### Spine involvement
- May cause localized pain or neurological symptoms, e.g. sciatica

### Acute inflammation
- May result from trauma or crystal-induced (CPPD or hydroxyapatite) deposition
- Bursal inflammation on the medial side of the metatarsal head may cause pain and swelling (a bunion)

## Diagnosis

OA is a clinical diagnosis aided by joint imaging. The main clinical features to note are:
- Characteristic pattern of joint involvement
- Early morning stiffness of 30 minutes or less
- Inactivity-associated joint stiffness (gelling)
- Use-related pain
- Absence of extra-articular manifestations

- Absence of wrist and MCP joint disease, which may distinguish it from RA
- Heberden's and Bouchard's nodes with swelling and erythema

## Investigation

Routine investigations are usually normal in primary OA but are helpful for evaluating associated conditions (e.g. haemochromatosis and Paget's disease) and the causes of secondary OA.

### Diagnostic imaging
- *Joint radiography:* X-ray may reveal specific changes in OA. These are loss of joint space, sclerosis, cysts, osteophytes, soft-tissue swelling, mineral deposits (e.g. CPPD deposition) and calcification within soft tissue deriving from ossicles or loose bodies. There may be complete discordance between radiography and clinical features.
- *MRI:* This is not necessary for most patients. It can identify OA at earlier stages of disease and can assess effusions, the synovium and ligaments.
- *Ultrasound:* This can identify OA-associated structural changes, e.g. synovial inflammation, effusion, osteophytes.

## Management

It is important to determine whether OA is the cause of the patient's complaint. Once this has been done, education and reassurance that the disease has a good prognosis are important. This may help alleviate anxiety and depression.

The treatment of OA is aimed at relieving pain and stiffness, increasing joint mobility, strengthening supporting muscles and helping the patient adapt to any disability. A summary is presented in **Table 4.3**. The following measures need to be considered:
- *Joint rest:* Use of a stick, crutches or walker may help. Weight loss and an occupational change may help too.
- *Physiotherapy:* This helps to relieve pain and stiffness as well as increasing joint mobility and strengthening supporting muscles.
- *Occupational therapy:* This is useful to help the patient adapt to disability, and to provide advice on minimizing joint stress in activities of daily living. Wearing shoes with shock-absorbent soles may be of appreciable benefit.
- *Drug treatment:* This includes analgesics for pain (**Table 4.4**), NSAIDs for inflammation and intra-articular corticosteroids for acute inflammation. Intra-articular hyaluronic acid may be useful to relieve joint pain.
- *Surgery:* This may be necessary to relieve pain, increase range of movement in severe disability or correct any mechanical derangement leading to OA. Total hip and knee replacement can successfully relieve pain but may not increase the range of movement.

**4**

## OSTEOARTHRITIS AT A GLANCE

OA is the most common condition to affect synovial joints and is a major cause of disability.
It is characterized by focal cartilage loss and bone regeneration.
OA has a characteristic pattern of hand, hip, knee and spine involvement.

### Clinical features

*Joint*

- Pain
- Gelling
- Crepitus
- Instability
- Limited movement
- Deformity
- Effusion

### Imaging

*Radiology*

- Loss of joint space, sclerosis, cysts, osteophytes, soft-tissue swelling, chondrocalcinosis

*MRI, CT*

- Useful for visualizing disc prolapse and the neural canal

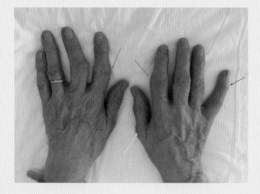

**Figure A** OA primarily affecting the DIP joints with Heberden's nodes (blue arrow), PIP joints (red arrows) and CMC joint (yellow arrow).

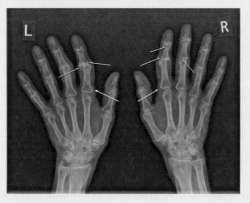

**Figure B** Plain radiograph erosive OA with bilateral symmetrical involvement of the PIP and DIP joints of both hands with splaying of the margins of the base of the middle phalanx of the index fingers (red arrows), central erosions (blue arrow) and marginal proliferation (green arrow) giving a classical 'gull wing appearance'. Well-defined subchondral cysts are noted at the heads of the proximal phalanges at the level of the DIP joints. There is associated soft-tissue swelling. Involvement of the MCP joints is also noted bilaterally (yellow arrow).

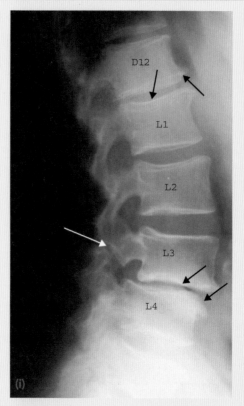

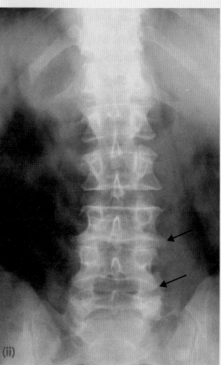

**Figure C** Lumbar spondylitis. **(i)** Anteroposterior and **(ii)** later radiographs of the lumbar spine. At L3/4 there is spondylolisthesis with approximately 1cm anterior displacement of L3 or L4. There is also spondylolysis (white arrow). Degenerative changes are noted in addition (reduction in height of the disc space and marginal osteophyte formation; arrows).

**Table 4.23** Microorganisms and arthritis

| Class | Infection known | Live microorganism | Microbial structures | Examples in joint tissue |
|---|---|---|---|---|
| Infective | Yes | Yes | Yes | Septic arthritides, viral arthritides |
| Reactive | Yes | No | Yes | Arthritides following infection with *Chlamydia*, *Salmonella*, *Yersinia* spp. |
| Inflammatory | No | No | Yes | RA, AS |

## Prognosis

OA progresses slowly and may stop altogether and remain static. Joint failure is rare.

## BONE AND JOINT INFECTION

Microorganisms causing joint and bone disease include bacteria, viruses, fungi and parasites. There are three mechanisms by which they can cause disease:

- Active infection with live organisms
- A reaction induced by inactive or degraded organisms (e.g. *Chlamydia*)
- Inflammation induced by autoactivation of the cellular and/or humoral immune system (e.g. possibly RA and Lyme disease)

For a summary of microorganisms and arthritis, see **Table 4.23**. Bone and joint infection require prompt recognition and treatment (**Table 4.24**).

## ACUTE BACTERIAL ARTHRITIS

Numerous pathogens can cause septic arthritis. The pathogen will depend in part upon the mechanism of infection and predisposing factors. Patients with RA are of greater risk of septic arthritis. Septic arthritis is usually monomicrobial. Staphylococcus aureus is the most common cause of septic arthritis in adults. TB should be suspected in the immunocompromised and if there is involvement of the spine.

### Epidemiology

In adults presenting with one or more acutely painful joints, prevalence has been estimated to be in the range of 8–27%.

**Table 4.24** Recognition and treatment of joint and bone infection

Most patients with septic arthritis present acutely with a red, hot, painful joint.
Gram-positive cocci are the likeliest cause (e.g. *Staphylococcus aureus*), except in very young or immunosuppressed patients.
Aspiration of synovial fluid, biopsy of resected tissue (e.g. bone) and blood cultures should be performed immediately.
Intravenous antibiotics should be given for 2 weeks and oral treatment for a further month if the diagnosis is confirmed.

### Disease mechanisms

- The common causes of infection are listed in **Table 4.23**.
- Infective arthritis is most common at the extremes of life and in immunosuppressed patients.
- Increased susceptibility is associated with diabetes mellitus, cancer, hypogammaglobulinaemia, chronic liver disease, damaged joints (e.g. resulting from RA, trauma or surgery), presence of prosthetic joint and treatment with corticosteroids or immunosuppressive drugs.

### Clinical features

- Patients usually present with a single swollen and painful joint, most commonly the knee, which may be warm with restricted range of movement.
- Most patients will be febrile, except the elderly.

### Diagnosis

- Nucleic acid amplification tests (e.g. polymerase chain reaction [PCR] and MALDI-TOF mass spectrometry) may be useful when routine cultures are negative. The likelihood of septic arthritis increases as the synovial fluid leucocyte count increases.
- Histology and microbiology of a synovial biopsy may be valuable, especially for diagnosing *Mycobacterium tuberculosis* infection, as these organisms are difficult to grow from synovial fluid. Needle biopsy of the spine or sacroiliac joint may be necessary if infection is suspected at these sites.
- Osteomyelitis should be suspected if the area of maximal tenderness extends beyond the joint. It is important to begin treatment early to prevent joint destruction.

### Management

Treatment consists of joint drainage and antibiotic therapy. Joint drainage may include needle aspiration, arthroscopy or open surgical drainage. Initial choice of empiric antimicrobial therapy should cover the most likely pathogens. The duration of therapy is tailored to individual clinical circumstances.

## ACUTE OSTEOMYELITIS

The metaphysis has a rich blood supply and a slow circulation time and phagocytic activity at sinusoid endothelial levels is reduced. Bacterial adherence and multiplication in the metaphysis are therefore favoured. Osteomyelitis is more common in children and young adults. The bone may be locally tender to touch and there may be swelling and warmth.

## CHRONIC OSTEOMYELITIS

### Clinical features

- Chronic osteomyelitis is usually post-traumatic or postoperative and the long tubular bones in the lower extremities are most often affected. In adults, chronic osteomyelitis usually occurs following trauma or surgery. The postoperative infection rate for prosthetic surgery is less than 2%.
- There is usually pain, swelling and increased temperature associated with the affected area, and there may be pyrexia. However, there may be pain without inflammatory signs or a sinus.
- Skeletal malformation is common.
- Subacute osteomyelitis is referred to as a Brodie's abscess (**Figure 4.34**).
- The recurrence rate is high (10–20%) and definitive healing is uncommon, even after adequate treatment.

### Diagnosis

- *Joint radiography:* This commonly shows soft-tissue swelling and joint distension, and later juxta-articular osteoporosis, periosteal elevation, joint space narrowing, bony erosions and possibly osteomyelitis (**Figure 4.35**). Spine changes may not be seen for a few months, but typically the disc space or vertebra is narrowed and there is bone proliferation at the vertebral margins. Lytic lesions in the vertebra may extend to the disc. Adjacent vertebrae may fuse during healing.
- *Chest radiography:* This is required to detect pneumonia.

- *CT and MRI:* When cord compression is suspected, CT/MRI can be helpful. MRI can provide multiplanar images of the spine and surrounding soft tissues.

### Management

The initial choice of antibiotics for treatment is based on the Gram stain. Treatment may change as culture and susceptibility results become available. For a summary of management of infective diseases, see **Table 4.24**.

### Prognosis

Full recovery without joint damage is usual if treated promptly.

## VIRAL ARTHRITIS

Some viral infections are accompanied by arthritis more often than others (e.g. rubella, parvovirus, hepatitis, arboviruses, mumps, chickenpox, HIV: see Chapter 3, Infectious disease).

### Rubella arthritis and arthralgias

- These may occur in up to 50% of infected women, compared with up to 6% of men; it is uncommon in children.
- Live virus and viral antigens have been detected in synovial fluid. The symptoms of arthritis occur within 1 week of the rash.
- The fingers, wrists, elbows, knees, and hip and toe joints are most commonly affected, usually asymmetrically. Tenosynovitis and carpal tunnel syndrome may occur. The arthritis usually resolves in approximately 30 days.

### Parvovirus B19

- This usually causes acute benign self-limiting disease, but it may be associated with rheumatoid-like polyarthritis.

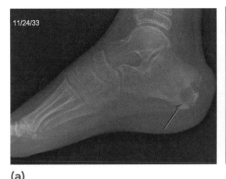
(a)

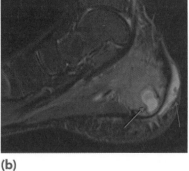
(b)

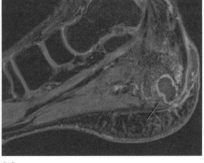
(c)

**Figure 4.34 (a)** Lateral projection plain radiograph of a paediatric foot. Intraosseous lucent foci on both sides of the calcaneal epiphysis (red arrow), typical of a Brodie's abscess. **(b)** Sagittal fat-suppressed MR image of a paediatric foot. Brodie's abscess in the calcaneus (red arrow) extending across the physis. Note further effusion in the subcutaneous calcaneal bursa (pre-Achilles bursa) – blue arrow. **(c)** Post contrast sagittal MR image in the same patient demonstrating enhancement of the periphery of the abscess in the calcaneus (red arrow).

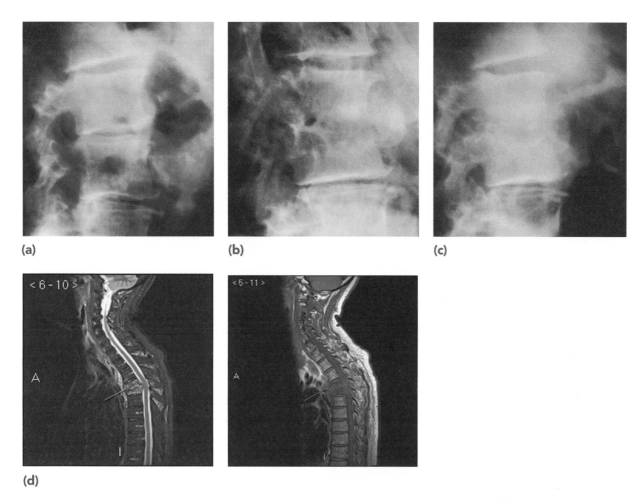

(a)                   (b)                 (c)

(d)

**Figure 4.35** Radiographs showing the development of infective discitis. The initial radiograph **(a)** shows early bony destruction of the anteroinferior aspect of L2 (arrow). Subsequent radiographs **(b,c)** show destruction of the end plates and adjacent vertebral bodies of L2 and L3. **(d)** Sagittal STIR and T1-weighted MR images of the upper spine. Severe discitis of the thoracic spine with end plate destruction (red arrow) and a large paravertebral large paravertebral mass/phlegmon (blue arrow). **(a–c)** reproduced from Axford JS. Joint and bone infections. *Medicine* 2002; 30:9 by kind permission of the Medicine Publishing Company.

**4**

- There may be symmetrical polyarthritis in association with erythema infectiosum (fifth disease), which gives a 'slapped-cheek' appearance.
- Rheumatic symptoms occur in 95% of infected children and may also affect adults; they are more common in women.

## PRIMARY TUMOURS OF BONE AND SYNOVIUM

Primary tumours of bone and synovium are rare (**Table 4.25**). Most are benign.

Secondary malignant tumours may be complications of primary bone sarcomas or metastatic tumours, or result from invasion by leukaemia, lymphoma or myeloma. Primary tumours of the lung, breast and colon are the most common sources, and pain is a common feature.

**Table 4.25** Common tumours of bone and synovium

| Type | Benign/ malignant | Tumour |
|---|---|---|
| Bone-forming | Benign | Osteoma |
| | | Osteoid osteoma |
| | Malignant | Osteosarcoma (**Figure 4.36**) |
| Cartilage-forming | Benign | Chondroma |
| | Malignant | Chondrosarcoma |
| Marrow tumour | Malignant | Ewing's sarcoma |
| | | Lymphoma |
| | | Myeloma |
| Synovial tumour | Benign | Pigmented villonodular synovitis |
| | Malignant | Synovial sarcoma |

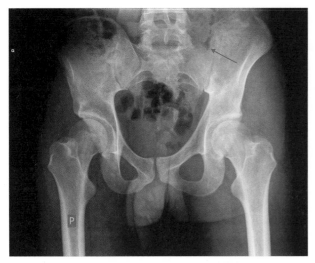

(a)

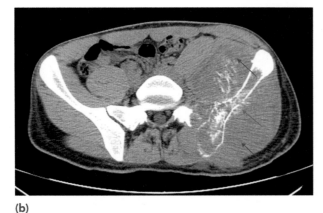

(b)

**Figure 4.36** Osteosarcoma of the ilium. **(a)** Plain AP radiograph of the pelvis. Bony destruction of the left sacral ala (red arrow). **(b)** Axial CT image of the pelvis of the same patient demonstrates a destructive lesion of the left ilium with 'sunburn' periosteal reaction (blue arrow) and a large extraosseous soft tissue mass extending into the left iliacus and gluteal muscles (red arrows).

## ISCHAEMIC BONE DISEASE

### OSTEONECROSIS

Osteonecrosis is a term given to cell death within bone and may be caused by a number of conditions, most of which lead to an impaired blood supply. The femoral head is commonly involved, although other bones may be affected (e.g. carpal scaphoid).

Osteonecrosis may be caused by trauma, but may also be associated with certain diseases (**Table 4.26**). There is an idiopathic group of conditions associated with osteonecrosis that occur predominantly in childhood.

**Table 4.26** Causes of ischaemic bone disease

**Traumatic**
- Head of femur
- Carpal scaphoid (wrist)
- Knee joint (osteochondritis dissecans)

**Non-traumatic (associated with specific diseases)**
- Drugs: corticosteroid, bisphosphonate
- Autoimmune disease: lupus, APS
- Acute lymphoblastic leukaemia
- Endocrine: Cushing's disease, corticosteroid therapy
- Storage disease (e.g. Gaucher's disease)
- Decompression sickness (e.g. Caisson's disease)
- Pancreatitis
- Haemoglobinopathies (e.g. sickle cell disease)
- Transplantation

**Conditions associated with childhood**
- Osgood–Schlatter disease (tibial tuberosity)
- Perthes' disease (hip)
- Sever's disease (os calcis)
- Slipped femoral epiphysis

### Clinical features

Symptoms include pain, swelling, crepitus and mechanical locking, depending upon location.

### Investigation

MRI and radiography may be diagnostic.

### Management

Management involves pain relief, physiotherapy and surgery.

## INHERITABLE DISORDERS OF CONNECTIVE TISSUE

Molecular biology has led to significant advances in our understanding of the aetiology of these primary connective-tissue disorders. Gene mutations for connective tissue proteins have been associated with a variety of disorders, which are classified according to their phenotype, as shown in **Table 4.27**.

## DISORDERS OF FIBROUS ELEMENTS

### Osteogenesis imperfecta

Osteogenesis imperfecta can be classified into four types using clinical and inheritance pattern criteria. All are characterized by bone, ocular, dental, aural and cardiovascular involvement, and brittle bones, to a varying degree. Limbs may be short and bent at birth. Blue sclera and deafness may also be features. The diagnosis can usually be made clinically (**Figure 4.37**).

**Table 4.27** Classification of inheritable disorders of connective tissue according to phenotype

| Phenotype | Inheritable connective-tissue disorder |
|---|---|
| Disorders of fibrous elements | Osteogenesis imperfecta |
| | Ehlers–Danlos syndrome |
| | Marfan's syndrome |
| | Pseudoxanthoma elasticum |
| Disorders of proteoglycan metabolism | Mucopolysaccharidoses |
| Osteochondrodysplasias | Achondroplasia |
| | Spondyloepiphyseal and metaphyseal dysplasias |
| Inborn errors of metabolism | Homocystinuria |
| | Ochronosis |

## Ehlers–Danlos syndrome

### Clinical features

These involve joints, skin, vessels and internal organs:

- *Joints:* There may be hyperextensibility of large or small joints, which can dislocate.
- *Skin:* This may be soft with a velvet-like texture and hyperextensible. 'Cigarette paper scars' may occur because of its fragility, and there may be easy bruising.

- *Vessels and organs:* There may be life-threatening arterial rupture and rupture of the colon or uterus.

## Marfan's syndrome

Marfan's syndrome was the first inheritable connective tissue disorder to be described.

### Clinical features

Marfan's syndrome is characterized by musculoskeletal, cardiovascular and ocular features:

- *Musculoskeletal:* This is characterized by tall stature and abnormal body proportions – a long arm span and an abnormally low ratio of upper segment to lower segment – and elongated digits (**Figure 4.38**). Other musculoskeletal features include anterior thoracic deformity (pectus excavatum and carinatum); abnormal vertebral column curvature (loss of thoracic kyphosis and scoliosis); hyperextensibility or contracture of peripheral joints; and pes planus, with long narrow feet.
- *Cardiovascular:* There is ascending aortic dilatation, which may result in aortic regurgitation and dissection; mitral valve prolapse resulting in mitral regurgitation.
- *Ocular:* There may be myopia and subluxation of the lens.

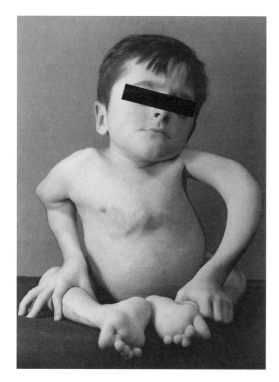

**Figure 4.37** A child with the skeletal features of osteogenesis imperfecta.

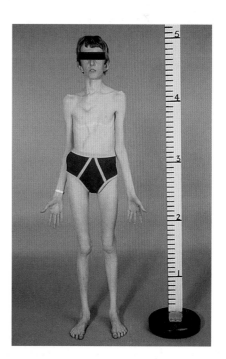

**Figure 4.38** Marfan's syndrome.

4

## MUST-KNOW CHECKLIST

- That there are genetic and environmental influences predisposing to arthritis
- The common major presenting clinical features of rheumatic diseases
- Blood tests used in diagnosis
- Imaging techniques used in diagnosis
- What analgesics and NSAIDs to use and their side effects
- When to use drugs that suppress rheumatic disease and their side effects
- How to diagnose and treat bone and joint infection
- Supportive treatment available for patients (e.g. educational resources, physiotherapy and occupational therapy)
- The importance of eye examination in JIA
- Important factors (red flags) in the diagnosis of back disease

**Questions and answers** to test your understanding of Chapter 4 can be found by clicking 'Support Material' at the following link: https://www.routledge.com/Medicine-for-Finals-and-Beyond/Axford-OCallaghan/p/book/9780367150594

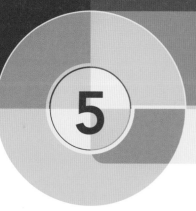

# Metabolic Bone Disease

JEFFREY LEE

## INTRODUCTION

Metabolic bone diseases are a group of disorders characterized by abnormal calcium metabolism and/or bone cell physiology leading to altered serum calcium concentration and/or skeletal failure.

## STRUCTURE AND FUNCTION

### STRUCTURE OF BONE

Bone consists of an extracellular matrix and cellular constituents which maintain bone formation and resorption throughout life with the net balance determining bone loss/growth.

### EXTRACELLULAR MATRIX

*Type I collagen and calcium/phosphate-containing crystals* provide most of the tensile strength and rigidity in bone.

### CELLULAR CONSTITUENTS

- *Mesenchymal-derived osteoblast lineage:* This consists of osteoblasts, osteocytes and bone-lining cells. Osteoblasts synthesize the organic matrix of new bone.
- *Osteoclasts:* These resorb bone tissue by local release of hydrolase enzymes.

### ANATOMY OF BONE

- *Cortical bone:* This is dense skeletal tissue on the external surface which contributes to most of the mechanical strength.
- *Trabecular bone:* Within the vertebrae and the ends of long bones, the trabecular (cancellous) bone acts as the body's reservoir for calcium.

### FUNCTION OF BONE

Bone has two main functions: to provide an endoskeleton and to act as a reservoir for body calcium.

### CALCIUM MEASUREMENT

Most calcium is bound to plasma proteins. To determine ionized serum calcium (biologically active):

- Add/subtract 0.02 mmol to the total calcium level for every g/L that the albumin is below/above 40 g/L.

### AGENTS IN BONE HOMEOSTASIS

#### Parathyroid hormone

Parathyroid hormone (PTH) is an 84 amino acid polypeptide secreted by the parathyroid gland in response to hypocalcaemia (**Figure 5.1**). It increases serum calcium by:

- Stimulating calcium release from bone by increasing osteoclast bone resorption

DOI: 10.1201/9781003193616-5

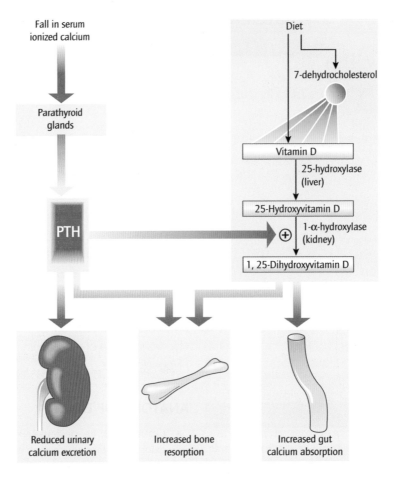

**Figure 5.1** Regulation of calcium metabolism by PTH and vitamin D. PTH and vitamin D are the principal hormones responsible for calcium homoeostasis. Note that these two regulatory mechanisms are interdependent because of the stimulatory action of PTH on renal 1-α-hydroxylase.

- Promoting renal tubular calcium reabsorption and phosphate excretion
- Enhancing renal conversion of 25-hydroxyvitamin D (25-OH-D) to 1,25-dihydroxyvitamin D $(1,25\text{-}(OH)_2\text{-}D)$

### Vitamin D

Vitamin D is a steroid hormone, which is largely produced in the skin from 7-dehydrocholesterol after exposure to sunlight.

The active form $(1,25\text{-}(OH)_2\text{-}D)$, produced by successive hydroxylations in the liver and kidney by the enzymes 25-hydroxylase and 1-α-hydroxylas respectively, increases serum calcium by:

- Increasing calcium and phosphate absorption from the proximal small intestine
- Stimulating calcium release from bone

### Other agents

- *Calcitonin:* Produced by thyroid gland parafollicular cells, this helps lower serum calcium and phosphate by mainly inhibiting osteoclast function. Its release is coupled to serum calcium.

- *Receptor activator of NFκB ligand (RANKL):* This is a protein produced by numerous cells which activates osteoclast differentiation and activation.
- *Sclerostin:* This is a protein produced by osteocytes inhibiting osteoblast function. Its production is inhibited by mechanical loading, PTH and stimulated by calcitonin.
- *Other hormones:* Steroids such as glucocorticoids, oestrogen and androgens have an important influence on bone metabolism (particularly with ageing).

## APPROACH TO THE PATIENT

### HISTORY AND EXAMINATION

In metabolic bone disease, the findings of the history and examination vary according to the metabolic bone disease in question (detailed individually in the following pages). In general, people with chronic diseases such as osteomalacia or osteoporosis present with features specific to the musculoskeletal system such as bone pain and deformity (**Table 5.1**). In contrast, people with disorders of short duration, such

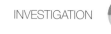

**Table 5.1** Musculoskeletal abnormalities in rickets and osteomalacia

Hypotonia, proximal muscle weakness and waddling gait
Impaired skeletal growth
Bowing deformity of long bones
Rib deformities:
• Prominence of costochondral junction (rachitic rosary)
• Indentation of the lower ribs (Harrison's groove)
Kyphosis and lordosis of the thoracolumbar spine
Skull abnormalities:
• Softened calvarium (craniotabes)
• Parietal flattening and frontal bossing
Delayed eruption of permanent dentition and enamel defects

as hypercalcaemia of malignancy, tend to present with an acute disturbance in calcium metabolism (**Table 5.2** and **Table 5.3**). Family history may reveal details of rare familial metabolic bone diseases as well.

## INVESTIGATION

### BIOCHEMISTRY

Serum biochemistry results are frequently diagnostic of the underlying metabolic bone disease (**Table 5.4**).

• *Serum creatinine:* This may be elevated in associated chronic renal failure, multiple myeloma, or dehydration from hypercalcaemia.

**Table 5.2** Clinical features of hypercalcaemia

| System | Feature |
| --- | --- |
| Neurological and psychiatric | Drowsiness and altered conscious level |
| | Headache |
| | Sleep disturbance |
| | Depression |
| | Muscle weakness |
| | Hyporeflexia |
| Renal | Polyuria |
| | Polydipsia |
| | Nephrolithiasis |
| | Nephrocalcinosis |
| | Renal impairment |
| Gastrointestinal | Constipation |
| | Nausea and anorexia |
| | Peptic ulceration |
| | Pancreatitis |
| Cardiovascular | Hypertension |
| | ECG abnormalities (shortened QT interval, first-degree heart block) |
| Articular | Chondrocalcinosis |
| | Gout |
| Miscellaneous | Pruritus and skin necrosis |
| | Bank keratopathy |

**Table 5.3** Clinical features of hypocalcaemia

| System | Feature |
| --- | --- |
| Neurological and psychiatric | Peripheral paraesthesia |
| | Circumoral numbness |
| | Tetany: |
| | • Cramp-like spasms |
| | • Laryngeal stridor |
| | • Chvostek's and Trousseau's signs |
| | Convulsions |
| | Anxiety |
| | Psychosis |
| | Basal ganglia and/or extrapyramidal calcification |
| Cardiovascular | ECG abnormalities (prolonged QT interval) |
| Ocular | Papilloedema |
| | Cataracts (if long-standing) |

• *Serum calcium, phosphate and PTH* (see **Table 5.4**): Serum calcium may be increased (hypercalcaemia, **Table 5.5**), normal (in osteoporosis) or decreased (hypocalcaemia, **Table 5.6**).
• *Serum alkaline phosphatase (ALP):* This is increased when there is osteoblastic hyperactivity (e.g. osteomalacia, hyperparathyroidism).
• *Serum 25-OH-D:* 25-OH-D serum levels are measured as it is a better indicator of vitamin D status compared to other vitamin D metabolites.
• *Bone markers:* Urinary and serum markers such as serum procollagen 1 N-terminal propeptide indicate the level of bone turnover and are used to assess response to treatments in osteoporosis and Paget's disease.

### DIAGNOSTIC IMAGING

#### Plain radiography

Fractures and characteristic features of conditions such as Paget's disease or Looser's zones may be seen.

#### Isotope bone scan

Skeletal scintigraphy involves injecting technetium ($^{97}$Tc) which is taken up by osteoblastic activity. Widespread uptake is most commonly due to bony metastases but also occurs in osteomalacia (Looser's zones) and Paget's disease; local uptake can be seen with fractures.

#### Bone densitometry

As there is a significant correlation between bone strength and bone mineral density (BMD), a number of techniques are used to quantify BMD as a surrogate marker for bone health/fragility. The current standard is dual energy X-ray absorptiometry (DXA). DXA measures BMD centrally (spinal BMD) and peripherally (hip and/or forearm BMD).

**Table 5.4** Serum biochemistry in metabolic bone disease

| Disease | Calcium | Phosphate | ALP | PTH |
|---|---|---|---|---|
| Osteomalacia | N or ↓ | ↓ | ↑ | ↑ |
| Osteoporosis | N | N | N | N |
| Hyperparathyroidism | ↑ | ↓ | ↑ | ↑ |
| Hypercalcaemia of malignancy | ↑ | N or ↓ | N or ↑ | ↓ |
| Hypoparathyroidism | ↓ | ↑ | N | ↓ |

↑ Increased; ↓ decreased; ALP, alkaline phosphatase; N, normal; PTH, parathyroid hormone.

## HISTOPATHOLOGY

### Bone biopsy

Because metabolic bone diseases generally affect the whole skeleton, a bone biopsy at the iliac crest can be carried out to determine underlying pathology. Its use is rare for metabolic bone diseases and tends to be for focal bone lesions.

## DISEASES AND THEIR MANAGEMENT

### RICKETS AND OSTEOMALACIA

Rickets and osteomalacia are childhood and adult diseases respectively due to vitamin D deficiency. Rickets results when defective mineralization during skeletal growth leads to impaired epiphyseal growth plate calcification and bony deformity (which does not occur in osteomalacia).

### Epidemiology

- Osteomalacia and rickets brought about by dietary deficiency are relatively common.
- They occur in childhood (rickets) and the elderly (particularly housebound).
- Osteomalacia is relatively common among Asian immigrants in the UK.
- Genetic involvement is rare, e.g. congenital renal 1-α-hydroxylase deficiency, hypophosphatasia, hereditary renal tubular disorders.

- Vitamin D deficiency is most frequently seen in countries where reduced sunlight exposure is common.

### Disease mechanisms

The cause of osteomalacia and rickets is usually a reduced serum level of 1,25-$(OH)_2$-D. This results in lowering of the calcium-phosphate product leading to impaired matrix mineralization.

There are many causes of reduced 1,25-$(OH)_2$-D levels (**Table 5.7**) with insufficient dietary intake of vitamin D associated with reduced skin synthesis from reduced sunlight exposure being the commonest reason. Rarely, rickets and osteomalacia can be due to non-vitamin D causes (e.g. excessive use of phosphate-binding antacids).

Childhood rickets is rare since the widespread supplementation of food and milk with vitamin D. However, osteomalacia is relatively common among the elderly, and the housebound and institutionalized.

Rickets leads to impaired epiphyseal growth in children; in osteomalacia, unmineralized osteoid compromises the mechanical strength of the skeleton.

### Clinical features

- The clinical features of rickets are impaired skeletal growth, bony deformities, weakness and symptoms of hypocalcaemia (see RICKETS AND OSTEOMALACIA: CLINICAL FEATURES AT A GLANCE, **Table 5.1** and **Table 5.3**).

**Table 5.5** Causes of hypercalcaemia

| |
|---|
| Primary hyperparathyroidism |
| Tertiary hyperparathyroidism |
| Solid and haematological tumours |
| Thiazides |
| Lithium |
| Theophylline toxicity |
| Vitamin A/D intoxication |
| Sarcoidosis |
| Tuberculosis |
| Histoplasmosis |
| Multiple endocrine neoplasia (MEN) 1 and 2 |
| Familial hypocalciuric hypercalcaemia (FHH) |
| Prolonged immobilization |
| Paget's disease of bone |

**Table 5.6** Causes of hypocalcaemia

| |
|---|
| Vitamin D deficiency or malabsorption |
| Impaired vitamin D metabolism: |
| • Chronic renal failure |
| • Chronic liver failure |
| • Phenytoin |
| • Congenital renal 1-α-hydroxylase deficiency |
| PTH resistance |
| Hypoparathyroidism |
| Hypomagnesaemia |
| Pseudohypoparathyroidism |
| Phosphate therapy |
| Acute rhabdomyolysis |
| Pancreatitis |
| Massive citrated blood transfusion |

**5**

**Table 5.7** Causes of rickets and osteomalacia

Increased vitamin D requirements in childhood because of skeletal growth

Poor diet combined with reduced sunlight exposure

Gastric surgery

Small bowel malabsorption syndrome (e.g. coeliac disease)

Chronic cholestasis

Chronic pancreatic insufficiency

Chronic renal failure

Chronic liver failure

Drugs (e.g. phenytoin, barbiturates)

Congenital renal 1-α-hydroxylase deficiency (vitamin D-dependent rickets)

Fluoride therapy

Bisphosphonates

Aluminium antacids

Hypophosphataemia

Isolated renal tubular defects in phosphate handling (e.g. X-linked hypophosphataemic vitamin D-dependent rickets)

Urinary phosphate wasting resulting from a generalized renal tubular defect (Fanconi's syndrome)

Distal renal tubular acidosis

Hypophosphatasia (inherited ALP deficiency)

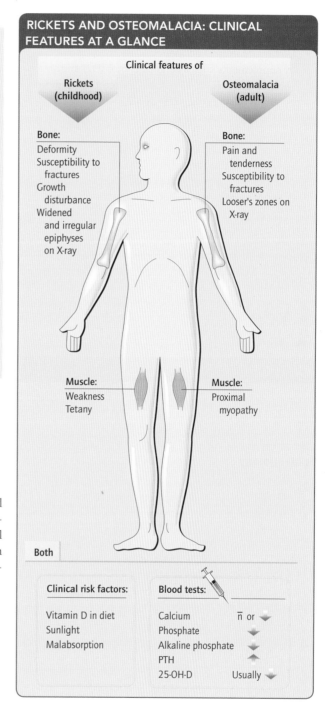

**RICKETS AND OSTEOMALACIA: CLINICAL FEATURES AT A GLANCE**

Clinical features of

Rickets (childhood)

Osteomalacia (adult)

**Bone:**
Deformity
Susceptibility to fractures
Growth disturbance
Widened and irregular epiphyses on X-ray

**Bone:**
Pain and tenderness
Susceptibility to fractures
Looser's zones on X-ray

**Muscle:**
Weakness
Tetany

**Muscle:**
Proximal myopathy

Both

| Clinical risk factors: | Blood tests: | |
|---|---|---|
| Vitamin D in diet | Calcium | $\bar{n}$ or ⬇ |
| Sunlight | Phosphate | ⬇ |
| Malabsorption | Alkaline phosphate | ⬇ |
| | PTH | ⬆ |
| | 25-OH-D | Usually ⬇ |

• Osteomalacia is characterized by widespread bone pain, muscle weakness, proximal myopathy and an increased fracture risk.

## Diagnosis

Childhood rickets can present with characteristic skeletal deformities. However, the clinical manifestations of osteomalacia in the adult are relatively non-specific (proximal myopathy, bone pain). Although radiographical changes such as Looser's zones may be seen, osteomalacia is most commonly diagnosed from serum biochemistry (see **Table 5.4**).

## Investigation

• If vitamin D deficiency is confirmed, further investigation to detect malabsorption is indicated if dietary deficiency and poor sunlight exposure is not found.

• If vitamin D levels are normal in a child with rickets, primary urinary phosphate wasting should be suspected and studies of renal tubular function should be carried out.

### *Biochemistry*

• *Serum calcium:* usually at the lower end, although can be normal due to compensatory secondary hyperparathyroidism

• *Serum phosphate:* reduced in the absence of renal failure

• *Serum ALP + PTH:* see **Table 5.4**

• *Serum 25-OH-D:* usually reduced; may be normal in abnormal vitamin D metabolism (e.g. in chronic renal failure)

### *Diagnostic imaging*

Plain radiography may show:

• Appearance of low density because of impaired mineralization

• Bone deformity and widened irregular epiphyses in rickets

• Pseudofractures (Looser's zones), which are insufficiency stress fractures in osteomalacia commonly seen at scapulae, ribs, pubic rami and proximal femur

## Management

### Dietary deficiency of vitamin D

- Dietary vitamin D deficiency is readily corrected by supplements such as ergocalciferol (D2) and cholecalciferol (D3), with cholecalciferol being more potent in raising serum 25-OH-D.
- Body stores of vitamin D can be replenished by administering oral doses of cholecalciferol (vitamin $D_3$), which has a high oral bioavailability.
- In vitamin D malabsorption, it can be given parenterally (intramuscular) or, alternatively, small doses of more potent metabolites such as calcitriol $(1,25\text{-}(OH)_2\text{-}D)$ and alfacalcidol $(1\text{-}\alpha\text{-}OH\text{-}vitamin\ D)$ may be used.

### Osteomalacia associated with renal disease

In chronic renal disease, there is often significant $1\text{-}\alpha$-hydroxylase deficiency and so $\alpha$-hydroxylated vitamin derivatives (e.g. calcitriol or alfacalcidol) should be prescribed.

**Table 5.8** Causes of secondary osteoporosis

| |
|---|
| Cushing's disease |
| Thyrotoxicosis |
| Hypogonadism |
| Hyperparathyroidism |
| Glucocorticoids |
| Heparin |
| Antiepileptics |
| Depot-progestogen injections |
| Antiretrovirals |
| Aromatase Inhibitors |
| Rheumatoid arthritis |
| Ankylosing spondylitis |
| Ulcerative colitis |
| Chronic obstructive pulmonary disease (COPD) |
| Low BMI |
| Primary biliary cirrhosis |
| Osteogenesis imperfecta |
| Chronic renal failure |
| Immobilization (e.g. long-term bed rest) |

## OSTEOPOROSIS

Osteoporosis can be defined as a decrease in the quantity of bone that compromises its mechanical function (as opposed to defective mineralization of bone matrix in osteomalacia).

### Epidemiology

- Worldwide, 1 in 3 women and 1 in 5 men over the age of 50 will suffer an osteoporotic fracture.
- Prevalence increases with age.
- Osteoporotic fractures at all sites are more common in women than men (female to male ratio of 1:6). However, men have a higher mortality rate with fragility fractures and there is an 80% chance of a secondary cause.
- The incidence of osteoporotic fractures is similar in different ethnic groups living in the same country, except in Afro-Caribbeans in whom it is relatively low.
- There may be a family history, and twin studies suggest a significant genetic component.
- Osteoporosis is most common in developed countries.

### Classification

#### Postmenopausal osteoporosis

Postmenopausal (or primary) osteoporosis accounts for the majority of cases. Bone loss is relatively rapid (up to 10–20%) in the first 5–6 years of menopause with loss mainly from trabecular bone (due to increased bone resorption from oestrogen deficiency) followed by a later slower loss of both cortical and trabecular bone, mainly due to reduced bone formation. A low adult peak bone mass further contributes to subsequent disease severity.

#### Secondary osteoporosis

Secondary osteoporosis develops as a result of a disorder known to cause osteoporosis. Premature ovarian failure and glucocorticoid treatments are commonest (**Table 5.8**).

#### Localized osteoporosis

Localized osteoporosis frequently develops where a limb is immobilized (e.g. after fracture, paraplegia). It may also occur in algodystrophy (reflex sympathetic dystrophy) after a precipitating event such as trauma.

### Disease mechanisms

Osteoporosis arises as a result of a low peak bone mass and/or excessive bone loss.

- *Low peak bone mass:* Insufficient bone tissue is formed during skeletal development. This may be because of genetic or environmental factors such as eating disorders and oestrogen deficiencies.
- *Excessive bone loss:* Bone loss may be excessive, resulting from elevated bone resorption and/or reduced bone formation (e.g. postmenopause, smoking, heavy alcohol intake).

### Clinical features

- *Vertebral body osteoporosis*: This leads to wedge fractures of the vertebral body to complete vertebral body collapse. Patients present either with sudden pain during an episode of vertebral collapse, or with a progressive kyphotic deformity ('silent vertebral fractures' leading to a dowager's hump). The cumulative effect of vertebral collapse may reduce mobility, restrict lung capacity and is a risk for further fractures.

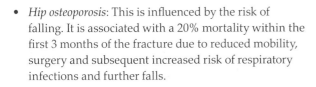

- *Hip osteoporosis*: This is influenced by the risk of falling. It is associated with a 20% mortality within the first 3 months of the fracture due to reduced mobility, surgery and subsequent increased risk of respiratory infections and further falls.

## Diagnosis

Osteoporosis should be considered when a person in a high-risk group for osteoporosis (e.g. postmenopausal women) presents with a fracture at the hip, wrist, humerus or vertebral bodies associated with relatively low levels of trauma (e.g. falling from standing height).

## Differential diagnosis

Secondary causes of osteoporosis should be excluded by further investigations, particularly in those with severe osteoporosis, young age (e.g. premenopausal women) or male gender.

## Investigation

### Biochemistry

Serum ALP may be marginally elevated if there has been a recent fracture.

### Diagnostic imaging

- *Plain radiography:* for the diagnosis of fractures
- *Isotope bone scan:* multiple areas of uptake throughout the skeleton may suggest malignancy; can be used to determine if a fracture is acute or chronic
- *DXA:* used as a means of assessing fracture risk in those with fragility risk factors for preventive therapy

### Fracture risk assessment tools

Online calculators have been developed since 2008 to further define the risk of fractures in an individual.

- *FRAX:* This is a 10-year probability of fracture based on clinical risk factors and BMD score. The calculator is region-specific worldwide.
- *Q fracture:* This is an online algorithm developed from the primary care database in the UK using clinical risk factors to calculate fracture risk.

## Management of acute vertebral collapse

Initially, this should be treated with rest and analgesia followed by early mobilization. Calcitonin or IV bisphosphonates may be given during acute episodes to relieve bone pain. In severe cases where conservative measures have failed to resolve, kyphoplasty is used successfully. Measures to prevent further osteoporotic is essential after dealing with the acute episode.

## Prevention of postmenopausal osteoporosis

### Lifestyle modification

Encouraging people to stop smoking, drink in moderation, take regular exercise and improve their dietary intake of calcium and vitamin D is essential in at-risk groups.

### Medical therapy

Several drugs are available for the prevention and treatment of postmenopausal osteoporosis.

- *Bisphosphonates:* These are the most widely used drugs to treat osteoporosis. They are antiresorptives inhibiting osteoclast function and are usually given for a limited number of years with a drug-free holiday due to the their long duration of action and association with side effects such as atypical femoral fractures.
- *Hormone replacement therapy:* This is used particularly in women with early menopause. Its use in older women is limited usually to those who have menopausal symptoms since the risk/benefits do not favour use for osteoporosis alone.
- *Selective oestrogen receptor modulators:* These are antiresorptive and have an increased risk for thromboembolism.
- *Denosumab:* This is a monoclonal antibody that binds RANKL and inhibits osteoclast function.
- *Anabolic agents:* These are normally used in clinical situations where antiresorptives have failed, led to antiresorptive side effects (e.g. atypical fractures) or when the underlying disease process is mainly due to poor bone formation.
- Teriparatide is a recombinant form of PTH. Although chronically elevated PTH in hyperparathyroidism leads to bone loss, intermittent daily boluses of teriparatide have an anabolic effect by activating osteoblasts.
- Romosozumab is a monoclonal antibody directed against sclerostin acting as both an anabolic agent and, indirectly, as an antiresorptive.

### Calcium and vitamin D supplementation

*Both supplements are essential,* particulary in the elderly who are frail or institutionalized (likely vitamin D-deficient) and patients on osteoporosis medications.

### Falls risk assessment and advice

In this population, there is not only increased skeletal fragility but an increased risk of falling.

## PAGET'S DISEASE OF BONE

Paget's disease of bone (**Figure 5.2**) is a focal disorder of bone remodelling that results in a disorganized structure of woven and lamellar bone.

### Epidemiology

- Paget's disease of bone affects approximately 3.6% of the population over 40 years of age in the UK. Its prevalence has been decreasing in the last decade, particularly in European countries.
- Patients are typically over the age of 55 years.
- 60% of patients are male.

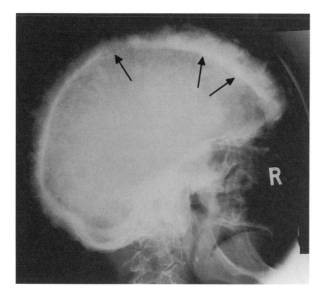

**Figure 5.2** Radiograph demonstrating Paget's disease of bone. There is thickening of the skull vault and regions of lucency and sclerosis (arrows).

- It occurs predominantly in populations of British descent (e.g. Australia, USA). It is rare in Scandinavian and Asian countries.
- 10–20% of patients have a family history of the disorder. The best known genetic association is with mutations in the *SQSTM1* gene.

### Disease mechanisms

- Skeletal lesions are characterized by initial focal increased osteoclastic bone resorption followed by accelerated bone formation leading to a mosaic of woven and lamellar bone.
- Measles virus and other viruses have been suggested as possible causative agents.

### Clinical features

- The main presenting symptom is bone pain. About 30% of pagetic lesions are associated with pain.
- The most commonly affected sites, in order of frequency, are the femur, spine, skull, sternum and pelvis, and the disease tends to be multifocal.

#### Limb involvement

This causes pain at the affected site. Deformity may be present such as the 'sabre tibia'. Long bone deformities can also cause osteoarthritis of adjacent joints. Paget's disease may result in fragility fractures because of localized skeletal fragility.

#### Skull involvement

Involvement of the skull leads to an increase in head size. Hearing loss may also occur (conductive and/or sensorineural). When the skull base is involved, this can lead to basilar invagination. Increased vascularization of skull lesions may

result in vascular steal syndrome, which causes blood to be diverted away from the cerebrum, leading to somnolence.

#### Facial involvement

This may cause facial deformity, leading to dental problems and a characteristic 'lion face' appearance (leontiasis ossea).

#### Osteosarcoma

The most devastating complication of Paget's disease, this occurs in approximately 0.2% of patients.

#### High-output cardiac failure

This is a rare complication of Paget's disease, which results from excess skeletal blood flow.

#### Hypercalcaemia

Hypercalcaemia rarely may occur during periods of prolonged immobilization.

### Diagnosis

- Paget's disease of bone is readily diagnosed on X-ray in patients presenting with localized bone pain.
- Alternatively, Paget's disease may be diagnosed incidentally in asymptomatic individuals with an elevated serum ALP.

### Investigation

#### Biochemistry

Serum ALP is nearly always elevated in active disease and is useful to monitor response to therapy. However, it can be normal in localized monostotic disease.

#### Diagnostic imaging

- *Plain radiography:* X-ray reveals generalized expansion and deformity of affected long bones, with a characteristic lytic leading edge ('blade of grass' appearance). There may also be areas of sclerotic bone at sites of osteoblastic reaction.
- *Isotope bone scan:* This is useful for showing the extent of pagetic involvement as well as determining active disease.

### Management

Bisphosphonates are the mainstay of treatment for Paget's disease of bone.

- Treatment should be offered to all symptomatic individuals, and can be considered in asymptomatic patients, particularly at locations where complications may develop (e.g. skull, near joints).
- Another indication for bisphosphonate treatment would be prior to orthopaedic surgery to active pagetoid bone, which reduces vascularity and excessive blood loss.
- More potent and longer-acting bisphosphonates, such as zoledronate, may lead to disease remission lasting years after a single dose. Alternatively, high-dose oral bisphosphonates and calcitonin may be used instead.

# HYPERPARATHYROIDISM

Hyperparathyroidism is defined as increased PTH secretion from the parathyroid glands.

## Epidemiology

- Approximately 1/1000 men and 2/1000 women at 60 years of age are affected.
- The incidence of primary hyperparathyroidism increases with age.
- Approximately 70% of patients are female.
- A small proportion of cases are familial, when primary hyperparathyroidism is usually a component of MEN 1 or 2.

## Classification

Hyperparathyroidism may be primary, secondary or tertiary:

- *Primary hyperparathyroidism:* This is usually caused by a single benign parathyroid gland adenoma (85% of cases). Carcinoma of a single parathyroid gland is rare, as are familial forms such as MEN 1 and 2.
- *Secondary hyperparathyroidism:* This is a physiological response to hypocalcaemia (eg. in chronic renal failure and osteomalacia). It is reversible following correction of calcium and phosphate levels.
- *Tertiary hyperparathyroidism:* This occurs when the increased PTH release of secondary hyperparathyroidism becomes autonomous. Raised PTH levels then persist, despite correction of calcium and phosphate levels, leading to hypercalcaemia.

## Disease mechanisms

In primary hyperparathyroidism, PTH release by the parathyroid gland is no longer under negative feedback control by serum calcium. This results in:

- Symptoms of hypercalcaemia
- Bone complications
- Renal damage due to nephrolithiasis and nephrocalcinosis
- Calcium deposition at other sites, such as joints, eyes and the skin

## Clinical features of primary hyperparathyroidism

Primary hyperparathyroidism most commonly presents as incidental hypercalcaemia on routine serum biochemistry. Symptoms of hypercalcaemia, remembered as 'bones, stones, abdominal groans and psychic moans' (see **Table 5.2**), are likely if the serum calcium concentration is higher than 3.0 mmol.

Older patients may present non-specifically with dehydration, drowsiness and confusion.

Clinical features are summarized in HYPERPARATHYROIDISM: CLINICAL FEATURES AT A GLANCE.

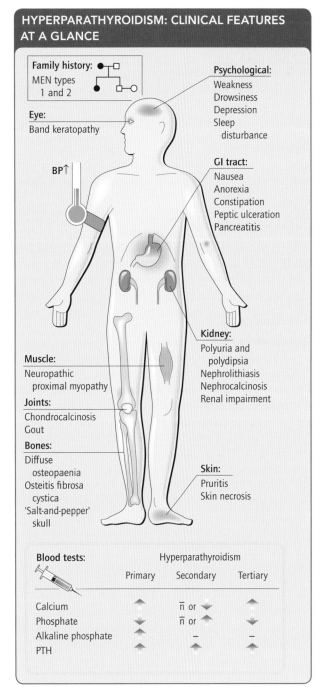

**HYPERPARATHYROIDISM: CLINICAL FEATURES AT A GLANCE**

| Blood tests: | Hyperparathyroidism | | |
| --- | --- | --- | --- |
| | Primary | Secondary | Tertiary |
| Calcium | ↑ | n̄ or ↓ | ↑ |
| Phosphate | ↓ | n̄ or ↑ | ↓ |
| Alkaline phosphate | ↑ | – | – |
| PTH | ↑ | ↑ | ↑ |

### Renal involvement

- This is the most common complication of primary hyperparathyroidism, affecting 20–40% of patients.
- It manifests as either nephrolithiasis or nephrocalcinosis (usually calcium oxalate stones).
- Primary hyperparathyroidism is detected in 5–10% of people with recurrent calcium-containing renal stones.

### Skeletal involvement

- Low bone density on bone densitometry is a fairly common finding.

- Osteitis fibrosa cystic, which typically affects the skull or phalanges and consists of bone cysts, fractures and deformity, may occur.

### Neurological complications

A syndrome of reversible proximal muscle weakness and wasting resulting from denervation and atrophy of type II muscle fibres can occur.

### Diagnosis

Increased PTH in the presence of raised serum calcium is considered diagnostic of primary and tertiary hyperparathyroidism.

### Differential diagnosis

Other causes of hypercalcaemia should be considered (see **Table 5.5**). It is particularly important to exclude malignancy, which, together with primary hyperparathyroidism, accounts for more than 90% of patients with hypercalcaemia.

### Investigation

#### Biochemistry

- *Serum creatinine:* increased, and creatinine clearance decreased if there is renal impairment
- *Serum calcium:* elevated in primary and tertiary hyperparathyroidism
- *Serum phosphate:* usually reduced in primary hyperparathyroidism (urinary phosphate wasting)
- *Serum ALP:* increased if there is associated bone disease
- *Serum PTH:* usually elevated; may be within a 'normal reference range' but still inappropriately high if hypercalcaemia is present (e.g. in mild primary hyperparathyroidism) as PTH production is normally suppressed in hypercalcaemia
- *Serum 25-OH-D:* reduced in secondary hyperparathyroidism
- *24-hour urinary calcium excretion:* is a vital investigation. FHH is due to loss of function in the calcium sensing receptors of the parathyroid gland leading to the same biochemical profile as primary hyperparathyroidism with the main difference being a low urinary calcium excretion (elevated in primary hyperparathyroidism)

#### Diagnostic imaging

- *Plain radiography:* Radiological evidence of osteitis fibrosa cystica is present in less than 5% of patients at diagnosis. It consists of subperiosteal bone resorption (best seen along the radial aspect of middle phalanges), erosions of the tufts of the terminal phalanges and mottling of the skull vault ('salt-and-pepper appearance'). There may also be radiological evidence of nephrocalcinosis.
- *DXA:* In primary hyperparathyroidism, DXA may indicate bone loss and should always include the distal radius due to the preferential loss of cortical bone.

- *Localization studies:* These are carried out to localize parathyroid adenomas prior to surgical removal.

### Management

#### Life-threatening hypercalcaemia

Life-threatening hypercalcaemia needs prompt treatment.
- Intravenous fluids such as 0.9% saline usually lower serum calcium effectively although the effects are transitory if saline is used on its own.
- Intravenous pamidronate or zoledronate may require 3–5 days post infusion to influence serum calcium. It can be very effectively used in combination with IV fluids.
- Calcitonin is a weaker agent than bisphosphonates but it acts quickly and can be used in combination with the above agents.

#### Symptomatic hypercalcaemia in people unfit for surgery and asymptomatic primary hyperparathyroidim

In people who are unfit for surgery and in those with mild hypercalcaemia with no evidence for organ involvement, a conservative approach may be used. Bisphosphonates are indicated for the prevention of bone loss and a calcimimetic such as cinacalcet is used to control hypercalcaemia.

#### Surgery

Surgery is the only curative treatment for primary hyperparathyroidism. It should be offered to patients with severe or symptomatic hypercalcaemia (e.g. more than 2.9 mmol/L), reduction in renal function, renal stones, osteoporosis, and in young patients (under 50 years).

Apart from eventual normalization of serum calcium after surgery, other important effects include:
- Transient postoperative hypocalcaemia, which is maximal 4–7 days postoperatively and persists for up to 2–3 weeks
- BMD improvement, which is dramatic in the first 1–2 years after surgery

## HYPERCALCAEMIA OF MALIGNANCY

Hypercalcaemia of malignancy is usually an indicator of advanced disease with secondary skeletal deposits.

### Epidemiology

There is a prevalence of around 5% of hospital inpatients with malignancy.

### Disease mechanisms

Nearly 50% of people with hypercalcaemia of malignancy have squamous cell carcinoma of the lung or adenocarcinoma of the breast.

Malignant hypercalcaemia is most commonly associated with secondary malignant deposits in the skeleton.

Such deposits stimulate osteoclast activity resulting in hypercalcaemia:

- *Release of local factors:* Skeletal metastases stimulate resorption of surrounding bone by releasing cytokines such as interleukin-1 and tumour necrosis factor.
- *Parathroid hormone related protein (PTHrP):* Malignant hypercalcaemia may resemble hyperparathyroidism despite reduced serum PTH level due to the release of PTHrP by tumour cells. PTHrP has PTH-like activity and is also responsible for the paraneoplastic hypercalcaemia that occasionally occurs from a non-metastatic malignancy.

## Clinical features

The elevated serum calcium that occurs in malignancy is frequently high enough to cause symptoms of hypercalcaemia (see **Table 5.2**).

- Bone pain from skeletal secondary deposits is common.
- There is often mild renal impairment because of dehydration, but significant renal failure is suggestive of multiple myeloma.

## Diagnosis

Hypercalcaemia of malignancy usually presents in patients with malignancy associated with metastatic bone disease. However, an occult tumour with paraneoplastic hypercalcaemia should be sought after causes such as primary hyperparathyroidism, sarcoidosis and FHH have been excluded.

## Investigation

### Haematology

Erythrocyte sedimentation rate (ESR) may be elevated, particularly in multiple myeloma.

### Biochemistry

- *Serum creatinine:* frequently elevated because of dehydration
- *Serum calcium + phosphate + PTH:* see **Table 5.4**
- *Serum ALP:* increased if there are bony metastases causing an osteoblastic response, but normal in the presence of osteolytic metastases (e.g. multiple myeloma)

### Diagnostic imaging

- *Plain radiography:* may reveal bone metastases
- *Isotope bone scan:* may reveal previously unsuspected secondary malignant deposits of the skeleton

## Management

Hypercalcaemia should generally be treated aggressively if there are associated symptoms. See 'Hyperparathyroidism: Management: Life-threatening hypercalcaemia' (above).

### Glucocorticoids

Glucocorticoids (e.g. prednisolone 30–60 mg/day) may be helpful in treating hypercalcaemia caused by haematological

tumours such as multiple myeloma and lymphomas and non-malignant causes such as sarcoidosis and vitamin D intoxication.

### Specific treatment

Malignant hypercalcaemia is usually caused by disseminated malignancy, in which case eradicating the primary tumour is not usually helpful in treating hypercalcaemia. However, if the hypercalcaemia occurred as a non-metastatic paraneoplastic manifestation, it may resolve following removal of the primary.

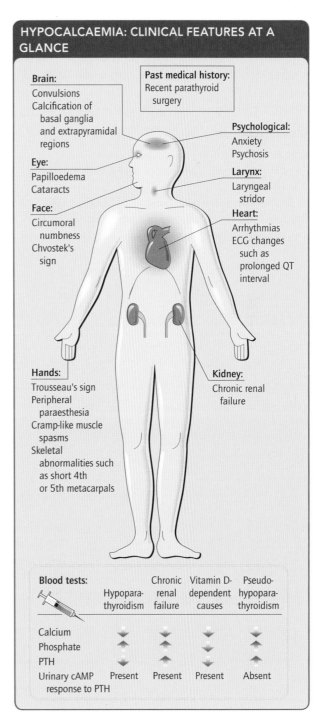

### HYPOCALCAEMIA: CLINICAL FEATURES AT A GLANCE

**Brain:** Convulsions; Calcification of basal ganglia and extrapyramidal regions

**Past medical history:** Recent parathyroid surgery

**Eye:** Papilloedema; Cataracts

**Psychological:** Anxiety; Psychosis

**Face:** Circumoral numbness; Chvostek's sign

**Larynx:** Laryngeal stridor

**Heart:** Arrhythmias; ECG changes such as prolonged QT interval

**Hands:** Trousseau's sign; Peripheral paraesthesia; Cramp-like muscle spasms; Skeletal abnormalities such as short 4th or 5th metacarpals

**Kidney:** Chronic renal failure

| Blood tests: | Hypoparathyroidism | Chronic renal failure | Vitamin D-dependent causes | Pseudo-hypoparathyroidism |
|---|---|---|---|---|
| Calcium | ↓ | ↓ | ↓ | ↓ |
| Phosphate | ↑ | ↑ | ↓ | ↑ |
| PTH | ↓ | ↑ | ↓ | ↑ |
| Urinary cAMP response to PTH | Present | Present | Present | Absent |

## HYPOCALCAEMIA

Hypocalcaemia is a less common clinical problem than hypercalcaemia.

### Disease mechanisms

Hypocalcaemia usually results from chronic renal failure or other vitamin D-dependent causes (see **Table 5.6**). Alternatively, it may be caused by hypoparathyroidism, which is most frequently seen as a postoperative complication of parathyroidectomy. There are a number of rare hypocalcaemic disorders characterized by hypoparathyroidism or PTH resistance.

Hypocalcaemia caused by chronic renal failure or hypoparathyroidism may result in hyperphosphataemia, which may lead to an increase in soft-tissue calcification (e.g. basal ganglia) from an increased calcium phosphate product.

### Clinical features

Clinical features of hypocalcaemia include:
- *Chvostek's sign:* Gentle tapping over the facial nerve causes twitching of the muscles. This is positive in 10% of people who do not have hypocalcaemia.
- *Trousseau's sign:* Inflation of a sphygmomanometer cuff above diastolic pressure for 3 minutes to obliterate the radial pulse causes distal tetanic spasm.

See **Table 5.3** and HYPOCALCAEMIA: CLINICAL FEATURES AT A GLANCE.

## DIFFERENTIAL DIAGNOSIS

If hypocalcaemia is not caused by chronic renal failure, severe osteomalacia (raised PTH and reduced serum phosphate) can be readily distinguished from hypoparathyroidism (reduced PTH and elevated phosphate) (**Table 5.9**).

## INVESTIGATION

### Biochemistry

- *Serum calcium:* reduced
- *Serum phosphate:* increased in chronic renal failure and hypoparathyroidism; decreased in vitamin D-dependent causes other than chronic renal failure
- *Serum PTH:* increased in chronic renal failure and other vitamin D-dependent causes; decreased in hypoparathyroidism
- *Serum magnesium:* hypomagnesaemia may be part of a general malabsorption leading to hypocalcaemia

### Diagnostic imaging

*Plain radiography:*
- Changes of renal osteodystrophy or osteomalacia/rickets may be found in chronic renal failure or vitamin D deficiency.
- In childhood hypoparathyroidism, radiographs may reveal skeletal abnormalities characteristic of pseudohypoparathyroidism.

## MANAGEMENT

### Acute life-threatening hypocalcaemia

Acute life-threatening hypocalcaemia is treated with slow IV infusion of calcium gluconate, adjusted according to the serum calcium. Patients receiving intravenous calcium should have cardiac monitoring because of the risk of arrhythmias.

**Table 5.9** Hypocalcaemic disorders caused by hypoparathyroidism or PTH resistance

| Cause | Description | Features |
|---|---|---|
| Idiopathic hypoparathyroidism | A rare autoimmune disorder | Often associated with cutaneous candidiasis and other autoimmune disorders such as Addison's disease<br>Usually presents in childhood<br>Also an adult-onset form |
| DiGeorge syndrome | Congenital absence of the parathyroid and thymus glands | Severe hypocalcaemia and T-cell immunodeficiency |
| Pseudohypoparathyroidism | Hereditary disorder characterized by end-organ resistance to PTH | Hypocalcaemia<br>Associated with intellectual impairment, short stature and skeletal abnormalities such as short 4th and 5th metacarpals and metatarsals (Albright's hereditary osteodystrophy) |
| Pseudopseudohypoparathyroidism | Hereditary disorder | Skeletal and developmental abnormalities of pseudohypoparathyroidism, but calcium metabolism is normal |
| Hypomagnesaemia | Most commonly caused by malabsorption | Causes hypocalcaemia by inhibiting PTH release and antagonizing its peripheral effects |

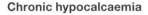
### Chronic hypocalcaemia

Chronic hypocalcaemia is difficult to manage. Recurrences of the symptoms of hypocalcaemia and complications of overtreatment are common.

- *Calcium:* This should be delayed until any associated hyperphosphataemia, and vitamin D deficiency has been treated. Oral calcium preparations are preferable in such cases.
- *Vitamin D formulations:* These are usually given in combination with calcium supplements and include ergocalciferol and cholecalciferol. Vitamin D metabolites such as alfacalcidol and calcitriol are used preferentially in chronic renal failure and liver failure (abnormal vitamin D metabolism) and will require regular monitoring of serum calcium to prevent intoxication.

**MUST-KNOW CHECKLIST**

- Useful investigations in metabolic bone disease
- Causes of secondary osteoporosis
- Diagnosis and treatment of osteoporosis
- Causes of rickets and osteomalacia
- Clinical features of osteomalacia
- Clinical features and causes of hypercalcaemia
- Clinical features and causes of hypocalcaemia
- Management of acute hypercalcaemia
- Clinical features of Paget's disease of bone

**Questions and answers** to test your understanding of Chapter 5 can be found by clicking 'Support Material' at the following link: https://www.routledge.com/Medicine-for-Finals-and-Beyond/Axford-OCallaghan/p/book/9780367150594

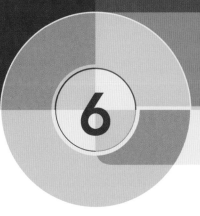

# Respiratory Disease

**6**

IAN PAVORD, NAYIA PETOUSI & NICK TALBOT

## APPROACH TO THE PATIENT

### HISTORY

The history commonly provides the most important clue to the cause of a respiratory disorder, and a systematic inquiry should be made (**HISTORY 6.1**).

## RESPIRATORY SYMPTOMS

### Cough and sputum

- Early morning cough with a small amount of sputum is common in smokers ('smoker's cough'). A change in character of a smoker's cough may indicate bronchial carcinoma.
- A *'bovine' cough* suggests left recurrent laryngeal nerve palsy, the most common cause being bronchial carcinoma.
- A cough may persist for several weeks after successful treatment of a lower respiratory tract infection due to bronchial hyperresponsiveness, and usually settles spontaneously.
- A *cough at night* may be the only symptom of asthma.
- A *dry cough* worse lying down, in the morning or after food suggests gastro-oesophageal reflux.
- Mucopurulent sputum (yellow or green) suggests lower respiratory tract infection. Copious quantities are seen in bronchiectasis and cystic fibrosis.
- Blood-stained sputum (haemoptysis) can have many aetiologies (**Table 6.1**). Ask about onset (acute or insidious), duration (days, weeks, months), whether it is mixed with sputum, and quantity (e.g. in teaspoons or cupfuls). Haemoptysis in a smoker should be investigated to exclude bronchial carcinoma.
- Massive haemoptysis can be a life-threatening manifestation of bronchial carcinoma, bronchiectasis, aspergilloma, Goodpasture's syndrome and systemic vasculitides, blood dyscrasias and idiopathic pulmonary haemosiderosis.

### Breathlessness

- Breathlessness or *dyspnoea* is the sensation of 'difficulty to breathe'. Causes according to rate of onset are given in **Table 6.2**.
- *Orthopnoea* (breathlessness lying flat) and *paroxysmal nocturnal dyspnoea* (waking at night with breathlessness) are suggestive of heart failure or pulmonary oedema.
- Breathlessness at night associated with cough, wheeze and chest tightness is suggestive of asthma.
- Breathlessness with haemoptysis and weight loss in a smoker could represent lung cancer.
- Breathlessness with fevers and sputum production suggests infection.
- Sudden-onset breathlessness with pleuritic chest pain may indicate pulmonary embolism (PE) or pneumothorax. If the chest pain is central, it may indicate a myocardial infarction.

### Chest pain

Pleuritic pain is the most common type of chest pain in respiratory disease, and is described as a localized, sharp ('stabbing') pain aggravated by coughing and inspiration.

DOI: 10.1201/9781003193616-6

## HISTORY 6.1

**Respiratory symptoms**

*General*

Time of day
Speed of onset and rate of progression
Continuous or intermittent
Duration (days, weeks, months)
Severity
Character
Exacerbating and relieving factors
Associated symptoms
Impact on life

*Cough*

When do you cough?
How long have you had the cough?
Is it dry or do you produce sputum? Do you ever cough up blood?
Is there associated wheeze?

*Breathlessness*

How far can you walk on the flat?
How many stairs can you climb?
Has it developed suddenly or slowly?
Does the breathlessness come and go?
Are you breathless lying flat?
Are you breathless at night?
Do you wheeze or pant?
Is there any associated pain?

*Pain*

Where is the pain?
How long have you had it?
Did it develop suddenly or slowly?
What kind of pain is it (sharp, dull, aching)?
What causes the pain? What relieves it?
Is it worse when you breathe in and out (pleuritic)?

**Disease impact**

Do your symptoms interfere with your work? How?
Do they interfere with your social activities? How?
Do they interfere with your daily life? How?

**Social history**

Have you ever smoked? If so, how much/how long?
Do you keep any pets (ask specifically about birds)?
What is your occupation?

**Drug history**

Are you taking any medications?
When were they started?

**Past medical history**

As a child did you have asthma/eczema/hay fever?
Have you had TB, pneumonia, blood clots, a heart attack, cancer, pneumothorax?
Have you ever had a tracheostomy?

**Family history**

Has anyone in your family had an allergy, cystic fibrosis, TB or cancer?

Pleuritic pain indicates pleural inflammation (e.g. caused by pneumonia or pulmonary infarction), and is also a feature of spontaneous pneumothorax or rib fracture (e.g. following trauma or a bout of coughing). Other causes of chest pain are given in **Table 6.3**.

**Table 6.1** Causes of haemoptysis

| **Common** |
| --- |
| Infection (e.g. pneumonia) |
| Bronchial carcinoma |
| Bronchiectasis |
| Pulmonary infarction |
| TB |
| **Rare** |
| Pulmonary aspergilloma |
| Benign bronchial tumour, e.g. carcinoid |
| Pulmonary haemorrhage, e.g. vasculitis, Goodpasture's syndrome |
| Chest trauma |
| Blood dyscracias |

### Wheeze, stridor

The emission of high-pitched noises (wheezes) when the patient exhales simply implies intrathoracic airway obstruction. Generalized wheezing (polyphonic) may be noted in chronic obstructive pulmonary disease (COPD) or asthma. Localized wheeze (monophonic) occurs when more central airways are obstructed (e.g. by a bronchial carcinoma or foreign body). The presence of a lower-pitched noise on inspiration (stridor) implies extrathoracic airway obstruction (e.g. obstruction of the trachea or a major bronchus).

## ASSOCIATED SYMPTOMS

Weight loss and night sweats may be features of bronchial carcinoma or pulmonary tuberculosis (TB), while painful wrists or ankles suggest hypertrophic pulmonary arthropathy (HPA). Ankle swelling may be a sign of congestive heart failure, or of cor pulmonale in a patient with COPD.

**Table 6.2** Causes of breathlessness according to rate of onset

| Rate of onset | Disorder |
| --- | --- |
| Acute (seconds–hours) | Pneumothorax |
| | Pulmonary embolus |
| | Asthma |
| | Pulmonary oedema |
| | Respiratory infection |
| | Cardiac tamponade |
| Paroxysmal | Pulmonary oedema |
| | Asthma |
| Weeks/months | Cardiac failure |
| | Recurrent pulmonary emboli |
| | Pleural effusion |
| | Pulmonary fibrosis |
| | Lung cancer |
| | Chronic airways diseases (asthma or COPD) |
| Years | COPD |
| | Pulmonary fibrosis |

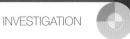

**Table 6.3** Causes of chest pain

| Pain characteristics | Disorder(s) |
|---|---|
| Local pain and tenderness | Fractures (simple or pathological) or pleural malignancy (e.g. mesothelioma) |
| Pain and swelling of costochondral junction, particularly of second ribs (Tietze's syndrome) | Perichondritis |
| Pain within the distribution of one dermatome | Herpes zoster of the thoracic nerves (often precedes vesicular rash) |
| Localized muscle pain | Breathlessness and coughing |
| Retrosternal 'raw' pain aggravated by deep inspiration | Inflamed trachea |
| Poorly localized, often dull, central chest pain | Large central tumours |
| Pleuritic pain | Pleural disease (effusion, malignancy, inflammation), pulmonary emboli, pneumonia, pneumothorax |
| Chest pain worsened by exercise | Ischaemic heart disease |
| Burning retrosternal discomfort | Gastro-oesophageal reflux |

## DRUG HISTORY

Important drugs to ask about are:
- *Beta-blockers, non-steroidal anti-inflammatory drugs (NSAIDs) and aspirin:* may worsen the symptoms of asthma
- *Amiodarone, cytotoxics* (e.g. bleomycin, busulfan) *and nitrofurantoin*: may cause pulmonary fibrosis
- *Steroids and other immunosuppressants*: increase the risk of infection
- *Contraceptive pill:* a risk factor for pulmonary emboli

## SOCIAL HISTORY

- *Smoking:* pipe, cigars or cigarettes; calculate number of pack years (20 cigarettes/day for 1 year is 1 pack year)
- *Alcohol abuse:* risk factor for pulmonary infection (e.g. pneumonia, abscess and TB); document number of units/week
- *Other substance abuse:* intravenous drugs (associated with staphylococcal pneumonia, TB, HIV infection), cannabis (associated with emphysema)
- *Pets:* dogs/cat allergy can exacerbate asthma; birds can cause hypersensitivity pneumonitis
- *Occupation:* may be relevant in occupational asthma, hypersensitivity pneumonitis and asbestos-related disease
- *Foreign travel:* relevant in Legionnaire's disease, histoplasmosis (e.g. the USA) and TB (e.g. Asia and Africa)

- *Ethnicity:* e.g. >30% of people with pulmonary TB in the UK are Asians; pulmonary sarcoidosis is rare in Asians but common in West Indians and young Irish women

## PAST MEDICAL HISTORY

- Childhood TB or whooping cough may cause bronchiectasis in adult life.
- Atopy (eczema and/or hay fever) is associated with asthma.

## FAMILY HISTORY

A family history of atopy, cystic fibrosis or cancer may give clues to the diagnosis.

## EXAMINATION

### GENERAL EXAMINATION

The patient should be positioned at 45 degrees. Note general well-being (e.g. mental alertness), as well as the presence of obesity, cachexia or jaundice. See EXAMINATION 6.2 and **Table 6.4**.

## INVESTIGATION

### LUNG FUNCTION TESTS

The aim is to detect and/or characterize abnormal lung function and allow monitoring over time. Results are usually expressed as a percentage of the predicted normal value based on age, height and sex ('% predicted').

#### Measurements during forced expiration

These measurements primarily assess large airway function. They are simple to perform and can be measured at the bedside.

- *Peak expiratory flow rate (PEFR)* is the greatest flow generated during a short sharp expiration, starting at full inspiration, and is a measure of large airway resistance. It is primarily used for assessing airway obstruction in patients with asthma, and can easily be monitored by patients at home, as part of a self-management plan.
- *Spirometry* is measurement of the volume expired in the first second of a forced expiration (forced expiratory volume in 1 second [FEV1]) and the total volume expired from full inspiration to full expiration (forced vital capacity [FVC]). FEV1 is normally >70% of the FVC (i.e. the FEV1/FVC ratio is >0.7). A low FEV1/FVC (<0.7) suggests obstructive lung disease. In restrictive lung disease, the FEV1/FVC ratio is normal or may even be elevated to the predominant fall in

**Table 6.4** Typical physical signs found in particular chest disorders

| Chest disorder | Chest wall movement | Mediastinal shift | Vocal resonance (and tactile vocal fremitus) | Percussion note | Breath sounds | Added sounds |
|---|---|---|---|---|---|---|
| Consolidation (e.g. lobar pneumonia) | None | None | Increased (whispering pectoriloquy) | Dull | Bronchial | Fine or coarse inspiratory crackles |
| Collapse or removal (e.g. lobectomy) | Reduced on affected side | Towards affected side | Reduced | Dull | Absent (or bronchial) | None |
| Localized fibrosis (e.g. previous TB or radiotherapy) | Reduced on affected side | Towards affected side | Increased | Dull or no change | Bronchial | Coarse or fine crackles |
| Generalized fibrosis (e.g. idiopathic pulmonary fibrosis [IPF]) | Reduced on both sides | None | Reduced or bronchophony | Dull or no change | Vesicular | Fine inspiratory crackles |
| Large pleural effusion | Reduced on affected side | Away from affected side | Reduced (aegophony) | 'Stony' dull | Reduced* | None |
| Large pneumothorax | Reduced on affected side | Away from affected side | Reduced | Normal or hyper-resonant | Absent or Reduced | None |
| Asthma or COPD | Reduced on both sides | None | Normal | Normal | Vesicular with prolonged expiration | Expiratory polyphonic wheezes |
| Bronchiectasis | Reduced on both sides | None | Normal | Normal | Bronchial | Expiratory wheezes, coarse inspiratory crackles, inspiratory and expiratory 'squeaks' |

\* Bronchial breathing may be heard at the upper level of the dull percussion note.

**6**

### General

*Examine the hands*

Note any tar staining, finger clubbing (**Table 6.5**), peripheral cyanosis or flap/tremor (indicates hypercapnia).

*Examine the face and neck*

Look at the conjunctivae for evidence of anaemia, and tongue/lips for central cyanosis.

Note the height of the jugular venous pressure (JVP) and observe the effect of respiration (e.g. JVP is raised in right heart failure; fixed and raised in superior vena cava obstruction).

Look for any facial features of systemic disease (e.g. telangiectasia) or drug side effects (e.g. Cushingoid appearance in long-term steroid users).

### Chest

*Inspection*

*Chest wall*

Note the shape of the chest.

Look for evidence of previous surgery or radiotherapy.

Look for engorged veins, subcutaneous nodules or use of accessory muscles.

Measure the respiratory rate.

*Palpation*

Determine the position of the trachea and apex beat.

Check the symmetry of movement of the two hemithoraces.

Palpate for cervical and axillary lymphadenopathy.

Test for vocal fremitus.

*Percussion*

Compare the percussion note of the two hemithoraces (not forgetting the apices).

*Auscultation*

Note the nature and intensity of the breath sounds.

Listen for added sounds (wheezes, crackles, pleural rub).

Note the character and intensity of vocal resonance.

**Table 6.5** Causes of clubbing

**Common**
- Bronchial carcinoma
- Bronchiectasis
- Cystic fibrosis
- IPF

**Rare**
- Bacterial endocarditis
- Inflammatory bowel disease
- Liver cirrhosis
- Cyanotic congenital heart disease
- Atrial myxoma
- Idiopathic

in the lungs after maximal expiration, measurement of total lung capacity (TLC), or its subdivisions residual volume (RV) and functional residual capacity (FRC), requires more complex techniques (e.g. helium dilution or body plethysmography) in a lung function laboratory. Patients with restrictive lung disease (e.g. fibrosis) may have reduced lung volumes, whereas those with obstructive lung disease may have hyperinflation (raised TLC and RV; **Table 6.8**).

### Measurement of gas exchange

Transfer factor of the lung for carbon monoxide (TLCO) is a measure of the transfer of gas from alveolar gas into capillary blood (**Table 6.9**). It is calculated by asking the patient to inhale a low concentration of carbon monoxide (e.g. 0.03%) and then hold their breath for 10 seconds at full inspiration. Not all patients can manage this. TLCO is the product of KCO and V$^A$. Its value depends upon multiple factors, including:
- Surface area available for gas exchange
- Thickness of the blood–gas barrier
- Pulmonary capillary blood volume
- Capillary blood haemoglobin concentration

## BLOOD GAS ANALYSIS

Arterial oxygenation can be monitored indirectly by pulse oximetry, which is widely available and non-invasive, but direct measurement of the arterial partial pressures of $O_2$ ($Pao_2$) and $CO_2$ ($Paco_2$) is important in many respiratory disorders. Samples of arterial blood are usually obtained from the radial artery.

FVC (**Table 6.6**; **Figure 6.1**). *Flow volume loops* can be generated during spirometry and the shape of these curves provides information about lung pathology. In particular, 'scalloping' of expiratory flow is common in obstructive lung disease, and may precede a fall in FEV$_1$ or FEV1/FVC (**Figure 6.2**).

### Measurement of lung volumes

A reduced FVC is an important finding (**Table 6.7**) and is detectable with spirometry. However, because gas remains

**Table 6.6** Classical changes in lung function during forced expiration in different diseases

| Lung disease | FEV$_1$ | FVC | FEV$_1$/FVC | PEFR | Increase after bronchodilator (%) |
|---|---|---|---|---|---|
| **Normal** | >80% predicted | >80% predicted | >0.7 | >80% predicted | 0 |
| **Obstructive** | | | | | |
| COPD | ↓↓ | Normal or ↓ | ↓ | ↓ | <12 |
| Asthma | ↓↓ | Normal or ↓ | ↓ | ↓ | >12 |
| **Restrictive** | | | | | |
| Pulmonary fibrosis | ↓ | ↓ | Normal or ↑ | Normal | 0 |

FEV$_1$, forced expiratory volume in 1 second; FVC, forced vital capacity; PEFR, peak expiratory flow rate.

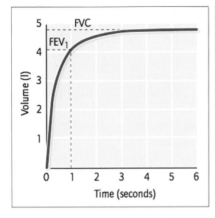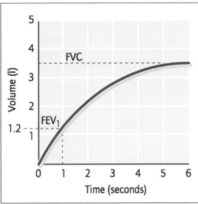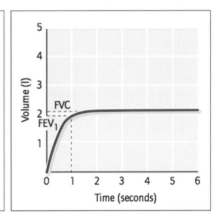

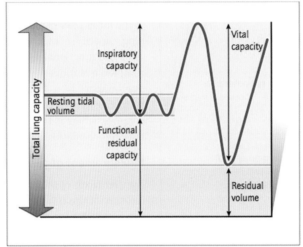

**Figure 6.1** Lung spirometry. **(a)** Spirogram of a normal adult (FEV1 4.1 L, FVC 4.9 L, FEV1/FVC 0.84). **(b)** Spirogram of a patient with airways obstruction, e.g. COPD (FEV1 1.2 L, FVC 3.5 L, FEV1/FVC 0.32). **(c)** Spirogram of a patient with a restrictive lung disease (FEV1 1.9 L, FVC 2.L L, FEV1/FVC 0.90). **(d)** Spirogram tracing showing static lung volumes.

Normal $PaCO_2$ is 4.8–6.0 kPa (35–45 mmHg). $Paco_2$ falls with hyperventilation, and rises with alveolar hypoventilation. Normal $Pao_2$ is 10.6–13.3 kPa (80–100 mmHg). Respiratory failure is defined as $Pao_2 \leq 8.0$ kPa (60 mmHg). Causes are given in **Table 6.10**. In patients with respiratory failure, calculation of the alveolar–arterial (A–a) $O_2$ difference can help distinguish gas exchange failure (type 1 respiratory failure; associated with an elevated A – a difference and normal or reduced $Paco_2$), from type II respiratory failure (ventilatory failure; in which the A–a difference may be

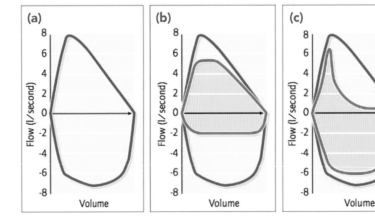

**Figure 6.2** Flow volume loops. In each curve, the volume above the zero line represents expiratory flow and the area below zero represents inspiratory flow. **(a)** Normal curve. **(b)** Extrathoracic large airway narrowing (e.g. due to a tracheal tumour) shown in red. **(c)** Intrathoracic airway narrowing with characteristic 'scalloping' of expiratory flow (e.g. asthma) shown in red.

**Table 6.7** Causes of reduced vital capacity

**Skeletal abnormality**
- Kyphoscoliosis

**Reduced lung volume**
- Diffuse pulmonary infiltration
- Pulmonary fibrosis
- Large pleural effusion
- Collapsed lobes/lung
- Pulmonary oedema

**Weak respiratory muscles**
- Myopathies
- Poliomyelitis
- Myasthenia gravis

**Severe airways obstruction***
- Asthma
- COPD
- Bronchiectasis

*Vital capacity can be measured during forced spirometry ('forced' vital capacity, FVC) or by asking the patient to exhale slowly from full inspiration to full expiration ('slow' vital capacity). These values are similar in health but, in obstructive lung disease, small airway collapse and gas trapping can occur during forced expiration, leading to a reduced FVC.

normal and the $Pa_{CO_2}$ is elevated). Alveolar $P_{O_2}$ ($PA_{O_2}$) is estimated using a simplified form of the alveolar gas equation:

$$P_{A}O_2 = P_IO_2 - (Pa_{CO_2} \div 0.8)$$

## IMAGING

The most common radiological investigation is the chest X-ray. Interpretation of the chest radiograph is therefore an essential skill for everyone involved in clinical medicine (**Figure 6.3**).

Computerized tomography (CT) is more sensitive than chest radiography and is a very common imaging modality in respiratory medicine. Common types of CT include:
- *CT thorax with contrast:* most approriate for identification and/or staging of malignancy or pleural disease; may be combined with positron emission tomography (PET) scanning
- *High resolution CT thorax (HRCT):* non-contrast scan providing higher resolution images but with gaps between imaged slices; useful for diffuse lung disease but may miss discrete lesions
- *CT pulmonary angiogram (CTPA):* image acquisition is timed to ensure maximum contrast in the pulmonary circulation; useful for excluding pulmonary emboli, but high contrast load makes it less suitable for investigating diffuse lung disease

**Table 6.8** Changes in lung volumes in different respiratory diseases

| Lung disease | TLC | RV | RV/TLC% |
|---|---|---|---|
| Obstructive (e.g. emphysema) | ↑ | ↑↑ | ↑ |
| Restrictive (e.g. pulmonary fibrosis) | ↓ | ↑ | Normal |

TLC, total lung capacity; RV, residual volume.

**Table 6.9** Changes in transfer factor in different diseases

| Disorder | Gas transfer (DLCO) |
|---|---|
| **Respiratory** | |
| Asthma | Normal or ↑ |
| COPD | Normal or ↓ |
| Pulmonary fibrosis | ↓ |
| Alveolar haemorrhage | ↑ |
| **Cardiovascular** | |
| Low cardiac output | ↓ |
| Anaemia | ↓ |
| Polycythaemia | ↑ |

DLCO, diffusing capacity of lung for carbon monoxide.

## BRONCHOSCOPY

The airways can be visualized down to the fourth or fifth divisions by fibre-optic bronchoscopy, during which the following may be performed:
- *Endobronchial biopsy/brushings:* These can be obtained from lesions in the larger airways and sent for histology/cytology.
- *Bronchoalveolar lavage:* For small airways pathology (e.g. infection, malignancy), saline may be introduced

**Table 6.10** Causes of hypoxia/respiratory failure

| Mechanism | Disorder | Cardinal features |
|---|---|---|
| Mismatching of pulmonary blood flow (Q) and alveolar ventilation (V) | Acute severe asthma or exacerbation of obstructive airways disease (most common cause of hypoxia) | Variable $Pa_{CO_2}$; increased alveolar–arterial $O_2$ gradient |
| Alveolar hypoventilation | Respiratory depression (e.g. sedatives), respiratory muscle weakness (e.g. myasthenia), thoracic cage abnormalities (e.g. kyphoscoliosis) | Increased $Pa_{CO_2}$; increased $FiO_2$ abolishes fall in $Pa_{O_2}$, normal alveolar–arterial $O_2$ gradient |
| Impaired gas transfer in lungs | Pulmonary fibrosis | Decreased $Pa_{CO_2}$, increased alveolar–arterial $O_2$ gradient, increased $FiO_2$ corrects fall in $Pa_{O_2}$ |
| Anatomical shunting | Extrapulmonary disorders (e.g. VSD) and intrapulmonary disease (e.g. consolidation) | Normal $Pa_{CO_2}$, increased alveolar–arterial $O_2$ gradient |

FiO2, inspired oxygen concentration; VSD, ventricular septal defect.

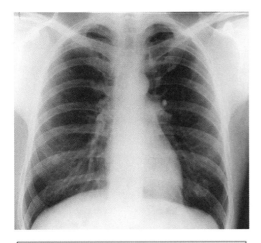

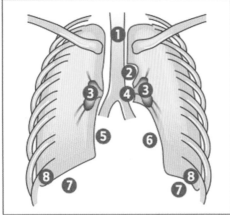

**Figure 6.3 (a)** Normal posteroanterior (PA) chest radiograph. **(b)** Line diagram of a PA chest radiograph. 1, trachea; 2, aortic arch; 3, hilar shadows (made up of bronchi, arteries and veins); 4, pulmonary artery trunk; 5, right atrium; 6, left ventricle; 7, diaphragms; 8, costophrenic recesses.

via the bronchoscope, before being aspirated and sent for microbiology/cytology.

- *Transbronchial needle aspiration:* Extrabronchial lesions (e.g. mediastinal and hilar lymph nodes) can be sampled through the bronchial wall, either by blind needle aspiration (guided by prior imaging) or using real-time endobronchial ultrasound (EBUS) guidance.
- *Transbronchial biopsy:* Blind biopsies taken using forceps inserted beyond the fifth division of the bronchial tree might include lung parenchyma, and can therefore be used to investigate suspected parenchymal lung disease (e.g. fibrosis or sarcoidosis). CT-guided percutanous biopsy is an alternative route for biopsy of abnormal parenchyma or peripheral lung lesions.

## PRINCIPLES OF MANAGEMENT

Most patients with chronic respiratory conditions are managed in the community. Despite exciting new treatments across the spectrum of respiratory disease, many conditions remain progressive and are associated with

considerable morbidity. In this setting, patient education about managing their illness, combined with community support from a multidisciplinary team including specialist nurses, physiotherapists and physicians, is very important. Multidisciplinary working is also of paramount importance for patients with lung malignancy, for whom close inter-action between chest physicians, oncologists and thoracic surgeons is essential for guiding management, and for patients with exacerbations of respiratory disease requiring admission to hospital. Inpatients may particularly benefit from specialist chest physiotherapy to clear secretions and encourage early mobilization.

# DISEASES AND THEIR MANAGEMENT

## RESPIRATORY INFECTIONS

### UPPER AIRWAY INFECTION

Most upper airway infections are caused by viruses, including echo-, adeno-, parainfluenzae, rhino- and respiratory syncytial viruses (RSV). They are highly infectious and transmitted by droplet spread. They can affect multiple parts of the upper airway simultaneously but may be more localized:

- *Rhinitis:* The 'common cold' causes rapid-onset coryzal symptoms (e.g. sneezing, nasal discharge), which typically resolve spontaneously in 2–3 days.
- *Pharyngitis:* Infection of pharyngeal lymphoid tissue (tonsils, adenoids). It is usually viral, but can be caused by β-haemolytic streptococci. If severe, a peritonsillar abscess requiring surgical drainage can develop (quinsy). It may be a manifestation of systemic infection (e.g. EBV).
- *Sinusitis:* Usually inflammatory/allergic, sinusitis can be complicated by bacterial infection (e.g. *Streptococcus pneumoniae* or *Haemophilus influenzae*). Chronic disease may respond to sinus washouts.
- *Laryngitis:* This presents with a hoarse voice. It is usually viral, but may be bacterial. If persistent, consider exclusion of laryngeal cancer or lung cancer with recurrent laryngeal nerve palsy.
- *Tracheitis/bronchitis:* This is most common in winter. It is usually viral but may be caused by *S. pneumoniae* or *H. influenzae*, particularly in chronic airways disease.
- *Bronchiolitis:* This usually occurs in children and is caused by adenovirus or RSV; in adults, it can be secondary to autoimmune disease (e.g. rheumatoid arthritis).

### COMMUNITY-ACQUIRED PNEUMONIA

This is acute inflammation of the lung caused by invasion by microorganisms. It may occur in a lobar or bronchopneumonic (patchy) distribution.

## Disease mechanisms

- Community-acquired pneumonia accounts for >1 million hospital admissions/year in the UK.
- Infection is usually by droplet inhalation or haematogenous spread.
- Risk factors are primarily related to impaired pulmonary defence mechanisms, and include older age, smoking, alcohol excess, diabetes, corticosteroid therapy/immunosuppression and chronic lung disease/airway obstruction.

## Clinical features

The classic clinical features are common to all pathogens:
- Fever
- Productive cough
- Shortness of breath
- Tachypnoea
- Pleuritic chest pain

A definitive microbiological diagnosis is made in fewer than 50% of patients, but common pathogens have characteristic features (**Table 6.11**).

## Investigations

Diagnosis is based on a typical clinical syndrome, including features on examination and radiological evidence (usually chest X-ray) of consolidation. The following investigations should be considered:

- *Radiology:* A chest X-ray should be conducted in all patients. CT imaging may be useful in non-resolving pneumonia or if lung abscess or underlying malignancy is suspected.
- *Blood tests:* Inflammatory markers are usually raised but white cell count (WCC) may be low in severe disease. Changes in C-reactive protein (CRP) are helpful for assessing trajectory. Liver function tests (LFTs) may suggest the underlying organism but may also be deranged secondary to antibiotics. Renal failure suggests severe illness.
- *Arterial blood gases:* These should be considered in all patients with decreased peripheral oxygen saturation (<92%). Acidosis suggests severe disease.
- *Urinary antigens:* Pneumococcal and *Legionella* antigens are detectable in the urine and are highly sensitive. Consider testing if available, to narrow the antibiotic spectrum.
- *Microbiology:* Bacteraemia is common, so blood cultures should be sent. Sputum microscopy and culture may be helpful in those with chronic lung disease and is essential when TB is suspected. Viral polymerase chain reaction (PCR) may be available

**Table 6.11** Characteristics of specific causes of community-acquired pneumonia

| Cause | Characteristics |
|---|---|
| *Streptococcus pneumoniae* | Most common cause of lower respiratory tract infection (60–75%) in all age groups, with peak rates in winter months |
| | Often a commensal in upper respiratory tract |
| | High fevers and pleuritic pain are classic |
| *Mycoplasma pneumoniae* | Causes pneumonia in autumnal epidemics, usually every 3–4 years |
| | Usually affects young adults and adolescents |
| | Onset may be insidious, and associated with extrapulmonary features, e.g. erythema nodosum, rash, myocarditis, pericarditis |
| *Haemophilus influenzae* | Usually bronchopneumonia in those with pre-existing lung disease (e.g. COPD) |
| | May chronically colonize those with airways disease |
| Viral pneumonia | Causes include influenza and SARS-CoV-2 (which causes coronavirus-19 [COVID-19]) |
| | Other causes are less common in the immunocompetent host, but viral respiratory tract infection may predispose to secondary bacterial infection |
| *Legionella pneumophila* | May contaminate air-conditioning systems, leading to outbreaks in hotels, with up to 10-day incubation period |
| | Multisystem disease is common (e.g. deranged LFTs, hyponatraemia, confusion) |
| | Mortality is high in the elderly |
| *Staphylococcus aureus* | Often coexistent with viral pneumonia (particularly influenza) |
| | Typically causes cavitating consolidation, and may be complicated by pneumothorax, empyema or metastatic deposits (e.g. pleura, spine) |
| | Risk factors include intravenous drug use or vascular procedures |
| *Chlamydia* species | *Chlamydia psittaci* is transmitted from birds and animals and there may be a long history prior to presentation |
| | *Chlamydia pneumoniae* is a rare cause of epidemics in the community |
| *Coxiella burnetii* (Q fever) | A rickettsial organism transmitted from cattle and sheep |
| | Typically runs a chronic course, complicated by headaches, myalgia or endocarditis |

(e.g. influenza, SARS-CoV-2, RSV) using upper airway swabs.

- *Serology:* Antibody titres may allow retrospective diagnosis of *Mycoplasma pneumonia*, Legionnaires' disease or psittacosis. Consider HIV testing in those with recurrent or severe infection, or unusual organisms.

## Management

Generic management of uncomplicated community-acquired pneumonia is given in **Table 6.12**.

## Prognosis

Pneumonia should respond rapidly to antibiotics, although full recovery may take months, particularly in the elderly. Mortality can be estimated using the CURB-65 score (**Table 6.13**). Failure to improve may result from inaccurate diagnosis, antibiotic

**Table 6.13** CURB-65 scoring system for stratifying risk of death in patients with community-acquired pneumonia. One point is given for each of the following criteria at presentation. A score of 0–1 signifies low risk (<3% mortality), 2 signifies intermediate risk (3–15%) and ≥3 signifies high risk (>15%)

| |
| --- |
| Confusion |
| Blood urea >7 mmol/L |
| Respiratory rate ≥30/min |
| Blood pressure ≤90 mmHg systolic *or* 60 mmHg diastolic |
| Age ≥65 years |

Reference: Lim WS *et al. Thorax* 2013; 58(5): 377–82.

**Table 6.12** Management of community-acquired pneumonia

**Antibiotics**
Send blood cultures before the first dose of antibiotics if possible, but do not delay treatment. Initial antibiotic choice is usually empirical, based on severity and local guidelines/antibiotic resistance, with spectrum then narrowed if organism identified. In the UK, suggested empirical management is:

- *Low severity:** 5 days of amoxicillin (in penicillin allergy, consider macrolide or tetracyline instead)
- *Moderate severity:** 7–10 days of amoxicillin *and* macrolide (e.g. clarithromycin)
- *High severity:** 7–10 days of co-amoxiclav *and* macrolide

**Oxygen**
Consider in those with SpO$_2$ <94%, unless there is pre-existing lung disease (in which case a lower target may be appropriate). Humidification may help if struggling with secretions.

**Rehydration**
Consider IV fluid to maintain blood pressure and preserve renal function, bearing in mind oral intake, urine output and insensible losses (including sweating, hyperventilation).

**Chest physiotherapy**
This is for sputum clearance, to encourage mobility and to optimize posture. It is particularly important in those with impaired clearance (e.g. neuromuscular weakness, bronchiectasis).

**Intensive care unit (ICU)**
Consider an urgent ICU referral in patients with severe hypoxia, rapidly increasing oxygen requirements, rising CO$_2$, hypotension or acidosis.

**Follow-up imaging**
Repeat the chest X-ray around 6 weeks after pneumonia, primarily to exclude an underlying lung malignancy.

*UK guidelines suggest assessing severity based on the CURB-65 score on admission (see **Table 6.13**).

resistance, non-adherence with therapy, or development of one of the following complications:

- *Lung abscess:* There may be a swinging fever and discrete cavitating lesions on chest X-ray. This often requires prolonged antibiotic therapy (4–6 weeks) and occasionally surgical drainage.
- *Pneumothorax:* This is particularly associated with *Staphylococcus aureus* pneumonia.
- *Parapneumonic effusion:* This is likely not to need additional treatment if small and the patient is improving. If the patient is deteriorating, consider sampling to exclude empyema.
- *Empyema:* This is infection of the pleural space. Infected fluid may be culture-negative but the pH will be low (<7.2). It usually requires intercostal drainage plus prolonged (4–6 weeks) antibiotics. Surgical washout may be required if not draining.
- *Metastatic infection:* This may include spinal abscess, endocarditis, joint infection. It is more common with *Staphylococcus aureus*.
- *Inflammatory pneumonia:* Organizing pneumonia can be triggered by infection and is treated with high-dose corticosteroids.
- *Acute respiratory distress syndrome (ARDS):* This is a severe inflammatory process affecting the lung parenchyma and vasculature. It may be triggered by pneumonia or be part of a systemic inflammatory response to infection elsewhere. Treatment is supportive, often including invasive ventilation, and mortality is high.

Viral pneumonia is considered mainly in Chapter 3, Infectious disease. It is most common in the context of epidemics, which may be seasonal (e.g. influenza) or sporadic (e.g. SARS-CoV-2, which causes COVID-19). The global pandemic of COVID-19 led to very large numbers of patients being admitted to hospital with severe viral pneumonia characterized by profound hypoxia. Hypercapnia and acidosis are uncommon. Hypoxia in COVID-19 is particularly resistant to simple supplementary oxygen. It may respond to treatment with continuous positive airway pressure (CPAP) or invasive ventilation, but mortality in severe disease is high.

## COMMUNITY-ACQUIRED PNEUMONIA AT A GLANCE

### Epidemiology

*Prevalence*

- At least 1 000 000 admissions/year in the UK

### Findings on investigation

*Blood tests*

- High WCC and CRP, particularly with *Streptococcus pneumoniae*; may be low in severe disease
- Deranged liver or renal function suggest severe disease/ systemic sepsis

*Immunology*

- Pneumococcal antigen in body fluids for *Streptococcus pneumoniae*
- Urinary antigen for early diagnosis of *Legionella pneumophila*

*Microbiology*

- Sputum and blood microscopy (Gram stain) and culture to confirm causative organism
- Treat empirically pending microbiological diagnosis (which is available in <50% of patients)
- Consider sampling parapneumonic effusion to exclude empyema and/or identify organism

*Chest radiograph*

- *Streptococcus pneumoniae:* patchy bronchopneumonia, lobar consolidation, pleural effusion
- *Mycoplasma pneumoniae:* lobar consolidation, patchy shadowing, sometimes normal
- *Haemophilus influenzae:* widespread inflammatory shadowing, scattered alveolar consolidation
- *Legionella pneumophila:* spreading inflammation
- *Staphylococcus aureus:* spreading bronchopneumonia, patchy consolidation, abscesses (may cavitate)
- Persistent consolidation after 6 weeks should raise a suspicion of underlying carcinoma

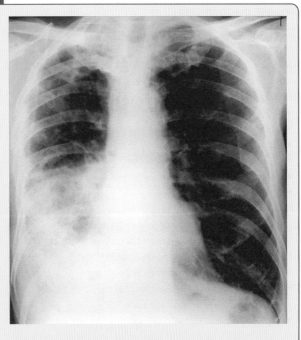

**Figure B** Posteroanterior chest X-ray showing bronchopneumonia in the right lower lobe, in this case secondary to *Mycoplasma pneumoniae.*

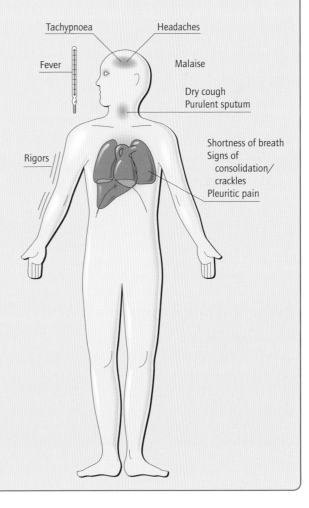

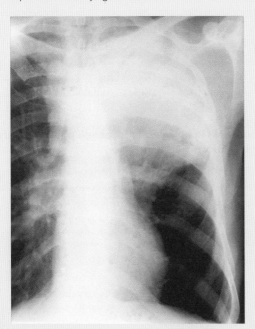

**Figure A** Posteroanterior chest X-ray showing lobar consolidation in the left upper lobe, secondary to *Streptococcus pneumoniae.*

## HOSPITAL-ACQUIRED PNEUMONIA

### Disease mechanisms

Hospital-acquired (nosocomial) pneumonia is pneumonia occurring 48 hours after admission to hospital, but also consider hospital-acquired pathogens in those admitted from nursing homes. Risk factors are those that impair host defence and/or ability to clear airway secretions:

- Pre-existing lung disease
- General anaesthesia and/or sedation
- Assisted ventilation
- Chest or upper abdominal surgery
- Steroids/immunosuppression
- Nasogastric feeding

The spectrum of bacteria overlaps with community-acquired pathogens, but hospital-acquired infection is more often caused by Gram-negative bacteria and anaerobes:

- *Staphylococcus aureus*, including MRSA
- *Escherichia coli* and *Proteus* spp.
- *Pseudomonas aeruginosa*, particularly in pre-existing lung disease or ventilated patients
- *Klebsiella pneumoniae*, particularly in the elderly, in whom it carries a high mortality

### Clinical features

Clinical features are similar to those of community-acquired pneumonia but patients are often more ill. *Klebsiella* infection is characterized by rapid-onset severe cavitating pneumonia, usually in the upper lobes.

### Investigation

Investigation is similar to that of community-acquired pneumonia, with particular emphasis on cultures to identify a pathogen.

### Management

Empirical antibiotic therapy should be guided by local microbiological sensitivities but usually includes broad-spectrum Gram-negative and anaerobic cover. Antibiotic side effects are common, hence the value of early identification of the pathogen, to allow targeted therapy. If not improving, consider MRSA or *Pseudomonas aeruginosa*, which are not usually covered by first-line empirical therapy.

## ASPIRATION PNEUMONIA

### Disease mechanisms

Aspiration pneumonia occurs when material is aspirated from the upper airway into the lower respiratory tract, typically into the right lower lobe. This may include stomach contents, upper airway secretions and commensal organisms. Clinical syndrome results from a combination of chemical pneumonitis, bacterial infection (often anaerobes) and airway obstruction. Risk factors include:

- Reduced conscious level (e.g. sedation, seizures, overdose)
- Poor swallow (e.g. neuromuscular disease, stroke)
- Abnormal upper gastrointestinal (GI) anatomy (e.g. hiatus hernia, nasogastric feeding)

### Clinical features

There is often a clear precipitant, such as an episode of vomiting, followed by rapidly developing breathlessess, hypoxia and fever, with progessive lower zone X-ray changes.

### Management

- Consider suction if upper airway material is still present.
- Give antibiotics early, including anaerobic cover.
- Have a low threshold for making the patient nil by mouth pending formal swallow assessment or increase in conscious level.

## PNEUMONIA IN THE IMMUNOCOMPROMISED

Patients with immunocompromise are more susceptible not only to the usual pathogenic organisms but also to a variety of opportunistic organisms. Management depends on the pathogen, so efforts should be directed towards microbiological diagnosis. This may include early bronchoalveolar lavage. Empirical treatment should be started while seeking the diagnosis.

### Pneumonia in HIV infection

Opportunistic lung infection is the most common presentation of AIDS. The most common life-threatening opportunistic infection is *Pneumocystis* pneumonia (PCP, see below), and empirical therapy should cover PCP, but other pathogens cause pulmonary disease in this setting (**Table 6.14**).

The clinical picture of pneumonia in HIV may be atypical. Look for other signs of opportunistic infection (e.g. oropharyngeal candidiasis, generalized lymphadenopathy or the skin lesions of Kaposi's sarcoma). Chest X-ray changes may be atypical, so have a low threshold for CT chest.

### Pneumonia in immunosuppressed patients without HIV infection

Immunosuppression with corticosteroids, cytotoxic agents or monoclonal antibodies is increasingly common in the

**Table 6.14** Pulmonary manifestations of HIV infection

| Cause | Uncommon | Common |
|---|---|---|
| Infection | *Legionella* | PCP |
| | Fungi | *Mycobacterium tuberculosis* |
| | Herpes viruses | Cytomegalovirus |
| | Toxoplasmosis | *Mycobacterium avium/ intracellulare* |
| | Cryptococcus | |
| | | Pyogenic bacteria |
| Tumour | Kaposi's sarcoma | |
| | Lymphoma | |

management of haematological malignancy, organ transplantation, autoimmune diseases and solid tumours. Immunosuppression also occurs in primary immunodeficiency syndromes (which should be excluded if unsure) and starvation.

Initial treatment is with broad spectrum antibiotics including Gram-negative cover. In the setting of neutropenia, pulmonary infection can progress rapidly to life-threatening systemic sepsis. If failing to improve despite empirical antibiotics, consider the addition of an antifungal agent.

## PNEUMOCYSTIS PNEUMONIA

### Disease mechanisms

Caused by the environmental pathogen *Pneumocystis jirovecii* (previously known as *Pneumocystis carinii*), PCP is one of the most commonly encountered opportunistic lung infections. Patients at particular risk are those on high-dose steroids or chemotherapy, or those with HIV and CD4 count $<200 \times 10^6$/L.

### Clinical features

This usually presents insidiously over 3–4 weeks, with a dry cough, dyspnoea and pyrexia. Examination is often unremarkable in the early stages, but clinical/radiological deterioration can be rapid.

### Investigation

- *Bloods:* The WCC may be normal; lactate dehydrogenase (LDH) is often elevated.
- *Chest X-ray:* Classically there are bilateral perihilar infiltrates, progressing to consolidation, but radiographs may be normal early on. CT typically shows widespread ground-glass changes with consolidation.
- *Microbiology:* Induced sputum may be positive in patients with HIV and high bacterial load, but bronchoscopy is often performed. Silver staining or immunofluorescence of lavage specimens has a high sensitivity, even after up to 2 weeks of treatment.

### Management

- *Antimicrobials:* Co-trimoxazole (trimethoprim and sulfamethoxazole) is the normal first-line drug, but it is often poorly tolerated. Intravenous administration carries a high fluid burden, and oral dosing may cause nausea and vomiting. Second-line agents include intravenous pentamidine.
- *Steroids:* High-dose corticosteroids (e.g. 40 mg prednisolone, weaned over 2 weeks) improve outcomes in patients with respiratory failure.

### Prognosis

Mortality is significant in all patient groups but particularly high (>50%) in HIV patients requiring mechanical ventilation.

## LUNG ABSCESS

### Disease mechanisms

A lung abscess is a cavitating lesion within the lung parenchyma caused by infection. They usually occur secondary to bronchogenic infection but can arise from septic emboli. They are uncommon, but alcoholics, the elderly, intravenous drug abusers and the immunocompromised are at greater risk. Causes of cavitating lung lesions are given in **Table 6.15**.

### Clinical features

Typically, there is subacute respiratory infection with productive cough and prominent fevers/night sweats, failing to respond to standard antibiotic therapy. Peripheral lesions may present with pleuritic pain. Central lesions may present with offensive sputum or haemoptysis, which can be massive.

### Investigation

- *Bloods:* Elevated inflammatory markers are slow to improve despite antibiotics. Platelets are usually high and albumin low, reflecting chronic inflammatory state.
- *Imaging:* Chest X-ray may show cavitation, with or without air–fluid level, and may provide clues as to organism. *Staphylococcus aureus* typically causes multiple thin-walled lung abscesses, while *Klebsiella* causes large upper lobe lesions.
- *Microbiology:* Obtain blood and sputum cultures. Consider bronchoscopy to identify the organism and exclude TB or malignancy. Percutaneous biopsy may provide a microbiological diagnosis but carries risk of pneumothorax/seeding.

**Table 6.15** Causes of cavitating lung lesions

**Infection**
- Pyogenic bacteria (e.g. *Staphylococcus aureus*, *Klebsiella pneumoniae*, *Pseudomonas* species)
- Mycobacteria (e.g. *Mycobacterium tuberculosis*, atypical mycobacteria)
- Fungi
- Parasites

**Cavitating tumours**
- Bronchogenic (usually squamous cell)
- Secondary deposits

**Pulmonary infarction**
- Thromboembolism
- Septic emboli
- Foreign body embolism (e.g. intravenous drug abuse)

**Bronchial occlusion**
- Bronchial tumour
- Inhaled foreign body (e.g. tooth, peanut)
- Localized bronchial stenosis

**Miscellaneous**
- Wegener's granulomatosis
- Infected bullae
- Pulmonary sequestration

## Management

Prolonged (4–6 week) courses of antibiotics are the main-stay, including anaerobic cover. If not resolving, consider percutaneous drainage or surgery. The feared complication is haemoptysis, which may require urgent surgery if massive.

# PULMONARY TUBERCULOSIS

Several mycobacterial organisms can cause disease in humans. The most important is *Mycobacterium tuberculosis*.

## Epidemiology

Pulmonary TB is common worldwide, with 10 million cases and more than 1 million deaths per year. In the UK, it is now relatively uncommon, with around 8000–9000 new cases per year (approximately 10/100 000). Risk factors include:

- Ethnicity
- Immunosuppression (HIV, diabetes mellitus, lymphoma, steroid, cytotoxic therapy)
- Anti-TNFα treatment
- Alcoholism and malnourishment
- Older age
- Silicosis

## Disease mechanisms

### Primary pulmonary TB

Spread is via droplet inhalation. *M. tuberculosis* settles in well-ventilated but poorly perfused areas of lung in the upper or middle lobe. Bacteria are taken up by macrophages and spread via lymphatics, leading to T cell activation and granuloma formation, classically consisting of central necrotic 'caseation' surrounded by Langerhans' giant cells. This is the Ghon focus. Hilar lymph nodes draining the affected lobe often enlarge. The combination of a Ghon focus and hilar lymph node enlargement is called the 'primary complex', which forms 3–8 weeks from the time of infection.

### Post-primary pulmonary TB

In the minority of cases, *M. tuberculosis* will overcome host defences and spread soon after infection, giving rise to pneumonia or pleural disease. More commonly (>90% of cases), granuloma formation prevents the spread of the bacilli, which become latent within the Ghon focus. The majority of active disease in adult patients is due to reactivation of latent TB (post-primary TB).

## Clinical features

### Primary pulmonary TB

Patients are usually asymptomatic, but there may be a mild illness with erythema nodosum. A small pleural effusion may develop and symptoms can arise if lymphadenopathy compresses a major bronchus, leading to distal collapse. Failure of lung reinflation after healing can cause bronchiectasis, particularly in the middle lobe.

### Post-primary pulmonary TB

This usually manifests over months, with malaise, weight loss, anorexia, night sweats and productive cough. There may be haemoptysis, breathlessness and chest pain, with or without pleural effusion. Some patients present with tender, enlarged cervical lymph nodes, usually in the anterior triangle, which may be the only manifestation of post-primary disease.

### Extrapulmonary disease

Pulmonary TB may present with extrapulmonary disease, which can also be seen in the absence of pulmonary manifestations. Common sites include:

- *Tuberculous meningitis:* typically presents with fevers, headache and altered conscious level or fits; CSF shows high protein, low glucose and lymphocytes
- *Spinal TB:* most common in the thoracic spine; may require prolonged antituberculous treatment and/or surgery
- *Tuberculous pericarditis:* presents with exudative pericardial effusion that might require drainage
- *Disseminated disease:* more common with underlying immunosuppression; usually involves the lung, with multiple tiny 'miliary' deposits, due to haematogenous spread

## Investigation

Definitive diagnosis requires direct visualization and/or culture of *M. tuberculosis*. In suspected cases, the priority should be obtaining a specimen for microbiological analysis.

- *Bloods:* These are often normal, but baseline tests are required prior to treatment.
- *Sputum microscopy and culture:* This is the first-line investigation in patients with a productive cough. Send at least two samples. If negative, consider bronchoscopy with lavage, pleural aspiration or lymph node biopsy.
- *Chest X-ray:* Classically there is upper-zone cavitating opacity with lymphadenopathy. There may be a pleural effusion. Miliary deposits are usually visible on X-ray but easily missed.
- *CT scan:* A scan is not required if the chest X-ray is classic, but it may be helpful to guide bronchoalveolar lavage. Cavitating consolidation and 'tree-in-bud' nodularity is typical of active disease.
- *Microbiology:* Ziehl–Neelsen staining is used to visualize mycobacteria. Conventional culture and drug susceptibility testing can take 4–6 weeks or longer as *M. tuberculosis* is slow-growing. PCR may be used for more rapid diagnosis and can identify genetic mutations predictive of resistance to rifampicin. Whole genome sequencing can provide rapid diagnosis and predict susceptibility across a wider range of drugs, but its use is not yet widespread.
- *HIV testing:* This should be offered to all patients with TB.
- *Mantoux test (tuberculin skin test):* This is not recommended in the investigation of active disease.

It is usually strongly positive in that setting, but a positive test can reflect latent TB or BCG vaccination. False negatives can occur in miliary TB or HIV.

- *Interferon-gamma release assay (IGRA):* A highly sensitive assay of the cellular response to TB, IGRA is useful in identifying latent TB but unable to distinguish between latent and active disease, so it is not recommended for investigation of the latter.
- *Histopathology:* Caseating granulomas are typical but not diagnostic. All specimens should also be sent for microbiological analysis (without fixative).

## Management

If possible, definitive diagnosis should be made prior to commencing treatment, but this should not delay therapy in a deteriorating patient.

- *Drug treatment:* Multidrug regimens are used to prevent the development of resistant strains (**Table 6.16**; **Table 6.17**). Uncomplicated pulmonary TB is usually treated for 6 months. In the UK, first-line therapy includes rifampicin, isoniazid (with pyridoxine), pyrazinamide and ethambutol for 2 months, then rifampicin and isoniazid (with pyridoxine) only for a further 4 months. A longer course is recommended for central nervous system (CNS) disease (e.g. 12 months).
- *Multidrug-resistant TB (MDR-TB):* This is defined as resistance to two or more first-line agents. More complex therapy regimens are required, with strict infection control measures for inpatients. Risk factors include previous TB, poor adherence to treatment and birth/residence in a high resistance area.
- *Contact tracing:* Screening of close contacts should be considered for all patients with active TB, and treatment for latent TB should be considered where appropriate.

**Table 6.16** Management of TB

**Prevention**
Vaccination with BCG
Contact tracing and screening
Treatment of latent TB

**Supportive treatment**
Good nutrition
Reduce alcohol intake

**Drug treatment**
Standard regimen for fully sensitive disease (6 months in total):
- Rifampicin, isoniazid (+ pyridoxine), pyrazinamide and ethambutol for first 2 months
- Rifampicin and isoniazid (+ pyridoxine) for a further 4 months
Consider DOT if concerns regarding adherence or in multidrug-resistant TB
TB involving the CNS will require longer duration of treatment (e.g. 12 months)

**Surgery**
To remove severely damaged bronchiectatic lobes (rare)

BCG, bacille Calmette–Guérin; TB, tuberculosis; DOT, directly observed therapy.

### Prevention

- *Vaccination:* Bacille Calmette–Guérin (BCG), a live attenuated strain of bovine TB, reduces the risk of developing TB by up to 70%. It may be offered to infants in high-risk groups or endemic areas, or to Mantoux-negative older children. It may be used in adults following exposure to TB or at high risk of exposure (e.g. healthcare workers).
- *Treatment of latent TB:* A positive Mantoux or IGRA with no symptoms and a normal chest X-ray suggests latent TB. Chemoprophylaxis (e.g. rifampicin and isoniazid for 3 months, or isoniazid for 6 months) is offered to those at high risk of active TB (e.g. those with recent exposure, HIV, solid organ transplantation, cytotoxic chemotherapy, anti-TNFα therapy).

**Table 6.17** Important characteristics of standard antituberculous drugs

| Drug | Pharmacological action | Side effects* | Contraindications | Monitoring of patients |
|---|---|---|---|---|
| Rifampicin | Bactericidal | Induces liver enzymes; Causes GI upset; Stains body secretions orange | Porphyria, jaundice; Note drug interactions (including with antiretroviral therapy) | Monitor liver function |
| Isoniazid | Bactericidal | Peripheral neuropathy (uncommon if given with pyridoxine); Hepatitis; Rash | Porphyria | Not necessary if pyridoxine is given as well |
| Pyrazinamide | Bactericidal | Liver failure; Anaemia | Liver disease; Porphyria | Monitor liver function |
| Ethambutol | Bacteriostatic | Optic neuritis | Renal disease; Poor vision | Monitor vision and renal function; Document visual acuity before starting |

*NB Patient should be warned that many antituberculous drugs have significant side effects.

## PULMONARY TUBERCULOSIS AT A GLANCE

### Epidemiology

*Prevalence*

- Around 8000–9000 new cases per year in UK (10/100 000 population); more common worldwide

*Ethnicity*

- Most common among those of Asian, West Indian and Chinese ethnicity in the UK

*Geography*

- Most common in developing countries

### Findings on investigation

*Haematology*

- May be normal, but may show anaemia

*Immunology*

- Mantoux test and IGRA positive, but does not distinguish active vs. latent disease

*Microbiology*

- Ziehl–Neelsen staining reveals acid-fast bacilli on microscopy
- Definitive diagnosis requires culture of *Mycobacterium tuberculosis*, which can take up to 6 weeks

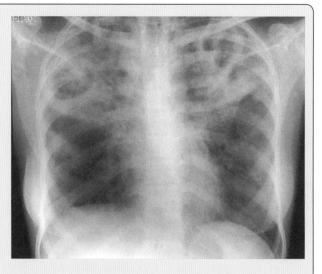

**Figure B** Post-primary pulmonary TB. Chest radiograph showing bilateral apical cavitating pneumonia.

*Histopathology*

- Pleural, lymph node or lung biopsy: histology reveals caseating granulomas (**Figure C**)

*Diagnostic imaging*

- Chest radiography: upper-zone soft shadowing, cavities

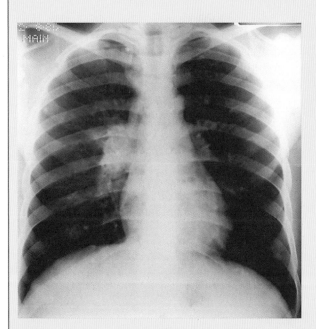

**Figure A** Primary pulmonary TB. Chest radiograph showing unilateral hilar lymphadenopathy. The Ghon focus is often not visible on the radiograph.

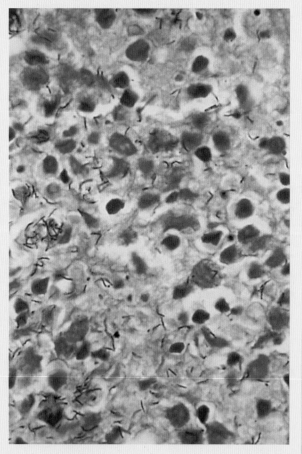

**Figure C** Ziehl–Neelsen-stained material obtained from a caseating mediastinal lymph node. Many acid–alcohol-fast bacteria are seen, with the typical red 'cording or clustering' appearance of *M. tuberculosis*. Reproduced from Bannister B *et al.* (1996) *Infectious Disease* (Wiley-Blackwell, Oxford) with the permission of the authors.

*Continued...*

DISEASES AND THEIR MANAGEMENT

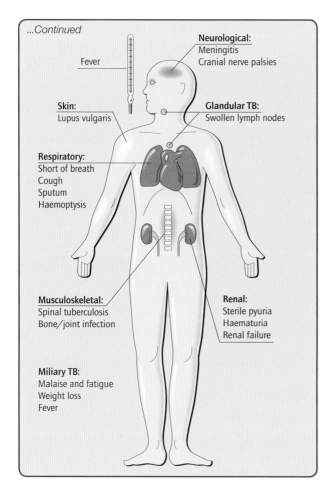

...Continued

**Fever**

**Neurological:**
Meningitis
Cranial nerve palsies

**Skin:**
Lupus vulgaris

**Glandular TB:**
Swollen lymph nodes

**Respiratory:**
Short of breath
Cough
Sputum
Haemoptysis

**Musculoskeletal:**
Spinal tuberculosis
Bone/joint infection

**Renal:**
Sterile pyuria
Haematuria
Renal failure

**Miliary TB:**
Malaise and fatigue
Weight loss
Fever

**6**

## Prognosis

The prognosis is good if the patient is not immunosuppressed.

## NON-TUBERCULOSIS MYCOBACTERIAL INFECTION

Non-tuberculous mycobacteria (NTM) are environmental organisms that rarely cause disease in healthy individuals but can colonize the airways and/or cause infection in susceptible patients.

### Epidemiology

- NTM is increasing in prevalence.
- Risk factors include chronic lung disease (particularly bronchiectasis, cystic fibrosis and COPD), increasing age and immunodeficiency.

### Disease mechanisms

Causative organisms are classified as either slow-growing (e.g. *Mycobacterium avium*, *M. intracellulare*) or rapidly growing (e.g. *M. abscessus*).

### Clinical features

Colonization may be asymptomatic. Infection typically presents as unexplained worsening of existing lung disease and/or systemic features of malaise and weight loss, with productive cough. Disseminated infection is rare outside the setting of severe immunodeficiency (e.g. HIV).

### Investigation

As for *M. tuberculosis*, sputum microscopy and culture are the first-line investigation, and culture is similarly slow. Given the possibility of asymptomatic colonization and/or contamination with environmental organisms, two positive sputum samples (or a single positive bronchoscopic lavage or biopsy specimen) are generally required prior to considering treatment.

### Management

- Multidrug regimens are used (e.g. rifampicin, ethambutol and a macrolide), and treatment is given for a minimum of 12 months. Risks of treatment should therefore be carefully weighed against severity of symptoms.
- Macrolide monotherapy should be avoided due to risk of resistance.

### Prognosis

It is not always possible to clear NTM infection, despite prolonged treatment (years).

## *ASPERGILLUS* LUNG DISEASE

### Epidemiology

- The fungus that most often produces lung disease is *Aspergillus fumigatus*. *Aspergillus* lung disease is nevertheless uncommon.
- Incidence is higher in the elderly or those with chronic lung disease.

### Disease mechanisms and clinical features

*Aspergillus* is ubiquitous and often cultured from the sputum of people in whom it is not pathogenic. There are, however, three distinct patterns of disease:

- *Aspergilloma:* A fungal ball forms in a pre-existing lung cavity (e.g. post-TB). It is often aysmptomatic and identified incidently, but it can be associated with haemoptysis due to erosion into vascular structures. This can be massive and life-threatening.
- *Allergic bronchopulmonary aspergillosis (ABPA):* An immunological response to *Aspergillus* causes airway inflammation and an asthma-like illness with episodes of cough, pyrexia and malaise. Yellowish sputum and bronchial plugs may be expectorated. Repeated episodes can lead to proximal bronchiectasis, more common in the upper lobes.
- *Invasive aspergillosis:* This involves direct invasion of the fungus into the lung parenchyma. It is uncommon without significant immunocompromise or neutropenia.

171

### Investigation

- *Blood tests:* There is usually a peripheral blood eosinophilia.
- *Immunology:* Total IgE and *Aspergillus*-specific IgE and IgG are usually elevated, with positive precipitans (precipitating IgG). Skin-prick tests to *Aspergillus* will be positive.
- *Microbiology and histopathology: Aspergillus* can be cultured in the sputum, and cytology reveals an excess of eosinophils, with or without fungal hyphae.
- *Imaging:* An aspergilloma may be visible as an ill-defined opacity within a lung cavity. ABPA is characterized by upper lobe bronchiectasis with bronchial wall thickening/oedema, which may create the classic 'finger-in-glove' appearance. Peripheral consolidation, ground glass and tree-in-bud nodularity may be present, and mucus plugging can cause lobar collapse.

### Management and prognosis

- *Aspergilloma:* This may remain stable for many years without treatment, but it seldom resolves. Progressive or symptomatic disease may be treated with antifungals, but with uncertain benefit. Large volume haemoptysis is treated by selective arterial embolization and/or surgical resection.
- *ABPA:* Oral corticosteroids are given in the acute stage, e.g. 0.5 mg/kg prednisolone, tapering over months. Maintenance oral and/or inhaled corticosteroids (ICS) may be required to prevent recurrent episodes, with or without antifungals (e.g. itraconazole) to reduce the antigenic stimulus. If well-controlled, long-term prognosis is good.
- *Invasive aspergillosis:* this is treated with systemic antifungal agents (e.g. amphotericin or voriconazole) and carries a very poor prognosis.

### Other fungal lung diseases

Other fungal lung infections are rare. *Candida albicans* and *Cryptococcus neoformans* can cause invasive pulmonary disease in the setting of immunosuppression, and they have a poor prognosis. *Actinomyces israelii* is an anaerobic gut bacterium, but it shares morphological features with fungi. It can be aspirated into the lungs, leading to abscess formation or invasive disease (actinomycosis), which normally responds to treatment with penicillin.

## OBSTRUCTIVE AIRWAYS DISEASE

## ASTHMA

Asthma is defined as reversible obstruction to airflow in the intrathoracic airways.

### Epidemiology

Asthma is common, affecting 10–15% of the population in the UK.

### Disease mechanisms

Symptoms and airflow limitation are due to a number of mechanisms including airway smooth muscle contraction, airway mucosal oedema and mucus plugging, often associated with eosinophilic airway inflammation orchestrated by the type-2 cytokines IL-5, IL-13 and IL-4. The last two mechanisms are particularly associated with non-bronchodilator responsive airflow limitation, and asthma attacks (EMERGENCY PRESENTATION 6.1).

### Clinical features

Airflow obstruction is typically episodic, worse after allergen exposure, at night, following exercise and with viral respiratory tract infections. It manifests as bouts of wheezing, chest tightness, cough and breathlessness.

- *Early-onset asthma* is typically associated with allergy to common aeroallergens (house dust mite, grass pollens, cat and dog epithelium, and fungi) and many patients have eczema or hay fever.
- *Adult-onset asthma* is usually non-allergic and is commonly associated with chronic rhinosinusitis and nasal polyposis. Both are now acknowledged to be heterogeneous conditions with respect to clinical presentation, severity, pathology and treatment responsiveness.

### Investigation

The diagnosis of asthma requires the demonstration of variable airflow limitation with associated symptoms.

- *Spirometry:* This may be obstructive (FEV1/FVC<0.7; see **Figure 6.1**) but may be normal when well, or show only subtle scalloping of the flow volume loop.
- *PEFR monitoring:* Significant (>20%) diurnal variability is suggestive of asthma.
- *Bronchodilator reversibility:* If spirometry is obstructive, the diagnosis of asthma is supported by reversibility after treatment with $\beta^2$ agonists or corticosteroids (an FEV1 increase of ≥12% and ≥200 mL constitutes significant reversibility).
- *Bronchial challenge testing:* If spirometry is normal, consider referral for inhaled methacholine or histamine challenge, which may demonstrate bronchial hyperresponsiveness.
- *Bloods:* These may reveal eosinophilia and/or elevated IgE. Specific IgE testing (or skin prick testing) may confirm environmental triggers if suspected.
- *Imaging:* Chest X-ray is often normal but may show hyperinflation. CT is not usually required but may reveal gas trapping.
- *Fractional exhaled nitric oxide (FeNO):* Increased exhaled nitric oxide is suggestive of eosinophilic airway inflammation.

## EMERGENCY PRESENTATION 6.1

### Management of asthma attacks

#### Diagnosis

The presence of one or more of the following features suggests acute severe asthma:

- PEFR <50% best or predicted
- Inability to talk in uninterrupted sentences
- Respiratory rate ≥25/min
- Tachycardia ≥110/min

#### Specific treatment

*At home*

Assess airway/breathing/circulation

Oxygen – high-flow

Nebulized $\beta_2$-agonists (e.g. salbutamol 2.5–5 mg, terbutaline 5–10 mg) or inhaled via spacer

Prednisolone 40 mg orally

*At hospital*

Reassess airway/breathing/circulation

Oxygen – high-flow

Nebulized $\beta_2$-agonists (e.g. salbutamol 2.5–5 mg) and muscarinic antagonist (e.g. ipratropium 0.5 mg)

Chest X-ray to exclude pneumothorax

Hydrocortisone 200 mg 4-hourly intravenously (or prednisolone if not yet given)

Antibiotics are not indicated unless there is radiological evidence of an infection

*Intravenous bronchodilators*

If no improvement or life-threatening features consider intravenous magnesium (1.2–2 g over 20 min) or aminophylline (e.g. 0.5–0.7 mg/kg/hour, with loading dose of 5 mg/kg over 20 min if not on oral maintenance therapy). Intravenous $\beta_2$ agonist is rarely indicated if the nebulized route is available.

#### Indications for intensive care

Patients with the following features of life-threatening asthma require intensive monitoring by experienced staff in the ICU:

- Hypoxia ($Pa_{O2}$ < 8 kPa) despite 60% inspired oxygen
- Hypercapnia ($Pa_{CO2}$ > 6 kPa)
- Cyanosis
- Exhaustion
- Bradycardia
- Hypotension
- Confusion or drowsiness
- Unconsciousness
- Respiratory arrest

### Management

The British Thoracic Society has published guidelines on the management of asthma (**Table 6.18**) and severe asthma attacks (see **EMERGENCY PRESENTATION 6.1**; **Figure 6.4**).

**Table 6.18** Management of asthma

**Supportive treatment**

Avoid precipitating causes

**Drug treatment**

The British Thoracic Society has produced guidelines (BTS/Sign Guideline 2019) for the pharmacological management of chronic asthma, based on stepping up when control is inadequate and stepping down when well-controlled, according to the steps shown below, to maintain the lowest controlling treatment burden:

*Regular preventer:*

- Regular low-dose inhaled corticosteroid (ICS)
- Short-acting inhaled $\beta_2$-agonist as required

*Initial add-on therapy:*

- Add inhaled LABA to low-dose ICS [fixed dose or MART (maintenance and reliever therapy)
- Short-acting inhaled $\beta_2$-agonist as required (unless using MART)

*Additional controller therapies:*

- Increase ICS to medium-dose OR add a leuokotriene receptor antagonist (LTRA)
- If no response to LABA, consider stopping LABA
- Short-acting inhaled $\beta_2$-agonist as required (unless using MART)

*Specialist therapies:*

- Refer patient to specialist care
- Increase ICS to high-dose OR add a LTRA (if not already trialled) OR consider adding tiotropium (long-acting muscarinic antagonist) OR consider adding theophylline.
- Short-acting inhaled $\beta_2$-agonist as required
- Consider use of daily oral steroid dose in lowest dose providing adequate symptoms control
- Patients with a high oral corticosteroid burden (either continuous or frequent use of oral steroid courses) are considered for treatment with biological ant-cytokine therapy, such as omalizumab (subcutaneous) or mepolizumab (subcutaneous) or reslizumab (intravenous) or benralizumab (subcutaneous), in specialized centres if they meet the eligibility criteria.

## CHRONIC OBSTRUCTIVE PULMONARY DISEASE

By definition, COPD is associated with fixed airflow limitation, as a result of increased airway mucus production, airway mucosal hypertrophy and loss of support of smaller airways by surrounding lung parenchyma (emphysema).

### Epidemiology/Disease mechanisms

- COPD causes approximately 30 000 deaths/year in the UK.
- It is strongly associated with cigarette smoking.

## ASTHMA AT A GLANCE

### Epidemiology

*Prevalence*

- 10–15% of the population

*Genetics*

- Associated with atopy

### Findings on investigation

*Haematology*

- Full blood count ( FBC): may show eosinophilia

*Immunology*

- IgE: may be increased in allergic asthma

*Imaging*

- Chest radiograph: usually normal
- Inspiratory/expiratory CT scan: may reveal gas trapping

*Spirometry*

- May be normal between exacerbations. Diurnal variation or an improvement in $FEV_1$ ≥12% (and ≥200 mL) following inhalation of a bronchodilator or a trial of corticosteroid is consistent with a diagnosis of asthma

*Bronchial provocation challenge*

- Methacholine or histamine may be used to demonstrate airway hyperresponsiveness if spirometry is normal

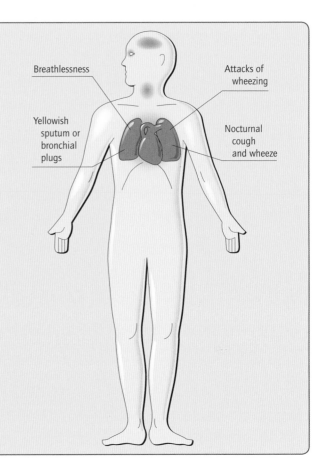

Breathlessness

Attacks of wheezing

Yellowish sputum or bronchial plugs

Nocturnal cough and wheeze

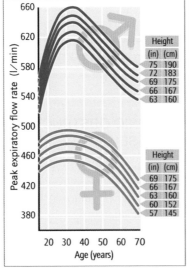

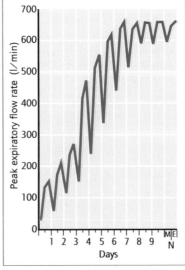

**Figure 6.4** Peak flow measurement in asthma. **(a)** Normal peak expiratory flow rate (PEFR) readings (males, blue; females, red). **(b)** Daily PEFR measurements in a patient with an episode of acute severe asthma at day 0, which improved with treatment over the subsequent 10 days. Note the diurnal variation in PEFR (M, N, E, morning, noon and evening).

- In most cases, the mechanism of susceptibility to cigarette smoke is unknown; a small percentage of patients are homozygous for the deficient alpha-1 antitrypsin gene (ZZ).

## Clinical features

Patients typically present with persistent cough, breathlessness, wheeze and chest tightness. Many patients are prone to exacerbations of symptoms associated with winter viral respiratory tract infections. Physical examination reveals use of the accessory muscles of respiration and a prolonged expiratory phase. The chest is overinflated and further chest expansion is poor. Breath sounds are typically diminished and polyphonic expiratory wheezes are often present.

People who have $CO_2$ retention have a bounding pulse and peripheral vasodilatation, and they may be cyanosed. Severe $CO_2$ retention is indicated by a coarse flapping tremor, confusion, headaches, an altered sleep pattern and papilloedema ($CO_2$ narcosis). Chronic hypoxia results in pulmonary vasoconstriction and vascular remodelling, and can be complicated by polycythaemia, pulmonary hypertension (PH) and right heart failure (cor pulmonale).

## Investigation

- *Bloods:* These may reveal polycythemia. A subset of patients has peripheral eosinophilia, which is a marker of eosinophilic airway inflammation.
- *Spirometry:* There is airflow obstruction (FEV1/FVC <0.7), often with limited reversibility. Gas transfer is reduced and lung volumes (RV and TLC) are elevated.
- *Imaging:* Chest X-ray may show emphysema and hyperinflation. CT may reveal emphysema (**Figure A** in CHRONIC OBSTRUCTIVE AIRWAYS DISEASE AT A GLANCE).

## CHRONIC OBSTRUCTIVE AIRWAYS DISEASE AT A GLANCE

### Epidemiology

*Prevalence*
- Common, affecting ~200 million people worldwide, predominantly aged >50 years
- Strongly associated with smoking
- Emphysema associated with $\alpha_1$-antitrypsin deficiency

### Findings on investigation

*Haematology*
- May reveal secondary polycythaemia in patients with persistent hypoxia

*Blood gases*
- Hypoxia and hypercapnia may be present

*Biochemistry*
- $\alpha_1$-antitrypsin deficiency may be present, particularly in non-smokers

*Chest X-ray*
- May be normal or show flattened diaphragms, altered rib angle, loss of lung markings, lung hyperinflation

*ECG*
- Right ventricular strain and p 'pulmonale' in cases of cor pulmonale

*Lung function*
- Spirometry: airflow obstruction (FEV1/FVC <0.7), air-trapping, increased RV
- Transfer factor is markedly diminished in those with underlying emphysema

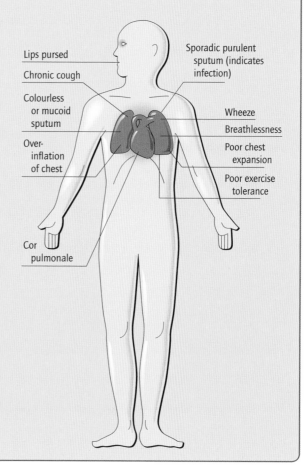

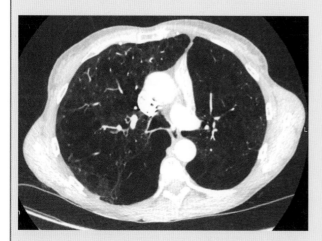

**Figure A** CT scan showing extensive emphysema in a smoker with COPD.

**Table 6.19** Management of COPD

**Supportive treatment**

*Physiotherapy*
- Little role unless there is overlying infection or secondary bronchiectasis

*Psychotherapy*
- Pulmonary rehabilitation classes can help severely affected individuals cope with their disability

**Specific treatment**
- Remove causal agent (cigarettes or occupational exposure)

**Drug treatment**
- Inhaled bronchodilators and ICS: the latter are more effective in patients with higher blood eosinophil counts
- Antibiotics: usually limited to the prompt treatment of acute infections
- Sometimes long-term rotating antibiotics or prolonged courses of low-dose macrolide antibiotics used to prevent recurrent infections
- Main infecting organism is *Haemophilus influenzae*, which is usually sensitive to doxycycline

## Management

Precipitating factors should be avoided and bronchospasm and acute infections should be treated (**Table 6.19**).

## BRONCHIECTASIS

Bronchiectasis is chronic dilatation of the bronchi. Mucus clearance is disrupted, secretions collect in the dilated bronchi and infection ensues. This damages the bronchi further, causing increasing sepsis, worsening bronchial inflammation and more secretion retention.

### Epidemiology

- Affects approximately 1/1000; more common in developing countries
- Onset usually in childhood but can affect any age
- Commonly an acquired condition but congenital causes include cystic fibrosis and IgA deficiency

### Disease mechanisms

The most common cause of bronchiectasis is damage to the bronchial tree after an infection in early life. Bronchiectasis may also complicate any condition where there is failure of normal mucus transport, autoimmune conditions and conditions associated with immunodeficiency (**Table 6.20**). No obvious cause is found in up to 50% of patients.

### Clinical features

- Symptoms include a chronic cough, and copious sputum, which is often purulent and offensive in severe disease.
- Exacerbations of infection are common and may be associated with haemoptysis.
- Examination may reveal coarse paninspiratory lung crackles that are widespread or localized to one area. Bronchospasm may be a feature. Other manifestations include finger clubbing and signs of the predisposing disease.

## Investigation

- *Bloods:* Haemoglobin is decreased in severe disease.
- *Imaging:* A definitive diagnosis is usually made on CT imaging, which typically shows bronchial wall thickening and cylindrical dilatation of the bronchi. More clinically important disease is often in the middle and lower lobes.
- *Immunoglobulins:* These usually show a non-specific increase but immunoglobulin deficiency (most commonly selective IgA deficiency) is a cause of bronchiectasis.
- *Sputum culture:* Culture may reveal *Haemophilus influenzae, Staphylococci* and *Pseudomonas* spp. NTM infection is rare but important as it is associated with progressive disease.

## Management

- Exercise and airway clearance techniques to remove retained bronchial secretions are important.
- Antibiotic therapy reduces bacterial load in the respiratory tree during acute infections. Inhaled (delivered by nebulizer) or continuous oral therapy can be used for chronic infection and more resistant pathogens (e.g. *Pseudomonas aeruginosa*).

**Table 6.20** Causes of bronchiectasis

| |
|---|
| Localized bronchial obstruction |
| Inhaled foreign body (e.g. peanut, tooth) |
| Enlarged hilar glands (which can compress the right middle lobe bronchus) |
| Bronchial tumours |
| Early-life infection (e.g. resulting from whooping cough, measles) |
| Recurrent infections resulting from immune defects (e.g. hypogammaglobulinaemia) |
| Autoimmune conditions (i.e. rheumatoid arthritis, inflammatory bowel disease) |
| Altered secretions (e.g. cystic fibrosis) |
| Ciliary dysfunction (e.g. Kartagener's syndrome or Young's syndrome) |

## BRONCHIECTASIS AT A GLANCE

### Epidemiology

*Prevalence*

- About 1/1000

*Geography*

- More common in developing countries

### Findings on investigation

*Haematology*

- FBC: haemoglobin may be decreased in severe disease

*Immunology*

- Often a polyclonal increase in immunoglobulins, unless primary aetiology is hypogammaglobulinaemia

*Microbiology*

- Sputum culture often positive for staphylococci and *Pseudomonas* spp.

*Diagnostic imaging*

- Chest X-ray: bronchial wall thickening, ring shadows
- CT scanning: airway dilatation and bronchial wall thickening

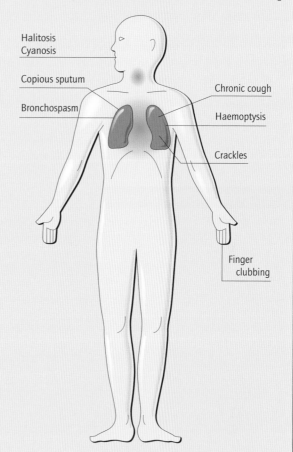

Halitosis
Cyanosis
Copious sputum
Bronchospasm
Chronic cough
Haemoptysis
Crackles
Finger clubbing

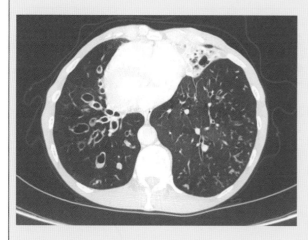

**Figure A** Severe bronchiectasis and mucous plugging in a patient with Kartagener's syndrome. Note dextrocardia.

- Bronchodilators are indicated for bronchospasm, which is often a concomitant feature. Inhaled and oral corticosteroid treatment is not usually indicated, except for cases associated with eosinophilia and aspergillus sensitization (ABPA).

### Prognosis

Bronchiectasis is a chronic disease that can be controlled by effective treatment.

## CYSTIC FIBROSIS

### Epidemiology

- Cystic fibrosis is a common autosomal recessive condition affecting 1/2000 births in white people, 1/20 000 in Afro-Caribbeans and 1/100 000 in Asians.
- Patients usually present at less than 1 year of age.

### Disease mechanisms

The cystic fibrosis (*CF*) gene is found on chromosome 7. It is very large, and to date >2000 mutations causing cystic fibrosis have been described. The most common mutation, *F508del*, is responsible for over 70% of cases of cystic fibrosis in the UK. The gene product is the cystic fibrosis transmembrane regulator (CFTR) protein. This regulates the chloride channel in the luminal surface of epithelial cells and its absence or dysfunction results in an abnormally high concentration of sodium in sweat and in a low water content in the mucus produced by airways, pancreas and intestine. Different gene abnormalities can cause differing degrees of CFTR malfunction and manifestation of disease.

### Clinical features

At birth, the infant is normal, but symptoms of organ dysfunction can occur soon after birth. Presenting features vary widely. Manifestations include:

- *Bronchiectasis* with recurrent airway infections and colonization with multiresistant *Pseudomonas*
- *Meconium ileus* in the neonate, due to abnormally viscid meconium obstructing the terminal ileum. (The adult equivalent is distal intestinal obstruction syndrome [DIOS])

- *Malabsorption and steatorrhoea* due to secretory dysfunction of the exocrine pancreas
- *CF-related diabetes* due islet cell damage secondary to chronic pancreatitis
- *Haemoptysis,* which can be massive and may require bronchial artery embolization
- *Pneumothorax*
- *Intrahepatic cholestasis and gallstones*
- *Altered fertility:* most men are infertile due to failure of vas deferens development; females may be fertile

### Investigation

- Sweat sodium and chloride concentrations are elevated (sweat sodium more than 60 mmol/L) in children over 10 years of age. With increasing age

there is an increasing incidence of diabetes mellitus, so regular screening is important.
- Sputum culture and sensitivity often reveal *Staphylococcus aureus* and *Pseudomonas* spp. NTM infection is an increasing problem.
- Genetic testing is increasingly important, as the specific genotype provides information about the nature of the underlying cellular defect, which may influence of the choice of novel targeted therapies.

### Management

Cystic fibrosis is best treated in a recognized CF centre where staff are experienced in the special needs of the patient. Each feature is treated according to its severity. Most patients require regular pancreatic supplements,

## CYSTIC FIBROSIS AT A GLANCE

### Epidemiology

*Prevalence*
- 1/2500 in the UK

*Age*
- Usually presents in infancy

*Race*
- Most common in white people

*Genetics*
- The classical CFTR mutation is *F508del*, but >2000 other mutations cause disease of varying severity

### Findings on investigation

*Biochemistry*
- Sweat test: raised sweat sodium and chloride concentrations
- Tests for diabetes mellitus positive in >20% of adult patients

*Immunology*
- Immune reactive trypsin positive in newborn (leading to screen for common CFTR mutations)

*Microbiology*
- Sputum culture commonly *Staphylococcus aureus*, *Haemophilus influenzae* and *Pseudomonas* spp.

*Diagnostic imaging*
- Chest radiography or CT scanning shows bronchiectasis

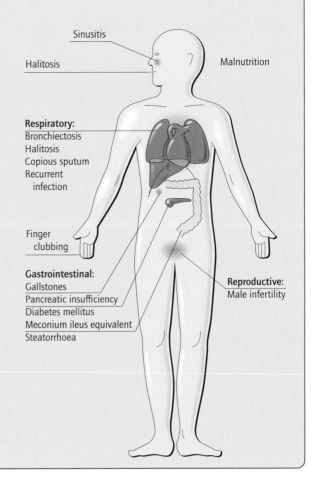

**Figure A** Chest radiograph showing widespread bronchiectasis in cystic fibrosis. Note the implanted venous access device for repeated intravenous antibiotic treatment.

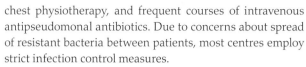

chest physiotherapy, and frequent courses of intravenous antipseudomonal antibiotics. Due to concerns about spread of resistant bacteria between patients, most centres employ strict infection control measures.

More than 90% of patients survive into adult life, when bronchiectasis is the main feature. Despite the best treatment, many patients develop progressive cardiorespiratory failure during adult life, but median age of survival is increasing, and is currently >40 years in developed countries.

The outlook for CF will likely be transformed over the next 5–10 years with the introduction of increasingly effective chloride channel correctors (CFTR modulators). These agents can normalize transepithelial chloride transport; they are associated with very large short-term clinical benefits and long-term use is anticipated to render CF a controllable chronic disease associated with a normal life expectancy.

## PLEURAL DISEASE

### PLEURAL EFFUSION

Pleural effusion is excessive accumulation of fluid in the pleural space.

#### Disease mechanisms

- Pleural effusion is common, with various aetiologies (**Table 6.21**).
- The commonest causes in the UK and US are heart failure (usually bilateral), infection (i.e. parapneumonic effusion) and malignancy.
- The effusion may be a transudate (protein <30 g/L) or an exudate (>30 g/L). When the distinction between transudate and an exudate is unclear, Light's criteria can be applied (**Table 6.22**).

#### Clinical features

- Breathlessness
- Pain (pleuritic or dull ache)
- Symptoms of the underlying cause (e.g. fever in parapneumonic effusions, orthopnoea in heart failure, haemoptysis and weight loss in bronchial carcinoma)
- On examination:
  o Stony dullness on percussion over the fluid, with absent or reduced breath sounds and vocal resonance
  o Bronchial breathing (in pneumonia) or fine inspiratory crackles (in heart failure) may be heard just above the effusion

#### Diagnosis and investigation

Following history and examination, initial tests should include:
- *Chest X-ray:* A pleural effusion is detectable clinically only when larger than 500 mL. Smaller effusions (>250 mL) are usually revealed by chest radiography.
- *Thoracic ultrasound:* This is more sensitive for detecting/characterizing small effusions.
- *CT scan:* Scan if the diagnosis is unclear.
- *Blood tests:* Test FBC, inflammatory markers, glucose, serum LDH and total protein (for comparison with pleural fluid) and consider autoimmune screen.
- *Pleural fluid aspiration:* Send for biochemistry (pH, LDH, glucose and protein as standard; consider amylase, triglycerides and cholesterol), microbiology (MC&S and mycobacterial culture, WCC differential, adenosine deaminase [ADA]) and cytology (including cell differential).
- *Pleural biopsy:* Take CT- or ultrasound-guided biopsy, or at thoracoscopy. Send for histopathology (in formalin) and microbiology (in saline).

#### Management

The aim is to relieve symptoms, treat the underlying cause and reduce risk of recurrence. The approach depends on the underlying cause and should be individualized according to patient preference and prognosis. Approaches can include:
- *Therapeutic aspiration:* 500–1000 mL of pleural fluid can be removed, aiming to relieve breathlessness.
- *Intercostal drain insertion:* A small (e.g. 12F) or large (>18F) drain can be inserted via a Seldinger technique or blunt dissection, with the aim of draining the effusion to dryness. Guidelines now recommend ultrasound guidance for intercostal drain insertion.
- *Pleurodesis:* A pleurodesis agent, usually talc, can be introduced either via an intercostal drain (talc slurry) or at thoracoscopy (talc poudrage). This is performed after an effusion is drained to dryness, with the aim of preventing recurrence (in malignant effusions). Success rates are variable.
- *Indwelling pleural catheter:* A long-term pleural drain is usually used for chronic or recurrent malignant effusions, in patients who either failed pleurodesis or have non-expanding lung. It allows repeated pleural drainage in the community.
- *Surgery:* Video-assisted thoracoscopic surgery (VATS) or thoracotomy and decortication may be required for infected effusions (empyema) not responding to intercostal drainage.
- *Intrapleural fibrinolytics:* In empyema not suitable for surgical treatment and failing conventional intercostal tube drainage, intrapleural fibrinolytic agents such as intrapleural alteplase (tPA) and dornase alpha (DNAse) may be considered.

### PNEUMOTHORAX

In pneumothorax, air collects between the visceral and parietal pleura, causing a real rather than potential pleural space. Air in the pleural space will allow the lung to move away from the

**Table 6.21** Causes of pleural effusion

| Type of effusion | Mechanism | Example(s) | Comment |
|---|---|---|---|
| Transudate (<30 g/L) | Haemodynamic failure | Cardiac failure | |
| | Hypoproteinaemia | Nephrotic syndrome | |
| | | Liver cirrhosis | |
| | | Starvation | |
| | Haemodynamic failure | Myxoedema | Rare |
| | Haemodynamic failure | Constrictive pericarditis | Rare |
| | Ascitic transfer | Meigs' syndrome | A rare syndrome of ovarian fibromas associated with a right-sided pleural effusion, which clears with removal of the tumour |
| | Urinothorax | Urinothorax | Effusion ipsilateral to obstructed kidney |
| Exudate (>30 g/L) | Simple parapneumonic effusion | Bacterial pneumonia | |
| | Complicated parapneumonic effusion | | pH <7.2 |
| | Empyema (collection of pus) | | Glucose <2.2 mmol/L<br>LDH >1000 IU/L<br>Common pathogens:<br>• *Streptococcus milleri* (30%)<br>• *Streptococcus pneumoniae* (15%)<br>• *Staphylococcus aureus* (10%) |
| | Carcinoma | Bronchial carcinoma<br>Metastatic carcinoma (e.g. breast carcinoma) | Often blood-stained |
| | Pleural inflammation | Pulmonary infarction | Often blood-stained |
| | Pleural inflammation | TB | Lymphocytosis present<br>Glucose low |
| | Pleural inflammation | Autoimmune rheumatic disease (e.g. RA, SLE) | Low glucose (<1.6 mmol/L)<br>Can have pseudo-chylothorax with high chylomicrons |
| | Pleural inflammation | Acute pancreatitis | Commonly left-sided<br>High amylase concentration<br>May be blood-stained |
| | Pleural inflammation | Subphrenic or hepatic abscess | Right-sided |
| | Primary pleural tumour | Mesothelioma | |
| | Pleural inflammation | Benign asbestos-related pleural effusion | |
| | Pleural inflammation | Post-cardiac surgery effusion | |
| | Blocked lymphatics | Yellow nail syndrome | Yellow nails, chronic lymphoedema and pleural effusions result from an abnormality of lymphatic drainage |
| | Fatty effusion | Chylothorax | Usually left-sided<br>Results from disruption of the thoracic duct by tumour or trauma<br>High in triglycerides |
| | Pleural bleeding | Trauma to the chest wall resulting in haemothorax | |

chest wall and the lung will partially deflate. A pneumothorax can be spontaneous or secondary to trauma (e.g. penetrating injuries to chest, rib fractures, central line insertions, thoracic biopsies) and can be classified as primary (in apparently normal lungs) or secondary (in lungs with underlying disease).

**Table 6.22** Light's criteria for exudate (one of the following)

Pleural fluid protein/serum protein ratio >0.5
Pleural fluid LDH/serum LDH ratio >0.6
Pleural fluid LDH >2/3 of upper limit of normal serum LDH

**6**

## PLEURAL EFFUSION AT A GLANCE

### Epidemiology

*Prevalence*

Common. More than 1 million cases/year in USA
Pleural effusion is most commonly a complication of:

- Left ventricular failure
- Bacterial pneumonia (parapneumonic effusion)
- Malignancy

### Findings on investigation

*Diagnostic imaging*

- Chest radiography: confirms site of effusion and may suggest cause
- Ultrasound: more sensitive than X-ray at detecting fluid, and used to guide pleural aspiration/drain insertion
- CT chest: may help to identify underlying cause (particularly malignancy)

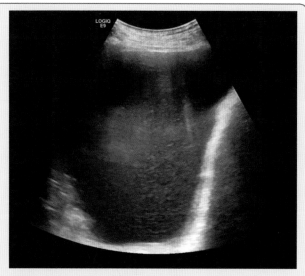

(iii)

**Figure A** **(i)** Large right pleural effusion on chest radiograph. **(ii)** Right malignant pleural effusion on CT imaging (note ipsilateral anterior pleural nodule). **(iii)** Large pleural effusion imaged with bedside ultrasound.

*Diagnostic pleural aspiration*

- Biochemistry: pleural fluid protein and LDH can be used to distinguish exudates and transudates; glucose typically low in empyema, TB, malignancy and rheumatoid arthritis; amylase may be high in pancreatitis
- Microbiology: low pH (<7.2) suggests empyema; microscopy and culture may reveal organism
- Cytology: may detect malignant/atypical cells
- If no diagnosis after aspiration, consider image-guided or thoracoscopic pleural biopsy

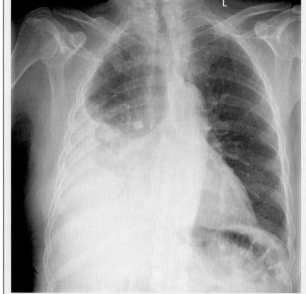

(i)

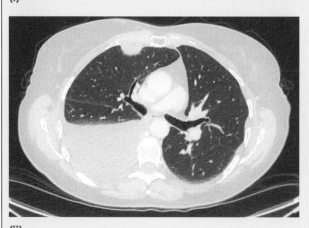

(ii)

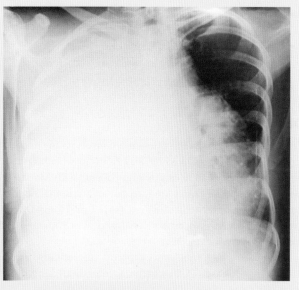

**Figure B** Massive pulmonary effusion. Note the displacement of the mediastinal structures (trachea, heart) to the contralateral side.

*Continued...*

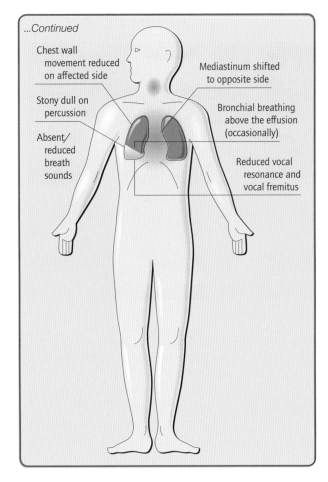

...Continued

Chest wall movement reduced on affected side

Mediastinum shifted to opposite side

Stony dull on percussion

Bronchial breathing above the effusion (occasionally)

Absent/ reduced breath sounds

Reduced vocal resonance and vocal fremitus

## Epidemiology

- The incidence of primary spontaneous pneumothorax is 9 in 100 000 per year.
- It is most common in males (5 : 1) than females, and is often seen in tall, thin young men.
- 20% of patients with primary spontaneous pneumothorax will have an ipsilateral recurrence. After a second and third episode, the recurrence rates are over 65% and 85% respectively.

## Disease mechanism

The pathogenesis in primary pneumothorax is poorly understood. There is a presumed air leak from apical subpleural blebs or bulla. It is more common in patients with Marfan's syndrome. Familial causes are rare, but an autosomal dominant mutation in the folliculin gene (as in Birt–Hogg–Dube syndrome, which also causes renal and skin tumours) is associated with pneumothorax.

Secondary pneumothoraces occur in patients with underlying disease: COPD, asthma, interstitial lung disease, TB, lung cancer, PCP, necrotizing pneumonia (e.g. staphylococcal), cystic fibrosis, lympangioleiomyomatosis (commoner in women), positive pressure ventilation in ICUs. Cigarette or cannabis smoking is a significant risk factor.

## Clinical features

- There is a sudden onset of sharp pleuritic chest pain and/or breathlessness.
- On examination: tachypnea, reduced expansion and breath sounds and hyper-resonant percussion on side of pneumothorax. Look for subcutaneous emphysema on the chest or neck (crackling sensation under the skin on palpation).
- Tension pneumothorax: A medical emergency that occurs when positive pressure builds up in the pleural space and results in mediastinal shift with breathlessness, hypoxaemia and eventually hypotension and shock secondary to impaired venous return. It is rare, but most commonly a complication of a traumatic pneumothorax or a pneumothorax during mechanical ventilation.
- A pneumothorax should always be considered in a patient with known lung disease with an unexplained increase in breathlessness.

## Investigation

- A chest X-ray confirms the diagnosis (**Figure 6.5**).
- Consider CT if there is uncertainty or complexity (e.g. partially tethered lung).

## Management

### Initial management

Initial management is outlined in EMERGENCY PRESENTATION 6.2 and **Figure 6.6**. A schematic of an intercostal drain and underwater seal is shown in **Figure 6.7**.

### Further management

*Outpatient follow-up*

- Repeat chest X-rays to ensure resolution, if still present on discharge.
- Advise the patient to avoid flying for at least 2 weeks following complete resolution on chest X-ray, and never scuba dive.

*Surgical management*

Indications for surgical referral include:
- Persistent air leak or failure to re-expand lung despite 3–5 days of intercostal drainage
- Second ipsilateral pneumothorax
- First contralateral pneumothorax
- Bilateral spontaneous pneumothoraces
- Professional pilots or divers who have a first pneumothorax

Surgical procedures include VATS for repair of apical blebs or bullae; talc poudrage; mechanical pleural abrasion and/or parietal pleurectomy.

## PLEURAL THICKENING

### Definition and disease mechanisms

Pleural thickening can be a result of:
- Fibrosis following pleurisy, recurrent/chronic effusions or empyema

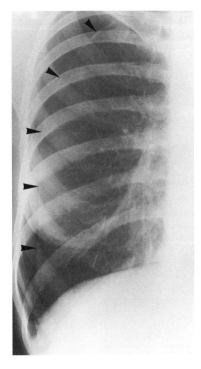 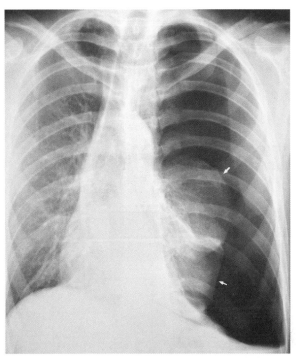

**Figure 6.5** **(a)** Small right pneumothorax on chest X-ray. Note clear space beyond pleural edge (arrowheads). **(b)** Large left tension pneumothorax, leading to depression of the left hemidiaphragm and shifting of the mediastinum to the right. Arrows indicate lung edge. Reproduced from Armstrong P & Wastie ML (1992) *Diagnostic Imaging*, 3rd edn (Wiley-Blackwell, Oxford) with the permission of the authors.

**EMERGENCY 6.2**

## Pneumothorax

### Diagnosis

Sudden pleuritic pain and breathlessness are the most common symptoms. A chest X-ray confirms the diagnosis.

### Assessment

*Airway*

*Breathing*

*Circulation*

### Supportive therapy

Oxygen

Analgesia

### Specific therapy

*Traumatic pneumothorax*

All require formal drainage as there is an increased risk of tension pneumothorax.

*Tension pneumothorax*

Rare. Clinical diagnosis in a patient with a pneumothorax with respiratory distress and cardiovascular compromise. Decompress with a 14G needle in the second intercostal space/ mid-clavicular line, then insert a chest drain.

*Other pneumothoraces*

Treatment depends upon:

* Size
* Symptoms of breathlessness
* Whether there is underlying lung disease (secondary)

An algorithm for generic management is provided by the British Thoracic Society (see **Figure 6.6**).

### Aspiration of a pneumothorax

Infiltrate local anaesthetic down to the pleura, in the second inter-costal space in the mid-clavicular line. The cannula should be 16G or less and at least 3 cm long. Having entered the pleural cavity, withdraw the needle. Connect a three-way tap to the can-nula and a 50 mL syringe (Luer lock) and an exit tube, fed under water to ensure correct direction of airflow.

Discontinue aspiration if:

* Resistance is felt
* The patient experiences excessive coughing
* More than 2.5 L (50 mL removed 50 times) have been aspirated

Repeat chest X-ray. If the pneumothorax is now only small or resolved, the procedure has been successful. (NB Failure to aspirate further may be because the cannula is being inadver-tently withdrawn from the pleural cavity or becoming kinked.)

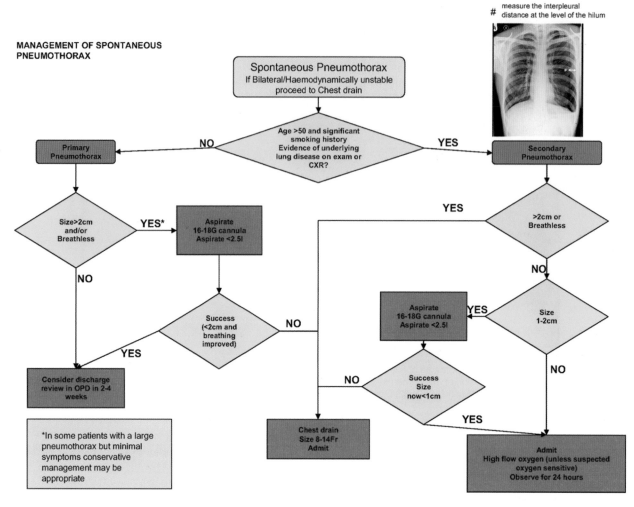

**MANAGEMENT OF SPONTANEOUS PNEUMOTHORAX**

# measure the interpleural distance at the level of the hilum

Spontaneous Pneumothorax
If Bilateral/Haemodynamically unstable proceed to Chest drain

Age >50 and significant smoking history Evidence of underlying lung disease on exam or CXR?

NO → Primary Pneumothorax

YES → Secondary Pneumothorax

Primary Pneumothorax:
Size>2cm and/or Breathless

YES* → Aspirate 16-18G cannula Aspirate <2.5l

NO

Success (<2cm and breathing improved)

YES

NO

Consider discharge review in OPD in 2-4 weeks

*In some patients with a large pneumothorax but minimal symptoms conservative management may be appropriate

Chest drain Size 8-14Fr Admit

Secondary Pneumothorax:
>2cm or Breathless

YES

NO

Size 1-2cm

Aspirate 16-18G cannula Aspirate <2.5l ← YES

NO

Success Size now<1cm

NO

YES

NO

Admit
High flow oxygen (unless suspected oxygen sensitive)
Observe for 24 hours

**Figure 6.6** British Thoracic Society (BTS) algorithm for management of spontaneous pneumothorax. From BTS pleural disease guideline; *Thorax* 2010; 65(2): ii18–ii31.

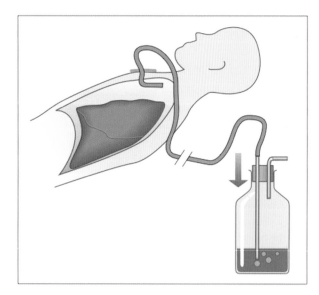

**Figure 6.7** Management of pneumothorax using an intercostal drain and underwater seal. The pleural air is usually expelled within a few days. If there is a persistent air leak, the application of low-pressure suction to the drain may help.

- Fibrosis following thoracotomy
- Fibrosis associated with asbestos exposure
- Asbestos-related pleural plaques (**Figure 6.8**)
- Secondary tumour metastases
- Malignant mesothelioma (**Figure 6.8c**)

## Clinical features

Pleural thickening is usually of no consequence unless it is severe, when it can cause pulmonary restriction and consequent breathlessness.

## Investigation

- *Chest radiography and CT scanning:* will show the extent of the disease
- *Lung function tests:* may reveal pulmonary restriction

## Management

Surgical pleurectomy is rarely indicated if there is no marked pulmonary restriction and the cause is benign.

## Prognosis

The prognosis is good if the cause is not malignant.

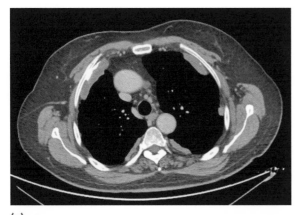

(a)

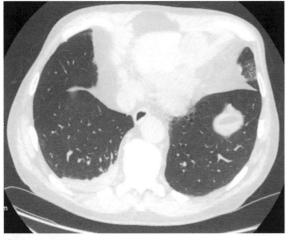

(b)

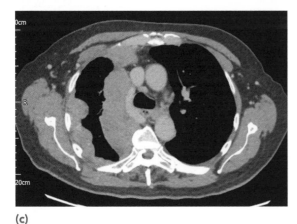

(c)

**Figure 6.8** Asbestos-related pleural changes. **(a)** Pleural plaques, which are a marker of asbestos exposure but are not considered pre-malignant. **(b)** Benign pleural thickening at the right lung base. **(c)** Right malignant mesothelioma, with extensive pleural tumour.

# MESOTHELIOMA

This is a rare malignant tumour of the mesothelial surfaces (usually pleura) resulting from asbestos exposure. There is no dose–response relationship and limited inhalation of asbestos can cause mesothelioma.

## Disease mechanisms

More than 90% of cases relate to occupational asbestos exposure that occurred >20 years previously, with mean latent interval between first exposure and death of 40 years. All types of asbestos can cause mesothelioma, but amphibole is the most potent.

## Clinical features

- Insidious onset of chest wall pain and weight loss
- Breathlessness if there is an associated pleural effusion
- Consider in a patient with pleural effusion or pleural thickening

## Investigation

- *Chest X-ray:* Radiographs may show pleural effusion or pleural thickening, or volume loss and rib crowding. There may be associated pleural plaques, highlighting previous asbestos exposure.
- *CT thorax (with pleural-phase contrast):* Look for nodularity and enhancement, pleural mass, pleural effusion or pleural thickening with uniform encasing of the lung (**Figure 6.8**). There may be diaphragmatic involvement, with local invasion of chest wall, ribs, heart, mediastinum and/or nodes.
- *MRI:* This can be helpful in assessing stage (as can CT-PET in assessing presence of metastases).
- *Thoracoscopy:* This allows direct visualization of the pleural surfaces, biopsy and therapeutic intervention (e.g. removal of fluid and talc pleurodesis).
- *Histology:* Biopsy can be achieved at thoracoscopy or via ultrasound/CT guidance. Histological subtypes include epithelioid (50% of cases; best prognosis), sarcomatoid and mixed (biphasic).

## Management

A multidisciplinary team approach is recommended, including radiologist, histopathologist, respiratory physician, thoracic surgeon, oncologist, specialist nurses, palliative care consultant. Aims are:

- *Supportive care,* including pain relief
- *Pleural fluid management*
- *Radiotherapy:* prophylactic radiotherapy to chest drain sites no longer recommended; palliative chemotherapy for localized pain is sometimes offered
- *Chemotherapy:* patients with good performance status (WHO 0-1) are offered first-line therapy with cisplatin and pemetrexed and, where licensed (not presently in the UK), bevacizumab may be added to this regime; immunotherapies and second-line agents are being examined in clinical trials
- *Surgery:* not currently recommended outside a clinical trial

## Prognosis

Most patients die within 18 months of presentation, with median survival 4–12 months.

# INTERSTITIAL LUNG DISEASES

## SARCOIDOSIS

Sarcoidosis is a multisystem granulomatous disorder of unknown aetiology. It most commonly affects the lungs, thoracic and mediastinal lymph nodes and skin but can also affect the eyes, brain and heart.

### Epidemiology

- Incidence varies across the world: in the UK, around 5–10 per 100 000 population; more severe and 16 times commoner in Afro-Caribbeans
- Usually presents in early adult life
- More common in women

### Disease mechanisms

It is characterized by non-caseating granulomata with activated T (CD4+) lymphocytes, which recruit monocytes and macrophages. The cause is unknown but it likely involves a combination of environmental and genetic factors, with an abnormal immunological reaction by the host.

### Clinical features

A number of clinical presentations are possible:
- *Lofgren's syndrome:* acute illness with pyrexia, malaise, bilateral hilar lymphadenopathy, erythema nodosum and polyarthralgia; usually self-limiting
- *Asymptomatic bilateral hilar lymphadenopathy Insidious progressive lung disease*, with symptoms of breathlessness, dry cough and chest pain and features of *extrathoracic disease:* hypercalcaemia, arthropathy, uveitis and keteroconjuctivitis, skin rash, generalized lymphadenopathy

Examination of the chest may reveal crackles (when fibrotic changes are present). Sarcoidosis can also affect the nervous system (with peripheral or cranial nerve involvement), the kidney with renal failure often related to nephrocalcinosis, and the heart with cardiomyopathy and conduction defect abnormalities (e.g. first-degree heart block).

### Investigation

- *Blood tests:* Lymphopenia is a sign of active disease. Erythrocyte sedimentation rate (ESR) may be increased. Serum angiotensin converting enzyme (ACE) is often increased (not a diagnostic test, but useful in disease monitoring). Serum calcium may be elevated, and renal function may be abnormal.
- *Chest X-ray:* More than 90% of patients have an abnormal chest X-ray and, in about a third of patients, sarcoidosis is picked up incidentally on chest radiograph. **Table 6.23** shows staging by chest X-ray appearance.
- *High-resolution CT (HRCT) thorax:* Scans may show hilar and mediastinal lymphadenopathy, nodules

**Table 6.23** Grading of pulmonary sarcoidosis according to its appearance on chest radiograph

| Grade | Chest radiograph |
|---|---|
| Stage 0 | Normal |
| Stage 1 | Bilateral hilar lymphadenopathy only |
| Stage 2 | Bilateral hilar lymphadenopathy plus pulmonary infiltration |
| Stage 3 | Pulmonary infiltration alone |
| Stage 4 | Fibrotic changes |

(large nodular opacities, micronodules or fissural nodularity), ground-glass shadowing (indicates active disease) and/or fibrosis.
- *Lung function tests:* A restrictive pattern is usually seen, with reduced FVC and reduced FEV1 and normal or high FEV1/FVC. If significant airways involvement, an obstructive pattern is possible. TLCO and KCO are reduced.
- *Bronchoscopy:* Bronchoalveolar lavage for differential WCC shows lymphocytosis (CD4 > CD8). Bronchial, transbronchial or lymph node biopsy reveals non-caseating granulomas.

### Management

Treatment of acute sarcoidosis is often unnecessary as it is self-limiting. Treatment of stage 1 disease is also not indicated.

Treatment is given if there is evidence of end-organ damage and active disease (e.g. reduced lung function, hypercalcaemia, skin, cardiac or CNS involvement). First-line treatment is with oral corticosteroids for a period of at least 6 months. Other immunosuppressant drugs used include azathioprine, hydroxychloroquine, mycophenolate mofetil and leflunomide.

### Prognosis

Young age, acute onset, erythema nodosum and hilar lymphadenopathy are good prognostic factors. Older age, insidious onset, extrapulmonary disease and pulmonary parenchymal involvement are poor prognostic factors. Acute sarcoidosis has a good prognosis, with the disease usually burning out either spontaneously or with treatment.

## HYPERSENSITIVITY PNEUMONITIS (EXTRINSIC ALLERGIC ALVEOLITIS)

This is lung disease related to inflammation in response to inhalation of common antigens.

### Disease mechanisms

The exact prevalence is unknown. It can be acute or chronic. Acute disease follows a short period of exposure to a high concentration of antigen, whereas chronic disease follows a longer exposure to a lower concentration of antigen. The antigen causes an inflammatory reaction in the bronchioles

**6**

## SARCOIDOSIS AT A GLANCE

### Epidemiology

*Prevalence*

- Approximately 1/20 000 in the UK; more common in women and in early adult life
- More common and more in Afro-Caribbeans than in white people

### Findings on investigation

*Blood tests*

- ESR may be increased
- Serum ACE and calcium may be increased

*Lung function*

- Reduced gas transfer and a restrictive defect on spirometry in chronic disease

*Diagnostic imaging*

- Chest radiograph can be normal or show only hilar lymphadenopathy
- Variable picture on CT imaging, with nodules and/or areas of fibrosis

*Histopathology*

- Lung biopsy: histology reveals non-caseating granulomas

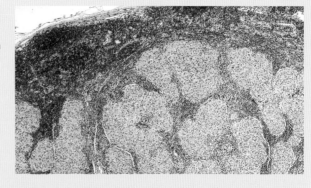

**Figure B** Lymph node biopsy showing non-caseating granuloma typical of sarcoidosis.

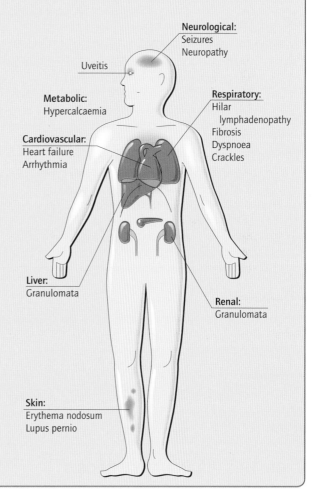

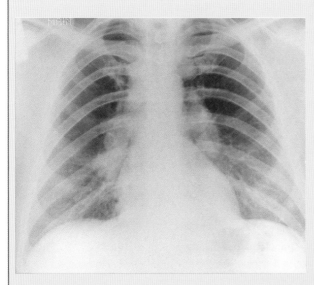

**Figure A** Chest radiograph of stage 1 sarcoidosis showing bilateral hilar lymphadenopathy and clear lung fields.

and alveoli (with neutrophils and lymphocytes) and can lead to formation of non-caseating granulomas. In chronic forms, it can progress to fibrosis. **Table 6.24** lists common causal antigens.

### Clinical features

- *Acute:* breathlessness, dry cough, fever, malaise, headache within hours of onset of exposure
- *Chronic:* slowly progressive breathlessness, dry cough, weight loss over months/years

On examination, the patient may be cyanosed and pyrexial, and have mid to late inspiratory crackles, heard mainly over the upper lobes. The presence of bronchiolar wall oedema may give rise to high-pitched mid-inspiratory monophonic wheezes and squeaks. In chronic disease with established fibrosis, there may be cyanosis and persistent crackles.

**Table 6.24** Causes of hypersensitivity pneumonitis

| Disease | Cause | Antigen(s) |
|---|---|---|
| Bird fancier's lung | Pigeons or budgerigars | Proteins in the 'bloom' of budgerigars, poultry |
| Farmer's lung | Mouldy hay | Thermophilic actinomyces, *Micropolyspora faeni* |
| Byssinosis | Cotton dust | Undefined contaminants |
| Humidifier lung/ fever | Contaminated humidifiers | A variety of bacteria and amoebae |
| Hot tub lung | Mould | *M. avium* complex |
| Malt worker's lung | Mouldy barley | *Aspergillus clavatis* |

### Investigation

- *Bloods:* increased neutrophil count
- *Immunology:* serum precipitins (IgG antibodies) for the offending antigen
- *Lung function tests:* restrictive pattern with reduced FEV1 and FVC with preserved/high FEV1/FVC ratio; TLC may be reduced; reduced gas transfer
- *Chest X-ray:* typically shows nodules, infiltrates, or ground glass in acute disease; in chronic disease, there may be upper/mid-zone reticulation and reduced thoracic volumes
- *HRCT thorax:* patchy diffuse ground-glass change, diffuse centrilobular nodules or micronodules and mosaic attenuation (see **Figure 6.9**, panel c); reticulation, honeycombing and/or traction bronchiectasis in chronic disease
- *Bronchoalveolar lavage:* typically reveals lymphocytosis
- *Histopathology:* may reveal granulomata

### Management

- Removal or reduction of exposure to antigen where possible
- Corticosteroids (e.g. prednisolone) for 3–6 months

### Prognosis

In acute disease, the prognosis is excellent if the offending antigen is removed. Permanent pulmonary damage may develop in chronic or recurrent disease.

## IDIOPATHIC PULMONARY FIBROSIS

IPF is a chronic interstitial pneumonia of unknown aetiology.

### Epidemiology

Prevalence is approximately 10/100000 population, but more common in older adults (median age at presentation is 66 years) and in men.

### Disease mechanisms

The aetiology is unknown. It is believed that chronic inflammation is followed by the development of fibrosis but the sequence of pathologic events is unknown. MUC5B polymorphisms have been implicated as genetic predisposing factors. Other causes of fibrosis are given in **Table 6.25**.

### Clinical features

- Insidious onset of breathlessness
- Cough (dry or productive of clear sputum)
- Fine basal end-inspiratory crackles
- Clubbing (in approximately 50%)
- Hypoxia, cyanosis and cor pulmonale in end-stage disease

### Investigation

- *Pulmonary function tests:* restrictive spirometry including reduced TLC and reduced gas transfer
- *Arterial blood gas:* type 1 respiratory failure (reduced $PaO_2$ with normal or low $PaCO_2$)
- *Chest X-ray:* reticular shadowing (predominantly basal and peripheral)
- *HRCT thorax:* reticulation, traction bronchiectasis, honeycombing; minimal or no ground glass (**Figure 6.9**, panel a)
- *Bronchoalveolar lavage:* usually neutrophilia
- *Histopathology:* 'usual interstitial pneumonia' (UIP) pattern on lung biopsy
- *Echocardiography:* may identify PH (secondary to hypoxic lung disease)

**Table 6.25** Causes of pulmonary fibrosis

**Idiopathic interstitial pneumonias**
- IPF
- Non-specific interstitial pneumonia (NSIP)
- Chronic organizing pneumonia (COP)

**Connective-tissue disorders**
- Rheumatoid arthritis
- Systemic sclerosis
- Polymyositis and dermatomyositis
- Sjögren's syndrome
- Ankylosing spondylitis

**Granulomatous diseases**
- Sarcoidosis
- Wegener's granulomatosis
- Previous TB

**Pneumoconioses**
- Asbestosis
- Coalworker's pneumoconiosis
- Silicosis

**Drug-induced**
- Methotrexate
- Nitrofurantoin
- Chemotherapy (e.g. bleomycin)
- Amiodarone

**Radiation-induced**

## HYPERSENSITIVITY PNEUMONITIS AT A GLANCE

### Epidemiology

*Prevalence*

- Prevalence unknown, but most common in bird owners and farmers

*Genetics*

- No known predisposition other than occupation (see **Table 6.24**)

### Findings on investigation

*Haematology*

- Acute disease: neutrophil leucocytosis
- ESR: may be raised

*Arterial blood gases*

- Hypoxia if severe acute episode or if progressive chronic disease

*Immunology*

- Serum antibodies (precipitins) usually positive for the offending antigen

*Diagnostic imaging*

- Chest X-ray: may be normal or show patchy nodular shadowing in acute disease, with reticulation and volume loss in chronic disease
- CT scanning: ground-glass, nodular changes acutely, progressing to fibrosis in chronic disease (**Figure A**, **Figure B**)

*Lung function tests*

- Restrictive spirometry, reduced lung volumes and reduced transfer factor

*Bronchoalveolar lavage*

- Usually lymphocytic

*Transbronchial or open lung biopsy*

- Acute disease: extensive lymphocyte and neutrophil infiltration of the alveoli on histology
- Chronic disease: classical granuloma and fibrosis

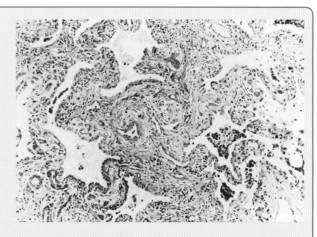

**Figure B** Chronic allergic alveolitis with fibrosis and obliteration of many alveolar spaces. Reproduced from Mygind N, (1995) *Essential Allergy*, 2nd edn (Wiley-Blackwell, Oxford) with the permission of the author.

6

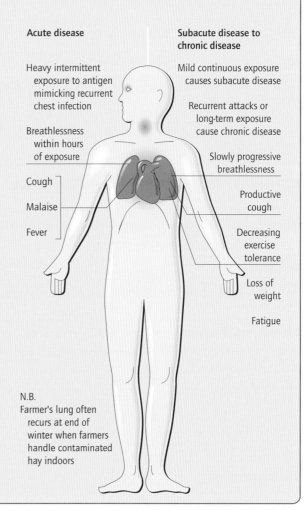

Acute disease

Subacute disease to chronic disease

Heavy intermittent exposure to antigen mimicking recurrent chest infection

Mild continuous exposure causes subacute disease

Recurrent attacks or long-term exposure cause chronic disease

Breathlessness within hours of exposure

Slowly progressive breathlessness

Cough

Productive cough

Malaise

Fever

Decreasing exercise tolerance

Loss of weight

Fatigue

N.B.
Farmer's lung often recurs at end of winter when farmers handle contaminated hay indoors

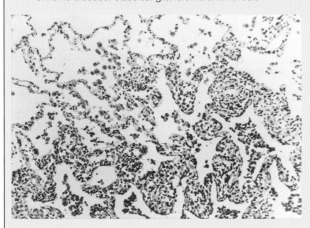

**Figure A** Acute allergic alveolitis with lymphocyte infiltration of alveolar walls and peribronchial tissue. Reproduced from Mygind N (1995) *Essential Allergy*, 2nd edn (Wiley-Blackwell, Oxford) with the permission of the author.

## Management

- Supportive treatment: Long-term oxygen therapy or ambulatory oxygen plus pulmonary rehabilitation are required.
- Minimize gastro-oesophageal reflux (with proton pump inhibitor; clinical trial evidence lacking).
- Disease-modifying treatment: Use antifibrotic agents such as pirfenidone or nintedanib (approved by NICE in the UK for a subset of patients with FVC 50–80% predicted).
- There is no evidence for the routine use of oral corticosteroids or other immunosuppressants.
- Evidence is lacking, but clinicians may use acetylcysteine for its antioxidant properties.
- In the case of acute deterioration/accelerated decline of IPF, prompt treatment of infection with antibiotics and exclusion/treatment of PE is paramount. High doses of oral steroids or pulsed methylprednisolone (intravenously for 3 days) are also used. In this situation, imaging may show new ground-glass opacification.
- Lung transplantation may be considered in symptomatic patients with severe and/or rapidly progressive disease.

## Prognosis

Prognosis is variable, but the median survival of patients is <5 years. In general, the earlier the onset of disease, the worse the prognosis. Poor prognostic factors include: low TLCO at presentation, PH, significant change in FVC or TLCO in the first 6–12 months.

# NON-SPECIFIC INTERSTITIAL PNEUMONIA

NSIP describes a histological pattern on lung biopsy, which is also associated with a clinical/radiological pattern (see below).

## Epidemiology

NSIP generally affects younger patients than IPF, with an age of onset 40–50 years.

## Disease mechanisms

NSIP probably encompasses a wide range of underlying pathology, including:
- Idiopathic
- Drugs
- Connective tissue disease (autoantibodies may be positive in NSIP without other features of autoimmune disease)

## Clinical features

- Gradual-onset breathlessness and cough (over months)
- Weight loss
- Fine crepitations at bases

## Investigation

- *Pulmonary function tests:* restrictive spirometry, reduced lung volumes (e.g. TLC) and reduced gas transfer factor
- *Immunology screen:* including ANA, anti-dsDNA, ENA, rheumatoid factor, anti-CCP, immunoglobulins and electrophoresis
- *Chest X-ray:* ground-glass or reticular shadowing
- *HRCT thorax:* ground-glass change (usually at bases), with or without reticulation or traction bronchiectasis (**Figure 6.9**, panel b); no honeycombing
- *Bronchoalveolar lavage:* lymphocytosis
- *Histopathology:* lung biopsy may show 'cellular' NSIP, characterized by mild interstitial inflammation with no fibrosis, or 'fibrotic' NSIP, characterized by fibrosis but without fibroblastic foci or honeycombing; there may be overlap

## Management

Lung biopsy is usually required for diagnosis (unlike IPF where radiological findings alone may suffice), except when NSIP occurs in the context of connective tissue disease. Prognosis can be good with appropriate immunosuppression, hence the importance of differentiating from IPF. Treatment is usually with corticosteroids (0.5 mg/kg) initially but other immunosuppressants can be used as steroid-sparing agents (e.g. azathioprine), in patients who fail to respond or in the context of specific connective-tissue disorders.

## Prognosis

Cellular NSIP has better prognosis than fibrotic NSIP, but fibrotic NSIP has better prognosis than IPF, with a 5-year survival of >50%.

# CHRONIC ORGANIZING PNEUMONIA

COP is a disease of unknown cause, characterized by multiple areas of lung consolidation.

## Disease mechanisms

Alveolar spaces are 'plugged' with granulation tissue (fibrin and inflammatory cells).

## Clinical features

The onset is over months (insidious) and can present as apparently slow-to-resolve respiratory tract infection despite multiple courses of antibiotics. Symptoms include:
- Breathlessness
- Dry cough
- Malaise and myalgia
- Fevers
- Weight loss

## Investigation

- *Bloods:* Findings are raised CRP and ESR, and high neutrophil count.

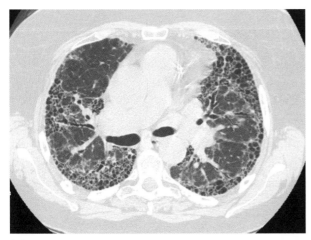

**(a)**

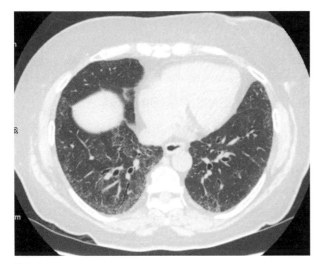

**(b)**

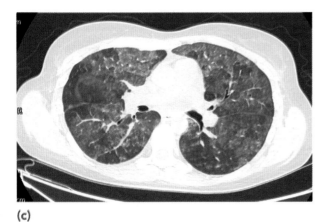

**(c)**

**Figure 6.9** Interstitial lung disease. **(a)** IPF, with predominantly subpleural reticulation and fibrosis (note 'honeycombing' appearance). **(b)** NSIP, with reticulation and fibrosis, but without honeycombing (note significant ground-glass change). **(c)** Acute hypersensitivity pneumonitis, with extensive ground glass but no established fibrosis.

- *Imaging:* Chest X-ray and CT show patchy consolidation (may be fleeting), possibly with ground-glass shadowing and nodularity.
- *Histology:* Transbronchial biopsy or CT-guided lung biopsy confirms the diagnosis by the presence of granulation tissue in alveolar spaces.

**Management**

COP usually responds to high-dose steroids (e.g. 1 mg/kg) for 3 months with a slow wean over 6–12 months.

**Prognosis**

Prognosis is good with treatment.

**6**

## OTHER IDIOPATHIC INTERSTITIAL PNEUMONIAS

- *Acute interstitial pneumonia (AIP):* This is similar to ARDS, with onset over days. Imaging shows diffuse ground-glass change and patchy shadowing. It can progress to pulmonary fibrosis.
- *Respiratory bronchiolitis-associated interstitial lung disease (RB-ILD):* This is smoking-related interstitial lung disease that develops over years, with mild symptoms. Imaging shows bronchial wall-thickening, ground glass and nodules. The prognosis is good upon smoking cessation.
- *Desquamative interstitial pneumonia (DIP):* A more severe and aggressive form of RB-ILD, DIP develops over weeks to months. The prognosis is good upon smoking cessation.
- *Lymphoid interstitial pneumonia (LIP):* The clinical course is variable. Imaging shows ground-glass, reticulation and cysts. Characterized by diffuse interstitial lymphoid infiltrates. Associated with autoimmune disease, lymphoproliferative disease and HIV.

## PNEUMOCONIOSES

### Asbestosis

This is chronic interstitial fibrosis resulting from asbestos inhalation. There is a dose–response relationship and asbestosis is usually seen in patients with many years of high exposure. It has a latency period of at least 15–20 years. Cigarette smoking increases risk and severity.

Clinical features include insidious onset of breathlessness, dry cough and bibasal fine inspiratory crackles on examination. Imaging is similar to IPF, with reticulonodular shadowing progressing to honeycombing. A differentiating factor is associated pleural thickening or pleural plaques in asbestosis. Pulmonary function tests show restrictive disease with reduced gas transfer.

There is no specific treatment. Management is supportive and prognosis is variable. Affected individuals are usually entitled to industrial compensation.

### Coalworker's pneumoconiosis

This is a chronic fibrotic illness caused by inhalation of coal dust. As with asbestos, there is a dose–response relationship. There are two types: simple and complicated (known as progressive massive fibrosis).

In simple pneumoconiosis, coal dust is engulfed by alveolar macrophages, which congregate around the respiratory bronchioles, chiefly in the upper lobes. These areas become fibrotic and centrilobular emphysema may develop in complicated disease. Coalescence of fibrotic lesions can lead to progressive massive fibrosis.

Simple coalworker's pneumoconiosis produces no symptoms or signs. Progressive massive fibrosis causes progressive breathlessness, cough and sputum (which can be black). Chest radiography may show nodular opacities in simple disease. In progressive massive fibrosis, there is coalescence of nodules (predominantly in the upper zones) with distortion, emphysema and cavitation. In simple disease there may be minor abnormalities in gas transfer. In massive pulmonary fibrosis, there may be obstructive or restrictive spirometry and impaired gas transfer.

Simple coalworker's pneumoconiosis does not cause disability or shorten life, whereas progressive massive fibrosis can result in respiratory failure. There is no specific treatment. Affected individuals are usually entitled to industrial compensation.

### Silicosis

This is a rare fibrotic lung disease caused by inhalation of silicon dioxide, such as during underground mining, stonemasonry, foundry work or sandblasting.

An insidious onset of progressive breathlessness that may continue even after exposure to silica dust has ceased. Concomitant TB is common because silicosis predisposes to this infection. If there has been an acute and intense exposure to silicon dioxide, there may be a rapid onset of breathlessness, cough and sputum (acute silicosis).

Chest radiography in uncomplicated silicosis shows fine nodular opacities (1–3 mm in diameter), predominantly in the upper zones. As the disease progresses, these may coalesce into larger opacities. Commonly, the hilar lymph nodes calcify at their periphery, producing the classical 'eggshell calcification'. In early disease, pulmonary function tests are normal, but as the disease progresses both lung volumes and gas transfer decrease.

Management involves removal of the patient from exposure and screening regularly for TB. Silicosis usually runs a benign course, but respiratory failure and cor pulmonale can result from acute silicosis or progressive massive fibrosis.

### Berylliosis

Berylliosis is a pneumoconiosis caused by beryllium. All forms of berylliosis are rare. Acute berylliosis follows intense exposure. Chronic berylliosis is associated with granulomatous lesions, similar in appearance and distribution to those of sarcoidosis (but ocular lesions do not occur).

Acute berylliosis is characterized by rapid-onset breathlessness accompanied by the production of blood-stained sputum and respiratory failure. Chest radiography shows patchy consolidation throughout the lung fields resulting from a chemical pneumonia. The main symptoms of chronic berylliosis are progressive breathlessness and lassitude, which may occur after only a brief exposure.

Treatment of acute berylliosis is oxygen and high-dose corticosteroids. Treatment of chronic berylliosis is long-term oral corticosteroids.

### Drug-induced interstitial lung disease

A number of different drugs can affect the lungs. The commonest presentations of drug-induced interstitial lung disease are:
- *Hypersensitivity pneumonitis:* nitrofurantoin, methotrexate, biologics (e.g. pembrolizumab)
- *Pulmonary fibrosis:* bleomycin, amiodarone, nitrofurantoin

## LUNG TUMOURS

## BRONCHOGENIC CARCINOMA

Bronchogenic carcinoma (lung cancer) refers to malignancy arising from the airways or lung parenchyma.

### Epidemiology
- Bronchogenic carcinoma is the most common cause of cancer death worldwide, with >35 000 deaths each year in the UK alone.
- Incidence increases with age.

### Disease mechanisms

More than 90% of lung cancer is smoking-related. Other risk factors include exposure to asbestos, ionizing radiation, heavy metals (e.g. arsenic, uranium) and air pollution.

Based on cell-type of origin, lung cancer is classified as small cell lung cancer (SCLC) or non-small cell lung cancer (NSCLC). The groups share clinical features, but management differs, related to the more rapid cell turnover and early metastasis seen in SCLC. Subtypes of NSCLC are given in **Table 6.26**.

### Clinical features

Lung cancer may be diagnosed in asymptomatic patients undergoing imaging for other reasons. However, most patients still present with symptoms, the majority of which are local. Smaller numbers present with symptoms of distant spread (~10%) or a paraneoplastic syndrome (10%, more common in SCLC).

#### Local symptoms
- *Cough:* with or without haemoptysis
- *Chest pain:* suggests pleural or chest wall involvement
- *Unresolving pneumonia:* may result from bronchial obstruction

**Table 6.26** Classification of bronchogenic carcinoma (based on WHO classification 2015)

| Histology | Proportion of lung cancer (%) | Comments |
|---|---|---|
| SCLC | 10 | Rapidly dividing cells |
| | | Metastasize early |
| NSCLC | | |
| Adenocarcinoma | 40 | Slow-growing |
| | | Metastasizes late |
| | | Often peripheral |
| Squamous cell carcinoma | 30 | Locally invasive |
| | | May cavitate |
| | | Often central |
| Large cell carcinoma | 15 | Intermediate between squamous and small cell |
| Miscellaneous | 5 | Includes adenosquamous carcinoma, carcinoid, etc. |

- *Breathlessness:* may be due to airway obstruction or pleural effusion
- *Hoarseness:* due to invasion of left recurrent laryngeal nerve
- *Stridor:* results from large airway obstruction
- *Diaphragm paralysis:* hilar tumour may cause phrenic nerve palsy
- *Superior vena caval obstruction (SVCO):* due to invasion of the superior mediastinum
- *Arm and shoulder pain:* invasion of brachial plexus by apical mass (Pancoast tumour)
- *Horner's syndrome:* invasion sympathetic chain by Pancoast tumour
- *Cardiac arrhythmia:* can occur due to direct invasion of the pericardium

### Distant spread

- *Lymphadenopathy:* cervical or supraclavicular nodes may be amenable to biopsy
- *Cerebral metastases:* may present with headache, seizure or stroke
- *Bone metastases:* may present with bone pain or pathological fracture
- *Liver metastases:* typically presents with hepatomegaly and jaundice
- *Adrenal metastases:* common, but rarely cause symptoms
- *Skin metastases:* skin nodules occur but are rare

### Paraneoplastic manifestations

- *Cutaneous:* e.g. clubbing, dermatomyositis/polymyositis, hypertrophic pulmonary osteoarthropathy
- *Endocrine:* e.g. hypercalcaemia due to excess production of parathyroid hormone-like peptide, hyponatraemia

due to syndrome of inappropriate antidiuretic hormone (SIADH), Cushing's syndrome due to ectopic adrenocorticotropic hormone (ACTH) secretion
- *Neuromuscular:* e.g. subacute cerebellar degeneration, limbic encephalitis, Lambert–Eaton myasthenic syndrome (autoantibodies against voltage-gated calcium channels)
- *Haematological:* e.g. anaemia, leukocytosis, thrombocytosis, hypercoagulability

### Initial investigation

- *Bloods:* including FBC, clotting, LFTs, sodium and calcium
- *Chest X-ray:* small and/or central lesions easily missed; look for lymphadenopathy, pleural involvement or rib lesions
- *CT thorax with contrast:* ideally including liver, adrenals and lower neck to allow preliminary staging; consider CT and/or MRI brain for those with neurological symptoms
- *CT-PET:* highlights metabolically active tissue to help distinguish benign and maligant lesions, and identify local or distant spread; used routinely in patients due for curative treatment, to exclude unidentified metastates
- *Lung function testing:* important for assessing suitability for lung biopsy or active treatment, which is higher-risk in patients with less respiratory reserve

### Tissue diagnosis

- *Sputum cytology:* This has low sensitivity and is generally reserved for those unsuitable for biopsy.
- *Bronchoscopy ± EBUS:* The common route for biopsy of primary lesion and/or associated lymph nodes, EBUS is simple to perform, with low morbidity. It allows safer lymph node biopsy. If nodes are inaccessible bronchoscopically, mediastinoscopy may be necessary.
- *Percutanous needle biopsy:* This may be necessary for peripheral lung lesions not accessible by bronchoscopy, or for central lesions not visible endobronchially (see **Figure B** in BRONCHIAL CARCINOMA AT A GLANCE).
- *Pleural aspiration/pleural biopsy:* This can provide a definitive diagnosis in those presenting with pleural effusion.
- *Genetic analysis:* Newer treatments for NSCLC are targeted to specific genetic phenotypes, including *EGFR* mutations or rearrangements in the *ALK* or *ROS1* genes in the tumour.

### Management

Treatment is curative in a minority of cases and is otherwise focused on limiting progression and/or improving quality of life. Management decisions should be made by a multidisciplinary team.
- *Surgery:* Lobectomy (open or thoracoscopic) and pneumonectomy are potentially curative, and may be combined with adjuvant chemotherapy.

## BRONCHIAL CARCINOMA AT A GLANCE

### Epidemiology

*Prevalence*

- Over 35 000 deaths/year in the UK

*Age*

- Commonly presents in late middle age

### Findings on investigation

*Biochemistry*

- Serum calcium may be increased and there may be hyponatraemia

*Diagnostic imaging*

- Chest radiography: may reveal lung nodule, lymphadenopathy and/or pleural effusion
- CT scanning: allows staging of disease and reveals involvement of lymph nodes, ribs or pleura

*Histopathology*

- Sputum cytology and biopsy reveal malignant cells

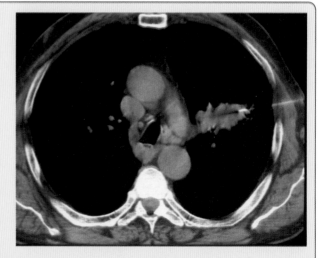

**Figure B** CT-guided biopsy of suspected left lung malignancy, with biopsy needle visible as it enters the lesion.

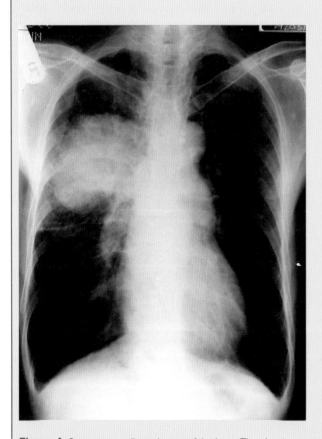

**Figure A** Squamous cell carcinoma of the lung. The chest radiograph shows a large round mass in the right midzone.

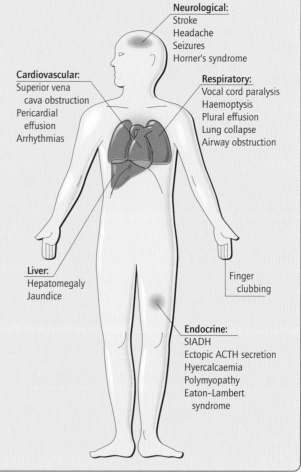

**Neurological:**
Stroke
Headache
Seizures
Horner's syndrome

**Cardiovascular:**
Superior vena
cava obstruction
Pericardial
effusion
Arrhythmias

**Respiratory:**
Vocal cord paralysis
Haemoptysis
Plural effusion
Lung collapse
Airway obstruction

**Liver:**
Hepatomegaly
Jaundice

Finger
clubbing

**Endocrine:**
SIADH
Ectopic ACTH secretion
Hyercalcaemia
Polymyopathy
Eaton–Lambert
syndrome

Metastatic disease should be robustly excluded and cardiorespiratory reserve assessed prior to offering surgery. SCLC is usually metastatic at presentation, so surgery is rarely an option.

- *Radiotherapy:* This may be used to limit progression and/or relieve symptoms, or to treat emergency presentations (e.g. SVCO). High-dose radical radiotherapy (with or without chemotherapy) may be

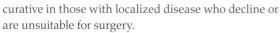

6

curative in those with localized disease who decline or are unsuitable for surgery.

- *Chemotherapy:* Conventional cytotoxic chemotherapy may be used as first-line therapy in advanced NSCLC, and is the treatment of choice in most patients with SCLC. It may be given after surgery, alongside radiotherapy, or with targeted molecular therapy/immunotherapy.
- *Targeted molecular therapy:* This is increasingly common for NSCLC with the appropriate genetic phenotype, e.g. tyrosine kinase inhibitors are used for tumours with EGFR mutations. It may be more effective and better-tolerated than conventional chemotherapy, but neither is curative.
- *Immunotherapy:* Immune checkpoint inhibitors may be suitable for some patients, e.g. pembrolizumab for patients with tumour expressing the cell surface protein PD-L1. This treatment enhances the ability of endogenous T-cells to recognize and destroy tumour.
- *Palliative care:* In frail patients and/or advanced disease, the focus may be on palliative care. Consider opiates for pain and dyspnoea, corticosteroids for severe cachexia, stenting of airway obstruction, radiotherapy for bone metastases and drainage of pleural fluid. Some patients benefit from hospice care.

## Prognosis

Prognosis remains poor but is improving. It varies according to subtype and stage of presentation, but overall survival in the UK is 30–35% at 1 year and around 10% at 5 years.

## BRONCHIAL CARCINOID TUMOUR

### Epidemiology

- Uncommon
- Seen predominantly in younger adults

### Disease mechanisms

Bronchial carcinoid tumours are neuroendocrine tumours that are only occasionally malignant.

### Clinical features

They typically present with bronchial obstruction or hae-moptysis, with or without a pulmonary nodule visible on imaging. The carcinoid syndrome is rare (1%).

### Investigation

Imaging is unable reliably to distinguish carcinoid from bronchial carcinoma. At bronchoscopy, carcinoids appear as highly vascular ('cherry-red') tumours growing into the airway lumen. Lung biopsy may be required if not classical in appearance, but there is a significant risk of bleeding.

### Management and prognosis

- Treatment is surgical resection.
- 5-year survival is 87–100% for typical carcinoid and 30–95% when there are atypical histological features.

## SECONDARY MALIGNANT TUMOURS

### Epidemiology and disease mechanisms

The lung parenchyma is a common site of spread for other tumours, including prostate, breast, bone, kidneys, uterus, ovary and GI tract. Over half of malignant lung lesions are secondary deposits.

### Clinical features

Patients may be asymptomatic despite large or multiple deposits. 'Cannon ball' lung metastases are characteristic of renal cell carcinoma.

### Management and prognosis

These depend on the primary tumour.

## MEDIASTINAL MASSES

The mediastinum is divided into four compartments, and masses in each compartment have characteristic aetiologies (**Figure 6.10**).

### Clinical features

Most patients are asymptomatic, in which case the risk of malignancy is low (~5%). Symptoms are generally caused by local compression, and are associated with increased likelihood of malignancy (~50%):

- *Airway compression:* stridor or unilateral wheeze
- *Oesophageal compression:* dysphagia
- *SVC compression:* headache, facial plethora, distended arm/neck veins
- *Nerve compression:* Horner's syndrome, recurrent laryngeal nerve palsy

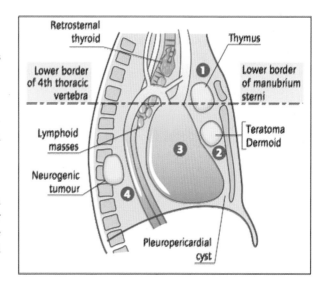

**Figure 6.10** To help in the differential diagnosis of mediastinal masses, the mediastinum is divided into four regions: 1, superior mediastinum; 2, anterior mediastinum; 3, middle mediastinum; and 4, posterior mediastinum. The locations of the common mediastinal masses are shown.

## Investigation

These should include chest X-ray and CT scan, plus thoracoscopy, mediastinoscopy or thoracotomy for biopsy.

## Management

Surgery is the preferred treatment for retrosternal, intrathoracic and thymic tumours. No treatment is required for stable pleuropericardial cysts, but monitoring is required.

# PULMONARY CIRCULATION

## PULMONARY EMBOLISM

### Epidemiology

PE is a common *de novo* presentation, but it may also complicate pre-existing disease. The reported incidence in the UK is ~70/100 000, but many more may go undiagnosed.

### Disease mechanisms

Most PEs arise from deep venous thrombosis (DVT) in the pelvic (15%) or femoral veins (70–80%), but other materials may embolize (e.g. amniotic fluid, fat). Key risk factors are listed in **Table 6.27**.

### Clinical features

The classic presentation of a small–moderate PE is abrupt-onset resting and/or exertional breathlessness and pleuritic chest pain, with or without cough and haemoptysis. Large PEs may present with collapse and/or haemodynamic instability. Clinical signs may include:

- *Tachypnoea* (particularly on exertion)
- *Tachycardia* (including new onset atrial fibrillation)
- *Pleural rub* (implies peripheral clot with lung infarction)
- *Split-second heart sound with loud P2* (implies right heart strain)
- *Hypotension with elevated JVP* (implies right heart failure)

### Investigation

Initial investigation is based on excluding alternative pathologies (important examples of which include pneumonia, pneumothorax, pleural effusion, musculoskeletal pain

**Table 6.27** Risk factors for PE

| |
|---|
| Pregnancy |
| Malignancy |
| Clotting disorder |
| Recent surgery (particularly orthopaedic) |
| Immobility |
| Oral contraceptive/hormone replacement therapy |
| Previous venous thromboembolism (VTE) |
| Indwelling venous catheter |

and anxiety) and establishing a pre-test probability, to guide the need for definitive investigations.

### Initial investigations

- *Chest X-ray:* Radiographs may be normal. Wedge-shaped consolidation suggests lung infarction.
- *ECG:* This often shows sinus tachycardia. The classic combination of S wave in lead I, Q wave in lead III and inverted T-wave in lead III ($S_1Q_3T_3$) signifies right heart strain but is rare.
- *Bloods:* Elevated inflammatory markers (WCC, CRP) are more suggestive of infection than PE, but they could reflect lung infarction. High troponin or brain natriuretic peptide (BNP) are poor prognostic markers.
- *Arterial blood gases:* Gas exchange is usually impaired, but $PO_2$ may be normal due to hyperventilation. Calculate the A–a gradient if unsure (which will usually be high).
- *D-dimer:* This is a sensitive but non-specific marker of recent thrombosis. If pre-test probability is low (Well's score; **Table 6.28**), a negative D-dimer effectively excludes PE. If pre-test probability is high, proceed to diagnostic investigations without measuring the D-dimer.

### Diagnostic investigations

- *CTPA:* This is easily accessible in most centres and, if negative, may provide alternative diagnoses. Disadvantages include exposure to contrast and radiation.
- *Ventilation-perfusion scan:* Advantages include higher sensitivity and lower radiation dose. Disadvantages are poor availability and higher rate of indeterminant result.
- *Doppler ultrasound:* Use this to look for DVT. If found, and there are typical symptoms of PE, this may be sufficient for diagnosis (e.g. in pregnancy, to avoid radiation).

## Management

- *Anticoagulation:* The mainstay of treatment, aimed at preventing propagation of existing thrombus and formation of new clots. Options include low molecular

**Table 6.28** Well's criteria for assessing pre-test probability in PE

| Clinical feature | Score |
|---|---|
| Clinical signs and symptoms of DVT | 3 |
| Alternative diagnosis less likely than PE | 3 |
| Heart rate >100 beats/min | 1.5 |
| Recent immobilization (>3 days, or surgery in previous 4 weeks) | 1.5 |
| Previous DVT/PE | 1.5 |
| Haemoptysis | 1 |
| Malignancy | 1 |

**Interpretation:** PE is *likely* if score >4 points, and *unlikely* if ≤4 points

Reference: Wells PS *et al. Thrombosis and Haemostasis* 2000; 83: 416–20.

## PULMONARY EMBOLISM AT A GLANCE

### Epidemiology

*Prevalence*

- Reported incidence 70/10 000; many more may go undiagnosed

### Findings on investigation

*Blood gas analysis*

- Hypoxia with elevated A–a $PO_2$ difference; worse on exertion
- $PCO_2$ normally low due to hyperventilation

*Chest radiography*

- May be normal

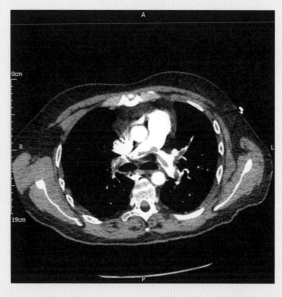

**Figure B** CT pulmonary arteriogram showing sub-massive PE. Note the large saddle embolus, with filling defects extending into the main and segmental pulmonary arteries bilaterally.

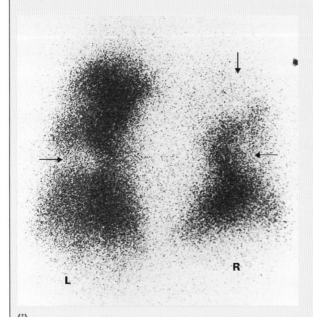

(i)

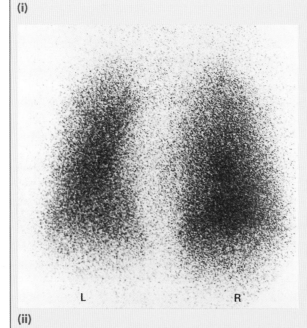

(ii)

**Figure A** Mismatched ventilation/perfusion defects on a 99mTc perfusion scan, in a patient with pulmonary emboli (note multiple wedge-shaped defects, arrows).

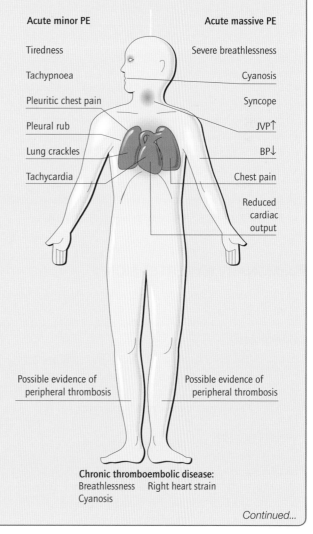

| Acute minor PE | | Acute massive PE |
|---|---|---|
| Tiredness | | Severe breathlessness |
| Tachypnoea | | Cyanosis |
| Pleuritic chest pain | | Syncope |
| Pleural rub | | JVP↑ |
| Lung crackles | | BP↓ |
| Tachycardia | | Chest pain |
| | | Reduced cardiac output |
| Possible evidence of peripheral thrombosis | | Possible evidence of peripheral thrombosis |

**Chronic thromboembolic disease:**
Breathlessness    Right heart strain
Cyanosis

*Continued...*

*...Continued*
- Look for pulmonary oligaemia in large acute PE
- Dilation of main pulmonary arteries in chronic thromboembolic disease

*CTPA*
- Widely available and may reveal clots as 'filling defects' outlined by intravenous contrast

*Radionuclide lung scan (V/Q scan)*
- Perfusion defects not matched by ventilation defects in minor PE. Large perfusion defects in large PE
- Widespread ventilation–perfusion (V/Q) mismatching in chronic thromboembolic disease

*Cardiac investigation*
- Acute right heart strain in acute massive PE (S1 Q3 T3 and right axis deviation)
- Elevated right ventricular pressure and right heart strain on echocardiogram in large PE

**Table 6.29** Classification of PH (summarized from WHO classification)

**Group 1: Pulmonary arterial hypertension (PAH)**
Includes idiopathic PH, heritable/genetic PH (e.g. BMPR2 mutation) and drug- or toxin-induced PH, and PH associated with e.g. connective tissue disease, HIV or schistosomiasis

**Group 2: PH due to left heart disease**
Includes systolic and diastolic dysfunction, valvular disease and congenital cardiomyopathy

**Group 3: PH due to lung disease and/or hypoxia**
Includes COPD, interstitial lung disease and sleep-disordered breathing

**Group 4: CTEPH and other pulmonary artery obstructions**
Includes CTEPH

**Group 5: PH with unclear and/or multifactorial mechanisms**
Includes PH secondary to haematological and metabolic disorders

weight heparin, warfarin or direct oral anticoagulants (DOACs). Duration of therapy for provoked DVT/ PE (e.g. postoperative) is normally 3 months. For unprovoked DVT, therapy may be continued for longer.

- *Thrombolysis:* Systemic thrombolysis (e.g. intravenous tissue plasminogen activator, t-PA) is reserved for large PE with haemodynamic instability. Catheter-directed thrombolysis (with or without embolectomy) may be safer and is becoming more common.
- *Inferior vena cava (IVC) filter:* This is usually considered only in patients with lower limb DVT and temporary contraindications to anticoagulation, or recurrent PE despite anticoagulation.
- *Cancer screening:* According to NICE guidelines in the UK, all patients with unprovoked PE should be screened for underlying cancer with chest X-ray, blood tests and urinalysis, plus abdominal/ pelvic imaging and a mammogram in those aged >40 years.

## PULMONARY HYPERTENSION

PH is defined as mean pulmonary arterial pressure ≥25 mmHg at rest.

### Epidemiology

Causes for PH are classified into five groups (**Table 6.29**). Group 1 includes idiopathic and heritable pulmonary arterial hypertension (PAH), which typically present in young people (mean age 35–40) with a female preponderance (2 : 1).

### Clinical features

Classic symptoms are exertional breathlessness, fatigue, chest pain and syncope. Clinical signs result mainly from right ventricular dysfunction and may include parasternal heave, loud P2, elevated JVP and peripheral oedema. Features of the underlying cause may be present.

### Investigation

#### Initial investigations
- *Chest X-ray:* enlarged pulmonary arteries, loss of peripheral vasculature (*'pruning'*) and right heart enlargement
- *Arterial blood gases:* $PO_2$ at rest may be normal due to hyperventilation but falls on exertion
- *ECG:* may show right ventricular strain pattern
- *Echocardiogram:* allows structural assessment of the right heart and estimation of systolic pulmonary artery pressure, but rarely sufficient for formal diagnosis
- *Pulmonary function tests:* reduced gas transfer (KCO and TLCO) in isolation may indicate PH, but features of associated lung disease may be present

#### Diagnostic tests
- *Right heart catheterization:* This is required for formal diagnosis, for direct measurement of pressures and pulmonary vascular resistance. Vasodilator studies may predict response to treatment.
- *Tests aimed at identifying underlying cause:* Once PH is confirmed, multiple tests will usually be required to assess the underlying cause.

### Management

For most patients (groups 2, 3 and 5), management focuses on treatment of the underlying condition. For patients with PAH (group 1) or chronic thromboembolic pulmonary hypertension (CTEPH, group 4), directed therapy is available. In the UK, such patients are referred to one of a small number of regional specialist centres:
- *General management:* Patients with PAH and CTEPH should normally be anticoagulated to prevent pulmonary emboli, and may benefit from diuretics

and digoxin to support right ventricular function. Long-term oxygen therapy is indicated if $PaO_2$ is <8 kPa. Pregnancy is associated with high mortality, so birth control is important.

- *Medical therapy:* In those responding to vasodilators at right heart catheterization, calcium channel blockers may be used. Other medical therapies include endothelin receptor antagonists (e.g. bosentan), phosphodiesterase inhibitors (e.g. sildenafil), and prostacyclin analogues (e.g. iloprost) or soluble guanylate cyclase stimulators (e.g. riociguat). Riociguat is the only medical therapy currently licensed for CTEPH.
- *Surgery:* In CTEPH with proximal thrombus, pulmonary endarterectomy conducted in a specialized PH centre is the treatment of choice.

## SLEEP-RELATED RESPIRATORY DISEASES

### OBSTRUCTIVE SLEEP APNOEA

Obstructive sleep apnoea (OSA) is repeated interruption of breathing during sleep due to collapse of the upper airway. Obstructive sleep apnoea syndrome (OSAS) is the presence of OSA with symptoms of daytime sleepiness.

#### Epidemiology

- More common in males (5 : 1) and in obese people
- Prevalence unknown but probably as high as 1% of the male population

#### Disease mechanisms

OSA is usually due to loss of muscular tone during sleep (particularly rapid eye movement [REM] sleep). An apnoea is defined as cessation of breathing for 10 seconds or more.

#### Clinical features

*History*
- Snoring
- Apnoeas (i.e. 'stopping breathing') witnessed by partner or family
- Arousals with choking sensation
- Nocturia
- Unrefreshed in the morning
- Excessive daytime somnolence
- Morning headaches
- Often seen in association with obesity. Other predisposing conditions include hypothyroidism, acromegaly or upper airway anatomy (enlarged tonsils, micrognathia or retrognathia)

*Examination*
- Elevated body mass index
- Nasal patency may be reduced

**Table 6.30** Example proforma for Epworth sleepiness score (ESS).

| Situation | Score (0–3) |
|---|---|
| Sitting and reading | |
| Watching television | |
| Sitting inactive in a public place (e.g. theatre or meeting) | |
| As a passenger in a car for an hour without a break | |
| Lying down to rest in the afternoon | |
| Sitting and talking to someone | |
| Sitting quiet after lunch with no alcohol | |
| In a car while stopped in traffic | |
| **Total** | |

For each situation, the patient is asked to score the likelihood of falling asleep on the following scale: 0 (would never doze), 1 (slight chance of dozing), 2 (moderate chance of dozing), 3 (high chance of dozing). A score of ≥10/24 indicates significant sleepiness

- Oropharynx: dental crowding, enlarged tonsils (document the Mallampati score)
- Increased neck circumference

#### Investigation

- Epworth sleepiness score (ESS; **Table 6.30**)
- Overnight sleep study: simple overnight oximetry ($SpO_2$ and heart rate), limited respiratory polygraphy or full polysomnography
- Markers of severity include the oxygen desaturation index (ODI) and apnoea–hypopnoea index (AHI); for the latter, AHI <15 per hour is mild, 15–30 moderate and >30 severe disease

#### Management

Treatment includes weight reduction and avoidance of sedatives (including alcohol). CPAP during sleep is the best treatment available. In milder forms of OSA, a jaw advancement device can be beneficial. Surgery such as tonsillectomy or orolaryngopalatoplasty is only useful in selected cases.

#### Prognosis

Prognosis is good if treated effectively.

### CENTRAL SLEEP APNOEA

Central sleep apnoea presents as repetitive cessation of breathing during sleep, with no evidence of upper airway obstruction. This is usually seen in the context of left ventricular failure or brain pathology. Treatment is aimed at improving the underlying condition (e.g. treatment of heart failure and relieving symptoms). For the latter, common approaches are CPAP (to treat any coexistent obstructive events), overnight oxygen or adaptive servoventilation (ASV; in patients with preserved ejection fraction).

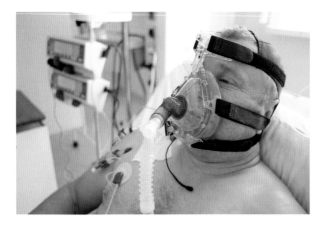

**Figure 6.11** Treatment with NIV in the acute setting. Home nocturnal NIV is also becoming increasingly common in the management of patients with chronic hypercapnic ventilatory failure (e.g. due to obesity hypoventilation or neuromuscular weakness).

## OBESITY HYPOVENTILATION SYNDROME

### Definition

Patients with obesity (e.g. BMI > 30) can have restrictive lung function tests and nocturnal hypoventilation. Some develop daytime ventilatory failure and hypercapnia. This is usually compensated (i.e. normal pH and bicarbonate) but can predispose to acute decompensation with respiratory acidosis when a further insult occurs such as infection.

### Clinical features

- Unrefreshed in the morning
- Morning headaches
- Excessive daytime somnolesence
- Breathlessness
- Snoring and OSA may coexist

### Investigation

- Spirometry
- Blood gas analysis
- Overnight sleep study

### Management

Treatment includes weight loss and domiciliary nocturnal non-invasive ventilation (NIV) with high inspiratory and expiratory pressures (IPAP and EPAP respectively; **Figure 6.11**).

## OTHER CONDITIONS CAUSING VENTILATORY FAILURE

A number of chest wall deformities and neuromuscular conditions can cause ventilatory failure (**Table 6.31**).

### Clinical features

Symptoms can develop slowly over years (e.g. in chest wall deformities or myopathies), progress rapidly over months (e.g. in motor neurone disease [MND]) or develop acutely (e.g. in myasthenic crises). Clinical presentation can be with:

**Table 6.31** Other causes of ventilatory failure (extrinsic to the lung itself)

**Chest wall deformities**
- Scoliosis
- Post-thoracoplasty (previously done for TB prior to availability of chemotherapy)
- Previous poliomyelitis (and also post-polio syndrome which is associated with reduced ventilatory drive)

**Neuropathies**
- MND/amyotrophic lateral sclerosis (ALS)
- Bilateral diaphragmatic paralysis (trauma, inflammatory neuritis or idiopathic)
- Spinal muscular atrophy
- High spinal cord transection

**Neuromuscular junction pathology**
- Myasthenia gravis
- Lambert-Eaton myasthenic syndrome

**Myopathies**
- Duchenne muscular dystrophy
- Acid maltase deficiency
- Myotonic dystrophy
- Limb-girdle myopathy

- *Features of the underlying disease:* e.g. limb weakness and gait abnormalities or bulbar symptoms (such as dysarthria or swallowing difficulties)
- *Symptoms of 'poor' cough:* including difficultly clearing secretions and recurrent lower respiratory tract infections (due to aspiration)
- *Symptoms of ventilatory insufficiency:* including shortness of breath (on exertion or at rest), orthopnoea, sleep disturbance (awakenings with breathlessness) and hypercapnic respiratory failure (e.g. morning headaches, excessive daytime sleepiness, cyanosis, ankle swelling)

### Investigation

Most are tests of respiratory function:
- *Lying and standing VC:* a fall of >10% on lying is abnormal
- *Mouth pressures:* maximum inspiratory and expiratory pressure (MIP and MEP) and sniff nasal inspiratory pressure (SNIP) may be reduced
- *Peak cough flow:* may be reduced
- *Overnight sleep study:* looking for desaturations or nocturnal hypoventilation
- *Blood gas analysis:* looking for arterial hypoxia, hypercapnia or raised bicarbonate

### Management

- If symptoms or signs of ventilatory insufficiency, consider non-invasive ventilation (see **Figure 6.11**)
- Cough assist adjuncts may be helpful

- Nutrition: a gastrostomy feeding tube may be inserted (e.g. in bulbar MND)
- Occupational therapy support is helpful

## LUNG DISEASE ASSOCIATED WITH SYSTEMIC DISEASE

### VASCULITIC LUNG DISEASE

#### Granulomatosis with polyangiitis (formerly Wegener's granulomatosis)

A rare and serious condition, more common in males. It is a systemic vasculitic disease characterized by necrotizing granulomas in the respiratory tract and focal necrotizing glomerulonephritis. Vasculitis lesions can occur in any tissue.

Patients typically present with a nasal discharge, respiratory symptoms (cough, pleurisy and perhaps haemoptysis) and general malaise. The lungs are involved in most cases. Chest radiography shows rounded opacities, which may

cavitate. There may also be pleural effusions and areas of infiltration. Antineutrophil cytoplasmic antibody (ANCA) is usually positive.

Haematuria, proteinuria and rapidly progressive renal failure can occur. The diagnosis relies on biopsy, which reveals typical granulomatous lesions. Treatment with high-dose prednisolone and cyclophosphamide is usually effective and long-term remission can occur.

#### Goodpasture's syndrome

This is a rare condition, usually seen in young males. There is pulmonary haemorrhage with associated nephritis. Pathogenic antibodies against the basement membranes in the lung and the kidney are found in the circulation and in the affected tissues.

It presents with episodes of haemoptysis. This may be preceded by acute glomerulonephritis. Non-specific malaise resulting from renal disease or iron-deficiency anaemia can occur. Chest radiography shows scattered patchy shadowing representing areas of alveolar haemorrhage.

**Table 6.32** Pulmonary involvement in rheumatological disease

| Disease | Pulmonary manifestations | Comments |
|---|---|---|
| Rheumatoid arthritis | Pleural effusion | The most common pulmonary manifestation of the disease |
| | | Usually unilateral |
| | | Pleural fluid has a low glucose and high rheumatoid factor |
| | Bronchiolitis obliterans | Rare |
| | | Progressive small bronchiole obliteration causes increasing dyspnea and irreversible airflow obstruction |
| | | Treatment is often ineffective |
| | Fibrosing alveolitis | Similar features as IPF |
| | | Runs a chronic indolent course, and shows little response to treatment |
| | Rheumatoid nodules | Asymptomatic |
| | | May be single or multiple and up to several centimetres |
| | | They frequently cavitate |
| | | Lesions are larger in association with pneumoconiosis (Caplan's syndrome) |
| Systemic lupus erythematosus | Pleurisy | A feature in 50% of patients |
| | | Often associated with small bilateral effusions |
| | | Responds to corticosteroids |
| | Basal atelectasis | Common |
| | | Caused by restricted chest wall movement |
| | Fibrosing alveolitis | An unusual manifestation |
| | | Has the same features as IPF and may respond to oral corticosteroids |
| | Shrinking lung syndrome | Uncommon |
| | | There is a diminution in lung size, but no evidence of parenchymal disease |
| | | Caused by chest wall or diaphragm malfunction |
| | | Shows little response to treatment |
| Systemic sclerosis | Pulmonary fibrosis | There is some degree of pulmonary fibrosis in most patients with systemic sclerosis, and parenchymal disease may be severe, with restricted lung volumes and poor gas transfer |
| | | Cyclophosphamide and steroid may help |
| | Aspiration pneumonitis | Common manifestation |
| | | Associated with oesophageal dysfunction |
| | Chest wall restriction | Causes breathlessness |
| | | Results from sclerosis of the chest wall |

Treatment is with plasmapheresis to remove the pathogenic antibody, and corticosteroids and other immunosuppressives (cyclophosphamide and then azathioprine) to suppress production of the pathogenic antibody. Patients may need oxygen therapy or ventilation and, if alveolar bleeding is substantial, blood transfusion may be necessary. Renal dysfunction may require dialysis. Most patients survive if plasmapheresis is started early.

### Idiopathic pulmonary haemosiderosis

This is a rare but serious condition affecting children and young adults associated with bouts of lung haemorrhage associated with anaemia and impaired gas exchange. The cause is unknown and optimum treatment unclear.

### Autoimmune rheumatic disease and the lung

Pulmonary involvement commonly occurs in rheumatoid arthritis, systemic lupus erythematosus and systemic sclerosis (**Table 6.32**).

## EOSINOPHILIC LUNG DISEASE

### Eosinophilic pneumonia

A number of conditions are associated with pulmonary infiltration and a marked peripheral eosinophilia (**Table 6.33**). Eosinophilic pneumonia is the most common. Patients present with malaise, weight loss, night sweats, cough and breathlessness. Physical signs of lung disease are often absent but chest radiography shows a striking peripheral ground-glass change (the so-called photographic negative of pulmonary oedema). The condition is exquisitely responsive to oral corticosteroids and usually resolves after a 6-month course of tapering oral prednisolone.

### Eosinophilic granulomatosis and polyangiitis

Eosinophilic granulomatosis and polyangiitis (EGPA; formerly known as Churg–Strauss syndrome) is less common than eosinophilic pneumonia. It is associated with a high eosinophil count, asthma and the presence of eosinophilic granulomatous vasculitis in most tissues. EGPA is treated with oral corticosteroids and other immunosuppressive drugs (azathioprine and cyclophosphamide)

### Hypereosinophilic syndrome

This is a very rare eosinophilic infiltration of many organs associated with arteritis. It usually presents with pyrexia, weight loss, abdominal pain and congestive cardiac failure resulting from myocardial involvement. Systemic corticosteroids shorten the duration of pulmonary eosinophilia and clear the pulmonary infiltrates. Hypereosinophilic syndrome is treated with oral corticosteroids and anti-IL-5 monoclonal antibodies.

**Table 6.33** Causes of eosinophilia and pulmonary infiltration

**Fungi**
- *Aspergillus fumigatus*
- *Candida albicans*

**Parasites**
- *Ascaris lumbricoides*
- *Strongyloides stercoralis*
- *Trichuris trichiura*
- *Wuchereria bancrofti* (tropics)

**Drugs**
- Aspirin
- Penicillin
- Para-aminosalicylic acid
- Nitrofurantoin
- Sulfonamides

**Autoimmune**
- Polyarteritis nodosa
- EPGA

## MUST-KNOW CHECKLIST

- Interpretation of simple spirometry and peak flow measurement
- Causes and classification of respiratory failure (type 1 and type 2)
- Diagnosis and empirical treatment of community-acquired pneumonia
- Diagnosis and treatment of TB
- Diagnosis and treatment of asthma, including acute severe asthma
- Diagnosis and treatment of COPD
- Causes and general management of bronchiectasis
- Clinical features and management of adult cystic fibrosis
- Investigation and classification of pleural effusion
- Clinical features, classification and treatment of pneumothorax
- Investigation and classification of interstitial lung disease
- Causes, investigation and treatment of lung cancer
- Clinical features, diagnosis and management of OSA

**Questions and answers** to test your understanding of Chapter 6 can be found by clicking 'Support Material' at the following link: https://www.routledge.com/Medicine-for-Finals-and-Beyond/Axford-OCallaghan/p/book/9780367150594

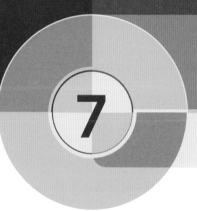

# Cardiovascular Disease

## 7

ALEXANDER LYON

## INTRODUCTION

Cardiovascular (CV) disease is the most common cause of death worldwide, accounting for 32% of all deaths in 2019. Of these 17.9 million deaths, 85% were due to acute myocardial infarction (MI) or stroke. In developed countries, approximately 30% of all deaths among men and 20% of deaths among women result from ischaemic heart disease, and the rate is rising in developing countries. CV disease is an important cause of premature mortality, accounting for 38% of death in people under the age of 70 years.

## APPROACH TO THE PATIENT

### HISTORY

#### ABOUT THE PATIENT

General information about patients is always important in putting their symptoms into context, e.g.:
- Age
- Gender
- Work status (e.g. employed/unemployed) and the nature of their work

- Risk factors: smoking status, hypertension, diabetes, hypercholesterolaemia, family history of CV disease, previous chemotherapy or chest radiotherapy

In contrast to a 55-year-old male diabetic or smoker, a non-smoking female of 35 complaining of chest pain is unlikely to have obstructive coronary disease.

### SYMPTOMS

Patients with CV disease usually present with well-defined symptoms (HISTORY & EXAMINATION 7.1 and HISTORY & EXAMINATION 7.2). These include pain, breathlessness, oedema, palpitations, dizziness, fainting and fatigue.

#### Pain

Chest pain is a common cause of admission to hospital. The patient should be admitted if they present with ongoing cardiac chest pain at rest to identify the cause (**Table 7.1**).

#### *Typical cardiac pain*

Typical cardiac pain, called angina, is centrally located and crushing in nature, and can radiate through to the back, up to the neck, or down one or both arms. It is commonly associated with exertion or emotional stress and usually arises when myocardial oxygen demand exceeds oxygen supply,

DOI: 10.1201/9781003193616-7

## HISTORY & EXAMINATION 7.1

### Questions to be addressed by the history and examination in cardiology

What are the patient's symptoms?
How long has the patient had these symptoms?
Have the symptoms changed with time, and if so, how?
How do the symptoms affect the patient's lifestyle?

## HISTORY & EXAMINATION 7.2

### Important questions to ask in cardiology

**About the patient**

How old are you?
What work do you do?

**Symptoms**

What symptoms do you get?

*Chest pain*

Where is it?
What does it feel like (a tight band, crushing, an ache, sharp)?
How long does it last?
Does it radiate into your arms, neck or back?
When do you get it (on exertion, at rest, when stressed)?
Is it painful to breathe deeply?
Do you have to take occasional deep breaths?

*Breathlessness*

When do you get it (on exertion, on lying flat, during the night)?
Is it painful to breathe deeply?
Do you have to take occasional deep breaths?

*Ankle swelling*

When do you get it (all the time, at the end of the day)?
What makes it worse?
What makes it better?

*Palpitations*

What are they like (fast or slow; regular or irregular)? Ask the patient to tap the beat onto the table
When do you get them?
What brings them on?
Do they stop suddenly or gradually?
Are they associated with dizziness, loss of consciousness or chest pain?

*Dizziness and fainting*

Describe what happens
What brings it on?
Do you have any warning?
Does chest pain or palpitations precede the dizziness?
Do you fall and hurt yourself?
Are you incontinent?

**Pattern of disease**

*Onset and progression*

How long have you had these symptoms?
Are the symptoms getting better or worse?

*Associated features*

Have you noticed any other associated symptoms (e.g. sweating, tiredness, pins and needles)?

**Drug history**

What prescribed and non-prescribed medicines, pills and potions do you take (including all those bought from health food shops such as vitamins)?

**Past medical history**

What illnesses have you had other than the usual childhood infections?
Have you had rheumatic fever?
What operations have you had?
Have you ever had treatment for cancer? What and when?

**Family history**

Does anyone in your family have (or has anyone had) a heart condition or high blood pressure? If so, what?
Is there any family history of premature CV disease or sudden death? Below age 50 years?

**Social history**

Do you smoke? If so, how much?
Do you drink alcohol? If so, what and how much?
Do you drink a lot of coffee?
How much exercise do you do?
Is your diet healthy or unhealthy?

usually as a result of a fixed coronary stenosis, and it is relieved by sublingual GTN. NICE guidelines define three characteristics for diagnosis:

- Central chest discomfort lasting <15 minutes
- Provoked by exercise or emotional stress
- Relieved by rest or sublingual nitrates

All three are required for the diagnosis of typical angina. Two out of three suggests atypical angina. Patients may describe it as a pain, but also a discomfort, sensation or pressure without referring to pain specifically. Alternative causes are microvascular ischaemia, uncontrolled hypertension with

**Table 7.1** Causes of chest pain

| **Cardiovascular** |
| --- |
| Angina: |
| • Obstructive coronary disease |
| • Microvascular ischaemia |
| • Hypertensive heart strain |
| Pericarditis |
| Aortic pathology: |
| • Dissection |
| • Aneurysm |
| **Non-cardiovascular** |
| Lung disease: |
| • Pleurisy |
| • Pneumonia |
| • Pneumothorax |
| • Embolism |
| Oesophageal disease |
| Musculoskeletal: |
| • Chest wall pain |
| • Intercostal muscle strain |
| Referred from cervical spine pathology |

**Table 7.2** Canadian Cardiovascular Society grading of angina

| | |
|---|---|
| Grade 1 | Angina on strenuous physical activity |
| Grade 2 | Angina on ordinary physical activity (e.g. walking uphill or climbing more than one flight of stairs) |
| Grade 3 | Marked limitation on ordinary physical activity (e.g. angina on climbing one flight of stairs) |
| Grade 4 | Angina on any physical activity and also at rest |

left ventricular hypertrophy (LVH), aortic stenosis (AS), hypertrophic cardiomyopathy and pulmonary hypertension with right ventricular (RV) strain. Occasionally, angina presents with epigastric pain on exertion or stress, usually due to inferior wall ischaemia, and should be considered in patients presenting with acute epigastric pain.

Angina has been categorized by the Canadian Cardiovascular Society according to the exercise limitation it imposes on the patient (**Table 7.2**).

### Atypical chest pain

Atypical chest pain does not fulfil the usual criteria for cardiac pain. It has a different character and occurs in any part of the chest or upper abdomen. It usually has no cardiac cause, but occasionally is caused by coronary spasm. Other cardiac causes of atypical pain are mitral valve prolapse (MVP) and mitral stenosis (MS), which may cause pain possibly because of expansion of the left atrium.

## Breathlessness

### Exertional dyspnoea

Exertional dyspnoea (or breathlessness) is a normal response to exercise. However, in heart disease it becomes exaggerated because of three mechanisms:

- Increased pressure in the left atrium and pulmonary veins with exercise causes stiffness of the lungs
- Inadequate cardiac output during exercise results in poor peripheral perfusion and an increased metabolic acidosis
- Impaired ventilatory efficiency due to respiratory muscle wasting and increased alveolar membrane fibrosis in chronic heart failure (HF)

Exertional dyspnoea can be an angina equivalent (myocardial ischaemia giving rise to poor ventricular function on exercise without chest pain). Distinguishing a cardiac cause from a respiratory cause for breathlessness can be difficult and requires measurement of natriuretic peptides and echocardiography. Exertional dyspnoea can be classified according to its effect on the patient's life (**Table 7.3**; **Table 7.4**).

### Paroxysmal nocturnal dyspnoea

Paroxysmal nocturnal dyspnoea (PND) is usually a symptom of poor LV function. The patient wakes from sleep acutely dyspnoeic because of a rise in left atrial pressure, and has to sit up or walk, the symptoms settling after a few minutes. This must not be confused with the nocturnal dyspnoea of asthma, which is not relieved by sitting forwards, is associated with wheeze and relieved by bronchodilators.

**Table 7.3** Differential diagnoses of exertional dyspnoea: distinction between cardiac and respiratory causes

**If cardiac:**

Dyspnoea may be associated with chest tightness (angina).

Dyspnoea will usually be exertionally related.

Lung fields on a chest X-ray may be normal or show pulmonary oedema or pleural effusions secondary to acute HF.

Brain natriuretic peptide (BNP) will be raised if secondary to LV and/or RV impairment, or if there is a large ischaemic territory.

A resting echocardiogram will identify LV dysfunction and/or valvular heart disease.

A stress test (exercise test or thallium scan or dobutamine echocardiogram) may be helpful.

### Orthopnoea

Orthopnoea is a symptom of LV failure or MS and is also caused by a rise in left atrial pressure. The patient is unable to lie flat because of breathlessness resulting from chronically raised left atrial pressure. Often patients report that they have increased the number of pillows they sleep on.

### Oedema

HF is one of the many causes of dependent pitting oedema, which is usually first visible at the ankles. If a patient is confined to bed, peripheral oedema usually occurs in the sacrum. Hepatomegaly and ascites develop in more severe right HF.

### Palpitations

Palpitation is a term to describe an awareness of a disturbance in the rhythm of the heart (irregular and/or accelerated) or an awareness of the force of the heartbeat. Patients also use phrases such as 'flutterings', 'skipped beats' or 'thumps' in their chest.

### Presyncope and syncope

Cardiac causes of dizziness (presyncope) and blackout (syncope) arise as a result of decreased cerebral perfusion. The most common causes are postural hypotension and vasovagal syncope. Other cardiac causes include arrhythmias (bradycardias and tachycardias), AS, hypertrophic cardiomyopathy and pulmonary hypertension.

### Fatigue

Fatigue is a relatively non-specific symptom of heart disease. It is often reported by patients with HF and also advanced

**Table 7.4** New York Heart Association (NYHA) grading of dyspnoea

| | |
|---|---|
| Grade 1 | No breathlessness |
| Grade 2 | Breathlessness on severe exertion |
| Grade 3 | Breathlessness on mild exertion |
| Grade 4 | Breathlessness at rest |

**7**

coronary artery disease. Some patients deny symptoms because they have adapted their way of life and take no exercise. A formal exercise test (or walk along the corridor with the patient) can be very helpful.

## RECREATIONAL DRUG HISTORY

Finding out whether the patient smokes and their alcohol intake and use of other drugs is important, as illustrated by the following examples:

- *Smoking:* a risk factor for coronary artery disease
- *Alcohol:* can cause HF and arrhythmias (particularly atrial fibrillation [AF])
- *Cocaine:* can cause vasospastic angina and acute myocardial infarction (AMI)
- *Methamphetamine (crystal meth):* a growing epidemic causing myocarditis and HF
- *Intravenous (IV) drug abusers:* risk of endocarditis

## PAST MEDICAL HISTORY

A history of previous cardiac disease (e.g. prior coronary stenting or coronary bypass surgery) increases the likelihood that new symptoms are cardiac. Other vascular disease (e.g. a cerebrovascular accident [stroke] or peripheral vascular disease [intermittent claudication]) makes the presence of coronary disease more likely. A history of rheumatic fever in childhood is relevant in patients with mitral valve disease who are older patients (>70 years) or patients from regions of the world where rheumatic fever is common (developing countries). Previous cardiotoxic anthracycline chemotherapy or radiotherapy to the mediastinal or left breast for previous cancer increases the likelihood of HF and coronary disease.

## FAMILY HISTORY

Some cardiac disorders have a clearly established pattern of inheritance: e.g. hypertrophic cardiomyopathy, familial hypercholesterolaemia and Marfan's syndrome are autosomal dominant diseases, so 50% of the children of a patient are likely to inherit the disease.

## EXAMINATION

### INITIAL EXAMINATION

When examining a patient, the following general points should be noted first:

- Is there a clear syndrome associated with CV disease (e.g. Marfan's, Down or Noonan syndrome)?
- How breathless is the patient walking into the consultation room?
- When the patient is relaxed and sitting at 45°, note whether the patient is cachexic, obese, anaemic, jaundiced, or has features of thyroid disturbance or renal failure

**Table 7.5** Signs of infective endocarditis

| |
|---|
| Fever |
| Anaemia |
| Heart murmur – may change |
| Splenomegaly |
| Nail bed splinter haemorrhages |
| Clubbing of nail bed |
| Petechial rash |
| Osler's nodes – painful nodules on the finger pads |
| Janeway's lesions on hand – maculopapular rash caused by immune complex deposition |
| Roth spots in retina resulting from retinal microinfarcts |
| Weight loss leading to cachexia |
| Haematuria |

### Cardiovascular signs

*Cyanosis* is a blue discoloration of skin and mucous membranes. It can either be central (with a blue tongue) caused by heart and lung disease, or peripheral because of poor peripheral perfusion.

The signs of endocarditis are listed in **Table 7.5** and those of rheumatic fever in **Table 7.6**.

### Pulse

Palpate the radial and carotid pulses and note their rate, rhythm, character and volume. If peripheral vascular disease is suspected, palpate the femoral, popliteal and pedal pulses.

#### Pulse rate

Compare the pulse rate with that of the apex. A deficit in the radial pulse can occur in AF or if there are ectopic beats. A *bradycardia* is a heart rate less than 60 beats/min; a *tachycardia* is a rate more than 100 beats/min.

#### Pulse rhythm

The rhythm may be:

- *Regular:* a normal increase and decrease in the heart rate with respiration–sinus arrhythmia

**Table 7.6** Features of rheumatic fever (Duckett–Jones criteria)

| |
|---|
| **Major** |
| • Carditis |
| • Polyarthritis |
| • Chorea |
| • Erythema marginatum |
| • Subcutaneous nodules |
| **Minor** |
| • Fever |
| • Arthralgia |
| • Previous rheumatic fever or rheumatic heart disease |
| • Elevated ESR or CRP |
| • Prolonged PR interval |

CRP, C-reactive protein; ESR, erythrocyte sedimentation rate.

- *Irregularly irregular:* as a result of AF or because of irregular atrial or ventricular ectopics or intermittent heart block
- *Regularly irregular:* because of regular atrial or ventricular ectopics

### Pulse character

The character of the pulse reflects the state of the outflow tract of the left ventricle (LV) (**Figure 7.1**). It may be:

- *Normal*
- *Slow rising:* resulting from AS and best felt at the carotid pulse
- *Collapsing:* resulting from aortic incompetence (or, very rarely, an arteriovenous fistula or PDA) and best felt at both the radial pulse, mid forearm as the 'muscle knock' when the forearm is raised and gripped firmly across the medial forearm muscles, and the carotid pulse
- *Bisferiens:* resulting from a combination of a slow rising and a collapsing pulse in mixed aortic valve disease
- *Sharp:* resulting from the abrupt ending of systole as in hypertrophic cardiomyopathy or mitral regurgitation (MR)

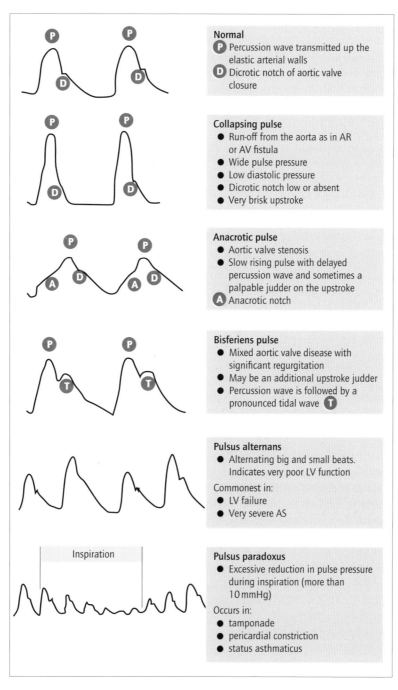

**Normal**
- **P** Percussion wave transmitted up the elastic arterial walls
- **D** Dicrotic notch of aortic valve closure

**Collapsing pulse**
- Run-off from the aorta as in AR or AV fistula
- Wide pulse pressure
- Low diastolic pressure
- Dicrotic notch low or absent
- Very brisk upstroke

**Anacrotic pulse**
- Aortic valve stenosis
- Slow rising pulse with delayed percussion wave and sometimes a palpable judder on the upstroke
- **A** Anacrotic notch

**Bisferiens pulse**
- Mixed aortic valve disease with significant regurgitation
- May be an additional upstroke judder
- Percussion wave is followed by a pronounced tidal wave **T**

**Pulsus alternans**
- Alternating big and small beats. Indicates very poor LV function

Commonest in:
- LV failure
- Very severe AS

**Pulsus paradoxus**
- Excessive reduction in pulse pressure during inspiration (more than 10 mmHg)

Occurs in:
- tamponade
- pericardial constriction
- status asthmaticus

**Figure 7.1** The types of arterial pulse which can be identified on clinical examination. AV, atriovenous; LV, left ventricular; AS, aortic stenosis.

### Pulse volume

The volume of the pulse may be:

- *Normal*
- *Increased:* as in high-output states such as anaemia, thyrotoxicosis and fevers
- *Decreased:* resulting from reduced cardiac output as in LV failure, AS and causes of reduced circulating blood volume such as haemorrhage

*Pulsus alternans* This occurs when, in the presence of a regular rhythm, the systolic blood pressure varies from beat to beat. It gives rise to an alternating weak and strong ('thready') pulse and is caused by the variable recovery time of weak heart muscle. It indicates a poor prognosis from LV failure.

*Pulsus paradoxus* This is an exaggeration in the difference in pulse pressure during inspiration and expiration. Normally this difference is less than 15 mmHg. In severe asthma, constrictive pericarditis or pericardial tamponade, inspiration results in a greater fall in systolic pressure (sometimes the systolic pressure disappears). RV filling, which is normally increased by the negative intrathoracic pressure of inspiration, then compromises LV filling because of the inability of the heart to expand in the fixed volume of the pericardium. Output from the LV and blood pressure therefore fall on inspiration.

### Blood pressure

The blood pressure is defined by the systolic pressure (when the pulse first becomes audible) and the diastolic pressure (when the Korotkoff sounds are no longer heard). Normal blood pressure at home is <130/85 mmHg and in the clinic is <140/90 mmHg. A wide pulse pressure is typical of aortic incompetence, PDA or a large arteriovenous fistula. A small pulse pressure can occur in severe AS.

### Jugular venous pressure

The jugular venous pressure (JVP) has the following characteristics to differentiate it from the carotid pulse:

- Impalpable
- Biphasic in each cardiac cycle (if in sinus rhythm)
- Falls with inspiration
- Blocked by pressure across the lower border of the anterior cervical triangle
- Increase with pressure on the liver (hepatojugular reflux)

The important clinical features of the JVP are height and character. There are two peaks and two troughs in a normal JVP in every cardiac cycle if the patient is in sinus rhythm (**Figure 7.2**):

- a *wave:* brought about by atrial contraction
- x *descent:* brought about by movement of the base of the heart towards the apex in systole
- v *wave:* brought about by right atrial filling against a closed tricuspid valve (TV)
- y *descent:* brought about by opening of the TV

### Abnormalities of the JVP

Abnormalities of the JVP are as follows:

- *Elevated JVP:* This indicates increased right atrial pressure – HF is the commonest cause.
- *Cannon waves:* These are huge a *waves* brought about by atrial contraction against a closed TV. They are seen intermittently during atrial tachycardias, complete heart block and ventricular tachycardia (VT) because, although the atria and ventricles contract independently, they occasionally contract at the same time. Cannon waves occur regularly with junctional tachycardias when the atria and ventricles usually contract simultaneously.
- *Systolic v waves:* These are brought about by tricuspid incompetence when blood regurgitates into the atrium during systole and obliterates the x descent and normal v peak.
- *Prominent y descent:* Constrictive pericarditis reflects rapid RV filling in early diastole.
- *Positive Kussmaul's sign:* An increase in JVP with inspiration may be due to cardiac tamponade or constrictive pericarditis.

## PALPATION OF THE PRECORDIUM

Four areas of the precordium should be palpated:

- Apex beat
- Left sternal edge
- Aortic area
- Pulmonary area

### Apex beat

The apex beat is the most lateral and inferior pulsation of the LV and is normally in the mid-clavicular line in the 5th intercostal space. It can be forceful in the normal location due to LVH, or displaced laterally, and over a wider area due to LV dilatation or rarely mediastinal shift. A double apical beat occurs in hypertrophic cardiomyopathy with outflow tract obstruction.

### Left sternal edge

A palpable impulse at the left sternal edge indicates either RV hypertrophy (RVH) or systolic expansion of the left atrium, as in MR.

### Aortic area

In AS, it is possible to feel a thrill (palpable murmur) to the right of the sternum when the patient sits forward.

### Pulmonary area

A palpable pulmonary component to the second heart sound in the second left intercostal space indicates pulmonary hypertension.

## AUSCULTATION OF THE HEART

Examination involves listening with both the bell and the diaphragm of the stethoscope at the apex, lower and upper

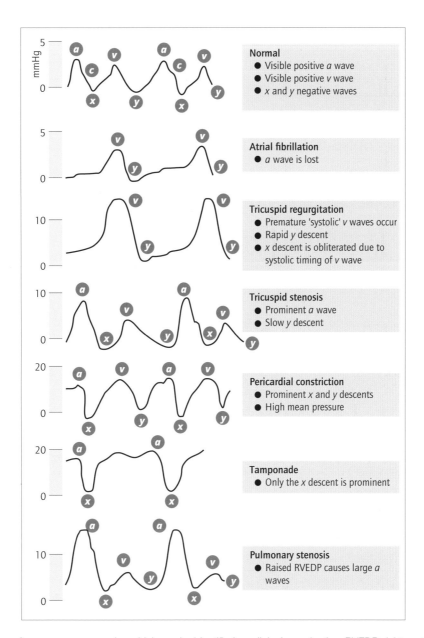

**Figure 7.2** The types of venous pressure pulse which can be identified on clinical examination. RVEDP, right ventricular end-diastolic pressure.

left sternal and upper right sternal edges with the patient at 45°. Sit the patient forwards and listen at the lower left sternal edge for aortic regurgitation (AR).

### Heart sounds

See **Figure 7.3**.

#### First heart sound

The first heart sound is caused by the consecutive closure of the mitral and tricuspid valves and is maximal over the apex beat. It is usually single but can be split, in which case the double click must be distinguished from either a fourth heart sound or an ejection click (EC). Normally, the valves are beginning to close before the onset of systole. Abnormal findings include the following:

- *Loud first heart sound:* This occurs in MS or when there is a short PR interval.
- *Soft first heart sound:* This results in advanced calcific MS, or MR with failure of mitral valve leaflet closure.

#### Second heart sound

The second heart sound is caused by closure of the aortic and pulmonary valves (PV) and is best heard in the second left intercostal space (the pulmonary area):

- *Physiological splitting of the second heart sound:* separation of the pulmonary component from the aortic component is increased by deep inspiration
- *Increased split of the second heart sound:* occurs with right bundle branch block (RBBB) or pulmonary stenosis

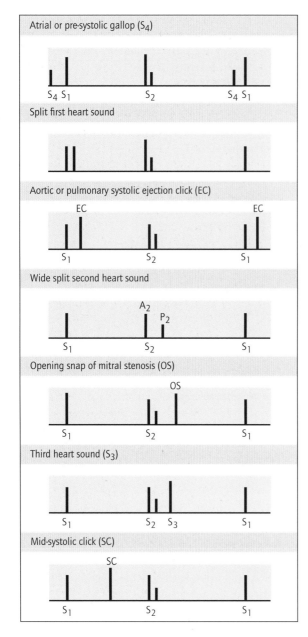

**Figure 7.3** The timing of the heart sounds in the cardiac cycle. $S_1$, first heart sound, mitral and TV closure; $S_2$ second heart sound, aortic and PV closure. (When noting heart sounds in the patient's records, the full cardiac cycle should be described and the height of the sound relates to its intensity.)

- *Fixed splitting of the second heart sound:* indicates an atrial septal defect (ASD)
- *Reverse splitting of the second heart sound:* caused by severe AS, left bundle branch block (LBBB) or advanced LV failure
- *Increased aortic sound:* A2 increases with systemic hypertension
- *Softer aortic sound:* occurs in AS
- *Increased pulmonary sound:* P2 is louder in pulmonary hypertension
- *Softer pulmonary sound:* pulmonary sound is soft in pulmonary stenosis

### Third heart sound

A third heart sound (S3) occurs after the second heart sound and is produced by high left atrial and LV filling pressures including volume overload and/or pressure overloaded ventricle. A left-sided S3 indicates LV failure, but it can be a normal finding in children, young adults and pregnant women.

### Fourth heart sound

A fourth heart sound (S4) occurs after the third sound and immediately before the first sound. It is brought about by LVH and atrial contraction against a stiff non-compliant ventricle.

### Ejection click

An EC occurs shortly after the first heart sound and indicates a bicuspid aortic valve.

### Mid-systolic click

A mid-systolic click indicates MVP and is often followed by a late systolic murmur.

### Pericardial knock

A right-sided S3 is due to constrictive pericarditis.

### Heart murmurs

Heart murmurs are described according to their timing in the cardiac cycle (**Figure 7.4**), so it is important to feel the carotid pulse while performing cardiac auscultation.

### Systolic murmurs

There are different types of systolic murmur:

- *Pansystolic murmur:* This is a sustained murmur throughout systole up to and including the aortic component of the second heart sound. It is a feature of MR, tricuspid regurgitation and ventricular septal defect (VSD).
- *Late systolic murmur:* This is a crescendo murmur in the latter part of systole. It is often preceded by a click and indicates MVP with regurgitation.
- *Ejection systolic murmur:* This is a crescendo/decrescendo systolic murmur caused by stenosis of the aortic or pulmonary valves.
- *Innocent (benign) systolic murmur:* Particularly common in children, this characteristically occurs early in systole. There is no underlying structural heart defect and it is of no importance.

### Diastolic murmurs

The different types of diastolic murmur are as follows:

- *Early diastolic murmur:* This is a decrescendo murmur in diastole that occurs immediately after the second heart sound. It is caused by aortic or pulmonary regurgitation.
- *Mid-late diastolic murmur:* A low-frequency rumble is only heard at the apex and often follows an opening snap (OS). It is due to either MS or tricuspid stenosis.

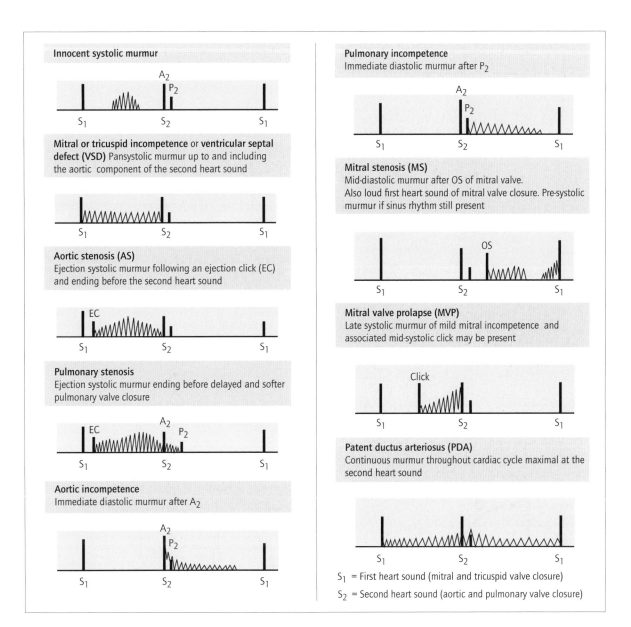

**Figure 7.4** The timing of the various heart murmurs.

***Continuous murmur (Gibson's machinery murmur)***
This is a continuous murmur throughout systole and diastole, resulting from continuous flow through a PDA.

CARDIAC INVESTIGATIONS

## THE ELECTROCARDIOGRAM

The standard 12-lead electrocardiogram (ECG) reflects the electrical activity of the heart from different angles (**Figure 7.5**). The components of an ECG complex are the P wave, the PR interval, the QRS complex and the ST segment (**Figure 7.6**).

- *P wave:* atrial wave in sinus rhythm triggering atrial contraction; best seen in standard lead II or V1

- *PR interval:* the interval between the onset of the P wave and the onset of the QRS complex; normal is 120–200 ms

- *QRS complex:* results from ventricular depolarization and consists of the Q wave (the initial negative deflection), the R wave (the first positive deflection) and the S wave (the subsequent negative deflection); normal width of the QRS complex is <120 ms

- *ST segment:* normally isoelectric

- *T wave:* usually in the same axis as the QRS complex because the wave of repolarization is in the opposite transmural direction to depolarization (from the epicardium to the endocardium)

- *U wave:* can be prominent in hypokalaemia and myocardial ischaemia

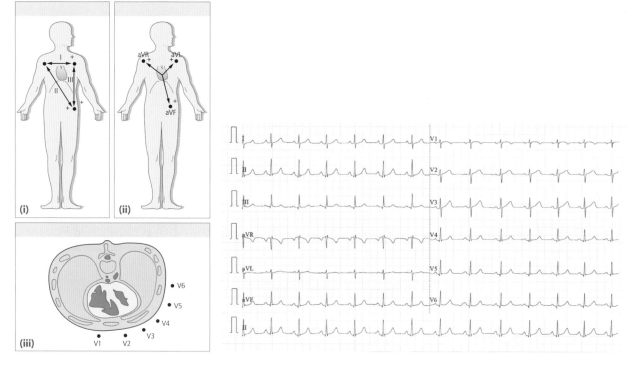

**Figure 7.5 (a)** The leads of the standard 12-lead ECG: **(i)** bipolar leads; **(ii)** unipolar leads; **(iii)** chest leads. **(b)** Example of normal 12-lead ECG.

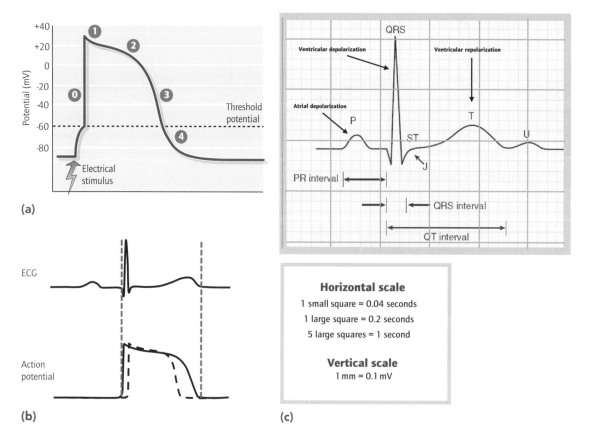

**Figure 7.6 (a)** The different phases of the action potential of the myocardial cell. **(b)** Temporal correlation of the surface ECG and the ventricular cardiomyocyte action potential. **(c)** The components of the surface ECG: P, QRC and T waves, and PR, QRS and QT intervals.

### The exercise ECG

The exercise ECG is useful for:
- Assessing exercise capacity in the context of ischaemic heart disease or HF
- Assessing with exercise-related arrhythmias

It is usually performed according to a standard protocol (e.g. Bruce or Naughton).

### Analysis of cardiac rhythm

- 24- or 48-hour ambulatory ECG (Holter monitor)
- 7- or 14-day ECG patch
- Implantable loop recorder (ILR): a long-term recorder implanted under the skin of the chest
- Phone apps for ECG recording using the patient's smartphone

## DIAGNOSTIC IMAGING

### Chest X-ray

A chest X-ray allows an assessment of heart size. The transthoracic cardiac diameter is normally less than 50% of the transthoracic diameter. The normal right heart contour consists of the inferior vena cava (IVC), the right atrial junction, the right atrial border at the junction between the right atrium and the superior vena cava (SVC). The normal left heart contour consists of the aortic arch, the pulmonary artery, the left atrium and the LV border (**Figure 7.7**).

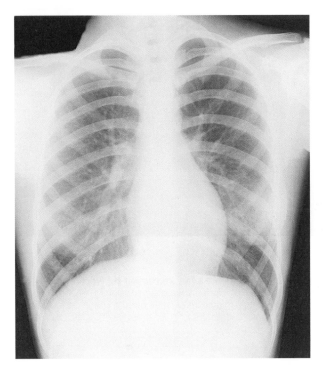

**Figure 7.7** Normal cardiac contour on a posteroanterior (PA) chest X-ray.

### Echocardiography

Transthoracic echocardiography is a non-invasive technique for analysing cardiac structure and function. It is particularly important for assessing ventricular function, presence of MI and valvular function, and can non-invasively assess pulmonary artery pressure. In patients with poor-quality images, IV contrast can be used to improve assessment of ventricular function. Advanced technologies, including strain imaging and 3D echocardiography, provide more detailed assessment of ventricular function.

#### Transoesophageal echocardiography

The heart can be imaged from the oesophagus using transoesophageal echocardiography (TOE) to evaluate heart valves, particularly prosthetic metallic heart valves, and abnormal cardiac masses in more detail. TOE is used in cases of suspected endocarditis or cryptogenic stroke.

### Nuclear cardiac imaging

Nuclear cardiac imaging can be used for the following indications:
- Myocardial ischaemia with myocardial perfusion imaging using thallium-201, technetium-99 SPECT or rubidium-82 PET-CT (**Figure 7.8c**)
- Myocardial inflammation using FDG-cardiac PET

### Cardiac magnetic resonance imaging

Cardiac magnetic resonance imaging (CMR) is useful for evaluating diseases of the myocardium. Injection of gadolinium allows assessment of MI, fibrosis and infiltrative diseases (**Figure 7.8d**). CMR can also assess for acute inflammation and myocarditis, myocardial iron levels in haemachromatosis and myocardial ischaemia with adenosine stress perfusion protocol. CMR also provides detailed anatomy of the great vessels, the pericardium and the thoracic aorta and assessment of abnormal cardiac masses.

### Computed tomography coronary angiography

Computed tomography coronary angiography (CTCA) has become a standard technique to non-invasively assess the anatomy of the coronary arteries and the presence of coronary artery disease (**Figure 7.8a**). It provides information on the presence, extent and location of coronary atheroma, calcification and stenoses. A new FFR-CT analysis technology can non-invasively assess if a coronary stenosis is likely to be flow-limiting (**Figure 7.8b**). CT can also quantify the degree of aortic valve calcification in patients with AS and access routes for patients requiring transcatheter aortic valve implantation (TAVI).

### Cardiac catheterization

This is a specialist procedure. Indications for its use are listed in **Table 7.7**.

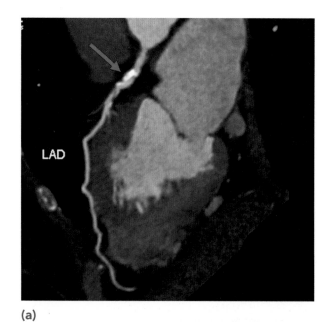

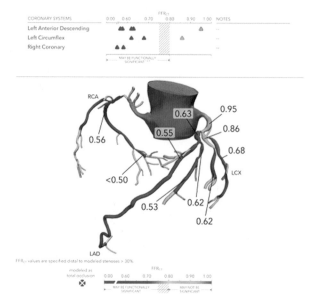

**(a)**

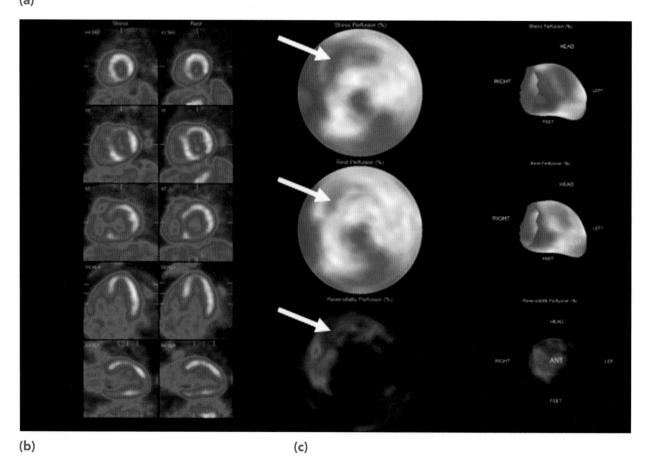

**(b)**          **(c)**

**Figure 7.8 (a)** CTCA showing calcified plaque in proximal left anterior descending coronary artery (red arrow). **(b)** Fractional flow reserve CT (FFR-CT) showing flow-limiting three vessel coronary artery disease. **(c)** Rubidium myocardial perfusion PET-CT showing reversible ischaemia in the anteroseptal myocardium (white arrows – top image stress, middle image rest, bottom image perfusion mismatch showing ischaemic territory). *(Continued)*

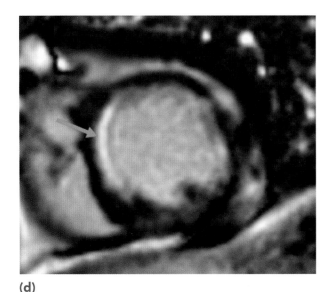

**(d)**

**Figure 7.8** (*Continued*) **(d)** CMR with late gadolinium enhancement in parasternal short-axis view showing subendocardial septal MI (blue arrow).

**Table 7.7** Indications for cardiac catheterization

To assess the presence and severity of coronary disease = coronary angiography

To assess valvular disease

To measure intracardiac pressures, oxygen saturation (assessment of intracardiac shunts) and calculate cardiac output and pulmonary artery resistance = right and left cardiac catheterization

### Electrophysiological studies of the heart

Introducing electrodes into the right atrium, RV and coronary sinus allows characterization of the electrical activity of the heart. The time delays in electrical activity of the heart can be measured and pathological arrhythmias can be stimulated.

## PRINCIPLES OF MANAGEMENT

CV 'healthy living' advice for all patients includes:
- Not smoking
- Avoiding too much fat (especially saturated fat) and complex carbohydrates in the diet
- Avoiding excessive weight
- Taking regular exercise – ideally 30+ minute sessions focused on aerobic exercise at least three times per week
- Minimizing stress
- Occasional 'screening' measurement of blood pressure and cholesterol level

## CARDIAC SURGERY

Cardiac surgery is an effective treatment for ischaemic heart disease and valve disease, relieving symptomatic angina and prolonging survival in selected patient groups. Standard indications for coronary artery bypass surgery include left main stem or triple vessel coronary artery disease, particularly in patients with diabetes and/or LV dysfunction where there is prognostic benefit. Surgery is offered for severe heart valve disease providing specific criteria are met, with either repair or replacement with bioprosthetic or mechanical valves. Surgical treatments for severe HF include cardiac transplantation or LV assist device implantation for eligible patients. Patients with complex congenital heart disease frequently require surgical correction.

All adults referred for cardiac valve surgery require preoperative coronary angiography to confirm if coronary disease requiring bypass is present in addition to the primary indication for surgery.

## INTERVENTIONAL TECHNIQUES

Interventional techniques whereby therapeutic procedures can be carried out using long catheters have been introduced over the last 30 years. These include:
- Percutaneous coronary intervention (PCI) usually with coronary stent insertion
- Radiofrequency ablation (RFA) for various arrhythmias
- TAVI for AS
- Mitral valvuloplasty for MS
- MitraClip™ and other mitral valve replacement technologies for MR
- Septal occluder device implantation for ASD, VSD and patent foramen ovale (PFO)
- Percutaneous PV implantation for pulmonary stenosis or regurgitation
- Left atrial appendage occluder device

## DISEASES AND THEIR MANAGEMENT

### ISCHAEMIC HEART DISEASE

#### Stable angina

Symptoms of stable angina develop when a coronary artery stenosis limits increased blood flow required for an increased demand for oxygen (e.g. during exercise or an emotional upset). Exertional angina is the typical presentation of ischaemic heart disease. Pain develops with physical exertion, particularly in cold weather, after meals or with an emotional upset, and resolves rapidly on rest or with sublingual nitrates.

Characteristically, angina is a central tightness in the chest. It radiates through to the back and shoulder or down one or both arms or into the neck and jaw. Occasionally, the only symptom is breathlessness because of increased pulmonary venous pressure resulting from the LV becoming stiff and failing to relax when ischaemic, particularly in patients with long-standing diabetes.

## Acute coronary syndromes

Atherosclerotic plaque rupture exposes the lipid and collagen content of the plaque to the bloodstream (**Figure 7.9**). This causes platelets to accumulate on the surface of the plaque forming a thrombus which rapidly reduces the diameter of the artery lumen, sometimes causing complete occlusion. This results in unstable (unpredictable) cardiac pain that can take three forms:

- Crescendo angina
- Unstable angina
- AMI

## ISCHAEMIC HEART DISEASE AT A GLANCE

### Epidemiology

*Prevalence*

- Main cause of death in developed countries. Incidence is falling in the USA and UK, with 30% of men and 20% of women dying from ischaemic heart disease

*Age*

- Incidence rises with age, particularly above 50 years

*Sex*

- Premature coronary disease is more common in men, but after the menopause the incidence in women increases to approach that of men of the same age

*Genetics*

- Premature coronary artery disease runs in families, but there is no established pattern unless familial hypercholesterolaemia is present. In the absence of other risk factors, a family history increases the risk in offspring by 20–30%

### Risk factors

- Hypercholesterolaemia
- Hypertension
- Cigarette smoking
- Family history
- Diabetes mellitus
- Sedentary lifestyle
- Psychiatric disease
- Previous radiotherapy of chest/thorax

### Findings on investigation

*Electrocardiography*

- *ECG:* often normal between episodes of angina, but may reveal previous MI

*Haematology*

- FBC to exclude anaemia

*Biochemistry*

- *Cardiac troponin (I or T) if unstable chest pain*
- *Cholesterol profile and HbA1c*
- *Thyroid function tests:* to exclude thyroid dysfunction
- *Urea and electrolytes:* to diagnose renal failure and confirm $K^+$, $Mg^{2+}$ and $Ca^{2+}$

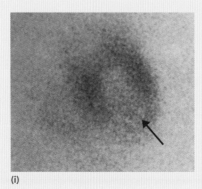
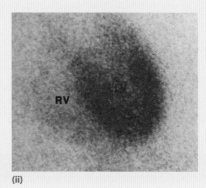

(i)  (ii)

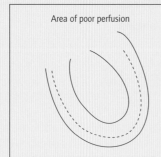
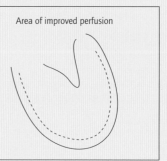

Area of poor perfusion    Area of improved perfusion

**Figure A** Thallium-201 myocardial perfusions scans. **(i)** Exercise scan showing an extensive area of poor perfusion in the apical region of the left ventricle (arrow). **(ii)** The same patient, following surgical revascularization, showing a normal appearance. Both figures reproduced from Armstrong P, Wastie ML, Diagnostic Imaging, 3rd edn., 1992 (Blackwell Scientific Publications, Oxford) with the permission of the authors.

*Continued...*

*...Continued*

*Diagnostic cardiac imaging*

- *Stable patients:* CT coronary angiography, myocardial perfusion scan (MPS), stress echocardiography or perfusion CMR
- *Stable patients:* diagnostic coronary angiography if prognostic disease is identified on CTCA or MPS, or if refractory chest pain despite anti-anginal drug therapy
- *Unstable patients:* cardiac catheterization with coronary angiography for patients with a suspected acute coronary syndrome and unstable angina
- *Resting echocardiogram:* review LV function, regional wall motion abnormalities, valvular function, pericardial effusion and pulmonary artery pressure

## Clinical features

*CV*

- Angina is typically described as central chest tightness (sometimes described as crushing) triggered by exercise or emotional stress which radiates through to the back and shoulder or down one or both arms or into the neck and jaw
- Breathlessness with exertion
- Hypercholesterolaemia
- Hypertension
- Reduced peripheral pulses
- Carotid artery bruits
- Signs of HF in severe cases

*Skin*

- Xanthelasma resulting from hyperlipidaemia
- Nicotine-stained fingers

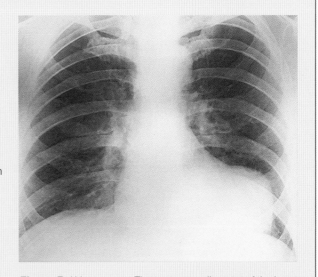

**Figure B** LV aneurysm. The transverse diameter of the heart is moderately enlarged. There is a bulge of the lower half of the left heart border extending down to the apex. This bulge is caused by the aneurysm itself.

7

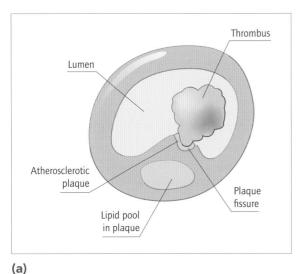

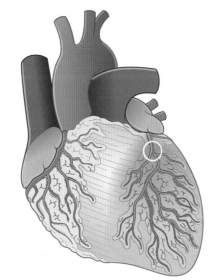

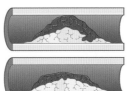

Plaque rupture/erosion with occlusive thrombus

Plaque rupture/erosion with non-occlusive thrombus

**(a)**      **(b)**

**Figure 7.9 (a)** Cross-section of coronary artery in acute coronary syndrome. **(b)** Schematic of a type 1 MI secondary to coronary atherosclerosis, plaque rupture and thrombosis. **(b)** From Thygesen K *et al.* (2019) Fourth universal definition of myocardial infarction. *European Heart Journal* 40: 237–69. https://doi.org/10.1093/eurheartj/ehy462. With permission.

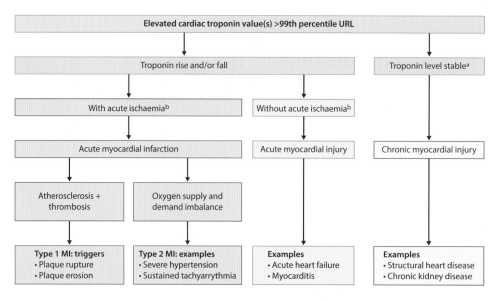

**Figure 7.10** Diagnosis algorithm for patients with elevated cardiac troponin. MI, myocardial infarction; URL, upper reference limit. <sup>a</sup> Stable denotes ≤ 20% variation of troponin values in the appropriate clinical context. <sup>b</sup> Ischaemia denotes signs and/or symptoms of clinical myocardial ischaemia. From Thygesen K *et al.* (2019) Fourth universal definition of myocardial infarction. *European Heart Journal* 40: 237–69. https://doi.org/10.1093/eurheartj/ehy462. With permission.

### Crescendo angina

Crescendo angina is either angina of recent onset or exertional angina with a deteriorating threshold. It implies that a coronary artery narrowing is becoming rapidly more severe.

### Unstable angina

Unstable angina is angina occurring at rest with a normal cardiac troponin. It can also occur at night when lying down (decubitus angina). It is caused by superimposed thrombus on a plaque, and up to 30% of people with this condition progress to have an MI.

### Acute myocardial infarction

AMI is defined as a rise and/or fall of cardiac troponin with at least one value above the 99th percentile upper reference limit (URL) *and* with at least one of the following (**Figure 7.10**):

- Symptoms of acute myocardial ischaemia
- New ischaemic ECG changes
- Development of pathological Q waves
- Imaging evidence of new loss of viable myocardium or new regional wall motion abnormality in a pattern consistent with an ischaemic aetiology
- Identification of a coronary thrombus by angiography including intracoronary imaging or by autopsy

## Diagnosis of ischaemic heart disease

Angina is diagnosed from the history and evidence of myocardial ischaemia on cardiac perfusion or stress imaging.

## Investigation

The investigation of angina involves two stages:

1  Confirming the diagnosis
2  Assessing the severity of the ischaemia and its prognostic significance

### Diagnostic imaging

- *CTCA:* This confirms coronary anatomy, presence or absence of any coronary at herosclerosis and if coronary stensoses are present.
- *MPS:* Nuclear MPS or stress echocardiography with exercise testing is used to diagnose myocardial ischaemia. Reduced tracer uptake in the ischaemic myocardium which returns during recovery confirms reversible ischaemia on a MPS. A fixed perfusion defect reflects a myocardial infarct.
- *Urgent invasive coronary angiography:* This is indicated for all patients presenting with AMI or unstable angina (see below).

## Management

Stable angina is managed by:

- Modifying lifestyle
- Controlling risk factors
- Drug treatment
- Revascularization by coronary stenting or coronary artery bypass surgery

### Drug treatment

*Disease-modifying drugs which improve prognosis*

- Statins
- Aspirin (or clopidogrel if aspirin-intolerant)
- ACE inhibitors

*Angina-relieving drugs (these control symptoms but do not alter prognosis)*

- GTN spray for immediate angina relief
- 1st line: beta blocker or calcium channel blocker (e.g. amlodipine, diltiazem)

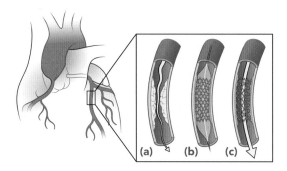

**Figure 7.11 (a–c)** PCI: direct coronary stenting with coronary balloon angioplasty.

- 2nd line: beta blocker and dihydropyridine calcium channel blocker (e.g. amlodipine) (NB Verapamil and diltiazem generally contraindicated with beta blockers)
- 3rd line: add oral isosorbide mononitrate or GTN patch
- 4th line: add nicorandil, ranolazine or ivabradine

### Interventional treatment

*PCI*, or coronary stenting, is conventionally offered to patients whose stable angina continues despite optimal medical therapy, or if prognostic disease is identified on CTCA or MPS (left main stem or proximal LAD on CTCA or >9% ischaemia on MPS) (**Figure 7.11**). Patients require dual antiplatelet therapy (DAPT) with aspirin and clopidogrel following coronary stenting to prevent in-stent thrombosis. The duration of DAPT depends upon the indication (ST elevation MI [STEMI], non-ST elevation MI [NSTEMI], stable angina), bleeding risks and consideration for the type and size of stent (bare metal vs drug eluting, size, length, location).

*Coronary artery bypass surgery* Bypass surgery (**Figure 7.12**) is indicated when:

- Antianginal medication does not provide adequate symptomatic relief from angina, and the coronary stenoses are not suitable for PCI.

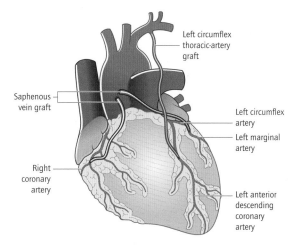

**Figure 7.12** Coronary artery bypass. Left internal mammary artery (LIMA) graft to the left anterior descending coronary artery (LAD), and saphenous vein grafts from the ascending aorta to the left obtuse marginal (OM) and right (RCA) coronary arteries.

- The anatomy of coronary disease suggests that the patient's prognosis can be improved by coronary surgery. Such patterns of narrowing are:
  - Left main stem coronary stenosis
  - Proximal stenoses in all three coronary arteries in the presence of previous MI and diabetes

### Acute coronary syndromes and unstable angina

All patients presenting with acute cardiac-sounding chest pain require an urgent 12-lead ECG and cardiac troponin. If the ECG shows ST elevation or new LBBB, the diagnosis is STEMI. If the ECG is normal or shows acute ST depression or T wave inversion, the diagnosis is either unstable angina if troponin levels are normal or NSTEMI if troponin levels are raised. If both serial ECGs and troponins are normal, non-cardiac causes of chest pain should be considered.

## MYOCARDIAL INFARCTION

Up to 30% of patients with unstable angina proceed to MI and so all patients require immediate treatment as an inpatient. Treatment includes dual antiplatelet drugs (aspirin and clopidogrel), subcutaneous low-molecular-weight heparin (LMWH), fondaparinux or glycoprotein 2b3 inhibitors. Patients with unstable angina should undergo early coronary angiography with a view to revascularization either by PCI or CABG surgery.

### Differential diagnosis of AMI

- *Pericarditis*
- *Aortic dissection*
- *Spontaneous pneumothorax*
- *Oesophageal rupture*
- *Pulmonary embolus*
- *Myocardial injury*: There are many causes of troponin elevation in the absence of acute coronary occlusion and MI. These are known as myocardial injury (see **Table 7.8**) and some are associated with chest pain.

### Investigation

#### Electrocardiography

The three phases in the ECG evolution of infarction are shown in **Table 7.9** and **Figure 7.13**.

*Inferior infarcts* are shown in leads II, III and aVF (**Figure 7.14**); *anterior infarcts* in leads V2–V5 (**Figure 7.15**); *lateral infarcts* in leads I, aVL, V5 and V6; and *true posterior infarcts* are seen with ST depression and dominant R waves in leads V1 and V2 with ST depression and dominant R waves and are confirmed using posterior ECG leads.

New LBBB (with 5+ mm ST elevation in praecordial leads) and concordant QRS and T waves in an acutely unwell patient with chest pain may reflect acute proximal LAD occlusion and is treated as a STEMI (**Figure 7.16**).

**7**

**Table 7.8** Causes of elevated serum cardiac troponin

**Myocardial infarction = cardiac troponin rise with evidence of myocardial ischaemia**
- Type 1: MI secondary to atherosclerotic plaque rupture
- Type 2: MI secondary to oxygen supply vs demand imbalance with ischaemia
- Coronary artery vasospasm
- Coronary artery dissection
- Coronary artery embolism
- Excessive demand with fixed stenoses or microvascular dysfunction:
  - ○ Hypertensive crisis with LVH
  - ○ Hypotension with fixed stenoses

**Myocardial injury = cardiac troponin rise without myocardial ischaemia**
*Cardiac conditions*
- HF
- Myocarditis
- Cardiomyopathy
- Takotsubo syndrome
- Catheter ablation
- Defibrillator shocks (DC cardioversion and defibrillation)
- Cardiac contusion
- *Systemic conditions*
- Sepsis, infectious disease
- Chronic kidney disease
- Stroke, subarachnoid haemorrhage
- Pulmonary embolism
- Pulmonary hypertension
- Infiltrative diseases, e.g. amyloidosis, sarcoidosis
- Cardiotoxic chemotherapy, e.g. doxorubicin
- Critically ill patients
- Strenuous exercise

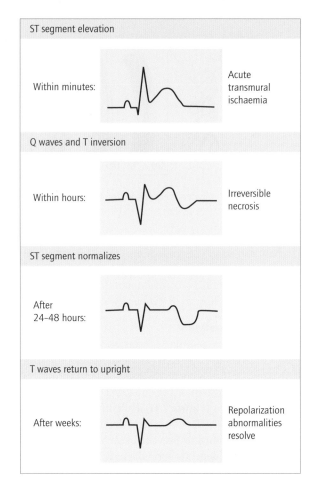

**Figure 7.13** The changing pattern of the ECG in the affected leads during the evolution of an MI.

## Management

If a patient presents with STEMI, they should be transferred by ambulance to a heart attack centre for primary PCI (PPCI). If for geographical reasons there is a predicted delay to access PPCI of >3 hours, thrombolysis either in the ambulance or at the admitting hospital may be indicated, followed by transfer to the heart attack centre. Patients presenting with NSTEMI or unstable angina should be admitted, started medical therapy and have urgent coronary angiography and PCI as appropriate, ideally within 48 hours of admission.

All acute coronary syndrome patients should be admitted to a coronary care unit with continuous ECG monitoring until stable and reperfusion completed.

### Complications of MI

#### Arrhythmias and their treatment
- *Ventricular fibrillation (VF):* defibrillation
- *VT:* beta blockers and/or amiodarone if haemodynamically stable; DC cardioversion if unstable with hypotension
- *AF:* beta blockers
- *Complete heart block:* can complicate inferior AMI caused by right coronary artery occlusion

### Acute HF
MI can lead to acute HF.

### Systemic thromboembolism
This is due to AF or LV apical infarction with associated apical thrombosis. There is no evidence for routine

**Table 7.9** The four phases in the ECG evolution of a Q-wave infarction

| Phase | Features |
|---|---|
| Hyperacute | ST elevation in infarct-related leads |
| Acute | ST-segment elevation in infarct-related leads, development of Q waves, and the beginning of T-wave inversion |
| Subacute | Q waves, loss of R waves and T-wave inversion |
| Chronic | Q waves, loss of R waves. T waves normal |

*Note:* that posterior infarcts cause ST depression in leads V1 and V2 (reciprocal of ST elevation) and R waves in these leads become more prominent, representing posterior Q waves.

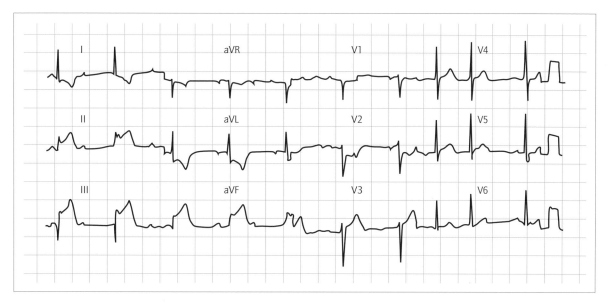

**Figure 7.14** ECG showing acute inferior myocardial infarction with complete heart block and reciprocal ST depression in V1–V2.

anticoagulation in all MI patients, but treatment of AF or apical thrombus with therapeutic anticoagulation is recommended.

### Ventricular septal defect, mitral regurgitation and cardiac rupture

These are rarer in the modern era of PPCI but are still observed in late presenters with established MI and patients receiving thrombolysis where PPCI is not available. If these complications occur, the patient's condition usually deteriorates suddenly with acute HF and cardiogenic shock.

### Dressler's syndrome

Dressler's syndrome is an autoimmune pericarditis which usually develops 1–6 weeks after infarction and is characterized by pericarditis, pleurisy and malaise. The patient may be febrile and anaemic and has a high erythrocyte sedimentation rate (ESR). The condition usually settles with colchicine and non-steroidal anti-inflammatory drugs (NSAIDs).

### Prognosis

### Stable angina

The prognosis in stable angina depends on the location of stenoses and extent of myocardial ischaemia. When pooled,

**7**

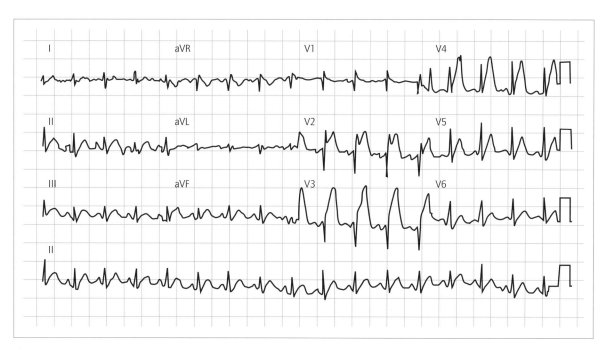

**Figure 7.15** ECG showing acute anterior myocardial infarction with ST elevation in V2–V4.

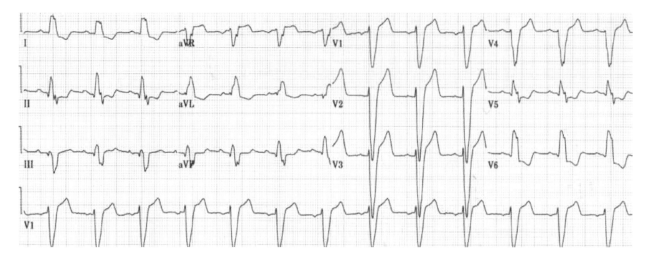

**Figure 7.16** ECG showing typical LBBB.

all patients with stable angina have a relatively good prognosis with modern risk factor management, and revascularization does not improve prognosis. In selected patients with ≥10% myocardial ischaemia, or if left main stem, proximal LAD, ostial RCA or ostial disease of a dominant circumflex coronary artery is identified, then revascularization improves prognosis.

### Myocardial infarction

Before routine PPCI, approximately 10–15% of patients admitted to hospital with AMI died while in hospital. This has fallen to 2–4% with PPCI and adjunctive medical therapy, and so the majority will have an uncomplicated course and be fit for discharge within 7 days of admission. The strongest predictor of death is the size of the infarct and degree of LV dysfunction. The mortality arises from HF, further infarction and malignant arrhythmias. Therefore, all patients should have an echocardiogram during admission and at follow-up.

All patients following MI should receive DAPT for 12 months and then long-term antiplatelet monotherapy (aspirin or clopidogrel), a high-dose statin (e.g. atorvastatin 80 mg) and an ACE inhibitor. If bleeding risk is high, 6 months DAPT is recommended. If LVEF is <40%, patients should receive a beta blocker and aldosterone antagonist. If LVEF is persistently <35% at 3–6 months follow up following MI despite effective medical therapy, then a primary prevention intracardiac defibrillator (ICD) should be considered if prognosis is >12 months.

## HEART FAILURE

### Definition

HF is a clinical syndrome characterized by typical symptoms (e.g. breathlessness, ankle swelling and fatigue) that may be accompanied by signs (e.g. elevated JVP, pulmonary crackles and peripheral oedema) caused by a structural and/or functional cardiac abnormality, resulting in a reduced cardiac output and/or elevated intracardiac pressures at rest or during stress.

### Classification

Patients with chronic HF are classified according to their LV ejection fraction (LVEF). This helps guide treatment decisions as trials assessed treatments in cohorts defined by their LVEF. It may provide some guide to pathophysiology, but these three groups contain many different types of HF, and there is a continuous spectrum between the different categories. Therefore, this classification based on LVEF has limitations. All patients have symptoms and signs of HF:

- HF with reduced LVEF (HFrEF): LVEF <40%
- HF with mildly reduced LVEF (HFmrEF): LVEF 40–49%
- HF with preserved LVEF (HFpEF): LVEF ≥50%

Patients with HFpEF and HFmrEF must have elevated BNP, and patients with HFpEF should have evidence of structural cardiac remodelling (LVH and/or LA dilatation) and/or diastolic dysfunction on echocardiography.

### Epidemiology

- HF is common, affecting 1–2% of the population, and its incidence is rising with increased survivorship following MI and cancer, and the ageing population.
- It affects approximately 10% of people over the age of 70 years.
- HFpEF is more common in the elderly.
- Cardiomyopathy causing gene mutations is identified in 20–30% of patients with dilated cardiomyopathy (DCM), with truncations on the *TITIN* gene responsible for 10% of cases of DCM.

### Prognosis

The prognosis of HF is poor, with 50% of patients who have severe HF dying within 5 years. Patients hospitalized with decompensated HF have a 10% in-hospital mortality. The mortality rate of patients in cardiogenic shock who are not given a heart transplant is 10–50% during the acute episode.

## Aetiology

### Acute and chronic HF

It is useful to distinguish between acute *de novo*, acute-on-chronic and chronic HF:

- *Acute HF:* Symptoms result from a sudden rise in either right or left atrial pressure causing acute pulmonary oedema and/or haemodynamic instability. It is a medical emergency requiring hospitalization for ECG monitoring and IV treatment. Severe cases are complicated by acute pulmonary oedema and/or cardiogenic shock (see below).
- *Chronic HF:* Fluid (oedema) accumulates in the lungs, abdomen and/or legs and is associated with adverse cardiac remodelling, inflammation and multiorgan dysfunction with many systemic complications.

The causes of acute and chronic HF are listed in **Table 7.10**.

### Acute HF

Acute HF most commonly results from MI.

- *Acute pulmonary oedema:* When the pulmonary capillary pressure rises above 24 mmHg, fluid filters first into the interstitial space of the lung

**Table 7.10** Causes of heart failure

| Cause | Comment |
| --- | --- |
| **Chronic HF** | |
| Ischaemic heart disease | MI, chronic ischaemia with myocardial hibernation |
| Primary heart muscle diseases: cardiomyopathies | Primary diseases of the heart muscle, usually with a genetic cause <br> Three types: dilated, hypertrophic and restrictive |
| Systemic hypertension | Uncontrolled hypertension causes LVH and the ventricle is slow to relax in diastole (non-compliant). This restricts ventricular filling and causes left atrial hypertension |
| Severe valvular disease | Severe AS, AR, MS and MR |
| Prolonged tachycardia (tachycardia cardiomyopathy) | Fast AF or flutter (>4 weeks) |
| Alcohol | |
| Cardiotoxic cancer drugs and radiotherapy | Anthracycline chemotherapy (doxorubicin, epirubicin, idarubicin, daunorubicin), trastuzumab, VEGF tyrosine kinase inhibitors, second-generation BCr-Abl tyrosine kinase inhibitors, proteasome inhibitors <br> Radiotherapy for mediastinal lymphoma and left breast cancer |
| Hypothyroidism | Classically presents with myxoedema and sinus bradycardia |
| Haemochromatosis | Inherited primary haemochromatosis and secondary to multiple blood transfusions (e.g. thalassaemia patients) |
| PPCM | Defined as occurring 4 weeks before or in first 5 months following delivery |
| Sarcoidosis with cardiac involvement | |
| **Causes predominantly affecting the RV** | |
| Chronic lung disease (cor pulmonale) | Causes pulmonary hypertension and RV dysfunction |
| Pulmonary hypertension | Caused by thromboembolism or primary pulmonary hypertension |
| Isolated RV infarction | |
| Arrhythmogenic RV cardiomyopathy (ARVC) | Caused by mutations of intercellular adhesion proteins |
| TV disease | Congenital (Ebstein's anomaly), endocarditis, carcinoid syndrome, pacemaker wires |
| PV disease | |
| **Acute HF** | |
| AMI | |
| Sudden valve regurgitation caused by IE or chordal rupture | |
| Viral myocarditis | |
| Giant cell or lymphocytic myocarditis | |
| Acute fast AF | |
| Takotsubo syndrome | |
| Acute pericardial tamponade | |
| Acute-on-chronic HF | Increased fluid congestion due to diuretic resistance, poor compliance, new arrhythmias, disease progression, concomitant non-cardiac illnesses (e.g. sepsis) |

(interstial oedema) and then, as the pressure rises, into the alveoli as well (alveolar oedema). This leads to dyspnoea, hypoxia and the sensation of drowning, which causes anxiety. It is a medical emergency.

- *Cardiogenic shock*: This is a specific syndrome where the patient is hypotensive, oliguric or anuric and confused because of poor cerebral perfusion secondary to HF. Patients with cardiogenic shock can be categorized as wet (acute pulmonary oedema ± peripheral oedema) or dry (no oedema). The prognosis is very poor with a high inpatient mortality. IV inotropes (dobutamine, milrinone, levosimendan) and

mechanical support with veno-arterial extracorporeal membrane oxygenation (VA-ECMO) or a temporary left ventricular assist device (LVAD) are required in eligible cases with reversible causes.

### Clinical features

The main symptoms of HF are shortness of breath, fatigue and reduced exercise tolerance. Dyspnoea severity can be graded according to the classification of the NYHA (see **Table 7.4**). Poor cardiac output causes skeletal muscle fatigue, wasting and generalized tiredness (**Table 7.11**). The principal symptoms of right HF are caused by fluid retention in the abdomen and peripheries (**Table 7.11**).

**Table 7.11** Symptoms and signs of HF

| Symptom/sign | Notes |
|---|---|
| **Symptoms** | |
| Exertional dyspnoea | Caused by increased pulmonary venous congestion and increased systemic acidosis (resulting from poor tissue perfusion during exercise) |
| Dyspnoea at rest, orthopnoea and PND | Caused by pulmonary venous congestion. When severe, the patient is unable to lie down (orthopnoea) and can experience PND |
| Fluid retention | Such as ankle swelling and abdominal distension (ascites) |
| **Signs** | |
| Resting tachycardia | |
| Pulsus alternans | |
| Displaced apex beat | Due to left ventricular dilatation (post MI, DCM, severe AR or MR) |
| A third heart sound | |
| A fourth heart sound | Caused by an audible atrial systole filling the stiff LV (does not occur in AF) |
| Inspiratory crepitations at both lung bases (rales) | Commonly caused by hypostatic pulmonary secretions and are particularly common in smokers |
| | Conversely, there may be no crepitations in severe pulmonary oedema |
| Pansystolic murmur of MR | As the LV dilates, the mitral annulus is stretched, papillary muscles are displaced laterally and chordae have increased tension resulting in secondary MR. It is a sign of severe ventricular dysfunction |
| Pulmonary oedema (usually acutely breathless, anxious, cold, clammy and cyanosed, and produce pink bloodstained sputum). Auscultation reveals crackles of alveolar oedema and the wheeze of bronchial congestion | Cold and clammy because of shut down of the peripheral circulation. Cyanosis caused by a fall in systemic oxygen, the $P_{CO_2}$ is also reduced because of the tachypnoea |
| Cardiogenic shock: cold, clammy and confused with hypotension and oliguria | The most severe form of ventricular failure: the cardiac output is so low that poor tissue perfusion leads to a systemic acidosis, oliguria and cerebral hypoperfusion, causing the patient to be confused. Sometimes, paradoxically, the pulmonary wedge pressure is not elevated, so the patient is not breathless from pulmonary congestion and may even require fluid to optimize the left atrial filling pressure and improve the output |
| Elevated venous pressure | Caused by increased RV diastolic filling pressure |
| | Signs of tricuspid regurgitation (systolic V wave in the neck, systolic murmur of tricuspid with an RV third sound, a pulsatile liver) |
| Ankle swelling | Often with tricuspid regurgitation because of functional TV annulus dilatation |
| Sacral oedema | Can extend up the legs to the abdominal wall |
| Hepatomegaly and ascites | |

PND, paroxysmal nocturnal dyspnoea; LV, left ventricle; RV, right ventricle.

## HEART FAILURE: INVESTIGATIONS AT A GLANCE

**Blood tests**

- Natriuretic peptide (BNP or NT-proBNP)
- FBC: to exclude anaemia
- ESR
- Serum electrolytes ($Na^+$, $K^+$, $Ca^{2+}$, $Mg^{2+}$)
- Kidney function (creatinine, eGFR)

- Thyroid function
- Liver function
- Iron profile to assess for iron deficiency and exclude haemachromatosis
- HbA1c (diabetes common in HF)
- Uric acid (if taking diuretics)
- Genetics – cardiomyopathy gene panel in cases of DCM and HCM

**Diagnostic imaging**

*Chest radiography:* This often shows a large heart. Upper lobe venous distension, Kerley B lines and/or pleural effusions (typically left sided or bilateral) reflect increased pulmonary venous pressure.

*Echocardiography:* Assess LV and RV volumes, systolic function including LVEF and diastolic dysfunction. Assess for structural heart disease (MI, hypertrophy) and valvular heart disease.

*CMR:* Assess LV and RV volumes, systolic function including LVEF, myocardial inflammation, infarction and fibrosis, myocardial iron loading and cardiac amyloidosis.

*Cardiac catherization:* This is to measure haemodynamic pressures in the cardiac chambers and coronary angiography to exclude significant coronary artery disease.

**Electrocardiology**

*12-lead ECG:* heart rate, rhythm, Q waves, LVH, T-wave inversion, QRS duration

24–48-hour Holter ECG to identify any propensity for arrhythmias

**Cardiopulmonary exercise test (CPEX)**

Measurement of functional exercise capacity, cause of exercise limitation and assessment for cardiac transplantation

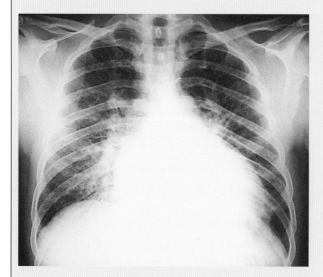

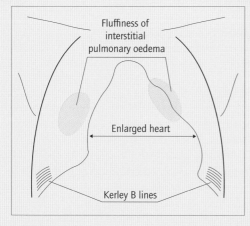

**Figure A** LV failure. The chest X-ray shows cardiac enlargement, dilatation of the upper lobe veins and interstitial pulmonary oedema. Kerley B lines are seen in the right costophrenic angle.

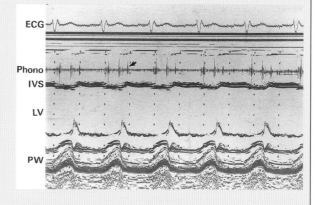

**Figure B** ECG and M-mode echocardiogram of HF with LBBB.

### Investigation

The investigation of HF should be directed at confirming the diagnosis of HF, identifying the cause(s), confirming the LVEF (determines treatment options) and identifying complications.

### Natriuretic peptides

Measurement of BNP or the N-terminal fragment of proBNP (NT-proBNP) is recommended to diagnose chronic HF. BNP and NT-proBNP have high sensitivity for HF, and therefore a normal result excludes HF in a treatment-naive patient.

Other blood tests which should be measured in patients with suspected or confirmed HF are summarized in HEART FAILURE: INVESTIGATIONS AT A GLANCE.

## MANAGEMENT OF CHRONIC HF

The care of patients with chronic HF should be provided by a multidisciplinary team including primary care, HF nurses and HF specialists.

## Drug treatment

### Neurohormonal blockade

The most important drugs which improve morbidity and reduce mortality in HFrEF are ACE inhibitors, beta blockers and aldosterone antagonists, known together as triple therapy.

#### ACE inhibitors

- These have a central role in treating HF, improving both symptoms and prognosis.
- ACE inhibitors inhibit conversion of the angiotensin 1 to vasoconstrictor peptide angiotensin 2 and therefore lower systemic vascular resistance and venous pressure. Treatment should be started at the lowest dose available and increased in steps providing blood pressure, renal function and $K^+$ are stable.
- Enalapril, ramipril and lisinopril are ACE inhibitors licensed for HF.
- ACE inhibitors cause a dry cough in 5–10% of patients. If cough occurs, the angiotensin receptor blockers (ARBs) candesartan or valsartan can be used in place of the ACE inhibitor.
- They can also cause hypotension. ACE inhibitors and ARBs should not be used in patients with renal artery stenosis because they can cause profound hypotension and renal failure.

#### Beta blockers

- Specific beta blockers improve symptoms and prognosis in patients with HFrEF, especially if there is a resting tachycardia.
- They reduce atrial and ventricular arrhythmias and sudden death in patients with HFrEF.
- Carvedilol, bisoprolol, nebivolol and slow-release metoprolol are licensed for HF.

#### Aldosterone antagonists

- Spironolactone and eplerenone are aldosterone antagonists which improve symptoms and prognosis in patients with HFrEF (LVEF <40%) despite ACE inhibitors and beta blockers.
- They can cause hyperkalaemia and renal impairment and so require monitoring of renal function and electrolytes after initiation.
- Spironolactone causes gynaecomastia in ~5% of men as it also inhibits oestrogen and progesterone metabolism. If this occurs, switch to eplerenone, which is 1000 times more selective for the aldosterone receptor.

#### Sacubitril–valsartan

- This is a combination of the ARB valsartan plus the neprilysin inhibitor sacubitril. Neprilysin inhibition increases BNP which increases its natriuretic, vasodilatory and anti-fibrotic effects.
- Sacubitril–valsartan is superior to enalapril in patients with HFrEF and resistant HF despite ACE inhibitors, beta blockers and aldosterone antagonists.
- It lowers blood pressure more potently than ACE inhibitors and ARBs, and should be avoided in patients with systolic BP below 100 mmHg.
- Patients with persisting symptomatic HFrEF despite triple therapy can be changed from their ACE inhibitor to sacubitril–valsartan providing the patient can tolerate at least 50% of target ACE inhibitor or ARB dose with a stable blood pressure.

#### Ivabradine

- Ivabradine is a selective sinus node inhibitor which reduces the heart rate if patients are in sinus rhythm.
- It improves symptoms and reduces HF hospitalization in patients with HFrEF who are in sinus rhythm with a resting heart rate >70 beats per minute despite triple therapy.
- Ivabradine should not be used in HF patients in AF.

#### SGLT2 inhibitors

- Two SGLT2 inhibitors, dapagliflozin and empagliflozin, are effective in reducing HF hospitalization and CV mortality in patients with HFrEF, including both diabetics and non-diabetics.
- They also reduce the risk of new HF in patients with type 2 diabetes.

### Diuretics

Diuretics are used for symptom relief in acute and chronic HF when pulmonary congestion, ascites or ankle oedema is present.

All diuretics cause the following metabolic disturbances:

- Potassium loss (unless the diuretic is specifically potassium-sparing): can be important in patients who have a tendency to arrhythmias; potassium supplementation is therefore indicated for most patients
- Hyponatraemia
- Hyperuricaemia
- Uraemia

There are three types of diuretic: loop diuretics, thiazide diuretics and potassium-sparing diuretics. Thiazide diuretics also cause glucose intolerance and worsen diabetes control.

## DEVICE THERAPIES FOR CHRONIC HF

### Cardiac resynchronization therapy

HF patients with symptomatic HFrEF despite drug therapy and who have widened QRS complexes on ECG benefit from biventricular pacing. Cardiac resynchronization therapy (CRT) is recommended for all symptomatic patients with HFrEF despite optimal medical therapy who have LBBB and a QRSd >150 ms, particularly if they are in sinus rhythm. It should be considered in symptomatic HFrEF patients in atrial fibrillation with wide LBBB (>150 ms), patients in sinus rhythm with LBBB QRSd 135–149 ms, and patients with RBBB and QRSd >150 ms.

If a patient with LV impairment (LVEF <50%) requires a pacemaker for bradycardia indication, a CRT device may be implanted if a high percentage of RV pacing is predicted, as RV pacing from a dual chamber pacemaker introduces dyssynchrony and often causes deterioration of a weakened LV.

CRT pacemakers can be a pacemaker alone (CRT-P device) or also include a defibrillator function (CRT-D device). The aim is for CRT to deliver pacing therapy to a minimum threshold of 95% of all heart beats, and ideally 100%.

### Implantable cardiac defibrillator

An implantable cardiac defibrillator (ICD) device improves the prognosis for patients with HF who have desynchrony and who have been successfully resuscitated following an episode of VF or haemodynamically unstable VT – a secondary prevention indication. ICDs are also recommended for patients at higher risk of sudden death from VT or VF (primary prevention), such as those patients with resistant HFrEF with LVEF <35% despite triple therapy, and particularly those patients with HFrEF caused by MI where the infarct scar increases the arrhythmia risk, and patients on a heart transplantation waiting list.

Patients recommended for an ICD and their families must be counselled that the ICD device will require inactivation at the end of their life, whether they are dying from cardiac or non-cardiac causes. Therefore, ICDs are not recommended for patients with a life expectancy <12 months.

### Left ventricular assist devices and cardiac transplantation

Eligible patients who have refractory HF despite optimal medical therapy and CRT, if appropriate, may be considered for a mechanical heart pump known as a left ventricular assist device (LVAD) (**Figure 7.17**) or cardiac transplantation (**Figure 7.18**). These patients are assessed at specialist transplant centres to ensure they are eligible and have no contraindications (pulmonary hypertension, irreversible renal failure, active infection or compliance concerns) as LVADs require mandatory anticoagulation with warfarin and mandatory immunosuppressive therapy is required after cardiac transplantation to prevent rejection.

## TAKOTSUBO SYNDROME

Takotsubo syndrome is an increasingly recognized cause of acute HF. The classical presentation is a postmenopausal woman who develops acute chest pain and dyspnoea following an unexpected shock (e.g. news of death of family member). It initially mimics an AMI with troponin elevated and ST elevation on resting 12-lead ECG (**Figure 7.19**). However, no culprit coronary occlusion or stenoses are present at invasive coronary angiography, and the LV has acute impairment with hypokinesia of the apical and mid-ventricular segments with a typical appearance on echocardiography or left ventriculography which resembles a vase or pot, named after the Japanese fisherman's octopus pot (the *takotsubo*).

Twenty percent of patients develop acute HF including pulmonary oedema, cardiogenic shock and there is a 5% mortality during the acute phase related to shock and ventricular arrhythmias secondary to severe prolongation of the QT interval. Cases can also be triggered by severe physical illnesses which activate the sympathetic nervous system and cause catecholamine storms including phaeochromocytoma, acute thyrotoxicosis, acute respiratory muscle paralysis (e.g. myasthenic syndrome, acute Guillain–Barré), acute subarachnoid haemorrhage and iatrogenic adrenaline administration. Although resting LV function appears to recover, 10–20% of patients are left with new cardiac problems (arrhythmias, breathlessness and chest pain due to long-term cardiac injury) and there is a 10% risk of recurrence in survivors, who then re-enter the high-risk phase.

## CARDIAC CONDUCTION DISEASE AND ARRHYTHMIAS

Abnormal heart rhythms can be classified as fast (tachycardia) or slow (bradycardia) and occasionally normal rate (e.g. idioventricular arrhythmias during acute MI).

## BRADYCARDIA

A bradycardia results from a heart rate of less than 60 beats/min. It may be normal (e.g. physiological bradycardia in athletes). Pathological causes of sinus bradycardia are listed in **Table 7.12**.

### Bundle branch block
Delayed conduction through the bundle branches can result in incomplete or complete bundle branch block (BBB), but does not cause a bradycardia.

**Table 7.12** Causes of sinus bradycardia

| |
|---|
| Sinus node disease |
| AMI (particularly inferior infarction) involving the sinus node |
| Drugs (e.g. beta blockers, verapamil, diltiazem, digoxin) |
| Degenerative changes in the sinus node known as sick sinus syndrome (common in the elderly) |
| Acute pain with increased vagal reflex |
| Other causes of increased vagal tone (e.g. bladder distension from outflow tract obstruction, intense coughing) |
| Non-cardiac (e.g. raised intracranial pressure, hypothermia, hypothyroidism) |

**Pulsatile-Flow LVAD**

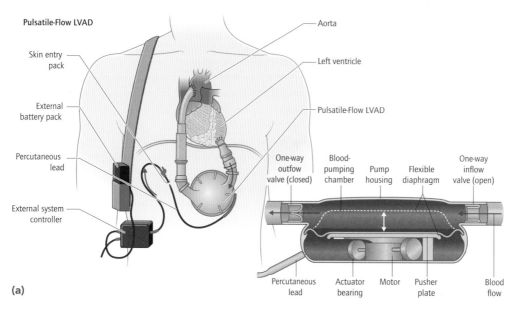

Aorta

Left ventricle

Pulsatile-Flow LVAD

Skin entry pack

External battery pack

Percutaneous lead

External system controller

One-way outflow valve (closed)

Blood-pumping chamber

Pump housing

Flexible diaphragm

One-way inflow valve (open)

Percutaneous lead

Actuator bearing

Motor

Pusher plate

Blood flow

**(a)**

**Continuous-Flow LVAD**

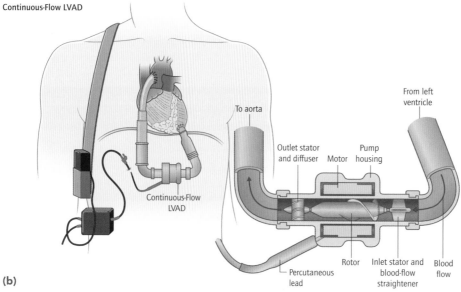

To aorta

From left ventricle

Outlet stator and diffuser

Motor

Pump housing

Continuous-Flow LVAD

Percutaneous lead

Rotor

Inlet stator and blood-flow straightener

Blood flow

**(b)**

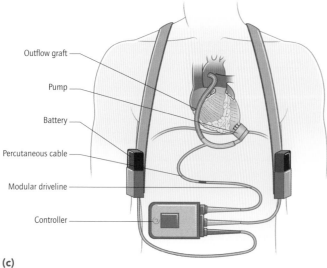

Outflow graft

Pump

Battery

Percutaneous cable

Modular driveline

Controller

**(c)**

**Figure 7.17** LVADs. **(a)** Pulsatile-flow LVAD; **(b)** continuous-flow LVAD; **(a,b)** adapted from *NEJM*: https://www.nejm.org/doi/full/10.1056/nejmoa0909938 **(c)** Example of a third-generation centrifugal continuous flow LVAD with external battery and controller unit.

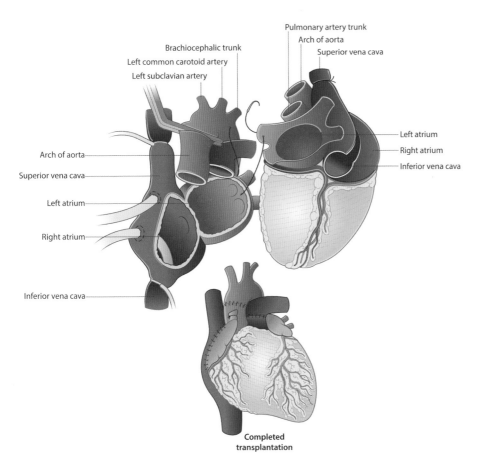

Completed
transplantation

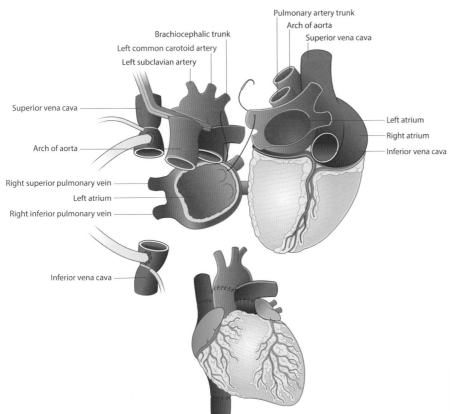

Completed
transplantation

**Figure 7.18** Heart transplantation.
**(a)** Standard biatrial heart transplantation; **(b)** orthotopic heart transplantation with bicaval technique. Adapted
from *NEJM*: https://www.nejm.org/
doi/pdf/10.1056/nejmp068048.

7

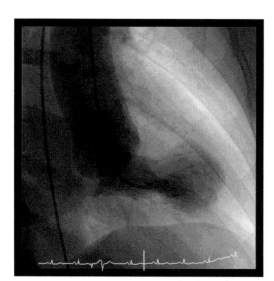

**(a)**

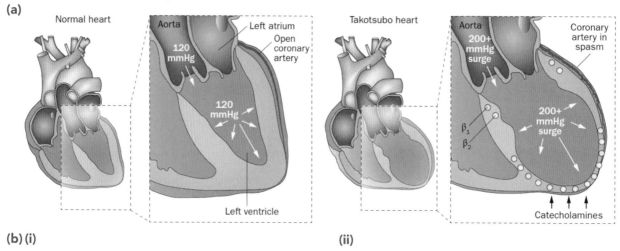

Normal heart

Aorta
Left atrium
Open coronary artery
120 mmHg
120 mmHg
Left ventricle

Takotsubo heart

Aorta
200+ mmHg surge
Coronary artery in spasm
β₁
β₂
200+ mmHg surge
Catecholamines

**(b) (i)**

**(ii)**

**Figure 7.19** Takotsubo syndrome. **(a)** Left ventriculogram at end-systole showing the typical apical variant of Takotsubo syndrome. **(b)** Schematic of the pathophysiology of Takotsubo syndrome comparing normal **(i)** and Takotsubo syndrome **(ii)**. Increased afterload, increased activation of apical β-adrenergic receptors and coronary vasospasm contribute to stress-induced Takotsubo syndrome. **(b)** From Akashi Y *et al.* (2015) *Nat Rev Cardiol* 12, 387–97. https://doi.org/10.1038/nrcardio.2015.39. With permission.

- *RBBB* (**Figure 7.20**): This is a normal finding in about 1% of the population but can be caused by conduction disease and diseases of the RV.
- *LBBB* (see **Figure 7.16**): This usually indicates conduction disease or disease of the LV.
- *Left hemi-block*: This is delayed conduction in either the anterior (giving rise to left axis deviation) or posterior (giving rise to right axis deviation) fascicle of the left bundle.
- *Bifascicular block:* This occurs when conduction to both the right bundle and either the left anterior or left posterior fascicle is delayed.
- *Trifascicular block:* This occurs when there is first degree heart block (PR >200 ms), RBBB and either left or right fascicle block (left or right axis deviation). This reflects advanced conduction disease and AV blocking drugs must be avoided.

### Atrioventricular block

There are three types of AV block: first-, second- and third-degree AV block.

*First-degree AV block* (**Figure 7.21a**) This is delayed conduction of the atrial impulse to the ventricles, usually within the AV node, with a prolonged PR interval (>200 ms). It can be normal in young people and athletes with increased vagal tone, is seen in patients taking AV node blocking drug (e.g. beta blockers) but otherwise is a sign of conduction disease. This does not cause a bradycardia.

*Second-degree AV block* This occurs when intermittently the P wave is not followed by a QRS complex. The block to conduction occurs in the AV node and can be of two types:

- *Mobitz type 1* (Wenckebach; **Figure 7.21b**): the PR interval increases with each beat until an atrial impulse is not conducted and then the PR interval

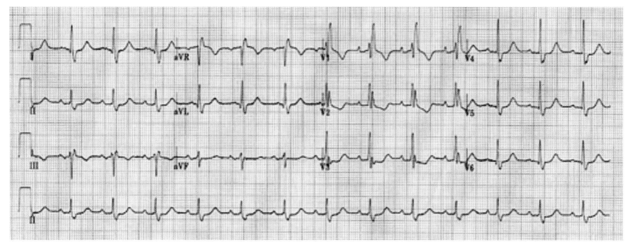

**(a)**

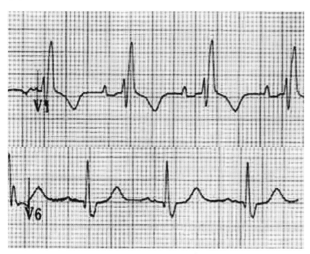

**(b)**

**Figure 7.20** RBBB. (**a**) ECG showing RBBB with left-axis deviation. (**b**) Typical RSR' pattern in V1 and QRs in V6 in RBBB.

7

returns to normal. This is usually physiological and due to high vagal tone.

- *Mobitz type 2* (second-degree AV block; **Figure 7.21c**): the PR interval does not change, but the QRS complex fails to follow the P wave because of a regularly or intermittently occurring block, which is usually below the AV node in the bundle branches or bundle of His. If there are two P waves to one QRS complex, it is a 2 : 1 block; if there are three P waves to one QRS complex, it is a 3 : 1 block. The degree of block can vary. A pacemaker is usually indicated.

*Third-degree AV block* (**Figure 7.22**) Also known as complete heart block, this occurs when there is a permanent dissociation between atrial and ventricular activity. A pacemaker is usually indicated.

- *When the block is in the AV node:* A subsidiary and usually reliable pacemaker takes over in the bundle of His, and the QRS complex is narrow.
- *When the block is below the AV node:* The residual pacemaker is in the bundle branches and gives a wide QRS complex. These pacemaker sites discharge at

slower rates and are less reliable, giving rise to fainting (a *Stokes–Adams attack*) and sudden death. *This is a medical emergency requiring urgent pacemaker implantation.*

**Management**

*Sinus bradycardia*

Sinus bradycardia does not usually need treatment, except in the acute setting of a vasovagal attack. Haemodynamically important sinus bradycardias are treated with IV atropine to inhibit vagal drive to the SA and AV nodes.

*Sick sinus syndrome*

Sick sinus syndrome may present with sinus pauses, inappropriate sinus tachycardias and bradycardias, and an intermittent wandering atrial pacemaker. A pacemaker may be required for severe chronic sick sinus syndrome with long pauses (>3 seconds).

*Atrioventricular block*

Both first and Mobitz type 1 second-degree AV block are usually asymptomatic. Mobitz type 2 AV block is more advanced and may cause dizziness or fatigue and reduced

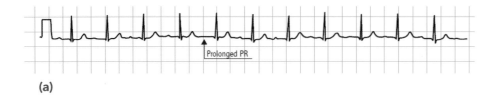

Prolonged PR

**(a)**

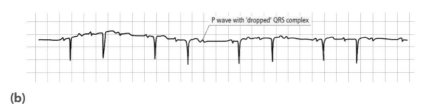

P wave with 'dropped' QRS complex

**(b)**

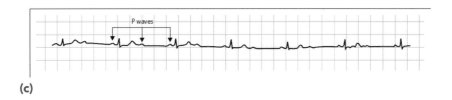

P waves

**(c)**

**Figure 7.21 (a)** First-degree heart block. Note long PR interval (more than 200 ms). **(b)** Second-degree heart block. Mobitz type 1 (Wenckebach). Note the lengthening PR interval on each successive beat until a P wave is not followed by a QRS complex. The next PR interval returns to normal. **(c)** Second-degree heart block. Mobitz type 2. Note there is a fixed relationship between the P wave and the QRS complexes. In this case, two P waves to one QRS complex (= 2 : 1 AV block).

exercise tolerance. Patients with third-degree AV block (complete heart block) are usually symptomatic with pre-syncope (dizziness) or syncope (blackouts) and usually require treatment with a pacemaker.

- *Temporary pacemaker:* A temporary device is used when complete AV block is brought about by a

cause that is likely to resolve, such as an inferior infarction. If the ventricular escape rhythm is fast enough, it may be possible to avoid a temporary pacemaker.

- *Permanent pacemaker* (**Figure 7.23**): This is usually required for Mobitz type 2 second-degree and

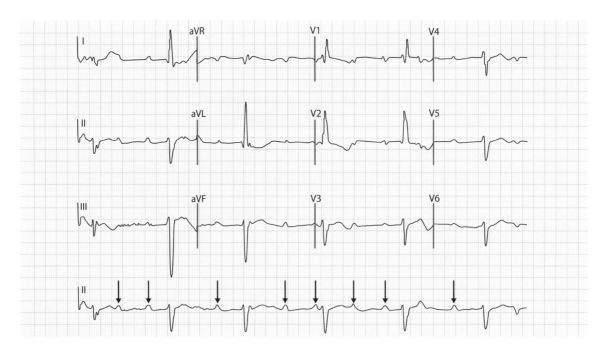

**Figure 7.22** ECG showing complete heart block. Ventricular bradycardia (wide QRS) and red arrows show P waves which are dissociated with QRS complexes.

third-degree complete AV block. For patients in sinus rhythm, this involves a dual chamber system in which both an atrial and a ventricular wire are implanted (known as a DDDR pacemaker). The atrial wire can sense atrial activity and then coordinate ventricular systole sequentially. For patients with permanent AF, a single-lead VVIR pacemaker is indicated.

There are a number of complications associated with pacemakers (summarized in PACEMAKERS: COMPLICATIONS AT A GLANCE).

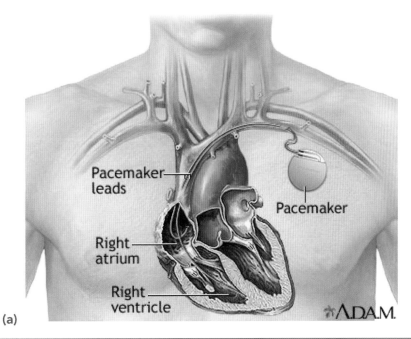

(a)

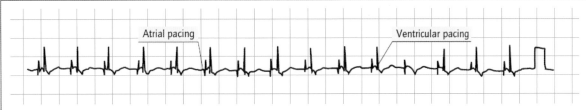

(b)

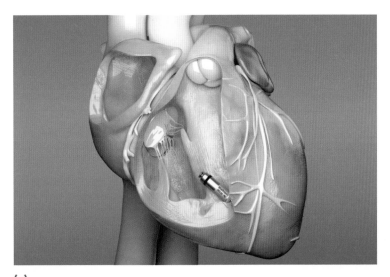

(c)

**Figure 7.23** **(a)** Schematic of a typical dual chamber pacemaker. **(b)** ECG of AV pacing. Note the two pacing 'spikes', one initiating the P wave, the other initiating the QRS complex. **(c)** Leadless RV pacemaker.

## PACEMAKERS: COMPLICATIONS AT A GLANCE

**Lead displacement**

This results in a sudden intermittent or permanent loss of pacing and the recurrence of symptoms.

**Infection**

This usually develops soon after pacemaker insertion and so prophylactic antibiotics are often used at implantation. If infection is established, the pacing system needs to be removed while the patient is maintained on a temporary pacing system. A new permanent pacing system can be installed when the infection has been fully treated and is no longer present off antibiotics.

**Erosion**

The generator or the pacing leads can erode through the skin, particularly in thin or cachexic patients. This requires device and lead explantation and a new pacemaker implanted.

**Pacemaker generator failure**

This is uncommon but requires replacement of the generator.

**Lead fracture**

This is rare but, if the pacing lead breaks, symptoms will return. The lead fracture can be identified on chest radiography.

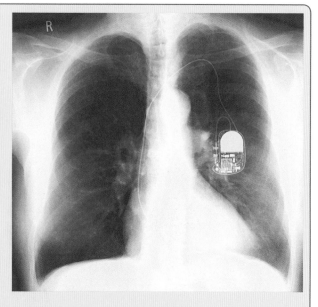

**Figure A** Pacemaker lead and generator appearance on chest X-ray. Note old pacemaker lead which has been cut short in the right cephalic vein.

## TACHYARRHYTHMIAS

A tachycardia is defined as a heart rate of more than 100 beats/min, and can be subdivided into sinus, atrial (supraventricular) and ventricular tachycardias.

### Sinus tachycardia

Sinus tachycardia is defined as a sinus rate of more than 100 beats/min. It is usually secondary to other causes (**Table 7.13**). Rarely, a primary sinus tachycardia can result from a sinus node re-entry mechanism.

### Atrial tachyarrhythmias

Atrial ectopics, atrial flutter, AF and atrial tachycardias all arise from the atrial myocardium and all have similar aetiologies.

### *Atrial ectopic beats*

Atrial ectopic beats can give rise to an awareness of a missed heart beat (**Figure 7.24**).

**Table 7.13** Causes of sinus tachycardia

| |
|---|
| Physiological – exercise, infection, fever, stress, pain |
| Thyrotoxicosis |
| Anaemia |
| Cardiac failure |
| Pulmonary embolus |
| Hypovolaemia |
| Hypoxia |
| Abnormal catecholamine stimulation (e.g. phaeochromocytoma, autonomic neuropathy) |
| Cocaine, amphetamines |
| Drug or alcohol withdrawal |

### *Atrial flutter*

Atrial flutter is a tachycardia in which the atrial rate is usually about 300 beats/min and there is a 2 : 1 AV block giving a ventricular rate of 150 beats/min (**Figure 7.25**). The ECG appearance has characteristic saw-tooth flutter waves. They are usually most obvious in leads III, aVF and V1. An atrial flutter ablation is usually curative. Anticoagulation is indicated.

### *Atrial fibrillation*

AF is an irregularly irregular rhythm: atrial foci discharge at very high rates (**Figure 7.26**). Not all impulses are transmitted by the AV node and so the ventricular rate is much slower and irregular. It is commonly caused by an associated cardiac abnormality including hypertensive heart disease, heart failure, previous MI and mitral valve disease, but there is no apparent cause in 5% of patients. There is an increased risk of thromboembolic stroke. A list of causes is given in **Table 7.14**.

### *Narrow QRS tachycardias*

Two atrial tachycardias are caused by automaticity: atrial tachycardia and junctional tachycardia. The other narrow QRS tachycardias are caused by re-entry circuits and are known as reciprocating tachycardias.

*Atrial tachycardia*
- This can be paroxysmal or chronic and is often associated with a degree of AV block.
- It is usually associated with underlying heart disease.
- The P-wave morphology is abnormal and may be unmasked by carotid sinus massage slowing AV conduction.

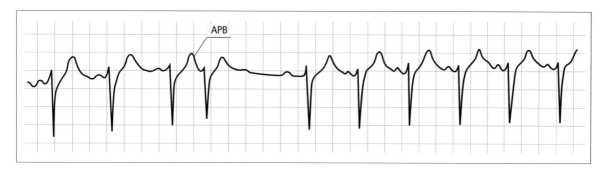

**Figure 7.24** Atrial premature (ectopic) beat (APB). Note the post ectopic compensatory pause.

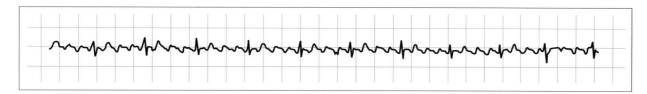

**Figure 7.25** Atrial flutter. Carotid sinus massage or treatment with adenosine can increase the degree of AV block. Note saw-tooth pattern of baseline with atrial rate of 300 beats/min and ventricular rate of 75 beats/min.

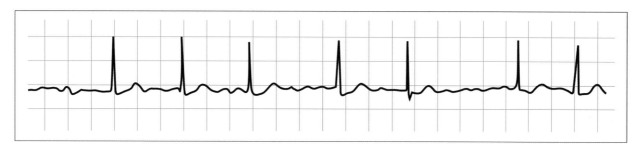

**Figure 7.26** AF. Note the irregular ventricular response (R–R interval) and absence of organized atrial activity.

**Table 7.14** Causes of AF

| |
| --- |
| **Normal heart and no systemic cause** |
| Lone AF |
| **Structural** |
| Mitral valve disease (stenosis or regurgitation) |
| Ischaemic heart disease |
| HF |
| Hypertrophic cardiomyopathy |
| Accessory pathways between the atria and ventricle (e.g. WPW syndrome) |
| **Hormonal** |
| Thyrotoxicosis |
| **Metabolic** |
| Acute and chronic alcoholism |
| **Other** |
| Pneumonia |
| Severe sepsis |
| Pulmonary embolism |
| Postoperative after cardiac or major non-cardiac surgery |

*Junctional tachycardia*

- This results from a junctional focus activating both atria and ventricles.
- It may be caused by digoxin toxicity or other forms of heart disease, such as coronary artery disease.

### Pre-excitation and atrioventricular re-entry tachycardia

Atrial activity is usually conducted to the ventricles only via the AV node. In pre-excitation, there is an extra muscle connection known as an accessory pathway between the atrium and the ventricles. Because this accessory pathway does not delay conduction, an impulse via the accessory pathway depolarizes the ventricles before the impulse via the AV node.

*Wolff–Parkinson–White (WPW) syndrome* WPW syndrome is caused by a congenital accessory bundle (bundle of Kent) between the atrium and ventricular myocardium. Early depolarization of the ventricular myocardium causes a short

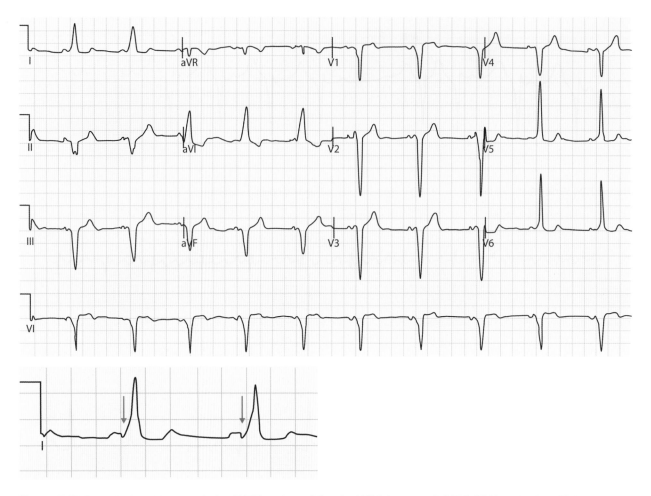

**Figure 7.27** Sinus rhythm with pre-excitation: WPW syndrome **(a)** 12-lead ECG from type B WPW. **(b)** Note the short PR interval and delta wave highlighted with red arrows in the expanded view.

PR interval and an initial deflection in the QRS complex, known as a delta wave (**Figure 7.27**). The anatomical abnormality of WPW syndrome provides a substrate for two types of tachycardia: AV re-entry tachycardia (AVRT) and AF (**Figure 7.28**).

- *AVRT* occurs when the circus movement tachycardia starts in the atrium, travels to the ventricle through the AV node, and then returns to the atrium from the ventricle via the bundle of Kent. The QRS complex is narrow unless there is an associated intraventricular conduction abnormality and there is no delta wave.
- *AF* impulses may be transmitted to the ventricles via both the AV node and the bundle of Kent. This can result in faster ventricular rates than usual in AF and may lead to VF and death.

A short PR interval does not always indicate an AV accessory bypass tract. Other causes of a short PR interval include small stature, increased sympathetic activity and a congenitally small AV node.

### Atrioventricular nodal re-entrant tachycardia

Approximately 1–2% of the population have dual AV node physiology with a second pathway between the atria

and ventricle within the AV node. A re-entry tachycardia (atrioventricular nodal re-entrant tachycardia [AVNRT]) (**Figure 7.29a**) occurs within the AV node due to fast and slow conduction. This precipitates a tachycardia by simultaneously activating both the atrium and ventricle.

AVRT and AVNRT can usually be distinguished on the ECG, especially when the tachycardia of AVRT is conducted through the concealed pathway and retrogradely through the AV node (antidromic AVRT) where the QRS complexes are broad. If the tachycardia is in AF, then a characteristic broad complex tachycardia that is irregularly irregular develops (pre-excited AF). Both AVRT and AVNRT can be provoked by specific stimuli such as exertion, caffeinated drinks and alcohol. Treatment involves a cardiac electrophysiology study and ablation of the accessory pathway (in AVRT) or one arm of the dual AV node pathways (in AVNRT).

### Ventricular ectopic beats

Ventricular ectopic beats (VEBs) are common and may be present with or without evidence of underlying heart disease. Sometimes they occur on a regular basis in relation to the normal beat. Alternation with a normal beat is

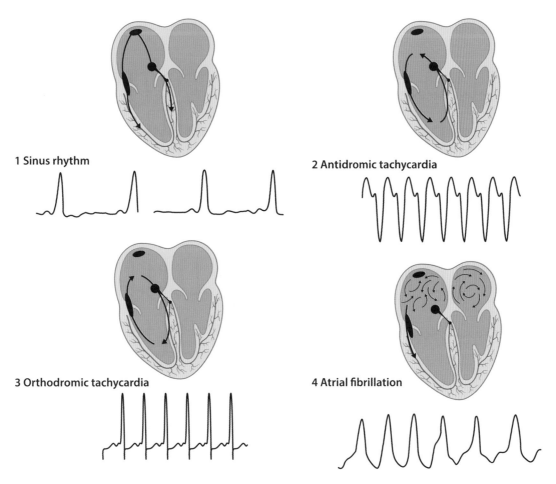

**Figure 7.28** Various arrhythmias observed in patients with accessory pathways. **(a)** Sinus rhythm with pre-excitation (delta wave). **(b)** Orthodromic tachycardia is a narrow complex tachycardia with re-entry circuit down the AV node and bundle of His and retrograde back up the accessory pathway into the atria. **(c)** Antidromic tachycardia is a broad complex tachycardia with conduction down the accessory pathway and retrograde up the His–Purkinje system and AV node to activate the atria. **(d)** AF with a broad complex tachycardia.

ventricular bigeminy, occurrence every third beat is ventricular trigeminy. High frequency of VEBs (>10% of all heart beats) can cause LV impairment, particularly if underlying HF, cardiomyopathy or infarction is present. The relationship between VEBs and risk of sudden cardiac death is not straightforward as many cases can be benign in the absence of underlying heart disease, and some trials suppressing VEBs with class 1 antiarrhythmic drugs increased mortality.

### Ventricular tachyarrhythmias

Ventricular tachyarrhythmias tend to be more serious than supraventricular tachyarrhythmias. They are usually a consequence of coronary artery disease, HF, severe valvular heart disease or a cardiomyopathy.

#### Ventricular tachycardia

VT is a broad complex tachycardia of more than four consecutive ventricular beats (**Figure 7.30**). In a structurally normal heart, it is usually well tolerated but, if HF, cardiomyopathy or previous MI is present, then usually it causes hypotension and

signs of cardiac decompensation. The ventricular rate is usually 120–250 beats/min. There may be signs of AV dissociation with intermittent cannon *a* waves in the JVP. The ECG shows a rapid heart rate with a wide QRS (>120 ms).

A diagnosis of VT needs to be distinguished from supraventricular tachycardia (SVT) with BBB. Review of a previous ECG for pre-existing BBB and the presence of dissociated P wave activity is extremely helpful in diagnosing VT. Other features that distinguish VT from SVT with aberration are listed in **Table 7.15**.

**Table 7.15** Broad complex tachycardia. QRSd >120 ms: variables increasing the probability versus SVT with aberrant conduction (BBB)

| |
|---|
| AV dissociation |
| QRS width >150 ms |
| History of ischaemic heart disease, cardiomyopathy or HF |
| Concordant QRS complexes in anterior leads (all QRS complexes in same direction) |

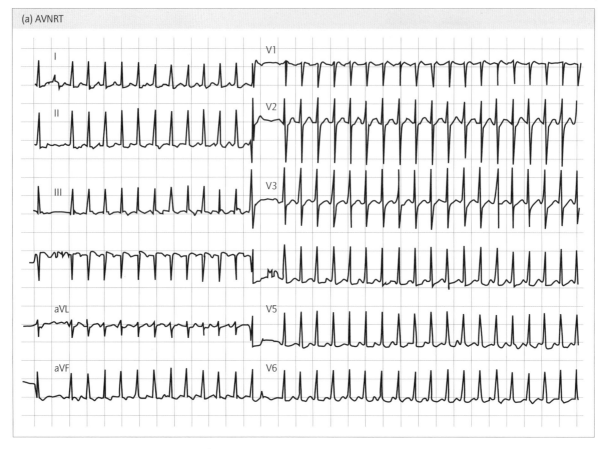

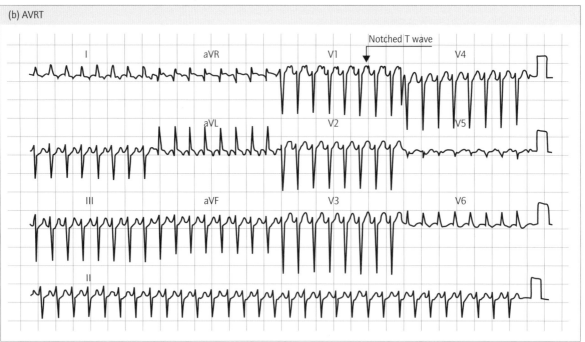

**Figure 7.29** Reciprocating tachycardia: **(a)** AVNRT; **(b)** AVRT. Note the notched T wave in lead V1 in AVRT in contrast to AVNRT due to the atrium being activated after the QRS complex. *(Continued)*

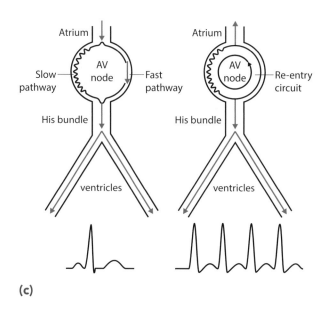

**(c)**

**Figure 7.29** (*Continued*) **(c)** Dual AV node physiology underlying AVNRT.

### Ventricular fibrillation

VF is a disorganized, rapid and irregular heart rhythm leading to a loss of cardiac output (**Figure 7.31a,b**). The patient rapidly becomes unconscious and stops breathing. The ECG shows no evidence of organized QRS complexes. Only rarely will it reverse spontaneously. Emergency resuscitation with defibrillation is required (see **Figure 7.32** for resuscitation algorithm). The common causes are AMI and HF. Rare causes include genetic syndromes such as Brugada syndrome which has a typical ECG appearance with RBBB with downsloping ST elevation in leads V1–V2 (**Figure 7.31c**).

### *Polymorphic ventricular tachycardia and torsade de pointes*

Polymorphic VT is characterized by wide complexes that change their axis from an upright to an inverted shape (**Figure 7.33**). This causes syncope and sudden death. The QT interval on the ECG when in sinus rhythm is prolonged after heart rate correction (QTc >500 ms). It may be genetic (long QT syndromes [LQTS]), or brought about by metabolic disturbances, cardiac and non-cardiac drugs, Takotsubo syndrome or other causes (**Table 7.16**).

### Clinical features of arrhythmias

Symptoms that can result from an abnormal heart rhythm are listed in **Table 7.17**. Some patients can be very aware of any change in rhythm, while others can have severe disturbances of rhythm without being conscious of any symptoms.

### Investigation

A precise diagnosis can only be made by documenting the rhythm disturbance on an ECG.

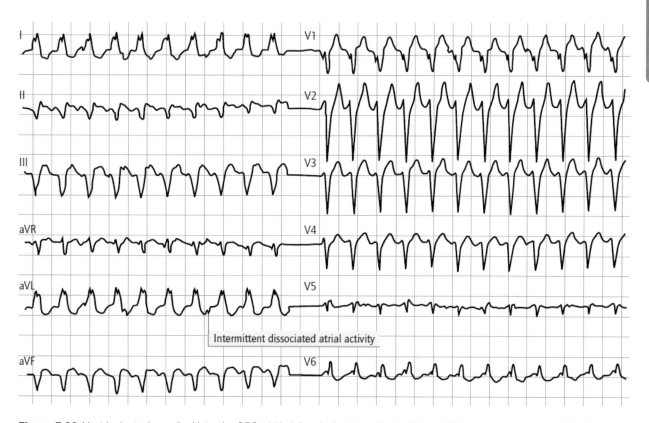

**Figure 7.30** Ventricular tachycardia. Note: the QRS width; left-axis deviation; the similarity of QRS morphology in leads V1–V5; and the dissociation of atrial and ventricular activity so an independent P wave can occasionally be seen.

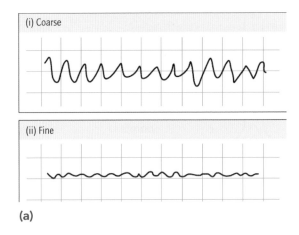

(i) Coarse

(ii) Fine

(a)

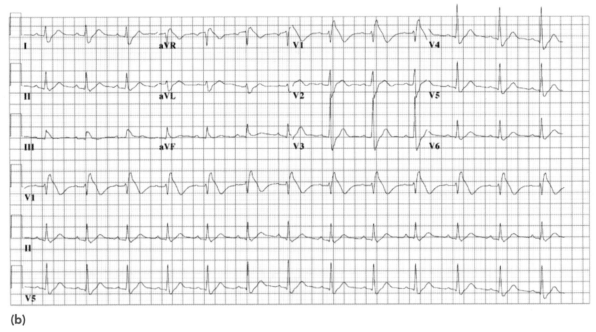

(b)

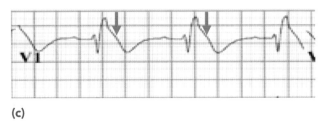

(c)

**Figure 7.31** **(a)** VF. **(b)** 12-lead ECG showing Brugada syndrome. **(c)** Down-sloping ST elevation in V1 in Brugada syndrome (highlighted with red arrows).

### Electrophysiology

- *Standard 12-lead ECG:* This is rarely helpful, although it may show the delta deflection of WPW syndrome. However, this can be intermittent and so a normal ECG does not exclude WPW.
- *24- or 48-hour ambulatory Holter ECG:* This is the mainstay for identifying a rhythm disturbance. However, with intermittent symptoms, a 24- to 48-hour Holter monitor is often negative, although, occasionally, asymptomatic markers of the rhythm

disturbance may be present (e.g. frequent atrial or ventricular ectopy, a tendency to long pauses or occasional ventricular ectopics).
- *7- or 14-day ECG recording patch:* These are single vector adhesive recording patches which are waterproof and record continuous rhythm for 7 or 14 days.
- *ILR:* An ILR is implanted below the skin with a battery life of 2 years. Data can be downloaded via radiofrequency transmission from the patient's home or in the pacing department.

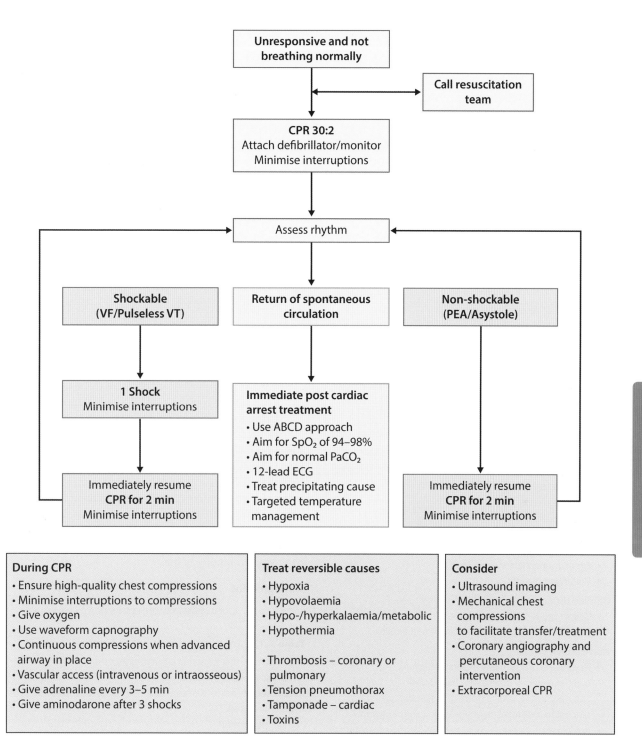

**Figure 7.32** Advanced life support algorithm. Source: Resuscitation Council UK.

**7**

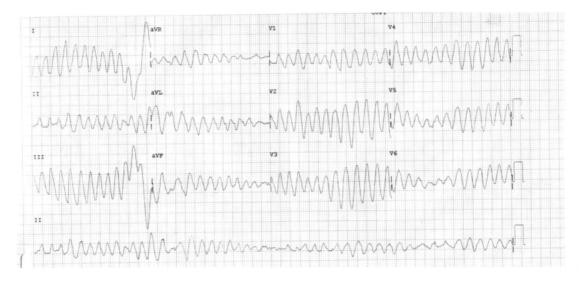

**Figure 7.33** Torsades de pointes.

**Table 7.16** Causes of a prolonged long QT interval and torsades de pointes

**Inherited long QT syndromes**
- Modern genetic studies have identified 16 different forms of LQTS – most involve mutations in the cardiac sodium and potassium channel genes
- Previously classified as Romano–Ward syndrome (autosomal dominant) and Jervell and Lange–Nielsen syndrome (autosomal recessive, associated with congenital deafness)

**Metabolic disturbances**
- Hypomagnesaemia
- Hypokalaemia
- Hypocalcaemia
- Hypothyroidism
- Organophosphate insecticides
- Prolonged dieting

**Cardiac drugs**
- Class I drugs such as quinidine
- Class III drugs such as amiodarone and sotalol

**Non-cardiac drugs**
- Psychiatric drugs: many including tricyclic antidepressants, quetiapine, thioridazine, chlorpromazine, and high-dose IV haloperidol
- Macrolide antibiotics: erythromycin, clarithromycin
- Antifungal antibiotics: fluconazole, ketoconazole, itraconazole
- Antimalarial drugs: quinine, chloroquine, mefloquine
- IV ondansetron
- Antihistamine drugs: terfenadine, astemizole
- VEGF tyrosine kinase inhibitors for cancer: sunitinib, sorafenib, pazopanib, vandetinib, lenvatinib
- Arsenic for AML
- Ribociclib for breast cancer

**Other**
- Takotsubo syndrome
- Bradycardia: physiological QT prolongation
- MVP

- *Electrophysiological studies:* It is possible to provoke arrhythmias by electrically stimulating the atria and the ventricles, but unless there is a documented arrhythmia with which to compare the result, it is not possible to be confident that the arrhythmia provoked during the electrophysiological study is clinically relevant.

It is important to confirm whether the arrhythmia is prognostically significant (is a marker of a life-threatening arrhythmia). If it is serious (e.g. if the patient is having episodes of VT), effective arrhythmia treatment is required. If the arrhythmia does not have prognostic significance, management depends on whether the patient is prepared to tolerate the symptoms or wishes to have treatment to improve their quality of life.

**Management**

See CARDIAC ARRHYTHMIAS: TREATMENTS AT A GLANCE.

**Table 7.17** Symptoms that can result from an abnormal heart rhythm

| |
|---|
| Presyncope and syncope |
| Palpitations |
| Breathlessness |
| Chest discomfort |

## PREVENTION OF STROKE AND THROMBOEMBOLIC COMPLICATIONS IN AF

Twenty percent of strokes in the UK are caused by AF. All patients with AF, whether paroxysmal, persistent or permanent, should have assessment of thromboembolic stroke risk using the $CHA_2DS_2VASc$ score (see **Table 7.18**) and therapeutic anticoagulation if their $CHA_2DS_2VASc$ score

**Table 7.18** CHA$_2$DS$_2$VASc score for estimating stroke risk in patients with AF

| Risk factor | Score |
|---|---|
| **C**ongestive heart failure / LV dysfunction | 1 |
| **H**ypertension | 1 |
| **A**ge ≥75 years | 2 |
| **D**iabetes mellitus | 1 |
| **S**troke / TIA / peripheral thromboembolus | 2 |
| **V**ascular disease | 1 |
| **A**ge 65–74 years | 1 |
| **S**ex – female gender* | 1 |
| **Total** | **Maximum 10** |

*Note:* If female gender is the only risk factor, CHA$_2$DS$_2$VASc is 0.

**Table 7.19** HAS-BLED score for bleeding risk in patients with AF

| Clinical characteristic | Points awarded |
|---|---|
| **H**ypertension | 1 |
| **A**bnormal renal and liver function (1 point each) | 1 or 2 |
| **S**troke | 1 |
| **B**leeding | 1 |
| **L**abile INRs | 1 |
| **E**lderly (age >65 years) | 1 |
| **D**rugs or alcohol (1 point each) | 1 or 2 |
| **Total** | **Maximum 9 points** |

score ≥2 and there is no history of major intracranial haemorrhage, recent major bleeding or any current bleeding. The benefits are based on annual and accrued 5- and 10-year stroke risk, and not short-term risk. Therefore, anticoagulation can be interrupted for 5–7 days for elective surgical and dental procedures, and possibly longer when the surgical site is high risk (e.g. spinal or neurosurgical procedures). Anticoagulation may be considered for patients with a CHA$_2$DS$_2$VASc score of 1 and is not indicated if the CHA$_2$DS$_2$VASc score is 0. There is no role for aspirin or other antiplatelets for stroke prevention in patients with AF.

Choices of anticoagulation for stroke prevention in AF are shown in **Table 7.20**. Direct oral anticoagulants (DOACs) have become standard care for many patients with AF due to their superior efficacy and/or lower bleeding risk compared to warfarin. For patients taking warfarin for AF, the target international normalized ratio (INR) range is 2.0–3.0. Their time in therapeutic range (TTR) should be reviewed regularly and if <65% then they should be switched to a DOAC.

## CONGENITAL HEART DISEASE IN ADULTS

### Epidemiology

Prevalence of congenital heart disease is 8/1000 live births. Bicuspid non-stenotic aortic valves are present in 2% of the population; some of these will become stenotic. Eight lesions are responsible for 70–80% of all congenital heart disease defects (**Table 7.21**).

## CYANOTIC AND ACYANOTIC CONGENITAL HEART DISEASE

Congenital heart defects are classified into cyanotic and acyanotic groups. Central cyanosis develops when the concentration of deoxygenated haemoglobin rises above 5 g/100 mL as a result of either mixing of systemic venous blood with systemic arterial circulation or a low pulmonary blood flow.

Differentiation between cyanotic and acyanotic conditions is important, although some acyanotic congenital heart diseases (e.g. ASD, VSD, PDA) can progress to cyanotic heart disease when pulmonary hypertension develops due to chronically increased pulmonary blood flow, and when the pulmonary pressure and therefore the right heart pressure increases above the left heart pressures, blood will shunt in reverse from right to left, introducing deoxygenated blood into the left heart and systemic circulation. This is known as Eisenmenger's syndrome.

The most common left-to-right shunts are listed in **Table 7.22**.

Causes of congenital heart disease are listed in **Table 7.23**.

### Clinical features

Depending on the defect, the major haemodynamic features are because of obstruction to flow and/or shunting of blood

**Table 7.20** Options for therapeutic anticoagulation for stroke prevention in AF

| **Vitamin K antagonists – target INR 2.0–3.0** |
|---|
| • Warfarin |
| • Coumarin |
| **Factor Xa inhibitors** |
| • Apixiban |
| • Endoxaban |
| • Rivaroxaban |
| **Direct thrombin inhibitors** |
| • Dabigatran |
| • Argatroban (IV) |

**Table 7.21** Common lesions responsible for 70–80% of all congenital heart disease defects

| |
|---|
| Biscuspid aortic valve |
| ASD |
| VSD |
| Persistent PDA |
| Coarctation of the aorta |
| Pulmonary stenosis |
| Tetralogy of Fallot |
| Transposition of the great vessels |

## CARDIAC ARRHYTHMIAS: TREATMENTS AT A GLANCE

### BRADYCARDIA

#### Sinus bradycardia

If haemodynamically important: IV atropine
If chronic: a pacemaker may be required

#### Sinus node disease (sick sinus syndrome)

*Chronic symptomatic sinoatrial disease*

- Permanent pacing

#### Inappropriate sinus tachycardia

Ivabradine, beta blockers or verapamil for sinus tachycardia

#### AV block

*Asymptomatic first- and Mobitz type 1 second-degree heart block*

- No treatment

*Symptomatic Mobitz type 1 second-degree heart block*

- EP study – permanent pacing may be required

*Mobitz type 2 second-degree heart block*

- Permanent pacemaker recommended

*Complete heart block (third-degree heart block)*

- Permanent pacing usually required unless reversible cause identified

#### Atrial tachyarrhythmia

*Atrial ectopic beats*

- Usually no treatment is required
- If very symptomatic, beta blockers or verapamil may be considered

*AF and atrial flutter*

All patients

- Treat any underlying cause (e.g. hypertension, HF, sleep apnoea, thyrotoxicosis)
- Correct electrolyte disturbance
- Assess thromboembolic risk ($CHA_2DS_2VASc$ score; see **Table 7.18**) and bleeding risk (HAS-BLED score; see **Table 7.19**):
- Anticoagulation indicated if score $\geq 2$
- If $CHA_2DS_2VASc$ score = 0, no anticoagulation is indicated
- If $CHA_2DS_2VASc$ score = 1, discuss risks and benefits with patient
- Classified as paroxysmal, persistent or permanent
- AF management options – rhythm or rate control

Rhythm control strategy (paroxysmal and persistent AF)

- Direct current (DC) cardioversion: patients undergoing elective DC cardioversion should be formally anticoagulated for at least 4 weeks pre cardioversion and 3 weeks post cardioversion
- Pharmacological cardioversion using class I or III antiarrhythmic drugs IV during acute presentation (requires an echocardiogram pre-treatment to exclude HF before IV flecainide)
- Beta blockers (licensed for HF) or low-dose amiodarone if HF or ischaemic heart disease present to reduce risk of recurrent paroxysmal AF
- Flecainide, propafenone, beta blockers (including sotalol) or low dose amiodarone if HF or ischaemic heart disease excluded as prophylaxis against recurrent paroxysmal AF
- AF ablation for recurrent symptomatic AF (especially paroxysmal AF)
- Flutter ablation for atrial flutter

Rate control strategy (permanent AF)

Control the ventricular rate in chronic AF with AV drugs – choice depends on whether LV function is normal or abnormal:

- Normal LV function: beta blocker, digoxin, diltiazem, verapamil
- Reduced LV function: beta blocker, digoxin

*Narrow QRS tachycardia AVNRT*

- Carotid sinus massage or modified Valsalva during acute presentation
- IV adenosine, verapamil or beta blockers during acute presentation
- Beta blocker or verapamil
- AVNRT ablation to remove dual AV node physiology

*Pre-excitation syndromes*

- Electrical DC cardioversion is recommended
- Ablation of accessory pathway to prevent AVRT
- AV node-slowing drugs (verapamil, digoxin, beta blockers) are contraindicated

#### Ventricular tachyarrhythmias

*Ventricular ectopics*

- When no structural heart disease is present, VEs can be ignored
- Treatment is indicated if they are high frequency (>10% of all heart beats), cause uncomfortable symptoms or proven to predispose to a more serious ventricular arrhythmia, such as VT or VF
- Treatment options include pharmacological (beta blocker, verapamil if normal LV function) or VE ablation

*Ventricular tachycardia*

- Treatment is usually urgent, particularly if there is severe haemodynamic collapse
- Immediate DC cardioversion (under short-acting general anaesthetic if the patient is still conscious)
- If the patient's condition is stable, IV metoprolol or esmolol may convert the rhythm back to sinus rhythm. If haemodynamically unstable, IV amiodarone (bolus of 300 mg over 1 hour followed by 900 mg over 24 hours) may restore and stabilize sinus rhythm
- Consider cardioversion early
- Treat underlying cause (acute MI, HF, prolonged QT interval)
- Specialist opinion regarding indication for ICD

*Ventricular fibrillation*

- Rarely reverses spontaneously and immediate cardiopulmonary resuscitation is required until defibrillation can be performed
- Treat underlying cause (acute MI, HF, prolonged QT interval)
- Specialist opinion regarding indication for ICD

*Torsade de pointes*

- Correct any electrolyte disturbance and discontinue proarrhythmic drugs
- Overdrive pace the atrium and ventricles with temporary dual chamber pacing
- IV isoprenaline may be helpful in the acute situation if pacing not immediately available
- Beta blockade is helpful in some of the genetic LQTS (LQT1 and LQT2)
- Specialist opinion regarding indication for ICD and genetic testing

**Table 7.22** Congenital heart lesions causing left-to-right shunts

| Level | Defect |
|---|---|
| Atrium | ASD |
| Ventricle | VSD |
| Great vessels | PDA (between aorta and pulmonary artery) Aortopulmonary window |
| Mixed | Aorta to atrium or ventricle (ruptured sinus of Valsalva aneurysm) |
| | Coronary artery to atrium or ventricle (coronary fistula) |
| | Ventricle to atrium (Garbode defect allowing shunting from the LV to the right atrium (rare, usually secondary to Down syndrome) |
| Multiple | Atrioventricular septal defects |

**Table 7.23** Causes of congenital heart disease

Chromosomal abnormalities
Down syndrome (trisomy 21)
Turner syndrome (45, X0)
Increased consanguinity (there is a 1–2% risk of congenital heart disease for siblings and a 5–10% risk for any offspring)
Rubella infection
Drugs (e.g. thalidomide, warfarin, phenytoin)
Irradiation
Maternal disease (e.g. diabetes mellitus, chronic alcoholism, systemic lupus erythematosus)

from one side of the heart to the other. Abnormal volume overloads or pressure loads on various chambers of the heart can ultimately cause heart failure, arrhythmias and sudden death. Patients with excessive pulmonary flow from left-to-right shunts (e.g. ASD, VSD and PDA) develop progressive pulmonary vascular disease, pulmonary hypertension and right HF.

Patients with shunts may develop paradoxical embolic events (passage of an embolus from the venous system across a shunt and into the systemic arterial circulation) and cerebral abscesses. They have increased risk of developing endocarditis and require antibiotic prophylaxis for dental procedures, and many are prone to recurrent chest infections. The cyanotic group also have abnormal coagulation, iron deficiency and thrombocytopenia. They may also develop hyperuricaemia.

In cyanotic congenital heart disease, desaturated blood in their arterial system leads to polycythaemia, iron deficiency, hyperviscosity syndrome (blurred vision, headaches, chronic fatigue), clubbing, small stature and poor dentition.

## Management

All patients diagnosed with congenital heart disease should be referred to a suitable cardiologist who specializes in adult congenital heart disease (patients over 18 years) or a paediatric cardiologist (under 18 years).

## COARCTATION OF THE AORTA

This is a fibrous constriction in the aorta. It is a rare finding. The condition is summarized in COARCTATION OF THE AORTA AT A GLANCE.

## TETRALOGY OF FALLOT

### Epidemiology

This is the most common cyanotic congenital heart defect.

## Disease mechanisms

The abnormalities in Tetralogy of Fallot (**Figure 7.34**) are:
- VSD
- An aorta overriding the defect and therefore receiving blood from both the RV and the LV
- Pulmonary stenosis (infundibular, valvar or supravalvar)
- RVH

Right-to-left shunting increases with lowering of the systemic vascular resistance and increased infundibular obstruction. This may occur with exercise or emotional upsets. Children with Tetralogy of Fallot often squat because this manoeuvre kinks the femoral arteries, increasing the systemic vascular resistance and decreasing the right-to-left shunt of blood through the VSD.

## Clinical features

Depending on the severity of the defect, mild cyanosis may be apparent in infancy. Children have decreased exercise tolerance and occasional hypoxic crises.

Physical signs are:
- Variable cyanosis and clubbing
- RVH
- A single second sound resulting from aortic closure (the pulmonary component is very late and too soft to hear)
- An ejection systolic murmur across the RV outflow tract (the VSD is large and does not generate a murmur)

## Management

All patients should be considered for surgery to increase blood flow to the lungs. Currently, children have corrective surgery. In the period from 1950 to the 1990s a systemic-to-pulmonary artery shunt may have been necessary for palliative surgery, and therefore adults may present with one of these operations (e.g. Blalock–Taussig shunt).

## COMPLEX CONGENITAL HEART DISEASE

Other rare forms of complex congenital heart disease are beyond the scope of this chapter and reference should be made to specialist texts.

7

## COARCTATION OF THE AORTA AT A GLANCE

### Epidemiology

*Sex*

- Twice as common in men

*Genetics*

- Associated with Turner syndrome

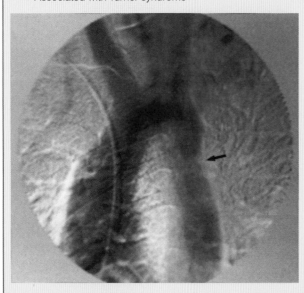

**Figure A** Coarctation of the aorta: aortogram. This digital subtraction aortogram shows a discrete coarctation (arrowed) in the thoracic aorta just beyond the left subclavian branch. Reproduced from Timmis AD & Nathan AW (1992) *Essentials of Cardiology*, 2nd edn (Wiley-Blackwell, Oxford), with the permission of the authors.

### Findings on investigation

*Diagnostic imaging*

- *Chest radiography:* shows a diminished aortic knuckle and dilatation of the left subclavian artery, and an indentation may be seen in the upper part of the descending aorta; rib-notching may be seen and is a result of the formation of collaterals
- *Echocardiography, CT, MRI* and *angiography:* all useful for further evaluation of the coarctation and collaterals
- ECG may show evidence of LVH

### Clinical features (often asymptomatic)

*CV*

- Leg fatigue or claudication
- Prominent upper limb pulses
- Small femoral pulses with radial–femoral delay
- Upper limb hypertension
- Congenital berry aneurysms in the cerebral circulation
- Bicuspid aortic valve (in 60%)
- An EC (if the aortic valve is bicuspid)
- An ejection systolic murmur
- A systolic murmur from the coarctation
- Bruits over collaterals
- Anomalous origin of the subclavian artery
- Features of LVH
- Palpable collaterals around the scapula

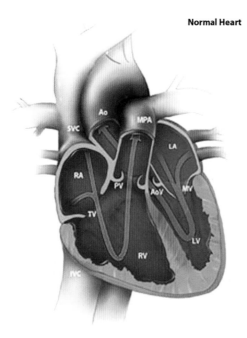

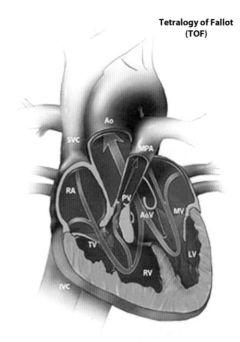

**Figure 7.34** Tetralogy of Fallot. **(a)** Normal cardiac anatomy and **(b)** anatomical changes in tetralogy of Fallot showing VSD, pulmonary stenosis, RVH and overriding aorta leading to right-to-left shunting of deoxygenated venous blood into the aorta and systemic arterial system.

# VALVULAR HEART DISEASE

## Epidemiology

In developed countries, the most common causes of valvular heart disease are acquired degenerative valve disease and congenital bicuspid AS. Rheumatic valvular heart disease is still the most common cause in developing countries and in people born in endemic areas who then move to other parts of the world.

The causes of heart valve disease are listed in **Table 7.24**.

## AORTIC STENOSIS

Conditions that can obstruct the outflow of blood from the LV include:

- *Aortic valve stenosis:* common (**Figure 7.35**)
- *Subvalvar AS:* rare – caused by a fibrous or muscular diaphragm situated below the aortic valve
- *Supravalvar stenosis:* rare – caused by a fibrous band above the aortic valve, which may be part of Williams' syndrome (elfin-like facies, hypercalcaemia and mental retardation)

The causes of AS are shown in **Table 7.25**.

**Table 7.24** Causes of heart valve disease

| |
|---|
| Valve calcification (associated with ageing) |
| Congenital valve disease e.g. Biscupid aortic valve |
| MVP |
| MR secondary to LV dysfunction |
| Endocarditis |
| Rheumatic fever |
| In association with other systemic disorders (e.g. ankylosing spondylitis, lupus, carcinoid syndrome) |

## Clinical features

AS results in a reduction in cardiac output, especially on exercise, and LVH. This pathophysiology gives rise to the three exertion-related symptoms of AS:

- Angina
- Breathlessness
- Dizziness (presyncope) or syncope on exercise

The signs are:

- A slow rising carotid pulse
- A soft or absent second heart sound (A2)
- An ejection systolic thrill palpable at the right sternal edge
- A thrusting apex beat from LVH

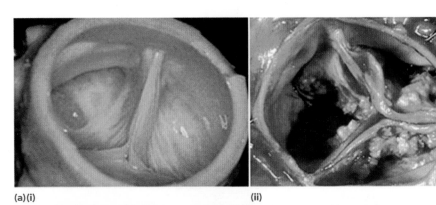

(a)(i)          (ii)

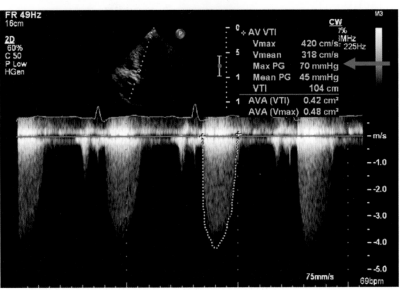

(b)

**Figure 7.35** AS. **(a)** Normal tricuspid aortic valve **(i)** and heavily calcified tricuspid aortic valve causing severe AS **(ii)**. **(b)** Continuous-wave Doppler echocardiography across the aortic valve demonstrating severe AS (peak transvalvular gradient 70 mmHg, mean gradient 45 mmHg).

- An ejection systolic murmur maximal at the left sternal edge and aortic area and radiating into the carotid arteries
- An ejection systolic click if a bicuspid valve

**Table 7.25** Causes of AS

Senile calcification of the aortic valve leaflets (does not usually cause severe AS unless the valve is congenitally bicuspid
Congenital, usually a bicuspid aortic valve (a bicuspid valve may not be stenotic, but may become so in later life because of calcification)
Rheumatic fever

### Investigation

#### Echocardiography

Echocardiography demonstrates a calcified valve (**Figure 7.35b**; **Figure 7.36**). Doppler is used to measure the pressure difference across the valve. If ventricular function is normal, a peak gradient up to 30 mmHg is mild AS, 30–63 mmHg indicates moderate AS, and a peak gradient greater than 64 mmHg indicates severe AS. AV area can be calculated and <1.0 cm$^2$ is severe AS. Mean AV gradients are also reported, and a mean AV gradient >40 mmHg indicates severe AS. If LV function is poor and cardiac output is reduced, the gradient will be less as transvalvular flow is reduced. A dobutamine stress echocardiogram is recommended in patients with suspected AS and LV dysfunction to assess the true severity of AS at increased flow rates.

#### Electrocardiography

ECG shows the LVH (increased QRS voltages) and may show the strain pattern of pressure overload (depressed ST segments and T-wave inversion in the lateral leads).

### Management

Surgical aortic valve replacement (sAVR) or percutaneous TAVI are the appropriate treatments for symptomatic severe AS (**Figure 7.37**). The decision of sAVR versus TAVI depends on fitness for cardiac surgery and also AV and root anatomy, which has to be suitable for TAVI. Current evidence suggests that sAVR has longer durability than TAVI and is currently recommended for patients with low surgical risk and severe AS. Children with severe non-calcified bicuspid AS can be treated by valvotomy when the valve cusps are split.

### Prognosis

Patients with symptomatic severe AS have a poor prognosis with a significant risk of sudden death. Patients with LV failure caused by AS have a 50% mortality rate within 2 years without surgery.

## AORTIC REGURGITATION

### Disease mechanisms

Blood leaking from the aorta into the LV during diastole leads to an increase in stroke volume and diastolic

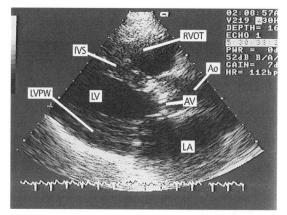

(a)

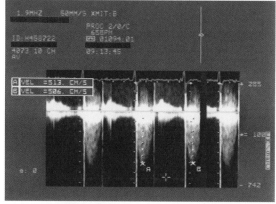

(b)

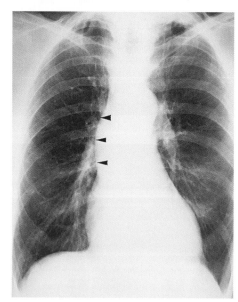

(c)

**Figure 7.36** AS **(a)** Severe AS in parasternal long-axis view showing calcified aortic valve and normal mitral valve. LV not enlarged, but very thick walls of interventricular septum (IVS) and posterior wall of LV (LVPW). RVOT, right ventricular outflow tract. **(b)** Echocardiogram of AS; Doppler estimate of velocity (>5 ms = >100 mmHg). **(c)** AS showing post-stenotic dilatation of the aorta (arrows). Note that there is little, if any, cardiac enlargement. Reproduced from Armstrong P & Wastie ML (1992) *Diagnostic Imaging*, 3rd edn (Wiley-Blackwell, Oxford), with permission of the authors.

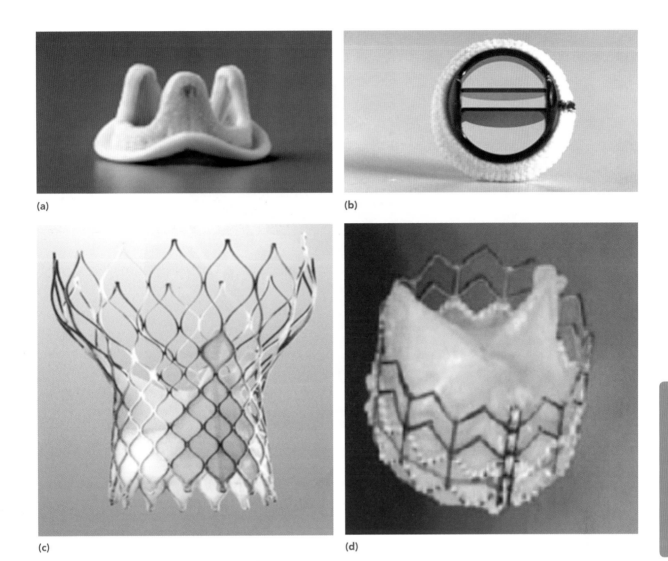

**Figure 7.37** Prosthetic heart valves. **(a)** Bioprosthetic (tissue) aortic valve. **(b)** Bileaflet mechanical prosthetic valve. **(c,d)** Percutaneous aortic valves for TAVI: **(c)** CoreValve; **(d)** Edwards SAPIEN valve.

dimensions of the ventricle (**Figure 7.38**). Causes of AR are listed in **Table 7.26**.

As the degree of regurgitation increases, end-diastolic pressure in the LV increases. Left atrial pressure is therefore increased, giving rise to pulmonary venous hypertension and exertional dyspnoea. Eventually, chronic LV dysfunction develops and the symptoms of LV failure occur at rest.

**Table 7.26** Causes of AR

| |
| --- |
| Bicuspid aortic valve |
| Dilatation of the aortic valve ring |
| Hypertension |
| Endocarditis |
| Mediastinal radiation |
| Bioprosthetic aortic valve failure |
| Rheumatic fever |
| Connective tissue disorders such as ankylosing spondylitis |
| Dissection of the aorta |
| Aneurysm of the aorta |
| Syphilitic aortitis |
| Marfan's syndrome |

**Clinical features**

The symptoms are exertional dyspnoea first, and later the symptoms of LV failure at rest (see **Table 7.11**). Occasionally, coronary perfusion diminishes as the arterial diastolic pressure falls and the ventricular diastolic pressure rises, giving rise to angina.

Signs are:

- *Collapsing pulse in the arm:* This is combined with a wide pulse pressure.
- *Early diastolic murmur:* This is maximal at the left sternal edge and towards the apex on auscultation. The diastolic murmur becomes shorter as severity increases, and the regurgitant jet of blood may

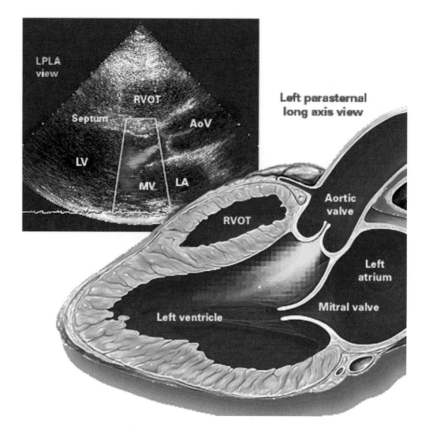

**Figure 7.38** AR.

cause the anterior mitral leaflet to vibrate, giving rise to a low-pitch mid-diastolic (Austin Flint) murmur.

The apex beat may be displaced laterally and volume loaded. There may be an accompanying fourth heart sound indicating atrial hypertension because of raised LV end-diastolic pressure.

### Investigation

#### Electrocardiography

ECG may show features of LVH and strain resulting from volume overload (increased voltages and T-wave inversion.

#### Diagnostic imaging

**See Figure 7.39.**

- *Chest radiography:* Radiographs show an enlarged transverse cardiac diameter and upper lobe blood diversion, indicating pulmonary venous hypertension.
- *Echocardiography:* This shows the regurgitant jet across the aortic valve, and can quantify the severity of the regurgitation. If chronic AR is present, it shows a volume-loaded LV. At first only the end-diastolic dimension is increased because compensatory increased systolic function preserves normal end-systolic dimension. If the condition deteriorates and

the LV begins to fail, the end-systolic dimension increases.
- *TOE:* This confirms anatomy and cause. In endocarditis, it can assess for aortic root abscess and vegetations.
- *Cardiac catheterization:* Use to assess for coronary artery disease in preparation for valve surgery.
- *CMR:* Use to measure aortic regurgitant volume, anatomy of aortic root and ascending aorta, and LV function and scarring.

### Management

Symptomatic AR is usually severe and requires surgical AVR (**Table 7.27**). This is indicated in asymptomatic patients with severe AR if there is evidence of ventricular decompensation such as an increase in the end-systolic dimension on serial echocardiography, which is recommended annually and, if the LV end-systolic volume or diameter starts to increase, then every 6 months. Vasodilators including ACE inhibitors may be used in asymptomatic patients to support ventricular function. Emergency surgical AVR is required if acute severe AR rapidly develops (e.g. secondary to *Staphylococcus aureus* endocarditis or a type A aortic dissection). Urgent AVR is required if a bioprosthetic AVR develops severe AR.

### Prognosis

Moderate and even severe AR in native valves is often well tolerated for many years without symptoms. Without surgery, 75%

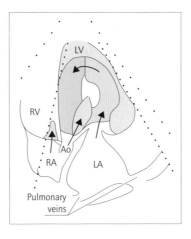
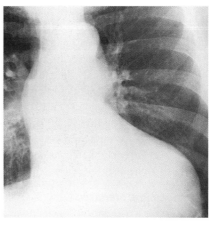

(a)                                                    (b)

**Figure 7.39** AR. **(a)** Colour flow Doppler in a patient with AR. Apical four-chamber view showing turbulent jet (white) of regurgitant blood impinging on anterior leaflet of mitral valve to mix with the stream (red) passing from left atrium to LV. Note change in colour to blue as the stream is directed by the ventricular apex towards the aortic valve. A small portion of right atrial to RV flow is depicted in red. **(b)** LV enlargement in a patient with aortic incompetence. The cardiac apex is displaced downwards and to the left. Note also that the ascending aorta causes a bulge of the right mediastinal border – a feature that is almost always seen in significant aortic valve disease. Both figures reproduced from Armstrong P & Wastie ML (1992) *Diagnostic Imaging*, 3rd edn (Wiley-Blackwell, Oxford), with the permission of the authors.

of patients with severe AR survive for 5 years. Furthermore, offloading of the ventricle with vasodilators in AR can improve the prognosis by limiting the deterioration in LV dysfunction.

**Table 7.27** Management of AR

**Specific treatment**

*Reduce afterload to the LV*

- Vasodilators such as ACE inhibitors to reduce peripheral vascular resistance in asymptomatic patients
- Diuretics and nitrates to reduce the end-diastolic pressure in the LV

*Surgery (AVR)*

- Symptomatic severe AR
- Indicated if there is evidence of ventricular decompensation such as increasing in the end-systolic dimension on echocardiography
- Emergency AVR – in acute severe AR with haemodynamic instability (e.g. *Staphylococcal aureus* endocarditis with leaflet destruction)
- Urgent AVR – rapidly progressing AR in bioprosthetic AVR failure

## MITRAL VALVE DISEASE

The mitral valve consists of two leaflets, the annulus (a muscular ring that contracts during systole to reduce the valve area), the chordae tendineae and two papillary muscles (**Figure 7.40**). The normal cross-sectional area is 5 cm².

## MITRAL STENOSIS

### Disease mechanisms

The main cause of MS is rheumatic fever, but it may be congenital stenosis, degenerative calcification in the elderly,

lupus or endocarditis via large vegetations. Lutembacher's syndrome is the combination of congenital MS and an ASD.

In rheumatic heart disease, the valve cusps become thickened and the commissures fuse. Similar thickening of the subvalvar apparatus with contraction of the chordae tendineae leads to reduced ventricular filling. The left atrium increases in size and often develops mural thrombus.

### Clinical features

Symptoms of MS usually occur when the valve orifice is reduced to less than 2 cm². Breathlessness is caused by

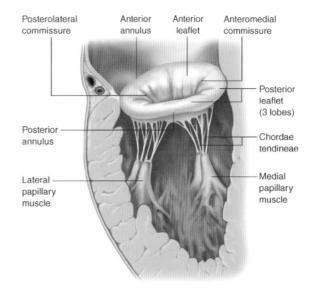

**Figure 7.40** Mitral valve anatomy. There are three components: mitral valve annulus, two mitral valve leaflets and the subvalvular apparatus (chordae tendineae and papillary muscles).

increased left atrial pressure and consequent pulmonary venous hypertension. Initially, the symptom is exertional dyspnoea but orthopnoea and PND develop with increasing stenosis, which eventually leads to pulmonary hypertension and signs of RV failure (peripheral oedema and ascites).

Other symptoms include exertional fatigue, recurrent chest infections and haemoptysis. Palpitations are caused by AF, and occasionally the first symptom is caused by a systemic embolus, often arising at the onset of AF. They occur as a result of clot development in the left atrium, giving rise to a stroke or a loss of peripheral pulse.

### Signs of mitral stenosis

- There is a malar flush consisting of a dusky discoloration of the cheeks.
- The pulse is either normal or irregularly irregular because of AF.
- Venous pressure is raised if pulmonary hypertension has developed. Sometimes there is a systolic $v$ wave of tricuspid regurgitation.
- The apex beat is not displaced and has a tapping quality because of a palpable first heart sound. If pulmonary hypertension has developed, there is a palpable RV heave and a palpable pulmonary component to the second heart sound in the second left intercostal space.
- A mid-diastolic murmur is the typical murmur, best heard using the bell of the stethoscope at the apex with the patient in the left lateral position. If the patient is in sinus rhythm, atrial systole accentuates the diastolic murmur immediately before the first heart sound, giving rise to presystolic accentuation.
- There is a loud first heart sound and an OS in early diastole immediately before the mid-diastolic murmur if the valve cusps are mobile in mild-moderate MS.

### Management

See **Table 7.28**.

**Table 7.28** Management of MS

| |
| --- |
| **Specific treatment** |
| *Anticoagulation with warfarin** |
| • Essential as prophylaxis against thromboembolism |
| *Lower left atrial pressure* |
| • Diuretics |
| *AF* |
| • Beta blockers and/or digoxin (monitor plasma digoxin levels) |
| *Surgery* |
| • To enlarge the mitral valve orifice as symptoms become more severe |
| • Balloon valvotomy, closed mitral valvotomy, open mitral valvotomy or mitral valve replacement |
| • Anticoagulation will be indicated after all procedures |

*DOACs are not indicated for AF secondary to MS.

### Prognosis

Without surgery, 70% of symptomatic patients with severe MS will survive for 5 years. However, even with surgery, the prognosis remains reduced. Following mitral valve replacement, only 60–70% of patients survive for 10 years, because of problems with the prosthetic valve such as thromboembolism and endocarditis, and progressive LV dysfunction.

## MITRAL REGURGITATION

Trivial and mild MR are very common and do not require treatment. Moderate MR requires regular follow up as treatment may be required if it progresses to severe. Severe MR usually requires treatment unless contraindications exist. Timing of treatment depends on either symptoms or evidence of early LV impairment in asymptomatic patients.

Acute MR secondary to acute chordal rupture or papillary muscle rupture can cause acute HF and is a medical emergency requiring urgent surgical repair.

### Pathophysiology

MR is classified as primary if caused by structural mitral valve leaflet abnormalities (e.g. MV prolapse, chordal rupture) or secondary if it results from LV dilatation or infarction leading to restricted motion of the MV leaflets and MV annular dilatation (**Table 7.29**; **Figure 7.41**). If the onset of MR is acute, the left atrium does not expand and the pressure wave is transmitted into the pulmonary veins. This causes acute pulmonary oedema. MR usually develops gradually, the left atrium expands and acts as a capacitance chamber absorbing the pressure wave generated by the regurgitant blood through the mitral valve. This causes only a small rise in pulmonary venous pressure and the patient is therefore not so breathless until the MR is very severe.

**Table 7.29** Causes of MR

| |
| --- |
| **Primary MR** (*caused by diseases of the mitral valve leaflets and/or chordae tendinae*) |
| • MVP |
| • IE |
| • Rheumatic heart disease |
| • Collagen disorders such as Marfan's syndrome or Ehlers–Danlos syndrome |
| • Connective tissue disorders (e.g. systemic lupus erythematosus) |
| • High-dose radiation to mediastinum |
| **Secondary MR** (*caused by diseases of the LV*) |
| • DCM |
| • MI – either papillary muscle or posterior MI causing restricted posterior mitral valve leaflet (PMVL) movement |
| • Hypertrophic cardiomyopathy |
| • Takotsubo syndrome (during acute phase) |

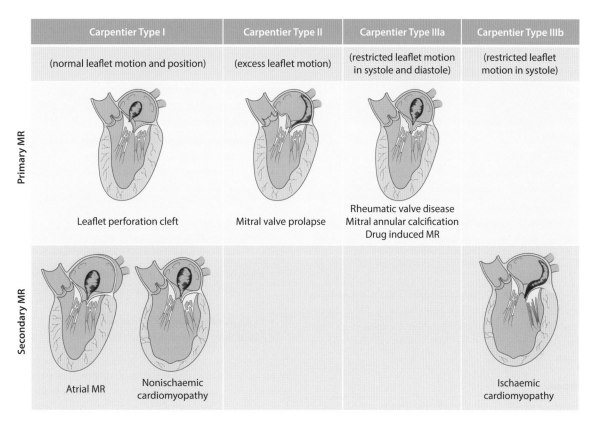

| | **Carpentier Type I**<br>(normal leaflet motion and position) | **Carpentier Type II**<br>(excess leaflet motion) | **Carpentier Type IIIa**<br>(restricted leaflet motion in systole and diastole) | **Carpentier Type IIIb**<br>(restricted leaflet motion in systole) |
|---|---|---|---|---|
| **Primary MR** | Leaflet perforation cleft | Mitral valve prolapse | Rheumatic valve disease<br>Mitral annular calcification<br>Drug induced MR | |
| **Secondary MR** | Atrial MR    Nonischaemic cardiomyopathy | | | Ischaemic cardiomyopathy |

**Figure 7.41** Different aetiologies leading to MR. First row is primary MR caused by diseases of the mitral valve leaflets. Second row is secondary MR resulting from dilatation of the mitral valve annulus or diseases of the LV (HF, MI). Adapted from El Sabbagh A *et al.* (2018) *J Am Coll Cardiol Img* 11(4): 628–43.

## Clinical features

Dyspnoea and orthopnoea are the typical symptoms of MR. As MR progresses, LV failure and then pulmonary hypertension and RV failure develop.

The physical signs of MR are as follows:

- *Apex beat may be displaced laterally and over a wider area:* The impulse may be overactive because of increased volume load on the ventricle.
- *Murmurs:* On auscultation there is a pansystolic murmur, which is typically maximal at the apex. If anterior mitral valve leaflet (AMVL) prolapse or restriction is present, the systolic murmur radiates to the axilla. If PMVL prolapse or restriction occurs, the murmur radiates to the left sternal edge. In MVP, the murmur may be late systolic and occur after a mid-systolic click.
- *The first heart sound is soft and there may be a third heart sound.*

## Investigation

### Electrocardiography

ECG may show an enlarged left atrium with P mitrale and LVH from volume overload.

### Diagnostic imaging

- *Chest radiography:* This shows an increased transverse cardiac diameter with left atrial and LV enlargement. Calcification in the mitral valve may be evident.

- *Echocardiography:* This shows features of a volume-loaded LV with vigorous systolic function of the LV and a dilated left atrium. The LVEF is supranormal (>65%) unless HF is present. The LV may be dilated. The aetiology of the MR may be evident. The colour wave Doppler signal demonstrates the regurgitation, and severity can be measured.
- *TOE:* This is recommended to confirm the anatomy and whether the valve may be suitable for surgical repair, or if the valve is suitable for the percutaneous MitraClip™ in patients with increased risk of cardiac surgery.
- *Right* and *left cardiac catheterization:* These may be helpful to confirm regurgitant *v* waves on the pulmonary capillary wedge pressure tracing and pulmonary artery hypertension, and exclude other causes of LV dysfunction or pulmonary hypertension.

## Management

When symptoms develop, diuretics and ACE inhibitors may be used while preparing the patient for MV surgery. If AF develops, digoxin and anticoagulation are required (**Table 7.30**).

Symptomatic patients with severe MR should be referred to a cardiac surgical centre for consideration of mitral valve surgery. Surgery depends on anatomy and comorbidities and is either a surgical repair or mitral valve replacement. In patients with very high perioperative risk

**7**

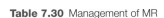

**Table 7.30** Management of MR

| Specific treatment |
| --- |
| Diuretics and vasodilators such as ACE inhibitors for symptoms while preparing for surgery |
| *AF* |
| • Digoxin |
| • Anticoagulation with warfarin or DOAC |
| *Surgery* |
| • If the symptoms are inadequately controlled by medical therapy or there is evidence of LV dysfunction |
| • Either open mitral valve repair or valve replacement |
| *Percutaneous MitraClip* |
| • Recommended for patients with severe MR (particularly primary MR) with suitable anatomy and prohibitive risk of open surgical repair |

**Table 7.31** Management of MVP

| Specific treatment |
| --- |
| *Prophylaxis against endocarditis* |
| • If moderate or severe MR is present |
| *Atypical chest pain and palpitations* |
| • Beta blockers |
| • Reassurance and explanation |
| *When symptoms of breathlessness develop* |
| • Diuretics will reduce left atrial pressure |
| • Vasodilators such as ACE inhibitors will encourage forward flow from the LV |
| *AF* |
| • Digoxin or beta blockers |
| • Anticoagulation with warfarin or DOAC |
| *Surgery* |
| • If MR becomes severe, if the symptoms are inadequately controlled by medical therapy or there is evidence of LV dysfunction |
| • Open mitral valve repair or valve replacement |
| • MitraClip in high-risk surgical patients |

due to comorbidities, a percutaneous MitraClip may be indicated. Guidelines provide thresholds of LV volumes and function at which surgery is recommended in asymptomatic patients with severe MR before LV dysfunction develops.

### Prognosis

Surgery has radically improved the prognosis of MR. Before surgery, however, approximately 80% of patients with severe regurgitation would survive for 5 years and 60% would survive for 10 years.

## MITRAL VALVE PROLAPSE (FLOPPY MITRAL VALVE)

### Epidemiology

- Up to 4% of women and 1% of men have MVP on routine echocardiography. In many ways, MVP can therefore be considered a normal variant, but sometimes the associated regurgitation causes symptoms and treatment is necessary.
- It is most commonly identified in young women.

### Disease mechanisms

MVP is usually associated with myxomatous degeneration of either:

- *Mitral valve leaflet:* allowing the leaflet to billow into the LV
- *Chordae tendineae:* which stretch and allow the leaflet to prolapse into the left atrium, resulting in MR

It is sometimes seen in association with an ASD, hypertrophic cardiomyopathy or Marfan's syndrome. There may be a family history as MVP is genetic in 35–50% cases.

### Clinical features

The most common symptom of MVP is palpitations, which on 24-hour ambulatory monitoring are shown to be caused by atrial or ventricular ectopics. Patients also complain of stabbing-like atypical chest pain, which usually causes severe anxiety because of the associated palpitations.

Typical signs are a mid-systolic click followed by a late systolic murmur. The click is caused by sudden tensing of the chordae tendineae during systole. The late systolic murmur can be variable and can become more evident with the Valsalva manoeuvre or on standing, both of which reduce ventricular filling increased afterload and increase the degree of prolapse.

### Investigation

#### Diagnostic imaging

- *Echocardiography:* confirms the aetiology of the MR, demonstrating malposition of the mitral valve leaflets with prolapse of one or other of the cusps into the left atrium
- *TOE:* indicated to evaluate the anatomy and determine suitability for repair

### Management and prognosis

Treatment is the same as for MR, but patients often present with atypical chest pain and palpitations, both of which can be difficult to control. Beta blockers are the first drugs to try, but reassurance and an explanation of the benign nature of the condition is essential (**Table 7.31**).

## TRICUSPID VALVE DISEASE

TV disease (tricuspid stenosis or tricuspid regurgitation) is rare in isolation and is usually a result of rheumatic fever in which case left-sided valve disease is usually present. Carcinoid syndrome is another recognized cause. Tricuspid regurgitation is most commonly caused by dilatation of the

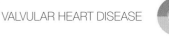

TV ring as a consequence of RV dilatation brought about by pulmonary hypertension. Tricuspid regurgitation occurs in Ebstein's syndrome when there is congenital displacement of the valve into the RV.

## Clinical features

Both tricuspid stenosis and incompetence cause right atrial hypertension and reduced cardiac output leading to hepatomegaly, ascites and dependent oedema. The hepatomegaly can be painful because of stretching of the liver capsule. The reduced cardiac output leads to fatigue and exertional dyspnoea.

### Signs of TV disease

- *Tricuspid stenosis*
  - Increased atrial component to the venous pressure pulse with a prominent A wave if the patient is in sinus rhythm
  - Rumbling diastolic murmur
- *Tricuspid regurgitation*
  - Systolic V wave in the venous pressure pulse
  - Pulsatile liver edge
  - Pansystolic murmur at the right sternal edge
  - Palpable RV

## Investigation

*Echocardiography* is the diagnostic test, recommended to evaluate the structure and severity of TV disease, RV function, PA pressure and IVC dimensions and variability (increased with reduced variability with high venous pressures).

## Management

For tricuspid stenosis, diuretics are the mainstay of medical therapy but valvotomy and, rarely, valve replacement may be necessary. For tricuspid regurgitation, treatment is as for congestive cardiac failure including the use of the diuretic spironolactone. Functional tricuspid regurgitation does not usually require surgery and can be managed medically but annuloplasty, where the TV is repaired, is often carried out in association with surgery on left-sided heart valves.

## PULMONARY VALVE DISEASE

PV disease (pulmonary stenosis and pulmonary regurgitation) is uncommon. Pulmonary stenosis is either congenital or acquired as a consequence of rheumatic fever or carcinoid syndrome. Congenital pulmonary stenosis can be an isolated lesion found at a routine examination or be part of a more complex defect such as tetralogy of Fallot. It is a feature of Noonan's syndrome. Pulmonary stenosis may be valvular, supravalvular or subvalvular and multiple stenoses in the pulmonary artery are a feature of rubella syndrome. Pulmonary regurgitation is most often seen following a

valvotomy for pulmonary stenosis. The other cause is pulmonary hypertension, commonly resulting from left-sided valve disease, particularly MS.

## Clinical features

### Pulmonary stenosis

Patients experience fatigue and syncope and symptoms of RV failure. Often the murmur is heard as part of a routine medical examination without symptoms. Unless severe, pulmonary regurgitation causes no symptoms and then those symptoms are caused by RV failure.

The clinical signs for pulmonary stenosis are:
- Ejection systolic murmur in the second left intercostal space
- A delayed soft pulmonary component to the second heart sound
- Pulmonary EC
- Fourth heart sound
- Prominent A wave in the venous pressure and RVH

### Pulmonary regurgitation

An early diastolic murmur is heard immediately after the pulmonary component of the second heart sound (Graham Steel murmur).

## Investigation

### Electrocardiography

ECG shows evidence of right atrial and RVH with P pulmonale and prominent R waves in the anterior chest leads. For pulmonary regurgitation, the ECG may show an RSR pattern in V1, V2 compatible with RV diastolic overload.

### Diagnostic imaging

- *Chest X-ray:*
  - In pulmonary stenosis, post-stenotic dilatation gives rise to a prominent pulmonary artery shadow.
  - In pulmonary regurgitation, there will be an enlarged heart and enlarged pulmonary arteries.
- *Echocardiogram:* Pulse Doppler measures RV systolic pressure and the gradient across the PV. For pulmonary regurgitation, the echocardiogram shows a dilated RV with reverse septal motion. Pulse Doppler detects a regurgitant jet.

## Management

In patients with pulmonary stenosis, if the RV systolic pressure rises above 60 mmHg, balloon dilatation and/or surgery of the valve is recommended (**Table 7.32**). No treatment is usually required for pulmonary regurgitation unless RV failure develops. Percutaneous pulmonary valve implantation is used, particularly in patients with PR following surgical repair of tetralogy of Fallot.

7

**Table 7.32** Summary of valve defects, symptoms, signs and management

| Valve | Defect | Symptoms | Murmur | Heart sounds | Management |
|---|---|---|---|---|---|
| Mitral | Stenosis | Breathlessness, palpitations | Mid-diastolic | Loud $S_1$ OS | Valvotomy |
| | Regurgitation | Breathlessness | Pansystolic | $A_2$ obscured | Diuretics, vasodilators, surgery |
| | Prolapse | Breathlessness, atypical chest pain, palpitations | Late systolic | Normal or mid-systolic click | Diuretics, vasodilators, surgery |
| Tricuspid | Disease | Swelling of ankles, swelling of abdomen (ascites), sacral oedema | Mid-diastolic | OS | Diuretics |
| Aortic | Stenosis | Angina, syncope, breathlessness | Ejection systolic | Reduced $A_2$ | Surgery |
| | Regurgitation | Breathlessness | Early diastolic | | Vasodilators, diuretics, surgery |
| Pulmonary | Stenosis | Fatigue | Ejection systolic | Delayed $P_2$ | Balloon dilatation |

# RHEUMATIC FEVER

## Epidemiology

- Less than 0.1% of the population in the UK are now affected by rheumatic fever, whereas 50 years ago it affected more than 10% of the population.
- Rheumatic fever is an illness of childhood, usually occurring in 5–15 year-olds.
- It is still common in sub-Saharan Africa, the Middle East and South Asia, affecting about 1% of the population. It reflects access to primary healthcare and antibiotics for paediatric pharyngitis.

## Disease mechanisms

Rheumatic fever results from a Lancefield group A streptococcal infection causing tonsillitis and scarlet fever. This gives rise to an autoimmune reaction with the development of antiheart antibodies and possibly an altered lymphocyte response.

The cardiac manifestations of rheumatic fever result in a pancarditis: a fibrinous pericarditis can develop. Aschoff nodules, which have a necrotic centre, develop in the myocardium. The endocardial lesions principally affect the valves, which become thickened causing stenosis and/or regurgitation. This process develops over many years with progressive valve calcification.

The mitral valve is more commonly involved than the aortic valve. The TV can be affected, but tricuspid regurgitation in rheumatic heart disease usually results from pulmonary hypertension and consequent RV dilatation. The PV is rarely involved.

## Clinical features

Acute rheumatic fever affects many systems, usually about 4 weeks after the history of sore throat.

### Heart involvement

Acute rheumatic carditis with valvitis causes acute regurgitation, myocarditis and/or pericarditis. Dilatation of the mitral valve ring can lead to MR. There may be a pericardial effusion and arrhythmias, particularly first-degree heart block, can occur. The heart involvement in the acute phase in rheumatic fever can be fulminant, leading to death, but this is rare in the UK. About 50% of patients who have rheumatic valvular heart disease have no history of acute rheumatic fever.

### Neurological involvement

Neurological manifestations include Sydenham's chorea or St Vitus' dance.

### Skin involvement

Skin manifestations include erythema marginatum, which is an erythematous rash with a raised edge found mainly on the trunk. It may fade over 24 hours, but keeps recurring. Nodules also develop over tendons and bony prominences. They are painless and can reach 1–2 cm in size.

### Joint involvement

Joint involvement of the larger joints, such as knees and elbows, can manifest as a temporary polyarthritis that moves from one joint to another. The joints are red, swollen and tender, but there is no long-term damage.

## Diagnosis

Diagnosis is based on the Duckett–Jones criteria (**Table 7.33**). Two or more major criteria or one major plus two or more minor criteria must be fulfilled to make the diagnosis.

## Investigation

### Haematology
- *FBC:* a normochromic normocytic anaemia develops
- *ESR* and *C-reactive protein (CRP):* increased

### Immunology
- *Antistreptolysin O antibody titre:* raised
- *Anti-DNAase antibody* and *antihyaluronidase antibody:* raised

**Table 7.33** Duckett–Jones criteria for diagnosing rheumatic fever

**Major**
- Polyarthritis
- Carditis
- Chorea
- Erythema marginatum
- Subcutaneous nodules

**Minor**
- Previous rheumatic fever or scarlet fever
- Arthralgia
- Fever
- Leucocytosis
- Increased ESR or CRP
- Increased ASO titre
- Prolonged PR interval on the ECG

ASO, anti-streptolysin O; CRP, C-reactive protein; ECG, electrocardiogram; ESR, erythrocyte sedimentation rate.

### Microbiology

Throat swab cultures for group A *Streptococcus* may be positive.

### Management

The management of rheumatic fever involves bed rest, antibiotics (usually high-dose IV benzylpenicillin and then oral penicillin V, aspirin and corticosteroids (**Table 7.34**). Bed rest is required until the fever settles and the cardiac manifestations resolve. If the patient is allergic to penicillin, a sulphonamide should be used instead. Prednisolone (up to 120 mg/day) is given for 1 week until the ESR settles and is then tailed off over the next 2–3 weeks. However, the effectiveness of corticosteroids is questionable.

**Table 7.34** Management of rheumatic fever

*Supportive treatment*
- Bed rest
- Specific treatment

*Drug treatment*
- Intramuscular or oral penicillin (or a sulphonamide if allergic to penicillin) for at least 1 week
- Aspirin in high dose
- Prednisolone (up to 120 mg/day) for 1 week until the ESR settles and then tail off over the next 2–3 weeks

*Prophylaxis*
- Long-term penicillin until at least 25 years old

### Surgery

Surgery to the valves is rare but may be necessary if severe HF develops because of valve regurgitation.

### Prophylaxis

Prophylactic treatment with long-term oral penicillin V is recommended, or with an alternative if penicillin-allergic. If the patient has no valvular heart damage, the prophylaxis should be for a minimum of 10 years, or up to 25 years of age. If valvular damage has occurred, it should probably be continued until 40 years of age.

### Prognosis

About 5% of patients with rheumatic fever die during the acute episode. The subsequent prognosis is affected by the tendency to repeated attacks of rheumatic fever. Patients are particularly vulnerable in the first few years after the initial attack.

## INFECTIVE ENDOCARDITIS

IE is a serious condition in which the cardiac valves or endocardium become infected. It may present either as a low-grade chronic illness (subacute endocarditis) or acutely with a fulminant course (acute endocarditis) when virulent organisms such as *Staphylococcus aureus* or fungi in immunosuppressed patients rapidly destroy the valves.

Diagnosis requires identification of affected valves and the causative organism.

### Epidemiology

Risk groups include patients with prosthetic heart valves, pre-existing valvular heart disease (e.g. MVP or AS), ill patients with prolonged hospitalization with indwelling IV lines, IV drug abusers (usually right-sided endocarditis of TV or PV), and immunosuppressed patients.

### Disease mechanisms

The infection is usually bacterial, but other organisms can be responsible (**Table 7.35**).

IE usually occurs on abnormal valves, but the acute form can involve valves previously thought to be normal. It can also occur in patients with congenital heart disease,

**Table 7.35** Organisms causing IE

| Organism | Percentage of cases and notes |
|---|---|
| *Streptococcus viridans* | 50% |
| *Staphylococcus aureus* | 20% of cases, but a more common cause of fulminant acute endocarditis |
| *Staphlylococcus epidermidis* | Following valve replacement surgery |
| *Enterococcus faecalis* | Patients with GI diseases, e.g. ulcerative colitis, colorectal cancer |
| Gram-negative organisms (e.g. *Haemophilus influenzae*) | A much less common cause of endocarditis and usually occurs following heart valve surgery or in drug addicts |
| *Coxiella burnetti* (Q fever) | Rare |
| Fungi, especially in immunosuppressed patients | Rare |

particularly on the low-pressure side of shunts with high pressure gradients (e.g. VSDs, PDA, arteriovenous fistulae).

IV drug abuse has led to a significant incidence of TV endocarditis. Prosthetic valves are particularly vulnerable and, once established, surgical resection of the infected valve and implantation of a new valve is required. Clumps of infecting organisms, fibrin and platelets, known as vegetations, develop on the affected valve. These vegetations can destroy the valve cusps, producing regurgitation and occasionally stenosis, and can lead to systemic embolization.

Infections of foreign material within the heart including pacemaker leads, indwelling IV catheters (central lines, PICC lines, Portacath lines) is an increasing cause of endocarditis.

### Clinical features

Endocarditis should be suspected in any patient with a fever and a heart murmur (see INFECTIVE ENDOCARDITIS: CLINICAL FEATURES AT A GLANCE). Anaemia, flu-like symptoms, night sweats and weight loss are common and the patient

has often been treated for influenza with antibiotics before a diagnosis of IE is established.

There is often a heart murmur, but the diagnosis of IE should be considered in appropriate circumstances, even if a murmur is absent. If a new murmur develops, or the character of a known heart murmur changes, endocarditis should be suspected.

Manifestations of IE outside the heart result from systemic embolization and immune complex deposition:

- *Systemic embolization:* This leads to splenic and renal infarcts, MI, embolic strokes and loss of peripheral pulses.
- *Immune complex deposition:* This gives rise to a vasculitis with manifestations in various parts of the body. These include small haemorrhages in the skin or mucosa (particularly the pharynx and conjunctiva), haemorrhages in the retina (Roth spots) or in the nail beds (splinter haemorrhages), small red macules on the hands (rare and called Janeway's lesions) and Osler's nodes (rare, small painful subcutaneous swellings in the pads of the fingers and toes).

Haematuria is common. It is usually caused by acute glomerulonephritis if microscopic, or renal infarction as a result of emboli if macroscopic. As in any chronic infection, splenomegaly is common. If there is splenic infarction, the spleen will be painful and there may be a friction rub. Clubbing of the digits is rare, but it can develop in the later stages of the chronic endocarditis. In right heart endocarditis, septic embolization to the lungs can cause pleuritic pain with haemoptysis. Pneumonia and lung abscesses can also develop.

### Investigation

#### Haematology

- *FBC:* a normochromic normocytic anaemia is common, and there is usually only a modest increase in the white cell count
- *ESR* and *CRP:* raised

#### Biochemistry

Urea and creatinine may be raised.

#### Microbiology

Multiple blood cultures are the key investigation. At least three sets of cultures should be taken over a 12–24-hour period from different sites (including IV line if present), before antibiotics are given. About 80% will prove to be positive, but 20% will be negative. Negative blood cultures are usually found in patients who have been exposed to antibiotics early on in the illness, or in those with a chronic history where high levels of antibodies have developed. Specific culture mediums and serological markers may be required for rarer organisms. Indwelling IV lines and catheters should be removed and sent for culture. Culture-negative endocarditis is associated with a poorer prognosis.

**INFECTIVE ENDOCARDITIS: CLINICAL FEATURES AT A GLANCE**

Fever

Roth spots in retina

Murmurs
Heart failure

Splenomegaly

Vasculitic rash

Haematuria

Janeway lesions

Clubbing
Nailfold infarcts
Splinter haemorrhages

Osler's nodes

Arthralgia
(i.e. joint pain)

Janeway lesions
(sole of foot)

### Diagnostic imaging

- *Chest radiography:* Radiographs may show evidence of HF. If there is right-sided endocarditis there may be pulmonary emboli or an abscess.
- *Echocardiography:* This may identify vegetations (**Figure 7.42**). These have to be at least 2 mm to be seen, so the absence of vegetations on echocardiography does not exclude the diagnosis.
- *TOE:* This approach may be more sensitive than transthoracic echocardiography for identifying vegetations, especially on prosthetic heart valves.

### ECG

ECG is usually not altered in endocarditis. Involvement of the conducting tissue in aortic valve endocarditis results in a prolonged PR interval and indicates a severe infection, possibly with an aortic root abscess.

### Management

Any underlying source of infection should be sought and treated; in particular, dental radiographs should be taken and tooth abscesses treated by immediate extraction (**Table 7.36**).

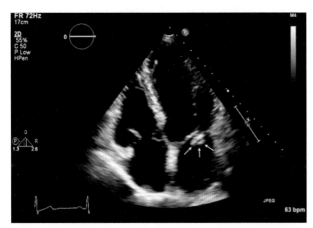

(a)

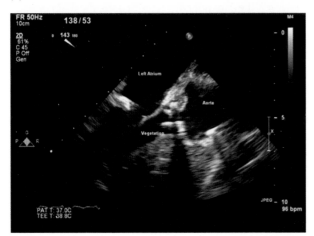

(b)

**Figure 7.42** Examples of endocarditis on echocardiography. **(a)** Mitral valve endocarditis with vegetation on the atrial side of the PMVL. **(b)** Aortic valve endocarditis with vegetation.

Management of IE involves a prolonged course of antibiotics (2–6 weeks) followed by surgical valve replacement if significant valve damage (severe regurgitation) has developed or if persisting infection requiring surgical resection of infected tissue is required.

Indications for urgent surgical valve replacement include acute HF (pulmonary oedema or cardiogenic shock), new severe AR, uncontrolled infection, aortic root abscess, high embolic risk (vegetation >15 mm) or recurrent emboli despite antibiotics. If neurological complications from infective emboli have developed, follow guidance regarding surgery versus medical management.

### Antibiotic prophylaxis

Antibiotic prophylaxis before dental procedures is recommended for the following patients:

- Prosthetic heart valves (metallic or biological including TAVI)
- Previous IE
- Cyanotic congenital heart disease defects
- Congenital heart disease with prosthetic material

Antibiotic prophylaxis for dental treatment is a single 2 g amoxicillin or 600 mg clindamycinn dose orally 30–60 minutes before the treatment.

**Table 7.36** Management of IE

*Specific treatment*

*Look for and treat any underlying infection*
- Refer for dental assessment
- Refer for gastroenterological assessment if *Enterococcus faecalis*
- Treat abscesses

*Antibiotics*
- Give high-dose IV benzylpenicillin and gentamicin (with blood level monitoring), once the blood cultures have been taken and before the results are available, but avoid gentamicin toxicity (measure gentamicin levels frequently)
- Change antibiotics according to the results of the blood cultures and sensitivities
- Measure antibiotic levels and perform back titration against the bacteria to ensure dose is sufficient
- If the blood cultures are negative, give ampicillin instead of penicillin
- Treat *Staphylococcus* endocarditis with three anti-staphylococcal antibiotics (e.g. flucloxacillin, fusidic acid and gentamicin)

*Surgery*

The criteria for urgent surgical valve replacement are:
- Acute HF
- New severe AR
- Uncontrolled infection
- Aortic root abscess
- High embolic risk (vegetation >15 mm) or recurrent emboli despite antibiotics

7

## Prognosis

The success of treatment can be measured by early normalization of the temperature, a fall in white blood cell count and a reduction in ESR and CRP. This will be accompanied by an improvement in the patient's overall condition.

The continued high mortality of 20% associated with IE in the UK is a result of the high incidence of prosthetic valve endocarditis, endocarditis in drug addicts and antibiotic-resistant organisms.

## MYOCARDIAL DISEASES

## MYOCARDITIS

### Epidemiology

Viral myocarditis is probably underdiagnosed because evidence of a viral infection such as influenza has usually disappeared by the time cardiac symptoms develop. Many viral illnesses are associated with ECG changes suggesting cardiac involvement.

### Disease mechanisms

Infections can damage the heart by direct infection of the myocyte (e.g. viruses) producing toxins (e.g. diphtheria), or inducing immune damage. Inflammation of the myocardium identified in biopsy has many causes (**Table 7.37**; **Figure 7.43**).

**Table 7.37** Causes of inflammation of the myocardium

| Cause | Example |
|---|---|
| Viruses | Coxsackie and parvovirus B19 |
| | Influenza |
| | Mumps |
| | Epstein–Barr virus |
| | SARS2-Coronavirus (COVID19) |
| Protozoa | Trypanosomiasis (endemic in Central and South America causing Chagas' disease), *Toxoplasma gondii* |
| Bacteria | Diphtheria |
| Rickettsia | *Coxiella* (causes Q fever) |
| Autoimmune disease | Cardiac sarcoidosis |
| | Polymyositis or dermatomyositis |
| | Rheumatoid arthritis |
| | SLE |
| Radiation | |
| Cancer therapies | Acute doxorubicin toxicity |
| | Acute cyclophosphamide toxicity |
| | Immune checkpoint Inhibitors |
| Chemicals and drugs of abuse | Chloroquine |
| | Lead poisoning |
| | Methamphetamines |
| | Cocaine |

## Clinical features

Myocarditis causes rapidly progressive HF, occasionally in association with a temperature. There may be history of a previous viral infection. The patient complains of fatigue, myalgia, shortness of breath and palpitations. Clinical examination reveals the signs of HF (raised venous pressure, bilateral basal crepitations and third and fourth heart sounds).

## Investigation

- *Cardiac troponin:* usually elevated
- *BNP or NT-proBNP:* usually elevated
- *WCC:* may be normal or elevated
- *CRP:* may be normal or elevated

### Electrocardiography

ECG usually shows a tachycardia and non-specific ST waves, which are usually transient. The ECG changes sometimes mimic those of MI, with Q waves and loss of R waves in the anterior leads.

### Diagnostic imaging

- *Chest radiography:* Depending on the severity of the illness, the heart may be enlarged and the lungs may show venous congestion and alveolar oedema.
- *CMR:* This is the gold standard imaging investigation and shows elevated $T_2$STIR signal of myocardial oedema in affected myocardium. During the acute phase, late gadolinium enhancement (LGE) may be present. At follow up, some patients have persistent LGE, typically in the epicardial layers or mid wall.
- *Cardiac FDG-PET-CT:* This may show increased myocardial uptake, suggesting inflammation.

### Immunology

Viral antibody titres may be raised and should be taken in the acute and convalescent phase to identify change. However, they are not critical for making the diagnosis.

### Histology

Endomyocardial biopsy may show white cell infiltration, and possible myocardial cellular death, but is often normal. At present, there is probably no indication for routine biopsy in patients presenting with suspected myocarditis, although endomyocardial biopsy is indicated in fulminant myocarditis with cardiogenic shock to diagnose giant cell myocarditis, cardiac sarcoidosis and lymphocytic myocarditis, as these three conditions require immunosuppressive drugs (high-dose IV steroids initially). Myocarditis is also a recognized complication of the new immune checkpoint inhibitors for various cancers, and biopsy is helpful.

## Management

The treatment of myocarditis includes:
- Bed rest
- Treatment of HF with diuretics and vasodilators

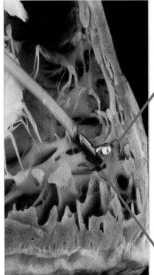
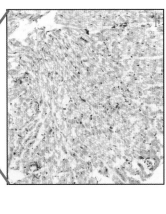

**CD45+ pos-cells: 59/mm²**

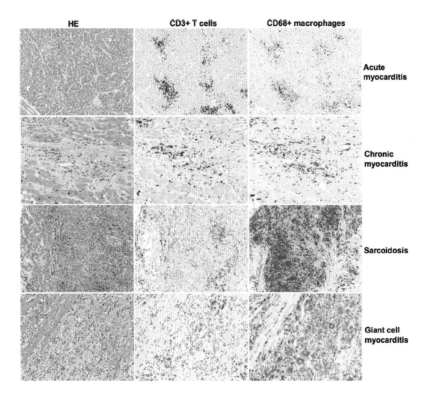

| | HE | CD3+ T cells | CD68+ macrophages | |
|---|---|---|---|---|
| | | | | Acute myocarditis |
| | | | | Chronic myocarditis |
| | | | | Sarcoidosis |
| | | | | Giant cell myocarditis |

**Figure 7.43** Causes of inflammation of the myocardium identified in biopsy.

- Treatment of arrhythmias (AF with digoxin, ventricular tachyarrhythmias with amiodarone)
- Role for beta blockers, ACE inhibitors (all routine in chemotherapy-induced myocarditis)
- Corticosteroids and other immunosuppressive drugs – not routinely but these are indicated in specific causes: giant cell myocarditis, lymphocytic myocarditis (including secondary to checkpoint inhibitors) and acute cardiac sarcoidosis

- Aciclovir or interferon, which may help if given early in the course of viral myocarditis but not routinely in all patients

**Prognosis**

There may be complete resolution and a return to normal heart muscle function. However, in the long term there is usually evidence of chronic ventricular damage, and myocarditis is a common cause of cardiomyopathy (**Figure 7.44**).

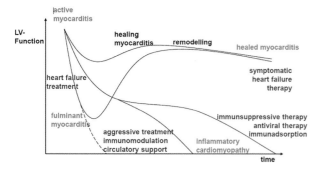

**Figure 7.44** Clinical outcomes following acute myocarditis.

# CARDIOMYOPATHY

Originally, cardiomyopathy was a term used to describe heart muscle disease of unknown cause. Cardiomyopathies are now classified according to distinctive pathological and haemodynamic parameters affecting the ventricles (**Table 7.38**). Genetic causes have now been identified for hypertrophic cardiomyopathy (sarcomeric gene mutations) and for an expanding subgroup of DCMs (e.g. ~10% have a mutation in the gene encoding the cardiac protein Titin) (**Figure 7.45**).

**Table 7.38** Causes of cardiomyopathy

| Mechanism | Condition |
|---|---|
| Dilatation | Genetic (familial) – including mutations of Titin, Laminin A3 |
| | Alcohol |
| | Myocarditis |
| | Cancer drugs |
| | Iron overload (1° haemachromatosis or 2° to multiple blood transfusions for inherited Hb disorders, e.g. thalassaemia) |
| | Uraemia |
| | Phaeochromocytoma |
| | Deficiency states such as beriberi and selenium deficiency (Keshar disease) |
| | Sarcoidosis |
| | Dermatomyositis and polymyositis |
| | Anomalous coronary arteries |
| | Idiopathic cardiomyopathy (when no cause is identified) |
| Hypertrophic | Hypertrophic cardiomyopathy with or without LV outflow tract obstruction |
| | Friedreich's ataxia |
| | Glycogen storage diseases |
| | Muscular dystrophy |
| Restrictive | Radiation |
| | Amyloidosis (AL and ATTR) |
| | Eosinophilic (Churg–Strauss syndrome) |
| | Pseudoxanthoma elasticum |
| | Carcinoid |
| | Methysergide |

- *DCM:* This is the most common and is characterized by dilatation of the ventricle with systolic malfunction. This results in a reduction of the ejection fraction from a normal 60%. An ejection fraction of less than 30% is associated with a poor prognosis.
- *Restrictive cardiomyopathy:* This is characterized by reduced ventricular filling and so there is diastolic dysfunction. The myocardium or endocardium may be involved and the ventricle does not dilate. Often there is an infiltration in the myocardium, which may be identified by myocardial biopsy (e.g. amyloidosis).
- *Hypertrophic cardiomyopathy:* This is characterized by hypertrophied myocardium, typically asymmetric septal hypertrophy (ASH), although other patterns including apical hypertrophy and severe concentric hypertrophy also occur (**Figure 7.46**). All have significant LV diastolic dysfunction predisposing to atrial arrhythmias and breathlessness.

# DILATED CARDIOMYOPATHY

## Clinical features

The symptoms and signs are those of progressive left and/or right HF. Dilatation of the annulus of both the mitral and tricuspid valves causing valve regurgitation may result from the ventricular dilatation. AF can develop and lead to systemic thromboembolism.

## Investigation

### Electrocardiography

ECG shows non-specific ST- and T-wave changes. Arrhythmias are also seen, in particular AF and ventricular tachycardias.

### Diagnostic imaging

- *Chest radiography:* shows cardiac enlargement with pulmonary venous congestion and possibly alveolar oedema
- *Echocardiography:* shows dilatation of the ventricles with poor systolic function (**Figure 7.47a**)
- *CMR:* important for confirming myocardial structure and function; the non-ischaemic mid-wall LGE can aid diagnosis (**Figure 7.47b**)
- *Cardiac catheterization:* excludes coronary artery disease and anomalies of the coronary circulation, which can be a rare cause of DCM

## Management

As for other causes of HF, bed rest, diuretics, vasodilators and antiarrhythmic drugs are indicated. Anticoagulants should be given because of the risk of systemic thromboembolism. Primary prevention ICD should be considered in patients with high risk of ventricular arrhythmias and SCD (e.g. specific genetic mutations, family history of SCD, severe LV impairment [LVEF <30%]).

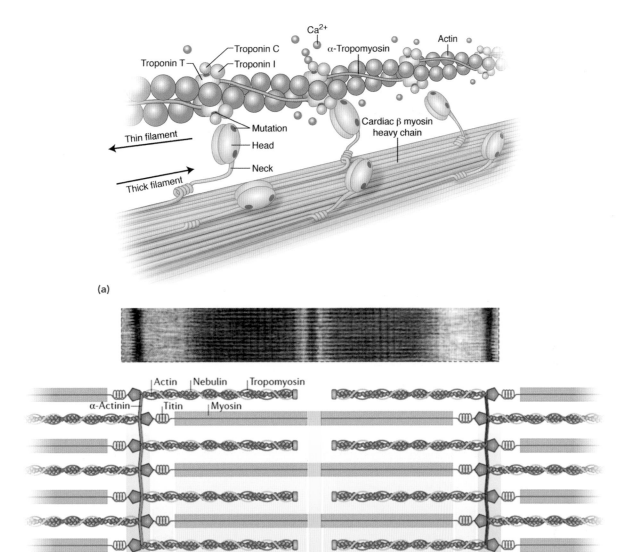

**Figure 7.45** Cardiac proteins where genetic mutations may lead to cardiomyopathy. **(a)** Myofilament proteins with mutations associated with hypertrophic cardiomyopathy. Source: https://hypertrophiccardiomyopathy.com/ **(b)** Sarcomeric proteins with mutations associated with DCM including Titin. Source: Ware and Cook *Nat Rev Cardiol* 2018 Apr;15(4):241-252.

A heart transplant should be considered for patients under 60 years of age.

## PERIPARTUM CARDIOMYOPATHY

It has long been recognized that HF can develop late in pregnancy or during the puerperium (HEART DISEASE IN PREGNANCY AT A GLANCE).

### Management

The treatment is as for a DCM, avoiding ACE inhibitors, aldosterone antagonists and ARNI in pregnant and breast-feeding women. Bromocriptine may be considered in peri-partum cardiomyopathy (PPCM) patients with cardiogenic shock.

## HYPERTROPHIC CARDIOMYOPATHY

### Epidemiology

- Hypertrophic cardiomyopathy usually presents by 30 years of age.
- A family history is common and a mutation in the sarcomeric genes (e.g. myosin heavy chain, myosin-binding protein C, troponin) is usually responsible. These genetic abnormalities are inherited in an autosomally dominant with variable penetrance.

### Disease mechanisms

Hypertrophic cardiomyopathy is characterized by sponta-neous hypertrophy of the myocardium of either the RV and/or the LV, and particularly in the septum (see **Figure 7.46**).

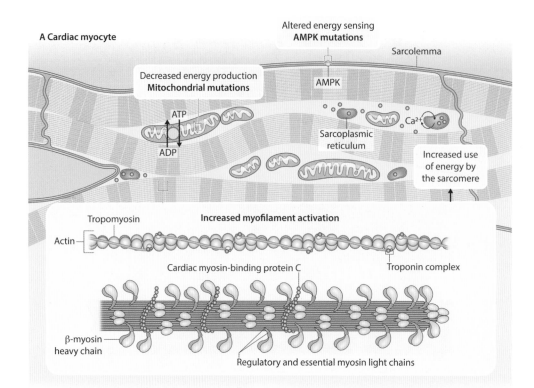

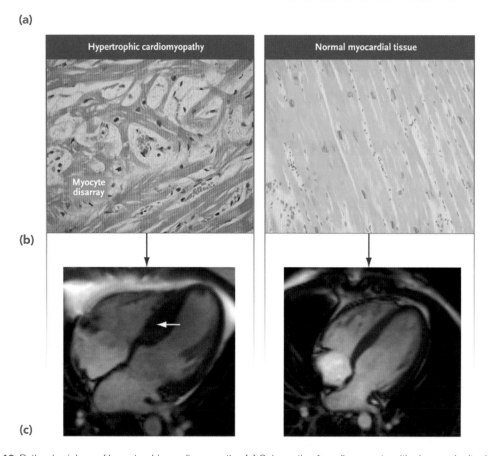

**Figure 7.46** Pathophysiology of hypertrophic cardiomyopathy. **(a)** Schematic of cardiomyocyte with abnormal mitochondrial function (mitochondrial protein mutations) leading to decreased ATP generation, altered energy store sensing (AMPK mutations) and/or increased ATP consumption by mutations in myofilament proteins leading to increased myofilament activation. **(b)** Myocyte disarray seen on endomyocardial biopsy. **(c)** ASH (white arrow) seen on CMR. Source: *NEJM*: https://www.nejm.org/doi/full/10.1056/NEJMra0902923.

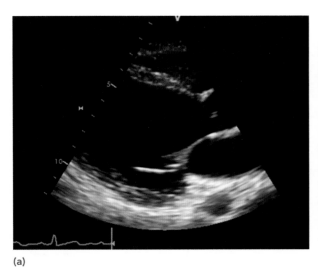

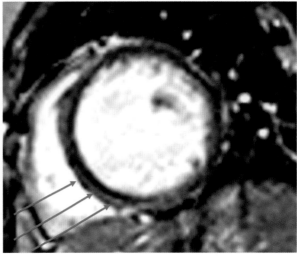

**(a)**

**(b)**

**Figure 7.47** DCM. **(a)** A parasternal long-axis echocardiographic image of DCM showing a dilated LV. **(b)** CMR with late gadolinium enhancement showing non-ischaemic mid-wall fibrosis (red arrows) in a patient with DCM.

## HEART DISEASE IN PREGNANCY AT A GLANCE

### Pregnancy may unmask asymptomatic cardiac disease

Cardiac output increases progressively during pregnancy reaching up to 50% higher than baseline at full term. This will unmask underlying heart disease (e.g. MS) and patients who are asymptomatic before pregnancy may become symptomatic with breathlessness and pulmonary oedema.

### Mortality associated with heart disease in pregnancy

5–10% of maternal deaths in England and Wales during pregnancy are brought about by heart disease.

### Indications for terminating pregnancy

Significant pulmonary hypertension of whatever cause is an indication, because the mortality associated with pregnancy in this condition is very high (40–50%).

Advanced heart disease also justifies a consideration of termination of pregnancy because of the risk to the mother.

### Anticoagulants in pregnancy

Warfarin has a teratogenic effect but this is now considered to be sufficiently small for patients to be encouraged to remain on oral anticoagulation while attempting to become pregnant. Anticoagulation during pregnancy increases the risk of placental bleeding and fetal mortality.

LMWH is the appropriate anticoagulant.

### Avoid endocarditis in patients with valvular heart disease

Bacteraemia during delivery can cause endocarditis in patients with underlying valvular heart disease. Prophylactic antibiotics are therefore required during the first stage of labour.

### Post-delivery cardiomyopathy

A rare form of cardiomyopathy can develop after delivery. It appears to be responsive to corticosteroids, sometimes with resolution of the condition.

The hypertrophy can be global, obliterating the cavity, or focal, causing ASH. The myocardial hypertrophy restricts diastolic filling of the LV. In many cases, an outflow tract gradient can develop late in systole, and this may be an important cause of symptoms. There may be associated MR.

### Clinical features

Symptoms include:
- *Syncope* or *presyncope:* often with exertion
- *Dyspnoea:* brought about by impaired filling of the LV causing dilatation of the left atrium and raised pressure in the pulmonary veins
- *Angina:* resulting from inadequate perfusion of the hypertrophied myocardium because of obstruction of blood flow from the ventricle and increased diastolic pressure inside the ventricle (reduced transcoronary gradient)
- *Cardiac arrhythmias*
- *Sudden death:* commonly caused by ventricular arrhythmias, but it can be by asystole

Signs include:
- *Sharp carotid pulse:* caused by the sudden abbreviation of systole from outflow tract obstruction
- *An a wave:* in the venous pressure pulse
- *Forceful apex beat:* not displaced and which can be 'double' because of an independent palpable fourth heart sound of atrial contraction as well as ventricular contraction
- *Fourth heart sound*
- *Systolic murmur:* caused either by MR or outflow tract obstruction (this can be altered by the Valsalva manoeuvre, which reduces venous return and ventricular filling and therefore increases outflow tract obstruction and the loudness of the murmur)

**7**

## Investigation

### Electrocardiography

- *ECG:* usually shows LVH and other repolarization abnormalities but may be normal in children
- *Holter 24- to 48-hour ECG monitoring:* may reveal atrial or ventricular arrhythmias

### Diagnostic imaging

- *Echocardiography:* This is usually diagnostic. The cardinal feature is a septal : posterior wall thickness ratio greater than 1.3 : 1. Great care must be taken to exclude the normal hypertrophy that can develop in athletes. Other characteristic echo features are a systolic anterior movement of the mitral valve, premature closure of the aortic valve because of outflow tract obstruction, and diastolic dysfunction with a characteristic dip and plateau movement to the ventricular wall in diastole.
- *CMR:* LVH with fibrosis is often seen in hypertophied segments. Microvascular ischaemia is seen on perfusion imaging.

### Histology

Histology shows disarray of the myocardial fibres, giving a whorled appearance (see **Figure 7.46**).

### Management and prognosis

Treatment can be difficult and is often ineffective. There is no clear evidence that any particular drug reduces the incidence of sudden death (**Table 7.39**).

Arterial vasodilators should be avoided because they can increase the outflow tract obstruction by reducing arterial pressure. This will also reduce the transcoronary gradient further and exacerbate angina.

**Table 7.39** Management of hypertrophic cardiomyopathy

**Specific treatment**

*Drug treatment*

- Beta blockers are indicated, particularly if there is angina or LV outflow tract obstruction (LVOTO)
- Avoid arterial vasodilators

**Options for symptomatic LV outflow tract obstruction**

*Septal myectomy surgery*

- A section of the septal myocardium is helpful (Morrow resection)
- Mitral valve replacement to reduce the outflow tract gradient
- *Percutaneous alcohol septal ablation* is an alternative
- *RV pacing*

**Treatment to prevent sudden death**

- *ICD* – indicated for patients with elevated 5-year risk of sudden cardiac death

**End-stage hypertrophic cardiomyopathy**

- Consider cardiac transplantation

**Genetic testing and family screening**

# RESTRICTIVE CARDIOMYOPATHY

## Epidemiology

- Restrictive cardiomyopathy is the rarest of the three types of cardiomyopathy.
- It is more common in countries such as in equatorial Africa where it is acquired secondary to endomyocardial disease.

## Disease mechanisms

Restrictive cardiomyopathies arise from loss of ventricular distensibility as a result of either myocardial or endocardial disease. The most common cause is endomyocardial fibrosis (EMF), which often occurs in association with eosinophilia (the hypereosinophilic syndrome). Other causes of restricted filling are amyloid disease and sarcoid. EMF usually affects both ventricular cavities, causing mitral and tricuspid regurgitation. Sometimes it can lead to the development of giant atria without the presence of mitral or tricuspid regurgitation.

### Hypereosinophilic syndrome

An eosinophil count higher than $1.5 \times 10^6$/L can cause heart disease. Such eosinophilia can be idiopathic (this is much more common in men) or secondary to parasitic infections (especially in the tropics), malignancy, Churg–Strauss type of polyarteritis nodosa, asthma and drug reactions. Thromboembolism is common.

### Cardiac amyloidosis

Amyloidosis refers to excessive deposition of protein in the extracellular matrix, leading to LV wall thickening, reduced myocardial compliance and restrictive cardiomyopathy. It is produced as either a primary condition due to deposition of the monomers of transthyretin, known as ATTR cardiac amyloidosis, or secondary to excessive light-chain deposition in patients with multiple myeloma or B-cell lymphoma known as cardiac AL amyloidosis.

## Clinical features

Shortness of breath is a predominant symptom associated with fatigue because of poor cardiac output. The elevated venous pressure on the right side gives rise to peripheral oedema, ascites and an enlarged liver, which can be painful. Signs include tachycardia, raised venous pressure with Kussmaul's sign (an increase in venous pressure on inspiration) and third and fourth heart sounds.

## Investigation

### Electrocardiography

ECG shows paradoxically small QRS complexes for the degree of LV thickening on echocardiography. Non-specific conduction changes, ST-segment and T-wave abnormalities may be present. AF is common.

### Diagnostic imaging

- *Chest radiography:* Usually there is no cardiac enlargement but left atrial dilation and pulmonary venous congestion may be present.
- *Echocardiography:* This shows restricted ventricular filling with LV and RV wall thickening and biatrial enlargement. Classically in cardiac amyloidosis the ventricular wall is thick but fails to thicken during systole. Long-axis function is reduced and may be absent in advanced cases.
- *CMR:* This is diagnostic when T1 sequences are abnormal, suggestive of raised extracellular volume (ECV). Other typical features are failure of dark blood pool suppression, increased LGE in a non-ischaemic pattern, and left atrial and/or LV thrombus may be present. It cannot differentiate cardiac AL amyloidosis from cardiac ATTR amyloidosis.
- *Cardiac $^{99m}$Tc-DPD scanning:* This is a radionuclide scan which is a very sensitive technique to detect cardiac ATTR amyloidosis.

### Blood tests

- Natriuretic peptides are always elevated, and a guide to prognosis.
- Serum immunoelectrophoresis and free kappa and lambda light chains should be measured in all patients with suspected cardiac amyloidosis.

### Histology

Endomyocardial biopsy is often indicated to establish a more precise diagnosis with positive staining for amyloid using Congo red staining in most cases.

### Management and prognosis

The treatment is as for cardiac failure and the underlying cause. If multiple myeloma and cardiac AL amyloidosis is confirmed, patients must be urgently referred to haematology and start multiple myeloma treatment, including proteasome inhibitors, which may be effective.

One specific drug, Tafamadis, has been assessed and shown to give improved survival, quality of life and slowed disease progression in ATTR amyloidosis. Systemic thromboembolism is common and anticoagulation is often required. A heart transplant may be considered.

## HF AND CV TOXICITY FROM CANCER TREATMENTS

The success and increased survival of cancer patients with modern cancer therapies has led to a large increase in the number of cancer patients with CV toxicity from their cancer treatments. The CV complications can occur early during treatment, potentially interfering with optimal cancer therapy if the treatment has to be interrupted or stopped, or following completion of cancer treatment in survivors, either in the first few years or late (>5 years after treatment).

Some treatments, including anthracycline chemotherapy and high-dose mediastinal radiotherapy for paediatric and young adults with cancers, lead to complex CV problems many (10+) years later (late CV toxicity).

The list of cancer therapies and their complications is summarized in **Table 7.40**. The increase in knowledge in this area has led to the development of the new medical field called cardio-oncology.

## PERICARDIAL DISEASES

## ACUTE PERICARDITIS

### Causes

Inflammation of the pericardium can arise from a number of causes. The most common is Coxsackie viral infection, which can occur in epidemics. Other causes include MI, uraemia, connective-tissue disorders (autoimmune rheumatic diseases), post-cardiac surgery, post-MI, trauma, tuberculosis, cancer and immune checkpoint inhibitors.

### Clinical features

The patient presents with severe substernal chest pain, which can radiate to the neck and shoulders and mimic the pain of MI. It is characteristically worse on lying flat and on inspiration, and can be relieved by sitting forward. There may be a history of a recent viral infection, and the patient may have a fever, particularly when the pericarditis is caused by infection, rheumatic fever or MI. The principal physical sign is a pericardial friction rub, which can be transitory.

### Investigation

- *ECG:* This shows characteristic concave upward ST-segment elevation, usually in all leads, rather than localized as in MI. Later, the ST segments return to normal and P-wave inversion develops, but this eventually normalizes.
- *Cardiac enzymes:* Troponin may be elevated if there is associated myocarditis (perimyocarditis).

### Management and prognosis

Bed rest is necessary, otherwise the illness can relapse. The cardinal treatment is anti-inflammatory medication with colchicine and either high-dose aspirin or ibuprofen.

## PERICARDIAL EFFUSION

### Epidemiology

Increased pericardial fluid above the normal 15–50 mL can occur with many conditions. Whether clinical symptoms develop depends on:

- Volume of fluid
- Rate of accumulation
- Response of the pericardium to the fluid

7

**Table 7.40** Cancer treatments associated with CV complications

| Treatment | Indication | CV complication |
|---|---|---|
| Anthracycline chemotherapy e.g. doxorubicin, epirubicin, idarubicin, daunorubicin | Breast cancer, lymphomas, acute leukaemias, sarcomas, paediatric solid tumours and paediatric leukaemias | • HF<br>• LV dysfunction |
| Trastuzumab (Herceptin™) | HER2+ breast cancer, HER2+ GI malignancies | • HF<br>• LV dysfunction |
| Radiotherapy to heart e.g. mediastinal radiotherapy including high-dose Mantle radiotherapy, left breast radiotherapy | Hodgkin's lymphoma with mediastinal LN Left breast cancer Paediatric cancers involving mediastinum / left chest | • Coronary disease<br>• Valvular heart disease<br>• Constrictive pericarditis<br>• HF<br>• Sick sinus syndrome<br>• Heart block<br>• Restrictive cardiomyopathy |
| VEGF tyrosine kinase inhibitors e.g. sunitinib, sorafenib, pazopanib, axitinib, cabozantanib, lenvatinib, vandetinib | Metastatic renal cancer, thyroid cancer, hepatocellular carcinoma, GIST | • Hypertension<br>• HF<br>• LV dysfunction<br>• QTc prolongation and arrhythmias<br>• Arterial thrombosis |
| BCr-Abl tyrosine kinase inhibitors e.g. ponatinib, nilotinib, dasatanib, bosutinib | Second- and third-line treatment for CML | • Accelerated atherosclerosis with MI/stroke/PVD<br>• HF<br>• LV dysfunction<br>• QTc prolongation and arrhythmias<br>• Hypertension<br>• Pulmonary hypertension<br>• Arterial thrombosis<br>• Peripheral arterial occlusive disease<br>• DVT and PE |
| Fluoropyrimidines e.g. 5-fluorouracil, capecitabine | GI malignancies, breast cancer | • Angina<br>• MI<br>• HF<br>• Cardiac arrest |
| Androgen deprivation therapies e.g. goserelin, leuprolide | Prostate cancer Metastatic ER+ breast cancer | • Diabetes<br>• Hypercholesterolaemia<br>• MI<br>• Peripheral vascular disease |
| Proteasome inhibitors e.g. carfilzomib, bortezomib | Multiple myeloma | • HF<br>• MI<br>• Ventricular arrhythmias<br>• DVT and PE |
| Bruton kinase inhibitors e.g. ibrutinib | chronic lymphocytic leukaemia | • AF<br>• Ventricular tachycardia |
| Immune checkpoint inhibitors e.g. ipilumimab, nivolumab, pembrolizumab | Metastatic melanoma, metastatic lung cancer (small cell and non-small cell), metastatic transitional cell bladder cancer, MMP-deficient cancers | • Myocarditis<br>• Pericarditis<br>• Coronary vasculitis<br>• MI<br>• Complete heart block<br>• HF |
| CDK4/6 inhibitors e.g. ribociclib | Metastatic ER+ HER2- breast cancer | • QTc prolongation |
| Raf-MEK inhibitors | Raf-mutant metastatic melanoma Raf-mutant thyroid cancer | • HF<br>• LV dysfunction |

## Disease mechanisms

Fluid can accumulate in the pericardium following:

- Viral pericarditis
- Tuberculosis
- Uraemia
- Myxoedema
- Neoplasia
- MI (Dressler's syndrome, myocardial rupture)
- Aortic dissection
- Radiotherapy
- Post-pericardiotomy (heart surgery)
- Perforation of the heart during cardiac catheterization

## Clinical features

When the pericardium cannot distend any further, ventricular filling is compromised, leading to a fall in cardiac output (*cardiac tamponade*) which is a medical emergency. The main symptom is breathlessness, but the patient may present acutely unwell, collapsed and hypotensive. Signs include a paradoxical pulse (the blood pressure falls by more than 15 mmHg during inspiration) and a raised venous pressure with a further increase on inspiration (Kussmaul's sign; normally, inspiration reduces venous pressure but increases it if there is restricted ventricular filling). The heart sounds are quiet.

## Investigation

### Electrocardiography

ECG shows reduced voltages with electrical alternans (varying amplitude of the QRS complex).

### Diagnostic imaging

- *Chest radiography:* shows cardiomegaly with a globular cardiac outline
- *Echocardiography:* identifies the pericardial effusion (**Figure 7.48**) and possible collapse of the RV in diastole if there is tamponade

## Management and prognosis

Pericardial drainage is required for tamponade. This can be carried out by direct puncture (pericardiocentesis), which can help in the diagnosis of a potentially infected pericardial effusion. Surgical drainage may be indicated for malignant pericardial effusions or when an effusion reaccumulates.

# CONSTRICTIVE PERICARDITIS

## Epidemiology

In 50% of cases the cause of constrictive pericarditis is unknown and is presumed to be a consequence of viral pericarditis. The causes of constrictive pericarditis are:

- Presumed postviral
- Post-cardiac surgery
- Post-mediastinal radiotherapy
- Chronic renal failure
- Connective-tissue disorders
- Pulmonary asbestosis
- TB

With the advent of heart surgery, constriction resulting from surgery is now recognized. Only 15% of cases in developed countries are caused by TB – although this is much more common in developing countries.

7

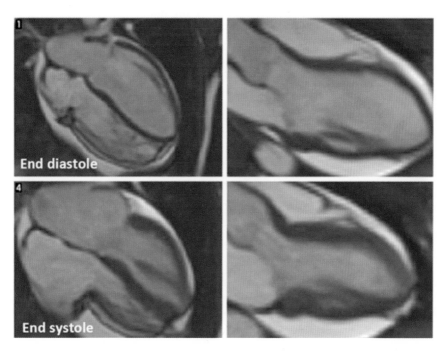

**Figure 7.48** Cardiac MRI in 4-chamber and 2-chamber views in systole and diastole showing pericardial effusion.

## Disease mechanisms

A thickened, fibrotic and calcified pericardium progressively embarrasses cardiac function, resulting in systemic venous congestion and reduced cardiac output. In developing countries, tuberculous pericarditis can present as early constriction, especially after an effusion has been drained.

## Clinical features

The patient presents with breathlessness, fatigue, dependent oedema, ascites and hepatomegaly. The physical signs are similar to those of tamponade (pulsus paradoxus and Kussmaul's sign). In addition, there may be a loud diastolic noise caused by rapid abbreviated ventricular filling (*pericardial knock*). AF is common.

## Investigation

### Diagnostic imaging

- *Chest radiography:* may show a normal-sized heart, and there may be calcification in the pericardium
- *Echocardiography:* may demonstrate thickened pericardium and restricted ventricular filling in diastole
- *CMR:* shows pericardial thickening, inflammation in some cases, and ventricular interdependence

## Management and prognosis

Surgical removal of the pericardium is possible. However, it is often difficult to separate the pericardium from the myocardium, and the perioperative mortality can therefore be as high as 10%. When the myocardium is involved in this way, symptomatic improvement is often disappointing.

## DISEASE OF THE AORTA

Aneurysms can develop in any part of the aorta.

## ABDOMINAL AORTIC ANEURYSM

- The abdomen is the most common site for aneurysm formation.
- This is the most common aortic aneurysm and routine screening by ultrasound is often recommended in people over 65 years.

## Disease mechanisms

Abdominal aortic aneurysms result from atherosclerosis but evidence of an active inflammatory process may be found.

## Clinical features

Abdominal aortic aneurysms present in one of three ways: as an asymptomatic finding on routine clinical examination, as a cause of epigastric pain or pain in the back, and a pulsatile mass found on examination, or if leaking, with acute pain, hypotension and a pulsatile mass in the abdomen.

## Investigation

### Diagnostic imaging

- *Abdominal ultrasound* and *CT angiography:* determines the size of the aneurysm and its relationship to branch vessels, particularly the renal arteries
- *Angiography:* occasionally helpful

## Management and prognosis

Treatment is by endovascular stenting or surgery with resection of the aneurysm and insertion of a dacron prosthesis. This depends on the anatomy of the aneurysm and risk of surgery. Treatment is indicated in asymptomatic patients with an aneurysm larger than 5.5–6.0 cm because of the risk of sudden rupture. The mortality rate of emergency surgery for a ruptured aneurysm is over 70%.

## THORACIC AORTIC ANEURYSM

### Disease mechanisms

Thoracic aortic aneurysms tend to arise in patients with hypertension, atherosclerosis, collagen disorders such as Marfan's syndrome, aortopathy associated with a bicuspid aortic valve, and rarely following chest trauma or syphilis.

### Clinical features

Commonly, patients are asymptomatic and the aneurysm is only revealed by a routine chest X-ray. Symptoms may result from compression of the SVC, oesophagus or bronchus. Pain may be a presenting symptom. Occasionally, patients are breathless because the aneurysm causes aortic incompetence. Very often, the first presentation is dissection, rupture and sudden death.

### Investigation

#### Diagnostic imaging

- *Cardiac ultrasound, CT aortography:* define the location, size and side branches compromised by the aneurysm
- *MR angiography:* provides valuable information for defining the extent of the aneurysm
- *Coronary angiography:* often considered to be helpful for identifying coexistent coronary artery disease, which may require coronary artery bypass grafting at the time of surgery

### Management and prognosis

Aneurysms larger than 5.0 cm are at risk of rupture and surgical reconstruction of the aorta is indicated. In collagen disorders such as Marfan's syndrome, thoracic aortic aneursyms >4.5 cm should be treated.

## AORTIC DISSECTION

### Disease mechanisms

Dissection of the aorta arises as a result of a tear in the aortic intima and is a medical emergency. The subsequent

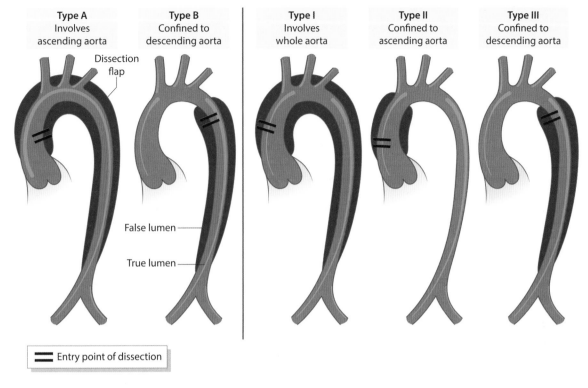

| Type A<br>Involves<br>ascending aorta | Type B<br>Confined to<br>descending aorta | | Type I<br>Involves<br>whole aorta | Type II<br>Confined to<br>ascending aorta | Type III<br>Confined to<br>descending aorta |

Dissection flap

False lumen

True lumen

≡ Entry point of dissection

**Figure 7.49** The two classification systems for dissection of the aorta.

dissecting haematoma can extend retrogradely towards the aortic valve. This can lead to acute AR and/or to the development of cardiac tamponade from blood leaking into the pericardium. The dissection can also extend progradely into the abdominal aorta and iliac vessels, and lead to avulsion of spinal and/or renal arteries. The dissection can occur in aortic aneurysms and in aortas of previously normal size.

Classically, thoracic aortic aneurysms are subdivided into those in the ascending aorta (type A) and those confined solely to the descending aorta (type B) (**Figure 7.49**).

The main risk factors for aortic dissection are hypertension, Marfan's syndrome, pregnancy, a bicuspid aortic valve and atherosclerotic disease (although the transmural nature of atherosclerosis is sometimes considered to protect against dissection).

### Clinical features

The patient presents with acute chest pain often radiating through to the back. If there is extravascular bleeding into either the pleura or pericardium, the patient will be shocked, with a low blood pressure and tachycardia.

About 50% of patients lose peripheral pulses because the dissection occludes a branch artery. This can include the spinal arteries, so patients can present with paraplegia. There may be AR if the dissection dislocates the aortic valve ring or MI if it involves a coronary orifice.

### Investigation

#### Diagnostic imaging
- *Chest radiography:* shows a widened mediastinum

- *Echocardiography:* may visualize on transthoracic and, if stable, TOE is required; also assess for pericardial effusion, AMI and tamponade
- *CT angiography:* confirms the diagnosis and extent of the dissection
- *MR angiography (if clinically stable):* helpful in defining the extent of the dissection and the site of the intimal tear

### Management and prognosis

All patients presenting with acute aortic dissection (types A and B) should be discussed with the acute aortic surgical service. Initial medical treatment involves controlling the blood pressure, aiming for a systolic pressure of less than 110 mmHg, provided that the urine output is maintained using IV labetalol, nitroprusside and/or nitrates.

#### Type A dissections
Emergency surgery is required to prevent cardiac tamponade. The risks of surgery are great, with a perioperative mortality of more than 20%, but mortality risk increases with every hour from presentation.

#### Type B dissections
The risk of paraplegia is high, and so attempts to stabilize the dissection with conservative treatment using hypotensive drugs are the preferred option. Endovascular stenting may be suitable depending upon anatomy. If type B dissections are managed conservatively at first, an aneurysm may subsequently develop requiring elective surgery or endovascular treatment later.

7

## CARDIAC TUMOURS

Cardiac tumours are rare. The different types are listed in **Table 7.41** and **Table 7.42**. The majority are secondary deposits involving the pericardium and occasionally the myocardium. Metastatic masses are 20–30 times more common than primary cardiac tumours. Benign primary tumours are 10 times more common than malignant primary cardiac tumours.

**Table 7.41** Types and relative incidence of benign cardiac tumours

| Tumour | Relative incidence (%) |
| --- | --- |
| Myxoma | 30 |
| Papillary fibroelastoma | 30 |
| Lipoma | 10 |
| Rhabdomyoma | 8.5 |
| Fibroma | 4 |
| Haemangioma | 3.5 |
| Other | 14 |

**Table 7.42** Types and relative incidence of malignant cardiac tumours

| Tumour | Relative incidence (%) |
| --- | --- |
| Angiosarcoma | 10 |
| Rhabdomyosarcoma | 6 |
| Fibrosarcoma | 3.5 |
| Malignant lymphoma | 1.5 |
| Other | 79 |

## EMERGENCY CARDIAC RESUSCITATION

### EMERGENCY PRESENTATION 7.1

#### Cardiac resuscitation

All doctors should be able to perform efficient basic life support (BLS), the objective of which is to provide oxygen to vital organs (brain, heart) until spontaneous effective ventilation and circulation can be restored by definitive medical treatment (advanced cardiac life support). In England and Wales, more than 100 000/year sudden deaths occur in the community alone. Most of these deaths will be the result of ischaemic heart disease, and the preterminal arrhythmia in over 80% of these cases will be VF. Studies from Seattle, where many of the local community can perform effective BLS, have shown that two factors determine survival when a patient collapses in the community with VF:

- The time elapsed before BLS is begun
- The time elapsed before defibrillation (advanced cardiac life support)

Early intervention with BLS can therefore help to save lives.

#### Basic life support

When confronted with a person who has suddenly collapsed, or on arriving at a scene where someone is unresponsive, the natural tendency is to panic. Panic can be minimized, and the chances of successful resuscitation maximized, if the ABC of resuscitation is adhered to:

- *Assessment and Airway*
- *Breathing*
- *Circulation*

*Assessment*

Assess the scene to ensure that you are not placing yourself in physical danger while caring for the patient. Minimize or remove any potential further risk to yourself and instruct someone to call for help.

Approach the patient and establish whether they are responsive by shouting 'Are you all right?', and gently shaking them by the shoulders, preventing movement of the head (**Figure A**). Responsive but obtunded/lethargic patients should be gently rolled over into the recovery position (**Figure B**), care being taken not to exacerbate any injuries. With unresponsive patients, shout for help and then attend to the airway.

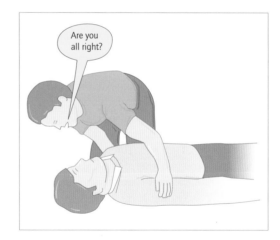

**Figure A** Approach the unconscious patient

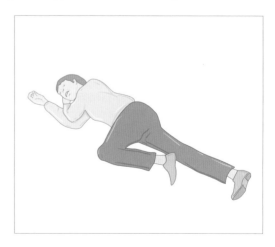

**Figure B** The recovery position

*Airway*

The mouth and oropharynx and should be cleared of any obvious foreign bodies, such as vomit or dislodged teeth, by sweeping an index finger around the oral cavity (**Figure C**). Excess vomit should be allowed to drain from the mouth by turning the patient onto their side.

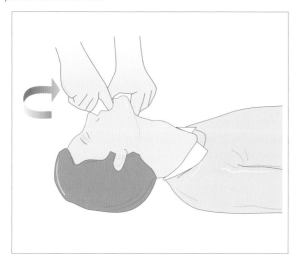

**Figure C** Clearing the mouth and oropharynx

Foreign bodies which are impacted can often be dislodged by the Heimlich manoeuvre (**Figure D**). Kneeling astride the patient, a fist is placed in the epigastrium, with the other hand on top of the fist. Both hands are then thrust up beneath the costal margin in an attempt to raise the intrathoracic pressure suddenly, and thereby expel foreign bodies obstructing the upper airway.

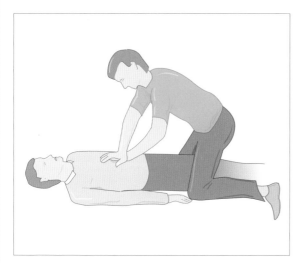

**Figure D** The Heimlich manoeuvre

When obstructions have been cleared, airway patency should be maintained by head tilt and the 'chin lift' manoeuvre (**Figure E**). In the unconscious supine patient, the tongue tends to flop back and obstruct the pharynx, and these two manoeuvres are designed to combat this (**Figure F**).

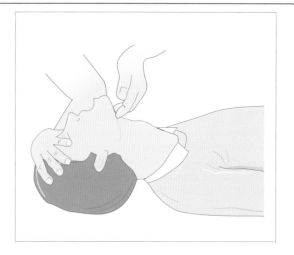

**Figure E** The 'chin lift' manoeuvre

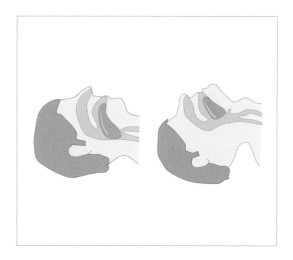

**Figure F** Avoiding obstruction of the pharynx by the tongue

*Breathing*

Having assessed and maintained the airway, evidence of spontaneous respiration should be sought. Place your cheek and ear over the patient's nose and mouth while watching the chest (**Figure G**).

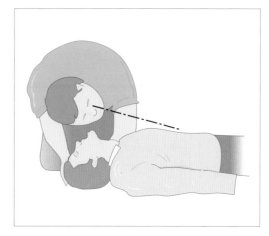

**Figure G** Checking for spontaneous expiration

7

Look for chest wall movements, listen and feel for exhalations. This can be very difficult to do in some circumstances (e.g. beside a busy road in the dark).

If you are unsure that there are spontaneous respirations, assume that there are not. Having cleared and maintained the airway, and assessed breathing, the circulation should be assessed.

*Circulation*

Feel for the carotid pulse (**Figure H**). Pulse pressure may be low, so allow 5–6 seconds to ascertain whether it is present or not.

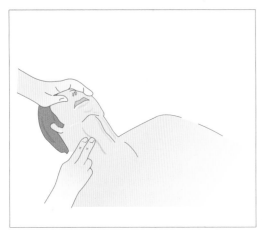

**Figure H** Checking the carotid pulse

**Action**

The sequence of resuscitation depends upon your assessment of the patient's Airway, Breathing and Circulation. **Figure I** summarizes the suggested sequence. Note the importance of telephoning for help. It is essential to obtain a defibrillator as quickly as possible.

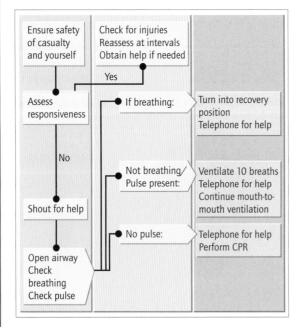

**Figure I** The sequence of resuscitation

*Cardiopulmonary resuscitation*

The absence of breathing necessitates artificial ventilation with mouth-to-mouth exhalations.

With one hand performing the chin lift, the other hand pinches the nose and maintains slight extension of the neck by gentle pressure on the forehead. Take a deep breath and apply your lips firmly around those of the patient, creating an airtight seal. Breathe out, observing the chest for movement.

Begin with two slow breaths, allowing the chest to deflate in between. If the chest does not rise, ventilation is inadequate, and you will need to adjust your technique and try again. If your technique is good and the chest still does not rise, perform the Heimlich manoeuvre, as the upper airway is likely to be obstructed.

In the absence of a pulse, external cardiac compression is necessary. Strict adherence to technique during this procedure allows maximum efficiency.

Feel for the xiphoid sternum. Place the heel of one hand two fingers' breadth above this point in the midline (**Figure J**). Place the heel of the other hand on the dorsum of the first and interlock the fingers (**Figure K**).

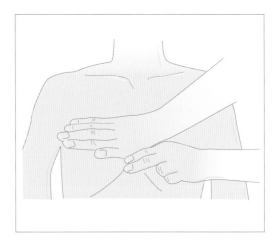

**Figure J** Hand positioning for cardiopulmonary resuscitation (CPR)

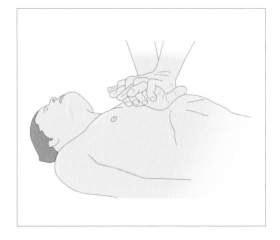

**Figure K** Interlocking of fingers for CPR

Keeping your elbows firmly extended, position your shoulders directly over your hands so that the weight of your body, and not flexion/extension at the elbow, produces the compressions (**Figure L**).

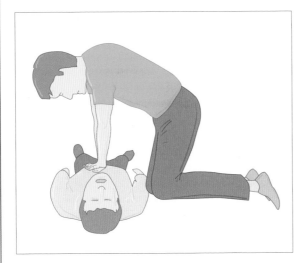

**Figure L** Position for compression in CPR

With a gentle rocking motion, depress the sternum 4–5 cm in a rhythmical fashion, counting 'one and two and three' for a total of 15 compressions. Then ventilate again with two breaths, followed by a further 15 compressions (**Figure M**). Continue with this method until help arrives. (The rate of compressions should be 60–80/min.)

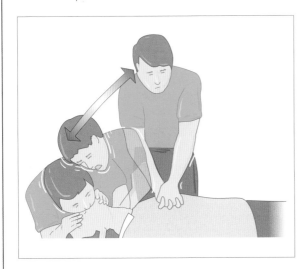

**Figure M** Use a sequence of 15 compressions followed by two ventilations in CPR

If two people are available (**Figure N**), the recommended sequence is one ventilation to every five compressions. The aesthetics of mouth-to-mouth resuscitation can be improved by an airway adjunct, such as a pocket face mask, as long as an adequate flow rate is achievable. Such devices will also protect against disease transmission. There have been no documented cases of HIV transmission following mouth-to-mouth ventilation.

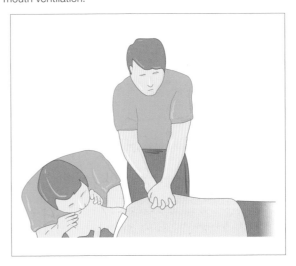

**Figure N** CPR with two people

*The precordial thump*

This manoeuvre should be employed only for witnessed or monitored arrests.

## Advanced cardiac life support (Figure O)

Sudden cardiac arrests may be precipitated by one of the following arrhythmias.

- VF/pulseless ventricular tachycardias are responsible for 80% of arrests and have the best prognosis.
- Asystole is responsible for 12–15% of arrests and has a poor prognosis.
- Electromechanical dissociation is responsible for less than 5% of arrests. It is diagnosed when the monitor shows a good quality ECG trace but there is no output.

*Priorities of management*

Continue BLS at all times. At no time should it be interrupted for more than 30 seconds, and then only to allow intubation.

Connect the patient to a monitor, and defibrillate immediately if VF is present.

Intubate and hyperventilate with 100% oxygen. Hyperventilation attempts to correct the acidosis.

Cannulate a large central vein; if this is not possible, a large peripheral vein. If venous access is impossible, the endotracheal route for drug administration may be used. Administer adrenaline 1 mg every 2–3 min.

Treat individual arrhythmias following the revised guidelines of the Resuscitation Council UK, as shown in **Figure 7.32**.

*Specific therapy*

*Tension pneumothorax:* If the patient has signs of a pneumothorax, insert a cannula into the second intercostal space to relieve any tension. Beware of the intubated patient who seems to be under ventilating the left chest. This is most likely to be caused by the passage of the tube into the right main bronchus.

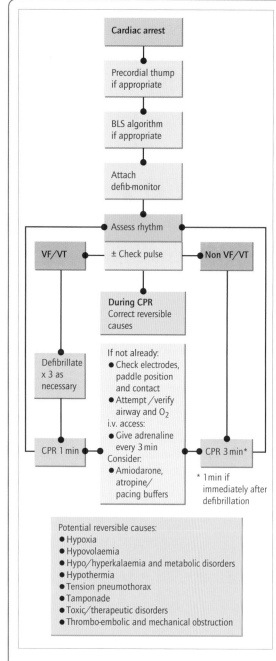

**Figure O** Advanced cardiac life support

*Hypovolaemia*: if this is suspected, continue BLS, give a 2 L fluid bolus, cross-match 10 units of blood and call the surgeon. Occult massive haemorrhage is the usual cause from either a leaking aortic aneurysm or an upper GI lesion.

*Cardiac tamponade*: In the absence of trauma, this condition is uncommon. However, it can present acutely when associated with pericardial disease or dissection of the aorta. It should be considered in any patient with electromechanical dissociation who has full neck veins and in whom a tension pneumothorax has been excluded. Relief of the tamponade can buy valuable time while waiting for definitive intervention. Using a wide-bore needle attached to a 60 mL syringe, insert the needle just to the left of the xiphisternum at an angle of 30° to the skin, aspirating as you proceed. Aim the tip of the needle towards the tip of the left shoulder. When blood flushes back, aspirate 100 mL; if tamponade is present, this should lead to a clinical improvement.

*Pulmonary embolus*: Without a thoracotomy, this situation is rapidly fatal. However, an external cardiac massage may help to fragment the embolus so that it moves more peripherally and therefore does not produce such a profound effect.

*Recommended adult drug doses:*

- *Adrenaline (epinephrine)*: 10 mL of 1 : 10000 (1 mg) or 1 mL of 1 : 1000
- *Atropine*: 1 mg
- *Lidocaine*: 100 mg (up to a total of 3 mg/kg)
- *Calcium chloride*: 10 mL of 10% solution
- *Sodium bicarbonate:* 50 mL of 8.4% solution
- *Bretylium tosilate*: 500 mg
- *Amiodarone*: 5 mg/kg IV

### Post-resuscitation care

All patients should be managed in a high-dependency unit. Correct:

- Hypoxia
- Acid-base disturbance
- Electrolyte imbalance

Monitor all vital functions, including urine output. Perform:

- Chest X-ray to check position of endotracheal tube and central venous pressure lines, and to exclude a pneumothorax
- ECG for signs of acute ischaemia, MI, etc.
- Continuing monitoring for arrhythmias

### MUST-KNOW CHECKLIST

- Diagnosis of cardiac pain
- Diagnosis of HF
- Interpretation of an ECG
- Causes of increased plasma troponin
- Management of cardiac resuscitation
- Management of cardiac emergencies

- Management of acute chest pain
- Management of acute HF
- Management of chronic HF
- Management of acute arrhythmia
- Identification of heart murmurs
- Diagnosis of endocarditis

**Questions and answers** to test your understanding of Chapter 7 can be found by clicking 'Support Material' at the following link: https://www.routledge.com/Medicine-for-Finals-and-Beyond/Axford-OCallaghan/p/book/9780367150594

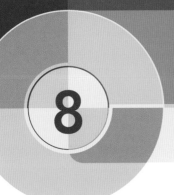

# Renal Disease; Fluid and Electrolyte Disorders

**8**

CHRIS O'CALLAGHAN

## RENAL DISEASE

### INTRODUCTION

The kidneys have multiple functions and are central to some of the most common medical conditions, including urinary tract infection, hypertension and the oedema caused by heart failure or liver disease. Kidneys are vulnerable to injury from certain drugs or inadequate hydration, and kidney function declines with age. In developed countries, there is a rising prevalence of around 1 in 1000 patients on renal replacement therapy (dialysis or transplantation). These patients have increased morbidity and mortality and their care is expensive. A key priority is to prevent avoidable kidney disease.

## STRUCTURE AND FUNCTION

There are two kidneys behind the peritoneum at the back of the upper abdomen. The right kidney lies below the liver and so is lower than the left kidney. The outer layer of the kidney is the *renal cortex* and the inner layer is the *renal medulla* (**Figure 8.1**). During development, kidneys form in the pelvis and move upwards. Sometimes one or both kidneys can remain in the pelvis. If both remain in the pelvis, they may fuse together to form a horseshoe kidney.

The kidney has many nephrons which each contain a glomerulus, tubules and blood vessels. Urine is formed in the *glomerulus* by filtration and modified along the *tubules* by the reabsorption and secretion of solutes and of water. Blood enters glomeruli from afferent arterioles and leaves

DOI: 10.1201/9781003193616-8

via efferent arterioles to flow around the tubules and then out of the kidney. Influences including hormones and neural input act on the nephron to regulate kidney function.

Key functions of the kidneys include (**Figure 8.2**):

- *Regulation* of body fluid ion content, acid–base balance and volume
- *Excretion* of unwanted compounds, ions, acid and water
- *Production of erythropoietin:* which promotes red blood cell formation
- *Production of vitamin D:* which influences calcium and bone metabolism

- *Production of renin:* which influences sodium and blood pressure

The kidney responds to:

- *Angiotensin II and aldosterone:* each promotes sodium retention
- *Vasopressin (antidiuretic hormone [ADH]):* promotes water retention
- *Parathyroid hormone (PTH):* promotes calcium reabsorption and phosphate excretion
- *Natriuretic peptides:* promote some sodium excretion

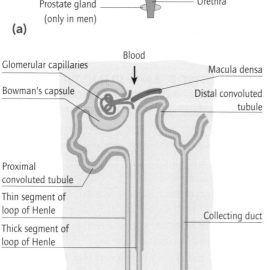

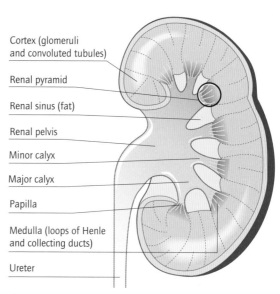

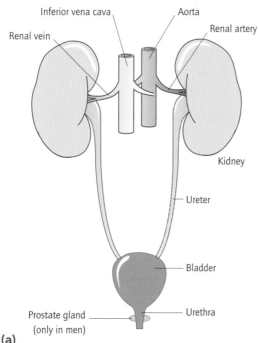

**Figure 8.1** Renal structure and function. **(a)** Overview of the renal and urinary system. **(b)** Section through a whole kidney. **(c)** A nephron. *(Continued)*

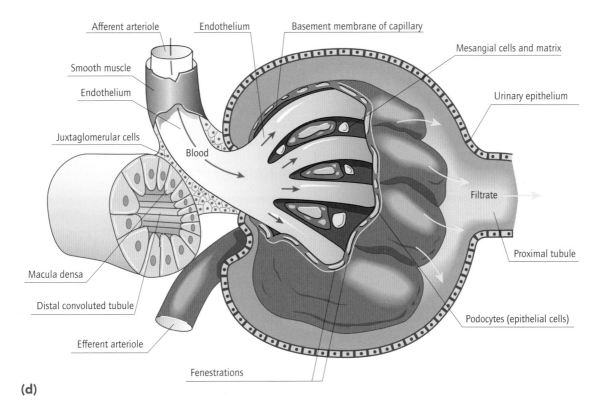

Figure 8.1 *(Continued)* **(d)** A glomerulus.

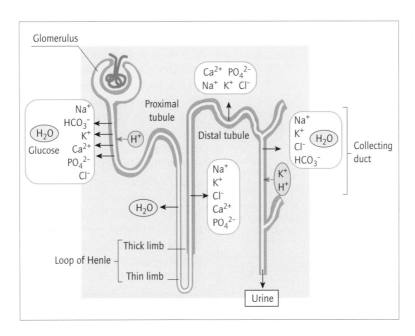

**Figure 8.2** Overview of nephron function. The figure shows in schematic form the key ion movements along the nephron. Most reabsorption of water and electrolytes is performed in the proximal tubule. Urine is concentrated in the loop of Henle and then final adjustment of urine composition occurs in the distal tubule and collecting ducts.

# APPROACH TO THE PATIENT

Kidney disease can occur without any symptoms or signs, so investigation of possible renal disease must include the biochemical tests of kidney function.

---

## HISTORY & EXAMINATION 8.1

### Kidney disease

#### Symptoms of kidney disease

*Changes in urine*

Is your urine ever discoloured, red or frothy?
Have you ever seen blood in your urine?
Have you ever passed a stone or any gravel?
Is your urine offensive smelling?

*Changes in micturition*

How often do you pass urine at night? During the day?
Do you pass urine more frequently than previously?
Do you pass normal amounts of urine?
Do you pass urine when you don't mean to?
Is it difficult to start or stop the flow of urine?
Does the urine come out in a normal stream or is the flow poor?
Do you have any pain, burning or discomfort when you pass urine?

*Salt and water retention*

Have your ankles or legs been swollen?
Have you noticed any shortness of breath? If so, is it worse when you lie flat?

*Uraemia*

Do you feel tired or weak?
Do you have difficulty sleeping?
Have you had any itching, muscle cramps or headaches?
Have you noticed any pins and needles, or numbness of your hands and feet?

*Pain*

Do you have loin pain or pain in the back, abdomen, pelvis or genitals?
When do you get this pain?
How severe is the pain, what is it like?
Does it go anywhere else?

#### General questions

Do you have any other symptoms such as painful joints, a rash, eye problems, cough?
Have you travelled or lived abroad? If so, where?

#### Drug history

Have you taken any medications either prescribed by a doctor or otherwise?
Have you taken painkillers, particularly non-steroidal anti-inflammatory drugs (NSAIDs) such as ibuprofen or indomethacin?

#### Past medical history

Have you ever had an operation or been in hospital. If so, what for?
Do you have any other medical condition?
Are you diabetic?
Do you have high blood pressure?
Have you had any recent infections or a sore throat?

#### Family history

Does anyone in your family have kidney problems, kidney stones or high blood pressure or deafness?

---

## HISTORY

### PAIN

Renal pain is uncommon but it can occur with renal obstruction or inflammation (usually resulting from infection). Urinary tract stones can cause referred pain from the loin down to the external genitalia.

### URINARY SYMPTOMS

Infection of the bladder can cause discomfort or burning on micturition, increased urinary frequency and offensive-smelling urine. Upper tract infection can cause loin pain, fever and rigors. Prostatic disease can result in a poor urinary stream, hesitancy, terminal dribbling and urinary frequency. Incontinence can arise for mechanical reasons or as a result of neuromuscular instability. Polyuria is an increase in total daily urine volume and is usually associated with a defect in the mechanism for controlling water excretion or with excess water intake.

### URINE APPEARANCE

Haematuria is the presence of blood in the urine and, when severe, may be visible as frank haematuria. Causes include renal stones, glomerulonephritis and urinary tract tumours. Frothy urine suggests a high protein content. Dark urine can occur with myoglobinuria because of muscle damage in rhabdomyolysis or haemoglobinuria when there is haemolysis.

## EXAMINATION

Check for signs of systemic disease, such as joint problems or neurological abnormalities. Cardiac valve lesions may suggest glomerulonephritis associated with infective endocarditis. Hypertension is common in renal disease, so it is important to measure the blood pressure properly (see Chapter 7, Cardiovascular disease). Vascular *bruits* may indicate vascular disease, which could also affect the renal arteries. Examine the kidneys by *bimanual palpation*. From the patient's left side, the right hand is placed over the upper abdomen on one side and the left hand is placed in the renal angle on the same side. The *renal angle* is formed by the 12th rib and the lumbar muscles. As the patient inspires, the left hand pushes into the renal angle and an enlarged kidney may be felt by the right hand as the kidney moves down the abdomen during inspiration and the left hand pushes it anteriorly (HISTORY & EXAMINATION 8.2; **Figure 8.3**).

## INVESTIGATION

### BEDSIDE TESTS

Urine should be dipstick tested for *protein, blood* and *glucose*. *Nitrites* and *leucocytes* may indicate infection.

## HISTORY & EXAMINATION 8.2

### Examination of a patient with renal disease

**General appearance**

Does the patient look well?
Does the patient look dehydrated or oedematous?
Do they have an unusual fishy smell (can occur in severe uraemia)?
Do they have a twitch, tremor or flap (check with the arms out-stretched and wrists extended)?
Is there any lymphadenopathy?

**Look at the skin**

Look for any rashes, purpura, jaundice
Does the patient look pale or anaemic?
Are there any wounds, pressure sores or ulcers? If so, inspect them for signs of infection

**Look at the eyes**

Look for signs of anaemia or jaundice
Look at the fundi, especially for hypertensive or diabetic changes

**Cardiovascular system**

Look for oedema
Feel the pulses
Measure the blood pressure
Listen for new murmurs or a pericardial rub
Listen for bruits (femoral, carotid, abdominal)

**Respiratory system**

Assess the breathing pattern. Is it laboured or rapid?
Listen to the chest for pulmonary oedema or other changes
Is the patient more breathless on lying flat?

**Abdomen**

Examine for enlarged or tender kidneys
Examine for a palpable bladder
Examine for hepatosplenomegaly
Inspect the external genitalia for congenital abnormalities (e.g. hypospadias, phimosis) and testicular inflammation or tumour
Palpate the prostate in men
Consider the need for a vaginal examination in women if pelvic disease is suspected

**Joints**

Examine for evidence of arthropathy

**Nervous system**

Examine for evidence of peripheral neuropathy, focal neuro-logical deficit and level of consciousness

**Urine**

Test the urine with a dipstick for protein and blood
Examine the urine under a microscope

## MICROSCOPY

See **Figure 8.4**.
- *Red cells:* indicate bleeding
- *White cells:* indicate inflammation, usually infection or interstitial nephritis
- *Casts:* form in the nephron and are cylindrical, usually containing protein, cells and sometimes lipid:
  - *Red cell casts* indicate glomerular bleeding and so glomerulonephritis

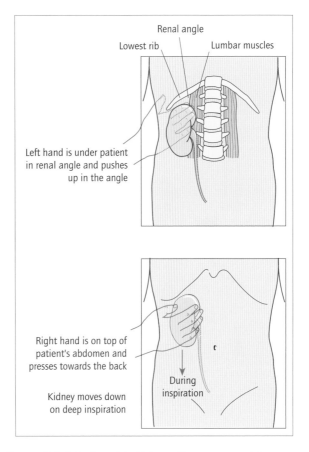

**Figure 8.3** Palpation of the kidneys. The upper panel shows the position of the left hand when palpating the right kidney. The lower panel shows the position of the right hand. On deep inspiration, the left hand pushes up in the renal angle and the kidney can be felt moving down by the right hand. The procedure is similar for the left kidney and the left hand is placed under the patient from the left side of the patient.

  - *White cell casts* usually indicate infection
  - Some non-cellular casts such as granular casts can be normal findings
- *Crystals:* can form after urine has been collected but, in fresh urine, can suggest a stone-forming tendency

## TESTS OF RENAL FUNCTION

*Urea* and *creatinine* are excreted by the kidney, so their blood levels rise if kidney function is impaired. As there is excess renal excretory capacity, the concentrations do not rise until there is a very substantial loss of renal function (**Figure 8.5**). Urea is a product of protein metabolism and urea levels rise after a protein meal. Glomerular filtration rate (GFR) can be assessed by calculating *creatinine clearance* using plasma and urinary creatinine concentration and urine volume, but this is inaccurate if the urine collection is not complete. Usually, an estimated GFR (eGFR) is calculated from the patient's blood creatinine, age, gender and ethnicity.

## RENAL DISEASE: CLINICAL FEATURES AT A GLANCE

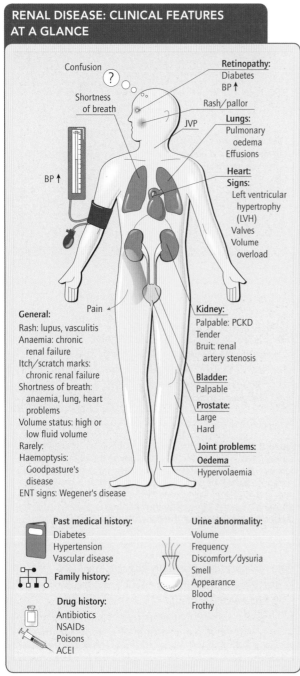

Confusion

?

Retinopathy:
Diabetes
BP ↑

Shortness
of breath

Rash/pallor

JVP

Lungs:
Pulmonary
oedema
Effusions

BP ↑

Heart:
Signs:
Left ventricular
hypertrophy
(LVH)
Valves
Volume
overload

Pain

Kidney:
Palpable: PCKD
Tender
Bruit: renal
artery stenosis

General:
Rash: lupus, vasculitis
Anaemia: chronic
  renal failure
Itch/scratch marks:
  chronic renal failure
Shortness of breath:
  anaemia, lung, heart
  problems
Volume status: high or
  low fluid volume
Rarely:
Haemoptysis:
  Goodpasture's
  disease
ENT signs: Wegener's disease

Bladder:
Palpable

Prostate:
Large
Hard

Joint problems:
Oedema
Hypervolaemia

Past medical history:
Diabetes
Hypertension
Vascular disease

Family history:

Drug history:
Antibiotics
NSAIDs
Poisons
ACEI

Urine abnormality:
Volume
Frequency
Discomfort/dysuria
Smell
Appearance
Blood
Frothy

## PROTEINURIA

Normally, only a very small amount of protein (<0.1 g/24 hours) is excreted in the urine but with renal damage, especially to the glomeruli, this can increase substantially. This can be quantified by measuring the amount of protein in a 24-hour urine collection, but it is more convenient to assess

**Figure 8.4** Appearances on phase contrast microscopy of red cells seen in urine: **(a)** dysmorphic red blood cells of glomerular bleeding; **(b)** non-dysmorphic red blood cells of lower urinary tract bleeding; **(c)** cellular casts; and **(d)** granular cast. Reproduced from Becker GJ *et al.* (1992) *Clinical Nephrology in Medical Practice* (Wiley-Blackwell, Oxford), with the permission of the authors.

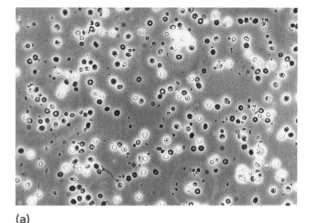

(a)

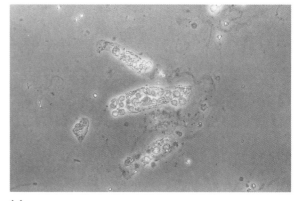

(b)

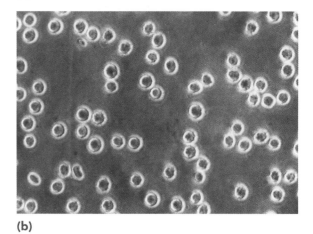

(c)

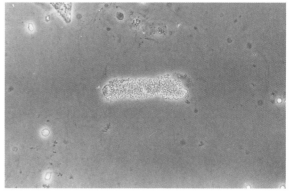

(d)

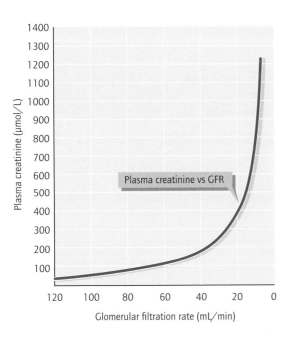

**Figure 8.5** Graph of plasma creatinine vs GFR.

the ratio of protein : creatinine in a single, random urine sample. Albumin can be measured accurately and albumin : creatinine ratios are widely used to assess for kidney damage. Microalbuminuria is the excretion of very low levels of albumin in the urine and is a sensitive test for renal damage.

## SPECIFIC DIAGNOSTIC BLOOD TESTS

Relevant tests can include:
- Antiglomerular basement membrane antibodies, which occur in Goodpasture's disease
- Antineutrophil cytoplasmic antibodies, which occur in systemic vasculitis
- Low complement levels and anti-double-stranded DNA (dsDNA) antibodies, which occur in systemic lupus erythematosus (SLE)
- A monoclonal band or free light chains, which can occur in myeloma
- A high creatinine kinase level indicates rhabdomyolysis

## ARTERIAL BLOOD GASES

Arterial blood gas analysis may be necessary to establish the patient's acid–base status. The kidney normally excretes acid, so kidney disease can lead to a metabolic acidosis.

## IMAGING

- *Ultrasound scanning:* Scans can assess kidney size and morphology, as well as obstruction and stones (**Figure 8.6**).
- *Computerized tomography (CT) and magnetic resonance (MR)* (**Figure 8.7**): These can provide detailed information and, with appropriate contrast, vessels can be studied.

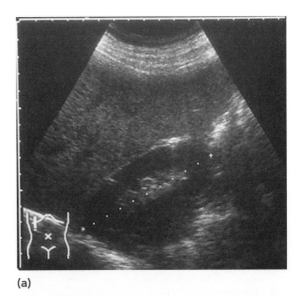

(a)

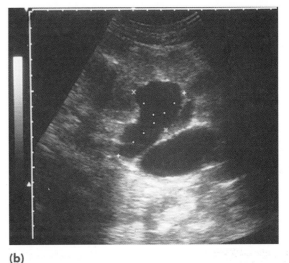

(b)

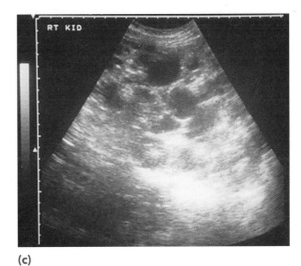

(c)

**Figure 8.6** Ultrasounds of the kidney. **(a)** Normal. The length of kidney is marked by a dotted white line. **(b)** Obstructed. The dilated pelvicalyceal system appears black. **(c)** Polycystic kidney. Cysts of different sizes are scattered throughout the kidney substance.

**8**

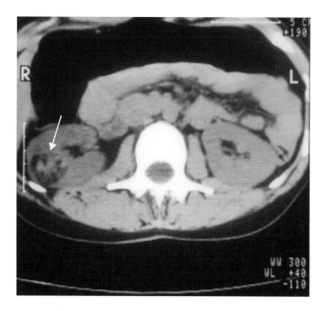

**Figure 8.7** CT scan of the kidney. A CT scan showing an angiomyolipoma in right kidney. Note the characteristic feature of fat within the lesion. This appears black (compare with subcutaneous fat in same picture).

## NUCLEAR TESTS

Radioactive markers can be injected and then the radioactivity in the kidney tracked over time to provide information about kidney function.

- $^{99M}$Tc-*DTPA* (diethylenetriamine penta-acetic acid): can provide information about renal blood flow and obstruction (**Figure 8.8**)
- $^{99M}$Tc-*DMSA* (dimercaptosuccinic acid): can provide information about the function in each kidney and its localization within the kidneys

## RENAL BIOPSY

This is the key test in many renal diseases (**Figure 8.9**). The appearances of a normal renal biopsy on light microscopy are shown in **Figure 8.10**.

# RENAL DISEASES AND THEIR MANAGEMENT

## GLOMERULAR DISEASE

### OVERVIEW AND CLASSIFICATION OF GLOMERULAR DISEASE

The effects of glomerular damage are relatively similar whatever the cause:

- Reduced glomerular filtration causing a rise in creatinine
- Proteinuria
- Haematuria

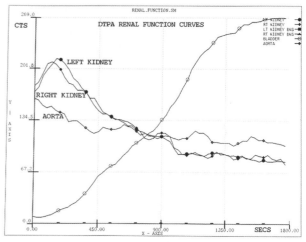

**(a)**

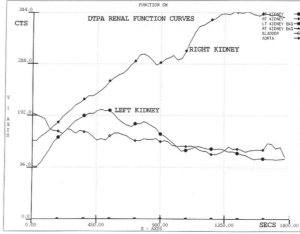

**(b)**

**Figure 8.8** Isotope renogram of kidney (Tc-DTPA). **(a)** Normal. A sharp peak of activity on the graph is followed by a rapid fall as isotope is cleared from the kidneys. **(b)** Obstruction of the right kidney. There is a continued rise of the right kidney graph as isotope is progressively trapped in the dilated kidney's collecting system.

- Hypertension
- Sodium retention causing oedema

The clinical results of glomerular disease can cause several different clinical syndromes:

- Asymptomatic haematuria or proteinuria
- Nephritic syndrome
- Nephrotic syndrome
- Chronic slowly progressive renal damage
- Acute rapidly progressive renal damage

Glomerular disease can be classified according to the clinical syndrome produced, the histopathological appearance or the underlying disease. Glomerular disease is *primary* if there is no other system affected and *secondary* if there is another system affected (the renal disease is considered secondary to the systemic condition). The glomerulus consists of the glomerular basement membrane, the glomerular

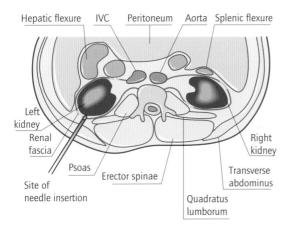

**Figure 8.9** Percutaneous renal biopsy. To perform a renal biopsy a needle is placed through the skin into the kidney using imaging guidance, usually by ultrasound. This procedure is usually only performed in specialist renal units as it carries a significant risk of life-threatening bleeding. Under local anaesthesia, a biopsy needle is passed through the back into the kidney and a core of kidney tissue is removed for histological examination, usually with immunostaining and sometimes electron microscopy.

cells, the intraglomerular blood vessels and the mesangium (the supporting connective tissue). Glomerular disease can affect one or more of these components.

## COMMON CLINICAL PRESENTATIONS OF GLOMERULAR DISEASE

These are listed in **Table 8.1**.

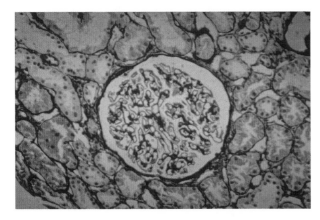

**Figure 8.10** A normal renal biopsy. A section of normal kidney viewed through a light microscope. The large circular structure in the centre is a glomerulus, which contains glomerular capillary loops. Around these loops is Bowman's space, which is the space into which the filtrate passes. Outside the glomerulus are multiple smaller roundish structures, which represent cross-sections of different types of renal tubules. These tubules are lined by pink tubular epithelial cells and the nuclei of these cells have stained dark purple. The tissue section has been stained with a silver stain which makes basement membranes a blue colour.

**Table 8.1** Common clinical presentations of glomerular disease

| Presentation | Condition to consider |
|---|---|
| A young person with nephrotic syndrome and no other disease | Minimal change nephropathy |
| A young person, typically male, with recurrent intermittent frank haematuria and hypertension or renal impairment | IgA nephropathy |
| An older person with nephrotic syndrome | Membranous nephropathy |
| A young man with haemoptysis and renal failure | Goodpasture's disease |
| A recent sore throat and renal disease | Postinfective glomerulonephritis (post-streptococcal if the infection is streptococcal) |
| A young woman with joint pains, rashes, neurological or psychiatric problems and renal disease | Glomerulonephritis secondary to SLE |
| Asymptomatic routine blood test showing blood and protein | Glomerular disease |

## NEPHROTIC SYNDROME

- Heavy urine protein loss (e.g. 5 g/day)
- Low plasma albumin levels (e.g. 20 g/L)
- Oedema
- Hypercholesterolaemia

Damage to the glomerular filtration barrier causes heavy proteinuria, which lowers blood albumin. Along with this, the kidney retains sodium and water and peripheral oedema develops. The nephrotic syndrome causes high lipid levels and predisposes the patient to venous thrombosis and infection, which are important complications. The underlying cause may be identified by renal biopsy and causes include:

- Minimal change nephropathy
- Focal segmental glomerulosclerosis (FSGS)
- Membranous nephropathy
- Amyloidosis
- Diabetes mellitus
- Drugs (e.g. non-steroidal anti-inflammatories, pencillamine)
- Systemic lupus erythematous (SLE)

### Treatment

The underlying glomerular disease is treated if possible. Diuretics help to control the oedema and lipid-lowering drugs are used for hypercholesterolaemia. In severe cases, anticoagulation is used to prevent venous thrombosis.

## NEPHRITIC SYNDROME

Acute aggressive inflammation in the glomeruli can cause:

- Hypertension
- Urine abnormalities: haematuria, red cell casts and proteinuria
- Oedema, caused by sodium and water retention
- Acute kidney injury (AKI) with reduced urine output and raised creatinine levels

Glomerular damage causes leakage of blood and protein into the urine. The damage also impairs kidney function so that urine output falls and creatinine rises. Renal inflammation provokes the release of substances such as renin, triggering angiotensin II and aldosterone production, which promote high blood pressure, sodium and water retention and oedema. Causes include:

- Diffuse proliferative glomerulonephritis, which is often a postinfective glomerulonephritis
- IgA nephropathy
- SLE
- Crescentic glomerulonephritis
- Systemic vasculitis
- Cryoglobulinaemia

### Treatment

This involves treatment of the underlying glomerular disease. Blood pressure should be controlled and diuretics can improve the oedema. Renal replacement therapy may be necessary if the renal impairment is severe. Antibiotics are given in postinfective glomerulonephritis to ensure that the infection is eradicated.

## PRIMARY GLOMERULAR DISEASE

### Minimal change nephropathy

*Epidemiology*

- The incidence is 2 per 100 000.
- It peaks in children, but all ages can be affected.

*Disease mechanisms*

Damage to the glomerular filtration barrier causes a protein leak and the nephrotic syndrome. Light microscopy and immunofluorescence are normal. Electron microscopy shows glomerular epithelial *podocyte foot process fusion* (**Figure 8.11**). The cause is unknown, but it can occur with SLE or use of NSAIDs.

*Clinical features*

- Nephrotic syndrome
- Frothy urine
- Oedema, which is often facial in children

*Investigation*

- High urine protein content
- High urine protein : creatinine or albumin : creatinine ratios
- Creatinine and eGFR are usually normal

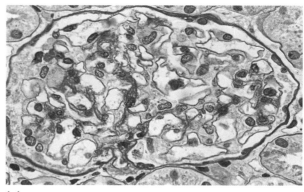

**(a)**

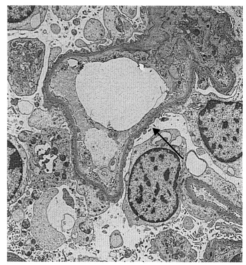

**(b)**

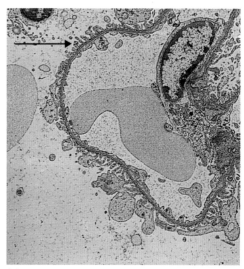

**(c)**

**Figure 8.11** Minimal change nephropathy. **(a)** The appearance on light microscopy is normal. Reproduced from Kincaid-Smith P & Whitworth JA (1987) *The Kidney: A Clinico-pathological Study*, 2nd edn (Wiley-Blackwell, Oxford), with the permission of the authors. **(b)** The appearance on electron microscopy shows the characteristic fusion of the foot processes. Compare with **(c)** an electron micrograph of a normal kidney.

- Low albumin; high lipids
- A biopsy is done in adults, but children are usually treated with a trial of steroids without a biopsy

## Management
- Steroids usually reverse the nephrotic syndrome, but it may relapse when they are stopped and cyclophosphamide or ciclosporin may be used.
- Diuretics are used for the oedema.
- Statins are used for hypercholesterolaemia.

## Prognosis and complications
- Most people respond to steroids, but relapse is common in adults.
- The main complications are thrombosis, including renal vein thrombosis, and infection.

## Focal segmental glomerulosclerosis
### Epidemiology
FSGS accounts for 15% of adult nephrotic syndrome.

### Disease mechanisms
This is similar to minimal change nephropathy, but can additionally cause kidney failure with a raised creatinine.

### Clinical features
- Proteinuria
- Nephrotic syndrome
- Hypertension
- Chronic kidney disease (CKD)

### Investigation
- Blood and protein are found in the urine.
- There may be hypoalbuminaemia and renal impairment with a raised creatinine.
- Renal biopsy is necessary to make the diagnosis.

### Management
- Steroids are now thought to be of benefit and cyclophosphamide or ciclosporin may be added to reduce the steroid dose.
- Blood pressure should be controlled.
- Angiotensin-converting enzyme (ACE) inhibitors help control blood pressure and have an antiproteinuric effect.

### Prognosis and complications
- The prognosis is not good and 40–60% develop end-stage renal disease within 10 years of diagnosis.
- The nephrotic syndrome remits in up to 40% of both adults and children in response to steroids.

## Membranous nephropathy
### Epidemiology
This is a common cause of adult nephrotic syndrome in the UK.

### Disease mechanisms
Most cases are idiopathic, but there are disease associations with hepatitis B, malignancy, SLE, mercury exposure and drugs, such as gold and penicillamine.

### Clinical features
Clinical presentation may include:
- Nephrotic syndrome
- CKD
- Hypertension
- Asymptomatic microscopic proteinuria or haematuria.

### Investigation
- Protein is found in the urine, often with blood.
- There may be hypoalbuminaemia and renal impairment with a raised creatinine.
- Renal biopsy is necessary to make the diagnosis.

### Management
- Treatment is with steroids and chlorambucil or cyclophosphamide or rituximab.
- Blood pressure should be controlled.

### Prognosis and complications
The prognosis is not good, and 30–50% of cases develop progressive kidney failure.

## IgA nephropathy
### Epidemiology
- IgA is a relatively common form of glomerulonephritis with a prevalence of 2 per 10 000.
- Peak incidence is in the second and third decades.
- More men than women are affected.

### Disease mechanisms
Deposition of IgA in the kidney occurs and is associated with inflammation and proliferation of mesangial cells (see **Figures 8.12** and **8.13**). There are associations with liver disease.

### Clinical features
The classic clinical presentation is with 'synpharyngitic' haematuria, which is macroscopic haematuria at the same time as, or 1–2 days after, a sore throat. Other features include asymptomatic microscopic haematuria, hypertension, renal impairment, the nephrotic syndrome and nephritic syndrome.

### Investigation
- There is often blood in the urine and there may also be protein.
- Blood creatinine may be raised and serum IgA levels are often elevated.
- A definitive diagnosis can only be made by renal biopsy (see **Figure 8.13**).

**8**

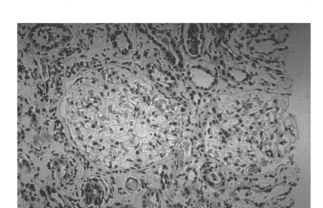

**Figure 8.12** Light microscopy of IgA nephropathy. Two glomeruli are seen in this section of tissue which has been stained with haematoxylin and eosin. The increased amount of mesangial matrix is visible as bright pink material in the glomeruli. There is also an increase in the number of mesangial cells in the glomeruli.

### Management

- ACE inhibitors are used to control blood pressure and steroids may be given for severe persistent nephrotic syndrome.
- Aggressive disease with crescent formation is treated with steroids and cyclophosphamide.

### Prognosis and complications

The prognosis is highly variable, ranging from remission to rapid progression to end-stage renal disease. Overall, 15% of patients develop end-stage renal disease by 10 years and 20–30% by 20 years.

## Membranoproliferative or mesangiocapillary glomerulonephritis

### Epidemiology

Incidence is declining in developed countries.

### Disease mechanisms

This may be idiopathic but there are associations with cryoglobulinaemia (which can be due to hepatitis C, SLE, complement deficiency syndromes and partial lipodystrophy).

### Clinical features

Clinical presentation can vary from asymptomatic haematuria or proteinuria to acute nephritis or severe nephrotic syndrome.

### Investigation

- There is blood and protein in the urine.
- Blood tests can indicate renal impairment, hypoalbuminaemia and low complement levels, especially C3.
- Renal biopsy provides a definitive diagnosis.

### Management

- Treatment must involve the treatment of any underlying cause.
- Blood pressure should be controlled.

### Prognosis and complications

- 50% develop end-stage renal disease by 10 years and 90% by 20 years.
- Complications include those of the nephrotic syndrome or of CKD if present.

## Diffuse proliferative glomerulonephritis

### Epidemiology

- Declining in developing countries
- Peaks in childhood

### Disease mechanisms

This can be idiopathic, secondary to infection (typically poststreptococcal infection) or associated with another condition such as IgA nephropathy or SLE.

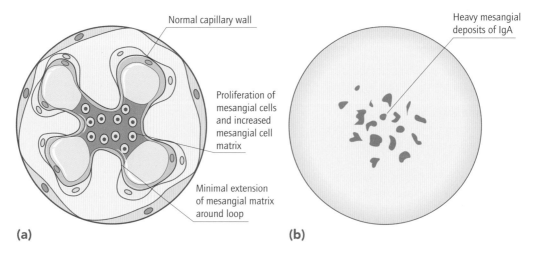

(a)                                              (b)

Normal capillary wall

Proliferation of mesangial cells and increased mesangial cell matrix

Minimal extension of mesangial matrix around loop

Heavy mesangial deposits of IgA

**Figure 8.13** IgA nephropathy. **(a)** Light microscopy. A schematic view of the changes seen in IgA nephropathy. **(b)** Immunostaining. This is the pattern of IgA deposition that would be seen in the glomerulus shown in **(a)**.

*Clinical features*

- Clinical presentation is typically 1–2 weeks after a streptococcal throat infection or 3–6 weeks after a streptococcal skin infection.
- Presentations vary from asymptomatic microscopic haematuria to acute nephritic syndrome.

*Investigation*

- There is blood in the urine in all cases and sometimes protein.
- Red cell casts are common.
- Blood creatinine may be elevated.
- There may also be serological evidence of infection such as raised antistreptolysin O titres (ASOT), which indicate streptococcal infection.
- Complement levels, especially C3, may be low.

*Management*

- Treatment is with antibiotics to ensure infection is eradicated.
- Blood pressure should be controlled and oedema treated with diuretics.

*Prognosis and complications*

- The prognosis is good as only 0.1–1% have progressive renal impairment.
- Complications include those of any ongoing infection or of uncontrolled oedema or hypertension.

## Antiglomerular basement membrane disease

### Epidemiology

The condition is rare, affecting only 0.5–1 per million, most of whom are White and male.

### Disease mechanisms

Autoantibodies to the alpha-3 component of type IV collagen in the basement membrane in the glomeruli and in the alveoli can cause damage to the kidneys and lungs.

### Clinical features

- Lung haemorrhage can cause cough, haemoptysis or shortness of breath.
- Renal involvement is initially asymptomatic but can cause loin pain, frank haematuria, oliguria and severe AKI.
- Respiratory signs may resemble those of pulmonary oedema or infection.

### Investigation

- Urine can contain blood, protein and red cell casts.
- Blood tests typically indicate AKI with raised creatinine levels.
- The key test is the detection of antiglomerular basement membrane antibodies in plasma.
- Radiologically, diffuse pulmonary haemorrhage may resemble pulmonary oedema or infection.
- Lung function tests may show an artefactual rise in gas transfer (KCO) due to absorption of carbon monoxide used in the test by blood that has leaked into the alveoli.

*Differential diagnosis*

- Systemic vasculitis
- Another glomerulonephritis with pulmonary oedema
- Pulmonary infection

*Management*

- Treatment is with plasma exchange to remove the pathogenic antibody and immunosuppression with steroids and cyclophosphamide to inhibit further antibody production and reduce inflammatory damage.
- Azathioprine may be substituted for cyclophosphamide in the later stages of treatment.

*Prognosis and complications*

- Untreated, most patients will die. Patients treated early may recover renal function, but others may not.
- Complications include respiratory failure, pulmonary infection and toxicity from the treatment, especially infection or bone marrow suppression.

## Crescentic glomerulonephritis (rapidly progressive glomerulonephritis, focal necrotizing glomerulonephritis or renal microscopic polyangiitis)

### Epidemiology

This is rare, affecting men more than women.

### Disease mechanisms

Causes are usually:

- Antiglomerular basement membrane antibodies
- Renal vasculitis, often but not always in the presence of systemic vasculitis
- A complication of a pre-existing glomerulonephritis, a systemic disorder or an infection

### Clinical features

- The condition may be asymptomatic or present with oliguria or extrarenal manifestations of associated systemic diseases including fever, weight loss and general malaise.
- Physical signs include manifestations of systemic disease, such as fatigue, malaise, rashes, eye or joint lesions.

### Investigation

- Urine can contain blood, protein and red cell casts.
- Blood tests typically indicate AKI with raised creatinine levels. Inflammatory markers, such as C-reactive protein (CRP), white cell and platelets may be raised.
- Immunological tests including antinuclear antibody (ANA), antineutrophil cytoplasmic antibody (ANCA) and antiglomerular basement membrane antibody may indicate a cause.
- Renal biopsy is undertaken to make the diagnosis.

**8**

**Table 8.2** Disease associations

| Disease | Association |
|---|---|
| Hepatitis B | Membranous nephropathy |
| | Mesangiocapillary glomerulonephritis |
| | IgA nephropathy |
| | Vasculitis |
| Hepatitis C | Mesangiocapillary glomerulonephritis |
| | Cryoglobulinaemia |
| HIV | Focal segmental glomerulosclerosis |
| Epstein–Barr virus | Microscopic haematuria and proteinuria |
| Streptococcal infection | Poststreptococcal glomerulonephritis (diffuse proliferative glomerulonephritis) |
| Staphylococcal infection (endocarditis, shunt infections, general sepsis) | Diffuse proliferative glomerulonephritis or focal segmental proliferative glomerulonephritis |
| Tuberculosis | Amyloidosis |
| Leprosy | Amyloidosis |
| | Diffuse proliferative glomerulonephritis |
| | Mesangiocapillary glomerulonephritis |
| Syphilis | Nephrotic syndrome, usually caused by membranous nephropathy |
| E. coli and other enteric infections | Haemolytic–uraemic syndrome |
| Leptospirosis | Acute tubulo-interstitial nephritis |
| Malaria | Acute kidney injury (blackwater fever) |
| | Glomerulonephritis and the nephrotic syndrome |

*Management and complications*
- Treatment is with immunosuppression, initially with prednisolone and cyclophosphamide or rituximab, but later azathioprine may be substituted for the cyclophosphamide. See above for treatment of antiglomerular basement membrane antibody disease.
- Complications include those of immunosuppression and of AKI.

## SECONDARY GLOMERULAR DISEASE

Glomerular disease can be secondary to many conditions such as diabetes mellitus (see Chapter 11, Diabetes mellitus, obesity, lipoprotein disorders and other metabolic diseases), hypertension, SLE, rheumatoid arthritis, systemic vasculitis (see Chapter 4, Rheumatic disease). Most patterns of glomerulonephritis can occur with cancer and may improve with treatment of the malignancy. Many patterns of glomerulonephritis can occur with infection (**Table 8.2**). Chronic infection or other causes of chronic inflammation can result in AA amyloid, which can cause CKD.

## TUBULO-INTERSTITIAL DISEASE

The differences between glomerulonephritis and tubulo-interstitial disease are summarized in **Table 8.3**. Diseases of the tubules and surrounding interstitium may present as:
- AKI
- CKD
- Abnormalities of tubular function
- Proteinuria

- Pyuria (pus in the urine)
- Haematuria

## ACUTE INTERSTITIAL NEPHRITIS

### Epidemiology

It accounts for up to 10% of acute kidney failure.

### Disease mechanisms

This is caused by an acute infiltration of inflammatory cells into the interstitium of the kidney and is often triggered by a drug or infectious agent. **Table 8.4** lists common causes.

### Clinical features

- Typically, there is AKI and flank pain may be present.
- Non-renal manifestations can include a maculopapular rash, fever, arthralgia and eosinophilia.

**Table 8.3** Differences between glomerulonephritis and interstitial nephritis

| Feature | Glomerulonephritis | Interstitial nephritis |
|---|---|---|
| Proteinuria | Usually >1 g/day | Usually <1 g/day |
| Hypertension | Usually present | Usually absent |
| Urinary deposit | Casts, red blood cells, pyuria | Pyuria, white cell casts |
| Renal biopsy | Glomeruli primarily affected | Glomeruli spared |

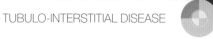

**Table 8.4** Causes of acute interstitial nephritis

| Antimicrobial agent | NSAID | Infection | Systemic disease | Other |
|---|---|---|---|---|
| Benzylpenicillin | Aspirin | HIV | Sarcoid | Phenytoin |
| Ampicillin | Naproxen | Hanta virus | SLE | Frusemide |
| Amoxicillin | Indomethacin | | Sjögren's syndrome | Allopurinol |
| Ciprofloxacin | Diclofenac | | | Cimetidine |
| Methicillin | Ibuprofen | | | Omeprazole |
| Sulphonamides | | | | |
| Co-trimoxazole | | | | |
| Rifampicin | | | | |

HIV, human immunodeficiency virus; NSAID, non-steroidal anti-inflammatory drug; SLE, systemic lupus erythematosus.

## Investigation

- There may be proteinuria and white cells or eosinophils in the urine.
- The blood eosinophil count may be raised.
- Renal biopsy confirms the diagnosis.

## Management

- If possible, the underlying cause should be removed.
- Idiopathic forms may respond to steroid therapy.
- The patient may need dialysis for severe AKI.

## Prognosis

Acute interstitial nephritis usually resolves but, if severe, may result in scarring with long-term kidney damage.

# CHRONIC INTERSTITIAL NEPHRITIS

## Epidemiology

Chronic interstitial nephritis is rare, but causes up to 10% of end-stage renal disease.

## Disease mechanisms

Chronic infiltration of the kidney with inflammatory cells can cause tubular atrophy, interstitial fibrosis and long-term renal damage. **Table 8.5** lists recognized causes.

## Clinical features

- There is usually low-level non-nephrotic range proteinuria with a variable degree of renal impairment.

- Damage to tubular function can result in a urinary concentrating defect, producing a dilute urine. There may also be other abnormalities of tubular function such as glycosuria, phosphaturia and bicarbonaturia (which causes renal tubular acidosis).

## Investigation

- Imaging of the kidneys can reveal macroscopic abnormalities such as papillary necrosis (see below) or obstructive nephropathy.
- Diagnosis is by renal biopsy.

## Management

The cause must be removed or treated.

## Prognosis and complications

In chronic interstitial nephritis there is, by definition, irreversible structural damage and scarring, but treatment of the cause may slow progression. *Papillary necrosis* (necrosis of the renal papillae) can arise particularly with drugs (notably the analgesic phenacetin, which is no longer available), sickle cell anaemia and infection (especially in diabetes mellitus or in combination with urinary tract obstruction). Imaging may reveal papillary damage.

# ABNORMALITIES OF TUBULAR FUNCTION

Tubular dysfunction can be caused by a single gene disorder or a disease causing more general structural damage (**Table 8.6**). Fanconi's syndrome describes loss of multiple

**8**

**Table 8.5** Causes of chronic tubulo-interstitial nephritis

| Drugs | Toxins | Systemic diseases | Other |
|---|---|---|---|
| Proton pump inhibitors | Lead | Sarcoid | Obstructive nephropathy |
| NSAIDs | Mercury | SLE | Ischaemic nephritis |
| Analgesics | Cadmium | Tuberculosis | Myeloma |
| Lithium | Other heavy metals | Sjögren's syndrome | Urate nephropathy |
| Ciclosporin | Solvents | Sickle cell disease | Radiation nephritis |
| Cisplatinum | Aristolochic acid (Balkan nephropathy) | | Chronic hypokalaemia |
| Aminoglycosides | | | |

**Table 8.6** Tubular syndromes

| Defect | Comment |
|---|---|
| **Proximal tubule** | |
| Aminoaciduria | Cystinuria (amino acids only): defective amino acid reabsorption causes excess urinary cystine which can form renal calculi |
| Renal glycosuria | Defective glucose reabsorption causing glucosuria with a normal plasma glucose |
| Phosphaturia | e.g. hypophosphataemic rickets |
| Bicarbonaturia | Defective bicarbonate reabsorption causing renal tubular acidosis |
| Chloride leak | Part of Bartter's syndrome |
| Multiple abnormalities | Fanconi's syndrome (defective proximal tubular reabsorption of multiple substances causing glycosuria, phosphaturia and bicarbonaturia) |
| **Distal tubule** | |
| Nephrogenic diabetes insipidus | Impaired water reabsorption resulting from defects in collecting ducts |
| Sodium-wasting nephropathy | e.g. chronic interstitial nephritis and any cause of interstitial damage |
| Bicarbonaturia | Defective bicarbonate reabsorption causing renal tubular acidosis |

substances from the proximal tubules, such as amino acids, glucose, phosphate, bicarbonate, sodium, potassium, calcium and water. It can be caused by genetic defects, chronic tubulo-interstitial disease or tubular toxins.

## SYSTEMIC DISEASES AFFECTING THE KIDNEY

### DIABETES MELLITUS

See also Chapter 11, Diabetes mellitus, obesity, lipoprotein disorders and other metabolic diseases.

#### Epidemiology

Diabetic nephropathy is responsible for 30–50% of patients with end-stage renal disease in developed countries. Type 2 diabetes mellitus is the fastest-growing cause of patients entering dialysis programmes.

#### Disease mechanisms

Diabetic nephropathy is clinically first detectable as albuminuria but can progress to end-stage renal disease.

#### Clinical features

- Hypertension is an early feature and accelerates the progression of renal failure.
- Salt and water retention may be marked and can cause oedema.

#### Investigation

- Renal biopsy is not usually necessary unless there is diagnostic uncertainty.
- Ultrasound can be used to check kidney size, bladder emptying and exclude obstruction.

#### Management

- Strategies to prevent or delay the development and progression of diabetic nephropathy include good glycaemic control and good blood pressure control.

- ACE inhibitors inhibitors or angiotensin II receptor antagonists have additional benefits to other antihypertensive agents in reducing proteinuria and slowing the progression of diabetic nephropathy.
- Control of cardiovascular risk factors is important.

#### Prognosis and complications

People with diabetes mellitus have a poorer prognosis on dialysis or after transplantation than non-diabetics because of the vascular disease and diabetic complications that they also suffer (see Chapter 11, Diabetes mellitus, obesity, lipoprotein disorders and other metabolic diseases).

### SYSTEMIC LUPUS ERYTHEMATOSUS

#### Epidemiology

The kidneys are affected in 35–75% of people with SLE.

#### Disease mechanisms

Renal disease in SLE (see Chapter 4, Rheumatic disease) can vary from mild to severe and the types of renal disease include:
- *Class 1:* minimal change nephropathy with normal light microscopy
- *Class 2:* mesangial changes
- *Class 3:* focal proliferative glomerulonephritis
- *Class 4:* diffuse proliferative glomerulonephritis
- *Class 5:* membranous glomerulonephritis
- *Class 6:* advanced sclerosing

#### Clinical features

- Renal disease in SLE can present as asymptomatic proteinuria, haematuria, nephrotic syndrome, acute nephritic syndrome or more slowly progressive chronic renal failure.
- Other features of the systemic disease are often present, such as skin rashes, joint disease or neurological or psychiatric disturbances.

### Investigation

- Blood, protein and red cell casts can occur in the urine.
- Renal biopsy is required to determine the type of glomerulonephritis and appropriate treatment.

### Management

Treatment depends on the type of the glomerulonephrits and clinical course.

- Steroids are often given in combination with a cytotoxic such as mycophenolate or cyclophosphamide.
- Plasma exchange is sometimes used for rapidly progressive glomerulonephritis.

### Prognosis and complications

These depend on the type of glomerulonephritis, which can change over time.

## MYELOMA

### Disease mechanisms

Renal manifestations of myeloma include:

- *Hypercalcaemia*
- *Myeloma kidney (or cast nephropathy):* Casts containing antibody light chain form in the tubules and provoke tubulo-interstitial damage.
- *Light chain deposition disease:* Antibody light chains deposit in the glomeruli and tubular walls.
- *Renal amyloid* (see below): There can be antibody light chains deposition in amyloid fibrils.

### Clinical features

- The usual presentation is with the features of myeloma such as bone pain or with renal impairment.
- The light chain deposition disease or renal amyloid may present with the nephrotic syndrome.

### Management and prognosis

- The treatment is that of the underlying myeloma plus supportive therapy (e.g. fluids or dialysis) as necessary.
- The prognosis of myeloma is worsened by the presence of renal disease.

## AMYLOIDOSIS

### Disease mechanisms

In amyloidosis there is extracellular deposition of protein fibrils in many organs (see Chapter 11, Diabetes mellitus, obesity, lipoprotein disorders and other metabolic diseases), including the kidney in up to 80% of patients. The fibrils contain antibody light chains in AL amyloidosis associated with myeloma or a paraproteinaemia (see Chapter 15, Haematological disease) or the acute phase reactant protein serum amyloid A protein in AA amyloidosis associated with chronic inflammatory disease.

### Clinical features

- Proteinuria is common and 25% of patients have nephrotic syndrome.
- Other systems such as the heart, liver and nerves may also be affected by amyloid deposition.

### Investigation

Biopsy of an affected organ such as the kidney demonstrates amyloid fibrils stains positively with Congo red stain.

### Management and prognosis

- Any primary or secondary cause should be treated.
- The renal prognosis is poor and the majority progress to end-stage renal failure.

## SYSTEMIC SCLEROSIS

Systemic sclerosis is characterized by progressive fibrosis (see Chapter 4, Rheumatic disease). Renal involvement can cause proteinuria and hypertension, a slow decline in renal function or, sometimes, a rapid decline in renal function with accelerated hypertension. Such a 'scleroderma renal crisis' is thought to result from renal arterial narrowing causing decreased renal perfusion and stimulating renin and subsequently angiotensin II production which with hypertension promotes renal vessel wall thickening, vasoconstriction and ischaemia.

Treatment with ACE inhibitors is used to reduce the likelihood of a renal crisis.

## SICKLE CELL DISEASE

### Disease mechanisms

In sickle cell disease, hypoxia promotes sickling of the red blood cells (see Chapter 15, Haematological disease) which can cause ischaemia, resulting in:

- Minor tubular dysfunction
- Tubulo-interstitial nephritis
- Papillary necrosis
- Frank haematuria
- Glomerular scarring, FSGS and proteinuria

### Clinical features

- Tubulo-interstitial nephritis can cause tubular dysfunction and urinary concentrating defects and so electrolyte or fluid balance abnormalities.
- The glomerulonephritis can cause nephrotic syndrome.
- End-stage renal disease can arise.

### Management

Good medical care to limit the number of sickling crises will reduce renal damage.

### Prognosis

End-stage renal disease occurs in 25% of people with homozygous sickle cell disease by 40 years of age.

**8**

## HAEMOLYTIC–URAEMIC SYNDROME

### Disease mechanisms

Most cases arise in children. Most patients have had a preceding diarrhoeal illness, and the toxin-producing *Escherichia coli* strain 0157 is a recognized cause.

### Clinical features

The characteristic triad is of:
- Intravascular haemolysis causing anaemia
- Thrombocytopenia
- AKI

### Investigation

- A blood film will show fragmented red cells, characteristic of a haemolytic anaemia and thrombocytopenia.
- There may be disseminated intravascular coagulation with raised fibrin degradation products, and a prolonged prothrombin time (PT) and activated partial thromboplastin time (APTT) are common.
- Renal biopsy demonstrates characteristic changes.

### Management and prognosis

- In children, the condition usually remits spontaneously; many affected adults require dialysis.
- Plasma exchange, intravenous (IV) methylprednisolone and fresh frozen plasma have been used in adults, but their benefit is unproven.

## GENETIC DISEASES

## POLYCYSTIC KIDNEY DISEASE

### Epidemiology

- The prevalence is 1 in 1000.
- Polycystic kidney disease (PKD) accounts for up to 10% of all end-stage renal disease.

### Disease mechanisms

Adult PKD is usually caused by a dominant mutation in the *PKD1* gene, which encodes the polycystin-1 protein. New mutations are common, so there may not be a family history. A minority of patients have mutations in the *PKD2* gene, which encodes polycystin-2. Cysts develop and enlarge, compressing and destroying normal renal tissue, resulting in a progressive decline in renal function. The cysts may bleed (into the cyst or urinary tract) and become infected.

### Clinical features

- Presentation is usually in adult life with features that may include haematuria, urinary tract infection and stones, renal abscess formation, hypertension and CKD.

- There are associations with cerebral artery aneurysms that can lead to subarachnoid haemorrhage.
- End-stage renal disease usually occurs in later adult life.

### Investigation

- Ultrasound, CT or MR scanning can all effectively diagnose the condition (ADULT POLYCYSTIC KIDNEY DISEASE AT A GLANCE, **Figure B**).
- Genetic diagnosis is possible within affected families.

### Management

- There is no treatment for the underlying disease although vasopressin analogues may slow progression in some cases.
- Good control of blood pressure, prompt treatment of infection and control of renal stones formation may help slow the progression to end-stage renal disease.

## ALPORT'S SYNDROME

This is a rare X-linked genetic disorder of type 4 collagen in basement membranes. It causes severe disease in males and mild, if any, disease in females. Microscopic and sometimes macroscopic haematuria progress to proteinuria and end-stage renal disease. Sensorineural deafness can also occur as can anterior protrusion of the lens in the eyes (anterior lenticonus).

## FABRY'S DISEASE

This is an X-linked genetic deficiency of the enzyme alpha galactosidase A (Gal A) resulting in intracellular accumulation of glycosphingolipid. Proteinuria occurs in adult life and progresses to end-stage renal disease. Systemic features include angiokeratomas (dark red papules) of the skin, coronary artery disease resulting from endothelial thickening and autonomic dysfunction.

## TUBEROUS SCLEROSIS

This is caused by mutations in the *TSC1* or *TSC2* genes, which are growth regulating genes. Mutations can be dominant, but the majority of cases represent new mutations without a family history. Affected individuals have a germline defect in one allele and, if a somatic mutation occurs in a cell in the other allele, then the cell can give rise to a proliferative lesion. The kidneys can be affected by renal angiomyolipomas (see **Figure 8.7**) or cysts and focal segmental glomerulosclerosis, renal carcinoma, urinary tract infections or end stage renal disease. Skin changes include hypomelanotic patches (white macules); angiofibroma (small red facial lesions) and shagreen patches (dark rough skin on hands and feet). Hamartomas and other proliferative lesions can occur elsewhere, including the brain, heart and lungs.

## ADULT POLYCYSTIC KIDNEY DISEASE AT A GLANCE

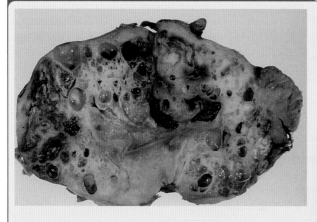

**Figure A** A polycystic kidney. There are multiple cysts of different sizes, some filled with blood.

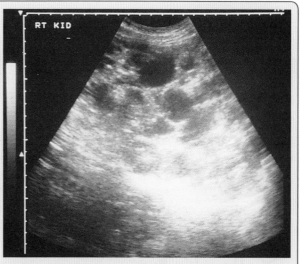

**Figure B** Ultrasound of a polycystic kidney. Cysts of different sizes are scattered throughout the kidney substance and can be seen as round black shapes.

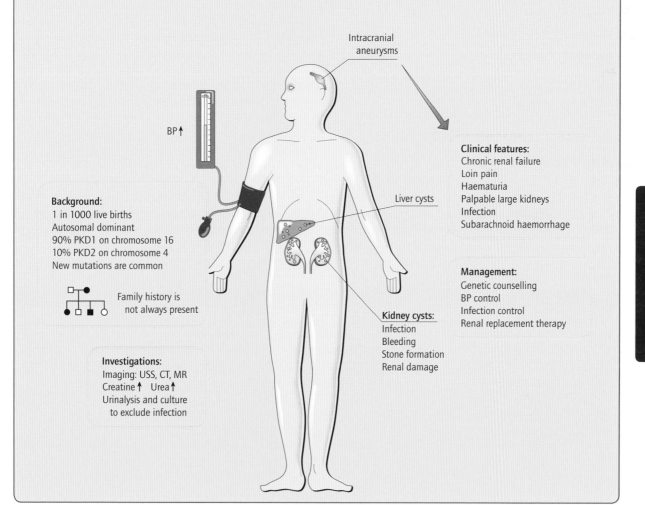

Intracranial aneurysms

BP↑

**Background:**
1 in 1000 live births
Autosomal dominant
90% PKD1 on chromosome 16
10% PKD2 on chromosome 4
New mutations are common

Family history is not always present

**Investigations:**
Imaging: USS, CT, MR
Creatine ↑  Urea ↑
Urinalysis and culture
  to exclude infection

Liver cysts

**Clinical features:**
Chronic renal failure
Loin pain
Haematuria
Palpable large kidneys
Infection
Subarachnoid haemorrhage

**Management:**
Genetic counselling
BP control
Infection control
Renal replacement therapy

**Kidney cysts:**
Infection
Bleeding
Stone formation
Renal damage

8

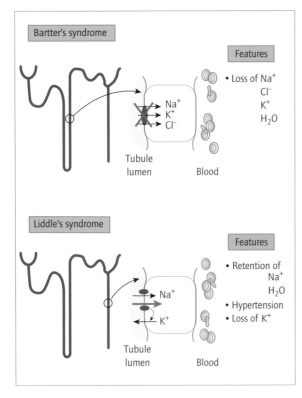

**Figure 8.14** Bartter's syndrome and Liddle's syndrome. In Bartter's syndrome, the NKCC2 cotransporter does not work properly. In Liddle's syndrome, the ENaC sodium channel is held open and the red arrow indicates the excessive sodium reabsorption that occurs.

## INHERITED TUBULAR SYNDROMES

### Bartter's syndrome

This is caused by an autosomal recessive mutation in the NKCC2 transporter in the loop of Henle and so *mimics furosemide* administration, with loss of sodium, chloride and potassium from the kidney (**Figure 8.14**). Long-term potassium chloride supplementation is necessary.

### Gitelman's syndrome

This is caused by an autosomal recessive mutation in the NCC transporter in the distal tubule and so *mimics thiazide* administration with loss of sodium, water, calcium and magnesium from the kidney.

### Liddle's syndrome (pseudohyperaldosteronism)

This is caused by an autosomal dominant activating mutation in the ENaC channel in the collecting ducts (**Figure 8.14**) and so *mimics aldosterone* administration, with sodium and water reabsorption causing hypertension, hypokalaemia and metabolic alkalosis. Amiloride blocks the channel and can be helpful.

## DRUGS AND THE KIDNEY

Some drugs can have damaging effects on the kidneys (**Table 8.7**).

Many drugs, or their metabolites, are excreted by the kidney so, if renal function is impaired, these drugs may accumulate to toxic levels. Dose reduction or avoidance of the drug may be required. Drugs may also have altered pharmacokinetics in severe renal impairment. It is important to check in a formulary whether a drug dose or dosing frequency should be adjusted in the presence of renal disease (**Table 8.8**; **Table 8.9**). In the presence of renal impairment:

- Loop diuretics may require high doses to reach the tubular site of action.
- Potassium-sparing diuretics can cause fatal hyperkalaemia.
- NSAIDs should be avoided as they reduce renal blood flow and GFR by opposing tonic prostaglandin-induced renal vasodilatation. This can result in ischaemic renal damage.

**Table 8.7** Renal damage caused by drugs

| Damage | Drug |
|---|---|
| **Idiosyncratic toxicity** | |
| Allergic interstitial nephritis | Proton pump inhibitors, penicillins, rifampicin, cephalosporins, fluoroquinolones, aciclovir, NSAIDs, thiazides, furosemide, mesalazine |
| Glomerulonephritis | Penicillamine, gold, captopril, phenytoin, penicillins, sulphonamides, rifampicin |
| Analgesic nephropathy (papillary necrosis) | Phenacetin, other analgesics |
| **Predictable toxicity** | |
| Crystalluria | High-dose aciclovir, anti-retrovirals, sulphonamides, acetazolamide |
| Renal calculi | Cytotoxics (urate release), possibly triamterene |
| Decreased creatinine secretion | Cimetidine, trimethoprim |
| Tubular damage | Lithium, ciclosporin, tacrolimus, gentamicin, foscarnet, amphotericin, cisplatin, radiographic contrast |
| Bladder damage leading to obstructive uropathy | Cyclophosphamide |
| Exacerbation of renal ischaemia | ACE inhibitors, angiotensin II receptor antagonists, NSAIDs |
| Miscellaneous | Tetracycline, clofibrate, cefradine (combined with frusemide), ACE inhibitors |

**Table 8.8** Drugs to avoid in renal impairment

| Drug | Reason |
| --- | --- |
| Chlorpropamide | Risk of prolonged hypoglycaemia |
| Lithium | Narrow therapeutic ratio, severe toxicity, causes nephrogenic diabetes insipidus with polyuria and dehydration |
| Metformin, phenformin | Increased risk of lactic acidosis |
| Nitrofurantoin | Renally excreted metabolites cause peripheral neuropathy |
| Tetracyclines | Can precipitate acute-on-chronic renal failure (except doxycycline and minoxycycline) |
| Acetazolamide | Metabolic acidosis |
| Phenylbutazone | Increased risk of toxicity |
| Procainamide | Increased risk of toxicity |
| Thiazides | Ineffective with GFR less than 30 mL/min |
| Bismuth | Danger of bismuth poisoning |
| Clofibrate | Renally excreted metabolites are toxic to skeletal muscle |
| Sodium aurothiomalate | Increased risk of gold toxicity |

**Table 8.9** Drugs to be used only with special care in renal impairment. Enhanced effects and increased toxicity are a result of retention of renally excreted drug or active metabolite in renal impairment

| Drug | Reason |
| --- | --- |
| Potassium-sparing diuretics | Danger of hyperkalaemia |
| Gentamicin, tobramycin and aztreonam | Increased toxicity |
| Nadolol | Enhanced effects |
| Vancomycin | Increased toxicity |
| Digoxin | Enhanced effects |
| Many cytotoxic agents | Enhanced effects |
| Ethambutol | Increased risk of optic neuritis and peripheral nephropathy |
| Allopurinol (especially in combination with azathioprine) | Enhanced bone marrow suppression |
| Sulphonamides | Increased prevalence of side effects, and crystalluria if low urine flow |
| Diazepam | Active metabolite causing enhanced effect |
| Opiates | Active metabolite causing enhanced effect |
| Sucralfate and other aluminium-containing antacids | Risk of aluminium toxicity |
| Sulphonylureas (except gliclazide) | Retained metabolites cause prolonged hypoglycaemia |

## RENAL VASCULAR DISEASE

### RENAL ARTERY STENOSIS

Narrowing of the renal arteries can cause hypertension, renal impairment from ischaemic damage or, rarely, flash pulmonary oedema from sodium and water retention. Most renal arterial disease is caused by atherosclerosis. In younger women, a condition known as fibromuscular dysplasia can occur which responds well to angioplasty. Sometimes, small fragments of cholesterol may be dislodged from atherosclerotic plaques, usually in the aorta, and these can lodge in small renal vessels (cholesterol embolization) causing ischaemia or an inflammatory response which may result in permanent damage.

### Epidemiology

The prevalence rises in parallel with that of atherosclerosis in other arteries and the risk factors are those of general atherosclerosis.

### Clinical features

Features may include:

- Hypertension
- Renal bruit
- Difference in renal size greater than 2 cm
- Renal impairment
- Deterioration in renal function following treatment with ACE inhibitors

**DRUGS AND THE KIDNEY AT A GLANCE**

Do not prescribe any drug until you know how it is handled in renal failure.

Use a source of drug information, e.g. *British National Formulary.*

Reduce the dose or increase the dose interval for renally excreted drugs.

Be extra careful with drugs having a narrow therapeutic ratio.

In unexplained renal damage, always consider drug toxicity as a cause.

**8**

- Episodes of pulmonary oedema not explained by ischaemic heart disease
- Severe atherosclerosis elsewhere in the vascular tree

### Investigation

- *Angiography:* Invasive angiography, CT angiography or MR angiography can all be helpful in the diagnosis (**Figure 8.15**). Angiography shows a beaded appearance of the renal artery in fibromuscular dysplasia.
- *Ultrasound:* This assesses renal size and asymmetry.

### Management

- Hypertension should be controlled and often responds well to ACE inhibitors or angiotensin receptor blockers, but renal function must be monitored closely for deterioration.
- The arterial stenosis can be angioplastied and stented, but as the renal damage is often irreversible, the benefit of this is unclear and hypertension often persists.
- Risk factors for atherosclerosis should be modified or treated where possible.

### Prognosis

- Stenosed renal arteries may progress towards complete occlusion.
- End-stage renal disease can result from chronic ischaemia.

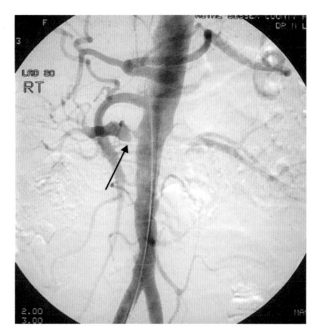

**Figure 8.15** Renal angiogram showing bilateral atherosclerotic renal artery stenosis. The stenosis of the right renal artery, seen on the left of the image, is over 75% and there is poststenotic dilatation; the left renal artery is completely occluded.

## RENAL VEIN THROMBOSIS

### Disease mechanisms

The most common cause of renal vein thrombosis is the nephrotic syndrome, which predisposes to venous thrombosis, but renal vein thrombosis can arise from other risk factors for venous thromboembolism.

### Clinical features

Presentation may be insidious with increasing proteinuria and/or pulmonary emboli resulting from partial occlusion of one or both renal veins. There will be leg oedema if the clot extends into the inferior vena cava. If there is an acute complete occlusion, there will often be flank pain and haematuria.

### Investigation

- *Creatinine and lactate dehydrogenase (LDH):* acute complete occlusion can cause a rise in creatinine and LDH, which is released from infarcted renal cells
- *CT or MR:* can be used to image the renal veins
- *Ultrasound:* sometimes gives useful information but often the renal veins cannot be clearly seen

### Management

- Anticoagulation should be continued as long as the underlying cause is still present.
- Thrombolysis may be needed for complete occlusion.

## HYPERTENSION

Hypertension is important because it can directly damage the heart, the kidneys and the eyes and is a major risk factor for vascular disease (**Figure 8.16**), especially cerebrovascular disease. The identification and treatment of hypertension is important because it improves the prognosis for these conditions. The kidney has a key role in blood pressure regulation and many drugs for hypertension act through the kidneys or the renin–angiotensin system. Most renal diseases can cause hypertension and hypertension itself can cause renal damage.

Hypertension is referred to as *'essential'* if no obvious cause is identified and *'secondary'* if the cause is known. *Most hypertension is essential.* The definition of hypertension is arbitrary and is usually diagnosed if clinic measurements are above 140/90 mmHg or home measurements are above 135/85 mmHg. The 140 refers to the systolic blood pressure resulting from contraction of the left ventricle and the 90 refers to the diastolic blood pressure present during ventricular relaxation when the aortic valve is closed.

### Epidemiology

- Hypertension is common, affecting 25% of adults globally and over 50% of people over 60 years of age (see **Figure 8.16**).

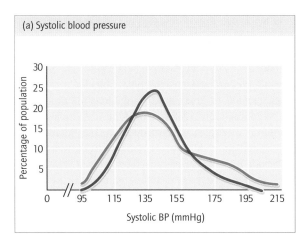

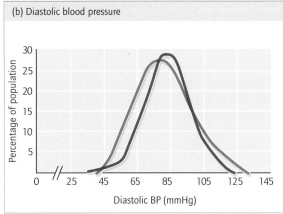

**Figure 8.16** Normal distribution of: **(a)** systolic; and **(b)** diastolic blood pressure (BP) in a white population (males, blue; females, red).

- The prevalence is similar in men and women and higher in people of African ethnicity.
- Risk factors for hypertension include a high alcohol intake and obesity. Salt intake has been correlated with blood pressure.

### Disease mechanisms

#### Essential hypertension

The causes of essential hypertension have not been well defined, but systemic vascular resistance is usually increased. The kidney can influence blood pressure in different ways including effects on systemic vascular resistance through the production of renin and the subsequent generation of angiotensin II and the regulation of body sodium and water content.

#### Secondary hypertension

- *Renal artery stenosis:* This reduces renal blood flow stimulating renin release and subsequent angiotensin II production. Angiotensin II causes hypertension by vasoconstriction and by stimulation of aldosterone release from the adrenal cortex, which promotes sodium retention by the kidney.
- *Drugs:* Those causing hypertension include steroids, ciclosporin and oestrogens in oral contraceptives.

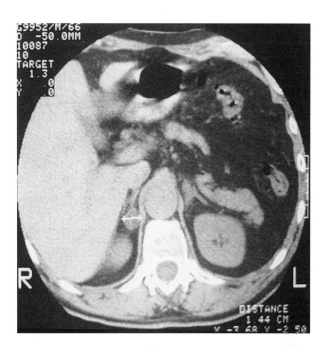

**Figure 8.17** CT scan of a right adrenal tumour (marked with a white line) in a patient with phaeochromocytoma.

- *Primary hyperaldosteronism (Conn's syndrome)* (see Chapter 12, Endocrine disease): Excess aldosterone increases renal sodium retention promoting hypervolaemia and hypertension.
- *Kidney disease:* This can cause hypertension.
- *Coarctation of the aorta:* This reduces renal perfusion and triggers renin secretion.
- *Catecholamine:* Release by a phaeochromocytoma causes systemic vasoconstriction and so hypertension (**Figure 8.17**).
- *Acromegaly:* This is associated with hypertension.

### Clinical features

- Hypertension is usually asymptomatic and is typically detected at a routine health check or medical examination for another clinical problem.
- It is usually diagnosed if blood pressure is ≥140/90 mmHg on three separate occasions.
- If it is unclear whether someone has genuine hypertension or is just anxious, home measurements or 24-hour ambulatory blood pressure monitoring may be useful.
- Evidence of end-organ damage from hypertension, such as retinopathy or left ventricular hypertrophy, can help confirm that the patient is hypertensive, so *fundoscopy* should be undertaken.
- Hypertension is often associated with obesity, excess alcohol intake, insulin resistance and gout.
- Peripheral bruits suggest vascular disease and raise the possibility of renal artery stenosis.
- The heart may display signs of left ventricular hypertrophy such as a left ventricular heave.

**8**

*How to measure blood pressure*

Blood pressure is usually measured with a sphygmomanometer, which uses an inflatable cuff around the arm.
Good automatic devices are available, but it is still important to be able to check the action of these devices with a
manual sphygmomanometer.

1 Choose a cuff of the right size. If the patient has a large
   arm, use a large cuff or the reading will be falsely high.
2 Wrap the cuff around the patient's arm and place a
   stethoscope over the brachial artery at the elbow.
3 Inflate the cuff until no sound is heard and then slowly
   deflate it.
4 When the first sounds start to be heard, this
   is the systolic pressure as indicated on the
   sphygmomanometer.
5 When the sounds finally disappear, this is the diastolic
   pressure.

If the patient is tense, allow them to relax and repeat the
measurements a few times.

### Investigation

Key initial investigations:
- *Urinalysis:* Protein may indicate hypertensive damage
  to the kidney.
- *Serum electrolytes:* Hypokalaemia can indicate
  hyperaldosteronism.
- *Urea and creatinine:* These may indicate renal disease.
- *Lipids:* Hypercholesterolaemia raises the possiblity of
  atherosclerotic renal aterial disease.
- *Glucose:* This is to assess for diabetes $\pm$ HbA$_{1c}$.
- *Electrocardiography, ideally with echocardiography:* This
  can identify left ventricular hypertrophy.

Further investigations might include plasma and urine
catecholamines or vanillylmandelic acid (VMA) levels to
exclude phaeochromocytomas, adrenal function tests to
check for steroid excess and imaging to exclude renal artery
stenosis.

### Management

In a well patient, elevated blood pressure is not an emergency and treatment should not be commenced until you
are sure that the blood pressure is truly elevated. Unless
there is severe hypertension (e.g. >180/110), papilloedema
or evidence of acute disease, treatment is not urgent and
can await full evaluation. Blood pressure can be improved
by exercise, reduced alcohol consumption and correction
of obesity. Reducing salt intake may help some patients,
especially if there is renal impairment. Other risk factors for
vascular disease, including smoking, should be modified to
reduce vascular complications. The commonly used antihypertensives are diuretics, beta blockers, ACE inhibitors,
angiotensin II receptor blockers, calcium-channel blockers
and alpha blockers.
- *Beta blockers:* These suppress renin secretion, reduce
  cardiac output and may have a centrally mediated

effect. Lowering cardiac output can worsen symptoms
of peripheral vascular disease. Beta blockers blunt
the catecholaminergic effects, which normally warn
diabetics of hypoglycaemia. Beta-1 selective blockers
avoid the bronchospasm of beta-2 blockade.
- *ACE inhibitors:* These inhibit angiotensin II production.
  They cause more dilatation in efferent arterioles than in
  afferent arterioles, which reduces the intraglomerular
  pressure and reduces proteinuria. Complications
  include hyperkalaemia caused by reduced aldosterone
  production and, in some cases, renal impairment
  worsens if renal artery stenosis is present. ACE
  degrades bradykinin, so ACE inhibitors cause high
  bradykinin levels, which can make patients cough.
- *Angiotensin II receptor antagonists:* These have similar
  effects to ACE inhibitors but cough is not a problem.
- *Calcium-channel blockers:* These cause vasodilatation
  and, in some patients, increase sodium excretion
  by poorly understood mechanisms. Verapamil and
  diltiazem reduce atrioventricular nodal conduction
  and should not be given with beta blockers.
- *Diuretics:* Mainly thiazides, these are ineffective if
  GFR is low. Furosemide may then be beneficial.
- *Alpha-1 antagonists:* Antagonists such as doxazosin
  block catecholaminergic vasoconstriction and can
  cause postural hypotension. They may increase urine
  flow rates when there is prostatic hypertrophy.
- *Direct vasodilators:* Examples including sodium
  nitroprusside, IV nitrates, hydrallazine, diazoxide and
  minoxidil cause peripheral vasodilatation directly.
  This usually causes reflex tachycardia.
- *Centrally acting drugs:* Examples are clonidine,
  methyldopa and guanethidine. They are seldom used
  because of multiple side effects.

### Complications of hypertension

*Renal complications*

Very low levels of albumin in the urine (microalbuminuria)
or heavier levels of proteinuria are consistent with hypertensive nephropathy. The groups most likely to develop
renal damage from hypertension are the elderly, the obese,
and people of African or South Asian ethnicity, especially if
they have diabetes. Hypertension can cause *glomerular sclerosis* and ischaemic atrophy.

*Cardiovascular complications*

The high vascular resistance strains the heart, causing left
ventricular hypertrophy with thickening of the myocardial
wall. Hypertension also increases atherosclerosis of coronary, peripheral and cerebrovascular arteries.

*Eyes*

Retinopathy is common and is graded according to severity.
Grade 3 or 4 indicates accelerated or 'malignant' hypertension (see HYPERTENSION AT A GLANCE, **Figure A**).
- *Grade 1:* arterial spasm, tortuous arteries, silver wire
  appearance

## HYPERTENSION AT A GLANCE

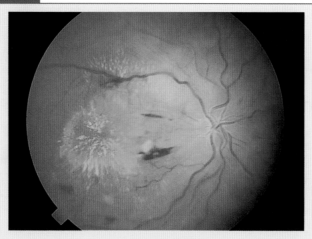

**Figure A** Grade 4 hypertensive retinopathy with exudates, flame haemorrhages and papilloedema.

**Background:**

Affects 5–10% of Western populations

BP $\geq \frac{140}{90}$ mmHg on 3 separate occasions

Can cause end-organ damage

Increases with:

  Age

  Obesity

  Alcohol intake

Secondary causes

  Renal artery stenosis

  Renal disease

  Primary hyperaldosteronism

  Phaeochromocytoma

  Drugs: contraceptive pill

        steroids

**Key questions:**

1 Is the patient truly hypertensive?
2 Is there end-organ damage?
3 Is there a treatable cause?
4 Will lifestyle changes help?
5 Is urgent treatment required?
6 Which drug is most appropriate?

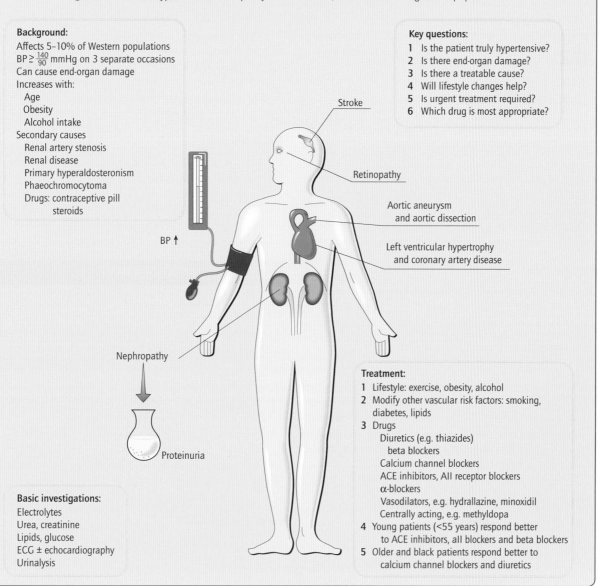

Stroke

Retinopathy

Aortic aneurysm
and aortic dissection

Left ventricular hypertrophy
and coronary artery disease

BP ↑

Nephropathy

Proteinuria

**Basic investigations:**

Electrolytes

Urea, creatinine

Lipids, glucose

ECG ± echocardiography

Urinalysis

**Treatment:**

1 Lifestyle: exercise, obesity, alcohol
2 Modify other vascular risk factors: smoking,
  diabetes, lipids
3 Drugs
    Diuretics (e.g. thiazides)
     beta blockers
    Calcium channel blockers
    ACE inhibitors, AII receptor blockers
    α-blockers
    Vasodilators, e.g. hydrallazine, minoxidil
    Centrally acting, e.g. methyldopa
4 Young patients (<55 years) respond better
  to ACE inhibitors, aII blockers and beta blockers
5 Older and black patients respond better to
  calcium channel blockers and diuretics

**8**

- *Grade 2:* arteriovenous nipping; veins appear narrowed where the arteries pass over them
- *Grade 3:* haemorrhage, including flame haemorrhage; lipid extravasation causes exudates, visible as white patches or spots
- *Grade 4:* papilloedema; a swollen optic disc

## ACCELERATED HYPERTENSION

Accelerated (or malignant) hypertension is characterized by severe hypertension (usually >180/110 mmHg) with retinal haemorrhages or papilloedema (grade 3 or 4 hypertensive retinopathy). It can occur *de novo* or as a complication of pre-existing hypertension and arises from a positive feedback loop:

- The central feature is *renal vessel damage*, usually caused by hypertension.
- This damage *reduces renal blood flow* and the reduction triggers renin secretion.
- *Renin secretion* triggers angiotensin II and aldosterone production causing further *hypertension* and sodium retention.

The clinical presentation can include:

- Headache
- Visual disturbance
- Shortness of breath because of cardiac problems
- Renal impairment, often with haematuria and proteinuria

Excess renin drives aldosterone secretion, which promotes renal potassium excretion and can cause *hypokalaemia*. Damaged blood vessels can harm red blood cells passing through them, causing a *microangiopathic haemolytic anaemia*.

### Management

Treatment is with ACE inhibitors, angiotensin receptor antagonists or beta blockers to block the renin cycle (beta blockers reduce renin output from the juxtaglomerular apparatus). Diuretics promote sodium excretion. Hypertensive encephalopathy, pulmonary oedema or severe acute disease may require IV treatment with sodium nitroprusside, hydralazine, labetalol or a nitrate preparation. IV sodium nitroprusside therapy allows minute-by-minute blood pressure control, but toxic cyanide metabolites can accumulate. If renal artery stenosis is present, a sudden reduction in blood pressure can reduce renal perfusion and worsen renal function.

## HYPERTENSION IN PREGNANCY AND PRE-ECLAMPSIA

Pre-eclampsia is increasingly common, occurring in up to 15% of first pregnancies. Pre-eclampsia arises in the third trimester or final 3-month period of pregnancy and is associated with *hypertension, proteinuria* and/or *oedema*. The incidence is higher with multiple pregnancies such as twins

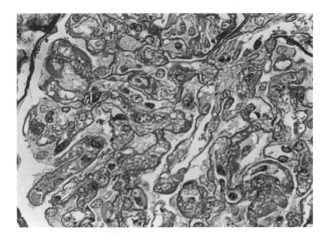

**Figure 8.18** Light microscopy of a renal biopsy from a patient with severe pre-eclampsia. There is endothelial cell swelling and vacuolation. Reproduced from Kincaid-Smith P & Whitworth JA (1987) *The Kidney: A Clinico-pathological Study*, 2nd edn (Wiley-Blackwell, Oxford), with the permission of the authors.

or triplets. Untreated, it can lead to seizures (eclampsia), coagulopathy and acute liver and renal failure (**Figure 8.18**). It is unlikely to arise in women in the first or second trimester, so hypertension, proteinuria and/or oedema in this context may represent intrinsic renal disease.

### Management

Hypertension in pregnancy may be managed with nifedipine, hydralazine, methyldopa or labetalol. If hypertension cannot be controlled in pre-eclampsia and other complications arise such as liver dysfunction, thrombocytopenia or seizures, the foetus is delivered immediately.

## ACUTE KIDNEY INJURY

AKI is common and represents a decline in renal function over hours or days from any cause. It is associated with significant morbidity and *mortality* (25%), but mortality increases with the severity of the AKI and not all those who survive will recover their lost renal function. AKI is diagnosed if:

- Serum creatinine rises by 26 µmol/L or more within 48 hours
- Serum creatinine rises by more than 50% within 7 days
- Urine output falls below 0.5 mL/kg/hour for more than 6 hours

## EPIDEMIOLOGY

The annual incidence of AKI is around 15 000 per million population in the UK. In developing countries the incidence is probably higher and obstetric complications and infections such as malaria are important causes of acute renal failure. People with CKD are at increased risk of AKI and

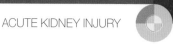

**Table 8.10** Drugs implicated in acute kidney injury

| Drug | Renal effect |
|------|--------------|
| Aminoglycosides | Tubular toxin |
| NSAIDs | Inhibit prostaglandin-mediated renal vasodilatation |
| ACE inhibitors | Reduce efferent arteriole tone and GFR |
| Cephalosporins | Tubular toxins |
| Amphotericin | Vasoconstrictor, causes membrane damage |
| Aciclovir | Precipitates in tubules and can form crystals in urine |
| Ciclosporin/tacrolimus | Indirect vasoconstriction |
| Radiocontrast | Vasoconstriction |

AKI in this context is sometimes referred to as acute-on-chronic kidney injury or disease.

## DISEASE MECHANISMS

AKI arises from three types of problem but it is often multifactorial.

- *Prerenal:* This arises from inadequate perfusion of the kidney due to loss of intravascular volume or low blood pressure. Causes include haemorrhage, reduced cardiac output or drugs that lower blood pressure or alter renal blood flow (e.g. NSAIDs).
- *Renal:* This arises from drugs (**Table 8.10**) or diseases (e.g. glomerulonephritis) that act directly on the kidney.
- *Postrenal:* This arises when there is an obstruction to urine flow. This can arise from outside the wall of the urinary system (e.g. a tumour or retroperitoneal fibrosis), within the wall itself (e.g. tumours or strictures) or within the lumen (e.g. stones, blood clots and detached tissue such as sloughed renal papillae or fragments of tumours).

### Renal causes of AKI

There are many disease processes that can result in acute kidney injury and they may affect the glomeruli, the tubules or both. Important causes include:

- Glomerulonephritis
- Interstitial nephritis
- Accelerated hypertension
- Cholesterol embolization
- Infection
- Drugs (see **Table 8.10** and also **Table 8.7**)
- Toxins including drugs, heavy metals or contrast media
- Rhabdomyolyis: myoglobin released from muscles causes tubular toxicity
- Haemoglobin: released during intravascular haemolysis and toxic to tubules
- Light chains of antibodies in myeloma: can cause tubular damage

- Calcium: not formally a toxin, but has negative effects on the kidney at high levels
- Urate: not formally a toxin, but damaging at high levels

## CLINICAL FEATURES

AKI in the community setting may be mild, arising from another illness such as gastroenteritis and only detected if blood tests are taken. AKI is common in hospital, commonly due to fluid depletion and detected by blood tests. Frank haematuria may suggest urinary tract stones or glomerulonephritis. Well-recognized scenarios include:

- *Haemoptysis:* suggesting a pulmonary-renal syndrome such as Goodpasture's syndrome or systemic vasculitis
- *A recent sore throat or infection:* suggesting postinfective glomerulonephritis
- *In men, a history of urinary symptoms such as a poor urinary stream, dribbling, hesitancy, nocturia and urinary frequency:* suggesting prostatic disease, which can cause obstruction and urinary tract infection
- *A history of recent trauma or very heavy exercise, or a long lie after a fall or crush injury, especially if associated with muscle pain:* raising the possibility of rhabdomyolysis
- *Recent gastroenteritis:* raising the possibility of infection with E. coli serotype 0157 and the presence of haemolytic–uraemic syndrome

The *past medical history* may highlight an underlying multisystem disease associated with renal disease, such as:

- SLE
- Vascular disease associated with renal artery stenosis
- Malignancy, which may be associated with hypercalcaemia
- Chronic infection such as osteomyelitis, which can be associated with amyloidosis affecting the kidney
- Abnormal or artificial heart valves, which are vulnerable to infective endocarditis associated with glomerulonephritis

Ask about symptoms such as joint pains or a rash that might suggest an underlying disease such as SLE. Enquire about any prescribed or recreational *drugs* that the patient may have taken and ask about self-poisoning with drugs or other toxic substances.

### Special considerations in hospitalized patients

Carefully check the medical records for evidence of renal insults, such as:

- Nephrotoxic drugs
- Radiological contrast media
- Hypotension, especially during anaesthesia/surgery
- Fever indicating infection
- Weight or fluid balance measurements indicating fluid depletion

8

Full examination is important.

- *A priority is the assessment of fluid status.* Is the patient dehydrated? Check skin turgor and jugular venous pressure, examine the heart, check for peripheral and pulmonary oedema and measure the pulse and the blood pressure lying down and standing up if possible.
- Look for a focus of current or previous *infection*. Check all over the patient's skin and under all bandages and dressings.
- Check all surgical or traumatic *wounds* and examine any bed sores on the buttocks, legs, feet and back and head.
- Examine *muscles* for any tenderness or swelling that might suggest rhabdomyolysis.
- Examine the *eyes* for changes of hypertension or diabetes mellitus.
- Upper airway disease or *ear, nose and throat* problems may indicate vasculitic disease.
- *Polycystic kidneys* may be palpable and a *large palpable bladder* suggests obstruction.
- *A rectal examination* may indicate prostatic or pelvic disease.

## INVESTIGATION

A range of useful specific immunological and other tests may provide diagnostic information (**Table 8.11**).

### Biochemistry

- *Plasma urea and creatinine:* Levels are elevated.
- *Potassium and acid:* These are excreted by the kidneys, so can accumulate causing dangerous hyperkalaemia and metabolic acidosis, both of which cause cardiac arrhythmias and cardiac arrest.
- *Creatinine kinase:* Rhabdomyolysis causes a major increase in the blood.
- *Arterial blood gases:* These must be checked to assess the extent of any metabolic acidosis.

### Haematology

- *Anaemia* may be present from blood loss, haemolysis or impaired red cell production.

- A high *eosinophil* count can occur with acute interstitial nephritis.
- In haemolytic–uraemic syndrome, there may be *haemolysis*, causing anaemia with damaged red blood cells on a blood film and a low platelet count.

### Urine

Urine dipstick analysis, microscopy and culture should all be performed.

- Although *haematuria* could indicate renal or postrenal disease, it can also be caused by urinary catheterization.
- Heavy *proteinuria* usually indicates a glomerular disease.
- Both *myoglobin and haemoglobin* can be measured in urine and indicate rhabdomyolysis and haemolysis, respectively.
- On microscopy, *red cell casts* are diagnostic of glomerulonephritis and white cells indicate infection or interstitial nephritis.
- *Eosinophils* in the urine are indicative of interstitial nephritis.

### Imaging

- *Ultrasound:* The kidneys should be imaged, usually with ultrasound, to exclude urinary tract obstruction and to establish the renal sizes. If the kidneys are small, CKD is likely. Other abnormalities such as polycystic kidneys will also be identified.
- *CT, MR or angiography:* These can provide further information if required.

### Histology

If the aetiology of the renal disease is unclear, renal biopsy should be undertaken to exclude a treatable intrinsic renal disease.

## DIFFERENTIAL DIAGNOSIS

The key differential diagnosis is of CKD. In CKD, there may be complications such as anaemia and bone disease, but the most obvious difference is that the kidneys are usually small on ultrasound or other imaging.

**Table 8.11** Renal causes of acute kidney injury

| Diagnosis | Clinical features | Investigations |
|---|---|---|
| Rhabdomyolysis | Muscle pain | CK ↑, myoglobulinuria |
| Glomerulonephritis | | Red cell casts |
| Goodpasture's disease | Pulmonary haemorrhage | Anti-GBM antibodies ↑ |
| Vasculitis | ± Systemic features, sinusitis, rash | ANCA ↑ |
| SLE | Joint/neurological signs, rash | Anti dsDNA ↑, antinuclear antibodies, low complement C3 and C4 |
| Interstitial nephritis | Drug cause | Eosinophils ↑ (in blood and urine) |
| Haemolytic–uraemic syndrome | Diarrhoea | Hb ↓, haemolysis, platelets ↓ |
| Acute tubular necrosis | Multiple factors, especially in hospitals | Granular tubular casts |

ANCA, antineutrophil cytoplasmic antibodies; CK, creatinine kinase; GBM, glomerular basement membrane; Hb, haemoglobin; SLE, systemic lupus erythematosus.

## MANAGEMENT

AKI, if severe, is a medical emergency as the patient can die from a cardiac arrest if there is severe hyperkalaemia or acidosis. It may be reversible if appropriate measures, such as rehydration, are taken. Any cause should be removed or treated if possible.

### General management

- Treatment on a *high dependency or intensive care unit* may be required.
- Hypoxia should be corrected with oxygen therapy and *ventilation* if necessary.

- Cardiac output should be maintained with *inotropic* drugs and fluids.
- Severe anaemia should be corrected by transfusion.
- Nutrition should be optimized with enteral or parenteral feeding if necessary.
- Infection should be treated.
- Hypertension should be controlled.

### Specific issues in management

An immediate priority is to prevent potassium levels rising too high and plasma pH falling fall too low as both are

## ACUTE KIDNEY INJURY AT A GLANCE

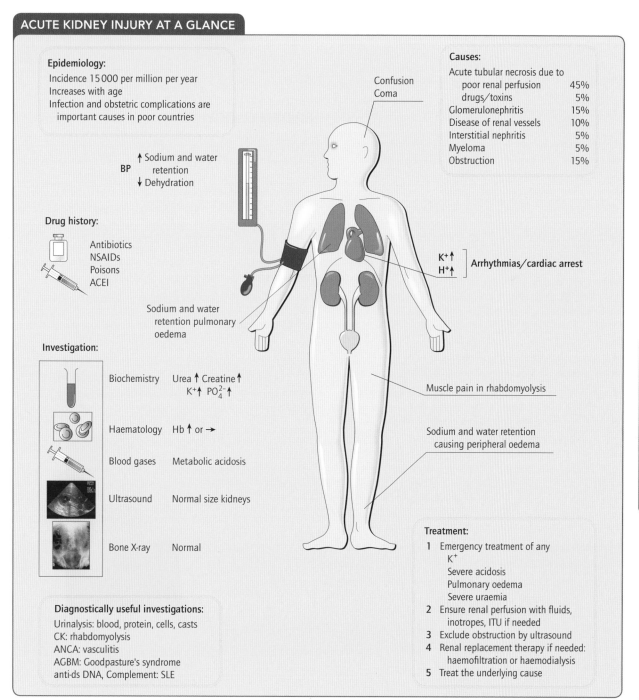

**Epidemiology:**
Incidence 15 000 per million per year
Increases with age
Infection and obstetric complications are important causes in poor countries

BP ↑ Sodium and water retention
↓ Dehydration

**Drug history:**
Antibiotics
NSAIDs
Poisons
ACEI

Sodium and water retention pulmonary oedema

**Investigation:**

| | | |
|---|---|---|
| | Biochemistry | Urea ↑ Creatine ↑ $K^+$↑ $PO_4^{2-}$↑ |
| | Haematology | Hb ↑ or → |
| | Blood gases | Metabolic acidosis |
| | Ultrasound | Normal size kidneys |
| | Bone X-ray | Normal |

**Diagnostically useful investigations:**
Urinalysis: blood, protein, cells, casts
CK: rhabdomyolysis
ANCA: vasculitis
AGBM: Goodpasture's syndrome
anti-ds DNA, Complement: SLE

Confusion
Coma

**Causes:**
| | |
|---|---|
| Acute tubular necrosis due to | |
| poor renal perfusion | 45% |
| drugs/toxins | 5% |
| Glomerulonephritis | 15% |
| Disease of renal vessels | 10% |
| Interstitial nephritis | 5% |
| Myeloma | 5% |
| Obstruction | 15% |

$K^+$↑
$H^+$↑ } Arrhythmias/cardiac arrest

Muscle pain in rhabdomyolysis

Sodium and water retention causing peripheral oedema

**Treatment:**
1. Emergency treatment of any $K^+$
   Severe acidosis
   Pulmonary oedema
   Severe uraemia
2. Ensure renal perfusion with fluids, inotropes, ITU if needed
3. Exclude obstruction by ultrasound
4. Renal replacement therapy if needed: haemofiltration or haemodialysis
5. Treat the underlying cause

8

strong risk factors for cardiac arrest. Electrolytes should be measured daily, or more frequently if the patient is very sick or unstable.

*Potassium* Potassium intake should be restricted. If hyperkalaemia arises, the standard methods of treatment for hyperkalaemia may be of some help, but if renal function is substantially impaired, dialysis or haemofiltration is required to remove the potassium from the body.

*Acid* Acidosis can impair metabolic processes and must be corrected. The only way to remove acid if the kidneys are not working is by dialysis or haemofiltration.

*Volume* Maintaining the patient's fluid status correctly helps prevent further renal damage:
- Regular clinical assessment of fluid status is essential at least once or twice daily.
- A reliable index of fluid replacement is daily weighing.
- Fluid balance charts documenting all input and output should be kept.
- When the patient is properly rehydrated, volume replacement should match output and insensible losses, which are usually approximately 500 mL (or greater if there is fever).
- If necessary, invasive monitoring with a central venous catheter may help guide fluid replacement.
- Urinary catheterization may be helpful to monitor urine output but it carries the risk of infection.

*Pulmonary oedema* If the patient has excess body water, they may develop pulmonary oedema. In renal failure, this is particularly dangerous because the kidneys may not be able to excrete the excess water in response to diuretic therapy:
- Sit the patient up and give them oxygen.
- If there is any renal function, give IV furosemide.
- If there is very poor renal function, arrange urgent dialysis or haemofiltration.
- In the meantime, IV nitrates will provide vasodilatation.
- If necessary and if renal replacement therapy cannot be arranged in time, venesect 200–500 mL blood and ventilate the patient with positive end-expiratory pressures (opposes the entry of fluid into the alveoli).

### Renal replacement therapy

Haemodialysis or haemofiltration is generally used; haemofiltration is slower but may be better tolerated in haemodynamically unstable patients. The absolute indications for starting renal replacement therapy in the presence of acute or CKD are:
- Acute hyperkalaemia
- Severe metabolic acidosis
- Pulmonary oedema
- Severe uraemic complications (e.g. pericarditis)

## CHRONIC KIDNEY DISEASE

CKD has been defined as abnormal kidney function or structure present for more than 3 months with implications for health. CKD is classified according to the eGFR and level of albuminuria (see **Table 8.12**). Kidney failure or *end-stage renal disease* occurs when the GFR is so low that life cannot be sustained indefinitely without some form of renal replacement therapy, such as dialysis or transplantation. CKD is common because renal function deteriorates with age, but most people with CKD will not progress to end-stage renal disease. However, CKD is associated with cardiovascular disease, so people with CKD should have their cardiovascular risk factors modified where possible. Stage G5 CKD represents serious kidney disease. Severe symptomatic untreated chronic renal failure is sometimes termed the 'uraemic syndrome'.

### EPIDEMIOLOGY

- CKD is common, with a prevalence of around 5–15% in some countries. End-stage renal disease is much less common, with around 1000 people per million receiving renal replacement therapy in the UK.
- There are global variations in the causes, e.g. schistosomiasis can cause renal obstruction in affected regions (see Chapter 3, Infectious disease).

**Table 8.12** Drugs used in kidney transplantation

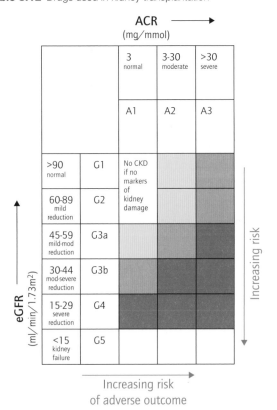

- Obesity and diabetes are contributory factors to a progressive global rise in CKD.
- CKD is more common in men and in people of African and South Asian ethnicity.

## DISEASE MECHANISMS IN ADVANCED CKD

- Reduced elimination of *potassium, acid and water* can cause hyperkalaemia, metabolic acidosis and hypervolaemia, which can cause systemic or pulmonary oedema.
- Reduced production by the kidneys of *erythropoietin* (which promotes red blood cell formation) causes a normochromic normocytic anaemia.
- Reduced production by the kidneys of vitamin D (which regulates calcium, phosphate and bone metabolism) causes *bone disease.*
- *Accumulation of toxic excretion products* can cause itching, pericarditis, neuropathy and other problems.

### Distinguishing acute and chronic kidney disease

The following features are characteristic of advanced CKD:

- Normochromic normocytic anaemia with no other obvious cause
- High plasma phosphate level and a low plasma calcium level; occasionally, high calcium levels if tertiary hyperparathyroidism is present (see Chapter 5, Metabolic bone disease)
- Bone imaging showing renal bone disease
- Features such as itch, tremor or pericarditis caused by accumulation of toxic substances
- Small *renal size* on imaging

## CLINICAL FEATURES

The clinical presentation of CKD varies from asymptomatic detection of biochemical abnormalities on blood tests taken for some other reason to symptomatic advanced CKD with the uraemic syndrome. The uraemic syndrome can cause confusion, tremor, itch, anaemia, anorexia and pericarditis. CKD can present with features of an underlying disease such as PKD, glomerulonephritis or diabetes mellitus.

### History

Key aims of the history are to establish the cause of the CKD and what complications are present. Ask about:

- *Past medical history* of conditions that will predispose to kidney disease, especially diabetes mellitus, hypertension, SLE, vasculitis, cancer (especially myeloma)
- *Family history* of kidney disease, especially PKD
- Features of vascular disease which might indicate renal artery stenosis

- Prostatic symptoms in men which might indicate urinary tract obstruction
- Haematuria which might indicate glomerulonephritis
- *General symptoms* of advanced CKD:
  - Tiredness
  - Confusion
  - Itch
  - Tremor
  - Loss of energy
  - Shortness of breath (from anaemia or acidotic breathing)
  - Nausea and vomiting
  - Pain from bone disease
  - Chest pain from pericarditis

### Examination

Check especially for:
- The fishy smell of uraemic breath
- Scratch marks indicating itch
- Pallor from anaemia
- Hypertension
- Fluid balance to exclude dehydration or fluid overload with pulmonary or systemic oedema
- Pericarditic rub
- Enlarged kidneys in polycystic kidney disese or renal cancer
- Distended bladder and in men an enlarged prostate

## INVESTIGATION

### Biochemistry

Plasma urea and creatinine levels are both elevated and eGFR is lowered. There may be hyperkalaemia and metabolic acidosis. Glucose levels may indicate diabetes. In advanced CKD plasma phosphate is raised and calcium lowered. If there is tertiary hyperparathyroidism, the calcium level may also be raised (see Chapter 5, Metabolic bone disease). Hyperlipidaemia is common.

### Haematology

In advanced CKD, normochromic normocytic anaemia is common from erythropoietin deficiency.

### Urine

Laboratory or dipstick analysis, microscopy and culture may indicate an underlying diagnosis.

### Imaging

In advanced CKD, the kidneys should be imaged, usually with ultrasound to exclude urinary tract obstruction and establish the size of the kidneys. If the kidneys are small, CKD is likely. Other abnormalities such as PKD can also be identified.

**8**

### Immunology and microbiology

Immunological tests are principally of use in monitoring any underlying disease such as SLE.

### Histology

If the kidneys are small, renal biopsy is not usually helpful as it may only show fibrosis.

## MANAGEMENT

The priority in CKD is to slow renal decline (**Figure 8.19**) by:
- Managing any underlying disease
- Controlling blood pressure
- Avoiding urinary tract infection
- Avoiding nephrotoxic drugs
- Avoiding dehydration

In the presence of severe CKD resulting in end-stage renal disease, the best option in an otherwise well patient is a kidney transplant. The alternative is a combination of:
- Dialysis to replace the excretory function of the kidney
- Erythropoietin administration to replace the erythropoietic synthetic function of the kidney
- Vitamin D administration to replace the vitamin D synthetic function of the kidney
- Various measures such as the restriction of water, sodium, potassium and phosphate intake to reduce the need for excretory function

### Haemodialysis

Haemodialysis is usually performed for around 4 hours three times a week. Blood is pumped past a semipermeable membrane and water, ions and small molecules pass across the membrane into dialysis fluid (**Figure 8.20**). By controlling the composition of this dialysis fluid, it is possible to control the removal of substances from the blood. If blood is forced past

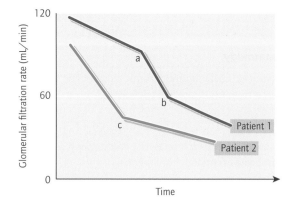

**Figure 8.19** Plots of change in renal function (glomerular filtration rate) with time. Patient 1 suffered a sudden accelerated decline of renal function at point a (resulting from a urinary tract infection and hypovolaemia) with recovery at point b because of their correction. Patient 2 enjoyed a deceleration in decline because of control of hypertension at point c.

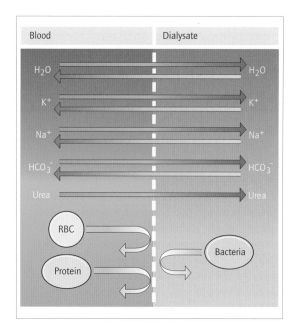

**Figure 8.20** The principles of dialysis across a semipermeable membrane. The semipermeable dialysis membrane is shown as white dashes. Small molecules pass through the membrane along a concentration gradient. Larger molecules (e.g. proteins) and cells cannot do so. RBC, red blood cell.

the membrane at a higher pressure, ultrafiltration of plasma also occurs. The membrane is usually in the form of small hollow fibres in a large cartridge and *heparin* is usually given to prevent blood clotting in the dialysis machine. Blood can be pumped from the body through large bore central venous catheters or needles placed in an *arteriovenous fistula*, which is formed by joining an artery to a vein in the arm.

Complications include infection and clotting of blood in the fistula or dialysis machine.

### Peritoneal dialysis

Fluid is placed in the peritoneal cavity through a tube tunnelled through the skin (**Figure 8.21**). Substances diffuse from the blood across the semipermeable peritoneal membrane into the fluid and are removed when the fluid is removed. Fluid can be pumped in and out overnight or the patient can run in bags of around 2 litres of fluid and empty them out every 4 hours. Altering the composition of the fluid influences the removal of substances by diffusion. Increasing the osmotic strength of the fluid increases the amount of water that is removed from the blood. The usual osmotic component in the bags is glucose.

The main complication is *infection*, either of skin and tissues around the tube or of the peritoneal cavity, causing peritonitis. This type of *peritonitis* is treated with antibiotics and repeated washing out of the peritoneum.

### Kidney transplantation

A kidney from a living or deceased donor can be transplanted into the pelvis of the recipient by attaching the kidney's blood vessels to the iliac vessels and implanting the ureter in the bladder. To reduce the chances of rejection of the kidney, the

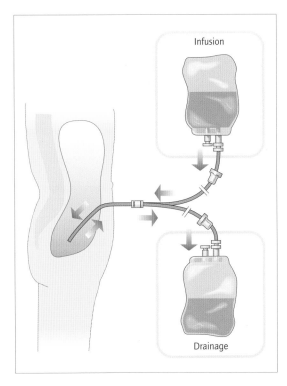

**Figure 8.21** Continuous ambulatory peritoneal dialysis. The patient's peritoneum acts as the semipermeable membrane between the dialysate and the plasma. A bag of fluid is allowed to drain into the peritoneal space, left there for several hours and then drained out.

donor and the recipient are matched whenever possible for their blood group and HLA types and the recipient is given immunosuppressive drugs. The drugs commonly include steroids, tacrolimus or ciclosporin and mycophenolate or azathioprine. Biological therapies such as the monoclonal

antibody basiliximab are also used. If transplant rejection occurs, immunosuppression is increased.

Complications of immunosuppression include infection (cytomegalovirus infection and Epstein–Barr virus are particular problems) and skin cancer. The major drugs used in transplantation are listed in **Table 8.13**.

## COMPLICATIONS OF KIDNEY FAILURE

### Anaemia

Anaemia arises because the kidney fails to produce adequate erythropoietin. *Recombinant erythropoietin (epoetin)* is usually given by subcutaneous injection every 1–2 weeks. Side effects include hypertension and polycythaemia. The response is poor in the presence of inflammation or deficiencies of iron, folate or vitamin $B_{12}$.

### Renal bone disease

Kidney failure reduces renal vitamin D synthesis and raises plasma phosphate. This lowers plasma calcium which triggers PTH secretion from the parathyroid glands. The high PTH level stimulates bone resorption and X-rays show subperiosteal resorption in the fingers, erosion of the phalangeal tufts and erosion of the heads of the clavicles (see CHRONIC KIDNEY DISEASE AT A GLANCE, **Figure A**).

Treatment includes:
- Reducing dietary phosphate intake
- Oral phosphate-binders to reduce phosphate absorption in the gut
- Dialysis to remove some phosphate
- Vitamin D replacement with 1,25-dihydroxy-vitamin-$D_3$ (calcitriol) or 1-hydroxy-vitamin-$D_3$ (alfacalcidol)

**8**

**Table 8.13** Drugs used in kidney transplantation

| Drug(s) | Action | Possible side effects |
|---|---|---|
| Steroids | Inhibit various immune cells | Infection |
| | | Osteoporosis |
| | | Hypertension |
| | | Hyperglycaemia |
| | | Hyperlipidaemia |
| Azathioprine | Inhibits purine metabolism and cell proliferation | Bone marrow suppression with low white cell counts and pancreatitis |
| Ciclosporin | Inhibits calcineurin and impairs T cell function | Renal toxicity |
| | | Hypertension |
| | | Electrolyte disorders, e.g. hyperkalaemia |
| Tacrolimus | Similar effects to ciclosporin | Hypertension |
| | | Nephrotoxicity |
| | | Impaired glucose tolerance |
| Mycophenolate | Similar effects to azathioprine | Gastritis |
| | | Oesophagitis |
| | | Diarrhoea |
| Sirolimus | Impairs cellular proliferation and so immune activity | Poor wound healing |
| | | Hyperlipidaemia |
| | | Proteinuria |

## SEVERE CHRONIC KIDNEY DISEASE AT A GLANCE

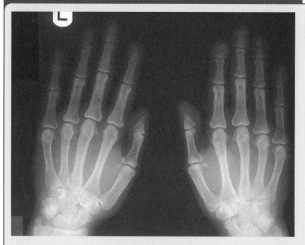

**Figure A** Renal osteodystrophy with hyperparathyroidism. Erosion of the terminal phalanges is accompanied by a loss of cortical structure and cyst formation, most marked on the radial sides of other phalanges.

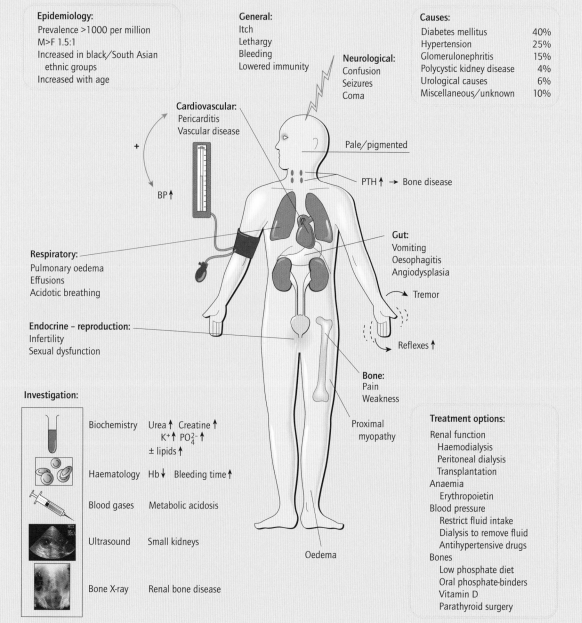

**Epidemiology:**
Prevalence >1000 per million
M>F 1.5:1
Increased in black/South Asian
  ethnic groups
Increased with age

**General:**
Itch
Lethargy
Bleeding
Lowered immunity

**Neurological:**
Confusion
Seizures
Coma

**Causes:**

| | |
|---|---|
| Diabetes mellitus | 40% |
| Hypertension | 25% |
| Glomerulonephritis | 15% |
| Polycystic kidney disease | 4% |
| Urological causes | 6% |
| Miscellaneous/unknown | 10% |

**Cardiovascular:**
Pericarditis
Vascular disease

BP↑

Pale/pigmented

PTH↑ → Bone disease

**Respiratory:**
Pulmonary oedema
Effusions
Acidotic breathing

**Gut:**
Vomiting
Oesophagitis
Angiodysplasia

Tremor

Reflexes↑

**Endocrine – reproduction:**
Infertility
Sexual dysfunction

**Bone:**
Pain
Weakness

Proximal
myopathy

Oedema

**Investigation:**

| | | |
|---|---|---|
| Biochemistry | Urea↑ Creatine↑ | |
| | $K^+$↑ $PO_4^{2-}$↑ | |
| | ± lipids↑ | |
| Haematology | Hb↓ Bleeding time↑ | |
| Blood gases | Metabolic acidosis | |
| Ultrasound | Small kidneys | |
| Bone X-ray | Renal bone disease | |

**Treatment options:**

Renal function
  Haemodialysis
  Peritoneal dialysis
  Transplantation
Anaemia
  Erythropoietin
Blood pressure
  Restrict fluid intake
  Dialysis to remove fluid
  Antihypertensive drugs
Bones
  Low phosphate diet
  Oral phosphate-binders
  Vitamin D
  Parathyroid surgery

### Other complications of kidney failure

- *Bleeding time:* (the time for bleeding from a cut to stop) is increased but measured clotting times are usually normal
- *Endocrine complications:* include growth retardation in children and loss of fertility and libido in adults
- *Skin:* dryness and itchiness
- *Nausea and anorexia*
- *Fatigue*
- *Peripheral neuropathy*
- *Muscle cramps or restless legs*
- *Depression and anxiety*
- *Pericarditis*
- *Increased vascular disease*
- *Hypertension*

## POSTRENAL PROBLEMS

## OBSTRUCTIVE UROPATHY

Obstruction to the flow of urine can arise at any point along the urinary tract and can cause kidney dysfunction (see **Figure 8.1a**). Lower tract obstruction is common in the elderly, mainly in older men with prostatic disease. The main causes of obstruction are:

- Benign or malignant prostatic disease
- Other tumours
- Stones
- Blood clots
- Retroperitoneal fibrosis

### Clinical features

- *Acute obstruction*, especially with stones, can cause severe pain in the areas to which the urinary tract refers pain, which is from the loin down to the external genitalia.
- *Chronic obstruction* can be asymptomatic.
- Symptoms of *prostatic obstruction* include poor stream, cause hesitancy, terminal dribbling and urinary frequency or nocturia.

### Investigation

- *Ultrasound:* used to identify obstruction
- *Blood tests:* may indicate impaired kidney function

### Management and prognosis

- Obstruction should be relieved by stenting, surgery or percutaneous drainage with a nephrostomy.
- If left untreated, obstruction can cause kidney failure.
- Obstruction must be relieved urgently if there is infection in the obstructed kidney.

## RETROPERITONEAL FIBROSIS OR PERIAORTITIS

This can be a manifestation of IgG4-related disease or associated with autoimmune diseases and results in inflammation around the aorta or periaortitis. This inflammation may be triggered by material leaking out of atheromatous plaques. The ureters can become embedded in fibrous tissue and so obstructed. It is often asymptomatic and diagnosed by CT or MR imaging.

Treatment is with steroids and other immunosuppressive drugs and stenting of ureters if required.

## URINARY TRACT STONES

If stone-forming substances in the urine, such as calcium phosphate, reach high enough concentrations to exceed their solubility, they come out of solution to form stones. Urinary stasis, infection and indwelling catheters all promote stone formation. Citrate, which is present in urine, inhibits stone formation by forming a soluble complex with calcium. *Nephrocalcinosis* describes diffuse renal calcium deposition, mainly in the medulla, and causes include hyperparathyroidism, distal renal tubular acidosis and medullary sponge kidney.

### DISEASE MECHANISMS

The major causes of stone formation are given in **Table 8.14**.

### Calcium stones

- Calcium stones are the most common stones, formed from calcium oxalate and/or calcium phosphate.
- Low urine volume, high urine calcium, high urine oxalate and low urine citrate levels promote their formation.
- *Hypercalciuria* occurs in 65% of all stone patients and is associated with increased intestinal calcium absorption, obesity, hypertension and sometimes primary hyperparathyroidism.
- *Oxalate* is a metabolite excreted in urine. *Hyperoxaluria* can arise from metabolic disorders, excess dietary oxalate intake in foods such as spinach, rhubarb and chocolate, and ileal disease.

### Urate stones

- Urate stones are radiolucent and form in acidic urine.
- *Treatment* involves reducing dietary purine intake (urate is a product of purine metabolism), and alkalinizing urine alkaline with sodium bicarbonate or potassium citrate. The drug allopurinol can be useful as it inhibits urate production.
- *Secondary causes* of urate stones include excess urate production from rapid cell turnover or death, especially during cancer chemotherapy.

**Table 8.14** Major causes of stone formation

| Stone type | Specific causes |
|---|---|
| **Calcium stones (80%)** | |
| Hypercalciuria | Causes of hypercalcaemia, especially primary hyperparathyroidism |
| | Idiopathic |
| Hyperoxaluria | Primary hyperoxaluria |
| | Excess intake |
| | Ileal disease and ileal bypass |
| Hypocitraturia | Distal tubular disease |
| **Uric acid stones (10%)** | |
| Acid urine causes uric acid precipitation | |
| High urate intake | |
| High cell turnover – tumours and tumour lysis | |
| **Cystine stones (2%)** | |
| Cystinuria | Autosomal recessive defect in dibasic amino acid transporter |
| **Infection stones (5%)** | |
| (*Magnesium ammonium phosphate and calcium phosphate*) | Chronic infection with urea splitting organisms |
| **Other stones (3%)** | |
| Xanthine stones in xanthinuria | |
| Rare renal chloride channel mutations can cause stone formation | |

### Cystine stones

- These are rare and caused by an *autosomal recessive mutation* in a renal amino acid transporter which results in raised urine cystine levels.
- Urine alkalinization and D-pencillamine can help prevent the stone formation.

### Infection stones

- These are often large staghorn calculi containing magnesium ammonium phosphate and calcium phosphate.
- Infection, usually with *Proteus* species, promotes stone formation.
- *Treatment* involves removal of the stones and antibiotics.

## EPIDEMIOLOGY

- Urinary tract stones affect up to 10% of men and 5% of women.
- 50% of patients have a recurrence.

## CLINICAL FEATURES

Urinary tract stones can present in a number of different ways:
- Acute obstruction
- Recurrent infection
- CKD
- Haematuria
- Passage of stones or gravel

Acute ureteric obstruction causes *renal colic* with acute and intense flank pain, often radiating to the groin, and sometimes nausea, vomiting, abdominal discomfort, dysuria, renal tenderness and haematuria. On examination, there may be renal tenderness on palpation if there is urinary

tract obstruction. Bladder stones can halt urine flow suddenly, with penile or perineal pain that may be relieved by lying down. There are three main sites where stones lodge in the ureter:
- *Pelviureteric junction:* Pain refers to the loin and back.
- *Pelvic brim:* Pain refers to the testis or labium majus.
- *Entry site of the ureter into the bladder:* Pain refers to the tip of the penis or perineum.

## ACUTE INVESTIGATION OF SUSPECTED STONES

- Urine should be tested by dipstick analysis for blood and microscopy for red blood cells. Urine infection should be excluded.
- Imaging by ultrasound or CT should be conducted to locate the stones.

## DIFFERENTIAL DIAGNOSIS

The differential diagnosis of an acute episode is:
- Obstruction by a clot (clot retention)
- Papillary necrosis
- Obstruction by a tumour or tumour fragment

## MANAGEMENT OF AN ACUTE STONE

If there is good renal function, NSAIDs are good analgesics. Obstruction must always be relieved as it can cause renal damage and can be life-threatening if the obstructed urine becomes infected. Stones less than 6 mm diameter usually pass spontaneously, but stones more than 1 cm will not. Stones can be broken up by extracorporeal shock wave lithotripsy (ESWL) or removed endoscopically, percutaneously

## URINARY TRACT STONES AT A GLANCE

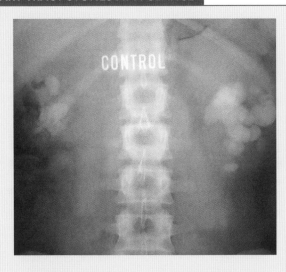

**Figure A** Bilateral staghorn calculi. No dye has been used in this study and the white radio-opacities seen on both sides are caused by large stones in the renal pelvices.

**Epidemiology:**

Affects
5% of women
10% of men
50% recurrence rate
Increased with obesity and hypertension
Increased in hot climates

Endemic areas of stone disease

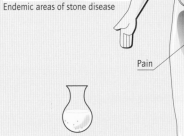

Pain

Pelviureteric junction
Brim of pelvis
Vesicoureteric junction
Bladder outflow

Sites where stones may lodge

**Urine:**
Haematuria
Gravel
Stones
Abnormal biochemistry

| Stone type | % of patients | Visible on X-ray | Treatment to prevent recurrence |
|---|---|---|---|
| Calcium | 80% | Yes | Thiazide diuretics / Potassium citrate – chelates calcium |
| Urate | 10% | No | Allopurinol / Potassium citrate – alkalinizes urine |
| Cystine | 2% | Weakly | D-penicillamine / Potassium citrate – alkalinizes urine |
| Infection | 5% | Yes | Remove stones / Eradicate infection |
| Others | 3% | Varies | Varies |

High fluid intake helps prevent all types

8

or by conventional surgery. ESWL aims shock waves at the stone through the skin, but it can be complicated by bleeding and infection.

## MANAGEMENT: INVESTIGATION OF PATIENTS WITH STONES

A full history and clinical examination should exclude bowel disease, diarrhoea and the use of antacids and diuretics. Diet should be assessed for fluid, protein, sodium, calcium, oxalate, purine and vitamin D intake and a family history taken. When available, the stones should be analysed to determine their constituents. Baseline investigations include:
- Urinalysis
- Serum calcium
- Phosphate
- Urate
- Creatinine and urea

Recurrent stone formation merits 24-hour urine collections for volume, osmolality, calcium, phosphate, oxalate, citrate, urate, sodium creatinine and pH as well as serum sodium potassium, chloride and bicarbonate.

### Prevention

- The key to prevention of all stone formation is increased fluid intake because this dilutes urine and so reduces the probability of stone formation.
- Dietary changes reduce the intake of relevant substances such as purines.
- Any metabolic defect, such as hyperparathyroidism, should be treated.
- Alkalinization of urine with potassium citrate or sodium bicarbonate may help prevent urate stone formation and the citrate chelates calcium which helps with calcium-containing stones.
- Thiazide diuretics can inhibit calcium excretion.
- Cystine stones are also prevented by urinary alkalinization and by D-penicillamine, which cleaves cystine to soluble cysteine products.
- Eradicate any chronic infection.

## COMPLICATIONS

The key complications of renal stone disease are infection and urinary obstruction, which can both lead to permanent renal damage.

## URINARY TRACT CANCER

Cancer can arise at any point along the renal tract and can bleed into the renal tract. It should always be considered if there is haematuria or altered urinary flow. Primary cancers of the ureter or urethra are rare. Children can develop Wilms' tumour of the kidney.

## RENAL CARCINOMA

In adults, renal cancer is known as renal carcinoma, renal cell carcinoma or hypernephroma. It spreads locally or via the lymphatic system to the renal hilum, retroperitoneum and para-aortic lymph nodes and often invades the renal veins and inferior vena cava. The left testicular vein drains into the left renal vein, so blockage of this vein by tumour can cause a left-sided varicocoele (dilated varicose vessels in the scrotum). Metastases typically arise in the lungs, liver, bones and brain.

### Epidemiology

- Accounts for only 2% of adult cancer
- Mainly in those over 50 years with an increased risk in men

### Clinical features

The usual presentation is with haematuria, but patients can also present with loin, back or abdominal pain. On examination, there may be an abdominal mass, groin or neck lymphadenopathy, skin metastases or a large liver or spleen. Renal cancers commonly cause systemic effects including weight loss, night sweats, fever, anaemia, nausea, malaise, polyneuritis and myositis. They can produce excess hormones such as erythropoietin (which can cause erythrocytosis), renin (which can cause hypertension), and PTH-related protein (PTHrP) (which can cause hypercalcaemia).

### Investigation

Investigations include urinalysis, urine cytology for malignant cells and imaging by ultrasound, CT or MRI and percutaneous biopsy or removal.

### Management

Treatment is surgical removal of the cancer and often the entire kidney. Chemotherapy or biological therapies may be used.

### Other renal tumours in adults

- Secondary renal tumours can arise from lung or breast tumours, melanomas or lymphomas.
- Von Hippel–Lindau disease is an autosomal dominant condition causing cancers in the kidneys, eyes, central nervous system, gonads, adrenals and pancreas.

## BLADDER CANCER

Most bladder cancers are transitional cell tumours, but a small percentage are squamous cell tumours, often arising from chronic inflammation. There may be local spread into the pelvis, but distant metastasis is uncommon.

### Epidemiology

- Bladder cancer is common and affects men more than women.
- Recognized risk factors include age, smoking, chronic bladder inflammation (especially that resulting from

schistosomiasis infection; see Chapter 3, Infectious disease) and exposure to industrial toxins from the dye industry.

### Clinical features and investigation

The typical presentation is painless haematuria. A bladder mass or obstructed kidney may be palpable. Investigation includes urine analysis and urine cytology, imaging using ultrasound, CT, MR and cystoscopy. Sterile pyuria (pus cells such as polymorphonuclear leucocytes in the absence of infection) can occur.

### Management

- Superficial cancers can be resected endoscopically and then followed up with repeated cystoscopic surveillance to detect recurrence.
- Deeper tumours may require surgery with radiotherapy or chemotherapy.
- If the bladder is removed, an artificial bladder may be constructed from small intestine.

## PROSTATE CANCER

Prostate cancer is a common cancer in men. Most cancers are adenocarcinomas and initially spread by local invasion and then involve pelvic lymph nodes, metastasizing to bone and less commonly lung and liver. Bone metastases are typically denser than normal bone on radiography.

### Clinical features

Presentation is usually with the symptoms of bladder outflow obstruction:
- Hesitancy
- Poor stream
- Terminal dribbling
- Frequency
- Nocturia
- Urinary retention or obstruction

The tumour is usually hard and irregular on rectal examination. The main differential diagnosis is benign prostatic hypertrophy.

### Investigation

Prostatic cells secrete prostate-specific antigen (PSA) and plasma levels are usually elevated in the presence of a cancer. Transrectal ultrasound can be used to identify and biopsy tumours.

### Management

Tumours can be treated with transurethral resection of the prostate (TURP) and regular follow up. Advanced tumours may require radical prostatectomy and radiotherapy. Tumour growth may be promoted by testosterone. Hormonal therapy of metastatic disease includes orchidectomy, synthetic oestrogens, androgen receptor antagonists (anti-androgens) such as bicalutamide or flutamide

and gonadotrophin-releasing hormone analogues such as buserelin.

## URINARY TRACT INFECTION

### Epidemiology

- Urinary tract infection is more common in women and peaks during the child-bearing years.
- In men, urinary tract infection peaks in later life in association with prostatic disease.

### Disease mechanisms

Most lower urinary tract infections are self-resolving, but ascending urinary tract infection can lead to severe life-threatening sepsis and permanent kidney damage. The usual organisms are the Gram-negative bacteria *Escherichia coli*, and *Klebsiella* and *Proteus* species.

- *Lower urinary tract infection:* This is restricted to the bladder and urethra. It usually involves only the superficial mucosa, is easily treated and has no long-term effects.
- *Upper urinary tract infection:* This affects the kidney or ureters, involves the deep renal tissue and can permanently damage the kidney. It can be difficult to treat and may recur.

The *shorter female urethra* provides easier access to the bladder for organisms that colonize the perineum from the bowel and genital tract. *Sexual activity*, especially initially or with a new partner, is associated with infection. During *pregnancy*, endocrine changes reduce the normal ureteric tone making reflux up the ureters more likely and increasing the risk of upper tract infection. Urinary stasis due to obstruction or incomplete bladder emptying promotes infection. Infection can also spread from a focus such as a chronically infected prostate gland or a urinary stone (typically *Proteus mirabilis* infection). Instrumentation or catheterization of the urinary tract can introduce infection. Infection of the urinary tract by *Mycobacterium tuberculosis* is uncommon in the UK but it is a cause of sterile pyuria (white cells in the urine, but no organism grown in standard culture conditions).

### Clinical features

- Lower urinary tract infection can produce discomfort or burning on micturition, increased urinary frequency and cloudy offensive-smelling urine.
- Upper tract infection or pyelonephritis can produce loin pain, fever, flank tenderness and rigors.
- In the elderly, upper or lower urinary tract infection can present without specific urinary symptoms, but can result in general malaise, confusion, drowsiness and sepsis.

### Investigation

- Urine can be dipstick tested for leucocytes and for nitrites indicating bacteria. Formal diagnosis requires urine culture.

8

- If upper tract infection is suspected, blood cultures should be taken and the urinary tract should be imaged, usually with ultrasound to exclude obstruction, stones or an anatomical abnormality.
- In men, the prostate should be assessed by rectal examination.
- If tuberculosis is suspected, early morning urine samples should be cultured for mycobacteria.

### Management and complications

- A key aspect of management is to maintain a high fluid intake, preferably more than 3 litres of fluid per day.
- Antibiotic therapy is required for upper urinary tract infection but may not be necessary for lower urinary tract infection, although it may help symptoms. Antibiotic choice should be based on known or predicted microbiological sensitivities.
- The probability of infection can be reduced by maintaining a good urine volume and, in women, by passing urine before and after sexual activity.
- Complications include AKI, stone formation and papillary necrosis.

### Differential diagnosis

The differential diagnosis of acute upper tract infection or pyelonephritis is of renal colic resulting from stones or renal infarction causing pain.

## FLUID, ELECTROLYTE AND ACID–BASE DISORDERS

### INTRODUCTION

The kidney is the key organ in the regulation of fluid, electrolyte and acid–base status. Electrolyte and fluid disorders can be dangerous (e.g. a high potassium level can cause cardiac arrest), so it is important to know how to respond to these situations as there may not be time to seek specialist advice.

### STRUCTURE AND FUNCTION

#### BODY FLUID

When clinicians refer to body fluid, they mean body water content. Sometimes, the terms body fluid volume and body volume are also used (e.g. 'volume contracted' or 'volume overloaded').

- Body water consists of water in cells (intracellular fluid) and water outside cells (extracellular fluid).
- Extracellular fluid consists of water in the circulation or vascular compartment (intravascular fluid) and

**Table 8.15** Normal constituents of body fluid compartments (in mmol/L)

|  | Extracellular fluid (mmol/L) | Intracellular fluid (mmol/L) |
|---|---|---|
| Na | 141 | 10 |
| K | 4.1 | 120 |
| Cl | 113 | 3 |
| $HCO_3^-$ | 26 | 10 |
| Phosphate | 2.0 | 140 (organic phosphate) |

water in the tissues or interstitial or extravascular compartment (extravascular fluid).
- Intravascular extracellular fluid is plasma.

Much confusion is generated by excessive attention to where the fluid is. The key issue is usually whether total body water content is too high or too low. The normal constituents of the different fluid compartments are shown in **Table 8.15** and **Table 8.16**.

Unlike many ions and molecules, water cannot be pumped directly in the body. Instead, water moves between sites by osmosis if there is an osmotic gradient and if the barrier separating the two sites contains pores or channels through which it can pass. Aquaporin molecules form water channels in most cell membranes. Intra- and extracellular fluid compartments are normally in approximate osmotic equilibrium. The $Na^+/K^+$ATPase pumps sodium out of cells and potassium into cells so:

- Intracellular fluid has high potassium and low sodium concentrations.
- Extracellular fluid has low potassium and high sodium concentrations.

### REGULATION OF BODY SODIUM AND WATER

As sodium is the major extracellular ion, it is the major determinant of body water content. Generally, *the body will maintain osmolality, even at the expense of volume changes.* This makes sense because a small change in body water content is tolerated by changes in vessel tone, but a change

**Table 8.16** Volumes of fluid in each fluid compartment and the percentage of body weight in each compartment

|  | Volume (L) in a 70 kg person | Percentage of body weight (%) |
|---|---|---|
| Total body fluid | 45 | 60 |
| Intracellular fluid | 30 | 40 |
| Extracellular fluid | 15 | 20 |
| Interstitial fluid | 12 | 16 |
| Plasma fluid | 3 | 4 |
| Total blood volume (plasma and blood cells) | 5 | 7 |

## URINARY TRACT INFECTION AT A GLANCE

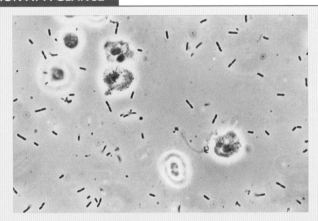

**Figure A** White blood cells and bacteria in urine from a patient with bacterial cystitis. Reproduced from Becker GJ *et al.* (1992) *Clinical Nephrology in Medical Practice* (Wiley-Blackwell, Oxford), with the permission of the authors.

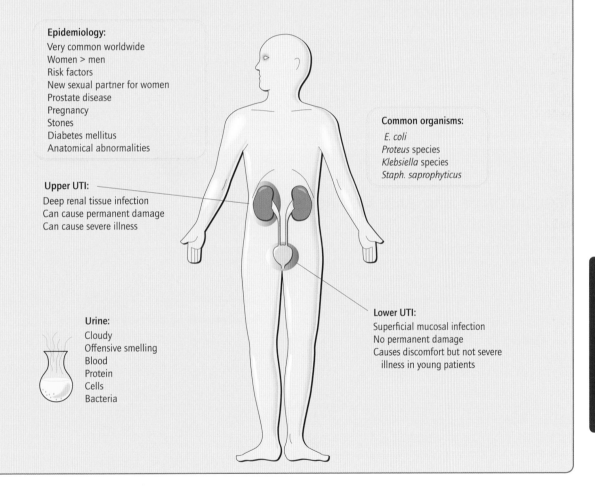

**Epidemiology:**
Very common worldwide
Women > men
Risk factors
New sexual partner for women
Prostate disease
Pregnancy
Stones
Diabetes mellitus
Anatomical abnormalities

**Common organisms:**
E. coli
Proteus species
Klebsiella species
Staph. saprophyticus

**Upper UTI:**
Deep renal tissue infection
Can cause permanent damage
Can cause severe illness

**Lower UTI:**
Superficial mucosal infection
No permanent damage
Causes discomfort but not severe
 illness in young patients

**Urine:**
Cloudy
Offensive smelling
Blood
Protein
Cells
Bacteria

8

in the osmotic gradient across cell membranes has severe effects on cells, such as causing seizures in the brain.

- *Control of osmolality:* Osmoreceptors in the hypothalamus detect changes in osmolality and trigger changes in water intake by thirst and in water excretion by altering vasopressin (ADH) secretion. *This maintains osmolality by changing*

*water handling* but does not control body osmolyte content.

- *Control of volume:* Volume receptors in the circulation detect stretch. Sodium handling by the kidney is influenced especially by angiotensin II and aldosterone. Because osmolality will normally be maintained, the total body water *volume is controlled by changing the amount of sodium in the body.* For example, if body volume is low, the kidney retains sodium, which increases plasma osmolality. The osmolality regulating system then causes more water to be drunk and less to be excreted by the kidney and the result is an increase in total body water.

## REGULATION OF BODY POTASSIUM

Body potassium is regulated by the adrenal gland and the kidney. A rise in potassium is detected by the adrenal cortex and stimulates aldosterone release. In the kidney, aldosterone promotes potassium secretion (and sodium reabsorption).

## REGULATION OF BODY CALCIUM, PHOSPHATE AND MAGNESIUM

The parathyroid gland senses calcium levels and, if calcium levels rise, PTH production falls (**Figure 8.22**). PTH causes bone resorption (destruction) with the release of calcium and phosphate. PTH acts on the kidney to increase phosphate excretion, to increase calcium reabsorption and to increase vitamin D synthesis. Vitamin D is synthesized in the kidney and acts on the gut, on bone and on the kidney to increase calcium and phosphate levels in plasma.

## REGULATION OF ACID–BASE METABOLISM

Normal metabolism produces acid, which must be buffered to prevent severe acidosis. The major soluble buffers are *bicarbonate, phosphate ions, ammonia, proteins and bone,* which can all combine with free hydrogen ions. The buffer systems are all in equilibrium with each other. In the bicarbonate buffer system, water and carbon dioxide combine and dissociate into hydrogen ions and bicarbonate ions (**Figure 8.23**). This reaction is catalysed by the enzyme carbonic anhydrase. As carbon dioxide is removed by the lungs, ventilation can affect acid–base status.

If the carbon dioxide concentration increases, the hydrogen ion concentration rises and the pH falls (**Figures 8.23, 8.24** and **8.25**). If the bicarbonate concentration increases, the hydrogen ion concentration falls and the pH rises. The body pH can be altered by regulating the ratio of carbon dioxide (acid) : bicarbonate ions (base):

- Carbon dioxide levels are controlled by altering ventilation.
- Bicarbonate levels are controlled by the kidney.

### Respiratory effects on acid–base balance

- If ventilation is reduced, carbon dioxide accumulates and the reaction in **Figure 8.23** shifts to the right. This produces hydrogen ions and a *respiratory acidosis.*

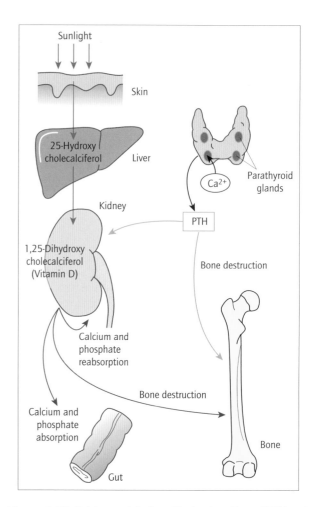

**Figure 8.22** Calcium metabolism. The basic actions of PTH and vitamin D are shown.

- If ventilation is increased, more carbon dioxide is removed and the reaction shifts to the left. This removes hydrogen ions and produces a *respiratory alkalosis.*

### Renal effects on acid–base balance

The kidneys control bicarbonate levels by controlling bicarbonate excretion. Changes in bicarbonate concentration alter the number of free hydrogen ions in body fluids.

- If the kidney reduces bicarbonate excretion, bicarbonate levels increase and shift the reaction to

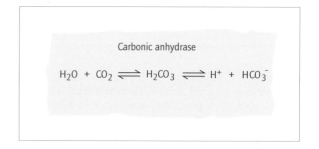

**Figure 8.23** The carbonic anhydrase reaction. This is reversible, but dissociation of $H_2CO_3$ to carbon dioxide and water is speeded up by the enzyme carbonic anhydrase.

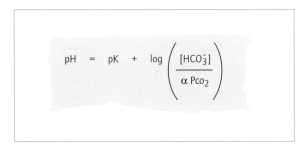

**Figure 8.24** The Henderson–Hasselbalch equation. α is the solubility coefficient of carbon dioxide in plasma, where pK is the dissociation constant for the $HCO_3^-$–$P_{CO_2}$ system in plasma.

the left, which reduces the number of hydrogen ions causing a *metabolic alkalosis*.

- If the kidney increases bicarbonate excretion (or bicarbonate is lost from the gut), bicarbonate levels fall and shift the reaction to the right, which increases the number of hydrogen ions causing a *metabolic acidosis*.

### Acid–base disturbances

- *A respiratory acid–base disturbance* arises when abnormal ventilation results in too little or too much carbon dioxide.
- *A metabolic acid–base disturbance* arises when bicarbonate levels are abnormal from a direct effect on the bicarbonate level itself (e.g. loss of bicarbonate from the kidney or gut) or by the addition of an acid or a base to the body.

### The anion gap

The anion gap is the difference between the positively charged measured cations ($Na^+ + K^+$) and the negatively charged measured anions ($HCO_3^- + Cl^-$). The body is electrically neutral, so this difference or gap is accounted for by other anions which are not measured. There is a normal anion gap of 6–16 mmol/L:

$$\text{Anion gap} = (Na^+ + K^+) - (HCO_3^- + Cl^-)$$

- If there is just simple loss of bicarbonate, bicarbonate levels fall but chloride levels rise to maintain electroneutrality and so the *measured anion gap is still normal*.
- However, if a new acid (such as salicylic acid in aspirin poisoning or ketoacids in diabetic ketoacidosis) is added to the body, *the measured anion gap increases*. The new acid dissociates into hydrogen ions and anions. The hydrogen ions ($H^+$) combine with bicarbonate to form carbon dioxide and water, so the bicarbonate level is lowered, but chloride levels are normal. The new anions take the place of the bicarbonate and contribute to the anion gap but are not measured so *the measured anion gap increases*.

## APPROACH TO THE PATIENT

### DIURETICS

Diuretics are commonly prescribed for hypertension and heart failure. They inhibit the reabsorption of electrolytes in the kidney leading to electrolyte and water loss, which can cause fluid and electrolyte disorders.

### Loop diuretics (principally furosemide and bumetanide)

These are strong diuretics that inhibit the NKCC2 cotransporter in the loop of Henle, increasing urinary loss of sodium, potassium and chloride as well as water. Secondary effects can include lowering of plasma calcium and magnesium.

### Thiazide diuretics (e.g. bendroflumethiazide)

These are weak diuretics that inhibit the NCC cotransporter in the distal tubule, increasing urinary loss of sodium, chloride and water. As some sodium is exchanged in the collecting ducts for potassium, potassium loss also occurs.

## POTASSIUM-SPARING DIURETICS

### Amiloride-type diuretics (amiloride and triamterene)

These are weak diuretics that inhibit the ENaC epithelial cell sodium channel in the collecting tubules. This slightly increases urinary sodium loss and, as sodium reabsorption is linked to potassium secretion in the collecting tubule cells, urine potassium loss is reduced. These drugs

| Disorder | pH | $P_{CO_2}$ | $HCO_3^-$ |
|---|---|---|---|
| **Respiratory acidosis** | | | |
| Acute | ↓ | ⬆ | ↑ |
| Chronic | N | ⬆ | ⬆ |
| **Respiratory alkalosis** | | | |
| Acute | ↑ | ⬇ | ↓ |
| Chronic | N | ⬇ | ⬇ |
| **Metabolic acidosis** | | | |
| Acute | ↓ | N | ↓ |
| Chronic | N | ⬇ | ⬇ |
| **Metabolic alkalosis** | | | |
| Acute | ↑ | ↑ | ⬆ |
| Chronic | N | ↑ | ⬆ |

**Figure 8.25** The main changes in the different types of acid–base disturbance. N, normal; blue arrows indicate the first change causing the disturbance; red arrows indicate the change in pH that this causes; small black arrows indicate a small compensatory change; large black arrows indicate a large compensatory change. This may not normalize pH.

are usually used with a loop or thiazide diuretic to reduce potassium loss.

### Aldosterone antagonist-type diuretics (principally spironolactone)

Aldosterone promotes sodium reabsorption and potassium secretion, partly by increasing the number of ENaC molecules in tubular cells. Spironolactone blocks aldosterone and so blocks this effect, which slightly increases urinary sodium loss and reduces urine potassium loss, as amiloride does. Side effects include gynaecomastia.

## LESS IMPORTANT DIURETICS

### Osmotic diuretics (mannitol)

Mannitol is filtered but not reabsorbed and osmotically opposes water reabsorption in the kidney. In the circulation, it has an osmotic effect, drawing water from cells, which is sometimes used to dehydrate brain cells if there is cerebral oedema.

### Carbonic anhydrase inhibitors (acetazolamide)

Carbonic anhydrase is required for bicarbonate reabsorption in the kidney, so if it is inhibited, bicarbonate ions in the renal tubules have an osmotic effect that opposes the reabsorption of water and increases urine volume.

## PRESCRIBING FLUIDS

Fluids can be prescribed as oral fluids, nasogastric or other tube-feeding fluids, or IV fluids. It is generally safer and easier to give fluids or water orally or nasogastrically. IV lines are a significant infection risk and may well be unnecessary.

## INTRAVENOUS FLUIDS

When a patient cannot drink or be given fluids or food via a feeding tube into the gut, they must be given IV fluids and electrolytes. First consider whether IV fluids are necessary. If a patient is nil-by-mouth for just a few hours and was normally hydrated beforehand, there is probably no need for IV fluid therapy. Usually 5% dextrose or normal saline with or without added potassium chloride is used:

- *5% dextrose* is 5 g of dextrose (dextrose is glucose) per 100 mL of water, which is a 278 mmol solution and approximately iso-osmotic with plasma.
- With 5% dextrose, the glucose is metabolized and the end result is merely the addition of water to the body. Therefore, if the patient only needs water, give 5% dextrose.
- *Normal saline* is a 154 mmol solution of sodium chloride in water (9 g of sodium chloride per litre) and is approximately iso-osmotic with plasma because there are both sodium and chloride ions in solution.

- With normal saline, the patient acquires 9 g or 154 mmol of sodium per litre of fluid administered and, in some diseases (e.g. heart failure, renal failure and liver failure), sodium excretion by the kidney may be reduced. If the sodium is retained, water will be retained with it, possibly resulting in oedema.

Anyone on IV fluids should have standard biochemistry (sodium, potassium and renal function) measured every day and have their fluid status assessed each day. Other electrolytes such as calcium, phosphate and magnesium should be assessed at least twice a week, or more frequently in sick patients.

### Prescribing potassium

Potassium chloride can be added to fluids to replace potassium loss. Kidneys excrete a certain amount of potassium each day, so, if a patient is not eating or drinking, this loss will need to be replaced. Rapid infusion of large amounts of potassium can cause fatal cardiac arrest. Generally, therefore, 20–40 mmol of potassium are added to 1 litre of normal saline or 5% dextrose and given over 4–8 hours.

### How much fluid to give

The amount of fluid required depends on the circumstances. Measure and replace urine output (and the output of any tubes, fistulae or drains) as well as the insensible losses, such as sweat and exhaled water vapour. Insensible losses are usually around 500 mL/day, but higher if the patient has a fever. Daily weight is a useful measure of fluid balance. Patients are usually given 2–3 litres of fluid per day, often consisting of 2 litres of 5% dextrose and 1 litre of normal saline with around 20–40 mmol/day of potassium.

### How to judge body fluid volume

Key features to pay attention to are:
- Blood pressure (especially a postural drop)
- Jugular or central venous pressure
- Presence of oedema in the lungs or the periphery

Listen to the bases of the lungs for pulmonary oedema.

---

# FLUID, ELECTROLYTE AND ACID–BASE DISORDERS AND THEIR MANAGEMENT

## UNDERSTANDING DISORDERS OF BODY FLUID VOLUME, OSMOLALITY AND SODIUM

## DISORDERS AFFECTING SODIUM AND WATER

Osmolality is controlled at the expense of volume and the kidney usually retains or excretes water to keep plasma osmolality normal, even if this causes an abnormal body fluid volume. For example, in heart failure the kidney retains sodium and the osmolality regulation system triggers the retention of water with it to maintain normal osmolality.

## DISORDERS OF BODY FLUID VOLUME

Changes in body sodium content cause changes in body volume, but usually osmolality is maintained and plasma sodium concentration is normal.

### Low body fluid volume – dehydration

- *Aldosterone deficiency:* This is usually caused by Addison's disease in adults (see Chapter 12, Endocrine disease). Aldosterone stimulates the kidney to retain sodium and excrete potassium, causing renal loss of sodium and with it water and hyperkalaemia.
- *Diuretics:* These cause renal excretion of sodium and with it water. Hyperglycaemia in poorly controlled diabetes mellitus can cause an osmotic diuresis and dehydration.
- *Renal disease:* Damage to tubular function in many kidney diseases can impair the ability of the kidney to reabsorb sodium from the tubules.

### Treatment

- Treatment is with fluid and electrolytes to replace losses.
- Underlying disease should be treated and causative drugs removed or their dose adjusted.
- Withhold diuretics until the patient is rehydrated.
- Aldosterone deficiency is treated by with the synthetic mineralocorticoid fludrocortisone.

### High body fluid volume – oedema

- *Aldosterone excess:* Excess aldosterone can be caused by adrenal hyperplasia or a tumour (Conn's syndrome) or by excess renin and angiotensin II. Excess aldosterone promotes excess retention by the kidney of sodium and with it water. Enhanced potassium excretion causes hypokalaemia.
- *Renal failure:* This impairs the ability of the kidneys to excrete sodium, water and other electrolytes.
- *Oedema states:* These have high levels of renin, angiotensin II aldosterone, vasopressin (ADH) and sympathetic nervous system activity, which all stimulate the kidneys to retain sodium and water, causing oedema. There three main oedema states are:
  o Congestive heart failure (see Chapter 7, Cardiovascular disease)
  o Liver failure (see Chapter 9, Liver, Biliary tract and pancreatic disease)
  o Nephrotic syndrome (see page 286)

### Treatment

- Treatment is with diuretics to stimulate sodium and water excretion by the kidney.
- ACE inhibitors or angiotensin II antagonists block the effects of angiotensin II.

- Spironolactone is used, especially in liver disease, to directly block the effects of aldosterone. In these conditions, fluid restriction and sodium restriction can also be helpful.
- Any underlying disease should be treated and any causative drug removed or the dose reduced.

## DISORDERS OF OSMOLALITY

The key disorders of osmolality are:
- *Syndrome of inappropriate antidiuresis (SIAD):* There is too much vasopressin and *low plasma osmolality*. Urine osmolality is inappropriately high.
- *Diabetes insipidus:* There is a deficiency of vasopressin or an inability of vasopressin to act on the kidney and *high plasma osmolality*. Urine osmolality is inappropriately low.

## LOW OSMOLALITY

There is excess water retention compared to sodium, usually caused by excess vasopressin in SIAD, resulting in excess reabsorption of water by the kidney. Causes include vasopressin secretion from a lung cancer, a postoperative rise in vasopressin as part of the stress response or lung disease, especially infection. *Urine osmolality is abnormally high compared to the low plasma osmolality.*

### Treatment

Treatment is with fluid restriction and sometimes demeclocycline, which causes a mild compensatory nephrogenic diabetes insipidus, or vasopressin receptor antagonists (vaptans).

Very rarely, patients may drink such vast quantities of water that they lower their plasma osmolality. This is sometimes termed 'psychogenic polydipsia', but urine osmolality may also be low.

## HIGH OSMOLALITY

There is inadequate water reabsorption by the kidney compared to that of sodium. *Urine osmolality is abnormally low compared to the high plasma osmolality.* It is usually caused by diabetes insipidus with dehydration and polydipsia. Diabetes insipidus can arise from:
- Inadequate vasopressin secretion from the posterior pituitary gland (cranial diabetes insipidus)
- Inadequate response of the kidneys to vasopressin (nephrogenic diabetes insipidus), which can be caused by genetic defects or as a side effect of a drug such as lithium, amphotericin or gentamicin

### Treatment

Treatment of cranial diabetes insipidus is with intranasal desmopressin (DDAVP), a synthetic vasopressin analogue.

RENAL DISEASE; FLUID AND ELECTROLYTE DISORDERS

Osmolality can also be high if there is excess ingestion or production of an osmotically active substance which causes water loss. This can arise with hyperglycaemia in uncontrolled diabetes mellitus.

## DISORDERS OF PLASMA SODIUM

The normal plasma sodium concentration is 135–145 mmol/L. As sodium is the major extracellular electrolyte, hyponatraemia is usually associated with hypo-osmolality and hypernatraemia is usually associated with hyperosmolality. Both plasma hypo-osmolality and hyperosmolality can have adverse effects on cells, especially neural cells. In each case, the diagnosis and treatment depends on an assessment of body fluid volume.

## HYPONATRAEMIA

### Disease mechanisms

Low plasma osmolality causes the osmotic entry of water into cells, especially brain cells, which swell. If another osmotically active substance is present at high levels, the body compensates by lowering sodium levels to maintain *normal osmolality*. This can occur if the plasma glucose level is very high.

#### Pseudohyponatraemia
This occurs when a substance such as lipid accumulates in plasma. The amount of sodium per 100 mL of plasma water is normal, but there is less sodium than normal per 100 mL of plasma volume, as some of that 100 mL of plasma volume is not water. It is the amount of sodium per unit of plasma water that matters and this is normal. *The osmolality of plasma water remains normal in pseudohyponatraemia.*

#### Hyponatraemia with low osmolality and low body volume
This is caused by fluid loss, with a greater loss of sodium than of water. The loss may be from the kidneys because of diuretics, tubular disease or inadequate aldosterone production in Addison's disease. Alternatively, the loss may be from outside the kidneys, usually from the gut or the skin.

#### Hyponatraemia with low osmolality and high body volume
This is caused by both sodium and water retention, such that there is more water retained than sodium. This can commonly arise and is usually a result of:
- Renal failure
- One of the oedema states (heart failure, liver failure or nephrotic syndrome)
- Excess water intake, especially from excess IV fluids

An important scenario in which hyponatraemia can arise is as follows. Initial fluid loss of both sodium and water

promotes vasopressin secretion. Treatment with IV 5% dextrose, which is equivalent to giving water, dilutes the sodium that is present. Young menstruating women are particularly likely to retain water in this way and dangerous hyponatraemia can occur – especially postoperatively – if they are given excess IV water in the form of 5% dextrose.

*SIAD* can cause a low sodium with a body fluid volume that is either normal or sometimes high. This is because of excess vasopressin secretion causing inappropriate water retention.

### Clinical features

Typically, neurological function is depressed with lethargy, confusion, cramps, reduced tendon reflexes and, ultimately, seizures and coma. However, initially there may be no symptoms or signs.

### Investigation

- Check renal function and electrolytes including plasma and urine sodium and osmolalities.
- If appropriate, investigate for an underlying cause. In SIAD, typically serum osmolality is <275 mOsm/kg, urine osmolality is >100 mOsm/kg and urine sodium concentration is >30 mmol/L.

### Management

Correct an underlying cause if possible. If the patient is otherwise well with no acute neurological change, treatment is not urgent.
- *If body volume is high*, treatment is usually to restrict fluid intake.
- *If body volume is low*, the missing sodium and water should be replaced, usually with IV normal saline.

Plasma osmolality should not be corrected too quickly because compensatory mechanisms alter intracellular osmolality, so that a sudden change to normality outside the cells can itself cause problems. If there is acute neurology, such as fitting, small volumes of 3% saline may be given to correct the sodium by around 5 mmol/L and then low volumes of normal saline (0.9% saline) with the aim to increase plasma sodium concentration by no more than around 8–10 mmol/L/day until it is above 130 mmol/L.

## HYPERNATRAEMIA

### Disease mechanisms

Hypernatraemia always causes hyperosmolality because sodium is the major extracellular cation.

#### Hypernatraemia with low body volume
This arises because there is loss of both water and sodium but a proportionately greater loss of water. As with hyponatraemia, the loss can be from the kidneys, because of diuretics or tubulo-interstitial diseases that reduce the kidneys' ability to produce concentrated urine. Alternatively, as with hyponatraemia, the loss may be from outside the kidneys,

322

usually from the gut or the skin. Normally, thirst corrects fluid intake, but in the sick and elderly this may not be possible. The hyperosmolality causes the osmotic exit of water from the cells, especially brain cells, which may shrink. There may even be tearing of blood vessels as a result of this shrinkage.

*Diabetes insipidus* can cause high sodium with a body fluid volume that is either normal or sometimes low. This is because of inadequate vasopressin secretion or action causing inappropriate renal water loss.

### Hypernatraemia with high body volume

This can arise with renal sodium retention in primary hyperaldosteronism when excess aldosterone promotes renal sodium retention in excess of water retention. Alternatively, it can be produced by excess administration of both sodium and water with relatively more sodium in IV fluids.

### Clinical features

Typically, neurological function appears initially increased with irritability, muscle twitches, brisk tendon reflexes and spasticity, but ultimately seizures and coma can occur. Initially, there may be no symptoms or signs.

### Investigation

Check renal function and electrolytes including plasma and urine sodium and osmolalities.

### Management

Any underlying cause should be corrected if possible. Water deficits should be replaced. Depending on the severity, this may be with oral water or IV 5% dextrose. However, plasma osmolality should not be corrected too quickly and plasma sodium levels should be checked regularly to monitor this. A rate of fall or no more than 12 mmol/L/day is usually considered acceptable.

## DISORDERS OF PLASMA POTASSIUM

The normal plasma potassium concentration is 3.5–5.0 mmol/L. Most potassium is inside cells and potassium is the main ion affecting the resting membrane potential of nerve and muscle cells. Abnormal plasma potassium levels can cause life-threatening cardiac arrhythmias including cardiac arrest and should be treated promptly. Abnormal plasma potassium levels can arise from changes in the total body potassium content or from shifts of potassium into or out of cells.

## HYPOKALAEMIA

### Disease mechanisms

#### Renal loss

- *Diuretics (loop diuretics and thiazides):* are the commonest cause of renal potassium loss

- *Aldosterone:* high levels promote renal potassium excretion
- *Magnesium depletion:* can increase renal potassium loss and should be corrected
- *Drugs such as penicillin, aminoglycosides and amphotericin:* can impair renal tubular function, causing potassium loss
- *Genetic defects in transporter channels:* can cause hypokalaemia (e.g. Bartter's syndrome)
- *Renal tubular acidosis:* can arise if there is abnormal tubular function and can cause hypokalaemia
- *Urine flow:* if very high, can promote potassium loss from the kidneys

#### Gut loss

Any potassium loss from the gut can cause hypokalaemia. Severe persistent vomiting of acid stomach contents can cause a metabolic alkalosis and promote renal potassium loss.

#### Shifts into cells

Insulin, beta-2 adrenergic agonists and metabolic alkalosis can all cause a shift of potassium into cells. Acute stress such as that of a myocardial infarction or surgery can cause catecholamine release and a shift of potassium into cells, causing some hypokalaemia.

#### Inadequate intake

Alcoholism, anorexia or starvation may be associated with poor oral intake.

### Clinical features

- There are usually no symptoms, although occasionally there may be lethargy, muscle weakness or reduced bowel activity with constipation or ileus of the bowel.
- Hypokalaemia can cause a resistance to the effects of vasopressin in the kidney and so a mild diabetes insipidus-like effect with polydipsia and polyuria may be seen.
- Cardiac arrhythmias including ectopic beats, atrioventricular block and atrial and ventricular fibrillation. Hypokalaemia can predispose patients to the toxic effects of digoxin on cardiac rhythm.

### Investigation

It is usually clear what the cause of the problem is, which in most cases is potassium loss from the kidney because of diuretics or from the gut because of loss of gut fluids. If there is doubt, exclude magnesium deficiency and consider drug effects other than those of diuretics. Unexplained hypokalaemia with hypertension raises the possibility of a high aldosterone level from, for example, a primary adrenal disorder (primary hyperaldosteronism) or renal artery stenosis, where the high renin level promotes aldosterone secretion. In the oedema states, diuretics can cause hypokalaemia but, even in the absence of therapy, the high aldosterone levels can cause hypokalaemia.

**8**

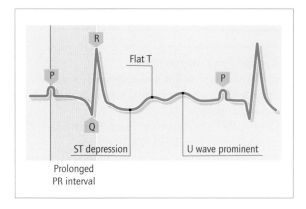

**Figure 8.26** ECG changes in hypokalaemia. Hypokalaemia is first evident as ST-segment sagging, T-wave depression and U-wave prominence. The QT interval remains normal. As hypokalaemia progresses, the T and U waves fuse.

### ECG changes

The classic changes of hypokalaemia on an electrocardiogram (**Figure 8.26**) are:

- Prolonged PR interval
- ST depression
- Flattened T waves and sometimes enhanced U waves

### Management

Any underlying cause should be treated:

- With severe hypokalaemia and a high risk of a cardiac arrhythmia (e.g. in a patient with digoxin toxicity or congestive heart failure), *cardiac monitoring* is important.
- Potassium levels should be corrected using oral therapy if the risk of arrhythmias is low, or IV therapy using fluids containing potassium chloride.
- If a diuretic is causing the problem but is necessary for the patient's underlying condition, a potassium-sparing diuretic such as spironolactone or regular oral potassium supplements may be used.

## HYPERKALAEMIA

### Disease mechanisms

Artefactual hyperkalaemia can arise if potassium is released from muscle during venesection (especially with a tourniquet or muscle constriction) or from red blood cells in a blood sample (especially if the sample is not analysed promptly). If there is doubt, take another sample, preferably without a tourniquet, and ensure that it is analysed promptly.

- Kidneys normally excrete potassium, so *kidney disease* either acute or chronic, can cause hyperkalaemia.
- *Drugs* that impair renal potassium excretion include the potassium-sparing diuretics, ACE inhibitors, angiotensin II receptor antagonists, trimethoprim, pentamidine and NSAIDs.
- Aldosterone promotes potassium excretion, so *aldosterone deficiency* can cause a rise in plasma potassium.

- Potassium can *leak out of cells* when there is cellular injury, as can occur with the muscle damage of rhabdomyolysis.
- Insulin promotes the movement of potassium into cells, so in diabetic ketoacidosis the deficiency of insulin can contribute to hyperkalaemia.
- Catecholamines promote the entry of potassium into cells, so beta blockers can cause hyperkalaemia.
- Metabolic acidosis causes hydrogen ions to enter cells where they are buffered and potassium ions leave the cells to maintain electroneutrality.

### Clinical features

Usually there are no symptoms, but there may be weakness and the effects of cardiac arrhythmias. Ultimately, *ventricular arrhythmias and ventricular fibrillation* can cause a cardiac arrest.

### Investigation

- Check the drugs the patient is taking for possible causes.
- Check the renal function and plasma glucose levels and acid–base status.
- If muscle injury is suspected, plasma levels of the muscle enzyme creatinine kinase will probably also be elevated.

### ECG changes

Initially, the P wave is narrow and peaked, then the QRS complex widens to meet the T wave (**Figure 8.27** and see Chapter 7, Cardiac disease). The typical changes are:

- Loss of the P waves
- Widening of the QRS complex
- Loss of the ST segment
- Tall wide T waves

Ultimately, a sine wave appearance may be seen and ventricular fibrillation may occur.

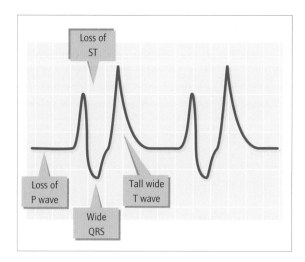

**Figure 8.27** ECG changes in hyperkalaemia. This is a very important and potentially dangerous rhythm with the characteristics shown.

**Treatment of hyperkalaemia**

Place the patient on a cardiac monitor and have resuscitation equipment to hand.

If there are ECG changes, give calcium gluconate. This dose can be repeated in 3–5 min if the ECG appearances do not improve.

Give dextrose intravenously with insulin. Monitor the patient's blood glucose after this as hypoglycaemia can occur and may require further glucose infusion.

If the patient has good renal function, a loop diuretic such as furosemide will promote potassium excretion and this can be given with IV fluid to enhance the diuresis.

Ion exchange resins are not of much use acutely but are often given with some oral fluid.

If the patient is acidotic, it may be necessary to give bicarbonate to correct the pH.

If the patient has poor renal function, dialysis or haemofiltration is likely to be necessary.

In the event of a cardiac arrest in a hyperkalaemic patient, give calcium intravenously.

## Management

Place the patient on a cardiac monitor under close observation in a coronary care or high dependency unit. If there are ECG changes, urgent treatment is required. In the immediate term, calcium chloride or calcium gluconate will antagonize some of the dangerous effects of the potassium on the heart and may reverse the ECG changes but the effect is short-lived. Plasma potassium can be lowered by giving IV insulin or nebulized salbutamol, both of which promote the movement of potassium into cells. Glucose is given with the insulin to prevent hypoglycaemia. This effect is also relatively short-lived.

Ultimately, the potassium must be removed from the body. If the patient's kidneys are functioning, this can be achieved by the administration of fluids and diuretics such as frusemide. If renal function is impaired, dialysis or haemofiltration can be used to remove the potassium. Oral or rectal administration of cation exchange resins is of minimal benefit and causes constipation, but it may bind potassium in the gut (EMERGENCY PRESENTATION 8.1).

## DISORDERS OF PLASMA MAGNESIUM

The normal range of serum magnesium is 1.4–1.75 mmol/L. Magnesium has an inhibitory effect on nervous tissue, increasing the depolarization threshold, and so is useful as an anticonvulsant, especially in eclampsia. It is also involved in regulating the intracellular content of other ions (e.g. $Ca^{2+}$ and $K^+$).

## HYPOMAGNESAEMIA

### Disease mechanisms

Magnesium can be lost through the kidneys (usually from diuretics) or from the gut.

### Clinical features

- Features include tremors, Chvostek's and Trousseau's signs, tetany and convulsions, muscle weakness and fasciculation.
- There may also be a change of personality, anxiety, delirium and psychosis.

### Investigation

- ECG changes include a *prolonged QT interval* and ventricular arrhythmias.
- Check for hypokalaemia, which is often present.

### Management

The treatment is with oral or IV magnesium chloride.

## HYPERMAGNESAEMIA

### Disease mechanisms

Hypermagnesaemia is rare. It is sometimes seen in patients with kidney failure, in Addison's disease or, in association with the use of magnesium-containing antacids.

### Clinical features

- Hypermagnesaemia causes *neurological depression*.
- Tendon reflexes are reduced and the patient may develop flaccid quadriplegia, difficulty swallowing and talking, and respiratory depression.
- There may also be bradycardia and hypotension.

### Investigation

- Plasma magnesium levels are high.
- ECG changes mimic hyperkalaemia.
- Check for hyperkalaemia – if the kidney has failed to excrete magnesium, it may also be unable to excrete potassium.

### Management

- The cause should be removed.
- Hydration and frusemide will promote renal excretion of magnesium, but if renal function is poor, dialysis may be required to remove the magnesium.
- Calcium can reverse some of the dangerous cardiac effects.

## DISORDERS OF PLASMA CALCIUM

## HYPOCALCAEMIA

Much of the calcium in plasma is bound to albumin, but it is the level of free unbound ionized calcium ($Ca^{2+}$) that

**8**

**Table 8.17** Causes of chronic hypocalcaemia

**With high phosphate level**

Chronic kidney disease

Acute kidney injury

Hypoparathyroidism (usually after parathyroidectomy)

**With normal or low phosphate levels**

Disorders of vitamin D metabolism

- Vitamin D deficiency
- Decreased 25-hydroxy-vitamin D production (liver disease, anticonvulsants)
- Decreased 1,25 hydroxy-vitamin D production (kidney failure)

Acute pancreatitis

Magnesium deficiency (inhibits PTH release and causes PTH resistance)

Postparathyroidectomy (hungry bone syndrome)

is important. For this reason, calcium values must be corrected for the amount of albumin in plasma or the free ionized calcium measured directly. Hypocalcaemia is a less common clinical problem than hypercalcaemia.

### Disease mechanisms

#### Acute hypocalcaemia

This can be caused by hyperventilation which reduces carbon dioxide levels causing a respiratory alkalosis. Hydrogen ions leave proteins to maintain the pH of the plasma and calcium ions then bind to the sites on proteins that the hydrogen ions have just left. The result is a fall in free ionized calcium levels.

#### Chronic hypocalcaemia

See **Table 8.17**. There are a number of rare genetic disorders that can cause hypocalcaemia, including pseudohypoparathyroidism which is caused by end-organ resistance to PTH.

### Clinical features

- Paraesthesia, particularly perioral and of the extremities, is common. If severe there may be tetany, laryngeal stridor and convulsions.
- Chvostek's and Trousseau's signs may be positive and, in chronic hypocalcaemia, there may be central nervous system effects such as confusion delirium or, depression.

### Investigation

- Plasma calcium and albumin levels must be measured to calculate the corrected calcium concentration (**Table 8.18**) or the free ionized calcium concentration measured.
- Phosphate, PTH, vitamin D and urinary calcium levels may be useful in establishing the cause.
- Check renal function and plasma magnesium.
- ECG changes include a *prolonged QT interval.*
- Bone radiography may show bone changes (e.g. with vitamin D deficiency).

### Management

- In acute hyperventilation, rebreathing into a paper bag elevates carbon dioxide levels and so corrects the alkalosis and hypocalcaemia.
- *Emergency treatment* of seizures or tetany requires prompt IV calcium gluconate with cardiac monitoring. Subsequently, or in less severe or chronic cases, identification and correction of the underlying cause is indicated.
- Chronic hypocalcaemia is usually treated with oral calcium salts with or without vitamin D.

## HYPERCALCAEMIA

### Disease mechanisms

Hypercalcaemia increases intracellular calcium which inhibits muscle relaxation, disturbs neurone function and impairs renal tubular function. In addition, it may cause calcification in tissues and hypercalciuria which promotes urinary tract stone formation. Causes are listed in **Table 8.19**.

### Clinical features

The signs and symptoms of hypercalcaemia include:

- *Gastrointestinal disturbance:* anorexia, nausea, vomiting, constipation, peptic ulceration and pancreatitis
- *Other muscular dysfunction:* hypertension, ECG changes (shortened QT interval) or cardiac arrest
- *Neurological dysfunction:* psychosis, confusion, stupor, coma
- *Kidney dysfunction:* polyuria (which can cause dehydration leading to AKI), nocturia, polydipsia, acute or chronic kidney disease, renal calculi.
- *Calcification:* in other tissues

**Table 8.18** Calculating corrected calcium levels

50% of plasma calcium is bound to plasma albumin, but it is the free calcium that is metabolically active and dangerous in hypercalcaemia.

Total plasma calcium should therefore be corrected, taking into account the concentration of albumin to assess this danger.

**The calculation**

Corrected calcium = measured total calcium + $0.02 \times (40 - \text{plasma albumin g}/\text{L})$

*A corrected calcium greater than 3.5 mmol/L is a medical emergency.*

**Table 8.19** Causes of hypercalcaemia

**Hyperparathyroidism** (see Chapter 5, Metabolic bone disease)
- Primary (usually adenoma)
- Tertiary: one or more glands may become autonomous

**Malignancy** (see Chapter 5)
- Metastatic resorption of bone (especially common in *myeloma*)
- Ectopic PTH production by tumour
- Non-metastatic effects (e.g. by tumour secretion of osteoclast activation factors)

**Vitamin D overdosage**

**Milk–alkali syndrome**
- Consumption of excess milk or antacids that promote enhanced calcium absorption from the gut

**Immobilization**
- Promotes bone demineralization
- Paget's disease of bone

**Endocrine disorders**
- Thyrotoxicosis
- Addison's disease

**Granulomatous disorders**
- Sarcoid
- Tuberculosis, histoplasmosis

## Investigation

Calcium levels need to be corrected for the plasma albumin concentration (see **Table 8.18**).
- Renal function should be checked.
- A raised alkaline phosphatase level may indicate bone disease.
- Measure PTH to exclude hyperparathyroidism.
- A raised serum ACE level is non-specific but may indicate sarcoidosis.
- Blood and urine should be checked for the presence of a monoclonal antibody band to exclude myeloma.
- Imaging may identify cancer or other systemic diseases.
- ECG changes include a *shortened QT interval*.

## Management

### Acute hypercalcaemia
- When hypercalcaemia is severe, either because of its symptoms and signs or if the corrected plasma calcium is more than 3.5 mmol/L, emergency measures should be taken (EMERGENCY PRESENTATION 8.2).
- Hydration is essential, but may not be possible if there is cardiac or renal failure and dialysis may be necessary.
- Bisphosphonates are useful, especially in hypercalcaemia associated with malignancy. They may be administered orally or intravenously.
- Hypercalcaemia resulting from hyperparathyroidism is often treated surgically by parathyroidectomy or by radiological injection of an ablative substance to destroy an adenoma.

---

**EMERGENCY PRESENTATION 8.2**

### Management of acute hypercalcaemia

**If plasma calcium is more than 3.5 mmol/L or there are serious clinical complications**

Give 0.9% saline intravenously to restore plasma volume.

Add furosemide 40–80 mg/hour intravenously if volume replete.

Measure urine volume, $Na^+$, $K^+$, $Mg^{2+}$ and replace losses.

**If plasma calcium is still more than 3.5 mmol/L**

Consider giving a bisphosphonate.

**If plasma calcium is still more than 3.5 mmol/L or patient cannot tolerate fluid load of above**

Consider dialysis.

---

### Chronic hypercalcaemia
- Treat the underlying cause if possible and maintain hydration.
- The mainstay of therapy in malignancy-related hypercalcaemia is the use of *bisphosphonates*.
- *Glucocorticoids* are sometimes useful for sarcoidosis, myeloma, vitamin D intoxication and immobilization. They inhibit calcium absorption by the gut, especially when stimulated by vitamin D. They also inhibit bone resorption by tumours. Their onset of action is within 2–3 days.

## DISORDERS OF PLASMA PHOSPHATE

## HYPOPHOSPHATAEMIA

Hypophosphataemia is rare.

### Disease mechanisms
- *Chronic alcohol use* is the most common cause of severe hypophosphataemia.
- Refeeding in malnourished people can cause substantial hypophosphataemia because of a shift of phosphate into the cells.
- Other causes include respiratory alkalosis, insulin therapy in diabetic ketoacidosis, excess PTH and genetic disorders such as familial hypophosphataemic rickets.

### Clinical features

The symptoms and signs of severe hypophosphataemia can be widespread:
- Red cell, white cell and platelet dysfunction
- Cardiomyopathy
- Acute respiratory insufficiency because of weakness of the diaphragm
- Encephalopathy
- Rhabdomyolysis
- Metabolic acidosis
- Osteomalacia

**8**

### Investigation

- Check PTH levels, and monitor and correct other electrolytes.
- A full blood count should exclude haemolysis, and liver and renal function should be checked.
- Creatinine kinase levels may indicate muscle damage.

### Management

Oral or, in an emergency, IV phosphate supplements should be given.

## HYPERPHOSPHATAEMIA

Hyperphosphataemia can result from phosphate release from damaged cells. This can occur with rhabdomyolysis or tumour lysis. However, the most common cause is kidney failure.

## ACID–BASE DISORDERS

## ALKALOSIS

### Respiratory alkalosis

Respiratory alkalosis is caused by hyperventilation, which removes carbon dioxide (**Table 8.20**). It is usually asymptomatic but may cause dyspnoea, dizziness, palpitations, sweating, carpopedal spasm, chest pain and fainting. Some of these symptoms result from hypocalcaemia.

### Metabolic alkalosis

Metabolic alkalosis is rare. The causes are listed in **Table 8.21**.

- *Low plasma potassium* causes excess $H^+$ loss in the distal tubule as potassium ions are reabsorbed instead of $H^+$.
- *Low plasma chloride* causes renal bicarbonate loss because chloride is reabsorbed in preference to bicarbonate.

**Table 8.20** Causes of respiratory alkalosis

| |
| --- |
| **Respiratory disease** |
| • Asthma |
| • Emphysema |
| • Pneumonia |
| • Pulmonary emboli |
| **Central nervous system** |
| • Midbrain lesion |
| • Psychogenic |
| **Metabolic** |
| • Aspirin poisoning |
| **Pregnancy** |

**Table 8.21** Causes of metabolic alkalosis

| |
| --- |
| **Prerenal causes** |
| *Extrarenal loss of acid* |
| • Vomiting |
| *Ingestion of alkali* |
| • Sodium bicarbonate as an antacid |
| **Deficiencies affecting renal tubular function** |
| • Low plasma potassium |
| • Low plasma chloride |
| **Other causes of renal tubular dysfunction** |
| • Hyperaldosteronism |
| • Bartter's syndrome |
| • Diuretics |

### Clinical features

Severe alkalosis causes cardiac arrhythmias, hypoventilation leading to hypoxia, especially if there is respiratory disease, and increased neuromuscular irritability (tetany, hyper-reflexia and seizures). Rarely, coma, respiratory depression and death can occur.

### Investigation

- Check arterial blood gases and electrolytes.
- Check *salicylate levels* to exclude aspirin overdose.

### Management

- Treatment of the underlying cause is usually the most effective and rapid way of correcting an alkalosis.
- Good hydration with IV sodium chloride and potassium chloride if necessary promotes bicarbonate excretion and $H^+$ ion retention.
- Carefully supervised rebreathing will raise $P\text{co}_2$ and can be used as a temporary emergency measure to stop cardiac arrhythmias.
- In the presence of kidney failure, dialysis may be necessary.

## ACIDOSIS

### Respiratory acidosis

Any cause of hypoventilation that increases $P\text{co}_2$ will lead to respiratory acidosis (**Table 8.22**).

**Table 8.22** Causes of respiratory acidosis

| |
| --- |
| **Neurological** |
| • Drugs |
| • Stroke |
| • Motor neurone disease |
| **Neuromuscular** |
| • Myasthenia gravis |
| • Guillain–Barré syndrome |
| **Respiratory** |
| • Any severe diffuse respiratory disease |

**Table 8.23** Classification of a metabolic acidosis

**Increased anion gap – gain of acid**
- Renal failure
- Lactic acidosis
- Diabetic ketoacidosis
- Poisoning (e.g. aspirin, ethylene glycol or methanol)

**Normal anion gap or hyperchloraemic – loss of bicarbonate**
- Gastrointestinal bicarbonate loss
- Renal bicarbonate loss (renal tubular acidosis)

## Metabolic acidosis

This is the most common and most dangerous acid–base disturbance. Its classification and causes are listed in **Table 8.23** and **Table 8.24**.

### Disease mechanisms

#### Metabolic acidosis

Metabolic acidosis is classified according to whether it causes an increase in the anion gap (see page 321) or not (**Table 8.23**). A metabolic acidosis caused by adding more anions to the plasma may increase the anion gap. Other causes of metabolic acidosis arise from loss of bicarbonate (from the gut or kidney) which is replaced by chloride ions to maintain electroneutrality and is known as a *normal anion gap acidosis* or *hyperchloraemic acidosis*.

The serum lactate level is normally ≤1 mmol/L and the causes of lactic acidosis are listed in **Table 8.25**. *Renal impairment* reduces the acid-excreting capacity of the kidneys and results in an increase in organic acids. *Diabetic ketoacidosis* results in the accumulation of acidic ketone bodies.

Renal tubular acidosis arises from loss of bicarbonate from the kidney.
- *Distal (type 1) renal tubular acidosis* can arise from various causes of renal damage including drugs and diabetes mellitus and results in minor bicarbonate loss, which can be replaced by oral therapy.

**Table 8.24** Causes of metabolic acidosis

**Renal**
- Renal impairment
- Renal tubular acidosis

**Extrarenal bicarbonate loss**
- Severe diarrhoea
- Bowel fistula

**Ingestion of acid**
- Ingestion of acids or aspirin (salicylic acid) or rarely rhubarb leaves (containing oxalic acid)

**Acid metabolized from exogenous substances**
- Methanol (forming formic acid)
- Ethylene glycol (forming oxalic acid)
- Ammonium chloride (forming hydrochloric acid)

**Disturbances of endogenous acid–base metabolism**
- Lactic acidosis
- Diabetic ketoacidosis

**Table 8.25** Causes of lactic acidosis

**Increased lactate production by anaerobic tissues**
- Any cause of decreased tissue perfusion/ischaemia
- Hypoxia
- Increased skeletal muscle activity (e.g. status epilepticus or marathon runners)
- Destruction of large tumour masses (e.g. lymphoma or leukaemia)
- Poisoning (e.g. carbon dioxide or cyanide)

**Decreased lactate transport**
- Decreased cardiac output

**Decreased lactate metabolism**
- Liver failure
- Metformin
- Alcohol
- Diabetes mellitus
- Liver hypoxia

**Miscellaneous**
- Haemofiltration or dialysis with lactate buffer
- Pregnancy

- *Proximal (type 2) renal tubular acidosis* is usually genetic and more severe and is often associated with loss of other ions in Fanconi's syndrome.

### Clinical features

- *Cardiovascular:* reduced myocardial contractility, decreased peripheral vascular resistance, low blood pressure and tissue hypoxia; pulmonary oedema; ventricular fibrillation
- *Respiratory:* rapid, deep breathing (Kussmaul's breathing)
- *Neurological:* confusion, seizures, coma

### Investigation

- *Blood gas analysis* will determine the pH, $Pco_2$, $Po_2$ and $HCO_3^-$, allowing definition of the severity and type of acidosis.
- Measure sodium, potassium, chloride and bicarbonate levels to calculate the anion gap. If the anion gap is raised, check plasma lactate and salicylate levels.
- Measure plasma creatinine and urea, liver function, ketones and glucose to determine the cause.

### Management of metabolic acidosis

- Treatment is urgent if the plasma pH is less than 7.2. IV hypertonic bicarbonate may be required and the cause corrected if possible. Milder degrees of acidosis may be corrected using either isotonic sodium bicarbonate intravenously or oral sodium bicarbonate.
- In renal tubular acidosis, potassium citrate mixture is effective in restoring plasma potassium levels to normal and helping to prevent renal calculi.
- If kidney function is poor, dialysis or haemofiltration may be required to remove acid.

**8**

**Prognosis**

The general prognosis for acidosis is good if it is treated before there are cardiovascular or neurological complications and if the underlying disease is amenable to therapy.

The prognosis for lactic acidosis is worse because it presents at a more advanced stage and the underlying cause may have a poor prognosis. If the acidosis is chronic, osteoporosis and osteomalacia can occur.

---

**MUST-KNOW CHECKLIST**

- Always measure blood pressure in anyone with kidney disease
- In acute kidney injury, always exclude dehydration
- In acute kidney injury, always exclude urinary tract obstruction
- Blood potassium levels can be elevated in acute or chronic kidney disease
- Type 2 diabetes mellitus is a major cause of chronic kidney disease
- Nephrotic syndrome consists of high urine protein loss, low blood albumin, oedema and hypercholesterolaemia
- NSAIDs should be avoided in patients with kidney disease
- Good blood pressure control slows the rate of decline of kidney function with most kidney diseases
- Renal artery stenosis can cause hypertension and chronic kidney disease
- The commonest genetic cause of chronic kidney disease is autosomal dominant adult polycystic kidney disease

---

**Questions and answers** to test your understanding of Chapter 8 can be found by clicking 'Support Material' at the following link: https://www.routledge.com/Medicine-for-Finals-and-Beyond/Axford-OCallaghan/p/book/9780367150594

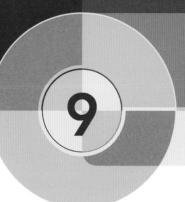

# Liver, Biliary Tract and Pancreatic Disease

## 9

JAMES NEUBERGER

## INTRODUCTION

The spectrum of liver disease varies from asymptomatic disease to jaundice and liver failure. In the West, alcoholic liver disease, non-alcoholic fatty liver and chronic infection with hepatitis C virus (HCV) account for most cases of cirrhosis. Disease of the gall bladder is usually related to stones and infection. Pancreatic disease, whether from inflammation, cancer or obstruction, may result in failure of the exocrine and/or endocrine function.

## STRUCTURE AND FUNCTION

### STRUCTURAL FEATURES OF THE LIVER, BILIARY TREE AND PANCREAS

The anatomical structure of the liver, biliary tree and pancreas is shown in **Figure 9.1** and hepatic functions in **Table 9.1**.

## FUNCTIONS

## APPROACH TO THE PATIENT

### HISTORY

As in other areas of medicine, diagnosis and management depend on a full and relevant history, clinical examination, appropriate blood tests and imaging (see HISTORY 9.1).

### EXAMINATION

Although many signs are associated with liver disease, very few are specific (see HISTORY & EXAMINATION 9.2; **Figure 9.2**).

The causes of hepatomegaly are listed in **Table 9.2**.

DOI: 10.1201/9781003193616-9

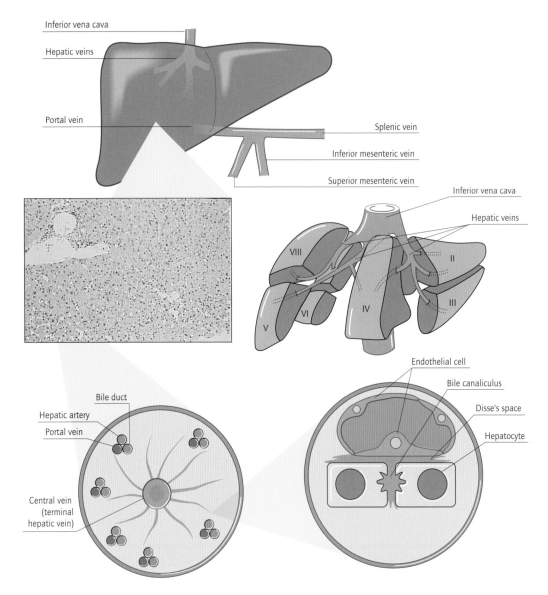

**Figure 9.1** Structure of the liver and segmental anatomy of the liver showing the eight liver segments. I, caudate lobe; II–IV, left hemiliver; V–VIII, right hemiliver.

**Table 9.1** Liver and pancreas functions

| Type | Function |
|---|---|
| **Liver** | |
| Metabolic | Carbohydrate metabolism (gluconeogenesis, glycolysis) |
| | Lipid metabolism |
| | Protein metabolism (synthesis of most plasma proteins, including albumin, most clotting factors, binding proteins) |
| | Bilirubin metabolism |
| | Bile acid metabolism |
| | Storage of glucose (as glycogen), fat, some vitamins |
| Immunological | The liver reticuloendothelial system acts as a barrier to infection |
| Toxicological | Metabolism and excretion of drugs and other xenobiotics |
| Hormonal | Synthesis of hormone-binding proteins and inactivation of hormones |
| Nutritional | Bile is important in digestion and absorption of fat-soluble vitamins |
| **Pancreas** | |
| Endocrine | Secretion of insulin (β cells), glucagon (α cells), somatostatin (D cells), pancreatic polypeptide (PP cells) |
| Exocrine | Secretion of proteases, lipase, bicarbonate and amylase |

## HISTORY 9.1

**Symptoms of liver and pancreatic disease**

Have you noticed any jaundice?
Any change in the colour and consistency of stools? Do they flush easily?
What colour is your urine?
Any pain: if so, what is its nature?
Any flu-like symptoms?
Any fever, rigors?
Any bruising?
Any increase in the size of your abdomen?
Any recent change in weight?
Any itching?

**Past medical history**

**Social and family history**

Age and occupation
Alcohol and smoking habits
Does anyone in your family have similar symptoms or any history of liver disease?
Have you had any recent contact with jaundice or liver disease?
Have you been abroad? Where? When?
Have you had any exposure to blood or blood products? If so, when and where?
What medications (prescribed and over-the-counter), tonics and herbal remedies are you or have you been taking?
Have you or are you using illicit drugs? If so what drugs, how do you take them and over what time?
Recent sexual activity

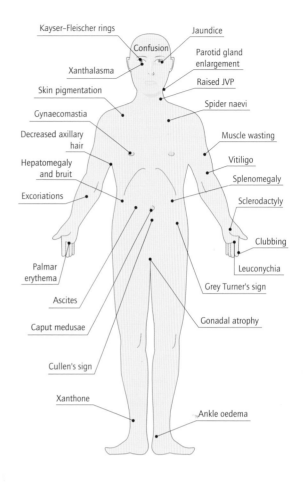

**Figure 9.2** Signs of liver, biliary and pancreatic disease.

**Table 9.2** Causes of hepatomegaly

**Inflammation**
- Hepatitis (alcoholic, viral or autoimmune)
- Abscesses (pyogenic or amoebic)
- Schistosomiasis

**Tumours**
- Benign or malignant primary or secondary disease
- Haematological malignancy

**Cysts**
- Hydatid disease
- Polycystic liver disease

**Biliary obstruction**
- Extrahepatic causes (e.g. carcinoma of head of pancreas)

**Venous congestion**
- Right ventricular failure
- Hepatic vein occlusion

**Metabolic**
- Fatty liver
- Amyloid
- Glycogen storage diseases

**Other mechanisms**
- Cirrhosis
- Myeloproliferative disorders

## SIGNS OF PANCREATIC DISEASE

If the gall bladder is palpable and there is jaundice, the cause of the jaundice is not gallstones (Courvoisier's law) because the gall bladder is usually fibrotic and shrunken if it contains gallstones.

## INVESTIGATION

### HAEMATOLOGY

#### Full blood count

- Pancytopenia from hypersplenism as a result of portal hypertension
- Macrocytosis caused by abnormal membrane lipids, or because of malabsorption of folate or vitamin $B_{12}$

#### Clotting

Clotting in patients with liver disease is complex with derangement in both anticoagulant and procoagulant processes. Traditionally, the INR has been used as a marker of coagulation, but functional tests such as thromboelastography and bleeding time are better markers of bleeding status.

## Prothrombin time

The prothrombin time (PT) is a sensitive marker of hepatocyte synthetic function because the liver synthesizes all the major clotting factors (except factor VIII).

## BIOCHEMISTRY

Urea may be low in liver disease because of impaired hepatic synthesis or poor protein intake. Hyponatremia may indicate impaired water excretion or effect of diuretics.

## Liver tests

### Serum bilirubin

This is elevated in most forms of liver disease. Bilirubin is derived primarily from the destruction of haemoglobin (see **Figure 9.3**).

- *Unconjugated bilirubin:*
  - Water insoluble (not excreted in urine)
  - Transported loosely bound to albumin to the liver
  - Conjugated by the hepatic enzyme UDP-glucuronyl transferase
- *Conjugated bilirubin:*
  - Water soluble
  - Excreted in the biliary system

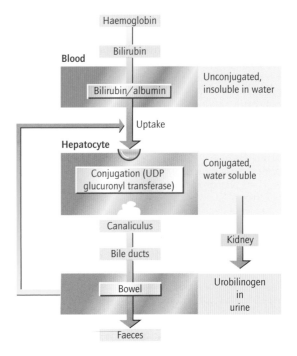

**Figure 9.3** Metabolism of bilirubin.

### Serum aminotransferases

- Aspartate aminotransferase (AST) is primarily mitochondrial; alanine aminotransferase (ALT) is mainly cytosolic.
- Increased serum levels indicate hepatocyte damage with leakage of the enzymes.
- In liver disease, ALT is usually >AST (except in alcoholic liver disease); both enzymes are found in other non-hepatocyte cells, especially cardiac and skeletal muscle.

### Serum albumin

This is low because of:

- Impaired synthesis by hepatocytes
- Poor dietary intake
- Malabsorption
- Increased loss through the skin, kidneys or bowel

### Serum alkaline phosphatases

- These are located in:
  - Canalicular and sinusoidal membrane of the hepatocyte
  - Biliary epithelium
  - Gut
  - Bone
  - Placenta
- Increased levels occur during growth spurts, bone fractures and some bone diseases and pregnancy.
- Increased levels of hepatic isoforms are seen in hepatitis, biliary obstruction, space-occupying lesions in the liver and bile duct damage.

### Serum gamma-glutamyl transferase

- The distribution of gamma-glutamyl transferase (GGT or gamma-GT) within the liver is similar to that of alkaline phosphatase.
- It is readily inducible and increased levels are a feature of some enzyme inducing drus detected in people taking drugs such as alcohol and phenytoin as well as liver damage.

### Oncofoetal antigens

- *Serum α-fetoprotein:* elevated in most liver cancers and during hepatic regeration
- *CEA and CA19-9:* increased in ascites

### Iron status

- *Saturation:* High iron saturation (iron : total iron binding capacity higher than 70%) suggests primary hereditary haemochromatosis.
- *Ferritin:* A high serum ferritin may indicate iron overload or hepatocellular disease. Ferritin is an acute phase protein and is elevated in conditions such as rheumatoid arthritis, some cancers such as Hodgkins lymphoma, hyperthyroidism as well as alcohol and non-alcohl related liver disease.

### Copper studies

Low serum copper and caeruloplasmin associated with high urine copper excretion suggest Wilson's disease.

### Serum α₁-antitrypsin levels

- Low levels suggest $\alpha_1$-antitrypsin deficiency, but serum levels in those with congenital deficiency may be within the normal range because it is an acute phase protein.
- Phenotyping is required to diagnose deficiency. The ZZ phenotype is associated with liver disease.

### Urine tests

The urine can be tested for bilirubin and urobilinogen.

### Tests in pancreatic disease

Conventional blood tests such as a full blood count (FBC) and biochemical profile are non-specific, but may reveal consequences of malabsorption:

- *Serum glucose:* In pancreatic insufficiency insulin levels fall, so glucose levels may rise.
- *Serum levels of insulin, glucagon and pancreatic polypeptide and glucose tolerance tests:* These provide an assessment of pancreatic endocrine function.
- *Serum amylase, fat absorption tests* (faecal fat, breath tests) and *tests of secretion* (collection and measurement of duodenal enzymes after hormone stimulation, food stimulation; *Lundh test*) or indirectly with the *para-amino benzoic acid (PABA) test:* These allow assessment of pancreatic exocrine functions.
- *PABA test:* PABA is formed by the action of chymotrypsin on orally administered

N-benzoyl-L-tyrosyl PABA; it is absorbed and excreted in the urine; thus, urine excretion is a good guide to pancreatic function.
- *Faeces:* Estimation of faecal fat content will document steatorrhoea; measurement of faecal elastase and chymotrypsin may help establish a diagnosis of pancreatic insufficiency.

## IMMUNOLOGY

### Immunoglobulins

Immunoglobulins (Ig) are often polyclonally raised in liver disease, but:

- IgG elevation is particularly associated with autoimmune hepatitis (raised levels of IgG4 in autoimmune cholangitis (AIC) and related conditions).
- IgA elevation is particularly associated with alcoholic liver disease but may also be elevated in viral hepatitis and non-alcoholic fatty liver disease (NAFLD).
- IgM elevation is associated with primary biliary cholangitis (PBC).

### Autoantibodies

Autoantibodies may help in the diagnosis of liver disease; titres >1 : 100 are usually significant.

- *Antinuclear antibodies (ANA):* associated with autoimmune hepatitis
- *Antimitochondrial antibodies (AMA):* diagnostic of PBC
- *Antiliver/kidney microsomal antibodies:* associated with some forms of autoimmune hepatitis and drug-induced liver injury (DILI)
- *Antineutrophil cytoplasmic antibodies (ANCAs):* have been associated with primary sclerosing cholangitis (PSC)
- *Anti-smooth muscle antibody (ASMA):* may be found in autoimmune hepatitis but also in PBC, HCV infection and some cancers (e.g. melanoma and breast cancer)

## MICROBIOLOGY

Microbiology is needed to identify causes of viral hepatitis, hydatid and amoebic infection (antibody tests), and sepsis.

## DIAGNOSTIC IMAGING

### Ultrasound

It is useful for detecting:

- Alterations in parenchymal consistency, tumours, cysts and dilatation of the intrahepatic biliary tree within the liver
- Dilatation of the biliary tree and stones within the gall bladder
- Pancreas visualization is often poor because of overlying gas but pancreatic tumours and cysts may be visualized

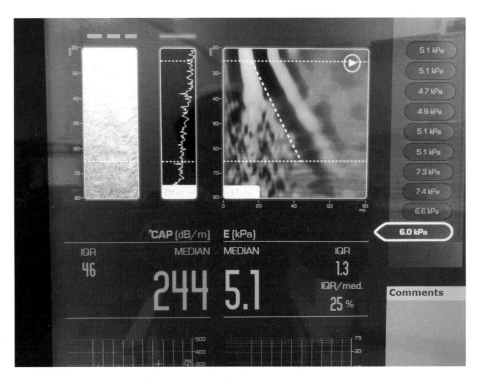

**Figure 9.4** Fibroscanning. Copy of readout of fibroscan showing no evidence of fibrosis (resistivity 5.1kPa) and mild steatosis (CAP 244 dB/m).

- The patency and direction of blood flow in all major arteries and veins
- Ascites

### Endoscopic ultrasound

This allows closer evaluation of the lower end of the common bile duct and in the diagnosis of stones in the common bile duct, abnormalities of the head of the pancreas and allows needle biopsy of abnormal nodes or other lesions.

### Fibroscanning

Fibroscanning (transient elastography; **Figure 9.4**) is a safe, non-invasive technique which measures both the degree of fibrosis and fat. It is both quantitative and reproducible and has largely replaced liver biopsy for the diagnosis of cirrhosis.

### Endoscopic retrograde cholangiopancreatography

Endoscopic retrograde cholangiopancreatography (ERCP) allows both visualization and therapeutic intervention of the biliary or pancreatic ducts after they have been cannulated using an endoscopic duodenoscope and injected with contrast (**Figure 9.5**). It allows biopsy or cytology of the pancreatic ampulla and some bile duct lesions. Diagnostic ERCP is being replaced by magnetic resonance cholangiopancreatography (MRCP).

Therapeutic manipulations include cutting the sphincter of Oddi, dilatation and stenting of biliary strictures and tumours (see **Figure 9.12**), removal of gallstones (see GALLSTONES AT A GLANCE, **Figure B**) and obtaining material for histology or cytology.

*Complications*
- Hyperamylasaemia (50%)
- Pancreatitis (mild 25%, severe 5%)
- Cholangitis (3%)
- Perforation (2%)
- Bleeding, after sphincterotomy (3%)
- Death (1%)

### Plain abdominal radiography

This is of limited value and rarely indicated. However, it may reveal some gallstones or calcification within the liver, gall bladder or pancreas.

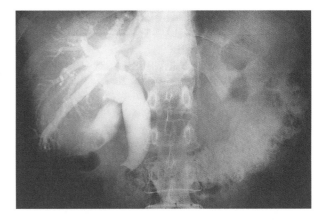

**Figure 9.5** ERCP showing a local stricture at the lower end of the common bile duct because of pancreatic cancer. There is dilatation above the stricture (the endoscope has been removed).

### Oral cholecystogram

Although rarely done, an oral cholecystogram provides information about the function of the gall bladder and may reveal the presence of gallstones.

### Percutaneous transhepatic cholangiography

Percutaneous transhepatic cholangiography (PTC) allows therapeutic intervention such as dilatation of strictures, insertion of stents or local irradiation.

### Computerized tomography

Computerized tomography (CT) gives higher resolution than ultrasound, and the use of intravenous contrast allows better visualization of vascular lesions (see **Figures 9.13** and **9.14**).

### Magnetic resonance imaging

Using appropriate techniques, arterial and venous vessels and bile ducts can be readily demonstrated. Magnetic resonance imaging (MRI) is also useful for defining and helping characterizing liver lesions.

### PET scanning

This is sometimes helpful for assessment of tumours (usually in conjunction with CT or MRI).

### Radioisotope scanning

Isotope scanning has been largely superseded by ultrasound, CT and MRI.

### Angiography

Angiography demonstrates the hepatic arterial and venous anatomy and tumour circulation. It also allows for blood sampling, pressure measurements and therapeutic intervention.

### Endoscopy

Upper gastrointestinal endoscopy is used to detect the presence of oesophageal and gastric varices and, where appropriate, to treat oesophageal varices by injection or banding.

## HISTOPATHOLOGY

### Liver biopsy

Liver biopsy is used to confirm the nature and severity of liver disease.

#### Risks
These include:
- Pain (up to 30%)
- Bleeding (moderate, requiring transfusion: 3%; severe, requiring surgery: less than 1%)
- Haemobilia (1%)
- Perforation of other organs (less than 1%)

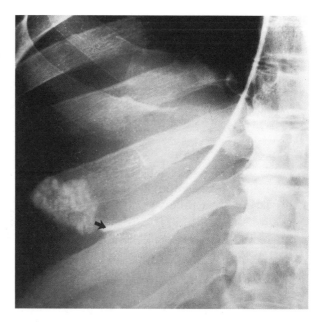

**Figure 9.6** Transjugular liver biopsy. The catheter is in the hepatic vein and contrast has been injected to show the wedged position. The Trucut needle is taking the liver biopsy (arrow). Contrast is present to identify the location of the catheter.

- Tumour seeding (2%)
- Death (0.15%)

#### Contraindications
Contraindications for *percutaneous liver biopsy* include:
- Inability to cooperate
- Abnormal blood clotting (INR >1.4 or platelets $<50 \times 10^9/L$)
- Difficulty in targeting the liver
- Abnormal anatomy
- Amyloidosis (increased risk of bleeding)
- Possible hydatid cyst (risk of shock)

If there is abnormal clotting, then a *transjugular liver biopsy* may be performed. A transjugular biopsy can be taken when a flexible needle is passed, under radiological imaging, through from the internal jugular vein to the hepatic vein and then into the liver (**Figure 9.6**). Complications of transjugular liver biopsy include liver perforation, sepsis, perforation of vessels and pneumothorax.

## GENERAL MANAGEMENT

### DIET IN LIVER AND PANCREATIC DISEASE

No specific dietary restrictions are required in liver disease unless there is:
- *Ascites:* restrict dietary sodium
- *Hyponatraemia:* restrict water intake
- *Encephalopathy:* protein may be restricted but will increase malnutrition
- *Steatorrhoea:* restrict fat (but can be supplemented by medium-chain triglycerides)

## DRUG PRESCRIBING

Drug pharmacokinetics and dynamics may be altered in patients with liver disease because of changes in:

- Absorption
- First-pass metabolism
- Metabolism
- Protein binding
- Drug distribution volume
- Excretion

Because of the complexity of drug handling in liver disease, prescribing must be performed with care and should always be checked in a formulary (e.g. *British National Formulary*).

## DISEASES AND THEIR MANAGEMENT

### JAUNDICE (NON-HEPATITIC, NON-OBSTRUCTIVE)

In the absence of hepatitis or obstruction, jaundice can be caused by congenital abnormalities or can be acquired. *Congenital non-haemolytic jaundice*:

- *Unconjugated:* e.g. Gilbert's syndrome, common; Crigler–Najjar syndrome
- *Conjugated:* Dubin–Johnson syndrome and Rotor's syndrome

*Acquired causes of jaundice*:

- Drugs
- Sepsis
- Enteral nutrition
- Some leukaemias and lymphoma

Cholestasis of pregnancy is discussed below.

Benign recurrent cholestasis is characterized by episodes of acute cholestasis, with jaundice, pruritus, steatorrhoea and weight loss.

### GILBERT'S SYNDROME

#### Epidemiology

- Affects 3–5% of the population
- Usually presents at 10–25 years of age
- Both males and females
- Usually autosomal dominant

#### Disease mechanisms

Changes in UGT1A1 lead to low levels of UDP-glucuronyl transferase.

#### Clinical features

- Jaundice is exacerbated by stress, illness and fasting.
- The urine is not pigmented.

#### Management

- The diagnosis is made by demonstrating an unconjugated hyperbilirubinaemia in the absence of haemolysis.

- Rarely, genetic studies can be used to test for homozygous *A(TA7)TAA* alleles.
- No treatment is required.

### ACUTE HEPATITIS

Acute hepatitis is a syndrome with many causes. The symptoms and signs are usually similar irrespective of the cause. However, it is important to establish the cause of the hepatitis to exclude treatable causes and to ensure resolution. In some cases, acute hepatitis may be the herald of chronic liver disease.

### VIRAL HEPATITIS

The viruses that commonly cause hepatitis are:

- *Hepatitis viruses:* hepatitis virus A (HAV), B (HBV), C (HCV), D, E and others, termed non-A and non-B
- *Other viruses:* cytomegalovirus, Epstein–Barr virus, adenovirus

Other causes include *Toxoplasmosis* (a protozoal infection).

The clinical pattern of viral hepatitis is broadly similar for all viruses (although HCV rarely causes an acute clinical illness). There is a prodromal period of flu-like symptoms, anorexia, nausea and muscular aches. This is followed by the appearance of dark urine, pale stools and clinical jaundice.

Usually, the symptoms resolve after 2–6 weeks and recovery is uneventful. Treatment is symptomatic.

### ACUTE LIVER FAILURE

Fulminant hepatic failure (FHF) is defined as hepatic encephalopathy occurring within 8 weeks of the onset of symptoms in a person with a previously normal liver.

The interval between the onset of symptoms and the development of encephalopathy is of prognostic importance: the shorter the interval, the better the prognosis.

The major causes of FHF are shown in **Table 9.4**.

### CLINICAL FEATURES

- Confusion, drowsiness and coma follow a prodromal illness with non-specific symptoms.
- Ascites is uncommon.
- Hypoglycaemia may occur.
- In the later stages, there is multisystem failure with cerebral oedema, renal failure, vasomotor disturbances, adult respiratory distress syndrome and often sepsis.

#### Grading of hepatic encephalopathy

1 Mild or episodic drowsiness; impaired concentration, rousable and coherent
2 Increased drowsiness; confusion and disorientation, rousable and conversant

## ACUTE VIRAL HEPATITIS AT A GLANCE

### Epidemiology

*Prevalence*

- Very common worldwide, exact figure unknown
- Hepatitis A (RNA virus): 30–40%
- Hepatitis B (DNA virus): 0.2% in UK
- Hepatitis C (RNA virus): 0.5%
- Hepatitis E (RNA virus): <3%

*Geography*

- Worldwide
- Hepatitis B: estimated 350 million carriers of hepatitis B virus (HBV) with prevalence reaching 10–15% of acute hepatitis infections in parts of Africa and Middle and Far East
- Hepatitis C: more common in Southern Europe and Japan

*Transmission*

- Hepatitis A: via faecal–oral route and contaminated food; overcrowding and poor sanitation facilitate spread
- Hepatitis B and C: from mother to child at birth (vertical transmission), or via blood transfusion, contaminated needles, sexual intercourse (particularly men who have sex with men) (horizontal)
- Hepatitis E: orofaecal route

### Clinical features acute hepatitis

*Hepatitis A, B, E (C is rarely symptomatic)*

- Nausea
- Vomiting
- Diarrhoea
- Anorexia
- Headaches
- Malaise
- Right upper quadrant discomfort
- Jaundice (after 14 days)

*Incubation (WHO)*

- Hepatitis A: 6 weeks
- Hepatitis B: 2 weeks to 6 months
- Hepatitis C: 4 weeks to 6 months

### Investigation

*Haematology*

- Hepatitis A: leucopenia with lymphocytosis is typical
- Hepatitis B and C: no specific changes

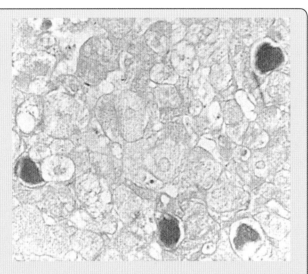

**Figure B** Orcein staining shows brown liver cells containing HBsAg. Reproduced from Sherlock S & Dooley J (1992) *Diseases of the Liver and Biliary System*, 9th edn (Wiley-Blackwell, Oxford), with the permission of the authors.

*Prothrombin time*

- Prolonged in severe cases

*Biochemistry*

- Elevated AST and ALT

*Immunology*

Serology:

- Hepatitis A: anti-HAV IgM antibodies indicate acute infection, anti-HAV IgG antibodies indicate past infection
- Hepatitis B: anti-HBsAg, anti-HBcAg, anti-HbeAg; HBV DNA for active infection (**Table 9.3**)
- Hepatitis C: anti-HCV and HCV RNA (RNA or ELISA)
- Hepatitis E: anti-HEV antibodies, HEV RNA

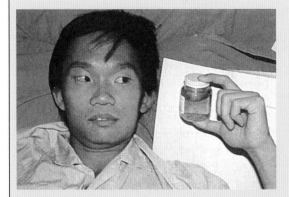

**Figure A** Hepatitis A. Typical appearance of jaundice and dark urine in viral hepatitis. Reproduced from Bannister B *et al.* (1996) *Infectious Disease*. (Wiley-Blackwell, Oxford), with the permission of the authors.

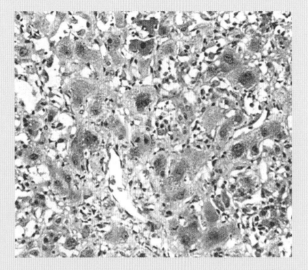

**Figure C** Viral hepatitis. There is marked necrosis, swollen cells and necrophilic bodies.

*Continued...*

...Continued

*Diagnostic imaging*
- Ultrasound to exclude bile duct obstruction

*Histopathology*
- Biopsy: only when doubt over diagnosis

**Management**

Primarily supportive: specific therapy is rarely required. Monitor for evidence of chronicity in B, C (and E in immunosuppressed)

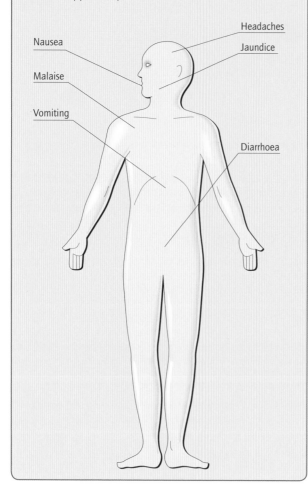

**Table 9.4** Causes of fulminant hepatic failure in the UK

| Cause | Proportion of cases (%) |
| --- | --- |
| Paracetamol overdose | 45 |
| Seronegative hepatitis | 40 |
| Viral hepatitis (A, B, E) | 20 |
| Drug-induced (such as halothane) | |
| Wilson's disease | <5 |
| Other causes including sepsis, pregnancy, malignancy, ischaemia | 5 |

3  Very drowsy, disorientated, response to simple commands
4  Response to painful stimuli only

## MANAGEMENT

Management includes:
- Treatment of the underlying cause
- Monitoring for and early treatment of sepsis, hypoglycaemia
- Avoidance of factors precipitating cerebral oedema such as stress and fluid overload
- Antibiotics and antifungal prophylaxis

## DRUG-INDUCED LIVER INJURY

The diagnosis of drug hepatotoxicity depends on taking a good drug history (including over-the-counter medicines, herbal remedies and vitamins).

The three 'golden rules' for DILI are:
- Any drug or medicinal compound should be considered as a potential cause of hepatotoxicity.
- Any type of liver disease can be caused by drugs.
- The diagnosis is one of exclusion of other causes and a suitable temporal relationship.

## VASCULAR ABNORMALITIES OF THE LIVER

### BUDD–CHIARI SYNDROME

#### Disease mechanisms

Budd–Chiari syndrome results from thrombosis of the hepatic veins. Causes include hypercoagulable states (polycythaemia, protein C or S deficiency, lupus anticoagulant, factor V Leiden mutation, malignancy, cysts, congenital webs, trauma, drugs (especially oral contraceptives) and idiopathic mechanisms.

#### Clinical features

Symptoms include acute, right upper quadrant pain, diarrhoea and rapid onset ascites.

**Table 9.3** Interpretation of HBV serology

| Antibody/antigen | Interpretation |
| --- | --- |
| Anti-HbsAg | Past history of infection or vaccinated |
| Anti-HbcAg (IgG) | Infected with HBV in past |
| Anti-HbcAg (IgM) | Recent history of HBV infection |
| HBsAg present | Currently infected with HBV |
| HBeAg present | Active viral replication |
| Anti-HbeAg | Little viral replication unless infected with a mutant virus |
| HBV-DNA | Active HBV replication |

An increasing number of mutant HBVs have been described in which the HBeAg is altered (and is very similar to the core antigens); hence anti-HBeAg antibodies may not be detected.

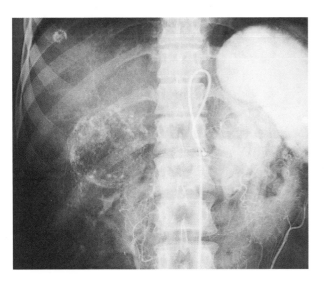

**Figure 9.7** Hepatic angiogram showing a vascular haemangioma.

## Investigation

The thrombus can be shown by Doppler ultrasound or CT/MR angiography.

## Management

Treatment is clot lysis with streptokinase or recombinant tissue plasminogen activator (TPA), shunting (portocaval (portal vein or peritoneovenous) or transjugular intrahepatic portosystemic shunt (TIPS) or transplantation.

## HAEMANGIOMAS

These benign vascular malformations occur in about 7% of the population. Small lesions are commonly revealed on screening for other conditions and are usually of no significance (**Figure 9.7**). The diagnosis is confirmed on imaging.

## LIVER ABSCESSES

### Disease mechanisms

#### Pyogenic liver abscesses

These abscesses are caused by infection, commonly with *Streptococcus milleri*, *Streptococcus faecalis* and *Escherichia coli*. Infection may arise from umbilical sepsis, biliary sepsis, abdominal sepsis (e.g. diverticular disease) or bacteraemia (often caused by dental sepsis).

#### Amoebic abscesses

These usually result from spread of amoebic dysentery from *Entamoeba histolytica* (see Chapter 3, Infectious disease). Hydatid cysts are caused by the larvae of animal tapeworms of *Echinococcus* species (see Chapter 3).

### Clinical features

- Pyogenic liver abscesses present with fever, anorexia, vomiting and abdominal pain.

- Ultrasound will confirm the abscess.
- Calcification is common in the wall of a hydatid abscess.

### Management

Treatment is with aspiration (unless amoebic or hydatid) and antimicrobial treatment.

## LIVER DISEASES OF PREGNANCY

### RECURRENT INTRAHEPATIC CHOLESTASIS

#### Epidemiology

Recurrent intrahepatic cholestasis is most common in Chileans and Scandinavians.

#### Disease mechanisms

It is closely associated with oral contraceptive-associated jaundice. Genetic mutations in the hepatocellular transport protein ABCB4 (*MDR3*), which controls biliary secretion of phosphatidylcholine, are present in 15% of cases of intrahepatic cholestasis of pregnancy (ICP).

#### Clinical features

The condition usually presents in the third trimester with pruritus followed 6–8 weeks later by mild jaundice. It usually recurs in subsequent pregnancies.

#### Management

- Treatment is symptomatic.
- Ursodeoxycholic acid (UDCA) 13–15 mg/kg/day is helpful but is not licensed in pregnancy.
- The disorder resolves spontaneously after delivery.
- There is no adverse effect on the mother, but there is an increased incidence of premature delivery.

### ACUTE FATTY LIVER OF PREGNANCY

#### Disease mechanisms

The syndrome is caused by disordered metabolism of fatty acids by maternal mitochondria resulting from long-chain 3-hydroxyacyl-coenzyme A dehydrogenase deficiency (LCHAD). LCHAD deficiency is autosomal recessive and mothers are often found to be heterozygous for the *E474Q* missense mutation. This leads to accumulation of fat in the hepatocytes (**Figure 9.8**).

#### Clinical features

This usually presents in the last trimester with vomiting, abdominal pain and jaundice, and may rapidly progress to FHF.

#### Investigation

This shows a fatty liver.

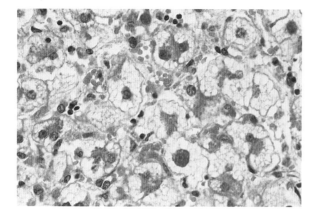

**Figure 9.8** Acute fatty liver of pregnancy. The liver cells are filled with fat.

## Management

Treatment is supportive, with rapid delivery of the foetus. It does not necessarily recur in subsequent pregnancies.

## CHRONIC LIVER DISEASE AND CIRRHOSIS

Chronic liver disease is usually defined as liver disease, of any cause, that lasts for more than 3 months. Ongoing liver inflammation usually leads to progressive fibrosis and eventually cirrhosis. Cirrhosis is a syndrome that is defined pathologically and characterized by fibrosis and nodule formation. There are many causes of cirrhosis (**Table 9.5**).

**Table 9.5** Causes of cirrhosis

| |
|---|
| **Viruses** |
| • HBV |
| • HCV |
| **Toxins** |
| • Alcohol |
| • Drugs |
| **Immune** |
| • Autoimmune hepatitis |
| • PBC |
| • PSC |
| **Metabolic** |
| • Wilson's disease |
| • Haemochromatosis |
| • $\alpha_1$-antitrypsin deficiency |
| • Fibrocystic disease |
| • Storage disorders (glycogen storage disease, galactosaemia, tyrosinaemia) |
| **Biliary disease** |
| • Chronic obstruction |
| **Outflow obstruction** |
| • Cardiac cirrhosis |
| • Budd–Chiari syndrome |
| • Veno-occlusive disease |

There are several measures for the severity of cirrhosis: the most commonly used is the Child–Pugh classification, which is based on:

- Grade of hepatic encephalopathy
- Severity of ascites
- Serum albumin
- Prothrombin
- Serum bilirubin

The MELD (Model for end-stage liver disease) is being used and is based on serum creatinine, bilirubin and INR.

In assessing and managing the patient with chronic liver disease, it is important to consider several aspects:

- *Cause of the liver disease:* Specific treatment may be indicated and family screening may be required.
- *Presence of portal hypertension:* This may lead to ascites and the development of varices that require screening and, where present, treatment to reduce bleeding.
- *Possibility of developing liver cancer:* Surveillance is therefore needed.
- *Effect on management of the patient:* Consider lifestyle, drug treatment and nutrition.

## AUTOIMMUNE HEPATITIS

### Epidemiology

- The two peak age ranges are 20–30 and 55–65 years.
- In younger patients it is more common in females.
- It is associated with the HLA phenotype B8, DR3 and DR4.

### Disease mechanisms

There is an autoimmune attack on the hepatocyte.

### Clinical features

Autoimmune hepatitis presents with asymptomatic abnormalities of liver tests, jaundice, acute hepatitis that fails to resolve, arthralgia or the complications of liver disease. Other autoimmune diseases may be present or develop, including thyroid disease, fibrosing alveolitis and glomerulonephritis. Examination reveals multiple spider naevi.

### Investigation

- *Serum aminotransferases:* elevated
- *Serum immunoglobulins:* especially IgG, increased
- *Serum autoantibodies:* present in increased titres

### Management

- The mainstay of treatment is corticosteroids (e.g. prednisolone or budesonide). Prednisolone should be started at 30–60 mg/day and reduced when the serum aminotransferases are within the normal range.
- Azathioprine should be introduced when the prednisolone dose is 20 mg/day if liver tests are normal.
- Lifelong treatment is usually necessary.
- Other drugs that are effective include mycophenolate, tacrolimus and ciclosporin.

### Prognosis

- Without treatment, the 5-year survival rate is 50%.
- If treatment is started before cirrhosis has occurred, the prognosis is good (90% 5-year survival).

## CHRONIC HEPATITIS B VIRUS INFECTION

### Epidemiology

- Prevalence varies from less than 0.1% in the UK to 15% in the Far East and Africa.
- It is more common in males than in females.

### Clinical features

Hepatitis B can be asymptomatic or with complications of liver disease.

### Management

Treatment when required is with either pegylated-IFN-2 for 1 year or with the oral nucleos(t)ide analogues such as lamivudine, entecavir, adefovir or tenofovir.

### Prognosis

- Without treatment, 3–5% of patients spontaneously seroconvert with loss of antigenaemia each year. This compares with 50% seroconversion among patients who are treated.
- Without treatment or spontaneous seroconversion, the disorder progresses to cirrhosis and hepatocellular carcinoma.

## CHRONIC HEPATITIS C VIRUS INFECTION

### Epidemiology

Hepatitis C accounts for about 50–70% of cases of what was previously termed cryptogenic cirrhosis.

### Clinical features

Disease progression is insidious; presentation is asymptomatic or with complications of cirrhosis.

### Management

Initial studies used pegylated-IFNγ with ribavirin. Now, oral treatments with protease inhibitors and NS5B polymerase inhibitors have meant that almost all patients can achieve a sustained viral response with a corresponding improvement in prognosis, irrespective of genotype.

## PRIMARY BILIARY CHOLANGITIS

### Epidemiology

- Prevalence is 1 in 5000 women in Europe but less common in Africa and India.
- It occurs predominantly in middle-aged women.

### Disease mechanisms

PBC is presumed to be an autoimmune disease.

### Clinical features

PBC may present with:
- Pruritus
- Asymptomatic
- Complications such as ascites, jaundice, gastrointestinal bleeding
- Lethargy (common)

Associated diseases include sicca syndrome with dry mouth and eyes, thyroid disorders, pancreatic insufficiency, vitiligo, coeliac disease, Raynaud's phenomenon, scleroderma, arthralgia and osteoporosis.

On examination, there is pigmentation and there may be xanthomas. Hepatosplenomegaly is common even in the early stages (**Figure 9.9**).

### Investigation

#### Immunology

- *Serum immunoglobulins:* These are increased, especially serum IgM.
- *Autoantibodies:* AMA and some ANA such as Gp210 are diagnostic.

#### Histopathology

Liver histology, rarely required to make a diagnosis, shows a lymphocytic infiltration around damaged middle-sized intrahepatic bile ducts or their remnants. It is useful where there is doubt about the diagnosis (e.g. when AMA and other PBC-specific antibodies are negative) or when there is suspicion of an overlap syndrome (as with RBC/autoimmune hepatitis [AIH] overlap).

### Management

UDCA (13–15 mg/kg/day) reduces the rate of progression: full responders usually have a good prognosis;

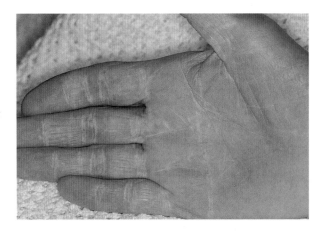

**Figure 9.9** Hand of a patient with primary biliary cirrhosis showing palmar erythema and xanthoma.

for non-responders, obeticholic acid should be offered (5–10 mg/day). Other drugs that may be of benefit include corticosteroids and fibrates.

Pruritus is treated with colestyramine (cholestyramine) (4–28 g/day as required). Non-responders, or intolerant patients, may benefit from rifampicin, sertraline, naltrexone or plasmaphoresis (all unlicensed indications).

### Prognosis

The median transplant-free survival is about 25 years from diagnosis.

## METABOLIC LIVER DISEASES

## WILSON'S DISEASE

The defect in copper transport results in copper deposition in various organs, most importantly the liver and the brain.

The disease is autosomal recessive, resulting from a mutation in the Wilson's disease protein (*ATP7B*) gene. Too many genetic abnormalities have been determined to allow for routine use of genetic markers in making the diagnosis.

### Clinical features

The disorder presents in childhood or young adulthood with either neurological or hepatic manifestations.
- *Neurological signs:* caused by copper deposition in the basal ganglia resulting in progressive decline in mental function, tremor, dysarthria, involuntary movements
- *Hepatic features:* range from mildly elevated liver tests to a chronic active hepatitis or FHF
- *Kayser–Fleischer rings:* caused by copper deposition on Descemet's membrane in the eye

### Investigation
- *Serum copper and caeruloplasmin:* low
- *24-hour urine copper levels:* elevated
- *Liver biopsy:* shows few diagnostic features, but allows the assessment of liver copper levels
- *Liver copper levels:* very high

### Management
- Copper chelation with D-penicillamine, trientine or zinc supplements reverses many of the complications and prevents progression.
- Relatives of a patient must be screened.
- Transplantation is needed in cases of acute liver failure or with end-stage cirrhosis.

### Prognosis

Prognosis is excellent if treatment is instituted before the development of irreversible organ damage.

## HEREDITARY OR PRIMARY HAEMOCHROMATOSIS

See PRIMARY HAEMOCHROMATOSIS AT A GLANCE.

## $\alpha_1$-ANTITRYPSIN DEFICIENCY

### Epidemiology

This is an autosomal dominant disorder.

### Disease mechanisms

$\alpha_1$-antitrypsin is a protease inhibitor. Deficiency is associated with emphysema because of unchecked protease activity and chronic liver disease because the hepatocyte fails to excrete $\alpha_1$-antitrypsin from the liver.

### Clinical features

$\alpha_1$-antitrypsin deficiency may present with neonatal hepatitis or with complications of cirrhosis.

### Investigation
- *Serum $\alpha_1$-antitrypsin levels:* These are usually low.
- *Phenotype measurement:* The diagnosis is confirmed by measuring the $\alpha_1$-antitrypsin phenotype. The *MM* phenotype is normal, the *Z* or *S* phenotypes are associated with disease.
- *Liver biopsy:* This may reveal a chronic active hepatitis or cirrhosis. Periodic acid–Schiff (PAS)-positive, diastase-resistant globules in the hepatocytes containing $\alpha_1$-antitrypsin are characteristic but not specific.

### Management

There is no specific treatment.

### Prognosis

The prognosis varies; only 25% with the *ZZ* phenotype will develop liver disease.

## ALCOHOLIC LIVER DISEASE

Excess alcohol consumption has major social, economic and medical consequences, including alcoholic liver disease. Alcohol consumption is rising in the UK and people are starting to drink at an earlier age. It is important that a full alcohol history is obtained and, where appropriate, multidisciplinary support given to encourage abstinence.

Liver damage associated with alcohol includes:
- Fatty liver
- Fibrosis
- Alcoholic hepatitis
- Alcoholic cirrhosis

See ALCOHOLIC LIVER DISEASE AT A GLANCE.

## PRIMARY HAEMOCHROMATOSIS AT A GLANCE

### Epidemiology

*Prevalence*
- 0.4%, but the prevalence of identified cases is much less

*Age*
- Usually 40–60 years of age

*Sex*
- Males usually present before females

*Complications of iron overload:*
- Liver: cirrhosis and liver cancer
- Skin: slate-grey discoloration
- Pancreas: diabetes mellitus
- Pituitary: gonadal atrophy and impotence
- Heart: arrhythmias and heart failure
- Joints: chondrocalcinosis

*Genetics*
- Fewer than 5% with genetic haemochromatosis develop iron overload

### Investigation

*Biochemistry*
- Liver tests may be normal
- Serum ferritin is increased, often exceeding 1000 µg/L
- Serum iron is high
- Iron saturation (serum iron : total iron binding capacity) exceeds 75%
- Liver iron exceeds 180 µg/g liver (dry weight)
- Genetics: shows *HFE* genes in >95% cases

*Genetics*
- Recognized mutations in *HFE* are C282Y and H63D

*Histopathology*
- Liver biopsy may reveal an established cirrhosis. There is excess iron deposition in the hepatocytes and biliary epithelial cells

### Management
Venesection

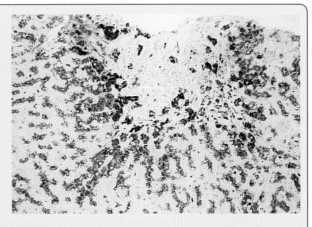

**Figure B** Perls' stain showing periportal deposits, heavier pigment and biliary epithelium.

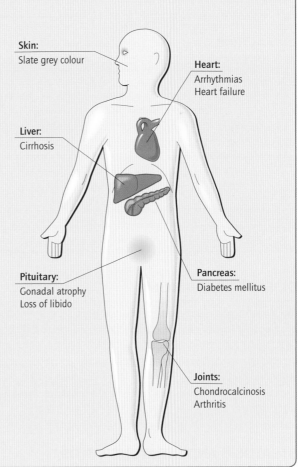

Skin:
Slate grey colour

Heart:
Arrhythmias
Heart failure

Liver:
Cirrhosis

Pituitary:
Gonadal atrophy
Loss of libido

Pancreas:
Diabetes mellitus

Joints:
Chondrocalcinosis
Arthritis

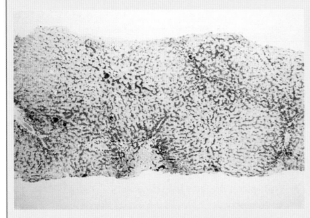

**Figure A** Perls' stain showing grade 4 siderosis with normal architecture.

## ALCOHOLIC LIVER DISEASE AT A GLANCE

### Epidemiology

- Most common cause of liver disease in UK with rising incidence
- Risk depends on the amount and duration of alcohol consumed (safe limit of 14 units/week)
- Other risk factors are:
- Gender (females more susceptible)
- Chronic hepatitis viral infection
- Obesity
- $\alpha_1$-antitrypsin deficiency
- Hereditary haemochromatosis

### Symptoms

- Range from nil to severe liver disease
- May present with extrahepatic manifestations, such as fits, neuropathy, pancreatitis, cardiomyopathy, Korsakoff's syndrome, Wernicke's encepaholpathy, dementia

### Examination

- Ranges from normal to signs of decompensated liver disease
- Note alcohol on breath

### Investigation

- No specific liver tests
- Raised GGT and mean corpuscular volume are suggestive but not diagnostic
- Serum IgA is high
- Carbohydrate-deficient transferrin may be a useful marker of excess alcohol intake
- Liver biopsy: liver cell necrosis, a heavy neutrophil infiltrate (in alcoholic hepatitis), steatosis, Mallory's hyaline and perivenular fibrosis. These features may be superimposed on cirrhosis

*Alcoholic hepatitis*

- Typical pattern with high WBC, very high serum bilirubin with alkaline phosphatase; serum transaminases may not be greatly elevated
- Consider blood/urine/breath alcohol testing
- Carbohydrate-deficient transferrin levels indicate chronic alcohol use (but are not totally specific)

### Treatment

- Non-specific
- Alcohol withdrawal may precipitate fits so give chlordiazepoxide
- Give vitamin replacement (especially thiamine)
- Supportive therapy as appropriate (addiction counselling, Alcoholics Anonymous or other)
- Treat infection aggressively
- Nutritional support
- Alcoholic hepatitis: corticosteroids if severe and no evidence of infection

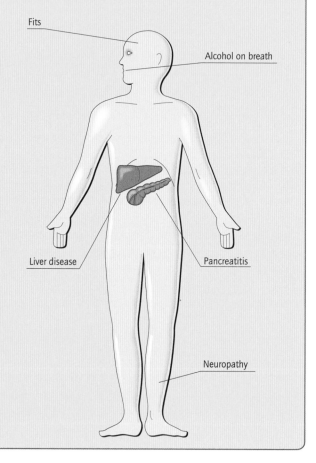

## DISEASE MECHANISMS

The hepatotoxic effects of alcohol are brought about largely by the main metabolite of ethanol, which is acetaldehyde (ethanol). There is a close relationship between the amount of ethanol consumed and the probability of developing severe liver damage. However, there is great variation. Current UK guidelines recommend a maximum weekly consumption of no more than 14 units (140 g ethanol).

## STEATOSIS AND STEATOHEPATITIS

NAFLD is becoming increasingly diagnosed. The term NAFLD includes NAFL (non-alcohol liver) where there is fatty infiltration but no inflammatory activity, hepatocyte damage (such as ballooning) or fibrosis. Non-alcoholic steatohepatitis (NASH) is associated with hepatocyte damage and fibrosis, which may progress to cirrhosis and liver cancer. There is a move to rename the condition 'metabolic associated liver disease'.

Risk factors for fatty liver are:

- Alcoholic fatty liver disease:
  - Alcohol
- Non-alcoholic fatty liver disease:
  - Obesity
  - Type 2 diabetes
  - Metabolic syndrome
  - Dyslipidemia
  - Less common: DILI, hypothyroidism, obstructive sleep apnoea, hypopituitarism, hypogonadism, polycystic ovary syndrome, pancreatoduodenal resection and psoriasis

## Clinical features

Clinically, the patient may be asymptomatic and the only abnormality on examination is hepatomegaly.

## Investigation

Investigations are not specific and blood tests may be normal.

- *Blood tests* are often normal and rarely differentiate between relatively benign fatty liver and steatohepatitis.
- In addition to a Fibroscan (see below), there are several non-invasive ways of assessing the degree of fibrosis:
  - The enhanced liver fibrosis (ELF) score which is derived from measurement of hyaluronic acid, amino-terminal propeptide of type III procollagen (PIIINP), and tissue inhibitor of metalloproteinase 1 (TIMP-1) is a measure of fibrosis and a score <10.51 means the patient is unlikely to have severe fibrosis.
  - The NAFLD fibrosis score (available at www.nafldscore.com) which is derived from six variables (age, body mass index, blood glucose, platelet count, albumin, and AST : ALT ratio). An intermediate or high score (> –1.455), suggests advanced liver fibrosis.
  - The Fibrosis (FIB) 4 score (available at www.gihep.com/calculators/hepatology/fibrosis-4-score/) includes age, AST, ALT, and platelet count. A score of >2.67 suggests advanced liver fibrosis.
- *Fibroscan:* This may show an increased CAP score (showing fatty infiltration). Elasticity measures fibrosis.
- *Liver biopsy:* This shows fatty infiltration of the liver with ballooning of the cells and nuclei, and fibrosis in steatohepatitis and cirrhosis. In NASH, there is liver cell necrosis, a heavy neutrophil infiltrate, steatosis, Mallory's hyaline and perivenular fibrosis. These features may be superimposed on cirrhosis.

## Management

- Underlying causes of NAFL should be treated actively.
- Agents that have been used to treat NAFL include metformin, pioglitazone, vitamin E, glucagon-like peptide 1, with many other agents being assessed.

## Prognosis

The prognosis of simple fatty liver is good; there is an increased mortality but this is associated primarily with cardio- and cerebrovascular disease. However, where there is evidence of a superimposed hepatitis (as in NASH), there is a higher probability of progression to fibrosis, cirrhosis and cancer.

The prognosis is poor if alcohol consumption continues. In severe cases, renal failure, increasing jaundice and prolonged clotting usually herald death. The severity of alcoholic hepatitis is assessed by several scores including Maddrey's Discriminant Factor, the Lille Score and the Glasgow Alcoholic Hepatitis Score:

$$(4.6 \times \text{prothrombin time} - \text{control PT}) + \text{serum bilirubin (mg/dL)}$$

Values >32 imply a poor prognosis.

## PORTAL HYPERTENSION

The major consequences of portal hypertension are variceal haemorrhage, ascites and hypersplenism. Hepatic encephalopathy may occur but can also occur without portal hypertension.

## VARICES

### Disease mechanisms

Varices are at risk of bleeding when the portal pressure exceeds 12 mmHg (EMERGENCY PRESENTATION 9.1). Portal

### EMERGENCY PRESENTATION 9.1

#### Variceal haemorrhage

**Presentation**

Haematemesis

Melaena

Shock

**Resuscitation**

Check airways, breathing circulation

Establish venous access with wide-bore cannula

Cross-match at least 10 units of blood; check FBC and clotting

If hypotensive, give colloid until blood available

If variceal bleeding is suspected, give terlipressin 2 mg every 6 hours (if no contraindications)

Start antibiotics (such as ciprofloxacin, co-amoxiclav)

If clotting abnormal, correct with fresh frozen plasma

If platelets less than $20 \times 10^9$/L, consider platelet transfusion

If drowsy and unable to protect airway, consider early ventilation

Monitor urine output

*Diagnosis*

Confirm at early endoscopy as 10% of patients with varices will bleed from sources other than the varices

**Management**

If oesophageal varices are bleeding, sclerotherapy or variceal banding

If this controls bleeding, monitor and repeat endoscopy in 1 week

If no control of bleeding, pass Sengstaken–Blakemore tube to control bleeding and repeat endoscopy 24 hours later to band/inject varices

If no control, urgent shunting by TIPS or mesocaval shunt to a mesenteric vein

If this fails, consider oesophageal transection

If gastric varices are present, either injection with histoacryl or thrombin or proceed to shunt (as above)

*Once bleeding controlled*

Look for precipitating causes: portal vein thrombosis, hepatoma development

Consider patient for prophylaxis with either propranolol or a banding programme

hypertension has various causes but in the UK most cases are the result of cirrhosis.

### Primary prophylaxis

All patients with cirrhosis should have an endoscopy to look for oesophageal and gastric varices. If these are absent, the endoscopy should be repeated in 3 years. If small varices are present, no treatment is indicated unless there is evidence of possible bleeding (such as cherry red spots). If middle or large varices are seen, the patient should be offered prophylaxis with banding and/or pharmacological treatment with non-selective β-blockers.

## ENCEPHALOPATHY

### Disease mechanisms

The cause of hepatic encephalopathy is not understood, but it is related to failure of the liver to remove toxic substances from the blood, absorption of nitrogen from the bowel and stimulation of the gamma-aminobutyric acid (GABA)–benzodiazepine receptor in the brain.

    *Precipitating factors* include:

- Sepsis (including spontaneous bacterial peritonitis [SBP])
- Drugs (especially sedatives or narcotics)
- Portal and/or hepatic vein thrombosis
- Gastrointestinal bleeding
- Electrolyte disturbances
- Constipation

### Clinical features

The clinical features of hepatic encephalopathy have been described above. The diagnosis is confirmed by electroencephalogram (EEG) and/or a number connection test (where the time taken to connect a series of numbered spots is measured).

### Management

Treatment comprises a search for and correction of any precipitating factors. Lactulose given in a dose to produce at least two soft bowel motions a day should be given and, if encephalopathy persists, rifaximin 550 mg twice daily is effective in some. A low-protein diet is sometimes indicated but the impact on nutrition usually outweighs the benefit. Unproven treatments include bromocriptine and flumazenil (benzodiazepine antagonist).

## ASCITES

### Disease mechanisms

The cause of hepatic ascites is not clear but the presence of ascites (**Figure 9.10**) is closely related to portal hypertension, which leads to splanchnic arterial vasodilation, reduction of the effective circulating volume, activation of endogenous vasoconstrictor systems, and avid sodium and water retention by the kidneys.

### Management

Selected patients with ascites (such as those with a previous history of SBP or who are at high risk of developing SBP, as evidenced by ascitic protein <1.5 g/dL and renal impairment) should be given prophylactic antibiotics (long-term treatment with ciprofloxacin, norfloxacin, co-trimoxazole or co-amoxiclav), which reduce the risk and mortality of bacterial infection.

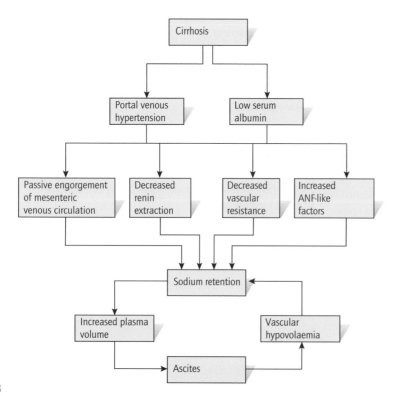

**Figure 9.10** Causes of ascites. ANF, antinaturetic factor.

Treatment includes:

- *Salt restriction:* Water restriction is required only if there is hyponatraemia as well. The most common cause for failure of treatment is not complying with salt restriction.
- *Diuretics* (e.g. spironolactone up to 800 mg/day with furosemide): Renal function must be closely monitored.
- *Paracentesis:* Ascites is directly drained from the abdomen; albumin should be given intravenously (8 g albumin per litre of ascites removed).
- *TIPS:* Recurrent ascites can also be treated by a TIPS.

Bacterial peritonitis may be fatal and should be considered in any patient who develops encephalopathy. It is diagnosed by showing the presence of organisms or a white cell count >250/mL indicates peritonitis requiring immediate antibiotic therapy. The most common organisms are *Escherichia coli*, *Klebsiella* and *Enterococcus* species.

## LIVER TUMOURS

Most tumours in the liver are secondary tumours. The most common primary liver tumours can be classified as:

- *Benign:* adenoma, focal nodular hyperplasia, haemangioma
- *Malignant:* hepatocellular carcinoma, cholangiocarcinoma

## BENIGN ADENOMA

### Disease mechanisms

Benign adenomas are associated with prolonged use of the oral contraceptive and other sex steroids.

### Management

If associated with pregnancy or sex steroids, a benign adenoma may regress when the drug is withdrawn or after the pregnancy. Surgery is indicated if the adenoma does not regress or the adenoma is large (>10 cm) or >5 cm and growing.

## HEPATOCELLULAR CARCINOMA

Hepatocellular carcinoma usually arises in a cirrhotic liver and may be solitary or multiple. Risk factors for hepatocellular carcinoma include a long history of cirrhosis, male sex, chronic infection with HBV or HCV, drugs (especially anabolic or contraceptive steroids), exposure to aflatoxin (a fungal metabolite found on mouldy ground nuts) and smoking. See HEPATOCELLULAR CARCINOMA AT A GLANCE.

## HEPATORENAL SYNDROME

### Disease mechanisms

Hepatorenal syndrome consists of functional renal failure in patients with advanced liver disease. The aetiology is not clear, but endotoxaemia and renal arterial vasoconstriction have been implicated. The urine sodium is very low.

### Management

- Hypovolaemia should be corrected, but treatment is otherwise directed at maintaining renal function.
- Intravenous terlipressin or midodrine may be of help but dopamine is usually of little value.
- A TIPS may be helpful in selected cases.
- Tolvaptan is an oral vasopressin receptor antagonist that can increase serum sodium concentrations by increasing electrolyte-free water excretion.

### HEPATOCELLULAR CARCINOMA AT A GLANCE

**Epidemiology**

*Prevalence*
- One of the most common cancers worldwide but rare in the UK

*Sex*
- 75% male

*Age*
- Varies with cause

*Geography*
- Most common in Africa and South East Asia (probable association with incidence of chronic HBV infection). Rare in Western hemisphere

**Investigation**

*Biochemistry*
- Serum α-fetoprotein is often raised
- Liver tests are not specific

*Diagnostic imaging*
- *Ultrasound:* hypoechoic (or mixed) shadow
- *CT:* early arterial enhancement with early washout
- *Radioisotope scanning:* shows a filling defect
- *Angiography:* shows tumour circulation
- *MRI scan:* space-occupying lesion with arterial phase enhancement

*Histopathology*
- Biopsy, under ultrasonic guidance, confirms diagnosis but risks tumour dissemination and is only performed if resection or transplantation is not planned (2% risk of dissemination)

**Management**
- Resection for small tumours or tumours in non-cirrhotic livers
- Chemotherapy
- Embolization, ethanol injection, cyrotherapy, radiofrequency ablation, chemoembolization (with/out irradiation), transplant

*Continued...*

...Continued

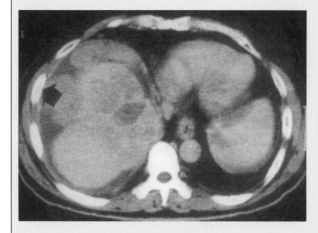

**Figure A** CT scan shows a low density tumour bursting through capsule (arrow). Ascites is also present.

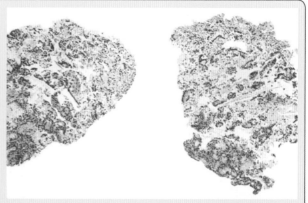

**Figure C** Fine-needle aspiration under ultrasound guidance yielded a clump of hepatocellular carcinoma. All figures reproduced from Sherlock S & Dooley J (1992) *Diseases of the Liver and Biliary System*, 9th edn (Wiley-Blackwell, Oxford), with the permission of the authors.

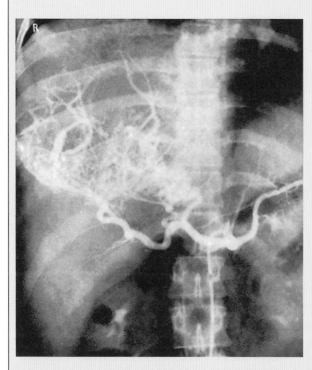

**Figure B** Hepatic angiography showing catheter in the bottom right-hand corner. The tumour is supplied by the hepatic artery and the lesion is an abnormal pattern.

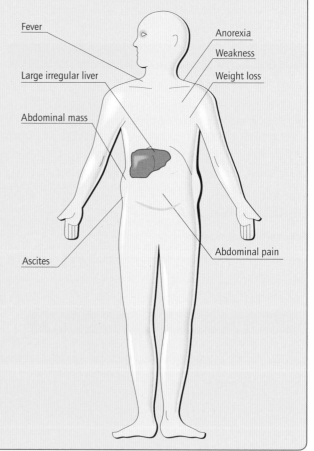

Fever

Anorexia

Weakness

Large irregular liver

Weight loss

Abdominal mass

Ascites

Abdominal pain

## LIVER TRANSPLANTATION

Liver transplantation is now the treatment of choice for patients with end-stage disease. The 1-year survival rate for elective liver transplantation exceeds 90% and 10-year rates are in excess of 70%. Most patients require long-term immunosuppression to prevent rejection of the graft. Many autoimmune diseases (e.g. PSC, PBC and autoimmune hepatitis) can recur in the graft.

Major causes of premature graft loss and/or death include *de novo* malignancy, recurrent disease, infection, renal failure and cardiovascular disease.

Most centres use a combination of corticosteroids, azathioprine and a calcineurin inhibitor (tacrolimus); newer drugs being used include mycophenolate and m-TOR inhibitors such as sirolimus.

# INDICATIONS FOR LIVER TRANSPLANTATION

Liver transplantation is an effective treatment with excellent long-term outcomes (>70% at 5 years) but, despite recent increases in both living and deceased donors, availability of suitable organs remains a problem.

- The indication for transplantation is that anticipated length of life or survival in the absence of transplantation is less than that obtained with a liver transplant.
- Projected 5-year survival after transplantation is >50%. Selection will be assessed secondarily on ability of transplantation to improve quality of life.

The prognosis of those with advanced liver disease is assessed by the MELD (Model for End-stage Liver Disease) score or UKELD (United Kingdom score for End-stage Liver Disease). Any patient who may be a potential candidate for transplantation should be discussed with the local transplant centre before the condition becomes terminal.

## GALL BLADDER DISEASES

### GALLSTONES

See GALLSTONES AT A GLANCE.

### EXTRAHEPATIC BILIARY CYSTS AND CAROLI'S SYNDROME

Extrahepatic biliary cysts (choledochal cysts) and Caroli's syndrome (intrahepatic biliary cysts) form a spectrum of disease characterized by cystic dilatation of the intra- or extrahepatic biliary tree. These rarely require treatment unless there is superimposed infection.

---

## GALLSTONES AT A GLANCE

**Epidemiology**

*Prevalence*
- Affects 15% of people

*Age*
- More common in older age

*Sex*
- More common in women (male : female 1 : 2)

**Stone types**

*Cholesterol stones (80%)*
- Usually in gall bladder
- Risk factors: female sex, oral contraceptives, obesity, rapid weight loss, some drugs, diabetes mellitus, gall bladder hypomotility, Crohn's disease, haemolytic diseases

*Brown pigment stones (10%)*
- Usually in bile duct
- Usually following surgery to biliary tree

*Black pigment stones (10%)*
- Gall bladder (or bile duct)
- Risk factors include chronic haemolysis

**Clinical features**
- Significant pain lasting more than 15 min to 5 hours
- Epigastric or right upper quadrant site; radiation to back
- Often occurs at night
- Recurrence at irregular intervals
- Jaundice, fever and rigors may be present
- Tenderness in the right upper quadrant

**Investigation**
- Blood tests may show leucocytosis and obstructive patterns of liver tests
- Ultrasound for gall bladder stones
- Endoscopic ultrasound, ERCP or MRCP for bile duct stones

**Treatment**

*General*
- Analgesia and antibiotics (if evidence of infection)

*Specific*
Gall bladder stones:
- If symptomatic: usually surgery (occasionally extracorporeal shock wave lithotripsy and gallstone dissolution)
- If asymptomatic: usually no treatment required

Bile duct stones: stone extraction at ERCP
- If obstructive and infected biliary tree, the bile duct must be decompressed (endoscopically or percutaneously as an emergency)
- Medical treatment (with UDCA) rarely indicated

**Complications**
- Pain and infection
- Perforation
- Pancreatitis
- Biliary obstruction
- Rarely, bowel obstruction
- Pancreatitis

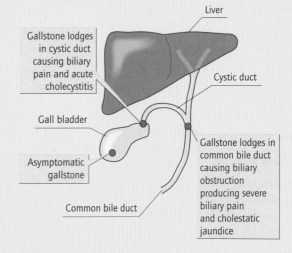

**Figure A** Gallstones.

*Continued...*

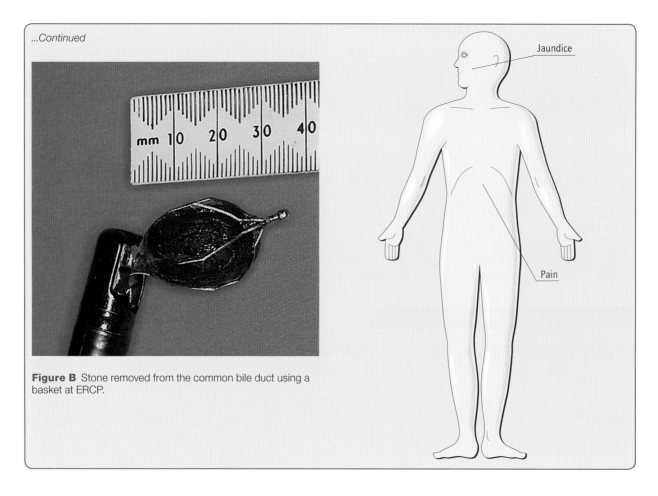

*...Continued*

**Figure B** Stone removed from the common bile duct using a basket at ERCP.

## PRIMARY SCLEROSING CHOLANGITIS

PSC affects both the intra- and extrahepatic biliary tree with diffuse inflammation, leading to stricture and dilatation. There is a strong association with inflammatory bowel disease, especially ulcerative colitis, but the extent of inflammation in one condition does not parallel the other. There is an increase in the probability of developing colon cancer, especially on the right side. PSC, like ulcerative colitis, is more common in non-smokers.

### Epidemiology

- Can affect any age
- About 67% of patients are male
- Associated with HLA-DR3

### Clinical features

- PSC may be asymptomatic, or may cause pruritus, jaundice or complications of cirrhosis. Examination usually reveals hepatomegaly.
- There is a significant risk of cholangiocarcinoma.

### Investigation

- *Liver tests:* Serum alkaline phosphatase and GGT are elevated and, in the later stages, serum bilirubin is also increased.

- *Autoantibodies:* Antineuclear antibodies may be present but are not specific.
- *MRCP:* Confirm the diagnosis, showing beading and dilatation throughout the biliary tree; ERCP is rarely done except when a dominant stricture or malignancy is suspected (**Figure 9.11**).

### Management

Treatment is symptomatic. The role of UDCA is uncertain. Most units will undertake surveillance for colon cancer and cholangiocarcinoma.

### Prognosis

Prognosis is variable with progression usual.

## AUTOIMMUNE SCLEROSING CHOLANGITIS AND AUTOIMMUNE PANCREATITIS

AIC and autoimmune pancreatitis (AIP) are chronic fibro-inflammatory diseases of the biliary tree and pancreas that belong to the spectrum of Ig G4-related diseases (IgG4-RD).

- The conditions present with obstructive jaundice. IgG4 levels are often elevated.
- Histologically, there is lymphoplasmacytic acinar inflammation and storiform.

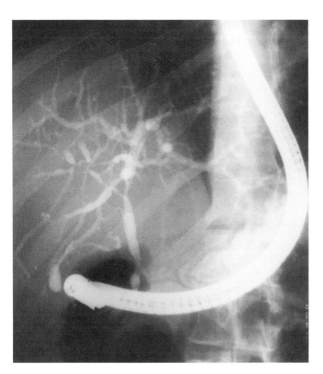

**Figure 9.11** ERCP of PSC, showing beading and dilatation in the biliary tree.

- Initial treatment of both is with high-dose corticosteroids for 4 weeks followed by a gradual taper. Relapses are common and often require treatment with immunomodulators and, more recently, rituximab.

## CHOLANGIOCARCINOMA

### Disease mechanisms

Cholangiocarcinoma can occur anywhere in the biliary tree. Risk factors include PSC and infestation with the liver fluke or trematode worm *Clonorchis sinensis*, which is common in the East (see Chapter 3, Infectious disease).

### Clinical features

Patients present with features of obstructive jaundice or a sudden deterioration in PSC.

### Investigation

- *Serum carcinoembryonic antigen and carbohydrate antigen (CA19-9):* elevated in about 20% of patients
- *Ultrasound or CT scanning:* commonly fail to reveal these tumours
- *Angiography:* tumours are usually hypovascular and cannot therefore be seen on angiography
- *ERCP, bile cytology and brushings of the stricture:* may provide the diagnosis

### Management

There is usually local spread by the time the diagnosis is made and so treatment is largely palliative, consisting of stenting or bypass surgery (**Figure 9.12**). Rarely cases can be treated with surgery, brachytherapy, chemotherapy and transplantation.

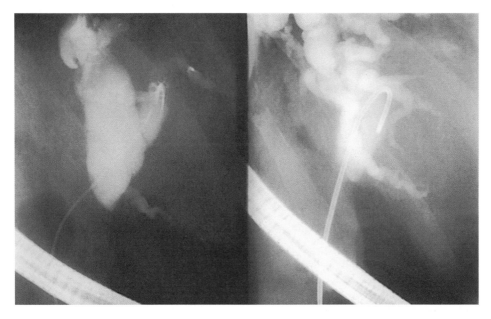

**Figure 9.12** Endoscopic stenting of a bile duct tumour resulting in palliative relief. There is gross dilatation of the intrahepatic ducts.

### Prognosis

Prognosis is poor, with a 1-year survival of less than 20%.

## GALL BLADDER CANCER

Gall bladder cancer is very rare. It is most common in people with gallstones.

## OTHER DISORDERS OF THE BILIARY TREE

- *Cholesterosis of the gall bladder:* This is characterized by deposits of cholesterol in the gall bladder wall. It is asymptomatic and no treatment is required.
- *Adenomyomatosis of the gall bladder:* This is often an incidental finding on cholecystography. There is thickening of the muscle layers and the gall bladder mucosa. Usually no treatment is indicated.
- *Acalculous cholecystitis:* This may occur in association with systemic diseases such as infection, polyarteritis nodosa and diabetes mellitus.

## DISEASES OF THE PANCREAS

## OVERVIEW OF PANCREATITIS

Pancreatitis may be classified as:
- Acute pancreatitis
- Recurrent acute pancreatitis
- Chronic pancreatitis
- Chronic relapsing pancreatitis

Acute and recurrent acute pancreatitis are associated with a full recovery, but chronic pancreatitis is associated with inflammation and fibrosis.

## ACUTE PANCREATITIS

### Disease mechanisms

The causes of acute pancreatitis are listed in **Table 9.6**. Gallstones and alcohol are the leading causes of acute pancreatitis in the UK.

### Clinical features

Acute pancreatitis presents with central or epigastric abdominal pain, radiating to the back or to between the shoulder blades. The pain may be mild or severe, and is associated with nausea and vomiting. In severe acute pancreatitis, the patient may be in shock.

There are several systems for assessing the severity of the attack:
- The Ransom system was developed for patients with alcohol-related pancreatitis.
- The APACHE II score is also helpful.
- SIRS and multi-organ failure (especially if developing after 48 hours) are markers of severity.

**Table 9.6** Causes of acute pancreatitis

| |
|---|
| **Mechanical obstruction** |
| • Gallstones |
| **Toxic effect** |
| • Alcohol |
| **Iatrogenic** |
| • Post-ERCP |
| • Surgery |
| **Drugs** |
| • Azathioprine |
| • Corticosteroids |
| **Infections** |
| • Mumps |
| • Coxsackie |
| **Autoimmune** |
| **Metabolic** |
| • Hyperparathyroidism |
| • Hyperlipidaemia |
| **Ischaemia** |
| **Trauma** |
| **Idiopathic** |

Examination may reveal shock, with abdominal tenderness and guarding. There may be bruising in the loins (Grey Turner's sign) and around the umbilicus (Cullen's sign). Jaundice and respiratory failure are features of severe inflammation.

### Complications

- *Local:* e.g. pseudocysts, abscesses, ascites, gastrointestinal bleeding, ileus and portal vein thrombosis
- *Systemic:* e.g. shock, respiratory failure, acute renal failure, hypocalcaemia, hyperglycaemia, disseminated intravascular coagulation (DIC) and fat necrosis
- *Early:* e.g. cardiac failure, renal failure, respiratory failure, DIC and venous thrombosis
- *Late:* e.g. pseudocyst, abscess, diabetes mellitus, fistula, ascites and stricture

### Investigation

#### Haematology

FBC may show evidence of complications such as DIC.

#### Biochemistry

- *Serum or urine amylase:* raised and confirms the diagnosis; serum amylase five times the normal upper limit is highly suggestive of acute pancreatitis
- *Serum pancreatic lipase:* may be increased but is less specific
- *Biochemical profile:* may reveal features of complications, such as hypocalcaemia, hypoglycaemia, hypoalbuminaemia or uraemia

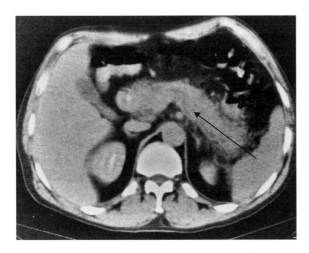

**Figure 9.13** Acute pancreatitis. CT scan showing diffuse enlargement of the pancreas with ill-defined edges.

### Diagnostic imaging

- *Contrast-enhanced CT or MRI:* remains the gold standard for diagnosis and is best done 48 hours after admission (**Figure 9.13**)
- *Ultrasound:* is helpful at presentation and can help diagnose a biliary cause

## Management

Management is largely supportive. Nutrition is important and enteral rather than parenteral nutrition is preferred. Maintaining adequate fluid balance is essential. Arterial blood gases should be measured.

Prophylactic antibiotics are not indicated except where there is severe necrotizing pancreatitis. It may be difficult to achieve analgesia, but opiates should be avoided as they are reputed to worsen the illness by increasing the tone of the sphincter of Oddi.

There is little evidence that early ERCP and sphincterotomy is helpful.

- *Pseudocysts:* These usually develop late and no treatment is required if they are small. Large and recurrent collections need drainage or surgical excision.
- *Pancreatic abscess formation:* Abscess is suggested by fever, neutrophil leucocytosis and deterioration about 1–2 weeks after the initial presentation. Intensive treatment with antibiotics and either surgical or percutaneous drainage is required.
- *Necrotizing pancreatitis:* Necrosectomy is usually indicated and can be done by laparoscopic necrosectomy, video-assisted retroperitoneal debridement (VARD), minimal access retroperitoneal pancreatic necrosectomy (MARPN) or the endoscopic transgastric route.

## Prognosis

The prognosis varies with the severity of the attack. Old age, a neutrophil leucocytosis, low serum albumin,

**Table 9.7** Markers of severe acute pancreatitis

| |
|---|
| Age >55 years |
| WBC >16 × 10⁹/L |
| Hypocalcaemia (calcium <2.2 mmol/L) |
| Renal impairment (urea increase >2 mmol/L) |
| Hypoxaemia ($Po_2$ <8 kPa/60 mmHg) |
| Acidosis (base deficit >4 mmol/L) |

WBC, white blood cell count.

hypocalcaemia, high CRP, hypoxia and uraemia suggest a poor outcome (**Table 9.7**).

## CHRONIC PANCREATITIS

### Disease mechanisms

Causes of chronic pancreatitis are:
- Alcohol (over 60% of cases)
- Hyperlipidaemia
- Malnutrition
- Cystic fibrosis
- Hypercalcaemia
- Hereditary (autosomal dominant)
- Idiopathic causes
- Genetic risk factors, including variants in cationic trypsinogen (PRSS1), serine protease inhibitor Kazal-type 1 (SPINK1) and carboxypeptidase A1 (CPA1)
- Autoimmunity

### Clinical features

The cardinal features of chronic pancreatitis are abdominal pain, weight loss and steatorrhoea. Less common presentations include jaundice, diabetes mellitus and portal hypertension. Examination is often unhelpful, revealing no specific physical signs.

### Complications

These include chronic abdominal pain, malabsorption, diabetes mellitus, pseudocyst, common bile duct strictures, intestinal obstruction, ascites, pleural effusions, aneurysm of arteries around the pancreas and splenic vein thrombosis.

### Investigation

- *Blood tests:* These are helpful for detecting early consequences of malabsorption.
- *Serum amylase:* This is usually normal.
- *Plain abdominal radiography:* Radiographs reveal pancreatic calcification.
- *Ultrasound (with or without contrast ehancement or endoscopic), CT or MRCP scanning and ERCP:* These show an irregular fibrosed gland. Calcification in chronic pancreatitis is mainly caused by small calculi within the pancreas that are obvious on CT scanning (**Figure 9.14**). CT is the preferred approach.

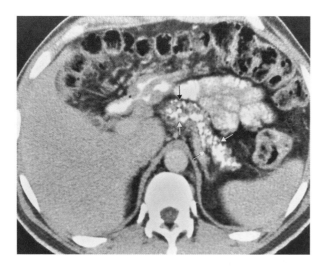

**Figure 9.14** Chronic pancreatitis. CT scan showing numerous small areas of calcification within the pancreas (arrows).

- *Pancreatic function tests:* Raised faecal fat levels (higher than 6 g in 72 hours), reduced faecal chymotrypsin, or an abnormal Lundh test (which measures duodenal trypsin after a standard meal) can be used to assess pancreatic function but have been generally replaced by measurement of faecal elastase.

### Management

There is no specific treatment. Alcohol and smoking must be avoided. It may be very difficult to achieve pain relief and, in extreme cases, surgical removal of some or all of the pancreas may be necessary. Pancreatic enzyme supplements (such as Creon or Pancrex) may help relieve symptoms of pancreatic exocrine insufficiency. Insulin may be required for diabetes mellitus

## PANCREATIC CARCINOMA

See PANCREATIC CANCER AT A GLANCE.

### Disease mechanisms

The aetiology is not clear, but pancreatic carcinoma is more common in smokers and alcoholics.

*Screening* should be offered for those at increased risk of pancreatic cancer. This should include people with hereditary pancreatitis and a *PRSS1* mutation, *BRCA1*, *BRCA2*, *PALB2* or *CDKN2A* (p16) mutations, and one or more first-degree relatives with pancreatic cancer and Peutz–Jeghers syndrome, two or more first-degree relatives with pancreatic cancer, across two or more generations, those with Lynch syndrome (mismatch repair gene [*MLH1*, *MSH2*, *MSH6* or *PMS2*] mutations) and any first-degree relatives with pancreatic cancer.

### Prognosis

Ampullary tumours carry a better prognosis, possibly because they present earlier and are amenable to excision. About 85% of patients with pancreatic cancer die within 1 year. Around 10% are amenable to surgery and the 5-year survival is about 25%.

## ENDOCRINE TUMOURS OF THE PANCREAS

Gastrinomas, insulinomas, glucagonomas and VIPomas are rare tumours that may arise in the pancreas.

---

### PANCREATIC CARCINOMA AT A GLANCE

#### Epidemiology

*Prevalence*
- 15 in 100 000 males in USA. Increasing in many Western countries, and now the fourth most common cause of cancer death in the UK and USA

*Age*
- Especially over 60 years of age

*Sex*
- More common in males (2 : 1)

Presentation:
- *Tumours in the body and tail:* present with abdominal pain and weight loss and, rarely, with diabetes mellitus; pain is central and classically relieved by sitting forward
- *Tumours in the head and ampulla:* present earlier with obstructive jaundice and weight loss and, in the early stages, without severe pain

#### Investigation

*Biochemistry*
- Serum alkaline phosphatase may be raised if biliary obstruction; CA19-9 and CEA of limited value

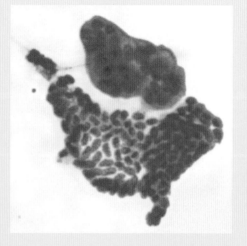

**Figure A** Brush cytology taken from a low common bile duct stricture. There is a sheet of benign biliary epithelial cells and above this a small group of large polymorphic cells characteristic of adenocarcinoma. Reproduced from Sherlock S & Dooley J (1992) *Diseases of the Liver and Biliary System*, 9th edn (Wiley-Blackwell), with the permission of the authors.

*Continued...*

**9**

*...Continued*

*Diagnostic imaging*

- CT or MRI and PET may confirm diagnosis and define extent of malignancy
- Ultrasound is useful for initial screening test; EUS may allow histology
- Duodenoscopy with ERCP may detect tumours at head of duct of the pancreas

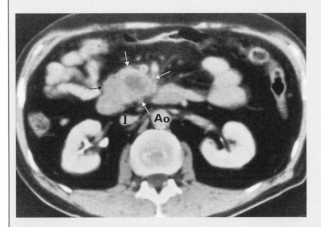

**Figure B** CT scan showing focal mass in head of pancreas (arrows). Ao, aorta; I, inferior vena cava. Reproduced from Armstrong P & Wastie M (1992) *Diagnostic Imaging*, 3rd edn (Wiley-Blackwell), with the permission of the authors.

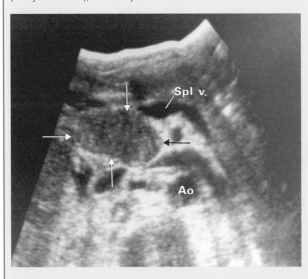

**Figure C** Ultrasound, transverse scan (different patient), showing a similarly situated mass (arrows). Ao, aorta; Spl v., splenic vein. Reproduced from Armstrong P & Wastie M (1992) *Diagnostic Imaging*, 3rd edn (Wiley-Blackwell), with the permission of the authors.

*Histopathology*

- Fine-needle aspiration biopsy (guided by endoscopic ultrasound, CT or ERCP) distinguishes from chronic pancreatitis
- Note risk of dissemination

**Treatment**

- *Surgical:* curative resection may be possible in a minority
- *Good palliation:* stenting may be helpful
- *Drug therapy:* folfirinox and gemcitabine may help

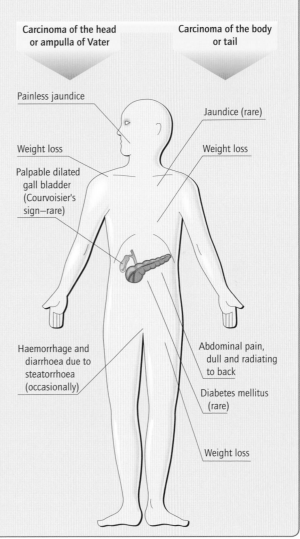

**MUST-KNOW CHECKLIST**

- Causes, signs and symptoms of acute hepatitis
- Diagnosis and early treatment of paracetamol overdosage
- Causes, signs and symptoms of cirrhosis
- Prevention and management of complications of cirrhosis
- Serology and treatment of hepatitis viruses (A, B, C)
- Investigation and management of gallstones
- Diagnosis and management of acute pancreatitis

**Questions and answers** to test your understanding of Chapter 9 can be found by clicking 'Support Material' at the following link: https://www.routledge.com/Medicine-for-Finals-and-Beyond/Axford-OCallaghan/p/book/9780367150594

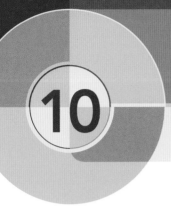

# Gastrointestinal Disease

## 10

GARETH DAVIES, CHRIS BLACK & KEELEY FAIRBRASS

## STRUCTURE AND FUNCTION

### STRUCTURE

The gut is a muscular tube running from mouth to anus, with three main layers (**Figure 10.1**), each region adapted for a specific function (**Table 10.1**; **Figure 10.2**). Via the ampulla of Vater in the duodenum, the pancreas and liver deliver enzymes and bile acids, respectively, to assist with digestion.

Arterial supply (**Figure 10.3**), lymph drainage and pain sensation broadly follow embryological origins and are of clinical relevance (e.g. in pattern of pain referral, cancer spread and vascular disease; **Table 10.2**). The watershed

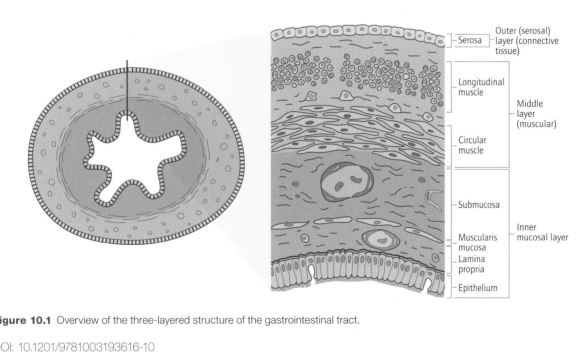

**Figure 10.1** Overview of the three-layered structure of the gastrointestinal tract.

DOI: 10.1201/9781003193616-10

**Table 10.1** Structural and functional features of different regions of the gut

| Region | Structural features | Special functions of each region |
|---|---|---|
| Oesophagus | Squamous mucosa as opposed to columnar type in rest of gastrointestinal tract<br><br>Two regions of increased muscle tone producing upper and lower oesophageal sphincters to help prevent acid reflux<br><br>Lower oesophagus is site of rich anastomosis between portal and systemic veins | Transport of food bolus to stomach<br><br>Glands producing bicarbonate in lower section to neutralize refluxed acid |
| Stomach | Additional transverse muscle layer | Mechanical breakdown of food<br><br>Parietal (also called oxyntic) cells secrete hydrochloric acid in response to vagal nerve stimuli and the hormones gastrin (secreted by gastric antrum), histamine (secreted by ECL cells in gastric body)<br><br>Columnar cells secrete thick layer of mucus, along with rapid mucosal turnover the main mechanism to stop stomach being digested by its own secretions<br><br>Protein digestion by pepsin (secreted as pepsinogen from specialized 'chief' cells in gastric mucosa – activated to pepsin by low pH)<br><br>Secretion of intrinsic factor, binds to B12 allowing its absorption in distal ileum<br><br>Secretion of gastrin by antrum in response to pH rise |
| Duodenum | Bile acids and pancreatic enzymes secreted into the duodenum via separate ducts joining at the ampulla of Vater (closed off when not required by the sphincter of Oddi) | Neuroendocrine function: arrival of food and gastric acid stimulates release of hormones co-ordinating digestive events:<br>• Secretin – stimulates pancreatic secretions<br>• Cholecystokinin – stimulates pancreatic secretions and gall bladder contraction<br>• Gastric inhibitory polypeptide (also known as the glucose-dependent insulinotropic peptide) – stimulates insulin secretion |
| Jejunum and ileum | Villi and microvilli (Figure 10.2) vastly increase the surface area (estimated as that of six tennis courts) | Main site of nutrient absorption; fluid and electrolyte secretion and reabsorption<br><br>Folic acid, iron and vitamins A, B, C and D are absorbed mainly by the jejunum and proximal ileum<br><br>Terminal ileum has specific receptors to uptake B12–intrinsic factor complex, and reclaim bile acids |
| Colon | Tight junctions between surface epithelial cells<br><br>Longitudinal muscle fibres for caecum to sigmoid form three separate bands (taenia coli) | Water absorption, formation and compression of a solid stool<br><br>Home of billions of bacteria essential to normal health (colonic microbiome) |
| Rectum | Internal and external muscle sphincters<br><br>Mucus glands<br><br>Site of rich anastomosis between portal and systemic vein | Maintain continence<br><br>Excretion of stool |

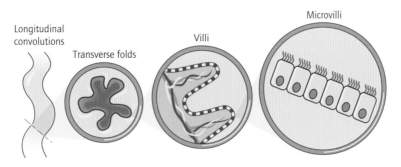

**Figure 10.2** Factors increasing the surface area of the small intestine.

10

between the superior mesenteric artery (SMA) and inferior mesenteric artery (IMA) supply near the splenic flexure is particularly susceptible to ischaemia.

Gut lymphatic drainage finally enters the circulation via the thoracic duct into the left subclavian vein: enlargement of the left subclavian lymph gland (Virchow's node) is associated with advanced abdominal cancers (Troisier sign).

The visceral nervous system, supplying motor and sensory fibres to internal organs, is separate in structure and function from the somatic, which supplies skin and skeletal muscles. Visceral pain sensation is limited to pressure (e.g. colicky pain in obstructed gut) and inflammation (often constant) and is more vaguely localized than somatic (**Table 10.2**). If inflammation involves the somatically innervated parietal peritoneum, pain becomes well localized (e.g. in appendicitis).

The gut has an intrinsic neural network (enteric nervous system) coordinating gastrointestinal (GI) motility

and secretions independent of central nervous control. In addition, the GI tract receives autonomic efferents throughout its length. Parasympathetic supply causes increased contractility and reduced sphincter tone; sympathetic effects are the opposite. The vagus nerve provides the main parasympathetic supply. Although it is best known for its efferent role in stimulating gastric acid output, 90% of vagal fibres are afferent (sensory). The autonomic nervous system provides stimuli for gastric and pancreatic secretion; however, hormonal stimuli are more important (see **Table 10.1**).

Abnormal gut visceral sensation (visceral hypersensitivity) is important in the pathophysiology of functional bowel disorders such as irritable bowel syndrome (IBS).

The venous drainage from most of the gut (stomach to rectum) is via a series circuit through the liver, to allow complete removal of digestion-derived toxins before blood returns to the systemic circulation (**Figure 10.4**). This anatomy underpins the complications of ascites and varices that can complicate cirrhotic liver disease (Chapter 9, Liver, biliary tract and pancreatic disease). Blood-borne spread of GI malignancies to the liver via this route is common.

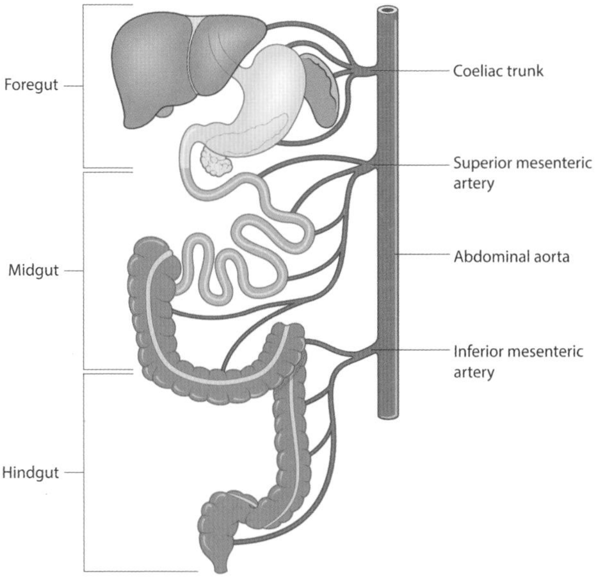

## FUNCTION

The main function of the gut is to absorb nutrients and liquids – achieved by a mixture of passive diffusion across concentration or osmotic gradients (water-soluble vitamins; water), active uptake systems (e.g. sodium and glucose) and complex systems where uptake is tightly regulated according to need (e.g. iron).

The processing of key dietary groups is as follows.

### FAT

The most important stage of fat digestion is coating fat droplets with phospholipids (bile-derived) so they are

**Figure 10.3** Arterial supply of the GI tract.

Foregut

Coeliac trunk

Superior mesenteric artery

Midgut

Abdominal aorta

Inferior mesenteric artery

Hindgut

**Table 10.2** Embryological regions of the gut and arterial supply. Lymphatic drainage and nerve supply follow the same distribution. Clinical relevance includes pattern of cancer spread, effects of arterial occlusion and typical location of pain

| Embryological group | Regions included | Arterial supply (lymphatic drainage follows same distribution) | Typical site of pain | Specific pain referral patterns |
|---|---|---|---|---|
| Foregut | Oesophagus, stomach, duodenum to level of ampulla, pancreas, liver and biliary tract | Coeliac axis | Retrosternal for oesophagus | *Gastro-oesophageal reflux disease:* rising burning behind sternum, usually helped by antacids/acid-lowering medication |
| | | | Upper abdomen for rest of foregut | *Oesophageal spasm:* severe central chest, radiates to back, often confused with myocardial pain |
| | | | | *Stomach:* epigastric, pain may alter up or down soon after eating |
| | | | | *Duodenum:* as part retroperitoneal, pain may radiate to back |
| | | | | *Gall bladder:* right upper quadrant radiating to right back, lower shoulder blade (T7–9 dermatome) level |
| | | | | *Pancreas* (retroperitoneal organ): epigastric –> back at same level |
| Midgut | Duodenum from ampulla, jejunum and ileum, colon to hepatic flexure | SMA | Mid abdomen | *Appendix:* initially visceral type mid-abdominal pain, until peritoneum involved, moves to right iliac fossa |
| Hindgut | Distal one-third of transverse colon, descending and sigmoid colon, rectum and upper two-thirds of the anal canal | IMA | Lower abdomen | *Colonic:* pain can refer to low back and upper thigh |

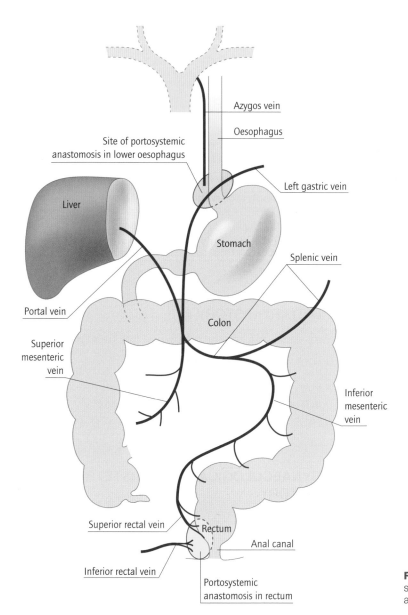

Azygos vein

Oesophagus

Site of portosystemic
anastomosis in lower oesophagus

Left gastric vein

Liver

Stomach

Splenic vein

Portal vein

Colon

Superior
mesenteric
vein

Inferior
mesenteric
vein

Superior rectal vein

Rectum

Anal canal

Inferior rectal vein

Portosystemic
anastomosis in rectum

**10**

**Figure 10.4** Venous drainage of the GI tract showing clinically important sites of portosystemic anastomoses.

water soluble, then enzymatic breakdown of triglycerides to monoglycerides and free fatty acids by pancreatic lipase. Dietary fat is almost completely absorbed in the proximal small bowel. The main cause of fat malabsorption is pancreatic disease; it can also occur with severe small bowel disease.

## CARBOHYDRATES

Pancreatic amylase breaks down starch to the disaccharide maltose, which along with other dietary carbohydrates (e.g. lactose, sucrose) is digested further by oligo- and disaccharidase enzymes located at the tips of the small bowel villi. Thus, disaccharide absorption is disrupted early in any process damaging the villi (e.g. coeliac disease [CD], infective gastroenteritis) with resulting diarrhoea as the unabsorbed large sugar molecules act as an osmotic laxative.

## PROTEIN

Protein is degraded to polypeptides by gastric secretions, then to oligopeptides and free amino acids and by peptidases (e.g. trypsin, chymotrypsin and elastase) secreted by the pancreas, and finally actively transported across the small bowel mucosa.

## WATER AND ELECTROLYTES

In addition to a typical oral intake of 1–2 litres, a further 6–7 litres of secretions enter the GI tract each day, yet on average only 200 mL fluid are lost in stool. The small bowel accounts for up to 80% of this fluid absorption, with water following sodium absorption. Sodium absorption is multifactorial, including by co-transport with glucose and amino acids, and particularly in the ileum by active transport systems across a high concentration gradient. Extensive small bowel resection has major consequences for fluid and electrolyte balance.

# APPROACH TO THE PATIENT

## HISTORY

### GENERAL COMMENTS

Gastroenterological presentations often have no specific cause or 'curative' treatment, so it is important to reassure and address concerns. Patients are often happy to live with symptoms if the physiological basis is explained and specific fears (e.g. cancer) addressed.

#### Age

Knowing the typical age of presentation of common conditions helps produce a sensible differential diagnosis. Some congenital conditions present exclusively in the first few weeks of life (e.g. pyloric stenosis) while others may also present later (e.g. cystic fibrosis, Hirschsprung's disease). GI cancers are rare in patients under 45 years, and this fact underpins many diagnostic and management strategies in gastroenterology.

#### Sex

Ratios are insufficient to allow a different approach based on gender.

#### Ethnicity

Some disorders are more common in certain ethnic groups:
- *Gastric cancer:* Japanese
- *CD, haemochromatosis:* White populations

Many such variations are caused by environmental factors such as diet, rather than ethnicity (e.g. gastric cancer rates rapidly reduce when ethnic Japanese migrate and adopt a Western diet).

### HISTORY OF THE PRESENTING COMPLAINT

Rapid progression (e.g. dysphagia) fits with malignancy, whereas recurrent symptoms with periods of normality in between or symptoms stable over many years argues for functional or benign disease. Establish how symptoms relate to activities such as timing and content of meals, posture (for reflux symptoms), timing of defaecation or to external stresses.

### PAST MEDICAL HISTORY

Many benign GI diseases relapse and remit over long timescales (e.g. inflammatory bowel disease [IBD], peptic ulcer). A past history of any malignancy may be relevant.

   Previous abdominal surgery may explain new presenting symptoms:
- *Gastrectomy:* iron-deficiency anaemia (IDA); recurrent ulceration; cancer; diarrhoea
- *Pancreatectomy:* diarrhoea
- *Small bowel resection:* short bowel syndrome
- *Post-cholecystectomy syndrome*
- *Any abdominal surgery:* increases risk of bowel obstruction due to adhesions.

### SOCIAL HISTORY

Smoking, alcohol and caffeine use are often relevant to gastro-oesophageal reflux disease (GORD) and dyspepsia, caffeine or alcohol use to diarrhoea. Stress commonly aggravates functional GI symptoms. Patients may be stressed by specific symptoms (e.g. fear of incontinence in conditions with diarrhoea and/or urgency), so addressing these concerns is useful in management. Traumatic childhood events may underlie functional symptomatology. Patients are often concerned about the effect of disease on sexual function.

### DIETARY HISTORY

Anaemia and weight loss can result from poor intake (e.g. vegetarians, the elderly living alone). A high-fibre diet may provoke symptoms in patients with mechanical bowel obstruction or IBS. Carbonated drinks, diet products and health products (e.g. multivitamins with iron) are among many dietary factors that may provoke GI symptoms.

### GYNAECOLOGICAL AND OBSTETRIC HISTORY

Symptoms from some gynaecological conditions (e.g. pelvic inflammatory disease, endometriosis) overlap with GI problems and, in particular, IBS – often dual investigation is indicated. Traumatic labour can cause pelvic muscle and nerve injury and lead to problems with defaecation (especially faecal incontinence). A history of gynaecological and obstetric interventions should be taken and any relationship of symptoms to menstrual cycle noted.

### DRUG HISTORY

Remember to ask about oral contraceptives, recreational as well as prescribed drugs, and note when drugs were started in relation to symptom onset.

### FAMILY HISTORY

Examples of increased disease risk with affected family members include IBD, CD and colorectal cancer.

## EXAMINATION

See GASTROINTESTINAL DISEASE: CLINICAL FEATURES AT A GLANCE.

## GASTROINTESTINAL DISEASE: CLINICAL FEATURES AT A GLANCE

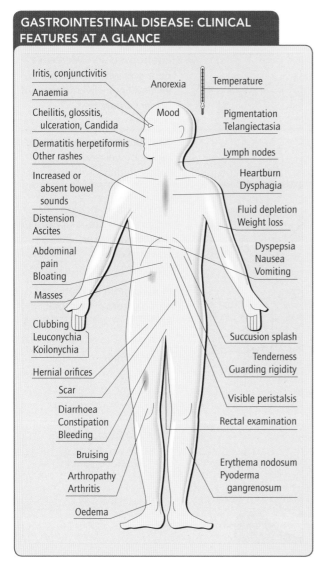

Iritis, conjunctivitis

Anaemia

Cheilitis, glossitis, ulceration, Candida

Dermatitis herpetiformis
Other rashes

Increased or absent bowel sounds

Distension
Ascites

Abdominal pain
Bloating

Masses

Clubbing
Leuconychia
Koilonychia

Hernial orifices

Scar

Diarrhoea
Constipation
Bleeding

Bruising

Arthropathy
Arthritis

Oedema

Anorexia

Mood

Temperature

Pigmentation
Telangiectasia

Lymph nodes

Heartburn
Dysphagia

Fluid depletion
Weight loss

Dyspepsia
Nausea
Vomiting

Succussion splash

Tenderness
Guarding rigidity

Visible peristalsis

Rectal examination

Erythema nodosum
Pyoderma gangrenosum

## GENERAL INSPECTION

- Ensure the patient is comfortable, lying flat with abdomen uncovered from pubis to xiphisternum
- Nutritional status:
  - Use body mass index (BMI)
  - Muscle loss (sarcopenia) often most evident in the small muscles of the hands
  - Obesity increases the risks of GORD, fatty liver and GI cancers
- Volume depletion may accompany GI bleeding, severe diarrhoea or intra-abdominal inflammation such as pancreatitis
- Fever
- Mood
- Anaemia and jaundice

## ABDOMINAL INSPECTION

- *Distension:* can be due to fat, fluid (ascites, large ovarian cyst or bladder), foetus, flatus (intestinal obstruction or ileus) or faeces; bulging of the umbilicus may occur in ascites
- *Visible peristalsis:* indicates intestinal obstruction
- *Striae:* indicate recent change in abdominal size because of pregnancy or ascites; purple striae are a feature of Cushing's syndrome
- *Scars* (**Figure 10.5a**)
- *Stoma:* the site can suggest the likely stoma type (**Figure 10.5b**)
- *Visible masses*
- *Bruising:* can signify retroperitoneal haemorrhage such as with severe pancreatitis; named patterns are Grey Turner's sign (flanks) and Cullen's sign (periumbilical)

## HANDS

- *Stigmata of chronic liver disease (SCLD)* (**Figure 10.6**): The most specific are spider naevi. Up to five can be physiological, usually small and on the hands. Spider naevi may occur anywhere in the drainage of the superior vena cava (SVC). Other SCLD are clubbing, palmar erythema, leuconychia (indicating hypoalbuminaemia) and, controversially, Dupuytren's contracture (most cases idiopathic).
- *Clubbing:* This may indicate IBD or liver disease.
- *Koilonychia:* This indicates severe iron deficiency (**Figure 10.7**).
- *Asterixis (or liver flap):* This indicates encephalopathy.

## MOUTH

- *Oral ulceration:* Causes include idiopathic (commonest), Crohn's, coeliac, Behçet's disease, ill-fitting dentures.
- *Candidiasis:* Causes include oral or inhaled steroids, immunosuppression, antibiotics, diabetes mellitus.
- *Telangiectasia:* This suggests hereditary haemorrhagic telangiectasia.
- *Angular cheilitis:* Causes include *Candida*, ill-fitting dentures, vitamin deficiencies (iron, vitamin B).
- *Glossitis:* Causes include iron and vitamin $B_{12}$ deficiency (**Figure 10.8**).
- *Erosions on the posterior surface of incisors:* These suggest frequent vomiting (e.g. bulimia) or severe GORD reflux.
- *Poor dentition:* This is an endocarditis risk factor.

## HEAD AND NECK

### Eyes

- Mild anaemia or jaundice may not be evident until close inspection of the conjunctiva or sclera, respectively.
- Xanthelasma are seen in hypercholesterolaemia and primary biliary cirrhosis (PBC).
- Uveitis is associated with IBD.

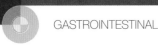
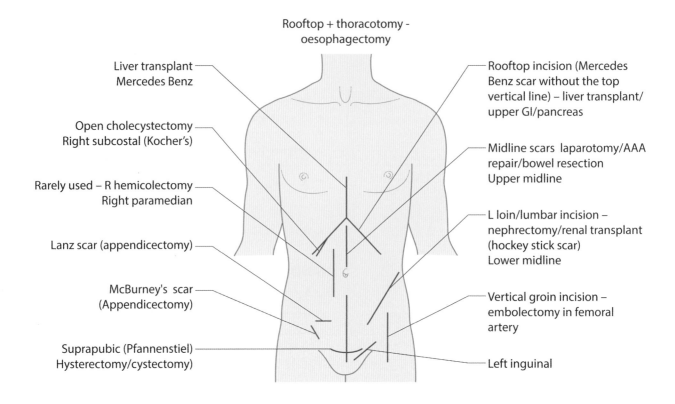

Rooftop + thoracotomy -
oesophagectomy

Liver transplant
Mercedes Benz

Open cholecystectomy
Right subcostal (Kocher's)

Rarely used – R hemicolectomy
Right paramedian

Lanz scar (appendicectomy)

McBurney's scar
(Appendicectomy)

Suprapubic (Pfannenstiel)
Hysterectomy/cystectomy)

Rooftop incision (Mercedes
Benz scar without the top
vertical line) – liver transplant/
upper GI/pancreas

Midline scars  laparotomy/AAA
repair/bowel resection
Upper midline

L loin/lumbar incision –
nephrectomy/renal transplant
(hockey stick scar)
Lower midline

Vertical groin incision –
embolectomy in femoral
artery

Left inguinal

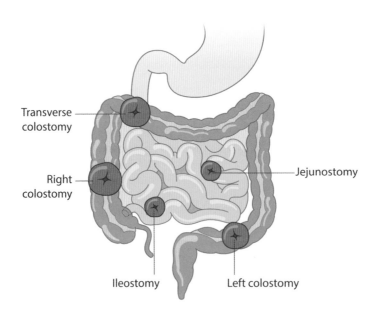

Transverse
colostomy

Right
colostomy

Jejunostomy

Ileostomy

Left colostomy

**Figure 10.5** Sites and common indications for surgical scars **(a)** and stomas **(b)**.

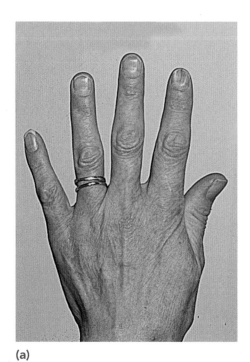

**(a)**

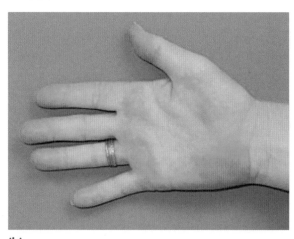

**(b)**

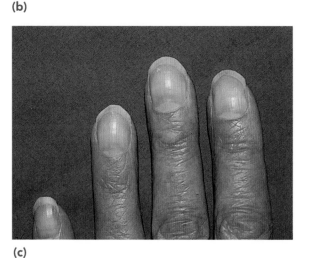

**(c)**

**Figure 10.6** Signs of chronic liver disease in the hand: **(a)** large spider naevus on the dorsum of the wrist; **(b)** palmar erythema; **(c)** leuconychia.

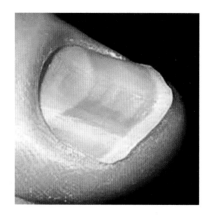

**Figure 10.7** Koilonychia.

### Neck

Enlarged neck or left supraclavicular nodes (*lymphadenopathy*) are associated with upper GI malignancy.

## ABDOMINAL PALPATION

Ask about abdominal pain and avoid these areas at first. The abdomen is conventionally divided into nine regions (**Figure 10.9**). Feel with the flat of the hand. Begin lightly, watch the patient's face, then palpate deeply if not painful. Feel for liver and spleen, moving the hand up as the patient breathes in. Feel bimanually (balloting) for kidneys, then for aortic aneurysm and bladder.

If an area is tender, note if there is resistance to pressure (guarding) or if pain increases when the hand is lifted (rebound tenderness) – both indicating peritoneal inflammation.

If tenderness is the same or worsens when the abdominal muscles tense, it is evidence of abdominal wall damage rather than visceral pain.

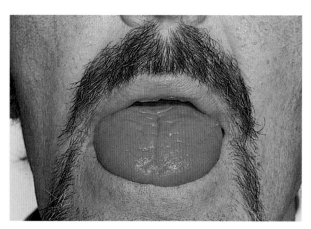

**Figure 10.8** Glossitis (smooth, red, raw tongue – causes include iron deficiency and $B_{12}$ deficiency).

10

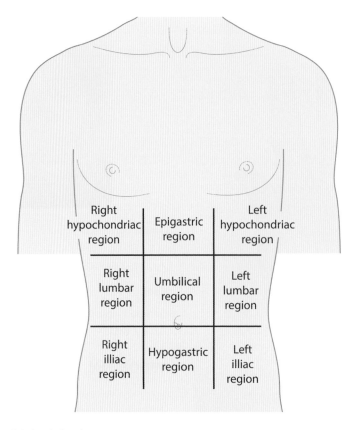

**Figure 10.9** Nomenclature of abdominal regions.

## PERCUSSION

This is typically dull over the liver and spleen and resonant over the kidneys.

Percuss the upper edge of the liver – in expiration usually in the fifth intercostal space, mid-clavicular line: if lower, then any hepatomegaly may be due to displacement (e.g. in chronic obstructive pulmonary disease [COPD] rather than enlargement).

Ascites produces shifting dullness – an area dull to percussion in the flank becomes resonant when the patient rolls to put that side uppermost, as the ascitic fluid sinks and gas-filled bowel rises. Abdominal percussion may be tympanic (hyper-resonant) when the bowel is distended with gas, as in intestinal ileus or obstruction.

## AUSCULTATION

Auscultation is of limited value in GI diagnosis. Bowel sounds may be accentuated in obstruction and diminished or absent in paralytic ileus. An aortic bruit may be normal in thin patients.

## RECTAL EXAMINATION

In patients presenting with acute abdominal pain, colorectal symptoms or GI bleeding, rectal examination is mandatory. Examine and note:

- Perianal disorders (tags, fistulae, external piles, fissures, excoriation)
- Mass lesions (e.g. cancer, polyp), oedema or induration (IBD) or abnormalities of the stool (constipation, diarrhoea)
- Prostate/cervix
- Localized tenderness (e.g. in appendicitis)
- Blood or pus, which may be seen on the glove after its withdrawal

## EXTERNAL GENITALIA

Testicular pain (e.g. from torsion or tumour) may refer to the lower abdomen.

## HERNIAL ORIFICES

These are best examined with the patient standing. This is particularly relevant in patients presenting with abdominal pain or signs of intestinal obstruction.

> A useful mnemonic for completion of a GI bedside assessment is 'SHRUG':
> **S**tool examination
> **H**ernial orifices
> **R**ectal exam
> **U**rinalysis
> External **G**enitalia

## GENERAL EXAMINATION

- *Chest:* Pleural effusions may indicate metastatic GI malignancies or portal hypertension; gynaecomastia – chronic liver disease.
- *Breast:* Metastatic breast cancer can present with weight loss, hepatomegaly or ascites.
- *Cardiovascular:* Atrial fibrillation (AF) is a major risk factor for intestinal ischaemia. Heart failure can cause ascites and hepatomegaly; endocarditis may present with weight loss and splenomegaly. Signs of peripheral vascular disease suggest an increased risk of bowel ischaemia, which may present with acute or chronic abdominal pain.
- *Skin:*
  o Erythema nodosum and pyoderma gangrenosum are associated with IBD.
  o Dermatitis herpetiformis, an itchy vesicular skin disorder, can occur in CD and responds to a gluten-free diet (GFD).
- *Joints:*
  o IBD, CD and some gut infections can be associated with a non-erosive arthropathy.
  o Isolated swelling of the first and/or second metatarsophalangeal (MTP) joints can be seen in haemochromatosis.

## INVESTIGATION

## BLOOD TESTS

These are frequently used to assess disease severity, but they rarely indicate a specific diagnosis.

## ENDOSCOPY

Flexible endoscopy is the major diagnostic tool in gastroenterology (**Figure 10.10**). The abilities to detect small or flat mucosal lesions and take biopsies are advantages over radiological imaging. Possibilities for delivering therapy are ever-increasing.

### Upper gastrointestinal endoscopy

Also known as gastroscopy or oesophagogastroduodenoscopy (OGD), this is the most commonly used investigation for upper GI symptoms. It is often performed without sedation, using lignocaine to numb the throat. If sedation is used, the most common agent is intravenous (IV) benzodiazepine; the main side effect is respiratory depression. A slim gastroscope can be introduced transnasally. This is easier to tolerate but has reduced diagnostic and therapeutic ability.

### Diagnostic indications
- Dyspepsia
- Dysphagia
- Nausea and vomiting
- Haematemesis and melaena
- Weight loss
- IDA (including duodenal biopsies for CD)
- Barrett's oesophagus

### Therapeutic indications and techniques
- GI bleeding: peptic ulcer, oesophageal varices
- Dilatation of oesophageal strictures
- Placing feeding tubes
- Percutaneous endoscopic gastrostomy

### Contraindications and precautions
Sedation is the major risk, especially in the elderly, and those with low BMIs, COPD or sleep apnoea. Patients with atlantoaxial subluxation (usually caused by rheumatoid arthritis) should have their neck supported in a hard collar. Avoid routine procedures within 6 weeks of myocardial infarction (MI) or cataract surgery. For routine diagnostic endoscopy, there is no need to stop aspirin or other antiplatelet agents; warfarin can be continued with an INR check before the procedure. Direct oral anticoagulants such as apixaban are omitted on the day. For therapeutic procedures, the risks of bleeding are higher and individual consideration is required.

Routine antibiotic prophylaxis for patients with cardiac risk factors is not necessary.

### Preparation and technique
A 6-hour fast is required (sips of water and essential medication allowed). Ideally, proton pump inhibitors (PPIs) should be avoided for 2 weeks before the procedure, as they may mask pathology and invalidate urease-based tests for *Helicobacter*.

### Complications
The overall incidence is 0.2%, mainly relating to oversedation or oesophageal perforation with therapeutic procedures in the acute setting; overall mortality is 0.01%.

### Endoscopic retrograde cholangiopancreatography

Endoscopic retrograde cholangiopancreatography (ERCP) is discussed in Chapter 9, Liver, biliary tract and pancreatic disease.

### Capsule endoscopy

Commonly used to examine the small bowel, a wireless capsule endoscope is swallowed and this records views of the jejunum and ileum (**Figure 10.11**). The technology can be modified to obtain views of the oesophagus or colon. The viewing angles cannot be altered and there is no therapeutic option.

### Double balloon enteroscopy

Intubation deep into the small bowel is now possible using a balloon system to pull the endoscope along. Biopsy and therapy of small bowel lesions is possible. General anaesthetic is usually required.

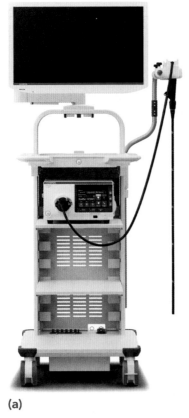

**(a)**

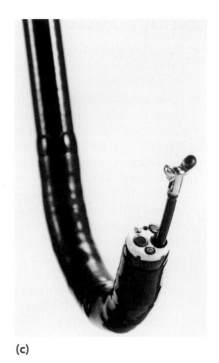

**(c)**

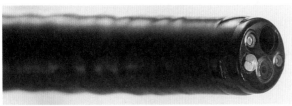

**(b)**

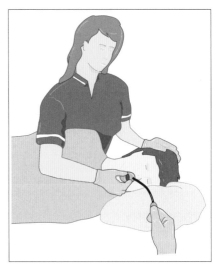

**(d)**

**Figure 10.10** Fibreoptic endoscopy. **(a)** General view of endoscope and video image processing unit. Equipment for producing hard copy photographs or video recordings of endoscopic views is shown under the monitor. Courtesy of Olympus UK & Ireland. **(b)** End view of endoscope. **(c)** Biopsy forceps exiting the endoscope's biopsy channel. **(d)** Patient position for the procedure – the nurse holds the mouthguard, aspirates the oral cavity as necessary and monitors the patient's overall condition.

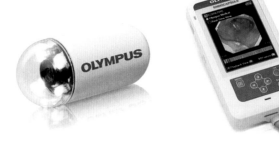

**Figure 10.11** Capsule endoscopy. Courtesy of Olympus UK & Ireland.

## Colonoscopy and flexible fibreoptic sigmoidoscopy

An endoscope is introduced via the anus and manipulated under direct vision around the colon. The bowel is prepared using a strong laxative and restricted low-residue diet. Iron-containing preparations are avoided for 1 week. Flexible fibreoptic sigmoidoscopy (FOS) only requires enema preparation and is used mainly for the investigation of anal canal type rectal bleeding.

### Colonoscopy indications
- Anaemia
- Change in bowel habit
- Surveillance for patients at increased risk of colorectal cancer
- Bowel cancer screening
- Monitoring of IBD

### Common therapeutic indications
- Removal of polyps
- Thermal treatment of angiodysplasia
- Dilation of benign strictures
- Stenting of malignant strictures
- Mechanically treatment of volvulus or intussusception

### Contraindications and complications
- Contraindications similar to those for OGD above
- Overall risk 1 in 1000 – main perforation or bleeding
- More common if therapy (e.g. polypectomy) has been undertaken

## Rigid endoscopy

This is a useful, quick, cheap, safe, outpatient technique for the initial examination (e.g. patients with diarrhoea, rectal bleeding or IBD). It is not safe to exclude organic disease by this procedure alone.

## Endoscopic ultrasound

Ultrasound views are obtained from a transducer on the end of an endoscope.

### Indications
- High-resolution views of mucosa (e.g. staging oesophageal cancer or assessing the pancreas)
- Distinguishing benign from malignant gut wall abnormalities
- Drainage of pancreatic cysts
- Assessment of common bile duct and ampullary lesions
- Facilitating access into the bile duct where ERCP has failed

## DIAGNOSTIC IMAGING

### Plain radiography

See **Figure 10.12**.

### Erect chest radiography

This may show:
- Air under diaphragm suggesting gut perforation
- Abnormal mediastinal/neck soft tissue air shadowing in oesophageal perforation
- Lung metastases
- Pulmonary tuberculosis (TB) (as a clue to the presence of abdominal TB)
- Pleural effusions (associations include oesophageal perforation, pancreatitis, or malabsorption states with low albumin)

### Supine abdominal films

These may show:
- Bowel obstruction
- Volvulus
- Faecal loading

## Barium studies

See **Figure 10.13**.

### Barium swallow

This assesses the oesophagus.

*Indications*
- Oesophageal motility disorders (although manometry is the 'gold standard')
- High dysphagia (e.g. due to pharyngeal dysmotility) or pharyngeal pouch

### Barium meal

This assesses the stomach but is now mostly superseded by gastroscopy.

*Indications*
- Demonstrating delayed emptying (gastroparesis), e.g. due to diffuse malignancy (linitis plastica), strictures or autonomic neuropathy
- Benign structural changes (e.g. postoperative stomachs, volvulus)
- Patients unwilling to undergo gastroscopy

### Barium follow-through/small bowel enema (enteroclysis)

This assesses the small bowel. MRI, ultrasound and enterostomy are now first-line.

*Indications*
- Steatorrhoea
- Abdominal pain

### Double-contrast barium enema

This assesses the colon. It is rarely used now: where colonoscopy fails or is not considered appropriate, CT colonography provides more accurate assessment of the colon and of other intra-abdominal organs.

### Ultrasound

See **Figure 10.14**.

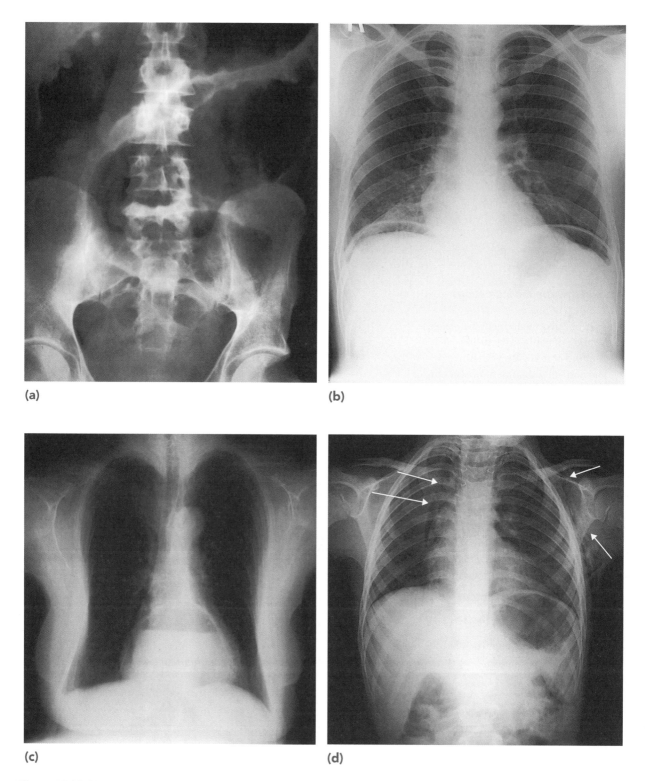

(a)

(b)

(c)

(d)

**Figure 10.12** Plain radiographs of the chest and abdomen revealing GI disorders. **(a)** Toxic megacolon. The colon is dilated throughout. Mucosal islands are visible (arrows): nodules of oedematous mucosa protruding into the dilated lumen, surrounded by ulcerated mucosa (e.g. at hepatic flexure). **(b)** Intra-abdominal perforation. Note the air under both diaphragms. **(c)** Hiatus hernia. Note the air–fluid level in the gastric lumen behind the cardiac shadow. **(d)** Oesophageal perforation in a 5-year-old child (after rigid oesophagoscopy). Note the mediastinal air on the right and subcutaneous air, particularly on the left. *(Continued)*

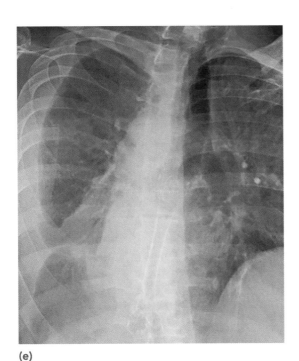

**(e)**

**Figure 10.12** *(Continued)* **(e)** Oesophageal stent in place for relief of dysphagia.

After endoscopy, ultrasound is the most common investigation used. Obesity and excessive luminal gas reduce the diagnostic yield.

*Indications*

- Abdominal pain
- Weight loss
- Suspected abnormalities of the liver, gall bladder, bile ducts, pancreas, spleen and small bowel

### CT and MRI scanning

See **Figure 10.15**.

These techniques are complementary to each other and to ultrasound: some liver lesions may be 'invisible' with one technique yet show up on another.

*Indications*

- Acute abdomen
- Pancreatic, biliary and liver disease
- Abdominal pain
- Weight loss
- Guided biopsy of masses
- Drainage of abscesses
- Cancer staging

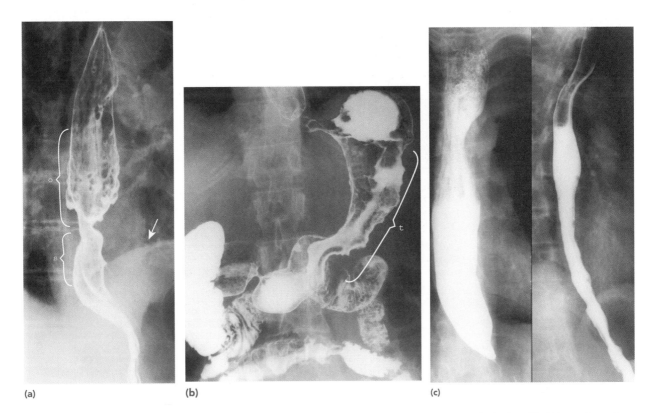

**(a)**          **(b)**          **(c)**

**Figure 10.13** Contrast radiology of the GI tract. **(a)** Barium swallow showing a hiatus hernia – note the barium-filled hiatus above the diaphragm (arrowed). **(b)** Contrast study showing advanced gastric carcinoma. Note the irregularity caused by tumour and ulceration along the greater curve (t). **(c)** Achalasia. Barium swallow showing excess food residue and dilated oesophagus tapering smoothly down to the cardia before (left) and after (right) pneumatic dilatation. Reproduced from Misiewicz JJ *et al.* (1994) *Diseases of the Gut and Pancreas*, 2nd edn (Wiley-Blackwell, Oxford), with the permission of the authors. *(Continued)*

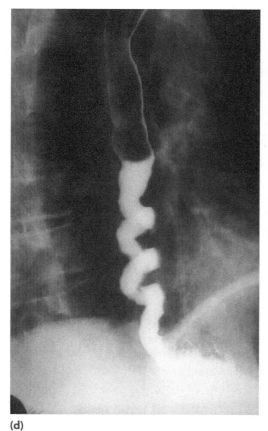

(d)

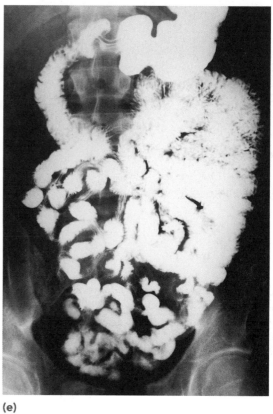

(e)

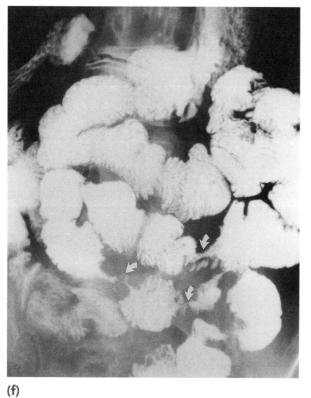

(f)

**Figure 10.13** *(Continued)* **(d)** Oesophageal spasm. The tertiary contractions in a normal calibre oesophagus give a corkscrew appearance. **(e)** Normal double-contrast barium meal and follow through. The lumen is distended with gas (introduced as an effervescent $CO_2$-releasing agent) while the mucosa is lined by a thin coating of barium. **(f)** Small bowel barium meal showing Crohn's disease of the small intestine with areas of stricturing (arrowed) and dilatation. Reproduced from Misiewicz JJ *et al.* (1994) *Diseases of the Gut and Pancreas*, 2nd edn (Wiley-Blackwell, Oxford), with the permission of the authors.

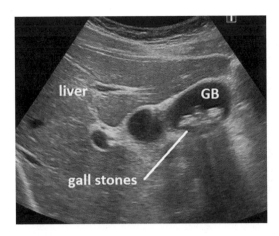

**Figure 10.14** Ultrasound examination of the upper abdomen showing three large stones (arrowed) in the gall bladder (GB). Image courtesy of Dr A Culverwell, Consultant Radiologist, Harrogate District Hospital.

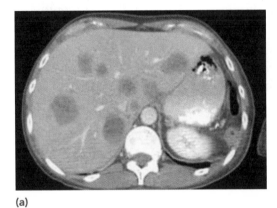

(a)

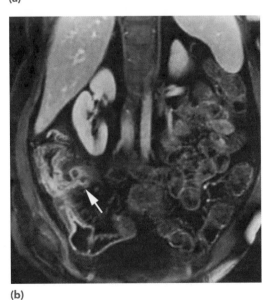

(b)

**Figure 10.15** Examples of cross-sectional imaging of the abdomen. **(a)** CT abdomen showing liver metastases (multiple hypodense lucencies throughout liver parenchyma, larger examples arrowed). **(b)** MRI small bowel showing typical features of terminal ileal Crohn's disease (thickened, inflamed small bowel mucosa in right ileac fossa [arrowed]). Images courtesy of Dr A Culverwell, Consultant Radiologist, Harrogate District Hospital.

## CT colonography

To obtain the detail equivalent to colonoscopy, the bowel needs laxative preparation and insufflation with gas prior to CT scanning.

### Gastrointestinal angiography

See **Figure 10.16**.

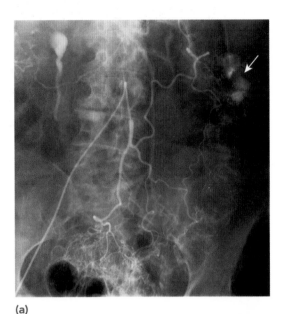

(a)

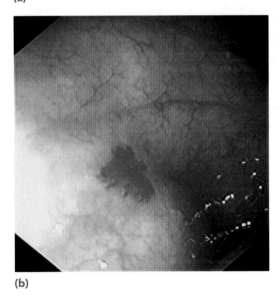

(b)

**Figure 10.16 (a)** Angiography of the mesenteric circulation in the investigation of obscure GI bleeding. The film shows contrast injected into the IMA. An angiodysplasia has been demonstrated in the region of the splenic flexure. Bleeding from the lesion shows as a 'blush' of contrast pooling in the lumen (arrow). **(b)** Typical endoscopic view of angiodysplasia.Once localized by angiography, most areas of the GI tract can now be reached with an endoscope (e.g. colonoscope or double balloon enteroscope) capable of delivering therapy such as thermal coagulation to stop bleeding. Reproduced from Cotton PB & Williams CB (1990) *Practical Gastrointestinal Endoscopy*, 3rd edn (Wiley-Blackwell, Oxford), with the permission of the authors.

*Indications*
- Active GI bleeding of unclear origin
- Angiomatous malformations
- Meckel's diverticulum

## BREATH TESTS

The general principles of breath tests are shown in **Figure 10.17**. Results need interpreting with caution as they can be affected by factors such as age, high-fibre meals and abnormal gastric emptying.

Examples include:
- *Lactose tolerance test:* lactase deficiency
- *Glucose or lactulose breath tests:* small intestinal bacterial overgrowth
- *Carbon 13-labelled urea breath test:* to detect *Helicobacter pylori* (HP)

## SURGICAL TECHNIQUES

### Conventional surgery

Conventional surgery (laparotomy) continues to have a major role in the management of the acute abdomen, persistent acute GI bleeding, GI neoplasia and IBD, although less invasive techniques, such as laparoscopy and endoscopic therapy, are increasingly used.

### Laparoscopy

Laparoscopy is now used routinely in preference to open abdominal surgery for cholecystectomy, inguinal and hiatus hernia repair, appendicectomy and limited colectomy. Diagnostic laparoscopy is now rarely used outside gynaecology.

Relative contraindications include previous abdominal surgery (adhesions increase the risk of intestinal perforation on insertion of the trochar) and coagulation disorders.

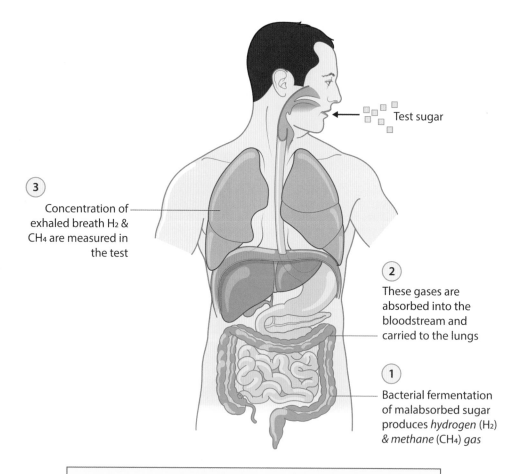

← Test sugar

**3** Concentration of exhaled breath $H_2$ & $CH_4$ are measured in the test

**2** These gases are absorbed into the bloodstream and carried to the lungs

**1** Bacterial fermentation of malabsorbed sugar produces *hydrogen* ($H_2$) & *methane* ($CH_4$) *gas*

*Concentrations of breath hydrogen and methane are used to indicate if the test sugar is malabsorbed or if proximal bacterial overgrowth is present*

**(a)**

**Figure 10.17 (a)** Principle of breath tests, in this example to detect small bowel bacterial overgrowth (SIBO). *(Continued)*

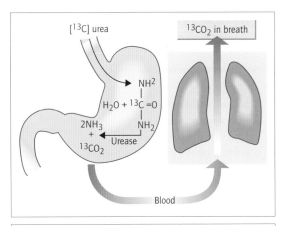

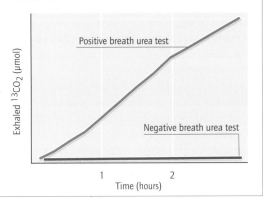

**(c)**

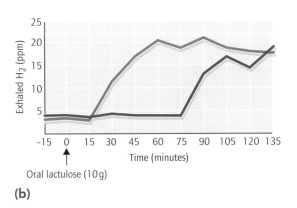

**(b)**

**Figure 10.17** *(Continued)* **(b)** Lactulose breath test result showing SIBO. The diagram shows normal exhaled hydrogen curve (blue) – orocaecal transit time is about 75–90 min; exhaled hydrogen curve of a patient with bacterial overgrowth (red) – the diagnosis is revealed by the early (at 15–30 min) rise of breath hydrogen concentration as lactulose is metabolized to hydrogen by bacteria in excess in the small intestine. **(c)** Principle of urea breath test for the diagnosis of HP infection. Urea labelled with carbon-13 isotope is ingested and hydrolyzed by urease of HP. Hydrolysis of urea produces labelled $CO_2$ which is absorbed rapidly into the bloodstream and detected in expired air.

## GASTROINTESTINAL EMERGENCIES

## UPPER GASTROINTESTINAL BLEEDING

### Overview

- Around 5% of medical admissions
- Mortality 7–10% (30% if initially admitted with other problems)
- Classic presentation: haematemesis and/or melaena, often with a sudden drop in haemoglobin or shock (contrast with chronic GI bleeding where presentation usually IDA)
- Occasionally no outward signs
- Abdominal pain unusual

### Causes

See **Figure 10.18**.
- Peptic ulcer
- Varices
- Gastritis, duodenitis and oesophagitis
- Mallory–Weiss tears
- No cause found (5–10% cases)
- Important rare cause: gastric malignancy

### Management

Initial management is the same whatever the cause.

## ACUTE LOWER GASTROINTESTINAL BLEEDING

### Overview

- Acute bleeding anywhere distal to the duodenojejunal junction

- 20% of all acute GI bleeds
- Usually stops spontaneously
- Less likely be haemodynamically unstable than upper GI bleeds
- Incidence increases with age

### Causes

Causes of lower GI bleeding are listed in **Table 10.4**.

### Clinical features

- The type of bleeding predicts the site:
  - *Fresh red rectal bleeding* commonly predicts anorectal pathology (e.g. haemorrhoids, anal fissure). This is usually obvious from the history (e.g. anal pain on defecation), or on rectal examination.
  - *Altered blood or black/digested blood (melaena)* suggests more proximal bleeding sites.
- Shock (5–10%)
- Anaemia
- Abdominal mass suggests neoplasia
- Tenderness ± vascular bruit suggests ischaemia

### Investigation

- Blood grouping and cross-matching
- FBC to identify chronic bleeding
- Prothrombin time
- A raised blood urea suggests a more proximal source

## EMERGENCY PRESENTATION 10.1

### Upper gastrointestinal bleeding

#### 1 Initial assessment and resuscitation

- ABC approach.
- IV access, insert two wide-bore cannulas.
- Assess volume needs and replace. Note blood pressure (BP) drop may be a late event in volume loss – tachycardia is usually the first sign (beware of blunted response if on beta blockers). If initial BP is normal, check lying and standing. Witnessed ongoing large volume haematemesis/melaena will require transfusion ± use of local major haemorrhage protocol and more invasive monitoring techniques in High Dependency Unit/Intensive Therapy Unit (HDU/ITU ). For more stable patients felt to be hypovolemic, fluid challenge with 250–500 mL crystalloid and reassess after 30 min. Over-transfusion can trigger re-bleeding, so transfuse only if haemoglobin (Hb) <7 and aim for 7-9 g/dL range (unless the patient has a cardiac history where higher values are appropriate to avoid aggravating ischaemic heart disease [IHD]/angina).
- Order full blood count (FBC), urea and electrolytes (U&E), liver function tests (LFTs), clotting, group and save (or cross-match four units if there is a significant bleed). If possible, obtain past blood results – low Hb or high urea is less relevant if chronically abnormal. Early Hb levels may be misleading – plasma expansion takes several hours after blood loss. Reassess Hb after a few hours if unstable. Transfuse platelets if <50 × 10$^9$/L and the patient is actively bleeding or haemodynamically unstable.
- Simultaneously gather key elements of history and examination (e.g. are there risk factors for cirrhosis or signs of chronic liver disease; possible causal drug use – aspirin, non-steroidal anti-inflammatory drugs [NSAIDs], anticoagulants?)
- Request senior medical/surgical help for unstable patients.
- GI bleeding may precipitate encephalopathy in cirrhosis. Consider anaesthetic assessment/intubation.
- Send stool for HP antigen (tests unreliable once PPIs started).
- Keep nil-by-mouth (NBM) in preparation for endoscopy.
- Do not place a nasogastric tube routinely.
- Do not place a urinary catheter routinely. However, this may be indicated in unstable cases to assess adequacy of volume replacement.

#### 2 Medication issues

- *Stop* aspirin and other antiplatelet agents, NSAIDs (including COX-2 inhibitors) and anticoagulants during acute bleeding phase.
- *Pause* antihypertensives and diuretics (as these increase the risks of acute kidney injury during an acute bleeding phase).
- Note steroids and selective serotonin reuptake inhibitors (SSRIs) increase the risk of bleeding if the patient is taking NSAIDs.
- Consider terlipressin before endoscopy if there is high suspicion for variceal bleeding.
- Give patients with suspected or proven variceal bleeding broad-spectrum antibiotics.
- Consider omeprazole (80 mg IV bolus then 8 mg/hour IV infusion) in *all* patients requiring admission *while awaiting* endoscopy.
- Consider erythromycin (250 mg IV 30–120 min before endoscopy). This encourages gastric emptying.
- Warfarin reversal: For actively bleeding patients, give fresh frozen plasma (FFP) if the prothrombin time >1.5× normal. If the fibrinogen level remains less than 1.5 g/L despite FFP, consider cryoprecipitate. For life-threating bleeding, reversal with prothrombin complex concentrate (e.g. Beriplex) is indicated; for stable cases, IV vitamin K is usually sufficient.
- Novel oral anticoagulant (NOAC) reversal: This is a complex and evolving field. Conventional laboratory tests do not help. If the patient is unstable, discuss with haematology. For stable patients, simply stopping the NOAC is usually adequate.

#### 3 Calculate risk scores

The Glasgow Blatchford score is most useful for immediate risk stratification (see below); the post-endoscopy Rockall score is better at predicting risk of re-bleeding and death.

#### 4 Based on risk scores *and* your overall clinical assessment, decide on the management pathway

*A EARLY DISCHARGE PATHWAY*

Criteria:

- Rockall 0, Blatchford 0–1
- No recent significant fall in Hb
- No postural drop in BP
- No coagulopathy
- No complex decisions required regarding restarting antiplatelet agents or anticoagulants
- No concern about varices

- Not an inpatient
- No social issues

Patients may be safely discharged for urgent outpatient endoscopy. Avoid NSAIDs. Restart aspirin, diuretics and antihypertensives. Oral PPI should usually be prescribed.

*B HIGH-RISK INPATIENT PATHWAY*

Any of:

- Cardiovascularly unstable
- Glasgow Blatchford score 7 or higher
- Likely variceal bleeding

Admit to an appropriate ward area familiar with management of potentially unstable GI bleed cases. Urgent discussion with the clinician responsible for emergency endoscopy, in UK NICE recommends endoscopy 'immediately after resuscitation'.

*C LOW-RISK INPATIENT PATHWAY*

If a patient does not fit into A or B above, admit them and organize endoscopy within 24 hours.

### 5 Immediate post-endoscopy management

- *High-risk peptic ulcer* (active bleeding, visible vessel, adherent clot): Continue IV PPI infusion for 72 hours.
- *All other diagnoses:* Stop IV PPI infusion. Convert to oral PPI if diagnosis responsive to acid suppression is found.
- If varices are found, manage as for variceal bleeding (Chapter 9: Liver, Biliary Tract and Pancreatic Disease).
- No need to remain NBM unless endoscopist has recommended early repeat endoscopy required.
- If malignancy suspected, refer for multidisciplinary team (MDT) discussion; if active treatment appropriate, organize staging investigations.
- Where repeat endoscopic therapy for bleeding/re-bleeding is not recommended, yet upper GI bleeding continues in a patient for active treatment, interventional radiology is usually preferred over laparotomy.
- Restart aspirin, diuretics and antihypertensives as soon as cardiovascularly stable.

### 6 Longer-term management

- HP eradication is indicated in all positive cases. Confirm success with stool antigen.
- For duodenal ulcer (DU) associated with HP, stop PPI after eradication treatment.
- For gastric ulcer (GU) associated with HP, continue PPI 6–8 weeks then repeat endoscopy to ensure ulcer healing (non-healing ulcers raise suspicion of malignancy)
- If ulcer linked to NSAID use, stopping the drug offers the best protection against recurrence: if this is not possible, combine low-dose COX-2 selective NSAID with a PPI (note avoid COX-2 inhibitors in patients with a history of cardiovascular events).
- Ulcers negative for both HP and NSAID have a high relapse rate. Note the possibility of false negative tests and consider retesting, otherwise use long-term PPI.
- Whether and when to restart ADP/P2Y antiplatelet agents (e.g. clopidogrel) and/or anticoagulants is often a difficult decision. Discuss with the team which prescribed the medications and the patient. Risk scoring systems can help, e.g. HAS-BLED for risk of GI bleeding in anticoagulated patients and $CHA_2DS_2$-VASc for risk of stroke in AF (**Table 10.3**).

**Table 10.3** $CHA_2DS_2$-VASc and HAS-BLED scoring systems

| CHA₂DS₂-VASc | Score | HAS-BLED | Score |
|---|---|---|---|
| **C**ongestive heart failure/LV dysfunction | 1 | **H**ypertension, i.e. uncontrolled BP | 1 |
| **H**ypertension | 1 | **A**bdominal renal/liver function | 1 or 2 |
| **A**ged ≥75 years | 2 | **S**troke | 1 |
| **D**iabetes mellitus | 1 | **B**leeding tendency or predisposition | 1 |
| **S**troke/TIA/TE | 2 | **L**abile INRs | 1 |
| **V**ascular disease (prior MI, peripheral arterial disease [PAD] or aortic plaque) | 1 | **E**lderly (e.g. >65 years) | 1 |
| **A**ged 65–74 years | 1 | **D**rugs (e.g. concomitant aspirin or NSAIDs) or alcohol | 1 or 2 |
| **S**ex – female gender* | 1 | | |
| Maximum score | 9 | | 9 |

*Note:* If female gender is the only risk factor, CHA₂DS₂VASc is 0.

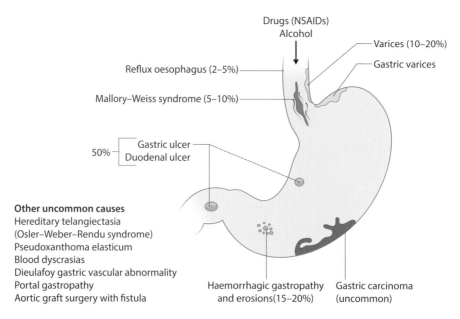

Drugs (NSAIDs)
Alcohol

Varices (10–20%)

Gastric varices

Reflux oesophagus (2–5%)

Mallory–Weiss syndrome (5–10%)

50% ⌐ Gastric ulcer
      ⌊ Duodenal ulcer

**Other uncommon causes**
Hereditary telangiectasia
(Osler–Weber–Rendu syndrome)
Pseudoxanthoma elasticum
Blood dyscrasias
Dieulafoy gastric vascular abnormality
Portal gastropathy
Aortic graft surgery with fistula

Haemorrhagic gastropathy
and erosions(15–20%)

Gastric carcinoma
(uncommon)

**Figure 10.18** Causes of upper GI bleeding.

### Endoscopy and diagnostic imaging

Using some or all of the techniques below, the cause of bleeding is identified in about 80–90% of patients.

- *Gastroscopy:* atypical upper GI bleed presentation
- *Colonoscopy:* preferably after adequate bowel preparation
- *CT angiogram:* usual next step if colonoscopy fails to identify bleeding source and bleeding continues; sometimes done as the initial investigation when unstable
- *Mesenteric angiogram:* allows selective imaging of smaller branches of mesenteric arteries, which can then be embolized if the bleeding source is found
- *Exploratory laparotomy:* if profuse, undiagnosed bleeding persists
- *Radiolabelled red cell scan, Meckel's scan, small bowel MRI and enteroscopy):* further investigations for undiagnosed cases, particularly where bleeding continues but the patient is haemodynamically stable

### Management

The steps taken depend on the haemodynamic state of the patient and local expertise. A typical scheme is shown in **Figure 10.19**.

### Specific treatment

- *Endoscopy:* Colonoscopic techniques such as clips, electrocoagulation and synthetic clot sprays can stop bleeding.
- *Topical treatment:* Radiation proctitis has been shown to respond to topical formalin, applied via soaked gauze.
- *Surgery:* Treatment for many of the causes of acute lower bowel haemorrhage is elective surgery.

- *Arteriography:* Vascular malformations can be selectively embolized.

## ACUTE ABDOMINAL PAIN/ACUTE ABDOMEN

### Overview

- Recent onset of severe continuous or colicky pain in a sick patient
- Often associated with vomiting, guarding, pyrexia, leucocytosis and raised inflammatory markers
- Requires urgent admission for surgical assessment

### Causes

Causes of abdominal pain are listed in **Tables 10.5** and **10.6**).

### Approach to the patient

#### History

The SOCRATES mnemonic provides a useful approach to ensuring the features of the pain are assessed.

> Use the SOCRATES mnemonic to ensure the following features of the pain are assessed:
> **S**ite
> **O**nset
> **C**haracter
> **R**adiation
> **A**ssociations
> **T**ime course
> **E**xacerbating/relieving factors
> **S**everity
> See **Table 10.7**.

**Table 10.4** Causes of painless lower GI bleeding

**Children** *(all rare)*
- Infections (A)
- IBD (A or C)
- Meckel's diverticulum (A)
- Haemangiomas (C)
- Intussusception (A)

**Adults**

*Common*
- Diverticulosis (A)
- Angiodysplasia/other vascular malformations (A or C)
- Cancer/polyps (C)
- IBD (A or C)
- Anorectal disease (e.g. haemorrhoids) (C)
- Endoscopic polypectomy (A)
- Ischaemia (A)

*Rare*
- Meckel's diverticulum (A)
- Benign solitary rectal ulcer (C)
- Radiation enterocolitis (A or C)

A, characteristically bleeds acutely; C, tends to cause chronic or recurrent, usually minor, or occult bleeding.

Obstructive pain is characteristically colicky (cramping, coming in waves) and causes the patient to be restless. By contrast, patients with inflammatory conditions tend to lie still. Note the diagnosis is often delayed as initially there are few signs despite severe symptoms.

### Examination

In addition to abdominal and rectal examination, remember cardiovascular disease (e.g. AF as a risk for mesenteric ischaemia) and testicular and gynaecological examination.

The common surface area markings for visceral pain from various organs are shown in **Figure 10.20**. Note, however, that there is a wide variation in practice.

### Investigation

### Bedside tests

Haematuria found on urinalysis supports a diagnosis of urolithiasis.

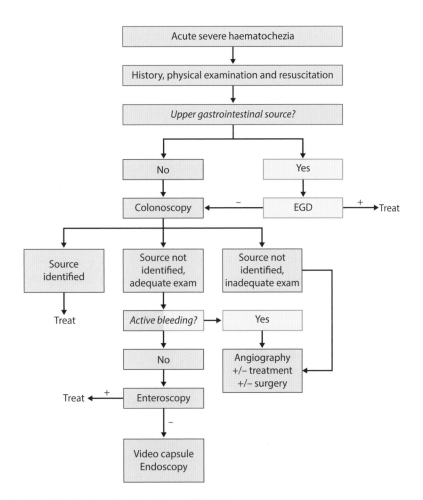

**Figure 10.19** Example of algorithm for investigation of lower GI bleeding.

**Table 10.5** Causes of abdominal pain resulting from disease of intra-abdominal organs (most common causes in capital letters)

| Type of disorder | Cause |
| --- | --- |
| **Distension/tension** | |
| Obstruction | |
| Intestinal | TUMOUR, HERNIA, ADHESIONS, volvulus, intussusception, faecal impaction |
| Biliary | GALLSTONE, TUMOUR, stricture, haemobilia |
| Ureteric | RENAL STONE |
| Motility/hypersensitivity | IBS |
| Hepatic capsule distension | HEPATITIS, Budd–Chiari syndrome |
| Gynaecological | Ectopic pregnancy |
| **Inflammation** | |
| Generalized peritonitis | PERFORATED VISCUS (peptic ulcer, diverticulum, gall bladder), ruptured ovarian cyst |
| Localized peritonitis | APPENDICITIS, DIVERTICULITIS, PANCREATITIS, CHOLECYSTITIS, SALPINGITIS, abscess |
| Other infection | ASCENDING URINARY TRACT INFECTION, abdominal TB |
| Inflamed viscus | PEPTIC ULCER, NSAID or other drug-induced mucosal injury, IBD |
| Mesenteric adenitis | |
| **Ischaemia** | |
| Mesenteric angina/infarction | Atheroma (thrombosis, embolus), arteritis |
| Splenic infarction | |
| Torsion | Ovarian cyst, testicle |
| Tumour necrosis | Hepatoma, fibroid/liver metastases |

### Blood tests

- *FBC:* raised neutrophil count in inflammatory or ischaemic conditions
- *C-reactive protein (CRP):* raised in inflammatory or ischaemic conditions
- *LFTs:* may be non-specifically abnormal with any severe intra-abdominal inflammatory pathology, but abnormalities suggest need for investigations to rule out hepatic biliary and pancreatic pathology
- *Amylase:* slight elevations can occur with a wide range of intra-abdominal pathology; levels over 3× normal suggest pancreatitis
- Pancreatic lipase: increasingly used as alternative to amylase as more specific

### Special investigations

- *Abdominal and chest X-ray:* for bowel obstruction or perforation
- *Electrocardiogram (ECG):* upper abdominal pain may be only symptom of MI
- *Ultrasound and computed tomography (CT):* both effective at ruling in and out a wide range of causes: which is used will depend on local practice and clinical suspicion (e.g. suspected cholecystitis: US; suspected intestinal obstruction or older patient where malignancy/bowel ischaemia more likely: CT)

**Table 10.6** Causes of abdominal pain referred from sites outside the abdominal cavity or caused by systemic disease

| Site/type of disorder | Cause |
| --- | --- |
| Retroperitoneal | Aortic aneurysm, neoplasia |
| Thoracic | Basal pneumonia, MI |
| Neurological | Herpes zoster, spinal arthritis, tabes dorsalis |
| Metabolic | Diabetic ketoacidosis, hypercalcaemia, hypoadrenalism, uraemia, porphyria, hypertriglycerideraemia, familial Mediterranean fever |
| Haematological | Sickle cell disease, paroxysmal nocturnal haemoglobinuria, haemorrhagic diathesis |
| Immunological | Angioneurotic oedema |
| Toxins | Lead poisoning |
| Drugs | Chronic high-dose usage of opiate drug, part of acute opiate withdrawal syndrome |
| Psychogenic | Depression, anxiety, Munchausen's syndrome, hypochondriasis |

**Table 10.7** Application of the SOCRATES system to different causes of the acute abdomen

| | Site | Onset | Character | Radiation | Associations (signs or symptoms) | Time course | Exacerbating factors/ Relieving factors | Severity |
|---|---|---|---|---|---|---|---|---|
| **Acute appendicitis** | Central abdomen, later: right iliac fossa | Gradual | Constant | No | Anorexia; Signs of sepsis | Typically a few hours, but can be subacute and diagnosis delayed | Movement, coughing, RIF palpation/Lying still | Moderate |
| **Acute diverticulitis** | Lower abdomen, usually LIF | Gradual | Constant | No | Signs of sepsis; Change in bowel habit; Mass in LIF | Hours to days | Movement, coughing, LIF palpation/Lying still | Moderate |
| **Perforated gut lumen** | Initially varies by organ, e.g. epigastric for perforated peptic ulcer, LIF for perforated sigmoid colon, then becoming generalized | Sudden | Constant | No | Signs of sepsis; Generalized peritonitis | Reaches maximal intensity quickly after onset | Movement, coughing, any abdominal palpation/Lying still | Severe |
| **Intestinal obstruction** | Central abdomen | Gradual | Colicky | No | Vomiting if high small bowel; Constipation if colonic; Not passing flatus | Comes and goes in waves | Eating/drinking | Severe |
| **Acute pancreatitis** | Upper abdomen, then generalized | Sudden | Constant | Back | Vomiting; Hypovolaemia (massive fluid loss into peritoneum); Signs of sepsis | Builds up over hours, may last days | Movement, coughing, epigastric palpation/Lying still | Severe |
| **Acute cholecystitis** | Right upper quadrant | Gradual | Constant | Between the scapulae | Murphy's sign; Vomiting; Jaundice; Signs of sepsis | Builds up over hours, may last days | Movement, coughing, RUQ palpation/Lying still | Moderate/ severe |
| **Acute salpingitis** | Lower abdomen | Gradual | Constant | Back, groin | Signs of sepsis; Vaginal discharge | Builds up over hours, may last days | Movement, coughing, lower abdominal or adnexal palpation/Lying still | Moderate |
| **Renal colic** | Unilateral flank | Sudden | Colicky | Ipsilateral groin/ lower abdomen | Nausea and vomiting; Haematuria | Typically settles after 4–12 hours | None | Severe |
| **Ruptured ectopic pregnancy** | Lower abdominal | Sudden | Variable, sharp dull cramping | Back/ shoulder | Missed period; Vaginal bleeding | Rapid onset of severe pain once ruptured | Abdominal/adnexal palpation | Severe |
| **Acute mesenteric ischaemia** | Depends on vascular territory affected | Gradual | Constant or cramping | No | Bloody diarrhoea; Bloating; Nausea and vomiting; Signs of sepsis | Typically progressively worse over hours/days | | Severe |
| **AAA/dissection** | Central abdomen (chest if dissecting thoracic aorta) | Sudden | Constant tearing/ ripping | Back (posterior thoracic if thoracic dissection) | Loss of arm pulses in thoracic dissection; Severe hypovolaemic shock in AAA rupture | Rapidly reaches maximal intensity. In dissection, intensity may vary over hours/days | None | Severe |

AAA, abdominal aortic aneurysm; LIF, left iliac fossa; RIF, right iliac fossa; RUQ, right upper quadrant.

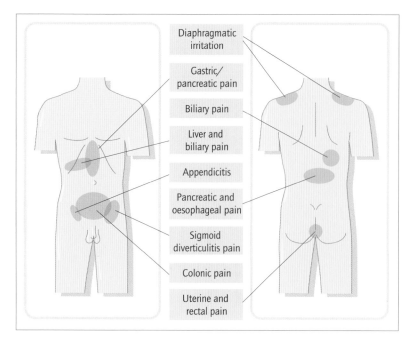

**Figure 10.20** Surface markings of radiation of pain from abdominal viscera.

## APPROACH TO COMMON GI SYMPTOMS

### DYSPHAGIA

- *Dysphagia* means difficulty in swallowing.
- *Odynophagia* means painful swallowing.
- Perception of the level of obstruction is often inaccurate.
- Dysphagia is a red flag symptom, highly predictive of oesophageal disease. Urgent investigation is required to exclude cancer.

#### Causes

See **Table 10.8**.

The main distinction is between:
- Mechanical (e.g. severe reflux oesophagitis, peptic stricture and malignancy)
- Dysmotility (e.g. oesophageal spasm or achalasia)

#### Approach to diagnosis

*Investigation*
- *Gastroscopy:* the first-line investigation unless a pharyngeal pouch suspected (where barium study undertaken first)
- *Manometry:* used to diagnose dysmotility

*Key aspects in the history*
- In malignant disease, symptoms progress over weeks to months: initially difficulty with solids, then softer food, liquids and finally saliva (absolute dysphagia).
- Intermittent dysphagia to solids, sometimes with long gaps between attacks, is typical of a benign stricture or eosinophilic oesophagitis (EO).

- In motility disorders, there may be trouble with liquids and solids form the outset, and regurgitation of liquids.
- Chronic heartburn suggests peptic stricture.
- If foreign body impaction is suspected, urgent endoscopy is indicated; if left untreated, it may erode through the oesophageal wall.

### HEARTBURN

- Heartburn is a burning retrosternal discomfort.
- When associated with regurgitation of gastric contents and relief with antacids, a diagnosis of GORD is extremely likely.

**Table 10.8** Causes of dysphagia (most common causes in capital letters)

| Type of disorder | Example(s) |
|---|---|
| Oral | Ulcers, stomatitis, neoplasm |
| Pharyngeal | Pharyngitis, pouch, neoplasm |
| Disorders causing extrinsic oesophageal compression | Lymphadenopathy (usually neoplastic), aortic aneurysm, neoplasms (usually bronchial carcinoma), left atrial enlargement |
| Mechanical oesophageal disorders | OESOPHAGITIS, PEPTIC STRICTURE, CARCINOMA, drug-induced injury (bisphosphonates, NSAIDs), foreign body impaction |
| Motility disorders of the oesophagus | Achalasia, oesophageal spasm |
| Stomach | CARCINOMA OF THE GASTRIC CARDIA |

**10**

## Approach to diagnosis

### Key aspects in the history

Symptoms are often worsened by:
- Increased intragastric pressure (stooping, lying down, straining, tight clothing, weight gain)
- Fatty food
- Smoking
- Alcohol
- Caffeine

## DYSPEPSIA

Dyspepsia is extremely common:
- It affects approximately 1 in 5 people in their lifetime.
- Most people do not consult their doctor.

Definitions of dyspepsia (or indigestion) are vague, referring to a range of upper GI symptoms including:
- Epigastric pain or burning
- Early satiety
- Post-prandial fullness
- Nausea
- Bloating

Dyspeptic symptoms:
- *Usually* associated with oesophageal, gastric, or duodenal disease
- May be triggered during or soon after eating and/or relieved by antacids or acid-suppressants – this pattern suggests a cause in the upper GI tract
- Can arise from the colon, biliary system, pancreas and small bowel: thus, differential is extensive (**Table 10.9**)

**Table 10.9** Causes of dyspepsia (most common causes in capital letters)

| Type of disorder | Example(s) |
|---|---|
| Oesophageal | OESOPHAGITIS, carcinoma, motility disorder |
| Gastric | ULCER, gastritis, motility disorder, carcinoma |
| Duodenal | ULCER, duodenitis |
| Gall bladder | Gallstones |
| Pancreas | Pancreatitis, carcinoma |
| Liver | Hepatitis, metastases |
| Intestine | IBS, ischaemia, transverse colon carcinoma |
| Lifestyle | Certain foods (e.g. fatty, spicy), alcohol, smoking, coffee |
| Metabolic | Hypercalcaemia |
| Psychogenic | Stress, depression, anxiety |
| Drugs | NSAIDs, corticosteroids, anticholinergics, antiparkinsonian drugs, antidepressants, antidiabetics, antibiotics, iron |
| Other | Functional* |

*No disease found to explain the symptoms.

## Causes

Causes are multifactorial:
- Mucosal damage (e.g. peptic ulcer, cancers)
- Mucosal inflammation (e.g. caused by HP infection, drugs, acid, bile)
- Disordered motility

However, in most cases, no organic cause is found during investigation. This is functional dyspepsia.

### Approach to diagnosis

#### Investigation

In the UK, NICE recommends urgent gastroscopy to exclude cancer if alarm features present:
- Dysphagia
- Aged >55 with weight loss and any of:
  - Upper abdominal pain
  - Reflux
  - Dyspepsia

Urgent clinic review is recommended for any upper abdominal mass suspicious for gastric cancer.

Other symptoms that may suggest upper GI cancer and usually warrant endoscopy, particularly in those over 55, include:
- Overt GI bleeding (haematemesis or melaena)
- Persistent vomiting
- Unintentional weight loss
- IDA

If there are no alarm features, it is reasonable to test for and treat HP infection and/or give a course of acid suppressant therapy, with gastroscopy reserved for patients unresponsive to empirical treatment.

Intermittent attacks of pain lasting a few hours and radiating to the back suggest biliary colic and abdominal ultrasound is required.

## CHRONIC ABDOMINAL PAIN

- A frequent presentation in hospital GI clinics
- Often difficult to diagnose; no organic illness found in a high proportion
- Differential diagnosis wide; overlaps with the causes of acute abdominal pain (see **Tables 10.5** and **10.6**), as some acute conditions (e.g. diverticulitis, pancreatitis) also have chronic or relapsing/remitting forms
- Site and nature of pain often give less diagnostic information than in the acute setting.
- Diagnostic clues (as to organ system/cause to consider) include:
  - onset during or soon after meals: gastric, biliary
  - response to antacids or acid-suppressant medication: oesophageal, gastric, duodenal disease
  - right upper quadrant pain lasting several hours with long symptom-free periods: biliary colic

o altered defaecation pattern or relief of pain with defaecation: IBS, colonic
o continuous pain, night waking, weight loss, anaemia, raised inflammatory markers: suggest serious organic disease

## NAUSEA AND VOMITING

### Causes

There is a wide range of causes: commonest are upper GI infectons/inflammation and drug side effects. Patients with persistent symptoms usually require gastroscopy.

### Approach to diagnosis

1 Whatever the cause – always assess for consequences, especially dehydration.
2 Ensure the patient is describing true vomiting, not regurgitation.
3 Many diagnoses may be suggested by basic clinical/laboratory assessment.
- *Medication:* including over-the-counter/recreational (especially cannabinoids)/herbal medicines; common causal prescription drugs are NSAIDs, aspirin, erythromycin, opiates, digoxin and cytotoxics
- *Gastroenteritis:* sudden onset, short-lived; ask about contacts; often associated diarrhoea
- *Upper GI tract inflammatory conditions* (e.g. pepetic ulcer): blood in vomit; relief by antacids/acid suppressants
- *Other inflammatory GI conditons* (e.g. pancreatits, appendicitis, cholecystitis): typical history (see **Table 10.7**); toxic patient; localizing tenderness; peritonism or raised amylase/CRP. Note at extremes of age, infections are more likley to present with non-localizing symptoms such as nausea/vomiting
- *Vesibular causes:* suggested if movement aggravates symptoms or if there is vertigo, deafness or tinnitus
- *Excess alcohol:* history; abnormal GGT/LFTs
- *Pregnancy:* menstrual history; pregnancy test
- *Myocardial ischaemia:* consider ECG in at-risk patients; ocasionally presents with epigastic pain ± nausea and no chest pain symptoms
- *CNS causes/raised intracranial pressure:* symptoms worse early morning; localizing CNS symptoms; past medical history of congenital or acquired neurological disorder; papilloedema (CT head required if suspected)
- *Cyclical vomiting syndrome:* history of severe and stereotypical attacks, with periods of normality in between
- *Mechanical or functional gastric outlet obstruction (gastroparesis):* large volume or projectile vomiting;

faeculant vomiting; signs of obstruction on imaging
- *Radiotherapy-induced:* any recent course raises possibility
- *Diabetic ketoacidosis, hypercalcaemia:* associated thirst and polyuria; urinalysis; basic biochemistry
- *Hyperthyroidism:* history and biochemistry
- *Uraemia:* known kidney disease; new hypertension; positive urinalysis; biochemistry
- *Hypoadrenalism:* hypotension; hyperkalaemia; skin pigmentation; low random cortisol
- *Migraine without headache:* rare and can be difficult to diagnose, one-third have prodromal aura; almost always cyclical attacks
4 If the above approach does not give a diagnosis, most patients require endoscopy, which will diagnose inflammatory disorders and proximal mechanical obstructive lesions, and can suggest other causes of gut obstruction if large volume gastric residue found.
5 If organic causes have been ruled out by 1–4, possible explanations are:
- *Gastroparesis* (abnormal gastric emptying due to neuromuscular pathology, one cause being diabetic autonomic neuropathy): Barium meal and follow-through will often demonstrate abnormal gastric emptying. Some centres offer specialized gastric emptying studies.
- *Mechanical obstruction of proximal small bowel* (beyond reach of gastroscopy): Barium meal and follow-through and abdominal CT are often diagnostic.
- *Psychological/psychiatric disease* (e.g. anorexia nervosa (AN)/bulimia, severe anxiety): Diagnosis is made on typical history and exclusion of organic causes.
- *Functional causes:* This is when the cause is unknown, but the key problem is disordered upper GI motility. Cyclical vomiting syndrome gives characteristic story (see 4 above), but otherwise diagnosis is by a process of elimination.

## ANOREXIA

Anorexia is diminution or loss of appetite. Lay people often wrongly consider it to be synonymous with AN: using plain English avoids communication difficulties.

### Causes

Common causes of anorexia and unexplained weight loss:
- *Chronic lung disease:* e.g. COPD
- *Upper GI pathology:* gastritis and all causes of dyspepsia (see **Table 10.9**).
- *Psychiatric:* stess, anxiety depression, AN
- *Neoplastic:* carcinoma of the stomach or oesophagus, metastatic cancer

- *Iatrogenic:* drugs, radiotherapy
- *Metabolic:* uraemia, hypercalcaemia, hypopituitarism
- *Infective:* many infections including viral hepatitis, TB
- *Lifestyle:* excess alcohol, smoking

### Approach to diagnosis

This will alter with age. Around 90% of eating disorders such as AN start between puberty and age 20 (with 90% cases female). They are usually diagnosable from the history. In older patients, malignancy, metabolic disease, and the side effects of drugs or alcohol are the key concerns. Anorexia can be a normal part of ageing. In dementia, a preference for sweet over savoury food may result in apparent anorexia until menus are altered.

### Key aspects in the history

- Associated weight loss, nausea or vomiting
- Drugs (including over-the-counter [OTC] and recreational)
- Past history of malignancy
- Smoking and alcohol use
- Stress
- Symptoms of infection elsewhere (especially at extremes of age where non-specific symptoms such as anorexia may be caused by urinary, chest and other infections)

### Examination

This is rarely helpful but, if localizing abdominal signs are found, a gastroscopy or abdominal ultrasound is usually ordered early.

### Investigation

First-line investigations:
- FBC (e.g. for blood loss, upper GI cancers)
- Renal function
- Calcium
- Thyroid function tests (TFT)
- LFT
- CRP
- HP stool antigen

If this initial assessment is negative and anorexia persists, gastroscopy and ultrasound are the usual next steps. If, however, if there is associated and progressive weight loss, consider CT chest, abdomen and pelvis in place of ultrasound.

## BLOATING/DISTENSION

- *Bloating* is the uncomfortable sensation of abdominal swelling.
- *Distension* is an actual increase in abdominal girth.

### Causes

The five 'F's mnemonic remains useful for possible causes of bloating/distension:
**F**at  **F**luid  **F**aeces  **F**latus  **F**oetus

### Approach to diagnosis

- A key concern of the patient is often of malignancy, in particular ovarian.
- If the abdomen swells up each day, becoming flat again in the morning, a functional disease is likely.
- Persistent distension suggests organic disease.

### Examination

Examination should determine if there is free fluid (urgent abdominal/pelvic ultrasound is the next step) or gas, where functional disease is common, but subacute bowel obstruction needs excluding.

### Investigation

- A negative CA125 is reassuring with regards to ovarian malignancy.
- CT abdomen/pelvis is the next test if an organic cause is suspected.
- A dietary trial of withdrawal of lactose, other disaccharides (fruit products), wheat and high-fibre foods can quickly confirm food intolerance as the cause.

## DIARRHOEA, STEATORRHOEA AND MALABSORPTION

### Diarrhoea

Diarrhoea is defined as passage of three or more loose stools a day, or more frequent and looser stool than usual.

- *Acute diarrhoea* is usually infective and self-limiting; cultures may be negative and are not routinely required. Any drug recently started must be suspect. A small percentage of patients will develop post-infective IBS.
- *Chronic diarrhoea* is defined as over 4 weeks of three or more stools a day with stool weight >200 g. People who pass frequent small hard pellets do not have diarrhoea.
- *Osmotic diarrhoea* is when the increased fluid is retained, caused by unabsorbed osmotically active molecules (e.g. lactose in lactase deficiency).

### Steatorrhoea

Steatorrhoea occurs when the pathology causing diarrhoea also causes small bowel fat malabsorption. Steatorrhoea stools *may be* pale, offensive smelling and difficult to flush, but in practice the nature of the stool is an unreliable guide. Significant fat malabsorption is usually accompanied by weight loss in addition to diarrhoea.

Causes include coeliac, small bowel Crohn's disease, pancreatic insufficiency, bile salt malabsorption and SIBO.

### Malabsorption

Malabsorption is defective absorption of one or multiple nutrients and *may* occur without associated diarrhoea or steatorrhoea (e.g. malabsorption of iron levels and resulting anaemia may be the only clinical sign of CD).

## Causes

Causes of diarrhoea/steatorrhoea are shown in **Table 10.10**.

## Approach to diagnosis

The common diagnostic challenges are excluding IBD and CD in younger patients, and colonic malignancy in older patients (**Table 10.11**).

**Table 10.10** Causes of chronic diarrhoea (those likely to include fat malabsorption/steatorrhoea are underlined)

**Common**

IBS

Bile salt malabsorption

Diet/intolerances

- Lactose
- Wheat/FODMAPs
- Artificial sweeteners
- Caffeine
- Alcohol

Carcinoma of the colon

Ulcerative colitis

Crohn's disease (steatorrhoea can develop if extensive small bowel involvement ± fistulae ± strictures)

Microscopic colitis

CD, tropical sprue, giardiasis, intestinal lymphangiectasia

Drugs (antibiotics (especially erythromycin) NSAIDs, magnesium containing antacids, metformin, gliptins, statins, cholestyramine, orlistat)

Anxiety

Severe constipation with overflow

**Rare**

SIBO

Chronic pancreatitis

Obstruction of bile or pancreatic duct (e.g. by tumour)

Pancreatectomy

Radiation enteropathy

Jejunal diverticulosis

Chronic bacterial/protozoal infections, giardiasis, parasitic/ fungal infections

Immunodeficiency syndromes (including HIV)

Lymphoma

Post bowel surgery (vagotomy, gastrectomy, blind loops, intestinal resection)

Thyrotoxicosis

Diabetic autonomic neuropathy

Cystic fibrosis

**Very rare**

Small bowel disease (Whipple's disease, tropical sprue, amyloid)

Endocrine tumours (VIPoma, gastrinoma carcinoid)

Addison's disease

Laxative abuse

**Table 10.11** Lower GI tract red flags for suspected colorectal cancer

>40 years with unexplained weight loss and abdominal pain

>50 years with unexplained rectal bleeding – all cases

<50 years with unexplained rectal bleeding if, in addition, patient has:

- Abdominal pain
- Change in bowel habit
- Weight loss
- IDA

>60 years and over with:

- IDA
- Change in bowel habit
- Occult blood in faeces

Rectal or abdominal mass

### Red flags

Red flag symptoms (require urgent referral – **Table 10.11**)

### Key aspects in the history

- Recent drug changes
- Family history (FH) of CD
- RIF pain and weight loss suggesting Crohn's disease
- Stool culture-negative bloody diarrhoea suggesting colorectal cancer
- In the absence of red flag features, patients over 60 with new diarrhoea warrant urgent referral to consider colonoscopy
- Diarrhoea alternating with constipation suggests IBS

### Investigation

In the UK it is recommended that, where there is suspicion for colorectal cancer but the above red flag criteria are not met, faecal occult blood testing is undertaken using an immunohistochemical assay (FIT test). Example patients include those *under* 60 years old with IDA or change in bowel habit or with a non-iron deficiency pattern anaemia but over 60.

The faecal calprotectin test has reduced the need for invasive procedures (in particular colonoscopy) where suspicion of organic disease is low, as a negative test has a >95% negative predicative value for IBD. The faecal elastase test is a quick non-invasive screen for pancreatic exocrine insufficiency. Coeliac serology has around a 98% negative predictive value.

Recent studies suggest around a third of patients labelled as diarrhoea-predominant IBS have bile salt malabsorption as the sole or contributory cause of their diarrhoea, and there should be a low threshold for diagnostic bile salt retention testing.

A suggested sequence for investigation of chronic diarrhoea is shown in **Figure 10.21**.

## WEIGHT LOSS

### Causes

Causes are shown in **Table 10.12**. Organic disease is found in around a third of cases.

**10**

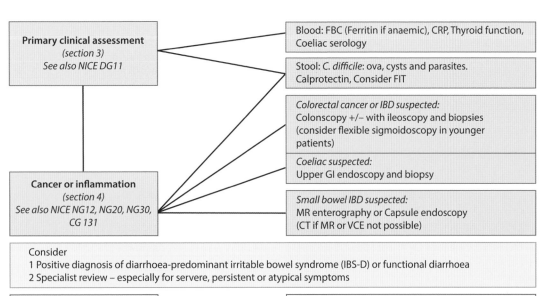

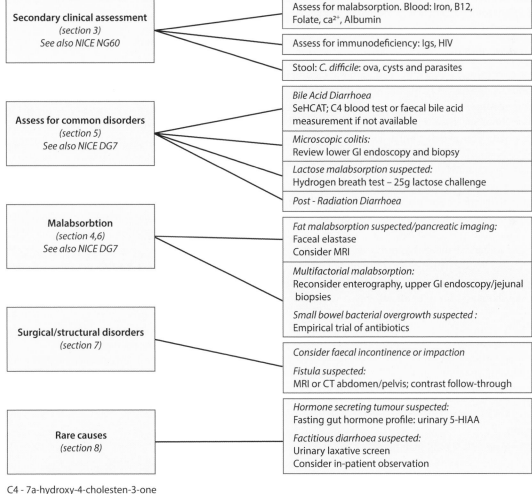

C4 - 7a-hydroxy-4-cholesten-3-one
HIV – Human immunodeficiency virus
Igs – Immunoglobulins
FIT – Faecal immunochemical test for haemoglobin
SeHCAT - selenium[75] homotaurocholate
VCE – Video capsule endoscopy
5-HIAA – Hydroxyindole acetic acid

**Figure 10.21** Example of algorithm for investigation of chronic diarrhoea.

**Table 10.12** Causes of unexplained weight loss

Cardiopulmonary (e.g. COPD, heart failure)

GI cancers (around half of all cancer causes)

All other cancer sites (e.g. lung, lymphoma, prostate, ovarian, bladder)

Non-malignant GI disease (e.g. dysphagia, CD, IBD, peptic ulcer, mesenteric ischaemia)

Depression/anxiety/stress

Medication side effects

Age-related issues (e.g. dementia, loss of smell/taste, poor dentition)

Endocrine disease (e.g. Addison's disease, diabetes, thyroid disease)

Infective disorders (HIV/AIDS, TB, subacute bacterial endocarditis [SBE])

Substance abuse (e.g. alcohol, cocaine)

Renal disease

Neurological (e.g. Parkinson's disease)

Systemic inflammatory disorders (e.g. rheumatoid arthritis)

## Approach to diagnosis

- Assess calorie intake. Appetite reduction is a common response to stress/anxiety (including health anxiety).
- Consider eating disorders in younger patients.
- Cardiopulmonary disease is a very common cause.
- In the elderly, consider dementia, social isolation, low mood, loss of taste and poor dentition.
- Localizing symptoms such as anorexia, dysphagia, dyspepsia, nausea, vomiting, abdominal pain and abdominal distension are investigated as above. Weight loss with diarrhoea suggests small bowel disease with fat malabsorption, and needs investigations as described under diarrhoea/steatorrhoea.
- SBE, thyrotoxicosis, diabetes and mesenteric ischaemia are non-malignant causes to consider.
- Consider dietetic referral for all patients.

## Examination

Examination may reveal relevant signs related to the cause of weight loss, such as organomegaly, abdominal mass or lymphadenopathy, or of the consequences of undernutrition such as anaemia, chelitis, poor skin/nail/gum condition, muscle mass loss, proximal weakness.

## Investigation

- *Baseline blood tests* should include FBC, U&E, LFTs, CRP, glucose and thyroid function.
- If there are no clues to the cause of the weight loss after the above considerations, further investigations are reasonable as a small percentage of patients with this presentation have an underlying malignancy. A first-line strategy should include *chest X-ray, gastroscopy with duodenal biopsy and abdominal ultrasound.*
- Thereafter, a 3-month *watch and wait period with dietetics support* is usually preferable to blind investigations.

- If weight loss continues with no localizing signs or symptoms developing, consider *CT of chest abdomen and pelvis.*
- Rarely, when no cause is found, patients with a low BMI are admitted for a trial of *nasogastric feeding* (with safeguards for refeeding syndrome) to avoid complications of malnutrition and as a weight gain response to provide reassurance that organic disease has not been missed.

# CONSTIPATION

Constipation is defined as infrequent stools (less than three per week) *or* difficult defaecation (hard stools, straining, feelings of obstruction or incomplete evacuation).

- It is extremely common.
- Colon cancer is the main concern in older patients.

## Causes

Causes are listed in **Table 10.13**.

## Approach to diagnosis

### Red flags

Current UK NICE guidance (see **Table 10.11**) does not discriminate between a change in bowel habit to constipation versus to diarrhoea. It recommends urgent referral of any patient with a change in bowel habit if over 60, and for younger patients with associated rectal bleeding, most of whom will undergo colonoscopy within 2 weeks.

### Key aspects in the history

If red flags are excluded, the history may suggest a cause.

- *Onset in early childhood:* Hirschsprung's disease or slow-transit constipation (diagnosis may be delayed to adulthood)
- *Traumatic labour* (e.g. forceps delivery causing damage to anorectal neuromusculature)
- *Congenital or aquired spinal cord injury*
- *Chronic neurological disease* (e.g. motor neurone disease, Parkinson's disease, MS)
- *Anal pain:* local anorectal cause
- *Alternating diarrhoea and constipation:* IBS or faecal impaction
- *Weight gain:* hypothyroidism
- *Low dietary fibre intake or certain drug treatments:* may be causal

### Examination

This is rarely helpful but signs of hypothyroidism may be found. Abdominal and rectal examination may suggest a cause.

### Investigation

- *Blood tests:* FBC (for anaemia), calcium and thyroid function
- *Colonoscopy:* for most patients over 40 to exclude organic causes.

If the history and investigations do not find a diagnosis, a diagnosis of IBS-constipation or slow-transit constipation is likely.

**Table 10.13** Causes of constipation (most common causes in capitals)

| Type of disorder | Examples |
|---|---|
| Large bowel organic disease | COLONIC OR RECTAL CARCINOMA, DIVERTICULOSIS, benign strictures (Crohn's, diverticular disease) |
| Perianal disease – causing obstruction or pain | Haemorrhoids, fissures, abscess, fistula, rectocoele |
| Abnormal motility | IBS, pseudo-obstruction, severe idiopathic constipation (also known as slow transit constipation) |
| Dietary | LOW-FIBRE DIET, WEIGHT-REDUCING DIETS, FASTING |
| Drugs | OPIATES, iron, anticholinergics, antidepressants |
| Lifestyle | Unaesthetic lavatory, too busy, inactivity, dehydration |
| Neurological disorders | Autonomic neuropathy, spinal cord disease, Parkinson's disease, multiple sclerosis, stroke, DEMENTIA |
| Metabolic disorders | Hypercalcaemia, hypothyroidism |
| Other | Pregnancy, old age |
| Psychiatric disease | DEPRESSION, AN |
| Pelvic floor muscle disorders | Anismus (inability of muscles to relax), dyssynergia (uncoordinated muscle movements), muscular weakness (e.g. after childbirth-related injuries to pelvic muscles/nerves) |
| Congenital | Hirschsprung's disease |

**10**

Occasionally, further tests are undertaken which include measuring bowel transit time using radio-opaque markers and assessing abnormal physiology of the anorectum/distal colon using manometry and/or defaecating proctography.

#### Complications
These include haemorrhoids, anal fissures and, rarely, stercoral perforation (in the elderly).

## IRON-DEFICIENCY ANAEMIA

IDA may be the presenting feature of malignant and benign GI disease. Daily blood loss into the gut lumen may not be evident clinically but, if it exceeds the body's ability to replace iron stores, it will cause IDA.

### Approach to diagnosis
#### Red flags
Urgent referral for suspected GI cancer is recommended for any patient >50 with isolated IDA.

#### Key aspects in the history
- Is there adequate iron in the diet? (Ask about vegetarian/vegan diet.)
- Can the iron be absorbed? (Consider FH of CD; symptoms of diffuse small bowel disease – weight loss, diarrhoea, steatorrhoea.)
- Are periods/pregnancy the likely cause of blood loss or excess iron stores use, respectively?
- Are there symptoms related to the source of blood (e.g. dyspepsia for peptic ulcer and diarrhoea for colorectal cancer)? Ask about anticoagulants and antiplatelet use.

#### Examination
- *Perioral telangiectasia* will suggest hereditary haemorrhagic telangiectasia (rare)

- *Oral ulceration* is occasionally seen in Crohn's disease and CD.
- *Abdominal and rectal examination* signs may suggest malignancy.
- *Aortic stenosis* is relevant as it is associated with bleeding from gut mucosal angiodysplasias (Heyde's syndrome).

#### Investigation
If red flags are excluded, UK guidance (updated 2021 guidelines) recommends:
- *Confirm with iron studies*
- *Urinanalysis for microscopic haematuria*
- *Coeliac serology*
- *Gastroscopy with duodenal biopsy:* for women <50 years still having periods
- *Colonoscopy and gastroscopy with duodenal biopsy:* for all postmenopausal women, women with severe anaemia (e.g. requiring blood or iron infusions), and any man with isolated IDA
- *Colonoscopy:* even if duodenal biopsy identifies CD, in patients >50 years

If advanced gastric cancer is found after OGD, it is reasonable not to proceed to colonoscopy (although many centres book patients in for both procedures at the same time rather than sequentially).

If gastroscopy, duodenal biopsy and colonoscopy are normal, it is reasonable not to investigate further unless:
- Anaemia becomes symptomatic despite oral iron supplements, requiring iron infusions or blood transfusions
- Features are suggestive of small bowel disease (abdominal pain, weight loss, diarrhoea, steatorrhoea)

A typical strategy would then be:

1 MRI or barium study to exclude small bowel stricturing
2 Capsule endoscopy.

If a localized small bowel source of GI bleeding is found, therapeutic balloon enteroscopy offers a minimally invasive way of treatment.

## MANAGEMENT OF COMMON GI SYMPTOMS

### GENERAL

All patients need detailed explanation and appropriate reassurance about their condition. This is particularly important when their problem:

- *Is chronic:* CD, IBD
- *Is potentially fatal:* cancer
- *Is complex to treat:* eradication of HP, IBD
- *Involves a major psychological component:* IBS

Such information may not only help patients cope with their disorder, but also alleviate symptoms, as in IBS.

Information to patients often needs to contain specific advice about changes in lifestyle (e.g. stopping smoking and avoidance of NSAIDs in peptic ulcer and IBD, postural measures in reflux oesophagitis).

For certain diseases, information leaflets and patient support groups (e.g. Coeliac Society, National Association for Colitis and Crohn's Disease) provide invaluable support.

### DIETARY TREATMENT

Wherever possible, nutritional support should centre on encouragement to eat the correct amount and range of normal foods, with oral supplements as necessary. Malnutrition is common in hospitalized patients and delays recovery from most illnesses and surgery. Sometimes patients are too unwell/anorexic to take in sufficient food, in which case enteral or parenteral feeding may be used.

- *Supportive dietary treatment* is very often helpful in gastroenterology:
  o High-fibre diet for constipation
  o Low-residue diet for small bowel stricturing
  o Low wheat/fibre or FODMAP* diet in IBS, particularly with bloating
  o Protein supplements for malnourished patients
- *Primary therapeutic dietary treatment* examples include:
  o Gluten-free in CD
  o Elemental/oligopeptide formulations for Crohn's disease in children

### ARTIFICIAL/INVASIVE NUTRITIONAL SUPPORT

#### Choice of route

Enteral should always be used in preference to parenteral nutrition if intestinal function is not severely impaired. This is because it is safer, simpler and cheaper.

#### Choice of technique

Nasogastric tubes (**Figure 10.22**) are suitable for short-term enteral feeding. If there is an obstructing lesion of the oesophagus or stomach, the fine-bore tube can often still be passed using guide wire techniques.

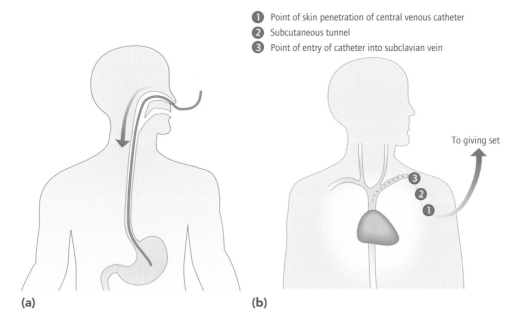

1 Point of skin penetration of central venous catheter
2 Subcutaneous tunnel
3 Point of entry of catheter into subclavian vein

To giving set

(a)          (b)

**Figure 10.22 (a)** Inserting an enteral feeding tube. A lubricated fine-bore tube stiffened by a guide wire is inserted through the nostril and passed gently down the oesophagus to the stomach; the guide wire is then removed. Its position in the stomach is confirmed if aspirate has a pH <5. If aspirate cannot be obtained, the position must be checked radiologically before commencing feeding.
**(b)** Inserting a central venous feeding line. The silastic feeding catheter is aseptically introduced via the subclavian vein into the SVC. Its proximal end is brought out through a subcutaneous tunnel to reduce the risk of infection.

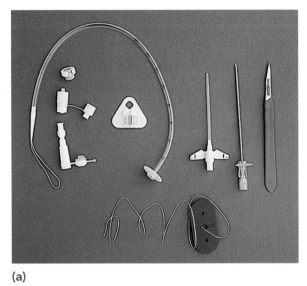

**(a)**

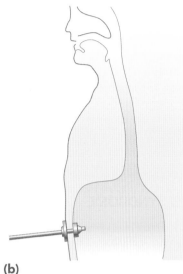

**(b)**

**Figure 10.23** PEG. **(a)** A kit for placement of a PEG tube. A cannula (right of figure) is introduced into the stomach – the site of puncture of the abdomen being guided by the prepositioned gastroscope. A nylon or metallic 'string' (bottom of picture) is passed through the cannula, grasped by a snare passed down the biopsy channel of the gastroscope, and pulled up out of the patient's mouth. The string is then attached to a loop on the end of the PEG tube (left of figure) and the tube pulled back down the oesophagus and out through the abdominal wall. A hard taper helps the leading end of the tube pass through the abdominal wall while a circular buffer stops the back end of the tube when it reaches the stomach wall. Once pulled through, the tapered end of the tube is cut off, and a valve attached to allow delivery of enteral feed. **(b)** Diagram showing the final position of a PEG tube.

If long-term (>2 weeks) enteral feeding is required, or where there is risk of aspiration (e.g. after a stroke), it is often preferable to insert a percutaneous endoscopic gastrostomy (PEG) (**Figure 10.23**). Very occasionally, the feeding tube is placed in the jejunum. A radiological technique may be required for gastrostomy (e.g. if the oesophagus is obstructed by a tumour).

### Choice and timing of enteral feed

There is a wide variety of nutritionally complete proprietary preparations (e.g. Fresubin, Ensure), referred to as *polymeric feeds* as whole protein is used. *Peptide feeds* contain the protein source as polypeptides, and *elemental feeds* deliver protein as free amino acids.

Enteral feeds can be administered continuously. Feeding only during the day reduces the risk of aspiration, but overnight regimens are more practical for ambulant patients.

Small amounts of ordinary food and drink can often be taken to add to quality of life. Progress should be monitored with a fluid balance chart and twice weekly measurements of weight, urea, electrolytes, glucose and albumin.

### Complications of enteral feeding

- *Diarrhoea:* e.g. due to the feed's hyperosmolarity, infected feed, or lactose intolerance (low osmolality or fibre-enriched feeds and slower infusion rates may help)
- *Pulmonary aspiration:* due to displaced tubes or regurgitation of rapidly administered feed
- *Inflammation of nose or oesophagus*
- *Metabolic problems:* fluid overload or depletion; glucose and electrolyte disturbances

## PARENTERAL NUTRITION

Because of its complexity, potential hazards and expense, patients requiring parenteral (or IV) nutrition should be managed by a specialist nutrition team.

### Indications

This is used when GI function is so severely impaired that enterally administered nutrients maintain or replace requirements. Examples include:
- Prolonged ileus or obstruction
- Massive intestinal resection
- Proximal enterocutaneous fistula
- Severe IBD
- Intra-abdominal sepsis and pancreatitis
- Perforated oesophagus

### Technique

IV nutrient solutions are irritant and usually given slowly into a large central vein. Tunnelled central lines (see **Figure 10.22**) or peripherally inserted central catheter (PICC) lines are placed aseptically in theatre and only used for feeds. Occasionally, peripheral veins can be used for short-term feeding, in which case a less hypertonic feed is used, and the drip site rotated every 24–48 hours to prevent irreversible venous damage.

### Complications of parenteral feeding

- *Local trauma:* pneumothorax, haemothorax, subclavian artery puncture or brachial plexus damage caused by catheter insertion

- *Air embolism*
- *Infusion of fluid* into the mediastinum or pleural cavity
- *Venous thrombosis*
- *Infection*
- *Metabolic problems:* hyperglycaemia; reactive hypoglycaemia; hypophosphataemia or refeeding syndrome; electrolyte or acid–base imbalance; deficiencies of trace elements, essential fatty acids, folate and vitamins; lipaemia; and jaundice
- *The most serious and frequent complication is line infection – and feeding often has to be discontinued as a result.*

## REFEEDING SYNDROME

In malnourished patients, providing increased calories without appropriate vitamins and trace elements can precipitate deficiency syndromes (e.g. of potassium, magnesium and phosphate). Refeeding syndrome is potentially fatal and prevented by a slow reintroduction of balanced nutrition and daily monitoring and replacement of micronutrients. Most secondary care Trusts will have an emergency refeeding policy to prevent harm; examples are also widely available online.

## GUT MICROBIOME

There are many trillions of bacteria in the healthy human gut, most in the colon.

Causal links have been proposed between an alteration in these bacteria (the gut microbiome) and many GI and non-GI conditions, including IBS, IBD, obesity, fatty liver, colon cancer, poor memory and HD.

A vast supplement industry has developed for probiotics (live bacteria) and pre-biotics (inert products encouraging 'good' bacterial growth) with the aim of restoring healthy gut bacteria.

Whether any of these proposed links to disease will translate into useful treatment for individuals is not yet clear.

Many patients with functional bowel disease such as IBS report improvements in symptoms such as bloating after short courses of probiotics. A placebo effect cannot be excluded; current costs are £70–80 a month.

Encouraging dietary changes (e.g. more volume and more variety of fruit and vegetable intake, reduced refined carbohydrate snacking) is a cheaper way of positively altering the colonic microbiome,

## DRUG MANAGEMENT

### Drugs for treating nausea and vomiting

All of these act on the vomiting centre/chemoreceptor trigger zone, located in the floor of the fourth ventricle. Metoclopramide and domperidone have additional prokinetic effects, stimulating gastric emptying.

If the cause of the nausea or vomiting is known, it can guide drug choice (**Table 10.14**).

Once dose and absorption of the initial choice are optimized (which may require IV/IM/sublingual/suppository routes if vomiting), it is logical to add a drug of a different class, avoiding interactions as indicated in **Table 10.14**.

### Drugs to suppress gastric acid production

Common indications are GORD and dyspepsia. Drugs to inhibit gastric acid secretion are listed in **Table 10.15**. Dosing strategies are discussed under specific conditions. PPIs are more potent than H2 receptor antagonists (H2RAs). PPIs are now available as generics and are a cost-effective first-line choice. PPIs significantly outperform H2RAs for reflux oesophagitis treatment and for prophylaxis and treatment of NSAID-induced upper GI injury.

Although by no means certain, recent data widely published in lay press have raised concerns over the long-term safety of PPIs (e.g. osteoporosis, increased risk of some GI cancers) and of H2RA formulations (possible carcinogen). Where there is risk of serious acid-related injury (e.g GORD, Barrett's oesophagus, complicated peptic ulcer), the benefits almost certainly outweigh these possible harms. For other conditions, it is good practice to use the lowest dose and duration of acid-suppressing drugs.

If possible, avoid PPIs prior to endoscopy as they may mask pathology and cause false negatives on HP tests.

Due to variable inhibition of the cytochrome enzyme systems, all PPIs could in theory increase plasma levels of some drugs (e.g. anticoagulants; antiepileptics) and reduce active metabolites of others (e.g. clopidogrel): however, PPI/antiplatelet interactions are unlikely to be clinically relevant.

### *H. pylori* eradication

Eradication of HP infection is indicated in peptic ulcer, dyspepsia and MALToma (a gastric lymphoma subtype).

Treating asymptomatic infected patients to prevent future peptic ulcer or gastric cancer is controversial, and not carried out routinely.

Resistant strains may be selected out by previous antibiotic use, so selecting a regimen where the patient is naive to all antibiotic components is ideal. Some hospitals produce guidance based on known local resistance patterns and/or sensitivity testing (requires gastric biopsies).

- *Example of first-line regimen* (1 week duration):
  Amoxicillin 1 g BD + clarithromycin 500 mg BD + omeprazole 20–40 mg BD
  Or where penicillin allergy:
  Metronidazole 500 mg TDS + clarithromycin 500 mg BD + omeprazole 20–40 mg BD
- *Second-line regimens* include first-line protocols but with metronidazole swapped from clarithromycin, or:
  Amoxicillin 1 g BD + omeprazole 20 mg BD + tetracycline 500 mg QDS or levofloxacin 500 mg BD
- There are *third-line protocols*, but these vary by unit and with local resistance patterns so are best discussed with local secondary care experts.

**Table 10.14** Drugs used in nausea and vomiting

| Drug class | Prokinetics | Antihistamines | Anticholinergics | Antipsychotics | 5-HT3 antagonists |
|---|---|---|---|---|---|
| Examples | Metoclopramide Domperidone | Cyclizine | Hyoscine | Phenothiazines (e.g. prochlorperazine) Butyrophenones (e.g. haloperidol) | Ondansetron |
| Pharmacological action | Central and peripheral dopamine (D2) antagonist | Centrally acting antihistamine | Central and peripheral anticholinergic actions | Predominantly centrally acting dopamine (D2) receptor antagonist, but also effects on wide range of other receptors (e.g. α serotonin, muscarinic, histamine) | Centrally acting 5-HT3 receptor antagonist |
| Side effects | Extrapyramidal (in young people – treated with IV antimuscarinics, e.g. benzatropine), hyperprolactinaemia | Drowsiness, dry mouth, blurred vision | Dry mouth, blurred vision, constipation, urine retention, confusion in elderly | Drowsiness, postural hypotension, dry mouth, extrapyramidal | Constipation, headache, flushing |
| Contraindications/cautions/interactions | Avoid chronic administration (risk of arrhythmias) Avoid combining with other drugs with anticholinergic (muscarinic) effects such as hyoscine and cyclizine which antagonize the therapeutic effect Avoid in Parkinson's disease and mechanical gut obstruction Avoid combining with 5HT3 antagonists (arrhythmias) | Glaucoma, prostatism | Glaucoma, prostatism | Extrapyramidal effects (e.g. parkinsonism), glaucoma, prostatism | Avoid combining with dopamine agonists (arrhythmias) Lactation and special care with pregnancy |
| Uses/comments | Especially useful where there is gastric stasis. Also useful in heartburn and IBS | Vestibular disease; motion sickness; bowel obstruction/compression Pregnancy (first-line) Radiotherapy; intracranial disease | Vestibular disease or post anaesthesia | Vestibular disease Post anaesthesia, chemotherapy and other drug-induced Pregnancy (first-line) Radiotherapy Metabolic causes | Prophylaxis and treatment of post anaesthesia, chemotherapy and radiotherapy Pregnancy (second-line) |

**Table 10.15** Inhibitors of gastric acid secretion

| Class | H2-receptor antagonists | Proton pump inhibitors |
|---|---|---|
| **Examples** | Cimetidine | Omeprazole |
| | Ranitidine | Esomeprazole* |
| | | Lansoprazole |
| | | Pantoprazole |
| | | Rabeprazole |
| **Pharmacological action** | H2 receptor blockade | Inhibit hydrogen/potassium exchange pump ('proton pump') |
| **Main indications** | Non-ulcer dyspepsia | Non-ulcer dyspepsia |
| | Reflux oesophagitis | Reflux oesophagitis |
| | Peptic ulcer healing | Peptic ulcer healing |
| | Peptic ulcer prophylaxis | Peptic ulcer prophylaxis |
| | Prophylaxis against bleeding in intensive care | Prophylaxis against bleeding in intensive care |
| | | Zollinger–Ellison syndrome |
| | | Treatment/prophylaxis of NSAID-induced gastroduodenal injury |
| | | Component of many HP eradication regimens |
| **Side effects** | Headache | Diarrhoea |
| | Confusion in the elderly | Nausea |
| | Gynaecomastia (cimetidine only) | Headaches |
| | Drug interactions | Rashes |
| | Loss of libido | Blurred vision |
| | Raised serum creatinine | Drug interactions |

*A preparation of omeprazole s-isomer, with the inactive r-isomer removed.

### Drugs for treating diarrhoea

Most diarrhoea is self-limiting and medication is best avoided (other than for rehydration and electrolyte/glucose replacement). Treatment with antidiarrhoeal drugs is indicated while awaiting diagnosis and definitive treatment of more persistent diarrhoea. The main contraindication is acute severe colitis (may precipitate toxic megacolon). Most antidiarrhoeals are opioid drugs. Loperamide is widely used as a first-line agent and rarely causes CNS side effects. Co-phenotrope combines an opiate and an anticholinergic. More potent opiates such as codeine or even slow-release morphine preparations are occasionally required.

The only other class of drugs commonly used for chronic diarrhoea are bile salt chelaters.

### Drugs for treating constipation

First exclude faecal impaction by rectal examination. If present, use suppositories (e.g. glycerol) and/or enemas (e.g. Microlax). Provide lifestyle advice for increased dietary fibre (or prescribe bulking agents such as ispaghula) and for adequate fluid intake. Bulking agents are contraindicated in mechanical bowel obstruction.

- *Faecal softeners* (e.g. docusate sodium) can be effective alone or in conjunction with colonic stimulants. Lactulose is a commonly prescribed softener but is expensive and may cause uncomfortable bloating; it has a specific role in the treatment of hepatic encephalopathy.
- *Magnesium sulphate* is a more potent osmotic agent, usually for short-term use.
- *Polyethylene glycols* (e.g. Movicol) do not cause bloating, are useful in resistant cases and are well tolerated in the long term.
- *Peripherally acting mu-receptor antagonists* (e.g. methylnaltrexone) block GI (constipating) effects of opioids without altering the central analgesic effects.
- *Other agents for resistant cases* (specialist use only):
  - Prucalopride ($5HT_4$ agonist – promotes increased GI motility)
  - Linaclotide (non-absorbed guanylate cyclase 2C agonist) and lubriprostone (activates gut wall chloride channels), the latter two drugs increasing intestinal water secretion and speeding up transit).

## DISEASES AND THEIR MANAGEMENT

### DISEASES OF THE OESOPHAGUS

GORD is extremely common, particularly in affluent societies. The lower oesophageal sphincter (LOS; **Figure 10.24**) is the main barrier preventing reflux of gastric contents into the oesophagus A hiatus hernia is one of several factors that may reduce LOS pressure and increase GORD. When

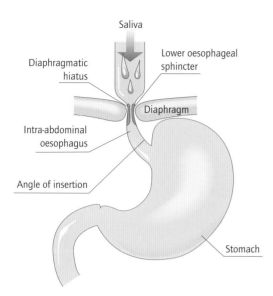

**Figure 10.24** Factors preventing gastro-oesophageal reflux. Gastro-oesophageal reflux is prevented by the action of: (i) the LOS, the pressure of which is normally 20 mmHg and is increased by cholinergic stimulation, gastrin and food in the stomach; (ii) the acute angle of entry of the oesophagus into the stomach; (iii) compression of the intra-abdominal segment of the oesophagus by intra-abdominal pressure; (iv) the diaphragmatic hiatus; and (v) neutralization of any acid reflux by swallowed saliva (approximately 1 L/day).

GORD is severe and prolonged, it can lead to Barrett's oesophagus, a risk factor for oesophageal adenocarcinoma.

## HIATUS HERNIA

Definition - part of the stomach above the diaphragm. There are two types (**Figure 10.25**):

- Sliding (most common)
- Rolling or para-oesophageal

### Epidemiology and risk factors

- Affects 30% of people aged over 50
- Incidence increases with age
- More common in women
- Lax diaphragmatic hiatus increases risk
- Increased intra-abdominal pressure if overweight or obese increases risk

### Clinical features

#### Common

- Frequently asymptomatic and incidental diagnosis at OGD
- May be associated with GORD
- Ulceration or erosions (Cameron lesions) where stomach is constricted at diaphragmatic hiatus

#### Rare

- Gastric volvulus and strangulation of a large hiatus hernia. Patients may complain of severe chest pain, vomiting or dysphagia.

### Investigation

#### Endoscopy

- *OGD:* shows gastric mucosa above the level of diaphragm

#### Diagnostic imaging

- *Barium swallow and meal:* rarely used, but will show hiatus hernia and associated reflux
- *Chest X-ray* (see **Figure 10.13c**): may reveal a large hiatus hernia (a retrocardiac gas-filled shadow, sometimes containing a fluid level)

### Management

- No treatment required if asymptomatic
- Any associated heartburn, reflux oesophagitis or Barrett's oesophagus should be managed accordingly (usually with PPIs)
- Gastric volvulus or obstructive symptoms will likely require surgery

## GASTRO-OESOPHAGEAL REFLUX DISEASE AND REFLUX OESOPHAGITIS

GORD is defined as symptoms (typically heartburn) suggestive of, or proven to be from, reflux.

Some patients with GORD have reflux oesophagitis, which is defined as inflammation/erosions/ulceration of the distal oesophageal mucosa, due to reflux of gastric contents. Sometimes inflammation is only detectable by taking oesophageal biopsies.

However:

- Many patients with GORD symptoms have a completely normal oesophagus, macroscopically and histologically.
- Conversely, some patients with typical reflux oesophagitis seen at OGD (**Figure 10.26**) have no GORD symptoms.

### Epidemiology

- About one-third of the normal population experiences monthly episodes of heartburn.
- It is common in affluent societies.

### Causes and risk factors

- Hiatus hernia
- Obesity
- Drugs, e.g. NSAIDs, antidepressants, anticholinergics, calcium-channel blockers
- Smoking, alcohol, caffeine and fatty foods can exacerbate symptoms

### Clinical features

#### Common

- Heartburn
- Non-cardiac chest pain

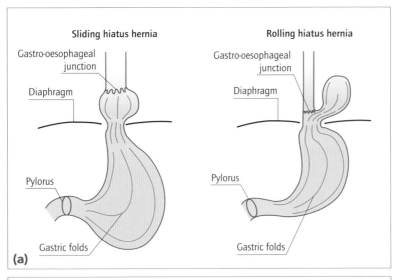

Sliding hiatus hernia

Rolling hiatus hernia

**(a)**

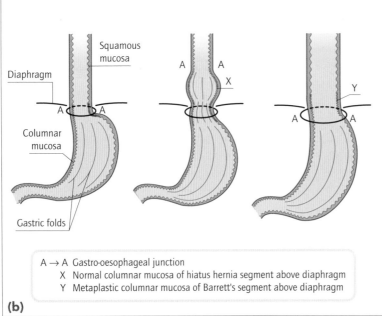

A → A Gastro-oesophageal junction
X Normal columnar mucosa of hiatus hernia segment above diaphragm
Y Metaplastic columnar mucosa of Barrett's segment above diaphragm

**(b)**

**Figure 10.25 (a)** Different types of hiatus herniae. **(b)** Differentiation of Barrett's columnar-lined oesophagus and a hiatus hernia. Note the presence of gastric folds in continuity with the columnar mucosa above the diaphragm in hiatus hernia.

- Dysphagia: caused by oesophageal ulceration, spasm or stricture
- Regurgitation of gastric contents into the throat, resulting in a bitter or acid taste

### Rare

- Chest pain, which can be difficult to distinguish from cardiac pain, particularly if there is associated oesophageal spasm.
- To add to the confusion, acid reflux may be worsened by exercise, and oesophageal spasm relieved by antianginal therapies such as glyceryl trinitrate spray.
- There are usually no physical signs.

### Differential diagnosis

- Other causes of dyspepsia
- Cardiac chest pain (should always be excluded before a diagnosis of non-cardiac chest pain or GORD is made)

### Complications

- Haematemesis or melaena
- Fibrotic stricture
- Barrett's oesophagus
- Aspiration of refluxate causing chronic cough, chest infections, aggravation of asthma

### Investigation

Many patients require no investigation; however, if there are red flag symptoms such as dysphagia or weight loss, if symptoms are severe, or if they persist despite treatment, then investigation is appropriate.

### Bloods

- Rarely, there may be anaemia due to bleeding oesophageal mucosa.

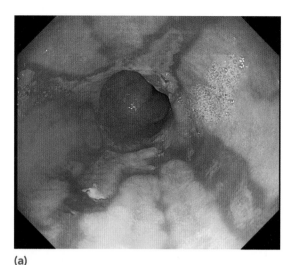

**(a)**

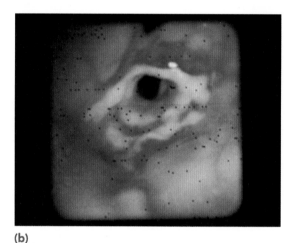

**(b)**

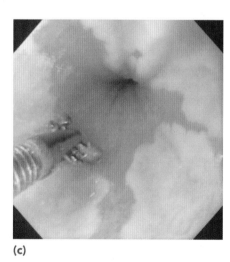

**(c)**

**Figure 10.26** Endoscopic views of oesophageal disease caused by acid reflux. **(a)** Linear hyperaemia with erosions: reflux oesophagitis. Image courtesy of Dr Bjorn Rembaken, Leeds Teaching Hospitals Trust. **(b)** Benign peptic oesophageal stricture. **(c)** Barrett's oesophagus. Note the tongues of orange–red columnar-type mucosa extending proximally up the distal oesophagus. The biopsy forceps are positioned at the junction of Barrett's mucosa and normal oesophageal mucosa. Reproduced from *Slide Atlas of Gastroenterology* with the kind permission of the author and Times Mirror International Publishers.

### Endoscopy
- OGD may show reflux oesophagitis (**Figure 10.26a**) (but is normal in 50%).

### Oesophageal 24-hour pH measurement (Figure 10.27)
- This is useful in patients with equivocal or refractory symptoms, or where there are typical GORD symptoms but normal endoscopy.
- A fine-bore tube with a pH sensor is passed into the oesophagus via the nose. Patients press a button to record the timing of symptoms. It allows 24-hour continuous assessment of oesophageal acid exposure and the relationship to symptoms.
- In some centres, wireless oesophageal pH probes are available. These are temporarily attached to the distal oesophagus and are more comfortable for the patient.

**10**

### Management

#### General and lifestyle measures
- Postural advice, e.g. avoid bending down
- Elevate the head of the bed
- Stop smoking and avoid alcohol
- Lose weight
- Avoid dietary triggers, e.g. fatty and spicy foods
- Avoid large meals and eating late in the evening
- Stop medications which may be contributing to symptoms

#### Drug treatment
- If lifestyle measures are insufficient, acid suppression should be tried using *PPIs* as first-line treatment.
- *H2RAs* may be sufficient for milder symptoms or added to PPI therapy for resistant cases.
- *Alginates* (e.g. Gaviscon) form a raft on top of the gastric contents and may offer additional relief.
- *Prokinetics* encourage gastric emptying and may reduce reflux.

#### Surgery
- A minority of patients who fail to respond require surgery, usually a laparoscopic Nissen's fundoplication, in which the gastric fundus is sutured around the distal oesophagus to create a lower oesophageal high-pressure zone to resist reflux.
- Peptic oesophageal strictures due to reflux can usually be treated using endoscopic balloon dilation.

### Other causes of oesophagitis (all rare)
- Drugs (NSAIDs, potassium, bisphosphonates)
- Corrosives
- Radiotherapy
- Candida oesophagitis (usually associated with oral/inhaled steroid use or immunocompromised patients, white mucosal plaques seen (**Figure 10.26b**)

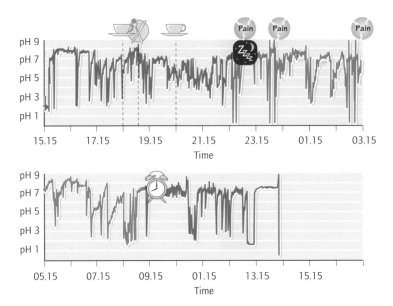

**Figure 10.27** 24-hour oesophageal pH study result. The *x*-axis shows time: this study was started at 15.15 in the afternoon and continued until the same time the following day. The *y*-axis shows the pH recorded in the distal oesophagus during the 24-hour period. The patient records major events as shown by the self-explanatory cartoons at the top of the trace, indicating drinking, eating, pain, going to bed and waking. The red trace shows the period the patient was supine in bed, the green period the awake and upright period. The greater the amount of time the trace dips below pH 4, the greater the potential for acid-induced damage to the oesophageal mucosa. This cumulative time where this patient's pH dropped below 4 was only marginally above the normal range at 4.7% of the 24-hour period. However, there is a strong symptom correlation. The patient awoke three times during the night as a result of reflux-type pain, clearly corresponding to periods of marked oesophageal acidification. The trace probably underestimated the normal situation, as this patient found the presence of the monitoring tube so uncomfortable he could only manage one light meal during the monitoring period. Oesophageal manometry showed him to have a grossly lax LOS. His symptoms were abolished by surgery to repair the valve.

## BARRETT'S OESOPHAGUS

This is an acquired condition due to long-term acid reflux where the stratified squamous epithelium that normally lines the distal oesophagus is replaced by columnar epithelium. This change, where one type of fully differentiated cell replaces another, is called metaplasia. It is a risk factor for oesophageal adenocarcinoma.

### Epidemiology and risk factors

- Prevalence in Western countries around 5%
- Like GORD, Barrett's oesophagus is more common in:
  - Developed countries
  - Men
  - Caucasian ethnicity
  - Smokers and obese patients
- Rare in Black and Asian populations
- Typical age at diagnosis is 50–60 years

### Clinical features

- Usually asymptomatic
- Patients may report co-existing reflux symptoms

### Investigation

Diagnosis is made by gastroscopy and biopsies.
- In Barrett's oesophagus, columnar mucosa is seen lining the distal oesophagus above the gastro-oesophageal junction. The different colours of

squamous (pink) and columnar (orange) mucosa allow differentiation by the endoscopist (**Figure 10.28a**).
- If biopsies of the distal oesophagus then confirm specialized columnar mucosa with intestinal metaplasia, a diagnosis of Barrett's can be made.

### Dysplasia and cancer risk

- Barrett's oesophagus is a premalignant condition. The overall incidence of cancer development is around 0.25% per year.
- Before becoming cancerous (neoplasia), cells first exhibit abnormal changes known as dysplasia. Dysplasia is described as low-grade or high-grade depending on severity.
- Not everyone with dysplasia will go on to develop cancer, but for patients with high-grade dysplasia, cancers occur at a rate of around 5% per year.
- Dysplasia can be detected using endoscopy and biopsy and treated to prevent cancer. This is the rationale for surveillance (see below).

### Management

#### Acid suppression
- Acid reflux promotes cancer development in Barrett's oesophagus, thus all patients should be offered PPI treatment, regardless of associated GORD symptoms or reflux oesophagitis.

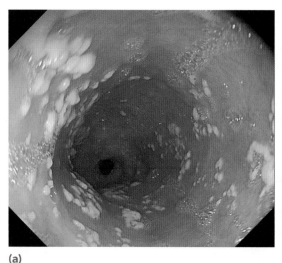

(a)

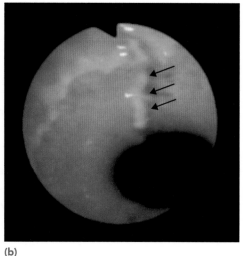

(b)

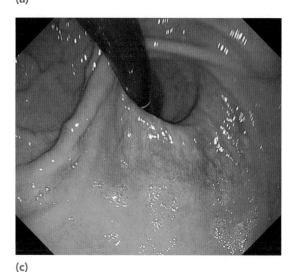

(c)

**10**

**Figure 10.28** Endoscopic views of benign oesophageal disease. **(a)** *Candida* oesophagus. Note ulceration and pseudomembranes. Image courtesy of Dr Bjorn Rembaken, Leeds Teaching Hospitals Trust. **(b)** Mallory–Weiss tear in the distal oesophagus. Note the linear tear (arrows) in the proximal gastric mucosa immediately distal to the gastro-oesophageal mucosal junction. **(c)** Hiatus hernia. The gastroscope is angled to look back upwards towards the head. The white band on the shaft of the endoscope is approximately at the level of the gastro-oesophageal junction. The oesophagus disappears into the centre of the picture. The rest of the mucosa seen is gastric and is above the level of the diaphragm (which can be judged by the endoscopist as it indents the mucosa) and is therefore by definition a hiatus hernia. The laxity of the valve between the stomach and oesophagus can be appreciated. Image courtesy of Dr Bjorn Rembaken, Leeds Teaching Hospitals Trust.

### Endoscopic surveillance

- Most patients undergo surveillance. The research evidence for overall benefit is still debated and protocols vary between countries.
- The histological diagnosis of dysplasia can be difficult and must be confirmed by two pathologists; treatment decisions should be guided by an MDT approach.
- If there is no dysplasia, surveillance endoscopy with biopsies is typically undertaken every 2–5 years (longer intervals for shorter lengths of Barrett's).
- If low-grade dysplasia is identified, options are radiofrequency ablation (RFA) treatment (see below) or more frequent surveillance.
- If high-grade dysplasia is found, endoscopic therapy is usually recommended.

### Treatments for dysplasia in Barrett's

#### Thermal ablation

- Heat can be used to destroy dysplastic cells. RFA is the most widely used modality.

- RFA uses a special balloon device via an endoscope to deliver radiofrequency (microwave) energy to the mucosa.

### Endoscopic resection

- Dysplastic areas can be resected using an endoscope.
- The mucosa is sucked into a special cap on the end of the endoscope captured using a rubber band, and cut away using a wire snare.

### Oesophagectomy

- Endoscopic treatments for dysplasia mean that oesophagectomy is rarely indicated.
- Oesophagectomy carries significant risk of postoperative complications and mortality.

## CARCINOMA OF THE OESOPHAGUS

Primary carcinoma of the oesophagus is the eighth most common cancer worldwide and has two main forms:

- *Adenocarcinoma:* associated strongly with Barrett's oesophagus
- *Squamous carcinoma:* associated with environmental carcinogens

## Risk factors

### Squamous carcinoma

- Smoking
- Alcohol
- Dietary factors (e.g. consuming hot drinks, N-nitrosamines [found in pickled foods]) have been implicated
- Achalasia (likely due to food stasis leading to chronic oesophageal inflammation)
- Possible association with human papilloma virus infection

### Adenocarcinoma

- Barrett's oesophagus and GORD
- Smoking (but *not alcohol*)
- Obesity

## Epidemiology

- Prevalence and geography:
  - Squamous carcinoma
    - Incidence is relatively stable over time in any one geographical area.
    - However, there are dramatic differences between areas. This probably reflects varying exposure to carcinogens rather than effects of race.

  - Adenocarcinoma
    - Previously uncommon, there has been a rapid increase in incidence over the last few decades.
    - The increase has been most marked in developed countries where incidence rates now exceed those of squamous carcinoma – a reversal of the situation 30 years ago.

- Incidence of both types increases with age (rare before age 50).
- Both types are more common in men.

## Pathology

- Squamous carcinoma occurs most commonly in the mid-oesophagus, while adenocarcinoma, because of the association with Barrett's, occurs mainly in the distal oesophagus.
- Both tumour types invade the submucosa at an early stage and extend locally.
- Local lymph node invasion occurs early because lymphatics are superficial in the oesophagus (lamina propria level) compared to elsewhere in the GI tract (beneath muscularis mucosa).
- Tumours can invade local structures, resulting in fistula formation to the trachea or aorta.
- Distant metastases are common at presentation.

## Clinical features

### Common

- Progressive dysphagia and weight loss
- Early disease is usually asymptomatic

### Less common

- Chest pain
- Cervical lymphadenopathy
- IDA

### Rare

- Pneumonia or pleural effusion due to oesophageal–respiratory fistula
- Massive upper GI haemorrhage due to oesophageal–aortic fistula

## Investigation

- *Blood tests:* may show anaemia
- *Gastroscopy and biopsy* (**Figure 10.29**): are the best tests - reveal the lesion and obtain diagnostic histology
- *CT scan:*
  - May suggest diagnosis due to finding of oesophageal thickening/mass/stricture, but gastroscopy would still be needed to confirm findings
  - Used to stage the disease and look for metastases
- *Endoscopic ultrasound (EUS):* may be used for more accurate local staging (e.g. depth of mucosal invasion; locoregional lymphadenopathy)

## Management

Decisions about treatment require multidisciplinary (surgeon; gastroenterologist; radiologist; pathologist; oncologist; palliative care) discussion in a specialist centre:

- Consider the tumour stage, type and anatomical location, as well as patient co-morbidities and preferences.
- In general:
  - Surgery is suitable for patients with localized (early-stage) disease.
  - Palliative care is recommended in patients with metastatic disease.
  - Patients who have a localized, but non-resectable, tumour may have chemotherapy and radiotherapy in combination:
    - As a stand-alone treatment
    - With the aim of down-staging the tumour so they can have surgery

### Surgery

- If CT scans suggest operability, use EUS to assess local spread.
- Oesophagectomy is most commonly performed using a thoracoabdominal approach (Ivor–Lewis oesophagectomy).
- 30-day postoperative mortality is high (around 2%).

### Chemotherapy and chemoradiotherapy

- Neoadjuvant (preoperative) chemotherapy is commonly used, and it improves outcomes, compared with surgery alone.
- Combined chemoradiotherapy can be used with curative intent in patients who cannot have surgery but can also be used as a neoadjuvant treatment.

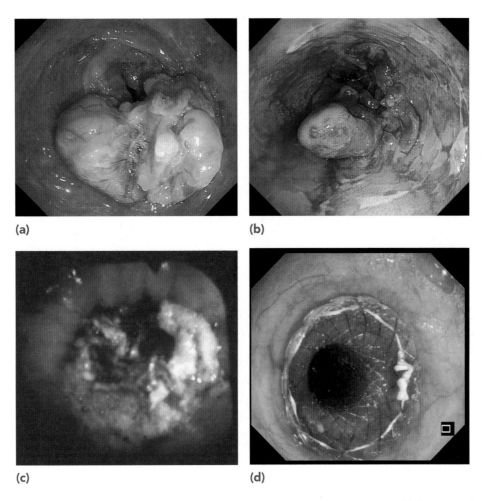

(a)

(b)

(c)

(d)

**Figure 10.29** Endoscopic views of oesophageal carcinoma. **(a)** Polypoidal oesophageal carcinoma. **(b)** Haemorrhagic oesophageal carcinoma. **(c)** Ulcerating oesophageal carcinoma. The blackened areas are caused by palliative laser therapy, which debulks the tumour, improving swallowing, and reduces bleeding from the ulcerated mucosa. **(d)** Oesophageal malignant obstruction relieved by a stent. Images **(a)**, **(c)** and **(d)** courtesy of Dr Bjorn Rembaken, Leeds Teaching Hospitals Trust; **(b)** reproduced from from Misiewicz JJ *et al.* (1994) *Diseases of the Gut and Pancreas*, 2nd edn (Wiley-Blackwell, Oxford), with the permission of the authors.

### *Radiotherapy*

- Neoadjuvant radiotherapy does not have a role.
- External beam radiotherapy can provide effective palliation. It is particularly useful for tumours in the upper third of the oesophagus where surgery is often impracticable.

### *Endoscopic resection*

- Very early-stage tumours (confined to the mucosa or submucosa with no lymphovascular involvement) can be resected endoscopically.
- Careful patient selection is key.
- The best outcomes are seen with smaller lesions.

### *Endoscopic ablation*

- This can be used for early-stage tumours using a range of modalities (e.g. RFA, cryotherapy).
- Recurrence rates are high.
- It is suitable for patients who are not surgical candidates, usually in conjunction with endoscopic resection.

### *Endoscopic stenting*

- Stents can be placed endoscopically across a tumour to restore a patent lumen and relieve dysphagia in patients with malignant oesophageal obstruction, where surgical resection is not possible.
- Self-expanding metallic stents offer the best results.

### **Prognosis**

Overall prognosis is very poor. Survival rates at 5 years are:

- 30% for patients with well-localized disease
- 10% for those with regional metastases or locally advanced disease
- Almost zero for those presenting with distant disease

## TRAUMA-INDUCED OESOPHAGEAL DISORDERS

### **Mallory–Weiss tear**

Mallory–Weiss tear occurs in the distal oesophagus or gastric fundus (see **Figure 10.28b**). It happens because of retropulsion of the gastric cardia into the chest during repeated retching or vomiting causing one or more short linear mucosal tears.

## Epidemiology
- One of the most common causes of minor upper GI bleeding
- Occurs mainly in young adults

## Clinical features
Patients usually present with a small, fresh haematemesis.

## Investigation
- Diagnosis is confirmed endoscopically.
- The mucosal tears heal rapidly and may not be visible if endoscopy is delayed.

## Management
- Usually, no treatment is necessary.
- Rarely, bleeding is ongoing or significant and requires endoscopic intervention or surgery.

### Acute oesophageal perforation
#### Causes
- *Common:*
  - Iatrogenic: during endoscopy, especially during oesophageal dilatation (1/100 risk)
- *Rare:*
  - Spontaneous (Boerhaave's syndrome): during vomiting
  - Ingestion of corrosives or foreign bodies
  - Secondary to chest trauma

## Clinical features
- *Pain:* e.g. chest, neck, back and upper abdomen
- *Surgical emphysema:* air in the subcutaneous tissue
- *Signs of infection and sepsis:* e.g. fever and shock; infection in the mediastinum (mediastinitis) is the main complication

## Investigation
- *Chest X-ray and CT scan:* diagnosis is confirmed radiologically
- *Contrast radiology:* e.g. water-soluble contrast swallow, may also be needed to look for a leak

## Management
This condition has high morbidity and mortality, so early and aggressive management is key.
- *General:*
  - Antibiotics
  - Analgesia
  - NBM; parenteral nutrition
- *Surgery:*
  - Large defects require early surgical repair.
  - An endoscopically placed fully covered stent can also be used for smaller defects.
  - Small defects often heal spontaneously with general conservative management, as above.

### Foreign bodies and food bolus
Foreign objects (e.g. coins, razor blades, batteries) may be swallowed accidently or deliberately, particularly by young children or people with mental health problems.

A food bolus can sometimes get stuck in the oesophagus once swallowed.

## Clinical features
Impaction at cricopharyngeal level or in the oesophagus may result in:
- Dysphagia
- Chest pain
- Perforation

Impaction may arise due to other oesophageal pathology (e.g. a stricture, EO).

## Investigation
Plain neck and chest radiography and, if necessary, contrast radiology along with the history will reveal most foreign bodies. If there is doubt, proceed to OGD.

## Management
- Oesophageal foreign bodies need prompt endoscopic removal.
- Objects already in the stomach often pass through the bowel without incident.
- However, sharp objects and batteries should be removed endoscopically to reduce the chance of mucosal damage.
- Impacted food boluses may pass spontaneously into the stomach; otherwise, antispasmodics such as hyoscine butylbromide may help, or endoscopic removal may be required.

# EOSINOPHILIC OESOPHAGITIS

EO is a chronic inflammatory condition of the oesophagus. Typical symptoms are dysphagia, chest pain and upper abdominal pain. Food bolus impaction requiring endoscopy occurs in up to 50% of patients.

## Epidemiology
- More common in men
- Annual incidence approximately 1/5000

## Disease mechanisms
- Poorly understood
- Associations with atopy
- Food allergy implicated as major contributor

## Differential diagnosis
Other conditions can lead to oesophageal eosinophilia, including:
- GORD
- Parasitic and fungal infections
- Drug-induced

## Pathophysiology

Diagnosis of EO requires finding significant oesophageal mucosal eosinophilia on biopsy, following adequate treatment with PPI (aiming to eliminate GORD as the cause of the eosinophilia).

## Investigation

- Gastroscopy may show typical concentric ring appearance (trachealization) of the oesophageal mucosa.
- Biopsies are taken to look for the presence of eosinophils.

## Management

- Dietary elimination of any food allergy triggers
- Topical steroids
- Oral viscous steroid tablets which dissolve on the tongue
- Even in absence of GORD, PPIs may offer some relief

# OESOPHAGEAL MOTILITY DISORDERS

These are rare but important to consider as causes of dysphagia and chest pain when common oesophageal and cardiac conditions have been excluded.

They may be:
- Primary:
  - Achalasia
  - Diffuse oesophageal spasm
- Secondary:
  - Scleroderma
  - Diabetes (because of autonomic neuropathy)

## Achalasia

Achalasia is characterized by:
- Failure of LOS relaxation after a swallow
- Loss of oesophageal peristalsis

### Epidemiology

The incidence is 1 in 100 000 in the UK.

### Disease mechanisms

- Results from a loss of ganglion cells in the myenteric (Auerbach's) plexus
- May be caused by an autoimmune process driven by latent infection with herpes simplex virus 1 (HSV-1)

### Clinical features

- *Dysphagia:*
  - May be intermittent at first and relieved by drinking, changes in position or regurgitation
  - Becoming more persistent later and is often worse for liquids than for solids
  - May cause nutritional deficiencies and weight loss
- *Occasional retrosternal chest pain:* from oesophageal spasm
- *Respiratory symptoms:* including cough and nocturnal wheezing

### Complications

- There is an increased risk of oesophageal carcinoma.
- Aspiration can cause recurrent chest infections or pneumonia.

### Differential diagnosis

This is as for dysphagia.

### Investigation

*Oesophageal manometry* This is the gold standard for diagnosis. Key findings are:
- Raised LOS resting pressure
- Failure of LOS relaxation on swallowing.
- A lack of peristalsis in the body of the oesophagus

*Diagnostic imaging*
- *Chest X-ray:* may be an oesophageal air–fluid level, and the normal gastric air bubble may be absent
- *Barium swallow:* often a smooth tapering down to the LOS and, in late cases, a dilated oesophagus containing food residue (see **Figure 10.14c**)

*Endoscopy* This is normal in the early stages. It is important for:
- Evaluation of the differential diagnosis
- Detection of complications (particularly biopsies for oesophageal dysplasia or carcinoma)
- Treatment (below)

### Management

- *Drug treatment:*
  - Smooth-muscle relaxing agents (e.g. calcium channel blocker and nitrates) provide temporary relief for some, but most require more invasive therapy.
- *Botulinum toxin:*
  - Injected into the LOS, reducing pressure to relieve symptoms
  - Temporary – repeat injection usually required by 6–12 months
  - Mainly reserved for older or frail individuals at high risk for definitive treatment
- *Endoscopic dilatation of the LOS:*
  - Was commonly undertaken using a pneumatic balloon
  - Less frequently performed now and carries a risk of perforation (1/100)
- *Heller's myotomy:*
  - The sphincter muscle at the lower end of the oesophagus is weakened by a longitudinal incision. The procedure can be performed laparoscopically.
  - Outcomes are good, with very few patients having ongoing problems with dysphagia.
  - An endoscopic method of performing a myotomy (per oral endoscopic myotomy (POEM)) appears to show comparable efficacy in some studies.

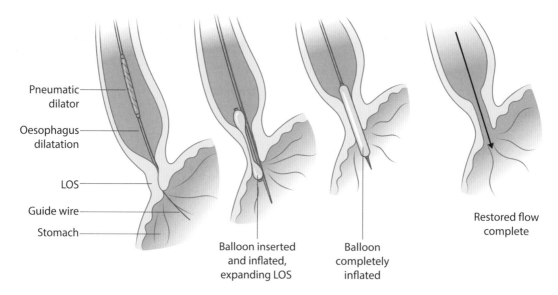

Pneumatic dilator

Oesophagus dilatation

LOS

Guide wire

Stomach

Balloon inserted and inflated, expanding LOS

Balloon completely inflated

Restored flow complete

**Figure 10.30** Technique and equipment for balloon dilatation of oesophageal strictures. For benign strictures, relief of dysphagia is often permanent, but the procedure can be repeated when necessary. If the stricture is malignant, an expanding metal stent can be inserted over the guide wire under radiological control, if necessary preceded by balloon dilatation. The most common immediate complications are pain and oesophageal perforation. Later problems include aspiration pneumonia, blockage of the tube by food or further tumour growth.

### Oesophageal spasm

Oesophageal spasm is an idiopathic motility disorder.

#### Epidemiology

Onset is usually in middle-age.

#### Clinical features

Intermittent non-propulsive repetitive oesophageal contractions which may cause:

- Chest pain
- Dysphagia

#### Differential diagnosis

The main differentials that must be excluded are:

- Cardiac ischaemia
- Achalasia
- GORD

#### Investigation

- *ECG:* to exclude IHD
- *Endoscopy:* to exclude reflux oesophagitis/other causes of dysphagia
- *Barium swallow:* may be helpful (see **Figure 10.14d**)
- *Oesophageal manometry:* can demonstrate characteristic dysmotility

#### Management

- Treatment can be difficult.
- Smooth-muscle relaxants (e.g. nitrates, calcium-channel blockers and phosphodiesterase inhibitors) may sometimes help.
- Balloon dilatation and even surgical cardiomyotomy may be necessary.

- Attacks precipitated by GORD may respond to acid suppression.

#### Benign oesophageal strictures

##### Causes

- Most are peptic (caused by acid).
- May complicate severe forms of any other cause of oesophagitis, with the exception of *Candida* when it is a rare complication.

##### Clinical features

- Strictures usually present with dysphagia.
- Weight loss is rare.
- Hiatus hernia often coexists.

##### Investigation

- *Contrast radiology:* may show stricture
- *Endoscopy and biopsy:* essential to confirm diagnosis and exclude malignancy and Barrett's oesophagus

##### Management

- Long-term high-dose PPIs to reduce GORD and prevent re-stricturing
- Endoscopic balloon dilatation of stricture if symptomatic (**Figure 10.30**)

## DISEASES OF THE STOMACH AND DUODENUM

### PEPTIC ULCER

A peptic ulcer is a break in the mucosa in (or close to) acid-secreting areas of the GI tract, where acid is involved wholly

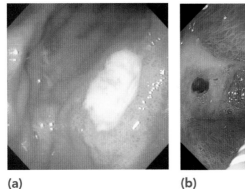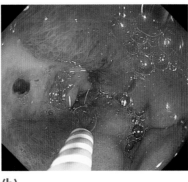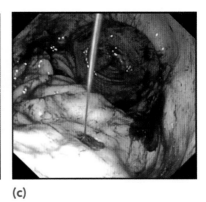

(a)                              (b)                              (c)

**Figure 10.31** Endoscopic appearances of peptic ulcers. **(a)** DU. **(b)** DU with visible but no bleeding vessel. Image courtesy of Dr Bjorn Rembaken, Leeds Teaching Hospitals Trust. **(c)** Peptic ulcer with arterial bleeding prior to treatment. Reproduced from Holster IL & Kuipers EJ (2011) *Curr Gastroenterol Rep.* 13(6):525-31. doi: 10.1007/s11894-011-0223-7. With permission from Springer.

**10**

or partly in the aetiology (**Figure 10.31**). The term is misleading as it is acid, not pepsin that is the significant factor in such ulcers (the term derives from the close association of pepsin and acid secretion).

Non-'peptic' causes of ulceration in these areas of the GI tract are rare (**Table 10.16**), the most important to consider being malignant GU. The term 'stress ulceration' refers to multiple small superficial ulcers, usually of the gastric mucosa, in patients with major organic stress (e.g. severe burns, ITU cases). Common locations of GUs and DUs are shown in **Figure 10.32**.

## Epidemiology

- 1-year prevalence 0.5–2%; lifetime prevalence 10–15% (20% if HP-positive)
- Point prevalence of 10–30% in NSAID users, of which GU : DU = 10 : 1.
- Commonest age is 20–60 years for DU, over 60 for GU
- DU slightly more common in men; GU in women

- No significant inheritable risks
- Higher overall rates of HP infection and earlier age of acquisition in resource-poor countries associated with higher incidence of peptic ulcer
- Falling incidence over time since 1950s in most studies, consistent with improving hygiene

## Disease mechanisms

The balance between factors attacking (e.g. acid) and defending the gastroduodenal mucosa is disturbed. Attacking factors may predominate in DU, and failed defence in GU. The main risk factors are HP infection and NSAID/aspirin use.

### Helicobacter pylori

HP (**Figure 10.33**) is causal in 50–70% of patients with GU and up to 95% of patients with DU; however, the majority of patients with HP do not develop GU or DU.

Two patterns of infection occur:

- *Antrum predominant:* leads to increased acid production, associated with DU

**Table 10.16** Causes of GUs and DUs

|  | Gastric ulceration | Duodenal ulceration |
|---|---|---|
| **Common** | *H. pylori* (pangastritis pattern) | *H. pylori* (antrum predominant pattern) |
| **(or requires excluding by biopsy** | NSAIDs /aspirin | NSAIDs/aspirin |
| **in all cases)** | Malignant ulcer (adenocarcinoma, lymphoma) | |
| **Rare** | Crohn's disease | Crohn's disease |
|  | CMV* | *CMV** |
|  | Vasculitis | Vasculitis |
|  | Upper abdominal radiotherapy | Upper abdominal radiotherapy |
|  | Crack cocaine | Crack cocaine |
|  | Bile reflux | Zollinger–Ellison syndrome |
|  | Stress ulcers | Renal dialysis |
|  |  | Primary hyperparathyroidism |
|  |  | CD |
|  |  | Malignant disease including lymphoma |

*Usually, immunocompromised patients.

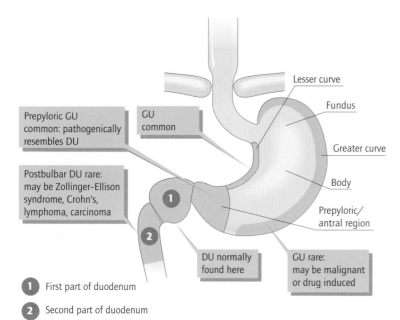

Figure 10.32 Sites of chronic peptic ulceration.

First part of duodenum

Second part of duodenum

- *Pangastritis:* untreated, mucosal atrophy develops with reduced gastric acid secretion and reduced ability of mucosa to defend itself; associated with GU and gastric cancer risk

### NSAIDs/aspirin
NSAID toxicity is due to:
- Inhibition of gastro-duodenal mucosal prostaglandin (PG) synthesis
- Direct drug toxicity to the mucosa

PGs are central to mucosal defence (e.g. by stimulating mucosal blood flow and mucus secretion). NSAIDs reduce PG production by inhibiting the enzyme cyclo-oxygenase (COX). The enzyme exists in two forms: COX-1 (PG production for mucosal defence) and COX-2 (PG production associated with pain in inflamed tissues). NSAIDs selectively inhibiting COX-2 (e.g. celecoxib) have a reduced risk of causing GU and DU.

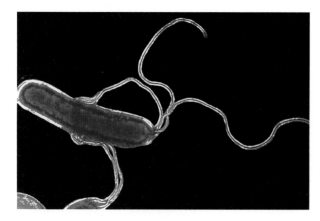

Figure 10.33 *Helicobacter pylori.*

## Clinical features
- Often asymptomatic, especially for NSAID-induced and in the elderly
- Dyspepsia and epigastric pain (note while some GU/DU patients have dyspepsia, most dyspeptic patients do not have ulcers)
- Classic descriptions are night waking with pain, relieved by antacids for DU, and post-prandial pain with nausea, vomiting and weight loss for GU: in practice, but there is a wide overlap and symptoms are poorly predictive

## Investigation
- *Uncomplicated dyspepsia/epigastric pain, under 55 years:* begin with non-invasive HP testing, triple therapy if positive, course of PPI if negative; gastroscopy only if symptoms persist
- *Dyspepsia/epigastric pain over 55 years, or at any age with alarms such as weight loss or vomiting:* direct to gastroscopy
- *Patients unable to come off NSAIDs/aspirin:* gastroscopy
- *Acute GI bleed:* urgent gastroscopy
- *Dyspepsia with IDA:* gastroscopy ± colonoscopy

### Testing for HP
Non-invasive detection typically uses a stool antigen. During gastroscopy, a urease biopsy test is standard, modern versions giving a result with a few minutes allowing targeted treatment at time of the procedure. PPIs and antibiotics cause false negatives for most HP tests and should be stopped for at least 2 and 4 weeks respectively.

## Management
### General
- Management of DU and GU is similar, the critical difference is need to repeat gastroscopy in GU to check healing and exclude cancer.

- Review medications. NSAIDs and aspirin cause ulcers. Corticosteroids, SSRIs, aldosterone antagonists and anticoagulants increase risk of haemorrhage. Calcium antagonists, nitrates and theophylline can aggravate dyspepsia. Bisphosphonates cause oesophageal ulceration. Immunosuppressives slow ulcer healing.
- Where an ulcer has led to a life-threatening complication, long-term maintenance with a PPI or H2RA is appropriate.
- It is controversial whether psychological stress, smoking or dietary factors contribute to peptic ulceration, but addressing these factors is good practice.

### HP-positive cases

- A 1-week course of HP therapy will lead to ulcer healing without the need for acid suppression drugs. However, HP eradication success at first treatment is in the range of 60–90%, so where patients have significant symptoms or complications, a 4- to 8-week healing course of acid suppression is given as well (usually PPI).
- HP eradication usually leads to lasting cure, with annual recurrence rates as low as 2%.
- For DU, treatment success can be assessed using non-invasive HP tests. However, this is unnecessary for uncomplicated DU cases asymptomatic after treatment.
- For GU, even if HP is found and successfully eradicated, repeat gastroscopy to confirm healing.

### NSAID/aspirin use associated cases

- Stopping causal drug and a 6–8-week course of PPIs heals the majority of ulcers.
- If the patient cannot stop the NSAID/aspirin, the safest strategy requires assessment of GI and cardiovascular risks (**Table 10.17**). Healing should be confirmed endoscopically.

### Peptic ulcers in patients taking NSAIDs/aspirin who are HP-positive

The interaction is controversial: a pragmatic approach is to assume both are relevant, stop the NSAID/aspirin therapy and eradicate HP.

### HP-negative and NSAID/aspirin negative cases

- Check for OTC NSAID/aspirin use, bearing in mind that some patients do not realize they are taking, or admit to taking, the drugs.

- Consider the possibility of a false negative HP result.
- There is a high risk of recurrence, so long-term PPI is often used is such cases, although the benefit is unproven.

### Resistant or relapsing ulcers

- Occasionally, symptoms persist or recur despite removal of causative factor(s).
- Repeat gastroscopy to check healing, and biopsy to exclude rare ulcer types and re-confirm HP status.
- Check serum calcium (to exclude primary hyperparathyroidism) and gastrin (to exclude Zollinger–Ellison syndrome).
- Long-term PPI or H2-blocker treatment can be used.
- Surgical resection may be indicated for the small number of patients who do not respond to these measures. Prior to the advent of PPIs in the 1980s, surgical management of peptic ulcer was far more common (**Figure 10.34**).

### Complications of peptic ulceration

- *Acute haemorrhage with haematemesis/melaena:* This can lead to occult bleeding and resultant anaemia.
- *Perforation:* This presents with sudden severe upper abdominal pain; peritonitis; air under the diaphragms on chest X-ray (**Figure 10.13b**). Half are associated with NSAID use. Treatment is urgent resuscitation, IV fluids, nasogastric suction, an NBM regimen, antibiotics and antisecretory agents (e.g. PPIs) and early surgical closure.
- *Pyloric stenosis with gastric outflow obstruction:* Patients present with large-volume stale vomiting, dyspepsia and weight loss. Examination reveals a succussion splash and fluid depletion. This can cause metabolic alkalosis with low plasma $K^+$ and $Cl^-$. It may respond to medical treatment or endoscopic balloon dilatation. Surgical intervention may be necessary.
- *Malignancy:* Around 5% of GU cases become malignant; almost never in DU.

## ACUTE GASTRITIS

This is sudden-onset and short-lived inflammation of the gastric mucosa.

**Table 10.17** NSAID use in patients at risk of GI bleeding

| | Low risk of GI bleeding (NO high-risk features) | High risk of GI bleeding (Presence of any risk feature: age >60; history of peptic ulcer or other cause of GI bleeding; use of antiplatelet agents, anticoagulants, steroids, SSRIs) |
|---|---|---|
| **Low cardiovascular risk** | Non-selective NSAID | COX2 selective NSAID (e.g. celecoxib) + PPI |
| **High cardiovascular risk** (e.g. history of cardiovascular event; diabetes) | Naproxen + PPI | Naproxen + PPI |

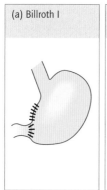
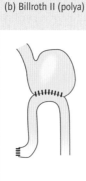
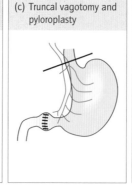
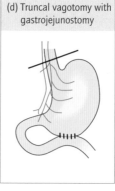
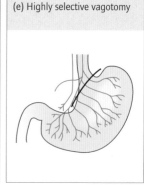

| (a) Billroth I | (b) Billroth II (polya) | (c) Truncal vagotomy and pyloroplasty | (d) Truncal vagotomy with gastrojejunostomy | (e) Highly selective vagotomy |

**Figure 10.34** Operations for peptic ulceration. **(a)** Partial gastrectomy with Billroth I anastomosis. The ulcer and the ulcer-bearing portion of the stomach are resected. **(b)** Partial gastrectomy with creation of a duodenal loop (Billroth II or polya). **(c)** Truncal vagotomy and pyloroplasty. The main nerves are divided to eliminate nervous stimulation of the stomach, reducing the acid secretory capacity, and gastric emptying is maintained with pyloroplasty. **(d)** Truncal vagotomy with gastrojejunostomy. The main nerves are divided and gastric emptying maintained with gastrojejunostomy. **(e)** Highly selective vagotomy. Innervation of the acid-producing area of the stomach is interrupted, leaving the nerve supply to the antrum and pylorus intact. This does not affect gastric emptying so a drainage procedure is not required.

### Risk factors

- HP
- Infections (e.g. norovirus and rotavirus)
- Alcohol
- Drugs (e.g. aspirin, NSAIDs)
- Severe systemic illness (e.g. burns)

### Clinical features

- Nausea and vomiting are typical, diarrhoea in addition if an infective cause also affects more distal gut (gastroenteritis).
- Drug- and alcohol-induced gastritis may be asymptomatic.
- Bleeding from extensive acute erosive gastritis in patients with serious illnesses (e.g. shock, sepsis, major trauma) can be severe and is often the terminal event.

### Investigation

Acute gastritis is usually self-limiting, with investigation rarely necessary.
- Stool samples can be sent for viral RNA or antigen testing.
- Endoscopy shows mucosal erosions and/or inflammation.

### Management

- Most infections self-limit and require no specific treatment
- Rehydration
- Treatment of associated GI bleeding
- Antibiotic treatment for HP infection
- PPIs, H2-blockers or sucralfate may ease symptoms, and are given prophylactically in high-risk patients (e.g. severe burns)
- Antiemetics

## CHRONIC GASTRITIS

This is long-term inflammation of the gastric mucosa, which is mostly asymptomatic. It can be classified and treated according to aetiology (**Table 10.18**).

## GASTRIC NEOPLASMS/GASTRIC CANCER

This section focuses on gastric adenocarcinoma (90% of gastric cancers): other types are lymphomas, gastro intestinal stromal tumours (GISTs) and carcinoid. Local invasion is common, with early spread to regional and distant lymph nodes, liver, lungs, brain and bones. Widespread submucosal involvement with a rigid stomach is termed *linitis plastica*. Presentation is usually late, and survival rates are poor.

### Risk factors

- Barrett's oesophagus: for proximal (cardia) adenocarcinoma, which often actually originates in the distal oesophagus
- HP: for non-cardia adenocarcinoma
- Dietary nitrate
- Salt/pickles used in food preservation
- Atrophic gastritis
- Smoking
- Alcohol
- Benign GU
- Previous partial gastrectomy

### Epidemiology

- Worldwide incidence falling since 1950 (possibly due to reduced *Helicobacter* prevalence and refrigeration for food preservation) though incidence of stomach adenocarcinoma is increasing (related to Barrett's oesophagus)
- Fourth most common cancer worldwide (seventeenth in the UK)

**Table 10.18** Chronic gastritis: classification, histology, clinical features and treatment

| Type | Pathology | Clinical features/associations | Treatment |
|---|---|---|---|
| Type A: autoimmune | Chronic atrophic gastritis | Hypergastrinaemia, antibodies to gastric parietal cells and intrinsic factor, malabsorption of vitamin $B_{12}$, increased risk of autoimmune thyroiditis, Addison's disease, vitiligo, gastric carcinoma | Vitamin $B_{12}$ for pernicious anaemia |
| Type B: bacterial | Chronic gastritis mainly affecting the antrum | HP, peptic ulceration | Eradication of HP |
| Type C: chemical | Chronic superficial gastritis | Alcohol, smoking, NSAIDs, previous gastrectomy (bile reflux) | Avoid cause, bind bile salts with colestyramine |

**10**

- Rare below 55 years (8% of cases); incidence rises sharply after age 65, peaking around age 80
- More common (up to twice) in men
- Very small increased incidence in first-degree relatives (FDRs)
- Incidence varies widely between and within countries: e.g. 77 per 100 000 in Japan and Korea and as low as 7 in 100 000 in India
- Japanese immigrants to the US adopting a Westernized diet and lifestyle have a much lower incidence

## Clinical features

- Presentation often late because small and potentially curable cancers usually asymptomatic
- Weight loss/anorexia
- Abdominal pain
- Nausea/vomiting
- Dysphagia (proximal tumours only)
- Epigastric mass
- GI blood loss (haematemesis, melaena, IDA)
- Occasionally jaundice, hepatomegaly, ascites, supraclavicular lymphadenopathy (Virchow's node)

## Investigation

- *Endoscopy with biopsy* (**Figure 10.35**)
- *Barium meal:* an option for patients unwilling to undergo endoscopy
- *Abdominal CT:* may show more advanced tumours
- *FBC:* microcytic anaemia
- *LFTs:* abnormality suggests metastatic disease

### Staging

Once diagnosed, assuming the patient is appropriate for active treatment, staging of the cancer by a tumour, nodes, metastases (TNM) classification is undertaken, usually by CT scan of the chest, abdomen and pelvis (**Table 10.19**). Further assessment can include PET CT, staging laparotomy and EUS.

## Management

- *General support:* This can be provided through MDT including cancer specialist and Macmillan nurses: explanation, pain control, nutritional replacement,

liaison with the primary care team and arranging palliative care if appropriate.
- *Surgery:* Subtotal or total gastrectomy offers the only chance of a cure: only 25% present with potentially resectable disease.
- *Chemotherapy:* Preoperative (neoadjuvant) chemotherapy can improve surgical outcome. For incurable but reasonably fit patients, palliative chemotherapy can increase survival times.
- *Biological therapy:* Where overexpression of human epidermal growth factor receptor 2 (HER 2) is detected in tumour biopsy, herceptin (trastuzumab) can be used.
- *Radiotherapy:* This is palliative (e.g. for debulking tumours to improve dysphagia/gastric outlet obstruction and reducing tumour bleeding).
- *Endoscopic treatment:* Oesophageal stents can be placed to relieve dysphagia and duodenal or pyloric stents to relieve gastric outlet obstruction.

## Prognosis

- Typical 5-year survival is up to 36%. However, in Japan, where population screening programmes are in place, 5-year survival rates for early gastric cancer of over 95% are being achieved.
- For unresectable disease, median survival is around 10 months.

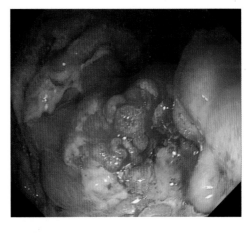

**Figure 10.35** Endoscopic appearance of gastric carcinoma. Image courtesy of Dr Bjorn Rembaken, Leeds Teaching Hospitals Trust.

**Table 10.19** TNM system for staging gastric cancers

| Primary tumour (T) | | Regional lymph nodes (N) | | Distant metastasis (M) | |
|---|---|---|---|---|---|
| TX | Primary tumour cannot be assessed | NX | Regional lymph node(s) cannot be assessed | M0 | No distant metastasis |
| T0 | No evidence of primary tumour | N0 | No regional lymph node metastasis | M1 | Distant metastasis or positive peritoneal cytology |
| Tis | Carcinoma *in situ*: intraepithelial tumour without invasion of the lamina propria | N1 | Metastasis in 1–2 regional lymph nodes | | |
| <>T1a | Tumour invades the lamina propria or the muscularis mucosae | N2 | Metastasis in 3–6 regional lymph nodes | | |
| <>T1b | Tumour invades the submucosa | N3 | Metastasis in 7 or more regional lymph nodes | | |
| T2 | Tumour invades the muscularis propria | N3a | Metastasis in 7–15 regional lymph nodes | | |
| T3 | Tumour penetrates the subserosal connective tissue without invasion of the visceral peritoneum or adjacent structures[a] | N3b | Metastasis in 16 or more regional lymph nodes | | |
| T4 | Tumour invades the serosa (visceral peritoneum) or adjacent structures* | | | | |
| T4a | Tumour invades the serosa (visceral peritoneum) | | | | |
| T4b | Tumour invades adjacent structures[†] | | | | |

*T3 tumours also include those extending into the gastrocolic or gastrohepatic ligaments, or into the greater or lesser omentum, without perforation of the visceral peritoneum covering these structures.

†Adjacent structures include the spleen, transverse colon, liver, diaphragm, pancreas, abdominal wall, adrenal gland, kidney, small intestine and retroperitoneum.

## DISEASES OF THE SMALL INTESTINE

The primary role of the small intestine is absorption of nutrients, and thus diseases affecting the small bowel may present with malabsorption.

## COELIAC DISEASE

CD is an auto-immune reaction to α-gliadin, a subunit of the gluten protein found in cereals such as wheat, barley and rye. This reaction in turn damages small bowel villi (villous atrophy; **Figure 10.36**). Treatment is a lifelong GFD.

Most patients reporting reactions to wheat have IBS/wheat intolerance and often only need to reduce, not avoid, wheat/gluten intake.

### Epidemiology

- Around 1% UK population have +ve serology; most not clinically diagnosed
- Common in Europeans (especially Celts); rare in Africa and Asia
- Presents at any age
- 10% risk in FDRs

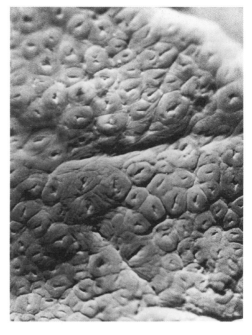

**Figure 10.36** Intestinal villous atrophy in CD.

## Clinical features

### Common

- Failure to thrive in children
- Diarrhoea/malabsorption
- IBS-type symptoms including bloating
- Anaemia
- Reduced bone mineral density

### Rare

- Dermatitis herpetiformis (responds to GFD)
- Other autoimmune disorders (e.g. diabetes, hypothyroidism, adrenal insufficiency)
- Hyposplenism
- Raised transaminases
- Infertility
- Small intestinal T-cell lymphoma and carcinoma of oesophagus or small bowel: strict GFD reduces risk

## Differential diagnosis

For other causes of diarrhoea, steatorrhoea and malabsorption, see **Table 10.10**.

## Investigation

- *Serology:* Positive tissue transglutamase ± endomyseal antibodies are nearly 100% specific for gluten allergy, but false negatives occur (sensitivity 95–98%). Where there is high clinical suspicion, duodenal biopsies should be obtained.
- *Duodenal biopsy* (see **Figure 10.37**): This is the gold standard for diagnosis. If serology is positive, biopsies are still recommended to assess disease severity.
- *FBC:* Anaemia is common due to iron ± folate ± (more rarely) $B_{12}$ deficiency.
- *Blood film:* Howell–Jolly bodies indicate associated hyposplenism.
- *Serum calcium, phosphate and alkaline phosphatase:* Phosphate may be low and alkaline phosphatase may be raised due to vitamin D malabsorption.

## Management challenges

1  *Duodenal biopsies suggestive of CD but negative serology:* Exclude causes of duodenal injury that can mimic CD: drugs (e.g. NSAIDSs), other food allergies, infecitons (e.g. *Giardia*), immunodeficiencies. A histological response to GFD trial ± relapse on re-challenge can help confirm or rule out CD.
2  *Positive serology but duodenal biopsies normal:* The commonest cause is latent CD, where the patient has the immunological marker for CD but no phenotypic expression in terms of mucosal damage. More rarely, the serology is truly false positive.

   In both situations, HLA DQ typing can be useful: a negative result for DQ2 and DQ8 makes CD very unlikely.
3  In non-coeliac gluten allergy, patients do not have the serological or histological features of CD but an immune

reaction seems to underlie the GI (e.g. diarrhoea/bloating) and systemic (e.g. fatigue, poor concentration) symptoms, which respond well to a GFD.

## Approach to proven coeliac disease

- Lifelong GFD, supported by specialist dietician
- Oat gluten seems safe in CD, often reintroduced once mucosal healing achieved
- Screening (serology) for FDRs
- Advice on obtaining gluten-free products on prescription (available in some UK areas)
- Join specialist society (e.g. Coeliac UK: local branches offer support and information, e.g. about GF restaurants)
- Bone mineral density at diagnosis
- Follow-up duodenal biopsy at 6–12 months
- Long-term follow up in a specialist clinic or primary care depending on local arrangements to include: diet reinforcement, screening for complications (e.g. TFT, glucose and LFTs to exclude some associated autoimmune conditions or nutritional deficiencies [including bloods for albumin and haematinics])

## Prognosis

Symptoms usually respond rapidly. Failure to respond is usually due to non-compliance with the diet, rarely due to incorrect diagnosis, secondary hypolactasia or small bowel neoplasia. True primary non-responders (definite CD but no response to GFD) are rare; remission can sometimes be induced with corticosteroids or immunosuppressives.

# SMALL BOWEL BACTERIAL OVERGROWTH

Bacterial counts in the small bowel are normally very low. Conditions leading to small bowel bacterial overgrowth (SIBO) usually present with diarrhoea ± malabsorption.

## Causes

- Small intestinal structural changes such as blind loops, fistulae, strictures, diverticula
- Abnormal small bowel motility
- Achlorhydria
- Hypogammaglobulinaemia

## Disease mechanisms

Excessive bacteria in the small bowel leads to:
- Inactivation of bile salts, causing steatorrhoea
- Reduced terminal ileal bile-salt absorption, causing diarrhoea as bile salts stimulate colonic water secretion

## Clinical and laboratory features

- Diarrhoea and/or steatorrhoea
- *FBC:* commonly reveals a macrocytic anaemia

- *Serum vitamin B$_{12}$* is often low; *folate* is often high because bacteria synthesize it
- *Serum calcium, phosphate and alkaline phosphatase:* may reveal biochemical osteomalacia
- Other clinical or laboratory features of malabsorptin (see **Figure 10.21**)

### Diagnosis

- *A hydrogen or lactulose breath test* is the usual way of confirming diagnosis (see **Figure 10.17**).
- Diagnsois is more likely if imaging such as barium study, CT or MRI has shown structural small bowel abnormalities such as blind loop, diverticula, fistula or stricture.

### Management

- Treat nutritional deficiencies.
- Where feasible, the underlying cause should be corrected (e.g. surgical excision of stricture).
- Antibiotics (e.g. tetracycline, amoxicillin) are given as intermittent or continuous courses.
- Give antidiarrhoeal agents.

## BILE SALT MALABSORPTION AND TERMINAL ILEAL RESECTION

Around 95% of bile salts are recycled by active uptake in the terminal ileum (TI) (**Figure 10.37**). The TI has other unique functions such as B$_{12}$ absorption, and resection can lead to significant clinical consequences (**Figure 10.38**).

If bile salt uptake is reduced, excess bile entering the colon stimulates water and electrolyte secretion and watery

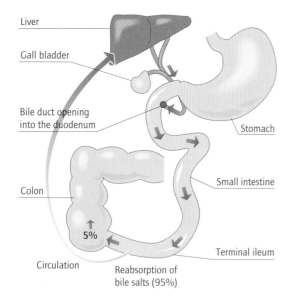

**Figure 10.37** The enterohepatic circulation of bile salts. Primary bile salts are synthesized in the liver from cholesterol, conjugated to make them water-soluble, and secreted into the small bowel after a meal to aid in fat absorption. Ninety-five per cent of conjugated bile salts are then actively reabsorbed in the terminal ileum and return to the liver for recirculation.

diarrhoea. In addition to surgical TI, resection causes include TI disease (e.g. Crohn's); diffuse small bowel damage (e.g. CD, SIBO); and post-surgical effects (cholecystectomy, gastrectomy). Around 10% patients labelled as diarrhoea-predominant IBS have BSM.

Diagnosis can be made by administering a radiolabelled bile acid ($^{75}$SeHCAT) and measuring retention at 7 days (normal >15%).

### Management

Treatment is with bile acid sequestering agents (e.g. colestyramine). Side effects include reduced absorption of fat-soluble vitamins and of many drugs, thus if used long-term, vitamin A and D supplements are recommended, and concomitant medication should be taken well before or after the colestyramine dose.

## SHORT BOWEL SYNDROME

In short bowel syndrome there is failure to achieve normal water and electrolyte and/or nutritional absorption due to small intestinal resection.

Symptoms depend on the length of small bowel remaining, and whether the colon is still in continuity (as the colon has a large capacity to absorb water and electrolytes). Without a colon, patients with less than 2 metres of small bowel remaining usually need some fluid and electrolyte support; under 1 metre enteral nutrition; under 50 cm parenteral nutrition. Adaptive changes can result in a functional improvement in the months following resection.

Indications for extensive small bowel resection include:

- Crohn's disease
- Mesenteric vascular occlusion
- Radiotherapy injury

### Clinical features

- Watery diarrhoea
- Fluid and electrolyte depletion, especially hyponatraemia
- Vitamin B$_{12}$ deficiency (due to loss of terminal ileum)
- Bile salt-induced diarrhoea (when colon in continuity)
- Bile salt deficiency with resulting steatorrhoea
- Gallstones
- Urinary oxalate stones

### Investigation

- Electrolyte (Na, Mg, urea, creatinine) and nutritional deficiencies
- Stool output
- Weight/BMI
- Fluid balance
- Bile-salt malabsorption, vitamin B$_{12}$ absorption and urinary oxalate excretion should be quantified

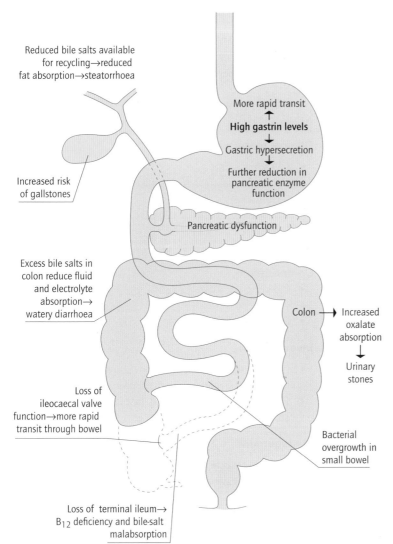

Reduced bile salts available for recycling→reduced fat absorption→steatorrhoea

More rapid transit

**High gastrin levels**

Gastric hypersecretion

Further reduction in pancreatic enzyme function

Increased risk of gallstones

Pancreatic dysfunction

Excess bile salts in colon reduce fluid and electrolyte absorption→ watery diarrhoea

Colon → Increased oxalate absorption

↓

Urinary stones

Loss of ileocaecal valve function→more rapid transit through bowel

Bacterial overgrowth in small bowel

Loss of terminal ileum→ $B_{12}$ deficiency and bile-salt malabsorption

**Figure 10.38** Consequences of surgery or disease affecting the terminal ileum. Terminal ileal disease (e.g. Crohn's disease) or resection leads to bile-salt malabsorption. This results in steatorrhoea (because of bile-salt deficiency in the small bowel), diarrhoea (because of colonic secretion of water and electrolytes), gallstones (because of bile-salt deficiency) and hyperoxaluria (because of bile salt-induced colonic hyperabsorption of dietary oxalate).

**10**

## Management

- Initially post-surgery, daily weight and fluid balance, IV restoration of fluid and electrolytes
- Specialist dietetic support for enteral ± parenteral nutrition
- Later, small frequent meals are introduced – low-fat diet for patients with marked steatorrhoea
- Long-term support may range from oral food and fluid supplements to total parenteral nutrition (TPN)
- Patients without a colon should use drinks iso-osmolar with tissue fluids (e.g. World Health Organization [WHO] formula); drinking hypotonic liquids such as water or tea causes sodium to move into the bowel lumen, and it is then lost in the jejunostomy output, worsening the situation
- Avoid excessive dietary oxalate
- Specific nutritional deficiencies (calcium, magnesium, zinc, folate, $B_{12}$, vitamins A, D and E) should be tested for and replaced
- Drugs to slow intestinal transit (e.g. loperamide, codeine phosphate)

- *After ileal resection:* colestyramine binds bile salts and reduces diarrhoea, sometimes at the expense of worsening steatorrhoea
- PPIs to reduce the gastric hypersecretion
- Antibiotics if there is SIBO
- *Patients with massive resections:* need to be referred to specialist centres: small-bowel transplantation offers a potential method for these patients to avoid lifelong parenteral nutrition

## DISACCHARIDE MALABSORPTION

Deficiency of intestinal mucosal disaccharidases (lactase, sucrose, maltase) can be either primary and irreversible or secondary to mucosal pathology such as CD or following gastroenteritis (thus potentially reversible). The undigested sugars cause an osmotic diarrhoea.

### Epidemiology

- Primary acquired alactasia is the most common disaccharidase deficiency worldwide (70% of non-White people). The enzyme disappears soon after weaning, but symptoms do not usually occur until the teenage years.

- Rare autosomal recessive congenital deficiencies present in childhood.

### Clinical features

- Only occur if the relevant sugar is ingested in large quantities (milk for lactase deficiency, fruit products for sucrase/maltase deficiency)
- Abdominal pain and diarrhoea
- Abdominal distension
- Flatus and borborygmi

### Investigation

- Breath testing
- Lactose challenge (1 pint milk): bloating, abdominal discomfort and/or diarrhoea soon after makes lactase deficiency likely

### Management

- Avoid the relevant sugar.
- Lactose-free dairy products avoid issues with calcium and vitamin D deficiency for patients with lactase deficiency.
- Use synthetic lactase preparations.
- Avoid lactose-containing medication.

## MECKEL'S DIVERTICULUM

This is a congenital anomaly of the mid-ileum (remnant of the umbilical cord). It is about 5 cm long, 60 cm from the ileocaecal valve.

### Epidemiology

- 2% of the population affected
- Male : female ratio 2 : 1
- 2% have complications
- Most present before 2 years of age

### Clinical features

- 98% are asymptomatic.
- There is bleeding from local ulceration because of acid secretion by the ectopic gastric mucosa in the diverticulum.
- Intestinal obstruction is caused by an associated band.
- Meckel's diverticulitis resembles appendicitis, except pain is usually localized to the *left* iliac fossa.

### Investigation

- Half of cases have ectopic gastric mucosa present, which can be demonstrated by an isotope scan ($^{99}$Tc pertechnetate).
- CT or barium studies
- Diagnostic laryngoscopy

### Management

If symptomatic, treatment is surgical resection.

## SMALL INTESTINAL NEOPLASMS

Neoplasms of the small intestine are very rare. Most are lymphomas (B- or T-cell origin) or adenocarcinomas.

### Clinical features

- CD a risk factor
- Symptoms often vague (malaise, anorexia, diarrhoea, weight loss)
- Investigations usually negative
- Mass often not palpable
- Bleeding, obstruction or perforation

### Complications

- Bleeding
- Obstruction
- Perforation

### Investigation

- *CT, MRI or barium studies:* may show non-specific ulceration, stricturing or mass lesions
- *Enteroscopy with biopsy:* may be possible
- *Laparotomy:* diagnosis and staging

### Management

- Surgical resection
- Chemotherapy and radiotherapy are alternatives

### Prognosis

Prognosis is poor: 5-year survival is 20%.

## IMMUNODEFICIENCY SYNDROMES

### Primary immunodeficiency syndromes

Selective IgA deficiency is the least rare (1 in 700) (**Table 10.20**).

**Table 10.20** Primary immunodeficiency disorders and their GI manifestations

| Immune deficiency | GI manifestations |
|---|---|
| **B-cell defects** | |
| Selective IgA deficiency | Diarrhoea, villous atrophy, giardiasis |
| Common variable acquired immunoglobulin deficiency | Diarrhoea, IBD-like, giardiasis, hepatitis |
| **T-cell defects** | |
| DiGeorge's syndrome (congenital thymic hypoplasia) | Candidiasis |
| **Combined defects** | |
| Wiskott–Aldrich syndrome | Colitis, malabsorption |
| Severe combined immunodeficiency | Diarrhoea, oral candida, IBD-like |

### Secondary immunodeficiency syndromes

AIDS is the most important example. GI effects include:

- *Oesophagus: Candida*, cytomegalovirus, herpes simplex infection
- *Small and large intestines: Cryptosporidia, Giardia, Entamoeba histolytica, Microsporidia, Mycobacterium, Campylobacter, Salmonella*
- *Anus and rectum:* gonorrhoea, syphilis, *Chlamydia*, cytomegalovirus and herpes simplex infections
- *Throughout the bowel:* Kaposi's sarcoma and non-Hodgkin's lymphoma

## FOOD ALLERGY AND INTOLERANCE

Adverse reactions to foods are common (**Table 10.21**); true food allergy is rare but can be life-threatening.

Of patients reporting reactions to food, wheat is the commonest culprit. A small proportion will have CD, the majority have non-immune-based intolerance, perhaps related to the high fibre content of wholegrains.

Reactions to dairy may be non-allergic (e.g. lactose intolerance) or immune-based (mostly in children).

Two main types of true allergic reactions to food occur:

- *Type I immediate hypersensitivity reactions:*
  - Can be triggered by small quantities of antigen (e.g. nuts, shellfish)
  - Symptoms within minutes to hours:
    - *GI:* swelling of the lips, vomiting, diarrhoea, abdominal pain
    - *Systemic:* rhinorrhoea, urticaria, angioedema, migraine, bronchospasm, eczema, anaphylaxis, cardiac arrest

**Table 10.21** Classification of adverse reactions to food

**Intolerance of fermentable fibres and sugars**
e.g. wheat, some vegetables

**Pharmacological**
Tyramine (cheese and wine); caffeine; histamine (mackerel)

**Toxic**
e.g. glutamates (Chinese food); acetanilide (rapeseed oil); sulphites (preservative added to some food and wine)

**Irritant**
Alcohol, very hot or cold drinks, some spices

**Enzyme deficiencies**
Disaccharidase deficiency

**Immunological-based reactions (true food allergy)**
Type I and II hypersensitivity
CD

**Psychological**
Reactions to specific foods due to patient beliefs, would not occur in blinded trial

**Psychiatric conditions**
Global avoidance of/reactions to foods (e.g. AN, bulimia)

- - *Diagnostics:* blood tests (elevated serum IgE; positive radio allergosorbent [RAST] test); skin-prick tests
  - *Self-management:* avoidance of the incriminated food; IM adrenaline (e.g. EpiPen®)
  - *Hospital management:* with ABC assessment, adrenaline, antihistamines, corticosteroids, IV fluids; intubation and ITU care may be required
- *Type II delayed hypersensitivity reactions:*
  - Cow's milk protein allergy in young children: symptoms include vomiting, diarrhoea, proctocolitis, failure to thrive, eczema, asthma
  - Egg, chicken, rice and soya proteins produce similar symptoms
  - No simple confirmatory tests; exclusion diets with re-challenge can be tried
  - *Treatment:* avoidance of implicated foods; oral disodium cromoglycate
  - *Desensitization:* cannot currently be recommended

## DISEASES OF THE LARGE INTESTINE

## COLORECTAL CARCINOMA

### Epidemiology

- Fourth most common cancer in the UK
- Most common in over 75-year-olds

### Pathology

- >90% adenocarcinomas
- 66% in rectosigmoid
- Spread is by direct invasion, to peritoneal cavity, lymphatic to local/distant nodes, or via portal vein to liver and lung
- Staging of resected tumour determines prognosis

### Clinical features

- IDA
- Change in bowel habit: diarrhoea, constipation or obstruction
- Rectal bleeding
- Weight loss
- Features of metastatic disease, e.g. jaundice or ascites

### Risk factors

- Adenomatous polyps
- FDRs, particularly if under 55 years old
- Poorly controlled IBD for >10 years
- Lifestyle: obesity, low dietary fibre
- Genetic: hereditary non-polyposis coli, familial polyposis coli.

### Genetics
*Sporadic colorectal carcinoma*

- Progression from normal mucosa →adenoma → carcinoma over a period of 8–10 years with serial mutations in growth regulating genes (**Figure 10.40**)

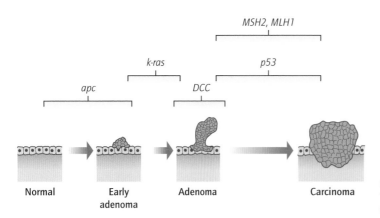

**Figure 10.39** The adenoma–carcinoma sequence for colonic neoplasia, showing the points at which associated gene mutations occur.

- Proto-oncogenes are activated (e.g. k-*ras* and c-*myc* oncogene)
- Tumour suppressor genes are inactivated

*Hereditary non-polyposis colon cancer syndrome (HNPCC) or Lynch syndrome*

- Autosomal dominant
- 2–3% of all colorectal carcinomas
- Usually occurs before the age of 50
- Lifetime colorectal carcinoma risk (usually right-sided) 80%
- Increased risk of other cancers, including endometrial, ovarian, upper GI, pancreatic, biliary, genitourinary and cerebral
- Caused by a mutation in DNA mismatch repair genes, one phenotypic result being development of DNA microsatellite instability

**Investigation**

- *FBC:* may be a microcytic anaemia
- *LFTs:* may be abnormal with hepatic metastases
- *Rectal examination:* essential to check for low rectal tumours
- *Colonoscopy* (**Figure 10.40**): biopsy of lesions; tattooing site to assist with location during surgical resection

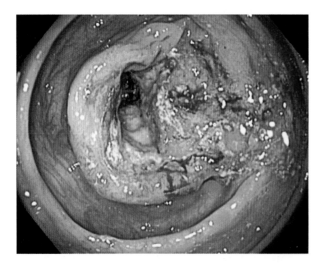

**Figure 10.40** Endoscopic view of colorectal cancer.

- If the patient is not fit for colonoscopy, CT colonography or unprepared CT are alternatives
- *Ultrasound and/or CT* (chest, abdomen and pelvis): to look for distant metastases

**Management**

MDT must discuss staging (**Table 10.22**) and treatment.

*Surgery*

- Endoscopic or transanal resection for potentially curable lesions (TNM stage I)
- Choice of surgery for more advanced tumours depends on site (**Figure 10.41**):
  o Low rectal: abdominoperineal resection
  o High rectal: anterior resection
  o Left colon: left hemicolectomy
  o Right colon: right hemicolectomy
- Panproctocolectomy or total colectomy for multiple polyposis or chronic extensive ulcerative colitis
- Temporary defunctioning colostomy in obstructive or more invasive carcinoma
- Resection of solitary hepatic metastasis

*Chemotherapy*

- Adjuvant chemotherapy (such as 5-fluorouracil, capecitabine, irinotecan or oxaliplatin) following resection (TNM stage II)
- Current trials for neoadjuvant chemotherapy in TNM stage III disease

*Radiotherapy*

- Palliation
- Prior to surgery in rectal disease

*Other*

- Palliative stenting for obstructing lesions (**Figure 10.42**)
- Community palliative and supportive care for advanced disease

**Bowel cancer screening programmes**

In the UK, people aged 60–74 years are offered a home faecal immunochemical test for occult blood (FIT) every 2 years: 2% are positive and offered colonoscopy. Flexible sigmoidoscopy at age 55 is also offered in some regions.

**Table 10.22** Staging and prognosis of CRC: the TNM classification has largely superseded Dukes'

| TNM classification | Modified Dukes' staging | 5-year survival (%) |
|---|---|---|
| Stage 0: carcinoma *in situ* | | |
| Stage I: no nodes or metastases, tumour invades submucosa (T1, N0, M0); tumour invades muscularis propria (T2, N0, M0) | A | 90 |
| Stage II: no nodes or metastases (T3, N0, M0); tumour invades other organs (T4, N0, M0) | B | 80 |
| Stage III: regional lymph nodes involved (any T, N1, M0) | C | 30 |
| Stage IV: distant metastases | D | 5 |

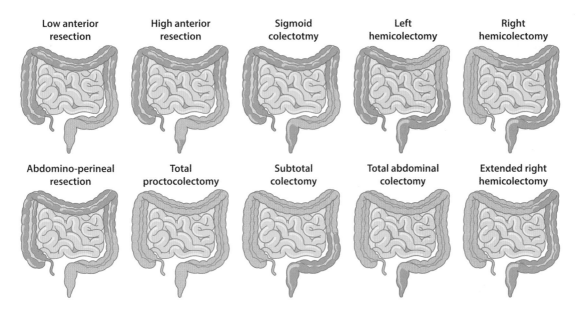

Low anterior resection · High anterior resection · Sigmoid colectotmy · Left hemicolectomy · Right hemicolectomy

Abdomino-perineal resection · Total proctocolectomy · Subtotal colectomy · Total abdominal colectomy · Extended right hemicolectomy

**Figure 10.41** Operations for colorectal cancer.

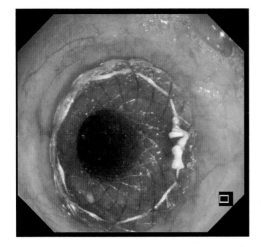

**Figure 10.42** Expanding metal stent placed to relieve malignant obstruction (in this case in the oesophagus, however the technology and endoscopic appearance is very similar in the colon).

Bowel cancer survival rates have doubled in the last 10 years due to better screening, early diagnosis and improved management.

In addition to the above screening programmes testing a whole population, certain groups identified as having above-average risk of colorectal carcinoma (CRC) should be offered planned colonoscopy at ages/intervals relevant to their risk (surveillance colonoscopy).

1 Premalignant polyps found during colonoscopy:
  2 or more polyps, at least one with high-risk features → one-off colonoscopy in 3 years
  5 or more polyps → one-off colonoscopy in 3 years
2 Following resection of colorectal cancer:
  → Colonoscopy at 1 and 3 years
3 FH of CRC:
  Moderate-risk FH (1 affected FDR <50, or 2 FDRs any age) → one-off colonoscopy at age 55
  High-risk FH (3 or more FDRs across >1 generation) → 5-yearly colonoscopy from age 40

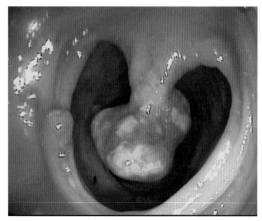

**(a)**

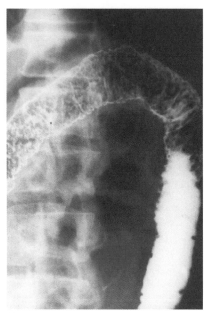

**(b)**

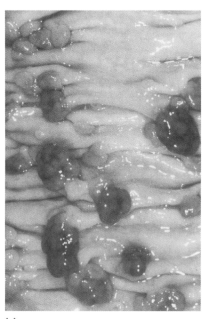

**(c)**

4 Genetic condition increasing CRC risk:
Lynch syndrome: recommendations vary by genetic testing, typical example → colonoscopy 2-yearly from age 25 to 75
Familial adenomatous polyposis (FAP) → colonoscopy 1–3-yearly from age 12
5 Long-standing IBD:
→ Commences after 8 years, then 1–5-yearly depending on extent and activity of disease and considerations such as FH of CRC. (Patients with IBD and primary sclerosing cholangitis are at particularly high risk and offered yearly surveillance from date of diagnosis)

## COLONIC POLYPS

Colonic polyps are tumours that project into the lumen of the colon (**Figure 10.43a**).

- *Neoplastic* (two-thirds of all polyps): These are usually adenomas, benign, but can transform into carcinoma.
- *Non-neoplastic* (one-third of all polyps): Most common are metaplastic rectal polyps, usually multiple and small (<5 mm). Others include inflammatory polyps seen in IBD and hamartomas, common in Peutz–Jeghers syndrome.

## ADENOMAS

### Epidemiology

Adenomas are common, occurring in 30–40% of people >60 years.

### Disease mechanisms

Adenomas may be single, multiple or part of a polyposis syndrome (**Table 10.23**).

Risk of malignant transformation is increased by:

- Older age
- Size (the most important factor, with risk of finding a cancer being 1% in an adenoma <1 cm, 1%, rising to 20–50% in adenomas >2 cm)
- Villous rather than tubular histological type
- Presence of severe dysplasia

### Clinical features

- Usually, asymptomatic
- Change in bowel habit
- Bleeding per rectum
- Mucous stools
- Rarely hypokalaemia or protein-losing enteropathy

**Figure 10.43** Colonic polyps. **(a)** Example of a large pedunculated adenomatous colonic polyp, with its stalk attached to the lumen at the 12 o'clock position: note the smaller flat (sessile) polyp on the mucosa at the 9 o'clock position. **(b,c)** Typical appearances of multiple colonic polyps in FAP syndrome. Images **(b)** and **(c)** reproduced from Misiewicz JJ *et al.* (1994) *Diseases of the Gut and Pancreas*, 2nd edn (Wiley-Blackwell, Oxford), with the permission of the authors.

**Table 10.23** Multiple adenomatous polyposis syndromes (all are premalignant)

| Syndrome | Associated clinical features |
|---|---|
| Familial polyposis coli | Polyps in stomach and small bowel |
| Gardner's syndrome | Osteomas, epidermoid cysts, soft tissue tumours, congenital hypertrophy of retinal pigment epithelium |
| Turcot's syndrome | Glioblastomas or medulloblastoma |

## Investigation

Colonoscopy is most sensitive and allows for definitive treatment by polypectomy.

## Management

- Polypectomy should be carried out at the time of initial colonoscopy for small polyps.
- Larger polyps may need referral to a specialist endoscopy service or surgical resection.
- Surveillance for recurrence with colonoscopy is required depending on findings.

# FAMILIAL POLYPOSIS COLI/FAMILIAL ADENOMATOUS POLYPOSIS

In familial polyposis coli, hundreds to thousands of polyps grow in the colon and can also occur in the stomach and small bowel. Colonic cancer develops at an average age of 40 years. FAP is shown in **Figure 10.43b,c**.

## Epidemiology

- Rare
- Usually presents in early adulthood (20s)
- Autosomal dominant
- Mutation of APC gene (tumour suppressor gene) on chromosome 5

## Clinical features

- Rectal bleeding
- Weight loss
- Abdominal pain
- Bowel obstruction
- FH and picked up on screening programme
- Features of Gardner's syndrome (see **Table 10.23**)

## Investigation

- *Colonoscopy and biopsy*
- *OGD:* to detect/remove upper GI polyps
- *Small bowel enteroscopy:* for small bowel polyps

## Management

- Early colectomy is required to prevent malignant transformation
- Gastroscopy and small bowel surveillance

- Colonoscopic screening of family members
- Research into genetic testing in progress

# DIVERTICULAR DISEASE (COLONIC DIVERTICULOSIS)

In diverticular disease, there is mucosal and submucosal herniation through the bowel wall at points of weakness where blood vessels enter (**Figure 10.44**). It commonly affects the sigmoid colon.

## Epidemiology

- Common
- Increased prevalence with age, affects approximately 50% of those >70 years old
- More common in women

## Clinical features

- Often asymptomatic
- Altered bowel habit
- Abdominal pain

### Complications
- Bleeding
- Infection (diverticulitis)
- Abscess
- Stricturing
- Perforation
- Fistulation

## Investigation

See **Figure 10.44**.
- *Bloods:* raised neutrophils and CRP in diverticulitis
- *Colonoscopy:* will detect colonic diverticula and allow biopsies of any associated stricture; risk of perforation is higher
- *Imaging:* CT colonography an alternative, and better for assessing complications of abscess and fistulation

## Management

- High-fibre diet
- Antispasmodics (mebeverine, buscopan)
- Acute diverticulitis is treated with fluids and antibiotics
- Localized perforation often managed with antibiotics ± drainage
- Surgical resection for serious complications (e.g. uncontrolled bleeding, fistula, perforation with generalized peritonitis)

# INFLAMMATORY BOWEL DISEASE

There are two main types of IBD: ulcerative colitis and Crohn's disease. These are described separately below.

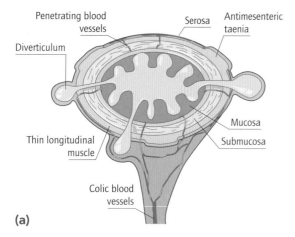

**(a)**

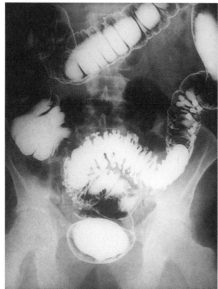

**(b)**

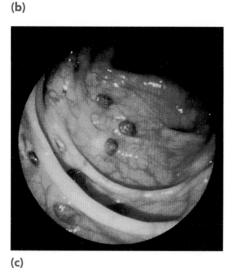

**(c)**

**Figure 10.44** Diverticular disease. **(a)** Colonic diverticula. Diagram showing the appearance of colonic diverticula. Note protrusion of the diverticula close to the blood vessels. **(b)** Barium enema showing multiple diverticula throughout the colon. **(c)** Colonoscopic view showing multiple diverticula in sigmoid colon. Reproduced from *Slide Atlas of Gastrointestinal Endoscopy* with the kind permission of the author and Times Mirror International Publishers.

### IBD and pregnancy/breastfeeding

Pregnancy outcomes are unchanged in quiescent IBD. However, there is higher risk of spontaneous abortion, premature delivery and stillbirth rates with active disease.

Overall, corticosteroids and amino salicylates have no adverse effects on pregnancy or breastfeeding.

Azathioprine is theoretically contraindicated in pregnancy although the outcome is usually satisfactory. They are not usually stopped.

Biological therapy should be discussed with the patient. Careful planning is required (e.g. infliximab should not be given in the third trimester).

## ULCERATIVE COLITIS

### Epidemiology

- More common in developed countries, prevalence is approximately 70 in 100 000
- Annual incidence about 5 per 100 000; peaks at age 20–40
- 10% risk for either UC or CD in FDRs
- 66% of HLA-B27 positive individuals with UC have associated ankylosing spondylitis

### Pathology

- Colitis begins in the rectum and spreads proximally.
- Mucosa shows hyperaemia, granularity, surface mucous and blood.
- As it heals, post-inflammatory polyps can form.

### Clinical features

- Disease activity relapses and remits over time.
- Triggers for relapse include emotional stress, infection, drugs (NSAIDs) and discontinuation of treatment.
- Symptoms vary according to the extent and intensity of mucosal inflammation (**Figure 10.45**):
  - *Proctitis:* There is rectal bleeding and mucous discharge, sometimes tenesmus and pruritus ani, and the stool is usually well formed. Well-being is maintained.
  - *Proctosigmoiditis:* Symptoms included rectal bleeding and mucus discharge accompanied by diarrhoea, urgency and sometimes abdominal pain. There may be malaise. Examination is usually normal.
  - *Extensive colitis:* There is profuse frequent diarrhoea with blood and mucus, fever, malaise, anorexia and weight loss, sometimes with extraintestinal manifestations. Often, the patient is systemically unwell with pyrexia and tachycardia.

### Complications

- *IDA* is common.
- *Carcinoma:* Incidence is increased in extensive disease >10 years; cumulative risk is about 20% at 30 years.

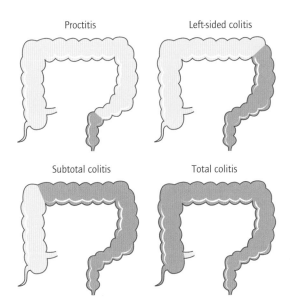

**Figure 10.45** Distribution of large intestinal involvement in ulcerative colitis.

- *Massive haemorrhage:* This will require urgent colectomy.
- *Extraintestinal manifestations:* These occur in both UC and CD (see IBD: EXTRAINTESTINAL MANIFESTATIONS AT A GLANCE).
- *Toxic megacolon:* Inflammation spreads to the muscularis mucosa and the colon dilates and may perforate. The patient deteriorates with tachycardia, fever and pain. The abdomen is distended and tender and there are no bowel sounds. Diagnosis is confirmed on abdominal radiography. Colectomy is usually required.
- *Colonic perforation:* This can occur with or without toxic megacolon; note steroids can mask the signs of peritonitis.

### Investigation

#### Bloods
- Markers of severity are IDA, high platelets, high CRP, low albumin

#### Microbiology
- *Stool microscopy and culture:* to exclude infective trigger
- *Calprotectin:* a stool marker of gut mucosal inflammation, like CRP, non-specific, but in known cases of UC a non-invasive way to assess total disease activity

#### Imaging
- *Colonoscopy/sigmoidoscopy with biopsy:* the main diagnostic modality (**Figure 10.46**) (avoid in acute severe disease, if possible, as increased risk of perforation)
- *Plain abdominal radiography:* used in hospitalized cases with severe disease to monitor for toxic megacolon (colonic dilatation)

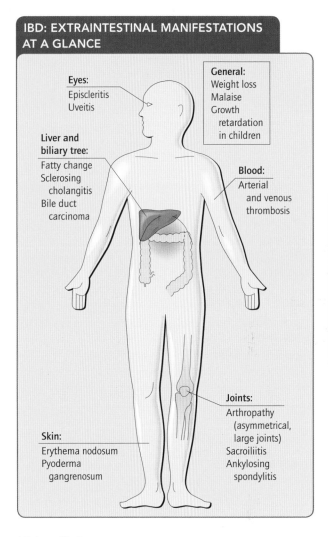

- **IBD: EXTRAINTESTINAL MANIFESTATIONS AT A GLANCE**

**Eyes:**
Episcleritis
Uveitis

**General:**
Weight loss
Malaise
Growth retardation in children

**Liver and biliary tree:**
Fatty change
Sclerosing cholangitis
Bile duct carcinoma

**Blood:**
Arterial and venous thrombosis

**Skin:**
Erythema nodosum
Pyoderma gangrenosum

**Joints:**
Arthropathy (asymmetrical, large joints)
Sacroiliitis
Ankylosing spondylitis

### Histopathology
- *Biopsy:* epithelial ulceration, acute and chronic inflammatory cell infiltration in lamina propria, crypt abscesses, goblet cell depletion, crypt atrophy; be aware of dysplasia: it is pre-cancerous

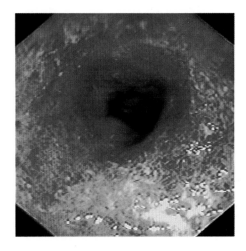

**Figure 10.46** Colonoscopic view of moderately severe UC, showing diffuse mucosal bleeding, oedema, granularity and ulceration.

**Table 10.24** Drugs commonly used in ulcerative colitis

| | Corticosteroids | Amino salicylates | Thiopurines |
|---|---|---|---|
| Example | Prednisolone | Mesalazine (asacol, pentasa, octasa) | Azathioprine |
| Formulations | Oral<br>Intravenous<br>Enema, suppository | Oral<br>Enema, suppository | Oral |
| Mechanism of action | Anti-inflammatory | Anti-inflammatory | Immunosuppressive |
| Indications | Active flare of IBD, avoid long-term use | Active and inactive UC: first-line maintenance therapy | Refractory IBD |
| Side effects | Facial mooning, diabetes, hypertension, hypokalaemia, osteoporosis, psychosis, myopathy | Rash, headache, diarrhoea, interstitial nephritis (all rare) | Nausea, rash, headache, bone marrow depression, pancreatitis, hepatitis |
| Contraindications | Uncontrolled diabetes or hypertension | Salicylate sensitivity | Sepsis, TB, viral hepatitis, skin cancer |
| Monitoring | Blood pressure, blood sugar, bone density | Serum urea and creatinine | FBC, LFTs |

## Management

### Supportive treatment

- Nutritional support from dietician
- Long-term specialist follow up in secondary care
- National Association for Colitis and Crohn's Disease (UK) and online information (e.g. https://www.crohnsandcolitis.org.uk/)

### Treatment

The aim of treatment is to induce and maintain remission of disease activity (**Table 10.24**).

*Immunosuppressive therapy*

- Examples include azathioprine and 6-mercaptopurine.
- Immunosuppressant drugs are reserved for those unresponsive to oral therapy or unable to wean off steroids. It can take weeks to months for the full benefits to be felt.
- Immunosuppressants increase the risk of infections and certain cancers. Patients are usually supported and monitored by IBD specialist nurses.

*Biological therapy*

Biological agents have transformed management of severe IBD. All agents down-regulate the inflammatory processes. Side effects include risk of infection and induction of autoimmune events including neurological. Antibodies may develop to these drugs, reducing or stopping the benefit: co-prescription of immunosuppressives can prevent such antibody formation. Assays are available to measure serum biological and anti-drug antibody levels to help guide treatment. Cost is a major issue (in the order of £10 000 a year, over 10 times more than conventional therapies), and healthcare guidance typically follows a step-up approach, with biological drugs only being sanctioned when conventional therapies have failed. However, given longer-term savings (e.g. associated with fewer hospital admissions, reduced risk of surgery), for some high-risk IBD cases biological therapies may be recommended as an initial treatment. Generic competitors (called biosimilars) are now entering the market with significantly reduced costs.

- Screening is necessary prior to receiving biologics (TB [quanteferon and chest X-ray], varacella zoster IgG, hepatitis B and C, HIV).
- FBC, renal and liver function should be monitored at least 3-monthly.
- Examples:
  o *Infliximab*: This is an anti-TNF agent, often first-line rescue in acute severe colitis, given by 2-weekly subcutaneous injection or IV infusion. Continued infusions may be needed every 8 weeks depending on response.
  o *Adalimumab*: This is an anti-TNF therapy injected subcutaneously. It can be stored and administered by the patient at home.
  o *Vedolizumab*: This is a gut-selective integrin blocker; fewer systemic side effects. It is administered intravenously.
  o *Ustekinumab*: Recently approved for IBD if unresponsive to oral and anti-TNF therapies, this is an anti-interlukin agent. The first infusion is IV followed by subcutaneous injections.
  o *Tofacitinib*: This is a JAK (Janus kinase) inhibitor, given orally twice daily. It is a small molecule thus less likely for drug antibodies to develop.

The treatment of UC and associated complications are summarized in **Table 10.25**.

*Surgery*

- A minority of patients require total colectomy. Elective surgery may be indicated for chronic intractable UC or colon carcinoma.
- Emergency surgery can be required in toxic megacolon, perforation, acute severe colitis unresponsive to treatment, or massive haemorrhage.

**Table 10.25** Treatment of ulcerative colitis and associated complications

| | Treatment | |
| --- | --- | --- |
| | Supportive | Specific |
| **Clinical features** | | |
| Proctitis | Treat constipation with a high-fibre diet and/or lactulose | Amino salicylate orally or rectally (enemas or suppositories) and short-term rectal corticosteroid |
| Left-sided colitis: mild–moderate attack – systemically well with less than six stools daily | Treat anaemia | Amino salicylate and prednisolone 40 mg orally and corticosteroid enemas daily, as outpatient<br>Prednisolone is reduced weekly as remission is achieved<br>Amino salicylate is continued indefinitely |
| More extensive colitis: severe – unwell, tachycardia, pyrexia with more than six bloody diarrhoeal stools daily | Hospital admission with close observation by physician and surgeon<br>IV fluids and monitor electrolytes<br>Prophylactic subcutaneous heparin | IV hydrocortisone with calcium for bone protection, oral amino salicylate<br>Surgery or IV biological therapy (e.g. infliximab) if no response in 5–7 days |
| **Complications** | | |
| Toxic megacolon | IV fluids, nasogastric suction | Medical treatment as for severe UC<br>If no improvement in 12–24 hours, colectomy |
| Colonic perforation | Antibiotics, IV fluids | Immediate colectomy |

10

- Preoperative counselling about ileostomy and advice from stoma care specialist nurses is mandatory.
- Surgical options include:
  o Panproctocolectomy with ileostomy: required for all patients on high-dose steroids prior to surgery; the option of stoma reversal can be discussed later
  o Panproctocolectomy with ileoanal pouch
  o Colectomy with ileorectal anastomosis

*Preventive treatment*
Surveillance colonoscopy is important to exclude dysplasia in those with UC over 8 years, as there is increased risk of bowel carcinoma. Follow up every 1-3 years depending on extent, activity (based on histology) and duration of the disease.

## CROHN'S DISEASE

### Pathology

- Crohn's disease can affect any part of the gut from the mouth to the anus, although in contrast to UC the rectum is typically unaffected. Common patterns are perianal; distal ileum/right colon; colon only; small bowel only.
- Affected gut segments are discontinuous (skip lesions).
- The cause is unknown but is likely to be a combination of genetic and environmental factors.

### Epidemiology

- Prevalence is 50–100 per 100 000 people
- Peak incidence around 15–30 years age range
- More common in White people and Jewish people of European descent
- Increased prevalence in FDRs (10%)

### Clinical features

- History of remission and exacerbations
- Diarrhoea ± bloody stool
- Weight loss and nutritional deficiencies
- Abdominal pain ± obstructive symptoms
- *Examination:* may show features of malabsorption, perianal disease (skin tags, fissures, fistulae, abscesses), abdominal mass and/or clubbing, abdominal mass

*Local complications*
- *Anal fissure, fistula and abscess:* common
- *Strictures:* obstructive symptoms, or malabsorption caused by proximal SIBO
- *Perforation*
- *Abscess and fistula:* form close to inflamed bowel and can discharge through fistulae into the skin, gut, bladder or vagina
- *Haemorrhage:* usually minor and recurrent from inflamed mucosa, contributes to anaemia
- Slightly increased incidence of small bowel and colorectal carcinoma
- *Extraintestinal manifestations:* occur in both CD and UC (see IBD: EXTRAINTESTINAL MANIFESTATIONS AT A GLANCE)

### Investigation

#### Bloods

- *Markers of severity:* include raised CRP and platelet count, low albumin
- *Iron, folate and vitamin B₁₂ deficiencies:* malabsorption or TI disease

#### Microbiology

- *Stool microscopy and culture:* exclude infection
- *Calprotectin:* a stool marker of gut mucosal inflammation, like CRP, non-specific, but in known cases of CD a non-invasive way to assess total disease activity

#### Diagnostic imaging

- *Colonoscopy/sigmoidoscopy* (**Figure 10.47**): useful for defining the extent of disease and distinguishing from UC (avoid if possible, during acute flare – risk of perforation
- *Ultrasound and CT scan:* detect inflamed bowel distribution and complications (e.g. abscess)
- *MRI:* gold standard imaging for small bowel disease and assessing fistulating CD

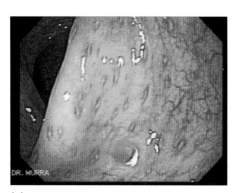

**(a)**

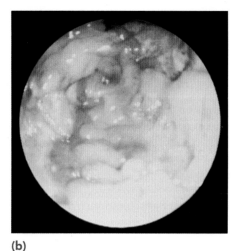

**(b)**

**Figure 10.47** Colonoscopic appearance of active Crohn's disease. **(a)** Mild colonic disease with aphthous ulceration. © 2000–2019 Gastrointestinalatlas.com. **(b)** Severe colonic disease with diffuse ulceration and cobblestoning. Reproduced from *Slide Atlas of Gastroenterology* with the kind permission of the author and Times Mirror International Publishers.

- *Small bowel wireless capsule endoscopy:* used in combination with MR to assess activity of small bowel Crohn's; small bowel stricture must be excluded pre-test

#### Histopathology

*Biopsy* can show transmural and patchy chronic inflammation with ulceration; micro abscesses; pathognomonic non-caseating granulomas. Aphthoid ulceration progresses to deep fissuring ulcers with cobblestoning, fibrosis, stricturing and fistulation (**Figure 10.47**).

#### Management

Treatment is aimed at inducing and maintaining remission (**Table 10.26**). As with UC, this starts with supportive explanation, nutritional guidance, specialist input and contact with the IBD team.

## IRRITABLE BOWEL SYNDROME

### Epidemiology

- Prevalence up to 20% adult population, with more likely undiagnosed
- Peak age of presentation 20–30 years
- More common in women (2 : 1)

### Disease mechanisms

- The cause is unknown. Possible aetiological factors include anxiety, food intolerances or triggered by acute GI infection.
- Abdominal pain is associated with abnormal intestinal motility and visceral hypersensitivity.
- Intestinal transit times are reduced in IBS-diarrhoea and increased in IBS-constipation.

### Clinical features: Rome IV criteria

- Abdominal pain for at least 1 day a week over 3 months
- Pain relieved by defaecation
- Associated with change in stool frequency or form (appearance) without red flag signs
- Symptoms persistent for at least 6 months
- *Other associated symptoms:*
  - Bloating, passing mucous, symptoms worse with eating or altered stool passage (e.g. incomplete evacuation, straining or urgency)
  - Lethargy, anxiety and depression, nausea, dyspepsia, headaches, dyspareurina and urinary symptoms
  - Associated with fibromyalgia in 20–50%, also chronic pain syndromes and chronic fatigue

### Investigation

- *Bloods:* FBC, ESR or CRP, antibodies for CD; consider TFTs and HbA₁C
- *Stool:* faecal calprotectin to exclude IBD; consider MC+S, ova, cysts and parasites

**Table 10.26** Treatment of Crohn's disease

| | Treatment | |
|---|---|---|
| | Supportive | Specific |
| **Clinical features** | | |
| Mild–moderate attack | Treat anaemia (iron, folate) if necessary | Prednisolone orally, as an outpatient, tailed off with remission |
| | | Consider azathioprine (2 mg/kg) if TPMT level normal |
| Severe attack | Hospital admission | IV hydrocortisone with bone protection |
| | Close observation by physician and surgeon | Oral azathioprine (optimal therapy takes 3 months) |
| | IV fluids and electrolytes | |
| | Prophylactic heparin | |
| Refractory Crohn's disease | | If refractory to/dependent on corticosteroids, and unresponsive or intolerant to immunosuppressives, consider biologics or surgery |
| **Complications** | | |
| Intra-abdominal abscesses, fistula | Nutritional support, prophylactic heparin, antibiotics | Surgical drainage/resection |
| Perianal disease | Local hygiene | Metronidazole/ciprofloxacin or azathioprine |
| | Salt baths | Abscesses require surgical drainage |
| | | Strictures may need dilatation |
| Stricture | IV fluids if total obstruction; low-residue diet if subacute | Obstructive episodes may settle with medical treatment (corticosteroids or liquid formula diet) |
| | Nutritional support essential | Surgery (resection or strictureplasty) often necessary |
| | Prophylactic subcutaneous heparin | |

- *Imaging:* not always required if bloods and faecal calprotectin are normal with a diagnostic history for IBS
- *Flexible sigmoidoscopy or colonoscopy:* particularly if >50 years, to exclude cancer, IBD and microscopic colitis

## Management

### Specific treatment

- *Lifestyle:*
  - Routine meals and increase exercise
  - Address stressful factors
- *Diet:*
  - Limit alcohol and caffeine; herbal teas may help (e.g. peppermint – an antispasmodic)
  - Low FODMAP diet: reduces intake of fermentable carbohydrates that contribute to bloating and discomfort
- *Drugs:*
  - *Pain predominant*: antispasmodics; low-dose tricyclics for resistant cases
  - *Diarrhoeal predominant:* antidiarrhoeals (e.g. loperamide)
  - *Constipation predominant:* bulk forming agents, laxatives (e.g. fybogel)
- *Other:* psychological therapies such as CBT and hypnotherapy may be beneficial in refractory IBS

### Prognosis

- There is a significant impact on quality of life, but no change in mortality.
- Around two-thirds of patients are asymptomatic at 5 years.

## NEUROENDOCRINE TUMOURS

Neuroendocrine tumours (APUDomas) are slow-growing and difficult to diagnose. Carcinoids are the least rare subtype.

## CARCINOID TUMOURS

- These are neuroendocrine tumours that secrete kinins, histamine, PGs and serotonin which are inactivated by the liver.
- They are most commonly found in small bowel and appendix.
- 95% have hepatic metastases. Hormones produced then bypass the liver leading to carcinoid syndrome.
- Carcinoid tumours can occur throughout the GI tract, as well as the lung, testis and ovary.

### Epidemiology

Prevalence is around 1–2 in 100 000.

**Table 10.27** Neuroendocrine tumours

| Tumour/pathology | Clinical features | Diagnostic factor |
|---|---|---|
| Gastrinoma (Zollinger–Ellison syndrome) Gastrin secretion leads to acid hypersecretion<br><br>About 25% have multiple endocrine neoplasia (MEN) type I | Dyspepsia, peptic ulceration, diarrhoea, steatorrhoea | *Serum gastrin:* fasting hypergastrinaemia >1000 pg/mL (normal <100 pg/mL) |
| Insulinoma VIPoma (Verner–Morrison syndrome) | Hypoglycaemia, neuropsychiatric Watery diarrhoea, hypokalaemia, achlorhydria | Whipples triad: 1. hypoglyaemia 2. neuroglycopenic symptoms 3. relief of symptoms after administeriing glucose. OR |
| | | biochemical tests (insulin, proinsulin, c-peptide) following prolonged fast (72 hours) |
| Arise in pancreatic islet D cells or, rarely, in duodenum or gastric antrum | | Vasoactive intestinal polypeptide (VIP) |
| Thyroid medullary carcinoma | Diarrhoea, flushing, local invasion | Calcitonin |

## Clinical features

- Flushing and facial telangiectasia
- Diarrhoea and urgency
- Wheezing
- Endocardial fibrosis (valve dysfunction with right ventricular hypertrophy and failure)
- Hepatomegaly

## Investigation

- *24-hour urinary excretion of 5-HIAA:* increased
- *LFTs:* hepatic metastases
- *Chest radiography, ultrasound, CT scan or MRI:* to localize primary and detect metastases
- *Radioisotope scanning (Octreoscan):* using radiolabelled octreotide or [131]I-meta-iodobenzyl guanidine ([131]I-MIBG) can locate and stage neuroendocrine tumours

## Management

- *Medication:* somatostatin derivatives (e.g. octreotide, lanreotide) or interferon alpha
- *Surgery:* only curative option, only in early stages of disease
- *Partial hepatectomy, arterial ligation or embolization:* can help symptoms in metastatic disease

## Prognosis

- Slow-growing despite metastases
- 40% survival at 5 years and 15% at 10 years

## OTHER NEUROENDOCRINE TUMOURS

All of these are very rare (**Table 10.27**).

### MUST-KNOW CHECKLIST

- Differential diagnosis and investigation of dyspepsia
- Medical treatment of peptic ulceration
- Investigation of dysphagia
- Assessment of nutritional status
- Causes and management of GI bleeding
- Investigation of IDA
- Investigation and management of diarrhoea
- Positive diagnosis of IBS
- Medical treatment of IBD
- Whom to screen for colon cancer

**Questions and answers** to test your understanding of Chapter 10 can be found by clicking 'Support Material' at the following link: https://www.routledge.com/Medicine-for-Finals-and-Beyond/Axford-OCallaghan/p/book/9780367150594

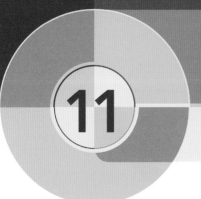

# Diabetes Mellitus, Obesity, Lipoprotein Disorders and other Metabolic Diseases

## 11

KEVIN BAYNES

# STRUCTURE AND FUNCTION

## INTERMEDIARY METABOLISM

### CONTROL OF GLUCOSE METABOLISM

#### Glucose production

Approximately 200 g of glucose is produced and used each day, but blood glucose levels are tightly regulated in health within the range of 3.5–8.0 mmol/L. The brain is an obligate consumer of glucose and uses approximately 100 g/day. After an overnight fast, peripheral tissues such as the brain, kidney and intestine are using glucose but, in contrast, skeletal muscle uses little glucose in the fasting state and derives most of its energy from fatty acid oxidation.

Total body glucose production is mostly hepatic: *glycogenolysis* (breakdown of glycogen to glucose) and *gluconeogenesis* (production of glucose from other molecules). Renal gluconeogenesis makes a small (5–10%) contribution to total daily glucose production.

#### Substrate supply when fasting

Liver glycogen is the major body store of carbohydrate for rapid release as glucose. Hormonal control of hepatic glycogenolysis = insulin, glucagon, catecholamines and cortisol. During fasting, insulin levels are low and glucagon levels are high, which stimulates glycogenolysis. Gluconeogenesis occurs using the gluconeogenic substrates alanine, glutamine, pyruvate, lactate and glycerol (**Figure 11.1**). Amino acids released by proteolysis are the major source of gluconeogenic substrates.

During prolonged fasting, lipolysis in adipose tissue releases fatty acids, which are increasingly used as a fuel supply. In the liver, fatty acids are converted into the ketone bodies acetoacetate and 3-hydroxybutyrate, which can be used by peripheral tissues including the brain. Insulin decreases ketone body production by the liver and glucagon increases ketone body production by the liver.

#### Postprandial changes

After feeding, blood glucose concentration rises because of absorption of carbohydrate from the intestine. To prevent an excessive blood glucose concentration, hepatic gluconeogenesis is inhibited, and glucose is taken up by peripheral tissues. The rise in blood glucose stimulates insulin release and inhibits glucagon release from the pancreas, thus altering the ratio of these antagonistic hormones. The incretin hormones glucagon-like peptide 1 (GLP-1) and glucose-dependent insulinotrophic polypeptide (GIP) are released from the gut after eating and increase insulin release.

- In the liver, insulin triggers a change from glucose production to glucose storage.
    - Insulin suppresses liver gluconeogenesis by inhibition of glycogen phosphorylasen (glucose itself inhibits this enzyme allosterically).
    - Insulin stimulates glycogen synthase to convert glucose to glycogen. Glucose is also used as a source of glycerol-3-phosphate for triglyceride synthesis.
- In skeletal muscle, insulin stimulates glucose uptake and increases the activity of muscle glycogen

DOI: 10.1201/9781003193616-11

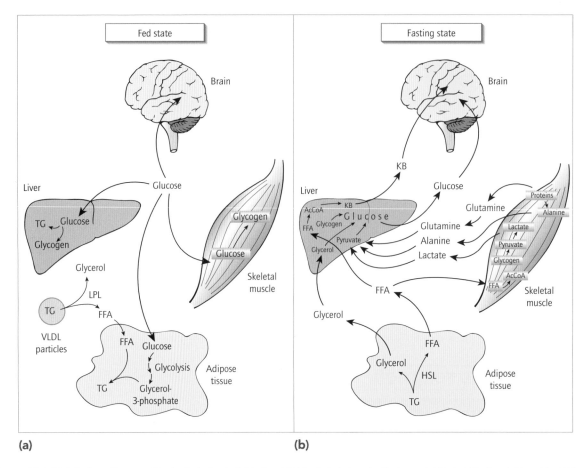

**Figure 11.1** Metabolic pathways of fuel substrates in **(a)** fed and **(b)** fasted states. Ac CoA, acetyl CoA; FFA, free fatty acids; HSL, hormone-sensitive lipase; LPL, lipoprotein lipase; KB, ketone bodies; TG, triglyceride; VLDL, very low-density lipoprotein.

synthase. After a meal, skeletal muscle absorbs more glucose than adipose tissue.

- In adipose tissue, insulin increases glucose uptake and suppresses lipolysis by inhibiting hormone-sensitive lipase. This suppression of lipolysis by insulin removes the supply of glycerol as a precursor for liver gluconeogenesis.

## CATECHOLAMINES AND CORTISOL

*Catecholamines* directly stimulate glycolysis in the liver. Catecholamines also stimulate lipolysis in adipose tissue, increasing the supply of fatty acids and glycerol to the liver where oxidation of fatty acids increases the supply of citrate, increasing hepatic gluconeogenesis. Glycerol is used as a substrate for gluconeogenesis.

*Cortisol* increases both proteolysis and lipolysis, thus increasing the supply of gluconeogenic substrates to the liver. Cortisol also reduces the sensitivity of tissues to insulin (insulin resistance), making the same amount of insulin less effective in controlling blood glucose concentrations.

A clinical consequence of these metabolic responses is that, in stress situations (e.g. sepsis or trauma), the increased release of corticosteroids and catecholamines may result in hyperglycaemia.

## METABOLIC DISEASES AND THEIR MANAGEMENT

### DIABETES MELLITUS

Diabetes mellitus (DM) is a cluster of conditions united by chronic hyperglycaemia (raised blood glucose). Untreated diabetes is characterized by excessive thirst ('polydipsia') and excessive urination ('polyuria'). DM is the most common endocrine disorder and has implications for both the individual and society. Morbidity and mortality are both increased in patients with DM because of macrovascular and microvascular complications (**Figure 11.2**). Life expectancy is reduced by ~15 years in type 1 DM and ~10 years in type 2 DM.

**Macrovascular complications**

- *Coronary artery disease:* angina, myocardial infarction, heart failure, arrhythmia

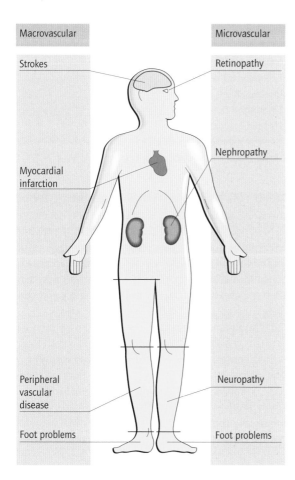

**Figure 11.2** Common macrovascular and microvascular complications of DM.

- *Peripheral vascular disease:* claudication, lower limb gangrene, amputation
- *Cerebrovascular disease:* stroke, transient ischaemic attack

### Microvascular complications

- *Retinopathy:* visual loss, blindness
- *Nephropathy:* chronic kidney disease, end-stage renal failure, nephrotic syndrome
- *Neuropathy:* affecting sensory, motor and autonomic nerves

## CLASSIFICATION AND TERMINOLOGY

### Type 1 diabetes mellitus

There is a loss of insulin-producing pancreatic islet β cells, resulting in absolute insulin deficiency. People with type 1 DM are prone to develop ketoacidosis and require insulin treatment for survival.

### Type 2 diabetes mellitus

This is relative insulin deficiency and/or insulin resistance, either of which may be predominant at the time of presentation. People with type 2 DM do not always require insulin for

**Table 11.1** Causes of secondary DM

**Iatrogenic**
- Corticosteroids
- Thiazide diuretics

**Endocrine**
- Cushing's syndrome
- Acromegaly
- Phaeochromocytoma
- Thyrotoxicosis

**Pancreatic disease**
- Cystic fibrosis related diabetes
- Chronic pancreatitis
- Haemochromatosis
- Pancreatectomy
- Fibrocalculous pancreatopathy
- Pancreatic carcinoma

survival but may be treated with insulin to improve symptoms of diabetes or for better metabolic control.

### Gestational diabetes mellitus

In this, glucose intolerance or diabetic hyperglycaemia develops during pregnancy. The condition usually resolves after the pregnancy, but not in all cases. Type 1 DM can present during pregnancy.

### Secondary forms of diabetes mellitus

If the specific cause of diabetes is known (e.g. post-pancreatectomy), it is classified under *secondary causes* or *other types of diabetes* (**Table 11.1**). Diabetes can arise in various endocrine disorders that should always be considered in a patient with newly diagnosed diabetes. Treatment of patients with secondary diabetes should be directed at the underlying disorder, as this may remove the cause of the hyperglycaemia.

### Genetic forms of diabetes

A number of gene mutations with a high penetrance and large effect on glucose metabolism can be thought of as monogenic forms of diabetes. The best described group is MODY ('maturity onset diabetes of the young'). These patients have a phenotype like type 2 diabetes (mild hyperglycaemia without ketosis) but are not obese and the onset of their diabetes is usually before the age of 25 years with autosomal dominant inheritance (**Table 11.2**).

**Table 11.2** Monogenic forms of DM

MODY (Maturity onset diabetes of the young)
  HNF 1-α
  HNF 4-α
  HNF 1-β
Glucokinase
Wolfram syndrome (DIDMOAD – Diabetes insipidus, DM, optic atrophy and deafness)
Neonatal diabetes
Alström syndrome

11

## DISEASE MECHANISMS

### Type 1 diabetes mellitus

Type 1 DM is almost always an autoimmune disease with selective destruction of the insulin-producing pancreatic β cells, leading to insulin deficiency (**Figure 11.3**). Evidence for this includes:

- Pancreatic tissue from patients shows infiltration of the islets by T cells ('insulitis') suggesting an autoimmune process.
- There is an association with various other autoimmune diseases, e.g. pernicious anaemia, coeliac disease, vitiligo, Graves' disease, Addison's disease.
- Autoantibodies are found in newly diagnosed patients, particularly against islets (islet cell antibodies [ICAs]) and glutamic acid decarboxylase (GAD), an enzyme found in pancreatic β cells.

Genome-wide searches for susceptibility genes for type 1 DM have revealed many chromosomal loci, some associated with the immune system. Those with the strongest effects are:

- Human leucocyte antigen (HLA) region on chromosome 6
- Insulin gene region on chromosome 11

### Type 2 diabetes mellitus

A large number of metabolic defects have been described in people with type 2 DM (**Table 11.3**). Obesity is a major risk factor and increases insulin resistance. In prospective studies, regular physical activity reduces type 2 DM risk. The effect is independent of any impact that exercise may have on body weight. Exercise increases whole body insulin sensitivity. There is an increased prevalence of type 2

**Table 11.3** Metabolic defects contributing to hyperglycaemia in type 2 DM

| |
|---|
| ↓ Insulin secretion |
| ↑ Glucagon secretion |
| ↓ Incretin effect |
| ↑ Lipolysis |
| ↑ Hepatic glucose output |
| ↓ Skeletal muscle glucose uptake |
| ↑ Renal glucose reabsorption |

DM in people born as low birth-weight babies. Poor foetal nutrition (caused by either poor placental development or lack of access to food by the mother during pregnancy) may result in defective pancreatic organogenesis *in utero*. Later in life, with increased demands on the pancreas from the insulin resistance of obesity, the pancreas may have a limited reserve; thus, relative insulin deficiency and clinical diabetes ensue.

Longitudinal studies suggest that insulin resistance can occur many years before the onset of clinical diabetes. However, the clinical onset of diabetes is associated with declining pancreatic release of insulin. Pancreatic tissue from people with type 2 DM shows infiltration with fibrils of amyloid.

Twin studies show concordance rates are greater in monozygotic than dizygotic twins suggesting that shared genes contribute to type 2 DM. Some populations have a very high prevalence of type 2 DM (e.g. Nauruans in the South Pacific, Pima Indians in the US). Genome-wide scans of populations with type 2 DM have shown many loci associated with diabetes, especially around genes that affect insulin secretion.

## EPIDEMIOLOGY

### Type 1 diabetes mellitus

- Children and adults under 30 years old with peak incidence 11–13 years of age, but may occur at any age
- Sex distribution equal
- Approximately 10% of adults with diabetes

### Type 2 diabetes mellitus

- Middle-aged or elderly adults; uncommon in children
- Sex distribution slight male excess (55% M : 45% F)
- Prevalence higher in South Asians and people of African ethnicity
- Higher prevalence in urban vs rural populations
- Obesity increases risk
- Prevalence increasing rapidly, probably due to obesity
- Approximately 90% of adults with diabetes

## CLINICAL PRESENTATION

DM should be *suspected* if:

- There are *symptoms* consistent with diabetes
- Blood tests demonstrate hyperglycaemia

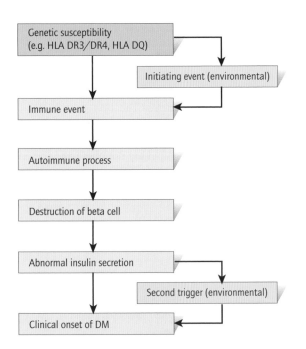

**Figure 11.3** Simplified representation of a possible mechanism for the development of type 1 DM.

## HISTORY 11.1

### Questions to ask a patient with diabetes

**Symptoms of hyperglycaemia**

Are you more tired than normal?
Do you feel abnormally thirsty?
Have you lost weight without trying to?
Is your eyesight blurred?

**Symptoms of ketoacidosis**

Are you feeling breathless?
Have you had sickness, vomiting or loss of appetite?

**Family history**

Does anyone in your family have diabetes?

**Past medical history**

Have you ever had pancreatitis?
Have you ever had heart problems, a stroke or circulation problems in your legs?

- Glycosuria is found on urinalysis
- A diabetes-associated complication is discovered
  See HISTORY 11.1 and HISTORY & EXAMINATION 11.2.

## Diabetes

Symptoms include:
- Thirst
- Polydipsia
- Dry mouth
- Polyuria
- Tiredness
- Blurred vision
- Unintentional weight loss

## HISTORY & EXAMINATION 11.2

**General appearance**

Does the breath smell of ketones?
Is the patient overweight or obese?
Are there features of secondary causes of diabetes (acromegaly, Cushing's syndrome, etc.)?
Are there skin changes – necrobiosis lipoidica, acanthosis nigricans?
Are there skin infections – abscesses and boils?

**Eyes**

Is there retinopathy?
Are there cataracts?

**Cardiovascular**

Are there bruits?

**Feet**

Are the peripheral pulses present?
Is sensation in the feet normal?
Are there foot ulcers?
Are there neuropathic changes?

**Urine**

Is there ketonuria?
Is there glycosuria?
Is there proteinuria?

If DKA is present, symptoms may include:
- Nausea
- Vomiting
- Abdominal pain
- Shortness of breath
- Drowsiness
- Coma

### Hyperglycaemia

*Fasting* plasma glucose >6.0 mmol/L or *non-fasting* >7.8 mmol/L is potentially abnormal and should be investigated further.

### Glycosuria

If the concentration of glucose is high in the blood, it will also be high in the filtrate formed in the kidney. The osmotic effect of this glucose retains water in the renal tubules and so increases urine volume (an osmotic diuresis) producing the symptoms of polyuria, dehydration and thirst. Glycosuria (glucose in the urine) does not always indicate diabetes (and the absence of glycosuria does not exclude diabetes). Glycosuria usually occurs when blood glucose values rise above a threshold of 10–13 mmol/L.

*Renal glycosuria* is glycosuria occurring with a *normal* blood glucose level. This occurs when glucose in the renal filtrate is incompletely reabsorbed because of reduced function of the glucose-reabsorbing transporters in the renal tubules. The class of oral diabetes drugs sodium-linked glucose transporter 2 inhibitors (SGLT2i) lower blood glucose by causing glycosuria.

## INVESTIGATION

### Diagnostic tests

#### Glycated haemoglobin assays

The glycated haemoglobin isoform used to monitor and diagnose diabetes is HbA1c. Since red blood cell lifespan is 120 days, the glycated haemoglobin assay provides information about the average glucose concentration for the previous 2–3 months. Glycated haemoglobin assays are not significantly affected by manipulating diet or treatment in the week before a clinic appointment but are altered if red cell lifespan is abnormal. In 2011, the World Health Organization (WHO) agreed the additional use of HbA1c testing for the diagnosis of diabetes.

#### Diagnosing diabetes and non-diabetic hyperglycaemia
(See **Table 11.4**).

*Criteria for the diagnosis of DM:*
- Symptoms of diabetes (see HISTORY 11.1) *and* blood glucose is significantly raised, *or*
- No symptoms of diabetes, but blood glucose is significantly raised on more than 2 days *and* there is no acute illness, *or*
- HbA1c is ≥48 mmol/mol and no other conditions apply (**Table 11.5**)

**Table 11.4** Diagnosis of DM and intermediate hyperglycaemia WHO guidelines 2006

| | Glucose (measured in mmol/L) | | |
|---|---|---|---|
| | Diabetes mellitus | Impaired glucose tolerance | Impaired fasting glucose |
| Fasting | ≥7.0 | <7.0 | 6.1–6.9 |
| 2 hour post-glucose load | ≥11.1 | >7.8 and <11.1 | <7.8 |

DM can be diagnosed on the basis of a non-fasting venous plasma glucose >11.0 mmol/L *if there are symptoms of diabetes*. If there are no symptoms of diabetes, it is important to repeat the blood glucose sample; transient hyperglycaemia may occur in stress situations, such as infections. If a non-fasting glucose is on the borderline of normal, a fasting blood glucose and HbA1c sample should be checked. The type of blood sample used (venous or capillary, plasma or whole blood) affects the reference values. Special considerations apply during pregnancy.

Once a diagnosis of DM has been established, the type of DM – and the possibility of secondary forms of DM – should be considered (**Table 11.6**).

A diagnosis of DM is usually lifelong (unless diagnosed during pregnancy or resulting from secondary causes) and has significant implications for driving, employment and life insurance premiums. It is therefore important to ensure the diagnosis is certain. Diagnosis should be based on laboratory blood samples rather than a capillary blood glucose monitor reading, and blood tests should be repeated in asymptomatic people. If there is diagnostic doubt, request a 75 g oral glucose tolerance test. *Urinalysis* should be performed in everyone with newly diagnosed DM since heavy ketonuria (≥3+) suggests diabetic ketoacidosis (DKA) and the need for urgent specialist assessment.

*Non-diabetic hyperglycaemia* Non-diabetic hyperglycaemia (NDH) (sometimes called *pre-diabetes*) is a blood glucose level outside the normal range but not high enough to diagnose diabetes. NDH includes impaired glucose tolerance, impaired fasting glucose and HbA1c values in the range 42-47 mmol/mol. People with NDH are at risk of future diabetes. Clinical trials show that lifestyle interventions reduce the progression to diabetes.

### Remission of diabetes

Complete remission is a return of glucose tests into the normal range (HbA1c <42, fasting glucose <5.6 mmol/L) of at least 1 year's duration in the absence of active therapy.

**Table 11.5** Assessing glycaemia by glycated haemoglobin assays

| Category | Normal glucose levels | Non-diabetic hyperglycaemia (NDH) | Diabetes mellitus |
|---|---|---|---|
| HbA1c (mmol/mol) | ≤41 | 42–47 | ≥48 |

**Table 11.6** Differentiating type 1 from type 2 DM

| Type 1 | Type 2 |
|---|---|
| Child or adult <30 years | Adult >40 years |
| Usually symptomatic | Often asymptomatic |
| Short history of symptoms – weeks | Ketosis infrequent |
| Ketosis frequent | Microvascular complications may be present |
| No microvascular complications at diagnosis | Population prevalence of pancreatic autoantibodies |
| Pancreatic autoantibodies | History of gestational diabetes (GDM) |
| History of other autoimmune diseases | Family history of type 2 diabetes – common |
| Family history of type 1 diabetes – sometimes | Overweight or obese |
| Slim or overweight | High-risk ethnic groups – South Asian, African, Caribbean, Hispanic, Polynesian |

*Remission of type 2 diabetes* Intensive lifestyle interventions may induce remission of type 2 diabetes. Success rates are higher with weight loss >10 kg. The DiRECT study using a very low-calorie diet achieved remission at 1 year in up to 50%. Metabolic (bariatric) surgery can induce remission in 30–60%, especially in younger patients with a shorter diabetes history. Median duration of remission after surgery is 8 years.

*Remission of type 1 diabetes* Up to 1 in 10 patients with type 1 diabetes experience a 'honeymoon' phase after starting on insulin therapy – blood glucose levels fall into the normal range and insulin doses either substantially reduce or even stop. This is thought to be due to elimination of any 'glucose toxicity' to the pancreas due to hyperglycaemia. In 90% of cases the honeymoon phase lasts <1 year. Transplantation of purified human pancreatic islet cells has been used to ameliorate type 1 diabetes, but the effect wanes, often over a few years. Pancreatic transplantation can reverse type 1 diabetes but, due to the surgical risks and need for immunosuppression, this is usually reserved for patients requiring a kidney transplant for diabetic kidney disease.

## GENERAL MANAGEMENT

See **Table 11.7**.
- Improve symptoms of hyperglycaemia.
- Slow or prevent the development of complications of DM.
- Minimize side effects from treatment.

Clinical trials have established that good long-term blood glucose control lowers the risk of *microvascular* complications of DM in both type 1 and type 2 DM. Good blood glucose control also lowers coronary heart disease (CHD) risk, tight blood pressure control reduces the incidence of

**Table 11.7** Management of DM

| | |
|---|---|
| **Supportive care** | **Macrovascular complications** |
| Education of patient, family and/or carers by nurses, dietitians, group education classes, cookery classes, diabetes charities (e.g. Diabetes UK, American Diabetes Association), summer camps for young people with DM | *Prevention* <br>• Stop smoking <br>• Seek and treat hypertension <br>• Seek and treat hyperlipidaemias <br>• Optimize weight <br>• Take adequate exercise <br>• Educate about foot care |
| **Specific treatment** | *Screening* |
| *Diet* | • Check for evidence of cardiac disease or peripheral vascular disease |
| • *Weight:* aim for 5–10% weight loss if obese, or ideal body weight if feasible | • Check footcare |
| • *Carbohydrates:* restrict intake of refined carbohydrates (e.g. sugar, jams, sweets, chocolate) and some restriction on complex carbohydrates (e.g. rice, pasta, potatoes) | *Specific treatment* <br>• Medical and/or surgical treatment of coronary artery disease |
| • *Proteins:* generally little restriction except for calorie control | • Prophylaxis for transient ischaemic attacks (aspirin) and surgery (endarterectomy) in selected cases |
| • *Fats:* reduce saturated fats and substitute with polyunsaturated or monosaturated vegetable oils | • Reconstructive surgery or amputation for peripheral vascular disease |
| • *Alcohol:* limit to sensible drinking guidelines of 1–2 units/day; avoid binge drinking | **Microvascular complications** |
| *Exercise* | *Prevention* |
| • Increase physical activity level if inactive and able to become more active | • Good blood glucose control <br>• Good blood pressure control |
| • *Oral hypoglycaemics* | • Eye examination (acuity, fundoscopy, retinal photography) |
| • Combination therapy often required | • Look for evidence of nephropathy (microalbuminuria or albuminuria) |
| *Insulin* | • Examine for evidence of neuropathy (reflexes, sensation, postural hypotension) |
| • Generally mandatory in type 1 DM | *Specific treatment* |
| • May be required for metabolic control in type 2 DM | • Photocoagulation for retinopathy |
| • Precise type of insulin and regimen depends on individual patient's lifestyle and requirements | • Cataract extraction <br>• ACE inhibitors/AT1 antagonists in microalbuminuric nephropathy |
| *Monitoring glycaemic control* | • Plan for renal replacement therapy |
| • Monitor with glycated haemoglobin and/or home blood glucose measurements | • Symptomatic measures to relieve neuropathic problems |
| • Feed back results to alter behaviour and/or medical therapy | |

**11**

stroke and heart failure and the progression of retinopathy. Cardiovascular disease risk is increased in DM and statin lipid-lowering therapy is beneficial.

## Education

• Symptoms of hypoglycaemia and how to treat it
• Symptoms of hyperglycaemia
• How to manage diabetes when unwell with another illness
• Role of medications and safe storage
• Healthy diet and effects of nutrients on blood glucose levels
• Self-testing of blood glucose ± blood/urine ketones
• Symptoms of DKA
• Safe driving with diabetes and local rules
• Smoking cessation
• Effects of diabetes on pregnancy
• Pregnancy planning
• Effects of diabetes on mental health
• Complications of diabetes
• Footcare

## Diet

All patients with DM should receive dietary advice. In type 2 DM, dietary change is as effective as medication in reducing hyperglycaemia. Maintaining dietary change is difficult and requires regular reinforcement. In overweight/obese type 2 DM, weight loss improves metabolic control, both by restricting the intake of carbohydrate and by increasing insulin sensitivity. Patients with type 2 DM are advised to follow a healthy eating plan of lower saturated fat, increased fibre and restricted carbohydrate intake. Increasing intake of vegetables, pulses and fruit, and reducing the amount of processed foods usually achieves this. In type 1 DM treated with multiple dose insulin or insulin pump, there is less need to restrict diet as insulin may be matched to food intake if the patient is carbohydrate-counting, but a healthy eating pattern is encouraged to avoid weight gain.

## Monitoring glucose control

### Glycated haemoglobin assays

HbA1c is the key test of glucose control and lower HbA1c values are associated with better outcomes in clinical trials.

## DIABETES MELLITUS AT A GLANCE

### Epidemiology

*Prevalence in UK*

- Type 1 DM 60 in 10 000
- Type 2 DM 600 in 10 000

*Age of onset*

- Type 1 usually under 30 years
- Type 2 usually over 30 years

*Genetics*

- Implicated in both type 1 and type 2 DM

*Geography*

- High prevalence of type 1 DM in Scandinavia and Malta; higher prevalence of type 2 DM in South Asians, Afro-Caribbeans, Polynesians

### Findings on investigation

Symptoms of DM
*plus*
Random venous plasma glucose ≥11.1 mmol/L
*or*
Fasting venous plasma glucose ≥7.0 mmol/L
*or*
HbA1c ≥48 mmol/mol

### Urinalysis

Urine should be tested in all people with suspected or newly diagnosed DM. Ketonuria 3+ suggests the possibility of keto-acidosis requiring emergency treatment with insulin

### Long-term complications

*Microvascular disease*

- Retinopathy
- Nephropathy
- Neuropathy

*Macrovascular disease*

- CHD
- Peripheral vascular disease
- Cerebrovascular disease

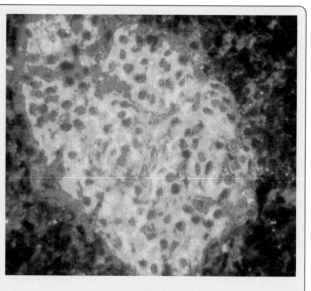

**Figure B** Human pancreas stained with anti-human IgG fluoresceinated serum: the cells within the islets are strongly positive.

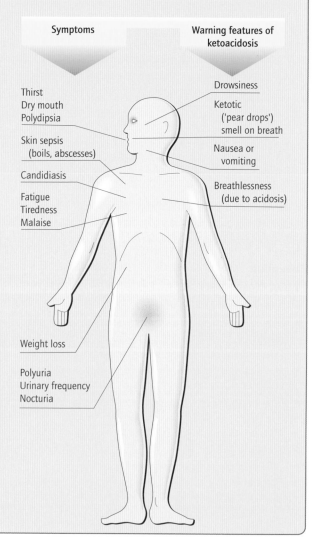

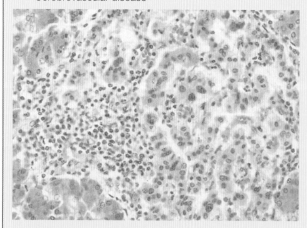

**Figure A** Infiltration of islets with chronic inflammatory cells, resulting in insulitis. In recent-onset type 1 DM most islets are insulin-deficient, with residual B cells showing 'insulitis' which could be a product of autoimmune destruction. H&E stain, magnification ×300. Both figures reproduced from Williams G & Pickup JC (eds) (1992) *Handbook of Diabetes* (Wiley-Blackwell, Oxford), with the permission of the authors.

Current UK guidance for type 2 DM is HbA1c <48 mmol/mol if on diet alone or metformin monotherapy, HbA1c <58 if on additional therapy including insulin. Current UK guidance for type 1 DM is HbA1c <53 mmol/mol.

### Self-testing of capillary blood glucose
Thsi is valuable for detecting hypoglycaemia, especially for patients with type 1 DM, who may alter diet, insulin or exercise. Blood glucose meters are most inaccurate at the extremes of their measurement ranges: glucose <3 mmol/L (hypoglycaemia) or >20 mmol/L.

### Continuous glucose monitoring devices
Increasingly used in richer countries, these devices detect interstitial fluid glucose levels rather than blood glucose, reducing the need for capillary blood glucose testing. They may send an alarm to the patient to alert them if glucose levels go out of range

### Ketone testing
- *Urine*:
  - Mild ketonuria (1+) occurs after fasting overnight because ketone bodies are used for gluconeogenesis.
  - Heavy ketonuria (3+) suggests DKA.
- *Blood*: Normal <0.5 mmol/L; 0.5–1.5 mildly raised, 1.5–3 moderately raised, >3 very raised.

In type 1 DM, ketones should be tested for if capillary glucose is persistently >17 mmol/L or there is nausea, vomiting or breathless as these symptoms may indicate incipient DKA.

### Oral hypoglycaemic agents
There are multiple oral therapies for treating type 2 diabetes (**Table 11.8**). Metformin is the first-line drug for type 2 diabetes and lowers mortality in overweight diabetic patients. Many patients with type 2 DM require more than one oral hypoglycaemic drug to achieve good glucose control. Current US/European guidelines recommend assessing cardiovascular and renal disease when choosing a second-line oral hypoglycaemic drug.

### Glucagon-like peptide 1 receptor analogues
GLP-1 is an incretin hormone which augments insulin release and inhibits glucagon release from the pancreas. GLP-1 has a short half-life because it is inactivated by proteases including dipeptidyl protease IV. A variety of drugs with GLP-1 receptor agonist activity are licensed for type 2 DM including exenatide, liraglutide, lixisenatide and semaglutide.

### Insulin and insulin analogues
Insulin is absolutely required in type 1 DM and may be used in gestational DM or type 2 DM. Insulin is mostly manufactured by a biotechnological process to produce a protein with the same amino acid sequence as native human insulin. Animal insulins are sometimes purified from the pancreas of the pig or cow. Insulin is usually administered by subcutaneous injection or infusion. The standard strength for insulin preparations is 100 units/mL (known as U100 insulin).

Insulins may be grouped as short-acting, rapid-acting, intermediate-acting, long-acting insulin analogues or mixtures of these.
- *Short-acting (soluble) insulins* are absorbed more slowly than expected as the insulin molecules form relatively stable hexamers.
- *Rapid-acting insulin analogues* have a faster onset of action because their altered amino acid sequences reduce hexamer formation.

**Table 11.8** Oral therapies for DM

| Class | Mechanism | Hypo risk | Weight change | Adverse effects | Examples |
|---|---|---|---|---|---|
| Biguanides | Activation of AMP kinase | Low | Neutral | Diarrhoea, dyspepsia, flatulence | Metformin |
| Sulphonylureas | Stimulate insulin release | High | Increase | Rash, taste disturbance, hepatic dysfunction | Gliclazide, glibencamide, tolbutamide |
| DPP IV inhibitors | Increase incretin levels | Moderate | Neutral | Rash, oedema, dyspepsia, pancreatitis | Alogliptin, sitagliptin, linagliptin |
| SGLT2 inhibitors | Increase renal excretion of glucose | Low | Neutral or decrease | Urogenital candidiasis, UTI, hypovolaemia, osteoporosis, euglycaemic ketoacidosis | Canagliflozin, dapagliflozin, empagliflozin |
| Thiazolidinediones | Increase insulin sensitivity | Low | Increase | Anaemia, osteoporosis, oedema, heart failure | Pioglitazone, rosiglitazone, lobeglitazone |
| Alpha glucosidase inhibitors | Inhibit digestion of disaccharides | Low | Neutral | Diarrhoea, flatulence, faecal incontinence | Acarbose, miglitol, voglibose |

UTI, urinary tract infection.

- *Intermediate-acting insulins* have a slower absorption into the bloodstream due to the addition of a protein and/or zinc; the protein protamine is commonly used.
- *Long-acting (basal) insulin analogues* have a prolonged duration of action due to factors that further slow the absorption from the injection site.

Many different brands of insulin are marketed, and the same insulin may be marketed under a different name in different countries. To avoid confusion, it is recommended that insulins are prescribed by brand name rather than by generic name.

### Starting insulin treatment

Insulin treatment can be started as an outpatient if the patient is well, and the patient can be trained to do the injections and blood glucose monitoring.

### Indications for insulin therapy

- DKA
- Hyperosmolar hyperglycaemic state (HHS)
- Established type 1 DM
- Gestational DM where diet is insufficient
- Type 2 DM where diet and oral hypoglycaemic agents are insufficient
- Major surgery in people with DM
- During any severe illness where there is a risk of DKA

### Choice of insulin

The choice of insulin regimen can be tailored to the patient and insulin is usually injected subcutaneously by the patient (**Figure 11.4**). Patients with impaired vision or cognitive problems may need insulin to be administered by carers. Patients with type 2 DM often start with a once-daily intermediate or basal insulin in addition to oral hypoglycaemic drugs. If this does not control their blood glucose adequately, they may move to a twice daily biphasic insulin mixture, containing both short-acting and intermediate-acting insulin, given before breakfast and before the evening meal (**Figure 11.5**). Insulin requirements are often higher in the morning because higher levels of cortisol, catecholamines and glucagon antagonize the action of insulin.

Patients with type 1 DM are frequently treated with a basal-bolus regimen of short-acting or rapid-acting insulin before meals and intermediate-acting or basal insulin at bedtime. The aim of a basal-bolus regimen is to try to mimic physiological insulin release. Alternatively patients with type 1 DM are treated with continuous subcutaneous infusion of insulin ('insulin pump') therapy.

## PREGNANCY AND DIABETES MELLITUS

DM that is already known about before the pregnancy is discussed below under 'Pregnancy and diabetes'. Hyperglycaemia discovered for the first time during pregnancy is known as *gestational diabetes* (GDM).

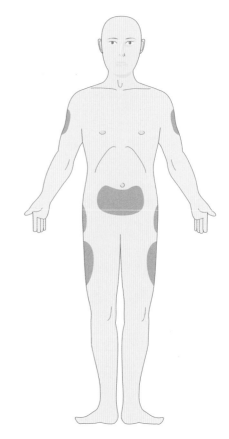

**Figure 11.4** Recommended sites for insulin injection.

### Pregnancy and diabetes

Most obstetric complications are increased in pregnant women with diabetes, especially:

- Congenital malformation
- Macrosomia (large fetus)
- Stillbirth

### Gestational diabetes mellitus

GDM is the appearance of glucose intolerance during pregnancy. Hormonal factors contributing to hyperglycaemia during pregnancy include placental lactogen, progesterone, prolactin and cortisol. Compared to the higher glucose values usually diagnostic of diabetes, the small degree of hyperglycaemia represented by impaired glucose tolerance is significant during pregnancy. Macrosomia and neonatal hypoglycaemia are increased in GDM. Congenital malformations do not appear to be increased with new-onset GDM, because the hyperglycaemia develops after organogenesis has started.

Risk factors for GDM include:

- Obesity
- Family history of type 2 DM
- Previous GDM
- Previous large baby (birth weight >4 kg)

GDM is usually asymptomatic and develops during the second trimester. Screening for GDM should be offered to all pregnant women. Initially, GDM is managed by diet, but if

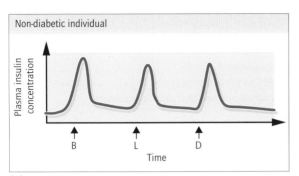

(a)

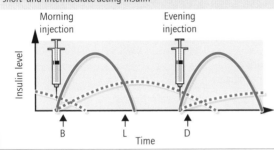

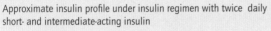

(b)

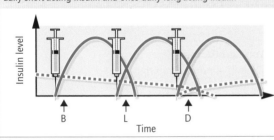

(c)

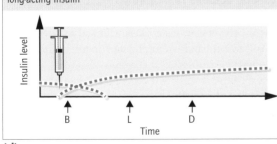

(d)

**Figure 11.5** Schematic representation of insulin profiles during a 24-hour period in: **(a)** a non-diabetic individual, and in three different insulin regimens; **(b)** twice daily mixture of short- and intermediate-acting insulin; **(c)** three times daily short-acting insulin with once-daily long-acting insulin (particularly useful in allowing flexibility in people with variable daily routines); and **(d)** once-daily long-acting insulin (does not allow good glycaemic control so unsuitable for young people, but may be appropriate occasionally in elderly people where convenience is paramount and good control not essential). B, breakfast; L, lunch; D, dinner.

glucose values remain high, metformin and/or insulin treatment is started. After delivery, GDM usually resolves as the hormonal changes reverse. A small proportion of women remain diabetic, so it is usual to arrange a diabetes screening test 6 weeks after delivery. Type 2 DM develops later in 30–50% of women with previous GDM.

## SURGERY AND DIABETES

There are four main concerns in patients with diabetes who are undergoing surgery:

- Hypoglycaemia during surgery and/or anaesthesia, impairing recovery from the anaesthetic
- Hyperglycaemia perioperatively, impairing the response to infection and impairing wound healing
- Increased risk of developing metabolic decompensation (DKA and lactic acidosis)
- Increased prevalence of cardiovascular disease in people with diabetes

### General guidelines for perioperative diabetes management

#### Emergency surgery

- There is a higher risk of metabolic decompensation due to release of stress hormones.
- It is safer to use variable rate intravenous insulin infusion (VRIII) for *all emergency operations* (**Table 11.9**).
- Stop metformin due to higher risk of acute kidney injury and lactic acidosis.
- Remember that DKA may cause severe abdominal pain (include in differential diagnosis of an acute abdomen).
- Surgery on patients with DKA has a high mortality so treat DKA before emergency surgery if at all possible.
- Protect patients at risk of foot ulcers during prolonged immobilization by doing a foot risk assessment and start pressure relief measures.

#### Elective surgery

- Plan diabetes management before admission. Your hospital should have detailed guidelines for managing diabetes around elective surgery – do consult them.
- Do not offer elective surgery to patients with poor metabolic control. Generally, if HbA1c >69 mmol/mol, try to optimize metabolic control.
- Before admission the patient should have a clear plan about what to do with their diabetes tablets and insulin around the time of surgery.
- Aim to have patients with diabetes at the start of a surgical list to reduce their duration of starvation.
- Aim to keep capillary blood glucose 6–10 mmol/L.
- Metformin can usually be continued if there is a short starvation period and normal renal function.
- Continue basal insulin, but use a 20% lower dose during the admission.
- Use VRIII if the patient is likely to miss more than one meal (i.e. have prolonged starvation, which increases risk of ketosis).

11

**Table 11.9** Surgery and DM

**Variable rate intravenous insulin infusion (VRIII)**

Start with 0.45% saline/5% glucose/0.15% potassium chloride **or** 5% glucose/0.15% potassium chloride at 125 mL/hour.

Slower infusions of 10% or 20% glucose may be used if fluid overload is a problem.

Start an IV infusion of 50 units of soluble insulin made up to 50 mL with 0.9% sodium chloride (1 unit/mL) in a syringe pump driver.

Deliver the following amounts of insulin according to the results of hourly capillary blood glucose measurements:

| Blood glucose (mmol/L) | Insulin dose (units/hour) | Comments |
| --- | --- | --- |
| ≤4.0 | 0.5 | Increase IV infusion of glucose by 30% |
| 4.1–7.0 | 1.0 | |
| 7.1–11.0 | 2.0 | |
| 11.1–14.0 | 4.0 | |
| 14.1–17.0 | 6.0 | |
| ≥17.1 | 8.0 | Check blood or urine for ketones |

**Special circumstances**

If blood glucose is not controlled, the dose of insulin used should be altered either up or down.

These suggested insulin doses are not suitable for use with children.

Patients with a history of heart failure or renal disease may need fluid restriction.

If there is hyperkalaemia ($K^+$ >5.5 mmol/L), KCl should not be added to the infusate.

### Stopping intravenous insulin infusions

The usual regimen can be restarted once the patient is eating and drinking normally. As intravenous (IV) insulin has a short half-life, subcutaneous insulin should be given at least 30–60 minutes *before* stopping an IV insulin infusion. The estimated glomerular filtration rate (eGFR) should be >45 mL/min before restarting metformin. After complex surgery in type 2 DM it may be necessary to use insulin temporarily.

## COMPLICATIONS OF DIABETES MELLITUS

### Diabetic retinopathy

Diabetic retinopathy is classified into different patterns of disease, but these do not necessarily progress from one to another:

- Background
- Maculopathy
- Preproliferative
- Proliferative
- Advanced

See **Figure 11.6**.

#### Background diabetic retinopathy

This is the commonest form of diabetic retinopathy. It is not usually seen for at least 10 years in type 1 DM but is present at diagnosis in up to 30% of people with type 2 DM. Features include:

- *Dots:* microaneurysms due to localized dilatation of the retinal capillaries
- *Blots:* small haemorrhages into the deep retinal layer
- *Hard exudates:* white hard-edged areas due to leakage of plasma containing proteins and lipid

#### Maculopathy

This is background diabetic retinopathy of the macula area and there may be associated retinal oedema. Macular oedema is difficult to detect with direct ophthalmoscopy and can cause permanent central visual loss if not treated.

#### Preproliferative retinopathy

This precedes the onset of new vessel formation, which is the characteristic of proliferative retinopathy (see below). Features include:

- Cotton wool spots due to axonal transport being interrupted by ischaemia
- Venous beading
- Dilated abnormal capillaries

#### Proliferative retinopathy

This is new blood vessel formation, due to growth factors released from ischaemic retina. The new vessels can bleed causing visual loss by vitreous or preretinal haemorrhage. New vessels on the optic disc are especially likely to bleed.

#### Advanced diabetic retinopathy

This is the end result of proliferative retinopathy, usually with irreversible visual loss. Clinical features include fibrous traction bands, retinal detachment and thrombotic glaucoma.

### Diabetic nephropathy

#### Factors influencing kidney function in diabetes

Kidney damage occurs in long-standing DM because of:

- Diabetic nephropathy (glomerular damage; **Figure 11.7**)
- Renal artery stenosis and ischaemia
- Ascending infection
- Papillary necrosis

#### Clinical features

Diabetic nephropathy is characterized by proteinuria, a fall in glomerular filtration rate and increasing blood pressure. In type 1 DM, the incidence of diabetic nephropathy peaks 10–20 years after diagnosis and about one-third of patients

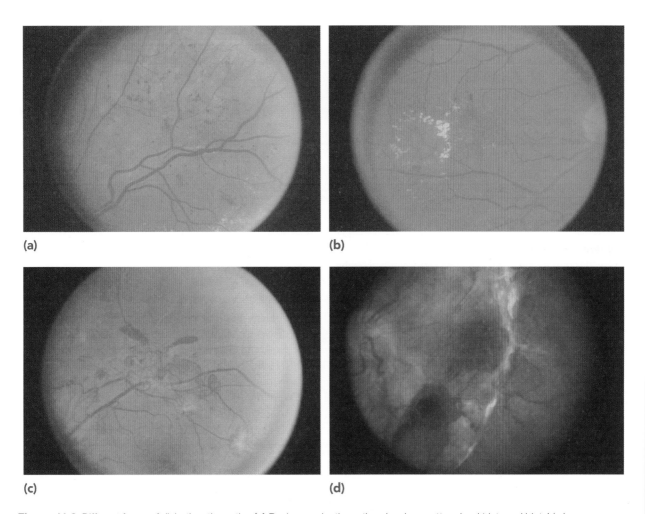

(a)

(b)

(c)

(d)

**Figure 11.6** Different forms of diabetic retinopathy. **(a)** Background retinopathy, showing scattered red 'dots and blots' (microaneurysms and haemorrhages), and exudates. **(b)** Maculopathy, showing hard exudates encroaching onto the macula. **(c)** Proliferative retinopathy, showing leashes of new vessels and haemorrhages. **(d)** Advanced retinopathy, showing retinal detachment. Reproduced from Pickup JC & Williams G (eds) (1991) *Textbook of Diabetes* (Wiley-Blackwell, Oxford), with the permission of the authors.

**11**

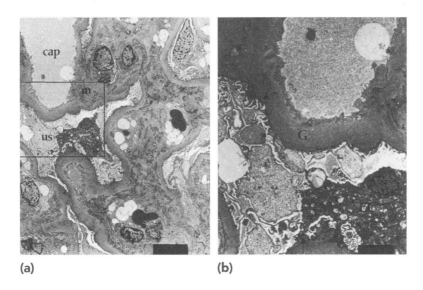

(a)

(b)

**Figure 11.7** Photomicrographs showing glomerular basement membrane thickening, and mesangial expansion in the kidney of a diabetic patient with nephropathy. **(a)** Magnification ×1700: m, mesangial cell and matrix; us, urinary space; cap, capillary lumen. **(b)** Magnification ×4300, enlargement of boxed area in **(a)**, foot processes are arrowed: G, glomerular basement membrane; EC, epithelial cell. Reproduced from Williams G & Pickup JC (eds) (1992) *Handbook of Diabetes* (Wiley-Blackwell, Oxford), with the permission of the authors.

eventually develop overt nephropathy. The first clinical feature may be proteinuria or worsening hypertension. Once diabetic nephropathy is established, glomerular filtration rate slowly declines, resulting in chronic renal failure and eventually end-stage renal failure.

## Diabetic neuropathy

Diabetic neuropathies fall into a number of clinical presentations:

- Symmetrical sensory polyneuropathy
- Mononeuropathy and multiple mononeuropathy
- Proximal motor neuropathy
- Autonomic neuropathy

### Symmetrical sensory polyneuropathy

This is the commonest form of diabetic neuropathy. There is usually gradual onset loss of sensation in the feet and occasionally hands ('glove and stocking' distribution). Patients may complain of 'walking on cotton wool'. Clinically, features include inability to feel a 10 g monofilament, loss of vibration sense and reduced/lost ankle and/or knee jerks. Loss of joint proprioception may cause difficulty in walking or loss of balance when visual cues are absent (e.g. walking in the dark, bending over to wash the face). Romberg's sign may be positive. Loss of peripheral nerve function can cause wasting of the small muscles of the feet and/or hands.

Less commonly, an acute painful form of sensory neuropathy presents with paraesthesiae, burning and electric shock-like pains in the feet and legs, often worse at night, disrupting sleep. Occasionally, acute painful sensory neuropathy may be associated with treatment for hyperglycaemia.

### Mononeuropathy and multiple mononeuropathy

Sudden-onset focal neuropathies of cranial nerves or peripheral nerves occasionally occur in patients with DM. Sometimes more than one nerve is affected (mononeuritis multiplex). The cranial nerves most often affected are the oculomotor (3rd) and abducens (6th). Fortunately they often recover spontaneously. Median nerve palsy (carpal tunnel syndrome), ulnar nerve palsy and common peroneal nerve palsy are all increased in patients with DM and have a variable clinical outcome.

### Proximal motor neuropathy (amyotrophy)

Amyotrophy is characterized by unilateral (or bilateral) pain and weakness in the quadriceps muscles. Typically, it affects older men with type 2 DM. There is often quadriceps muscle wasting, weakness or difficulty in walking, reduced or absent knee jerks and sometimes extensor plantar reflexes. Poor glucose control is common and the condition usually responds to better glucose control. If extensor plantar responses are present, spinal cord compression should be excluded.

### Autonomic neuropathy

Autonomic nerve damage is common in long-standing DM and effects can include:

- *Cardiovascular:* There may be loss of vagal (parasympathetic) tone – resting tachycardia and loss of sinus arrhythmia – and loss of sympathetic activity in arterioles – peripheral vasodilatation and postural hypotension.
- *Gastrointestinal:* There is delayed gastric emptying – early satiety or, rarely, recurrent vomiting (gastroparesis). Diarrhoea, typically nocturnal, may be associated with faecal incontinence.
- *Atonic bladder:* Loss of bladder smooth muscle tone results in incomplete emptying, stasis and an increased risk of urinary tract infection (UTI). In severe cases, the bladder is atonic, painlessly distended, and overflow incontinence occurs.
- *Gustatory sweating:* This is an unusual symptom whereby eating causes excessive facial sweating.
- *Erectile dysfunction:* Autonomic dysfunction contributes to erectile dysfunction (ED).

## Foot disease

Foot problems in diabetes can be caused by peripheral vascular disease, peripheral neuropathy or both. The severity of each should be assessed with a problem diabetic foot (**Table 11.10**). The most common clinical problem is a non-healing foot ulcer. Ulcers occur because of increased pressure at points on the foot and/or reduced skin nutrition from poor blood supply. Once an ulcer has formed and the epithelial barrier is breached, infection can occur, further reducing the likelihood of healing.

### Neuropathic foot ulcer pathophysiology

Peripheral neuropathy can cause small-muscle wasting with weakness of the interosseous muscles in the foot. Over time, unopposed action of the long flexors in the foot causes clawing of the toes and a high foot arch. These changes redistribute pressure over the foot and cause high pressure over the metatarsal heads. Callus (hard skin) builds up over the metatarsal heads, but paradoxically this increases shear pressure in the underlying soft tissues, leading to haemorrhage and an inflammatory exudate. Rupture of this region through the overlying skin produces the ulcer (**Figure 11.8**).

### Ischaemic foot ulcer pathophysiology

A poor blood supply results in reduced epithelial cell turnover and thinner, flaky skin (**Figure 11.9**). Smoking

**Table 11.10** Comparisons between purely neuropathic and purely ischaemic diabetic feet

| | Neuropathic foot | Ischaemic foot |
|---|---|---|
| Symptoms | Painless | Claudication |
| | Neuropathic pain | Rest pain |
| Signs | Full, bounding pulses | Weak/absent pulses |
| | Normal capillary return | Poor capillary return |
| | Warm skin | Cool skin |
| | Clawed toes | |
| | Dry (lack of sweating) | |
| Ulcer site | Metatarsal heads | Toes |
| | | Heels |

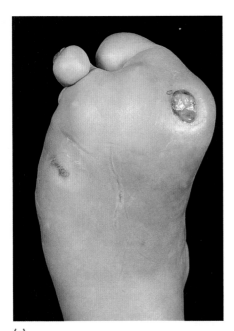

**(a)**

bed-bound patients, the heel is particularly at risk (e.g. postoperatively).

*Charcot's arthropathy*

This is an unusual complication of neuropathic feet presenting as a red, hot, swollen foot with or without pain. Blood flow to the foot is increased due to autonomic neuropathy. Peripheral neuropathy may contribute to unnoticed trauma. An excessive local inflammatory response results in focal osteolysis and osteoporosis. Sustained mechanical stress deforms the foot with fracture-dislocations of forefoot bones and mid-foot collapse. Once foot deformity has

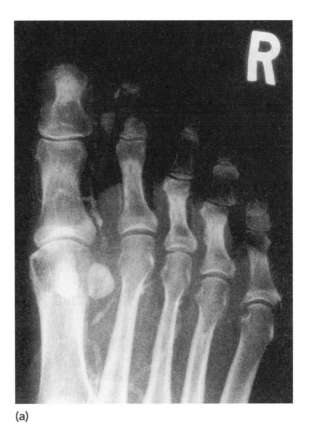

**(a)**

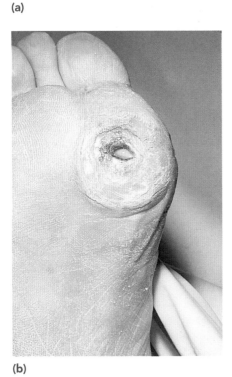

**(b)**

**Figure 11.8** Neuropathic ulcers. **(a)** Typical punched-out' ulcer under first metatarsal head. Note previous amputations. Reproduced by kind permission of Dr Ian Casson, Broadgreen Hospital, Liverpool. **(b)** Note particularly thickened callosities caused by high pressure area. Reproduced from Williams G & Pickup JC (eds) (1992) *Handbook of Diabetes* (Wiley-Blackwell, Oxford), with the permission of the authors.

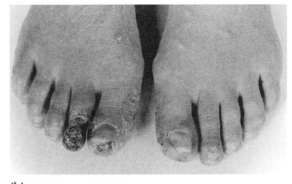

**(b)**

further reduces the oxygen-carrying capacity of the blood. Weakened skin is easily damaged if external pressure causes further hypoperfusion and anoxic tissue necrosis. External pressure from new shoes is a common cause of ischaemic ulcers around the margins of the foot. In

**Figure 11.9** Ischaemic diabetic feet. **(a)** Radiograph showing medial artery calcification, a well-recognized feature in diabetics. **(b)** Digital gangrene typical of diabetic vascular disease. Reproduced from Williams G & Pickup JC (eds) (1992) *Handbook of Diabetes* (Wiley-Blackwell, Oxford), with the permission of the authors.

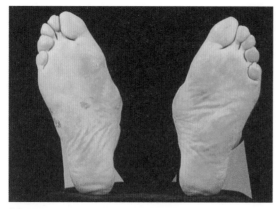

**(a)**

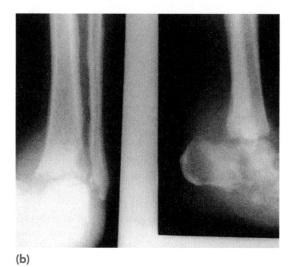

**(b)**

**Figure 11.10** Advanced Charcot's arthropathy. **(a)** Gross disorganization of small joints in foot. **(b)** Radiograph of advanced Charcot's arthropathy showing destruction of the ankle and foot joints. Reproduced from Williams G & Pickup JC (eds) (1992) *Handbook of Diabetes* (Wiley-Blackwell, Oxford), with the permission of the authors.

occurred, the risk of foot ulceration is high and with it the risk of soft tissue and bone infection. Charcot arthropathy is often misdiagnosed as cellulitis but, if not recognized, serious complications are likely.

- *Plain radiographs* are initially normal, but later show fracture, osteolysis, new bone formation and disorganization of the joint by subluxation.
- *MRI scans* may show bone marrow oedema in the mid-foot region, but may be difficult to differentiate from osteomyelitis (**Figure 11.10**).

## SURVEILLANCE AND MANAGEMENT OF COMPLICATIONS

### Diabetic eye disease

Annual eye checks are needed, including visual acuity and retinal examination – ideally by retinal photography if resources allow. Screening is valuable because treatment

may be started before visual loss occurs. Visual loss is caused by macular oedema (maculopathy) or retinal haemorrhage (proliferative retinopathy). Hyperglycaemia may affect vision by causing swelling of the ocular lens. Cataracts are more common in people with diabetes.

Unexplained visual loss in a patient with diabetes should be assessed by an ophthalmologist, because macular oedema is difficult to detect by direct fundoscopy. Sight-threatening diabetic retinopathy is treated by either intra-vitreal injections of anti-VEGF (vascular endothelial growth factor) antibodies or retinal laser. Focal laser burns to the retina reduce secretion of endothelial growth factors by the ischaemic retina. Extensive laser treatment may restrict peripheral vision but aims to preserve central vision.

### Diabetic nephropathy

#### Surveillance

Make annual measurements of urine proteinuria and plasma creatinine/eGFR. Proteinuria has other causes, including UTI. Diabetic retinopathy increases the chance that diabetic nephropathy is the underlying diagnosis. In the absence of diabetic retinopathy, and the presence of significant persistent proteinuria, other causes of proteinuria such as glomerulonephritis should be considered.

#### Microalbuminuria

In established diabetic nephropathy, the urinary albumin excretion can be >300 mg/24 hour (the normal range is <3 mg/24 hour). Patients with intermediate albumin excretions of above 3 mg/24 hour (microalbuminuria) have an elevated risk of developing established diabetic nephropathy. Microalbuminuria suggests early-stage glomerular damage, although not all will progress to established diabetic nephropathy. Screening with urine albumin : creatinine ratio (UACR) in a single urine sample is simpler than a 24-hour urine collection to estimate urinary albumin excretion. Microalbuminuria in diabetes is associated with slightly higher blood pressure and higher rates of cardiovascular disease compared to normoalbuminuric diabetics. Better glucose and blood pressure control reduce progression of microalbuminuria to diabetic nephropathy. Angiotensin-converting enzyme (ACE) inhibitors and angiotensin II receptor blockers have been shown to be beneficial.

#### Established diabetic nephropathy

Tight control of blood pressure and a low protein diet slow the progression of established diabetic nephropathy to end-stage renal failure. Drugs acting on the renin-angiotensin system (ACE inhibitors, angiotensin II receptor blockers) are more effective than older antihypertensive drugs with similar effects on blood pressure. Multidrug treatments are often needed to reduce blood pressure. Low protein diets are not often used due to the potential for protein malnutrition. Patients should be monitored for problems related to advanced chronic kidney disease (e.g. fluid overload, anaemia and renal bone disease). Regular attendance at a specialist renal clinic is useful to plan for renal replacement therapy.

## Diabetic neuropathy

### Preventive care

Regular chiropody is helpful for neuropathic feet, as minor trauma (e.g. incorrect toenail cutting) may introduce infection. Callus over points of high pressure should be debrided to reduce shear forces in the tissue beneath. Patients with neuropathy should be advised to avoid walking barefoot and should inspect their feet daily for evidence of trauma, as they may not experience pain. Footwear should fit well and not constrict the feet. High heels increase pressure over metatarsal heads and should be avoided.

### Neuropathic foot ulcers

Infected ulcers require broad-spectrum antibiotics. Infected ulcers with >3 cm surrounding cellulitis may require IV broad-spectrum antibiotics and sometimes bed rest. Tissue culture samples from the ulcer base (rather than superficial swabs) are recommended to guide antibiotic therapy. In the absence of infection, healing is promoted by local debridement of callus, reduced walking and redistribution of weight over the foot by surgical shoes.

### Charcot's arthropathy

- *Acute phase:*
  - Plaster cast or removable plastic cast to offload pressure on foot
  - Watch out for fractures of foot bones
- *Non-acute phase:*
  - Bespoke shoes to redistribute foot pressure, especially if foot deformity
  - Internal fixation of foot bones with metal pins is sometimes used to reduce deformity

### Painful neuropathy

Symptoms may be improved by drugs such as tricyclic antidepressants, duloxetine, gabapentin, pregabalin or carbamazepine. Response rate is often below 50%.

## Diabetic ischaemic feet

### Preventive care

Stop smoking. Any new shoes should not be tight-fitting and should not be worn for more than an hour initially. Trauma from a blister can easily deteriorate into an ulcer.

### Ischaemic ulcers

Treat infection promptly and drain pus. Inspect footwear and change it if inappropriate. Surgical intervention can be used to improve the proximal blood supply if appropriate. Note: Peripheral vascular disease in diabetes is often 'distal' in smaller vessels and less amenable to bypass surgery or angioplasty.

### Critical ischaemia

Rest pain or gangrene in the foot requires urgent vascular surgical assessment. Check foot radiographs for evidence of gas in the soft tissues, because gas gangrene requires urgent surgical debridement to prevent progression.

## Blood pressure and lipid-lowering agents

Hypertension is more common in patients with DM; approximately 50% are hypertensive. Many secondary causes of diabetes are associated with hypertension (see **Table 11.1**). People with DM gain greater benefit from treatment of hypertension due to their increased risk of macrovascular disease. Strict blood pressure control reduces the chance of stroke, heart failure and the progression of diabetic retinopathy in patients with type 2 DM. Blood pressure targets in type 1 DM are currently <130/<80 mmHg and in type 2 DM are <140/80 mmHg or <130/<80 if the albumin : creatinine ratio is >70 mg/mmol or there is chronic kidney disease. Control of hypertension is an important part of diabetic nephropathy management.

National guidelines on treating diabetes recommend routine statin therapy as primary prevention for cardiovascular disease in patients with type 2 diabetes because of the high cardiovascular risk. Statin therapy should also be considered in type 1 diabetes if there is evidence of the microvascular complications of microalbuminuria or retinopathy.

## Erectile dysfunction

ED – the inability to maintain an erection sufficient for sexual intercourse – is relatively common in men over 60 years, but more prevalent in men over 60 years with diabetes. It may occur in much younger men with long-standing type 1 DM. A combination of autonomic nerve dysfunction and/or a reduced vascular supply makes ED more prevalent in men with diabetes.

Treatment options include phosphodiesterase 5 inhibitors (e.g. sildenafil, tadalafil), intracavernosal injections (of prostaglandins or α-blockers) and vacuum pump devices.

# DIABETIC EMERGENCIES

## DIABETIC KETOACIDOSIS

DKA is a medical emergency with a reported mortality rate of up to 5%. It is the leading cause of death in patients with type 1 DM under the age of 20 years. Mortality from DKA is high in the elderly as a result of coexisting morbidities.

### Disease mechanisms

#### Risk factors for diabetic ketoacidosis

DKA results from absolute or relative insulin deficiency. It may occur because of undiagnosed type 1 DM, omission of insulin or infection. Infections can precipitate DKA because stress hormones and cytokines antagonize the action of insulin. Patients with type 1 DM should never omit their insulin completely, even if they are eating less or vomiting, because DKA will inevitably ensue. Patients with type 2 DM

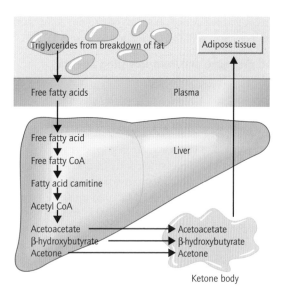

**Figure 11.11** Ketogenesis.

may also develop DKA under major stress, such as postoperatively, after myocardial infarction or with sepsis.

### Metabolic changes in diabetic ketoacidosis

Insulin inhibits glucose production in the liver and lipolysis in adipose tissue. In the absence of insulin, these processes are uninhibited, which results in hyperglycaemia and increased fatty acid release. The fatty acids released by adipose tissue are converted into ketone bodies in the liver (**Figure 11.11**). Ketone bodies are strong organic acids and dissociate at physiological pH to produce hydrogen ions (H+) and ketone anions. The resulting metabolic acidosis stimulates the brainstem vomiting and respiratory centres. Dehydration is produced by both the hyperglycaemic osmotic diuresis and vomiting.

### Clinical features

DKA usually develops over a period of a few days. Advice from a telephone helpline increases the use of early preventive action during intercurrent illnesses and may reduce the incidence of DKA.

#### Symptoms
- Thirst and polyuria caused by hyperglycaemia
- Vomiting, shortness of breath and abdominal pain caused by acidosis
- General malaise and drowsiness
- Symptoms from any underlying infection

#### Signs
- Smell of acetone on breath (like 'pear drops' or 'nail varnish remover')
- Hyperventilation (Kussmaul's respiration) caused by acidosis
- Dehydration
- Hypotension and tachycardia caused by hypovolaemia
- Signs of any underlying precipitating illness

### Management

See EMERGENCY PRESENTATION 11.1.
Treatment of DKA has three main features:
- Correction of hypovolaemia
- Maintaining potassium homeostasis
- Correction of insulin deficiency

Insulin is best given intravenously by a pump as subcutaneous insulin may be poorly absorbed into the blood because of hypovolaemia with reduced peripheral blood flow. The primary aim of insulin therapy in DKA is to switch off lipolysis, the main source of the metabolic acidosis. Rapid correction of hyperglycaemia using high doses of insulin may be harmful. The high blood glucose in DKA raises the osmolality of both the plasma and the brain, so if plasma glucose falls more quickly than brain glucose, water will flow from plasma into brain tissue. This can cause brain swelling or cerebral oedema and coma. This is a particular risk when treating DKA in children and adolescents. When treating DKA, blood glucose should not be lowered by more than 3–5 mmol/L/hour.

## HYPEROSMOLAR HYPERGLYCAEMIC STATE

HHS is characterized by a very high plasma glucose (usually >30 mmol/L) and a significantly raised plasma osmolality. Ketosis and acidosis are mild or absent.

### Epidemiology
- Usually elderly or middle-aged
- More common in people of African ethnicity

### Disease mechanisms

In patients with HHS, ketone body levels are not excessively high as in DKA; this may be because severe hyperglycaemia can inhibit excessive lipolysis or because there is enough endogenous insulin (in type 2 DM) to inhibit lipolysis. High glucose concentrations inhibit pancreatic insulin release (glucose toxicity).

### Clinical features

HHS presents with thirst, polyuria, confusion, collapse or reduced consciousness. Intercurrent infection (e.g. pneumonia) is frequently present. Ketosis is usually mild (blood ketones <1.5 mmol/L; urine ketones 1+ to 2+) and acidosis absent or mild (pH >7.3). The high plasma glucose concentration can cause hyperviscosity and thromboembolic disease is increased.

### Management

See EMERGENCY PRESENTATION 11.2.
The management of HHS resembles that of DKA, but there are important differences.
- *Fluid replacement:* Impaired consciousness arises from fluid movement from the brain to the hyperosmolar blood. Treatment of HHS aims to lower the

## EMERGENCY PRESENTATION 11.1

### Diabetic ketoacidosis

#### Establish the diagnosis

Triad of:

1. *Hyperglycaemia:* glucose usually more than 15 mmol/L
2. *Metabolic acidosis:* pH lower than 7.35, $HCO_3^-$ less than 17 mmol/L
3. *Ketosis:* blood ketones >3.0 mmol/L or ketonuria 3+ or more

#### Main metabolic features

*Hyperglycaemia:* leading to dehydration from osmotic diuresis
*Metabolic acidosis:* caused by elevated ketone bodies from insulin deficiency
*Hyperkalaemia:* secondary to acidosis; whole-body potassium stores will be low

#### Mainstays of treatment

IV rehydration
IV insulin
Replacement of low body potassium stores
Most acute hospitals will have their own treatment protocol so look for and use this if available

#### Initial treatment

1 litre 0.9% saline over 30 min
Actrapid insulin 6 units IV (or actrapid insulin 20 units intramuscularly if no IV access)
Consider treating an underlying cause

#### Insulin

Start fixed-rate IV infusion of soluble insulin at 0.1 units//kg/hour. If blood glucose does not fall, first check patency of IV lines and that infusion apparatus working; if these are satisfactory, increase prescribed dose of insulin. Aim to reduce blood glucose by no more than 3–5 mmol/L/hour. Continue fixed-rate insulin infusion until ketosis has resolved.

#### Fluid

As a guide, infuse 1 litre over first 30 min, then 1 litre over 1 hour, then 1 litre over 2 hours, then 1 litre over 4 hours, then 1 litre over 6 hours. Consider central venous pressure monitoring in the elderly, and those with heart failure or renal failure.
When blood glucose falls below 14 mmol/L, add in a second infusion of 10% glucose at 125 mL/hour while continuing 0.9% saline and fixed rate insulin infusion.

#### Potassium

Potassium should usually be given from the second bag of fluid, unless the patient is oliguric or $K^+$ is more than 5.5 mmol/L. Give 20–40 mmol/L with each litre of fluid (maximum rate of 20 mmol/hour). Increase rate of potassium replacement if $K^+$ falls below 4 mmol/L. Plasma potassium should be measured after 60 min, and then every 2–4 hours until stable.

#### Alkali

Consider giving 250 mL of 1.4% sodium bicarbonate if pH is lower than 7.0, after seeking specialist advice.

#### Precipitating causes

Stopping insulin deliberately or running out
Infections increasing insulin resistance
Myocardial infarction
New diagnosis of diabetes

11

hyperosmolality of the blood slowly to allow water to move back into the brain slowly. Too rapid a shift may cause cerebral oedema which can worsen the level of consciousness. Normal saline has a lower osmolality than the hyperosmolar plasma of patients with HHS so will gradually lower the plasma osmolality in addition to the lowering of the plasma glucose by insulin. Initial fluid replacement volumes are similar to those in DKA. If severe hypernatraemia (sodium >160 mmol/L) persists after starting treatment, then half normal saline (0.45% saline) is sometimes used.

- *Insulin:* This should *not* be started immediately when treating HHS as this will lower plasma glucose rapidly causing an undesirable rapid fall in plasma osmolality. HHS is more sensitive to insulin than DKA, so less insulin is usually required. A fixed rate of 0.05 units/kg/hour is often used, started once plasma glucose stops falling with IV fluids only.

---

**EMERGENCY PRESENTATION 11.2**

### Hyperosmolar hyperglycaemic state

#### Diagnosis

- *Hyperglycaemia:* blood glucose often >30 mmol/L
- *No/minimal acidosis:* pH >7.3, $HCO_3^-$ >17 mmol/L
- *Minimal ketosis:* blood ketones <1.5; ketonuria 2+ or less
- *Hyperosmolarity:* usually >330 mOsm/L

#### Treatment

IV insulin does not need to be started immediately.

Fluid replacement will lower blood glucose due to dilution.

Start low-dose IV insulin infusion 0.05 units/kg/hour when glucose stops falling.

Prescribe antibiotics for intercurrent infection.

Hypernatraemia is frequent. Consider using 0.45% saline if plasma Na >160 mmol/L

Anticoagulation is with prophylactic heparin dosing due to high risk of thromboembolism.

Patients are more often elderly, with type 2 DM, and can usually be managed long-term with oral hypoglycaemic drugs and diet.

---

- *Anticoagulation:* Venous thromboembolism prophylaxis is used routinely, and treatment dose heparin given if there is active thromboembolism (e.g. pulmonary embolus).

#### Prognosis

HHS has a mortality of up to 30%. Factors include:

- Older age
- Electrolyte abnormalities (particularly sodium concentration)
- Thrombotic complications caused by hyperviscosity
- General complications of being unconscious
- Infection
- Any underlying condition precipitating HHS

People who survive HHS do not necessarily require continued insulin treatment. They usually have type 2 DM, and some may be managed by diet, with or without oral hypoglycaemic drugs. HHS can arise in type 2 DM if patients have not adhered to their diet and/or medication. Testing for cognitive deficit should take place on recovery and an education package started as needed.

## HYPOGLYCAEMIA

Capillary (or arterial) blood glucose concentration <3.5 mmol/L is generally taken to indicate hypoglycaemia. Venous blood glucose concentrations <3 mmol/L may occur in normal people during an oral glucose tolerance test because of a high arteriovenous difference in blood glucose. Hypoglycaemia most commonly occurs as a result of drug treatment for hyperglycaemia in people with DM but may also occur spontaneously or through inappropriate use of

**Table 11.11** Causes of hypoglycaemia

**Drug-related**
- Diabetes treatment (insulin/sulphonylureas)
- Deliberate self-harm using insulin or sulphonylureas
- Alcohol intoxication
- IV quinine therapy

**Liver disease**
- Liver failure
- Primary hepatic carcinoma

**Physiological**
- Reactive hypoglycaemia
- Dumping syndrome after gastrectomy or gastric bypass surgery
- Starvation
- Prolonged exercise

**Endocrine**
- Hypoadrenalism
- Hypothyroidism
- Insulinoma

**Infection**
- Septicaemia

**Congenital**
- Neonatal hyperinsulinism (nesidioblastosis)
- Hereditary fructose intolerance
- Galactosaemia
- Glycogen storage disease

hypoglycaemic drugs in non-diabetic individuals. Causes of hypoglycaemia are listed in **Table 11.11**.

### Hypoglycaemia in diabetes mellitus

Hypoglycaemia is a side effect of treatment in diabetes. It is more common with insulin than with oral hypoglycaemic drugs. A capillary blood glucose of 4.0 mmol/L is usually taken as the cut-off for hypoglycaemia ('four is the floor') due to variability in the accuracy of portable glucose meters (usually at least 10%). Hypoglycaemia can significantly affect cognitive and mental function and so influence work performance. Decreased motor coordination during hypoglycaemia can be hazardous if operating machinery or driving. The benefit of reducing overall glycaemia to prevent long-term complications of diabetes needs to be balanced against the risk of an unacceptable degree or frequency of hypoglycaemia. The main causes are insulin and suphonylureas. The risk of hypoglycaemia is low with metformin, SGLT2 inhibitors, GLP-1 agonists, alpha-glucosidase inhibitors, DPP IV inhibitors and pioglitazone.

### Disease mechanisms

Symptoms are variable and depend on the individual and the degree and speed of onset of the hypoglycaemia (**Figure 11.12**). In people *without* diabetes, mild symptoms of hypoglycaemia start with capillary blood glucose <3 mmol/L, and significant symptoms arise when this falls

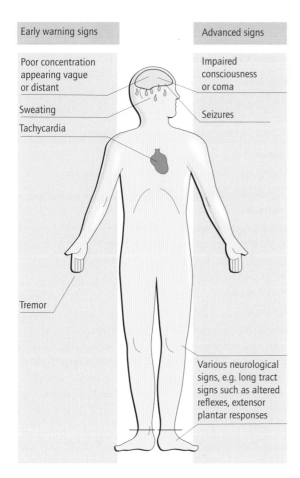

**Figure 11.12** Warning signs in hypoglycaemia.

Early warning signs

Poor concentration appearing vague or distant

Sweating

Tachycardia

Tremor

Advanced signs

Impaired consciousness or coma

Seizures

Various neurological signs, e.g. long tract signs such as altered reflexes, extensor plantar responses

**Table 11.12** Treatment of mild hypoglycaemia

If the patient is fully conscious and able to eat, they should take a rapidly absorbed form of carbohydrate supplying 16 g of glucose:
- ✓ A small glass (150 mL) of soft drink containing glucose or sucrose
- ✓ 2–4 glucose (dextrose) tablets
- ✓ Confectionary (candy) containing glucose syrup

Liquid solutions are more rapidly absorbed than solid forms. If there is no improvement after 5–10 min, this should be repeated.

A snack containing a source of more slowly absorbed carbohydrate (e.g. fruit, slice of bread, biscuit) should be taken to maintain blood glucose levels if the next meal is not due within 1 hour.

to <2 mmol/L. Hypoglycaemic symptoms have been classified as 'autonomic activation' and 'neuroglycopenia'.

### Autonomic activation

Hypothalamic autonomic centres are activated by blood glucose concentrations ≤2 mmol/L and stimulate both sympathetic and parasympathetic pathways; the resulting release of catecholamines, cortisol, glucagon and growth hormone raises blood glucose concentrations. Autonomic activation produces symptoms of cold sweat, tachycardia, tremor, blurred vision, hunger and altered salivation.

### Neuroglycopenia

Mild hypoglycaemia (blood glucose 2–3 mmol/L) causes subtle defects in higher cognitive function such as reasoning ability. More severe hypoglycaemia (blood glucose <1 mmol/L) causes neuroglycopenic symptoms including aggression, confusion, slurred speech, double vision and ataxia. Identity bracelets showing the patient uses insulin may help bystanders to recognize a hypoglycaemic attack which might otherwise be wrongly attributed to alcohol intoxication. If severe hypoglycaemia is sustained, impaired conscious level, fitting, coma and neurological damage can ensue.

## Diagnosis

Most episodes of hypoglycaemia are mild, recognized by the subject and self-treated (**Table 11.12**). Hypoglycaemia should always be considered in the differential diagnosis of an unconscious or confused patient. In a patient with diabetes, sweating, confusion and tachycardia suggest hypoglycaemia. Hypoglycaemia produces transient neurological signs (e.g. extensor plantar responses) that resolve when it is treated. If possible, test capillary blood glucose with a portable meter and send blood for laboratory glucose estimation. If there is any doubt, treat immediately for hypoglycaemia without waiting for laboratory results.

Prolonged or severe hypoglycaemia may be followed by a long period of recovery. A headache or 'hung over' feeling may last for many hours afterwards.

Hypoglycaemia occurs because of a mismatch between carbohydrate intake and insulin action. Insulin analogues have a lower prevalence of hypoglycaemia compared to soluble or intermediate insulins but are more expensive.

Nocturnal hypoglycaemia is a particular problem because the early warning symptoms are not recognized and the degree of hypoglycaemia is usually more severe before sweating, restlessness or even fitting wakes the patient. A bedtime snack may reduce the chance of nocturnal hypoglycaemia.

Factors that increase the risk of hypoglycaemia are intensive insulin regimens aiming for normoglycemia (e.g. during pregnancy), increased physical activity, alcohol use and duration of diabetes (**Table 11.13**).

## Hypoglycaemia unawareness

Patients with long-standing diabetes may lose the warning symptoms of hypoglycaemia. In part, this may reflect the loss of symptoms of autonomic activation due to autonomic neuropathy. Repeated episodes of hypoglycaemia cause adaptation of hypothalamic centres so that the same degree of hypoglycaemia produces a smaller autonomic activation. Loss of autonomic activation symptoms means that action to correct hypoglycaemia is not taken, resulting in

11

**Table 11.13** Factors increasing hypoglycaemia in people using insulin

**Excessive insulin dose**
- Dose recommended by doctor is too high
- Intentional injection of larger or extra dose of insulin
- Accidental injection of larger dose

**Insufficient carbohydrate**
- Late meal
- Missed meal
- Dieting

**Increased speed of insulin absorption**
- Exercise
- Altered site of injection
- Increased skin temperature from hot bath

**Concomitant hypoglycaemic factors**
- Alcohol
- Exercise

more severe hypoglycaemia. Loss of higher mental function and confusion with severe hypoglycaemia will also prevent individuals from treating themselves.

## Management

See EMERGENCY PRESENTATION 11.3.

Mild hypoglycaemia is almost inevitable in people treated with insulin and may occur in those taking sulphonylureas. People with diabetes at risk of hypoglycaemia should be educated in self-treatment of hypoglycaemia (see **Table 11.12**). Everyone treated with insulin should carry readily absorbable carbohydrate with them at all times (e.g. glucose tablets). Mild hypoglycaemia can be treated with oral ingestion of carbohydrate, ideally glucose (see **Table 11.12**). In unresponsive patients, glucagon is a useful treatment as non-clinicians can easily be taught to give an IM injection whereas IV glucose needs to be administered by trained personnel. Coma from hypoglycaemia usually responds within minutes to restoration of blood glucose concentrations. However, severe and/or prolonged hypoglycaemia may take longer to respond.

## Prevention

The risk of hypoglycaemia may be minimized by:
- *Diet:* Nocturnal hypoglycaemia can often be prevented with a bedtime snack.
- *Education:* Late or missed meals, insufficient carbohydrate intake or increased physical exercise increase the risk of hypoglycaemia.
- *Therapeutic changes:* Changing the dose of insulin and/or sulphonylureas, altering the type of insulin used or the timing of injections also increase the risk.

## INSULINOMA

Insulinomas are rare tumours of the pancreas that cause hypoglycaemia because of unregulated secretion of insulin.

---

**EMERGENCY PRESENTATION 11.3**

### Severe hypoglycaemia

**Diagnosis**

Blood glucose less than 3.5 mmol/L

*plus*

Help from a third party required for treatment

**Causes**

Patients with diabetes taking insulin or sulphonylureas

Other causes are listed in **Table 11.11**

**Treatment**

If fully conscious and safe swallow:
- Give oral carbohydrate (**Table 11.12**)

If impaired conscious level or unsafe swallow:
- IV glucose, *or*
- IM glucagon

*IV glucose*

100–150 mL 20% glucose IV (= 20–25 g glucose)

These are recommended doses for adults only. Children should be given smaller doses. High-concentration glucose should be given into a large vein and flushed with saline afterwards to reduce the risk of thrombophlebitis. **Care**: High-strength glucose may cause skin necrosis if extravasated

*IM glucagon*

Glucagon 0.5–1 mg intramuscularly

May be given by paramedical staff or trained family members. No risk of thrombophlebitis. May cause vomiting. Ineffective in chronic liver disease and prolonged starvation as glycogen stores are depleted

**Aftercare**

After recovery, ensure that oral carbohydrate is taken,

Consider the cause for the hypoglycaemic episode.

If the conscious level does not improve rapidly with correction of hypoglycaemia, consider the possibility of another cause of coma such as head injury, stroke, deliberate self-harm (e.g. overdose).

---

Symptoms of hypoglycaemia may be wrongly attributed to anxiety or to neurological disease. Insulinomas classically cause *fasting* hypoglycaemia which typically occurs at night, but daytime symptoms may also occur. Because anxiety is common and insulinomas are rare, an algorithm (Whipple's triad) should be used to suggest the diagnosis. Whipple's triad states that:

1 Symptoms should be associated with fasting or exercise.
2 Hypoglycaemia is demonstrated to be present during the symptoms.
3 Glucose relieves the symptoms.

The diagnosis requires demonstration of inappropriately high or non-suppressed insulin levels during hypoglycaemia. This can be done by fasting the patient for a prolonged period (48–72 hours) and monitoring blood glucose concentrations. An important differential diagnosis is factitious hypoglycaemia secondary to insulin injection or use of sulphonylureas. Insulin for injection does not contain C-peptide so elevated C-peptide in the presence of hypoglycaemia suggests either insulinoma or sulphonylurea use. Sulphonylureas may be detected in blood or urine samples. Most insulinomas are benign tumours and surgical excision is usually curative. Preoperatively, the tumour may be localized by a number of techniques including CT/MRI scanning, PET scans and pancreatic angiography. Diazoxide, which inhibits insulin release by pancreatic β cells, may be used to prevent hypoglycaemia in preoperative patients or in those unfit or unwilling to undergo surgery.

## OBESITY AND OVERWEIGHT STATES

Body weight is determined by genetic, environmental, cultural and psychosocial factors. Obesity is a condition in which excess body fat accumulates, such that health may be affected. In healthy adult men of average weight, body fat = 15–20% and for women = 25–30% of total body weight. It is difficult to measure body fat directly, so the body mass index (BMI) is usually used as an indirect measure.

$$BMI = [weight(kg)] / [height(m)]^2$$

Obesity in adults is BMI of ≥30 kg/m² (**Table 11.14**). Epidemiological studies show an increased morbidity and mortality as BMI increases above the desirable range. Special scales may be required to accurately weigh very heavy patients. Fat mass can be estimated using scales that measure bioelectrical impedance. Skin-fold thickness, measured over the triceps or subscapular areas, may be used in specialist centres.

### SIMPLE OBESITY

When obesity is not secondary to another disorder, it is classified as simple obesity. Eating in excess of energy requirements is the primary cause; the origin for this is

**Table 11.14** WHO classification of overweight

| BMI (kg/m²) | WHO class | Popular term |
| --- | --- | --- |
| <18.5 | Underweight | Thin |
| 18.5–24.9 | Normal range | Healthy, acceptable |
| 25.0–29.9 | Pre-obese | Overweight |
| 30.0–34.9 | Obese grade 1 | Obese |
| 35.0–39.9 | Obese grade 2 | Obese |
| >40 | Obese grade 3 | Morbidly obese |

BMI, body mass index.

**Table 11.15** Causes of secondary obesity

Hypothyroidism
Cushing's syndrome
Drug treatments:
- Corticosteroids
- Phenothiazines
- Atypical anti-psychotics
- Lithium
- Tricyclic antidepressants
- Sodium valproate
- Insulin

Monogenic syndromes associated with hypogonadism:
- Prader–Willi syndrome
- Laurence–Moon–Biedl syndrome

Pituitary and hypothalamic disorders

multifactorial with both biological and psychological mechanisms driving overeating.

## SECONDARY OBESITY

Obesity occurs as an associated feature of a number of conditions, and weight gain may be exacerbated by drug treatments (**Table 11.15**). These differential diagnoses should be considered in any subject presenting with obesity.

## EPIDEMIOLOGY

There have been significant trends in obesity prevalence in many countries (**Table 11.16**). Between-country differences in obesity rates are not completely explained by affluence (e.g. Japan and India have similar obesity prevalence figures). Obesity is more prevalent in women and increases with age up to 50–60 years.

## DISEASE MECHANISMS

Day-to-day food intake needs to be closely matched to energy expenditure for the maintenance of stable body

**Table 11.16** Prevalence of obesity in different countries in adults >18 years old (male and female combined). (Source WHO data repository)

| Country | 1996 | 2006 | 2016 |
| --- | --- | --- | --- |
| Australia | 18.1% | 23.5% | 29.0% |
| Brazil | 12.7% | 17.3% | 22.1% |
| Egypt | 20.3% | 25.5% | 32.0% |
| France | 14.5% | 17.9% | 21.6% |
| India | 1.3% | 2.3% | 3.9% |
| Japan | 1.8% | 2.7% | 4.3% |
| Mexico | 18.9% | 23.8% | 28.9% |
| Nigeria | 3.2% | 5.4% | 8.9% |
| Samoa | 34.0% | 40.8% | 47.3% |
| UK | 16.6% | 21.9% | 27.8% |
| US | 22.6% | 29.7% | 36.2% |

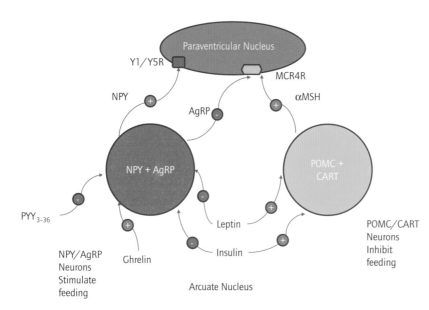

**Figure 11.13** Hypothalamic control of appetite. NPY, Neuropeptide Y; Y1/Y5R, NPY receptor subtypes 1 and 5; AgRP, agouti-gene related peptide; $PYY_{3-36}$, peptide $YY_{3-36}$; POMC, pro-opiomelanacortin; CART, cocaine and amphetamine regulated transcript; αMSH, α-melanocyte stimulating hormone; MCR4, melanocortin receptor 4.

weight. When energy intake exceeds expenditure, the excess calories are stored as adipose tissue. Fat is stored subcutaneously, around internal organs, within the omentum and in intramuscular spaces. Fat storage confers a survival value when food is in short supply, allowing a person of normal weight to survive 2 months of total starvation. A plentiful food supply and overconsumption can lead this physiological mechanism to become a health risk.

### Hypothalamic control of eating

The physiological urge to eat and the perception of being satiated are controlled centrally by the hypothalamus (**Figure 11.13**). The hypothalamus sends signals to the cerebral cortex to stimulate eating and as feeding progresses this stimulus is inhibited. The activity of these neural centres is regulated by several peripheral factors, including:

- Rise in plasma glucose and/or insulin
- Leptin released from adipose tissue
- Humoral substances released from the gut
- Autonomic nervous system input from stretch receptors in the stomach

#### Genetics

Twin studies suggest a genetic contribution to body weight. A number of rare genetic changes can affect feeding behaviour and cause obesity even in infancy. Genome-wide association studies have identified many loci associated with obesity and, in most people, any genetic influence on obesity is probably polygenic.

### Cognitive control of eating

Psychological theories of obesity emphasize the role of learned and cognitive influences on eating behaviour. Hunger is related not solely to metabolic status (time since last meal) but also to anticipation of nutritional requirements. An early 'psychosomatic theory' of obesity regarded overeating as a response to emotional stimuli. Obesity was

thus a result of a learned behaviour (overeating) adopted as a coping response. The 'externality theory' has suggested that obese people are more responsive to external cues to eating such as palatability of food and less responsive to internal satiety and hunger cues ('interoception'). More recent theories have emphasized the role of voluntary restriction of food intake. A proportion of people identified as 'restrained eaters' consciously limit their food intake; however, if given an amount of food thought to exceed their self-imposed limit, they abandon restraint and overeat. Such a cognitive loop might occur in people with bulimia nervosa.

### Energy intake and expenditure

For adults to maintain a stable weight, their daily energy intake (food) needs to match their daily energy expenditure. Total daily energy expenditure combines:

- Energy used to maintain the resting metabolic rate: 60–70%
  This is unchanged in obesity. However, it is lowered in untreated hypothyroidism.
- Thermic effect of food: 10%
  After eating, energy is required to power the digestion, absorption and storage of nutrients. No changes significant enough to cause weight gain have been identified in obese people.
- Energy cost of physical activity: 20–30%
  Physical activity is the only variable under voluntary control that affects total energy expenditure. Obese people are less physically active than lean people. Prospective studies indicate that low physical activity at baseline weight is a risk factor for later weight gain.

## CLINICAL FEATURES

Clinical examination of obese people should be directed to identifying associated comorbid conditions (**Table 11.17**) and clinical features of disorders causing secondary obesity

**Table 11.17** Comorbidities associated with obesity

**Metabolic**
- Type 2 DM
- Hyperlipidaemia
- Insulin resistance

**Cardiorespiratory**
- Hypertension
- CHD
- Sleep apnoea (obesity hypoventilation syndrome)
- Thromboembolic disease
- Cerebrovascular disease

**Rheumatological**
- Osteoarthritis
- Back pain
- Ligament/tendon injury

**Gastrointestinal**
- Gallstones
- Reflux oesophagitis
- Hepatic steatosis (fatty liver)

**Psychological**
- Depression
- Anxiety
- Low self-esteem

**Cancer risk increased**
- Endometrium
- Breast
- Colorectal
- Prostate
- Ovary

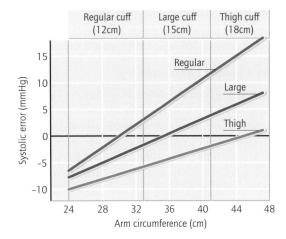

**Figure 11.14** Relationship between arm circumference and blood pressure cuff size as related to systolic error of blood pressure measurement. Reproduced from Swales JD (1994) *Textbook of Hypertension* (Wiley-Blackwell, Oxford), with the permission of the author.

**11**

(see **Table 11.15**). Obesity may present with symptoms of these comorbid conditions. An assessment of the mental state should be included; morbidly obese people have higher rates of anxiety and depression. Breathlessness may be due to the increased work associated with walking with an increased mechanical weight load and compounded by lack of physical fitness. Consider other causes of breathlessness, including obesity hypoventilation syndrome. Body temperature regulation is more difficult in the obese because of the insulating effect of fat causing problematic sweating. Ascites may present as 'obesity' and should be considered as a differential diagnosis in people with an increasing waist size.

## Complications of obesity

### Metabolic
These include insulin resistance, NDH, type 2 diabetes, hyperlipidaemia (raised triglycerides, raised low-density lipoprotein (LDL)-cholesterol and low high-density lipoprotein (HDL)-cholesterol). Obesity is a major risk factor for type 2 diabetes, but most moderately obese people do not develop diabetes.

### Cardiovascular
This is the principal cause of death among obese people. Modifiable risk factors for cardiovascular disease (smoking, hypertension, hyperlipidaemia, physical inactivity) should be addressed. Blood pressure should be measured with a correctly sized cuff – an inappropriately small cuff size produces spuriously raised blood pressure readings (**Figure 11.14**). There is a correlation between degree of obesity and blood pressure. Weight loss improves both hypertension and hyperlipidaemia associated with obesity.

### Cancer
Obesity increases the risk of a number of cancers (**Table 11.17**). It is also a major factor in the increasing incidence of certain cancers. Significant *unintentional* weight loss in an obese person may be the first symptom of any cancer.

## INVESTIGATION

Obese people should be assessed by thyroid function tests, HbA1c or fasting glucose, lipid profile and ECG. Overweight (BMI 25–29.9 kg/m$^2$) and obesity (BMI ≥30 kg/m$^2$) have a combined prevalence of 40–65% in European countries; specialist investigation is restricted to those with features to suggest a secondary cause or where the rate of weight gain is rapid. The gonadal axis should be investigated if there is a lack of androgenization in men or menstrual disturbance in women. Patients suspected to have Cushing's syndrome, hypothalamic or pituitary disease should be assessed by an endocrinologist. Sleep apnoea should be suspected in the very obese.

## MANAGEMENT

### Treatment choices and goals

Treatment of obesity aims to improve health and reduce associated complications of obesity. Success is usually reduction in severity of obesity rather than return to an 'ideal' body weight. Modest weight loss of 5–10% body weight improves blood pressure, dyslipidaemia and hyperglycaemia. Long-term changes in lifestyle, both in diet and in physical activity, are required for weight maintenance.

### Dietary treatment of obesity

Estimated energy requirement = 30–35 kcal/kg/day. Dietary treatment of obesity involves reducing daily energy intake. An energy deficit diet that supplies 500–1000 kcal/day less energy than the estimated requirement energy usually results in weight loss. It is difficult to maintain a 1000 kcal/day energy deficit long-term. Energy restriction more severe than this causes excessive loss of lean tissue and should be discouraged.

The diet should be balanced and take into account the patient's tastes and lifestyle. Initial weight loss on an energy-restricted diet is more rapid because of loss of glycogen stores and their associated water content. Weight loss >0.5–1 kg/week should not be expected from a fairly restricted diet of 1000 kcal/day deficit. Patients may expect to lose more weight than this and will abandon a diet that was working well for 'lack of efficacy'. Support from a slimming club, family members and a professional dietitian can aid motivation.

### Cognitive–behavioural treatment

Cognitive–behavioural treatment increases weight loss when used as an adjunct to diet treatment alone. Food diaries may identify situations or emotions that lead to uncontrolled eating. Behavioural treatments aim to reduce exposure to these situations (stimulus control). Cognitive therapy aims to identify false beliefs about body image. Psychotherapy or drug treatment for depression may be required before a diet treatment plan is adopted.

### Exercise

Regular exercise increases daily energy expenditure and aids weight loss so long as energy intake is not similarly increased. People who increase physical activity, as well as adhere to a calorie-restricted diet, experience greater weight loss. Importantly, people who continue their increased level of physical activity are more likely to maintain their weight loss after stopping calorie restriction.

### Drugs

Drug treatment for obesity is considered if obesity is accompanied by other factors that accentuate the health risks from obesity (e.g. hypertension, sleep apnoea, diabetes). Most drug treatments report weight losses of 5–10% of initial body weight, but weight is often regained when the drug is stopped. Drugs currently licensed for weight loss are listed in **Table 11.18**, but licensing varies between countries.

### Metabolic (bariatric) surgery

Lifestyle change and drug treatments for obesity have limited effectiveness, but metabolic surgery is highly effective and may produce relatively long-lasting weight loss

**Table 11.18** Drugs licensed for treating obesity, mechanisms and possible side effects

| Name | Mechanism of action | Side effects |
|---|---|---|
| Orlistat | Inhibits intestinal lipases | Fat malabsorption diarrhoea, faecal incontinence |
| Liraglutide | GLP-1 receptor agonist | Nausea, vomiting, diarrhoea, rash |
| Lorcaserin | Serotonin 2C agonist | Dizziness, headache, insomnia |
| Phentermine + Topiramate | Noradrenaline releaser + anti-convulsant | Dizziness, headache, insomnia |
| Naltrexone + Bupropion | Opiod antagonist + Aminoketone antidepressant | Nausea, constipation, headache, dry mouth |

compared to drug treatments. Some procedures are associated with improved metabolic parameters and overall reduced mortality. Specialist surgical centres and laparoscopic techniques now have 30-day mortality rates <0.1% in developed countries. Four main procedures are used:

- Adjustable gastric band
- Roux-en-Y gastric bypass
- Vertical sleeve gastrectomy
- Hepatobilary bypass

Adjustable gastric banding is the least effective procedure for weight loss and is not associated with remission of diabetes. The other three procedures may all induce remission of type 2 diabetes, but the mechanisms for this are unclear.

## PLASMA LIPID AND LIPOPROTEIN DISORDERS

Plasma lipid and lipoprotein disorders – the dyslipidaemias – are associated with increased risks of atherosclerosis-related disease, particularly coronary artery disease (CAD). Severe hypertriglyceridaemia is a risk factor for pancreatitis.

Treatment of dyslipidaemia is an important component of secondary prevention of CAD and of primary prevention of CAD in those at high risk. Familial lipid disorders are associated with a high relative risk of CAD and merit therapy in their own right. Relatives of individuals with premature CAD and of those with known familial lipid disorders should be screened for lipid abnormalities.

## LIPID AND LIPOPROTEIN METABOLISM

Cholesterol and triglyceride are relatively insoluble in aqueous plasma and are transported in lipoproteins, which

## OBESITY AT A GLANCE

### Epidemiology

*Prevalence in England (2019)*

- Obesity 27% of men; 29% of women
- Overweight 41% of men, 31% of women

*Age*

- Incidence increases with age between 20 and 60 years

*Genetics*

- Twin and adoption studies suggest a genetic contribution

*Geography*

- Higher prevalence in developed countries

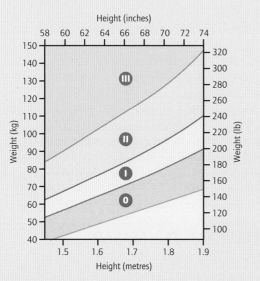

**Figure A** Height/weight relationships indicating boundaries of desirable weight (0), mild (I), moderate (II) and severe (III) obesity. Reproduced from Grossman A (1992) *Clinical Endocrinology* (Wiley-Blackwell, Oxford), with the permission of the author.

### Findings on investigation

*Anthropometry*

- Body mass index (BMI) ≥30 kg/m$^2$

*Biochemistry*

- Role of biochemical investigations to exclude secondary causes of obesity
- Impaired glucose tolerance
- Hyperlipidaemia

*Differential diagnosis*

- Hypothyroidism
- Cushing's syndrome

### Associated features

*Metabolic*

- Hyperlipidaemia
- Insulin resistance
- Type 2 DM

*Cardiorespiratory*

- Hypertension
- CHD
- Stroke
- Thromboembolism
- Sleep apnoea

*Gastrointestinal*

- Hiatus hernia
- Gallstones

*Rheumatological*

- Osteoarthritis
- Back pain

**11**

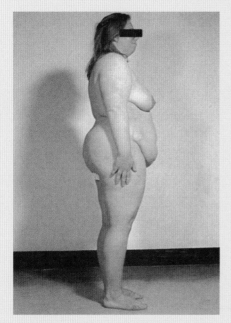

**Figure B** Moderately obese female who has a significant risk of heart disease.

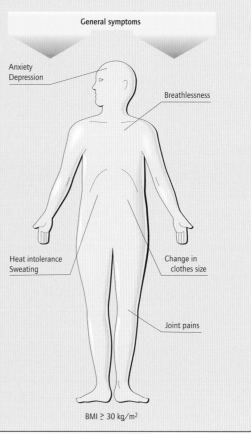

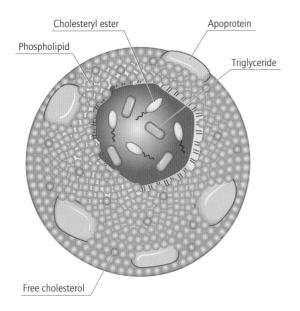

Cholesteryl ester
Apoprotein
Phospholipid
Triglyceride
Free cholesterol

**Figure 11.15** Structure of lipoprotein particles.

are multimolecular micelle-like particles (**Figure 11.15**). Insoluble cholesterol ester and triglyceride form a lipid droplet at the centre of the lipoprotein with more polar molecules such as free cholesterol, phospholipid and apoproteins on the surface, at the interface with plasma. Apoproteins have both structural roles and regulatory functions in lipoprotein metabolism (**Table 11.19**).

Lipoprotein metabolism may be simplified to three main pathways (**Figure 11.16**):

- *Exogenous pathway:* lipids from food
- *Endogenous pathway:* lipids synthesized by the liver
- *Reverse cholesterol transport:* return of cholesterol from tissues to liver

## LIPIDS, LIPOPROTEINS AND ATHEROGENESIS

The classification of lipoproteins is summarized in **Table 11.20**.

Increasing plasma cholesterol concentrations are strongly and independently related to risk of atherosclerosis-related disease, particularly CAD (**Figure 11.17**). LDL-cholesterol determines the relationship of total plasma cholesterol to CAD risk.

HDL-cholesterol is inversely related to CAD, probably because it plays a role in reverse cholesterol transport.

The relationship between plasma triglycerides and CAD is less clear. Hypertriglyceridaemia can be associated with the accumulation of remnant particles, which are considered to be highly atherogenic. In addition, when triglycerides are raised, LDL subclass distribution is altered towards smaller denser particles, which are thought to be more atherogenic.

Lipoprotein(a) (Lp(a)) is a form of LDL with an additional apoprotein (apoprotein(a)) attached to it. Apoprotein(a) has structural similarity to plasminogen. Lp(a) concentrations are largely genetically determined and are a risk factor for CAD when plasma cholesterol is raised.

## DYSLIPOPROTEINAEMIAS

Lipid disorders are classified as primary or secondary (**Tables 11.21** and **11.22**). The primary disorders are named, where possible, on the underlying metabolic and/or genetic abnormality. Lipid and lipoprotein concentrations are normally measured in the fasting state. In routine clinical practice total cholesterol, total triglyceride and HDL-cholesterol are measured directly

**Table 11.19** Classification and function of apoproteins

| Type | Molecular weight (kDa) | Origin | Lipoprotein distribution | Principal function |
|------|------------------------|--------|--------------------------|--------------------|
| A-I | 29 | Liver, intestine | HDL, chylomicrons | LCAT activator |
| A-II | 17 | Liver, intestine | HDL, chylomicrons | Structural protein in HDL |
| A-IV | 44 | Liver, intestine | HDL, chylomicrons | Non-specific LCAT cofactor |
| $B_{48}$ | 241 | Intestine | Chylomicrons, chylomicron remnants | Mediates chylomicron formation and secretion by enterocytes |
| $B_{100}$ | 513 | Liver | VLDL, LDL | Mediates hepatic VLDL formation / Ligand for LDL receptor |
| C-I | 6.6 | Liver | Chylomicrons, VLDL, HDL | Inhibitor of chylomicron uptake |
| C-II | 9 | Liver | Chylomicrons, VLDL, HDL | LPL activator |
| C-III | 9 | Liver | Chylomicrons, VLDL, HDL | Inhibitor of LPL |
| D | 19 | Liver | HDL | ?Involved in cholesteryl ester transfer |
| E | 34.1 | Liver | Chylomicrons, VLDL, HDL | Ligand for chylomicron receptor and LDL receptor |

HDL, high-density lipoprotein; LCAT, lecithin–cholesterol acyltransferase; LDL, low-density lipoprotein; LPL, lipoprotein lipase; VLDL, very low-density lipoprotein.

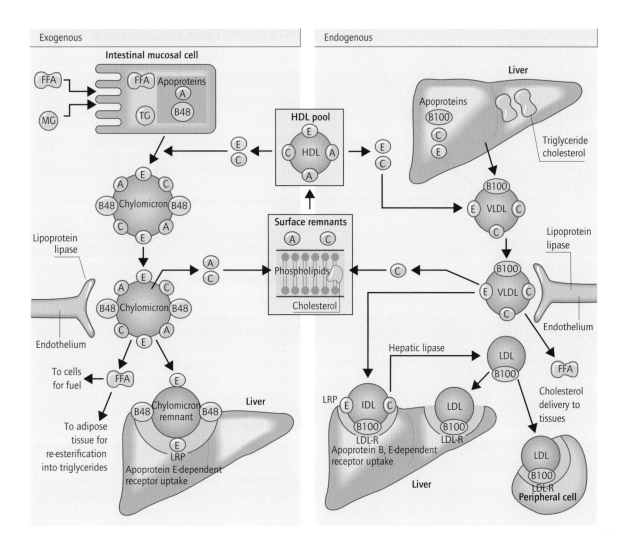

**Figure 11.16** Overview of lipoprotein metabolism: exogenous and endogenous pathways. FFA, free fatty acids; LDL-R, LDL receptor; LRP, LDL receptor-related protein; MG, monoglycerides; TG, triglycerides; letters A, B48, B100, C and E refer to apoproteins A, $B_{48}$, $B_{100}$, C and E, respectively.

**Table 11.20** Classification of lipoproteins

| Class | Diameter (nm) | Density (g/mL) | Electrophoretic mobility | Chemical composition (% of dry mass) | | | | |
|---|---|---|---|---|---|---|---|---|
| | | | | | Cholesterol | | | |
| | | | | Triglycerides | Esters | Cholesterol | Phospholipids | Proteins |
| Chylomicrons | 75–1200 | 0.93 | $\alpha_2$ | 86 | 3 | 2 | 7 | 2 |
| VLDL | 30–80 | 0.96–1.006 | Pre-$\beta$ | 55 | 12 | 7 | 18 | 8 |
| IDL | 25–35 | 1.006–1.019 | Slow pre-$\beta$ | 23 | 29 | 9 | 19 | 19 |
| LDL | 18–25 | 1.019–1.063 | $\beta$ | 6 | 42 | 8 | 22 | 22 |
| HDL$_2$ | 9–12 | 1.063–1.125 | $\alpha_1$ | 5 | 17 | 5 | 33 | 40 |
| HDL$_3$ | 5–9 | 1.125–1.210 | $\alpha_1$ | 3 | 13 | 4 | 25 | 55 |

HDL, high-density lipoprotein; IDL, intermediate-density lipoprotein; LDL, low-density lipoprotein; VLDL, very low-density lipoprotein.

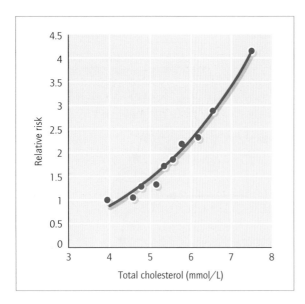

**Figure 11.17** Relationship of plasma cholesterol to CHD mortality in the Multiple Risk Factor Intervention Trial (MRFIT) study. Adapted from Stamler J *et al*. Is relationship between serum cholesterol and risk of premature death from coronary heart disease continuous and graded? *JAMA* 1986; 256: 2823–8.

and LDL-cholesterol is calculated by the Friedewald formula:

$$\text{LDL-cholesterol [mmol/L]} = \text{total cholesterol} \\ - \text{HDL-cholesterol} - (\text{total triglyceride}/2.19)$$

If triglycerides are >4.5 mmol/L, the formula is invalid.

## FAMILIAL HYPERCHOLESTEROLAEMIA

Familial hypercholesterolaemia (FH) is associated with a high risk of premature CAD.

### Epidemiology

- Approximately 1 in 250–500 of the UK population are heterozygotes, so the homozygous form is very rare
- Average age of onset of CAD in untreated heterozygous cases: men early forties; women early fifties
- Autosomal dominant
- More common in some populations (e.g. South Africans of Dutch ethnicity, Lebanese, Ashkenazi Jews, Finns)

### Disease mechanisms

Genetic defects identified in:
- *LDL receptor gene* (80% cases): absent or defective LDL receptor activity causing reduced hepatic removal of LDL-cholesterol
- *Apolipoprotein B gene* (5% cases): helps LDL receptor bind LDL; mutations can reduce hepatic removal of LDL-cholesterol

### Clinical features

Typical features are high plasma total cholesterol and high LDL-cholesterol, premature CAD and tendon xanthomas (**Figure 11.18**). Individuals *homozygous* for FH can develop CAD in adolescence. Adult heterozygotes usually

**Table 11.21** Classification of primary hyperlipidaemias

| Type | WHO phenotype | Typical lipid levels (mmol/l) | | | |
|---|---|---|---|---|---|
| | | Cholesterol | Triglycerides | Lipoproteins | Clinical signs |
| Polygenic hypercholesterolaemia | 2a | 6.5–9.0 | <2.3 | LDL ↑ | Xanthelasma, corneal arcus |
| FH | 2a | 7.5–16.0 | <2.3 | LDL ↑ | Tendon xanthoma, arcus, xanthelasma |
| Familial defective apoprotein B$_{100}$ | 2a | 7.5–16.0 | 2.3 | LDL ↑ | Tendon xanthoma, arcus, xanthelasma |
| FCH | 2a, 2b, 4 or 5 | 6.5–10.0 | 2.3–12.0 | LDL ↑, VLDL ↑, HDL ↓ | Arcus, xanthelasma |
| Remnant particle disease | 3 | 9.0–14.0 | 9.0–14.0 | IDL ↑ | Palmar striae, tuberoeruptive xanthomas |
| Familial hypertriglyceridaemia | 4, 5 | 6.5–12.0 | 10.0–30.0 | VLDL ↑ | Eruptive xanthomas, lipaemia retinalis, hepatosplenomegaly |
| Lipoprotein lipase deficiency | 1 | <6.5 | 10.0–30.0 | Chylomicrons ↑ | Eruptive xanthomas, lipaemia retinalis, hepatosplenomegaly |
| **Primary HDL abnormalities** | | | | | |
| Hyperalphalipoproteinaemia | – | HDL >2.0 | – | HDL ↑ | – |
| Hypoalphalipoproteinaemia | – | HDL <0.9 | – | HDL ↓ | – |

HDL, high-density lipoprotein; IDL, intermediate-density lipoprotein; LDL, low-density lipoprotein; VLDL, very low-density lipoprotein.

**Table 11.22** Factors contributing to secondary hyperlipidaemias

**Hormonal factors**
- Pregnancy
- DM
- Hypothyroidism

**Nutritional factors**
- Obesity
- Anorexia nervosa
- Problem drinking

**Liver disease**
- Primary biliary cirrhosis
- Extrahepatic biliary obstruction

**Renal dysfunction**
- Nephrotic syndrome
- Chronic renal failure

**Iatrogenic**
- Antiretroviral drugs
- High-dose thiazide diuretics
- Retinoids
- Corticosteroids
- Exogenous sex hormones
- β-Adrenergic receptor antagonists (some)

have total cholesterol >7.5 mmol/L and LDL-cholesterol >5.0 mmol/L.

Tendon xanthomas are typically seen in the extensor tendons on the backs of the hands, over the knuckles and in the Achilles tendons. Development of xanthomas is a function of age; approximately 70% of patients have xanthomas by the age of 30 years.

It is important to make the diagnosis, as aggressive lipid-lowering therapy is required given the high CAD risk. Family screening is important to identify affected individuals.

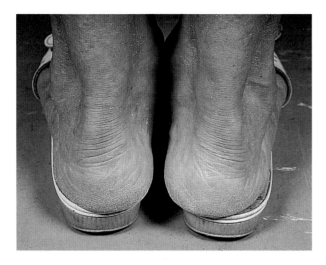

**Figure 11.18** Tendon xanthoma in a patient heterozygous for FH.

# FAMILIAL COMBINED HYPERLIPIDAEMIA

## Epidemiology

- Approximately 1 in 200
- Genetics uncertain; three chromosomal regions are associated with the condition, but no specific gene defects have been described

## Disease mechanisms

Overproduction of apolipoprotein B-containing lipoproteins by the liver results in high cholesterol and/or triglycerides, reduced HDL, raised apo B and increased small, dense (atherogenic) LDL. Obesity and insulin resistance are more common in familial combined hyperlipidaemia (FCH) and contribute to the phenotypic variation.

It has been estimated that FCH accounts for 10–15% of premature myocardial infarction in Europe and North America. Affected family members have multiple lipoprotein phenotypes.

## Clinical features

FCH is associated with increased CAD risk. There are no agreed criteria for diagnosis and no specific clinical stigmata; affected individuals may have corneal arcus and xanthelasma, but these signs are not specific. Tendon xanthomas do *not* occur. The diagnosis is often presumptive in a patient with mixed lipaemia and a family history of primary hyperlipidaemia. Clinically there is overlap with the metabolic syndrome.

# REMNANT PARTICLE DISEASE

## Epidemiology

- Rare, affecting 1 in 5000–10 000 individuals
- >90% of patients with remnant particle disease are homozygous for apoprotein $E_2$

## Disease mechanisms

Remnant particles are produced from the processing of chylomicrons that deliver lipids from the gut. Apoprotein E is involved in the uptake of remnant particles in the liver via the LDL receptor-related protein (LRP) receptor (see **Figure 11.16**). Apoprotein E has three common genetically determined isoforms: $E_2$, $E_3$ and $E_4$. About 70% of individuals are homozygous for $E_3$ (the normal allele). Around 1% of the UK population are homozygous for apoprotein $E_2$, which is a less efficient ligand for the LDL and LRP receptors. For the remnant particle disease phenotype to develop, further genetic factors (e.g. FH, FCH) or environmental factors (e.g. obesity, DM, hypothyroidism) are required, which 'stress' the apoprotein E-mediated removal of remnant particles.

## Clinical features

The clinical hallmarks are palmar xanthomas and tuberoeruptive xanthomas (**Figure 11.19**) and there is a high risk

11

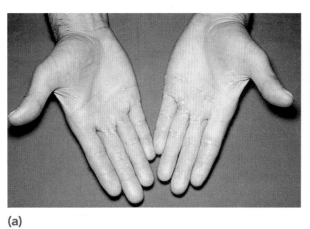

**(a)**

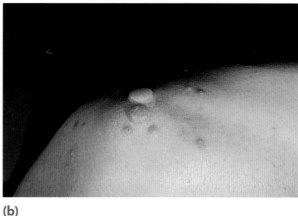

**(b)**

**Figure 11.19 (a)** Palmar and **(b)** tuberoeruptive xanthomas in a patient with remnant particle disease.

of premature CAD and peripheral vascular disease. Due to accumulation of remnant particles, both plasma cholesterol and triglyceride are markedly raised. Remnant particles produce a characteristic broad β band on lipoprotein electrophoresis. Apoprotein $E_2$ homozygosity can be demonstrated by electrophoresis of apoproteins or by sequencing the apoprotein E gene.

## COMMON POLYGENIC HYPERCHOLESTEROLAEMIA

This diagnosis applies to the *majority* of patients with hypercholesterolaemia.

### Epidemiology

- Common. Frequency depends on dietary intake of saturated fat and cholesterol.
- Polygenic. Common polymorphisms in different gene loci (e.g. apoprotein E, apoprotein B, LDL receptor gene) influence plasma cholesterol level.

### Clinical features

There are no specific clinical features, although corneal arcus and xanthelasma may be present. Diagnosis made after exclusion of secondary causes and monogenic primary disorders.

## CHYLOMICRONAEMIA SYNDROME

This syndrome is characterized by severe hypertriglyceridaemia (fasting triglyceride >11 mmol/L) due to persistence of chylomicrons in the fasting state. Cholesterol may be normal or raised. Usually the syndrome occurs in patients with alcohol excess, DM or on antiretroviral therapy, who often have another genetic hyperlipidaemia such as FCH. Very rarely, it is caused by inborn errors of lipid metabolism such as LPL deficiency.

Clinical features include eruptive xanthomas (**Figure 11.20**), hepatosplenomegaly and lipaemia retinalis (white discoloration of retinal vessels). Severe hypertriglyceridaemia may

affect other laboratory measurements (e.g. haemoglobin, bilirubin, liver transaminases). Measured hyponatraemia (approximately 2–4 mmol/L per 10 mmol/L triglyceride) occurs because of the decreased water volume of the plasma, but the sodium concentration in plasma water is normal (pseudohyponatraemia).

Chylomicronaemia increases the risk of pancreatitis and patients can experience intermittent episodes of abdominal pain without full-blown acute pancreatitis. Severe hypertriglyceridaemia may interfere with amylase assays producing falsely low levels.

## LIPOPROTEIN LIPASE DEFICIENCY

### Epidemiology

- Rare: approximately 1 in 1 million
- Autosomal recessive defects in the LPL gene

### Clinical features

Patients exhibit extreme hypertriglyceridaemia (triglyceride 50–100 mmol/L). Fasting plasma refrigerated overnight shows a characteristic cream layer. Symptoms and signs are

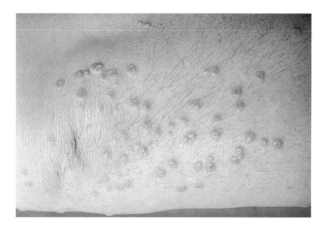

**Figure 11.20** Eruptive xanthomas in a patient with chylomicronaemia syndrome.

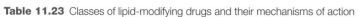

**Table 11.23** Classes of lipid-modifying drugs and their mechanisms of action

| Drug class | Mechanism of action | Metabolic effects | Plasma lipoproteins | | |
|---|---|---|---|---|---|
| | | | LDL | HDL | VLDL |
| HMG-CoA reductase | Inhibit early stage of cholesterol synthesis | Increased clearance of LDL from plasma by LDL receptors | ↓↓↓↓ | ↑ | ↓ |
| Fibrates | Increased lipoprotein lipase activity, reduced hepatic VLDL production | Increased VLDL catabolism Increased synthesis of HDL | ↓↓ | ↑↑ | ↓↓↓ |
| Bile acid sequestrants | Interruption of entrohepatic circulation of bile salts increases hepatic bile acid synthesis from intracellular hepatic cholesterol upregulating hepatic LDL receptors | Increased clearance of LDL from plasma by LDL receptors | ↓↓↓ | ↑ | → |
| PCSK9 inhibitors | Reduced degradation of LDL receptors | Increased clearance of LDL from plasma by LDL receptors | ↓↓↓↓ | ↑ | ↓ |
| Nicotinic acid | Inhibition of lipolysis in fat tissue, reducing free fatty acid flux to liver | Decreased VLDL and LDL synthesis Decreased clearance of HDL | ↓↓↓ | ↑↑↑↑ | ↓↓↓↓ |
| Fish oils | Inhibit VLDL synthesis | | → | → | ↓↓↓ |
| Ezetimibe | Inhibits intestinal absorption of dietary and biliary cholesterol | Reduced delivery of cholesterol to liver in chylomicra | ↓↓ | ↑ | ↓ |

as for chylomicronaemia (see above). A similar phenotype is seen in people who lack apoprotein $C_2$, which is required for activation of LPL.

## MANAGEMENT OF DYSLIPIDAEMIA

The most common reason for the treatment of dyslipidaemia is the secondary prevention of vascular disease in people with established atherosclerotic disease and the primary prevention of vascular disease in those at high risk (**Table 11.23**). Less often, therapy is given to reduce the risk of pancreatitis. Eruptive xanthomas in chylomicronaemia and palmar and tuberoeruptive xanthomas can disappear with therapy.

Nutritional counselling (**Table 11.24**) and other lifestyle measures such as exercise and smoking cessation are important in all patients (**Table 11.25**).

### Statins

The major therapeutic agents are the statins, which are specific competitive inhibitors of 3-hydroxy-methylglutaryl coenzyme A (HMG-CoA) reductase, the rate-determining enzyme in cholesterol synthesis. Their major site of action is the liver where they reduce cholesterol synthesis which causes upregulation of LDL receptors. This increases LDL uptake by the liver and plasma LDL-cholesterol concentrations fall by 30–60%.

#### Secondary prevention of vascular disease
Statins lower the risk of death from CAD, CAD events and stroke in people with a wide range of plasma cholesterol concentrations who have established CAD. Therefore, all patients with established vascular disease, irrespective of cholesterol level, should be offered statins unless contraindicated.

**Table 11.24** Basic principles of lipid-lowering diet

| Principle | Amount | Food sources |
|---|---|---|
| Decreased total fat; decreased saturated fat | <30% of energy 7–10% of energy | Avoid butter, hard margarine, whole milk, cream, ice cream, high-fat cheese, fatty meats and poultry, sausages, pastries, coffee whitener, products containing hydrogenated oils, palm oil and coconut oil |
| Increased use of high-protein food (low in saturated fat) | | Fish, chicken and turkey; veal, game, spring lamb |
| Increased complex carbohydrate; increased fruit and vegetable fibre; increased legumes | About 35 g/day of fibre, half derived from fruit and vegetables | All fruit, including dried fruit; all fresh and frozen vegetables; lentils, dried beans, chick peas; unrefined cereal foods, including oats |
| Decreased dietary cholesterol | <300 mg/day | Allowance of up to two egg yolks/week; liver up to twice monthly, other offal avoided |
| Moderately increased use of mono- and polyunsaturated | Mono: 10–15% of energy Poly: 7–10% of energy | Olive oil, sunflower oil, corn oil and products based on these oils and products |

**Table 11.25** Management of hyperlipidaemias

**Exclude secondary causes of hyperlipidaemia**
- Glucose tolerance
- Thyroid function
- Urea and electrolytes
- Liver function

**Secondary causes of hyperlipidaemia**
- Treat the primary condition

**If lipid abnormality persists**
- Lipid abnormalities may persist in DM and renal impairment despite the best endeavours and contribute to morbidity from atherosclerosis-related disease
- Treatment should then be as for a primary lipid abnormality

**Nutritional counselling**
- Weight loss if overweight
- Modify total fat content of the diet, particularly saturated fat
- Lipid-lowering modifying diet (**Table 11.24**)

**Chylomicronaemia syndrome**
- Reduce dietary fat intake to less than 20% of calories; supplementation with medium-chain triglyceride makes the diet more palatable

**If dietary and lifestyle measures fail to lead to acceptable lipid levels**
- For individuals at high risk of premature vascular disease, hypolipidaemic drug therapy (**Table 11.23**)

### Primary prevention of vascular disease

Statin therapy also reduces the risk of death resulting from CAD, CAD events and stroke in individuals without symptomatic vascular disease (**Figure 11.21**). Guidelines for primary prevention stress calculation of *absolute* risk for the individual based on population data. A number of online CAD risk calculators (e.g. QRISK) are available for this purpose. The absolute risk at which statin therapy is warranted for primary prevention of vascular disease is largely determined by economic considerations and has fallen over time. Current UK guidelines suggest prescribing statins for those with >10% 10-year risk of CAD.

Risk calculators should not be used for familial dyslipidaemias (FH, FCH, remnant particle disease) as these conditions should be treated in their own right given the very high CAD risk.

### Other drug treatments

Patients with severe familial dyslipidaemias sometimes need combination drug therapy. In heterozygous FH patients, anion-exchange resins, ezetimibe or PCSK9 inhibitors added to statins can lower LDL cholesterol further. In homozygous FH, plasma apharesis may be required to sufficiently lower LDL cholesterol. In FCH, statins are first-line drugs, but combination therapy with a fibrate may be used. This has an increased frequency of side effects, particularly myopathy. Patients should be warned to stop statins if they experience severe muscle pain and tenderness.

Severe hypertriglyceridaemia is best treated with high-dose omega-3 fatty acid-rich fish oil and fibrates in addition to a low total fat diet.

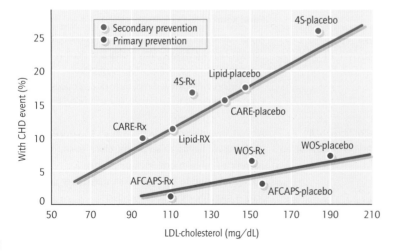

**Figure 11.21** Important clinical trials using statin drugs. The graph shows the reduction in CHD events with some of the different trials. The benefit of each trial is shown in the reduction in events from the placebo group to the treatment (Rx) group. The slope of the lines indicates the magnitude of the benefit, and it can be seen that the benefit is greater in secondary prevention than in primary prevention.

## THE PORPHYRIAS

The porphyrias are caused by defects in the enzymes involved in haem synthesis and can result in accumulation of porphyrins, which are intermediate compounds in haem synthesis. Excess production of porphyrins occurs either in the liver (hepatic porphyrias) or red cells and bone marrow (erythropoietic porphyrias) (**Table 11.26**). The result is a spectrum of clinical manifestations, especially neurological symptoms and skin photosensitivity, summarized in **Table 11.27**. All porphyrias (except acute intermittent porphyria) are associated with photosensitivity.

## PATHOPHYSIOLOGY

Haem biosynthetic pathways are complex (**Figure 11.22**).

- In all acute porphyrias, aminolaevulinic acid (ALA) and porphobilinogen (PBG) accumulate and cause acute neuropsychiatric and gastrointestinal symptoms. Urinary ALA and PBG are raised. Further distinction is based on other porphyrin metabolites in urine and faeces:
  - *Acute intermittent porphyria*: no elevation of coproporphyrinogen (COPRO PG)
  - *Hereditary coproporphyria*: COPRO PG in urine and faeces
  - *Variegate porphyria*: COPRO PG and protoporphyrinogen (PROTO PG) in faeces
- In non-acute porphyrias, neither ALA nor PBG levels are raised.

## HEPATIC PORPHYRIAS

### Acute intermittent porphyria

#### Disease mechanisms
- Enzyme deficiency: hydroxymethylbilane (HMB) synthase
- Autosomal dominant

#### Clinical features
- Abdominal pain, nausea, vomiting and constipation
- Polyneuropathy: sensory or motor

**Table 11.26** Classification of porphyrias

| Type | Hepatic | Erythropoietic |
|---|---|---|
| Acute | Acute intermittent porphyria | |
| | Hereditary coproporphyria | |
| | Variegate porphyria | |
| Non-acute | Porphyria cutanea tarda | Congenital porphyria |
| | | Erythropoetic protoporphyria |

- Cardiovascular: tachycardia and hypertension
- Psychiatric symptoms: anxiety, depression, disorientation, hallucinations, paranoia
- Other pain symptoms: affecting the limbs, head, neck and chest
- Genitourinary: dysuria and urinary retention
- Often a family history of porphyria

Heterozygous patients usually remain asymptomatic unless exposed to factors that increase the production of porphyrins. Symptoms rarely occur before puberty.

Common precipitating factors are:
- Alcohol
- Synthetic oestrogens and progestrogens
- Porphyrinogenic drugs (e.g. sulphonamide antibiotics, barbiturates, succinimides)

#### Investigation
- ALA and PBG are increased in plasma and urine during acute attacks.
- Urine turns red-brown on standing during acute attacks.
- Faecal porphyrins are usually normal or minimally increased.
- Red cell HMB synthase measurement confirms the diagnosis outside acute attacks and can be used to screen asymptomatic family members.

#### Management
- Avoid drugs known to precipitate porphyria, including alcohol and the oral contraceptive pill.

**Table 11.27** Clinical manifestations of porphyrias

| Clinical manifestation | GI | PNS | CNS | CVS | GUS | Photosensitivity | Bone marrow |
|---|---|---|---|---|---|---|---|
| **Hepatic porphyrias** | | | | | | | |
| Acute intermittent porphyria | Yes | Yes | Yes | Yes | Yes | No | No |
| Variegate porphyria | Yes | Yes | Yes | Yes | Yes | Yes | No |
| Hereditary coproporphyria | Yes | Yes | Yes | Yes | Yes | Yes | No |
| Porphyria cutanea tarda | Hepato-megaly | No | No | No | No | Yes | Splenomegaly |
| **Erythropoietic porphyrias** | | | | | | | |
| Congenital erythropoietic porphyria | No | No | No | No | No | Yes, in infancy | Anaemia Splenomegaly |
| Erythropoietic protoporphyria | Chronic liver disease | No | No | No | No | Yes, in early childhood | Anaemia Splenomegaly |

GI, gastrointestinal; PNS, peripheral nervous system; CNS, central nervous system; CVS, cardiovascular system; GUS, genitourinary system.

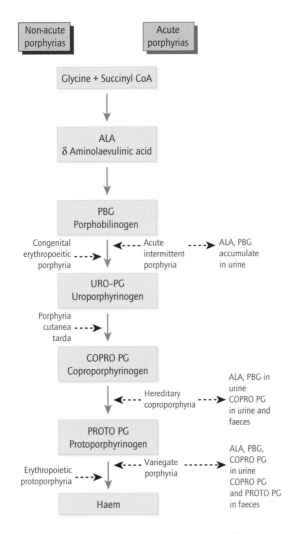

**Figure 11.22** The haem biosynthetic pathway and the acute and non-acute porphyrias. If there is a block in the pathway, metabolites above the block tend to accumulate. Both PBG and uroporphyrinogen can be present in the urine and later metabolites can also accumulate in faeces.

- Opiates can be given for abdominal pain and phenothiazines for nausea, vomiting, anxiety and restlessness.
- High carbohydrate intake reduces hepatic ALA synthase activity, so IV glucose or parenteral nutrition is used.
- IV haem reduces porphyrin precursor excretion and is thought to lead to more rapid recovery.

### Variegate porphyria and hereditary coproporphyria

#### Disease mechanisms
- Autosomal dominant
- Enzyme deficiency:
  - *Variegate porphyria:* protoporphyrinogen oxidase
  - *Hereditary coproporphria:* coproporphyrinogen oxidase

#### Clinical features
Symptoms are similar to acute intermittent porphyria plus photosensitivity. Hereditary coproporphyria is rare.

#### Investigation
Urinary ALA and PBG are raised during acute attacks. In variegate porphyria, there is increased faecal protoporphyrin and coproporphyrin, as well as increased urinary coproporphyrin during attacks. In hereditary coproporphyria, coproporphyrin is increased in urine and faeces.

#### Management
Manage as for acute intermittent porphyria.

### Porphyria cutanea tarda

#### Disease mechanisms
This is an acquired or inherited deficiency of hepatic uroporphyrinogen decarboxylase. Iron and transferrin levels can be raised, and mild hepatic iron overload can occur.

#### Clinical features
Cutaneous photosensitivity causes bullous eruptions on sun-exposed areas that heal with scarring. Hirsutism, hyperpigmentation and hepatomegaly may occur. Neurological manifestations do not occur. The most common contributory factor is excessive alcohol intake, although associations with iron, oestrogen and polychlorinated hydrocarbons have been described.

#### Investigation
Urinary uroporphyrin is increased, but urinary ALA and PBG are normal.

#### Management
Contributory factors, especially alcohol use, should be discontinued. Repeated venesection reduces hepatic iron content. Hydroxychloroquine forms complexes with the excess porphyrins and promotes their excretion.

## ERYTHROPOIETIC PORPHYRIAS

### Congenital erythropoietic porphyria

#### Disease mechanisms
- Autosomal recessive (very rare)
- Enzyme deficiency: uroporphyrinogen synthase

#### Clinical features
There is severe skin photosensitivity, beginning in early infancy. There may be secondary infection. Porphyrins are deposited in teeth and bones.

### Erythropoietic protoporphyria

#### Disease mechanisms
- Autosomal dominant
- Enzyme deficiency: partial deficiency of ferrochelatase

#### Clinical features
There is skin photosensitivity in childhood. Accumulation of protoporphyrin may cause chronic liver disease leading to liver failure and death. Protoporphyrin levels are increased in bone marrow, circulating erythrocytes, plasma, bile and faeces.

## OTHER METABOLIC DISEASES

## LYSOSOMAL STORAGE DISEASES

### Disease mechanisms

Lysosomes are cytoplasmic organelles which contain enzymes. Their major function is the degradation of macromolecules, but they are also involved in the uptake of molecules such as vitamin $B_{12}$, lipoproteins, peptides, hormones and growth factors. Lysosomal storage diseases are rare and are usually autosomal recessive or X-linked recessive disorders. They are characterized by progressive deposition of metabolic substrates in organs including brain, liver, spleen and bone.

Lysosomal storage diseases have been classified into groups according to the type of macromolecule affected (**Table 11.28**). These groups include:

- Sphingolipidoses
- Mucopolysaccharidoses
- Mucolipidoses

### Clinical features

These are varied and include learning disability, epilepsy, hepatosplenomegaly and bony abnormalities. In sphingolipidoses, retinal degeneration can cause a diagnostic 'cherry red spot' appearance at the macula. Mucopolysaccharidoses are associated with coarse facies, thickened skin, clouded corneas and skeletal abnormalities. Mucolipidoses are clinically similar to mucopolysaccharidoses.

### Investigation

Diagnosis depends on demonstrating enzyme deficiency in tissue biopsies or genetic investigation. Parental consanguinity is frequently found in the autosomal recessive disorders.

## DISORDERS OF CARBOHYDRATE METABOLISM

### Glycogen storage diseases

#### Disease mechanisms

A failure to catabolize glycogen or an abnormal glycogen structure causes an abnormal increase in glycogen storage. These are mostly autosomal recessive conditions that present in childhood. Type 1 (von Gierke's disease) and type 5 (McArdle's disease) are the most common forms (**Table 11.29**).

#### Clinical features

There are two main presentations:

- Infants with hypoglycaemia and hepatomegaly: hypoglycaemia because the liver cannot maintain gluconeogenesis in the fasting state and hepatomegaly because of excess glycogen storage
- Children with muscle weakness, hypotonia and muscle wasting

#### Investigation

Diagnosis may require liver or muscle biopsy to demonstrate defective enzyme activity or genetic investigation. In McArdle's disease, muscle enzymes (creatine

**11**

**Table 11.28** Lysosomal storage diseases

| Disease | Enzyme deficiency | Stored material | Genetics | Specific manifestations |
|---|---|---|---|---|
| **Sphingolipidoses** | | | | |
| $G_{M1}$ gangliosidosis | β-galactosidase | Ganglioside $G_{M1}$ | AR | Coarse facies, blindness |
| $G_{M2}$ gangliosidosis (Tay–Sachs disease) | Hexosaminidase | Ganglioside $G_{M2}$ | AR | Macrocephaly, cherry red spot Increased prevalence in Ashkenazi Jews |
| Gaucher's disease | β-glucocerebrosidase | Glucocerebroside | AR | Mental retardation, hepatosplenomegaly Increased prevalence in Ashkenazi Jews |
| Fabry's disease | α-galactosidase | Trihexoside | X-linked recessive | Paresthaesiae Cutaneous angiokeratoma Renal failure |
| Niemann–Pick disease | Sphingomyelinase | Sphingomyelin | AR | Hepatosplenomegaly, foam cells in liver and bone marrow |
| **Mucopolysaccharidoses** | | | | |
| Hurler's disease | α-iduronidase | Dermatan sulphate Heparan sulphate | AR | Coarse facies, corneal clouding, deafness |
| Hunter's disease | Iduronate sulphatase | Dermatan sulphate Heparan sulphate | X-linked recessive | Coarse facies, deafness |
| **Mucolipidoses** | | | | |
| Mucolipidosis I | N-acetyl-neuraminic hydrolase | Sialic acid-rich glycoproteins | AR | Myoclonus, cherry red spot, foam cells in blood/bone marrow |

AR, autosomal recessive.

**Table 11.29** Glycogen storage diseases

| Type | Disease | Affected tissues | Clinical features | Prognosis |
|---|---|---|---|---|
| 1 | von Gierke's | Liver, kidney, intestine | Hepatomegaly, hypoglycaemia, lactic acidosis | High mortality in infant years, good prognosis if survive |
| 2 | Pompe's | Liver, skeletal and cardiac muscle | Heart failure, hypotonia | Usually die in first year of life |
| 3 | Forbes' | Liver, muscle | Similar to type 1, but milder phenotype | Good |
| 4 | Andersen's | Liver | Hepatomegaly, failure to thrive, liver cirrhosis and portal hypertension | Usually die in first 3 years of life |
| 5 | McArdle's | Muscle | Muscle cramps, proximal muscle wasting | Normal life expectancy |

phosphokinase, lactate dehydrogenase) are raised after strenuous exercise and myoglobinuria may occur.

### Management

Dietary therapy with frequent feeding can help with hypoglycaemia. Muscle cramps in McArdle's disease may be prevented by taking glucose before exercise or avoiding strenuous exercise. Glucagon is usually an ineffective treatment for the hypoglycaemia because the liver cannot mobilize the glycogen stores.

### Galactosaemia

#### Disease mechanisms

Lactose in milk is a disaccharide containing galactose and glucose. After ingestion, it is hydrolyzed by intestinal lactase and the absorbed galactose is converted to glucose in the liver (**Figure 11.23**). Galactose-1-phosphate uridyl transferase (GALT) deficiency causes classic galactosaemia with autosomal recessive inheritance.

#### Clinical features

Classic galactosaemia usually presents within days to weeks of birth with reluctance to take breast milk or milk formulas, dehydration, hypoglycaemia and dehydration. Jaundice, hepatomegaly and ascites may develop. Cataracts develop over weeks to months. The infant dies within weeks in the absence of treatment.

Galactokinase deficiency results in cataract formation caused by galactitol deposition in the lens, but no other clinical features.

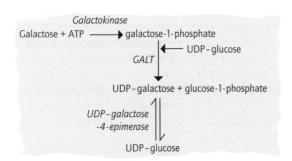

**Figure 11.23** Metabolism of galactose. Classic galactosaemia results from GALT deficiency.

### Investigation

- Raised blood galactose and galactose-1-phosphate
- Assay of red blood cell GALT activity

### Management

Stop breastfeeding. Use milk substitutes that do not contain galactose instead. Survivors require long-term follow-up because they remain at risk of hepatic damage and cataracts.

#### Hereditary fructose intolerance

- Autosomal recessive
- Enzyme deficiency: fructose-1-phosphate aldolase

Defects of fructose metabolism lead to raised blood fructose, hypoglycaemia and vomiting soon after fructose ingestion. In children, vomiting, hepatomegaly, jaundice, proteinuria, aminoaciduria and failure to thrive may occur. Avoiding fructose-containing foods removes the symptoms so children learn to avoid sucrose- and fructose-containing food.

## INHERITED DISORDERS OF AMINO ACID METABOLISM AND STORAGE

Eight of the 20 different amino acids required for protein synthesis are essential and must be obtained from dietary sources because humans cannot synthesize them. There are many amino acid disorders, which are typically due to catabolic defects or transport abnormalities.

### Epidemiology

These disorders are rare, affecting approximately 1 in 500–1000 live births/year.

### Disease mechanisms

Disorders of amino acid breakdown (catabolism) can cause the accumulation of intermediary compounds in the blood or urine (**Table 11.30**). This may be the parent amino acid (aminoacidopathy) or products in the catabolic pathway (organic acidaemia).

### Clinical features

Clinical manifestations vary from being asymptomatic to being lethal in the untreated neonate (e.g. ornithine

**Table 11.30** Inherited disorders of amino acid metabolism

| Amino acid affected | Disorder | Enzyme defect | Clinical manifestations |
|---|---|---|---|
| Phenylalanine | Phenylketonuria | Phenylalanine hydroxylase | Mental retardation, neuropsychiatric dysfunction, hypopigmentation of skin and hair, eczema |
| Tyrosine | Alkaptonuria | Homogentistic acid oxidase | Dark urine stains nappies, blue-grey cartilage (ochronosis), arthritis |
| Tyrosine | Albinism | Tyrosinase | White hair, pale skin, pink eyes, easy sunburn |
| Homocystine | Homocystinuria | | |
| | Type 1 | Cystathione-β-synthase | Mental retardation, Marfan-like syndrome, thrombotic tendency |
| | Type 2 | 5,10-Methylene tetra-hydrofolate reductase | Mental retardation |
| Ornithine | Hyperammonaemia | Ornithine transcarbamylase | Mental retardation, neuropsychiatric dysfunction, protein intolerance, ammonia intoxication |
| Branched chain amino acids (valine, leucine and isoleucine) | Maple syrup disease (branched chain ketoaciduria) | Branched chain keto-acid decarboxylase | Neonatal acidosis, fits, mental retardation, protein intolerance, maple syrup odour |
| Glycine | Hyperoxaluria (type 1) | Alanine glyoxylate aminotransferase | Recurrent renal calculi (calcium oxalate stones), renal failure |

carbamoyltransferase deficiency). Central nervous system dysfunction may occur, resulting in developmental retardation, seizures, alterations in sensation and behavioural disturbances. Protein-induced vomiting, neurological dysfunction and raised plasma ammonium levels (hyperammonaemia) occur in disorders of the urea cycle intermediates (e.g. ornithine carbamoyltransferase). Metabolic ketoacidosis is frequent in branched-chain amino acid metabolism disorders (e.g. maple syrup urine disease). There is sometimes focal tissue or organ involvement (e.g. liver disease, renal failure, cutaneous abnormalities or eye lesions).

### Management

Diagnosis and appropriate treatment can prevent or reduce the effects of these disorders. Treatment often involves reducing the intake of the amino acid that cannot be effectively metabolized. Screening programmes to detect phenylketonuria in newborns have been established in most developed countries. Aminoacidopathies and organic acidaemias can be screened for in the newborn using blood or urine. Genetic defects have been determined for many of these disorders, allowing prenatal diagnosis in affected families.

### INHERITED DEFECTS OF MEMBRANE TRANSPORT

Many molecules require transporters to cross cell membranes (**Table 11.31**) and there are many inherited disorders of membrane transport, which particularly affect the gut and/or the kidney. The molecules affected include amino acids, lipids, sugars, cations, anions and water. These disorders have specific phenotypes and usually have autosomal recessive or X-linked inheritance. The phenotypes vary from benign disorders with no pathological consequences (renal glycosuria) to life-threatening multisystem disorders (cystic fibrosis). The genetic defects associated with these disorders have largely been determined.

## AMYLOIDOSIS

The amyloidoses are a heterogeneous group of disorders caused by extracellular protein deposition which results in organ dysfunction. Patients may present with nephrotic syndrome, chronic kidney disease, heart failure, autonomic neuropathy, peripheral neuropathy, malabsorption or synovitis.

### EPIDEMIOLOGY

Amyloid light-chain (AL) amyloidosis, the commonest type of amyloidosis, complicates 5–10% of cases of myeloma and other monoclonal B-cell dyscrasias. Amyloid A (AA) amyloidosis develops in 1–5% of patients with chronic inflammatory disorders. $\beta_2$-microglobulin amyloid deposition in the bones and joints can arise with long-term dialysis. Hereditary systemic amyloidosis can be caused by mutations in various genes and accounts for up to 5% of cases.

### DISEASE MECHANISMS

Amyloid deposits contain proteins that are produced either in abnormal *quantity* or in abnormal *forms* and produce fibrils (**Table 11.32**). The deposits contain serum amyloid P (SAP) protein combined with *either*:

- An antibody protein in AL amyloid, *or*
- The acute phase protein serum amyloid A protein in AA amyloid

**Table 11.31** Genetic disorders of membrane transport

| Disorder | Substrate(s) | Tissue manifesting defect | Molecular basis of defect | Major clinical manifestation | Genetics |
|---|---|---|---|---|---|
| **Amino acid** | | | | | |
| Cystinuria | Cystine, lysine, arginine, ornithine | Proximal renal tubule, jejunal mucosa | Mutation of shared di-basic cystine transport protein | Cystine nephrolithiasis | Autosomal recessive |
| Hartnup's disease | Neutral amino acid | Proximal renal tubule, jejunal mucosa | Neutral amino acid transport protein | Aminoaciduria, pellagra | Autosomal recessive |
| **Sugar** | | | | | |
| Renal glycosuria | D-glucose | Proximal renal tubule | Mutation of D-glucose transporter | Glycosuria with normal blood glucose | Autosomal recessive |
| **Anion** | | | | | |
| Familial hypo-phosphataemic rickets | Inorganic phosphate | Proximal renal tubule, jejunal mucosa | Mutation of inorganic phosphate transport protein | Rickets/osteomalacia | X-linked dominant |
| Cystic fibrosis | Chloride | Lung, pancreas, sweat glands | Mutation of ion channel protein | Bronchiectasis, pancreatic failure | Autosomal recessive |
| **Cation** | | | | | |
| Renal tubular acidosis | Hydrogen ion | Distal or proximal renal tubule | Mutation of hydrogen ion pump carrier protein | Hyperchloraemic acidosis | |
| | | | | Type 1: hypokalaemia | Autosomal recessive |
| | | | | Type 2: bicarbonate wasting | Autosomal recessive |
| **Water** | | | | | |
| Nephrogenic diabetes insipidus | Water | Distal renal tubule | Defective vasopressin receptor | Polyuria, polydipsia | X-linked recessive |
| | | | Defective aquaporin channel | | Autosomal dominant and recessive |

**Table 11.32** Classification of the most common types of amyloid and amyloidosis

| Type | Fibril protein precursor | Clinical syndrome |
|---|---|---|
| AA | Serum amyloid A | Reactive systemic amyloidosis associated with acquired or hereditary chronic inflammatory diseases |
| | | Formerly known as secondary amyloidosis |
| AL | Monoclonal immunoglobulin light chains | Systemic amyloidosis associated with myeloma, monoclonal gammopathy, occult dyscrasia |
| | | Formerly known as primary amyloidosis |
| ATTR | Normal plasma transthyretin | Senile systemic amyloidosis with prominent cardiac involvement |
| | Genetically variant transthyretin | Familial amyloid polyneuropathy, usually with systemic amyloidosis |
| | | Sometimes prominent amyloid cardiomyopathy or nephropathy |
| $A\beta_2 M$ | $\beta_2$-Microglobulin | Periarticular and, occasionally, systemic amyloidosis associated with renal failure and long-term dialysis |
| $A\beta$ | $\beta$-Protein precursors (and rare genetic variants) | Cerebrovascular and intracerebral plaque amyloid in Alzheimer's disease Occasional familial cases |
| AIAPP | Islet amyloid polypeptide | Amyloid in islets of Langerhans in type 2 DM and insulinoma |

Amyloid deposits disrupt the structure and function of normal tissues, although accumulation sufficient to cause symptoms may take many years. Organs may be markedly enlarged, especially the liver, spleen, kidneys, heart and tongue. The variety of organs that may be involved, especially in AL amyloidosis, produces a wide spectrum of clinical features.

## CLINICAL FEATURES

Amyloidosis is typically diagnosed following a biopsy for organ dysfunction (e.g. of the kidneys, liver, heart or gut). The diagnosis should be specifically considered in certain situations (e.g. proteinuria in a patient with a chronic inflammatory disorder or with a monoclonal gammopathy). Certain signs are highly characteristic of AL amyloid, including peri-orbital bruising and macroglossia (large tongue).

Typical features of amyloid organ involvement (**Figure 11.24**):

- *Kidney:* mild proteinuria to nephrotic syndrome with progressive renal failure
- *Heart:* restrictive cardiomyopathy
- *Skin:* diffuse waxy infiltration with nodules and plaques; purpura caused by vascular fragility, characteristically around the eyes in AL amyloidosis
- *Liver:* hepatomegaly, but function is often well preserved; cholestasis can occur
- *Gut:* weight loss, dysmotility, bleeding, altered bowel habit and malabsorption; more often resulting from autonomic dysfunction than from severe amyloid infiltration

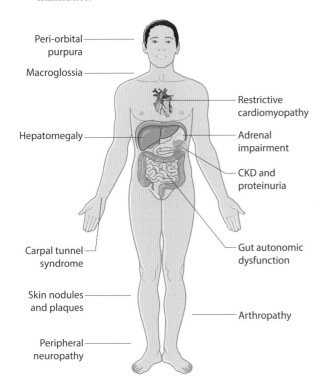

**Figure 11.24** Clinical features of amyloidosis.

- *Endocrine:* mild adrenal impairment common in all systemic types
- *Nervous system:* peripheral neuropathy (sensorimotor) and autonomic neuropathy (postural hypotension, diarrhoea, bladder dysfunction)
- *Joints:* painful arthropathy with swelling, typical in $\beta_2$-microglobulin type and occasionally in AL amyloidosis
- *Miscellaneous:* carpal tunnel syndrome, macroglossia, acquired clotting factor IX and X deficiencies all characteristic of AL amyloidosis

### AL amyloidosis

This often involves the heart, kidneys, skin, gut, liver, muscle (e.g. tongue) and peripheral and/or autonomic nerves. The immunoglobulin light chain amyloid precursor protein differs in every patient, and the deposits may be localized or diffuse.

### AA amyloidosis

This presents with proteinuria and/or renal impairment in 95% of cases. The spleen and adrenal glands are commonly affected, and the liver in about 25%. Clinically significant cardiac and neuropathic amyloid is very rare, but patients with advanced disease often have gastrointestinal dysfunction.

## INVESTIGATION

When stained with Congo red dye amyloid fibrils show red-green birefringence under polarized light in tissue biopsy histochemistry samples. The type of amyloid fibril is determined by immunohistochemical staining using specific antibodies. Measurement of serum free light chains may point to a diagnosis of amyloidosis. Radiolabelled SAP is used as a nuclear medicine tracer for imaging of amyloid deposits *in vivo* to provide a whole-body survey and for serial monitoring (**Figure 11.25**).

## MANAGEMENT

Studies in several different forms of amyloidosis have shown that therapy that succeeds in reducing the supply of the amyloid fibril precursor protein helps to preserve organ function and can prolong survival substantially. For AL amyloidosis, this is treatment of the antibody producing plasma cell disease such as myeloma. For AA amyloidosis, it is treatment of the underlying inflammatory disorder. Supportive therapy for failing organ function can include dialysis and sometimes organ transplantation.

## PROGNOSIS

- AL amyloidosis: median survival <2 years
- AA amyloidosis: median survival 5–10 years

11

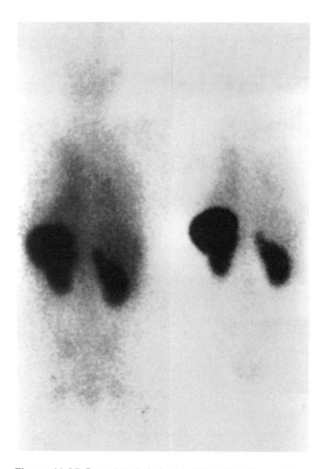

**Figure 11.25** Posterior whole-body scintigraphs following IV injection of radiolabelled serum amyloid P component ($^{123}$I-SAP) of a patient with AA amyloidosis complicating rheumatoid arthritis. **(a)** At presentation with proteinuria, the spleen, kidneys and adrenal glands are infiltrated with amyloid. **(b)** 12 months later, a follow-up scan shows more intense uptake into the same organs, indicating that the quantity of amyloid has increased. The remainder of the image is because of tracer in the circulation.

## MUST-KNOW CHECKLIST

- A random venous plasma glucose >11 mmol/L is abnormal and suggests a diagnosis of DM.
- HbA1c should not be used to diagnose DM in children or pregnant women.
- Microvascular complications of DM may be present at diagnosis.
- Patients with DM are most likely to die from macrovascular complications.
- Intensive treatment aiming to normalize blood glucose concentrations reduces the appearance of diabetic microvascular complications in both type 1 and type 2 DM.
- Obesity increases the risk of cardiovascular disease, hypertension, type 2 diabetes and some cancers.
- Polygenic hypercholesterolaemia is the most common form of hypercholesterolaemia but is a diagnosis of exclusion.
- Statins (HMG-CoA reductase inhibitors) reduce total cholesterol by upregulating hepatic low-density lipoprotein receptors.
- Inherited metabolic diseases are frequently associated with learning disability and epilepsy.
- Amyloidosis frequently presents with renal disease, but multiorgan involvement is common.

**Questions and answers** to test your understanding of Chapter 11 can be found by clicking 'Support Material' at the following link: https://www.routledge.com/Medicine-for-Finals-and-Beyond/Axford-OCallaghan/p/book/9780367150594

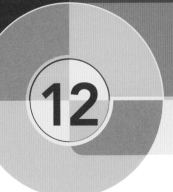

# Endocrine Disease

## 12

PIERRE-MARC BOULOUX

## STRUCTURE AND FUNCTION

The endocrine system is a network of hormone-secreting glands reaching their targets via the bloodstream, regulating growth, development and metabolism. Endocrinopathies result from inadequate or excessive production of hormones, resulting in perturbations of homoeostasis (the internal balance of body systems), metabolism (body energy levels), reproduction and response to stressful or injurious stimuli.

- The glands include the hypothalamus, pituitary, pineal, thyroid, parathyroids, adrenals, endocrine pancreas and ovaries/testes (**Figure 12.1**).
- Hormones specifically interact with surface membrane, cytoplasmic or nuclear receptors in target tissues.
- Hormonal secretion is subject to *negative feedback regulation* (e.g. the hypothalamo-pituitary-target organ axis, in which changes in hormone concentrations secreted by peripheral endocrine organs are regulated by the hypothalamo-pituitary [HP] axis).
- A gland may sense and respond to changes in the variable it regulates (e.g. parathyroid and ionized calcium).
- Endocrine glands must be distinguished from exocrine glands, which secrete substances onto an epithelial surface by way of a duct. Examples include the sweat, salivary, mammary, ceruminous, lacrimal, sebaceous, prostate and mucous-secreting glands.

## PRINCIPLES OF ENDOCRINOLOGY

### HORMONES AND THEIR ACTIONS

#### Protein and polypeptide hormones

- Mostly single-chain polypeptides
- Insulin looped into a ring before excision of C peptide leaving two chains linked by two disulphide bridges (**Figure 12.2**)
- Glycoprotein family (human chorionic gonadotrophin [hCG], luteinizing hormone [LH], follicle-stimulating hormone [FSH], thyroid-stimulating hormone [TSH]) has sugar moieties attached and comprises $\alpha$ (constant), $\beta$ subunit (variable)
- Released in regular and pulsatile bursts (insulin, LH, FSH). Growth hormone (GH) and prolactin (PRL) have a tonic level of release, with additional superimposed bursts
- Released rapidly and rapidly metabolized

#### Cholesterol derivatives

These include adrenal and gonadal steroids (**Figure 12.3**) and vitamin D.

#### Tyrosine and tryptophan derivatives

- Thyroid hormones formed by conjugation of two tyrosine molecules and iodine
- Tyrosine made into norepinephrine (NE) and epinephrine (E)
- Tryptophan precursor of serotonin (5-hydroxytryptamine)

DOI: 10.1201/9781003193616-12

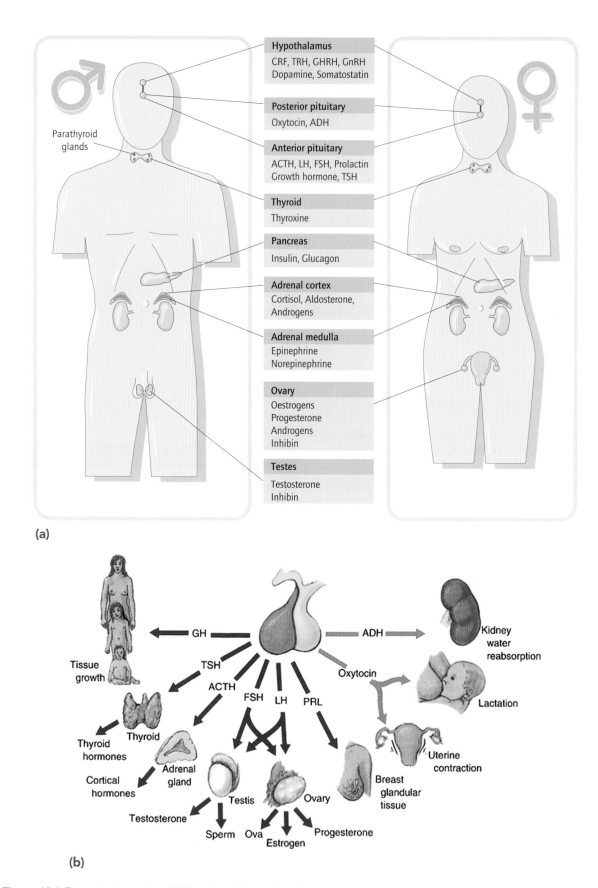

**Figure 12.1** The endocrine system. **(a)** Overview of the major endocrine organs and the hormones they produce. **(b)** The anterior and posterior pituitary gland and its peripheral targets.

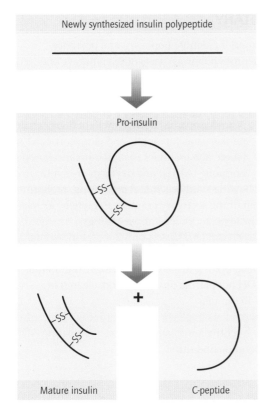

**Figure 12.2** The nascent insulin protein is looped into a ring with the formation of disulphide bridges, and mature insulin formed with the cleavage of the C-peptide.

### Lipid and phospholipid derivatives

Eicosanoids include prostaglandins, prostacyclins, thromboxanes and leukotrienes.

## HORMONE TRANSPORT

- More than 90% steroid and more than 99% thyroid hormones circulate as complexes bound to specific plasma globulins or albumin
- Hydrophobic in contrast to hydrophilic protein peptide hormones
- Only free hormone biologically active
- Assays of total hormone concentrations do not reflect changes in free hormone concentration
- Free hormone measurement preferable

## HORMONE RECEPTORS

Protein and peptide hormone receptors are G protein-coupled receptors (GPCR).

- Hormone–receptor interaction leads to dissociation of intracellular G protein, allowing opening of membrane ion channels or activation of enzymes promoting/inhibiting secondary messenger production (e.g. cyclic adenosine monophosphate [cAMP])
- Second messengers activate protein kinases/phosphatases triggering other intracellular events
- Insulin receptor: transmembrane protein with tyrosine kinase activity

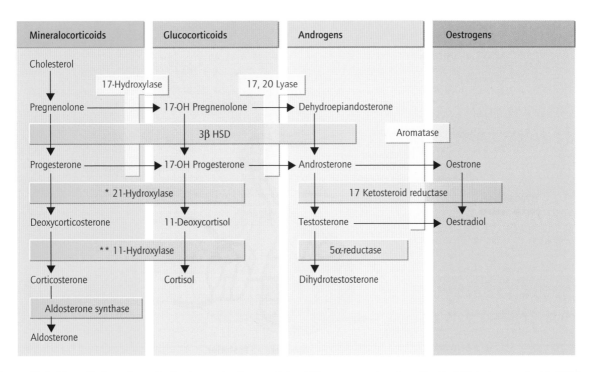

**Figure 12.3** Biosynthetic pathway for the four main classes of steroid hormones: mineralocorticoids (MCs), glucocorticoids (GCs), androgens and oestrogens. The key enzymes involved in steroid biosynthesis are shown.

- Steroid hormones lipid-soluble and diffuse easily across cell membranes with intracellular receptors classified by location
- Effect of hormone–receptor interaction influenced by: receptor number, hormone concentration, affinity of hormone for receptor.

## THE HYPOTHALAMO-PITUITARY AXIS

### HYPOTHALAMUS

- Produces releasing and inhibiting hormones, neurosecreted into the medial eminence capillary plexus and reaching the adenohypophysis via long portal vessels (**Figure 12.4**)
- Influences autonomic nervous regulation of heart rate and blood pressure (BP), body temperature
- Affects fluid/electrolyte balance, thirst, appetite, body weight, glandular secretions of stomach and intestines
- Influences sleep cycle
- Links nervous system to endocrine system

### PITUITARY

- Anterior (adenohypophysis) and posterior (neurohypophysis) parts of the pituitary of different embryological origin:
  - *Adenohypophysis:* outgrowth of primitive pharynx (Rathke's pouch)
  - *Neurohypophysis:* downgrowth of diencephalon; perikarya in supraoptic and paraventricular nuclei, where nonapeptides vasopressin (antidiuretic hormone [ADH]) and oxytocin are synthesized
- Following synthesis/initial processing, prohormone-containing secretory granules migrate by axoplasmic flow to posterior lobe nerve endings
- *Vasopressin (ADH)* acts on V2 receptor on renal collecting tubular cells, increasing water reabsorption, concentrating urine and reducing urine volume
- ADH not plasma protein-bound, cleared in 5–10 minutes
- Increments in plasma osmolality (PO) detected by hypothalamic osmoreceptors stimulating ADH secretion and thirst

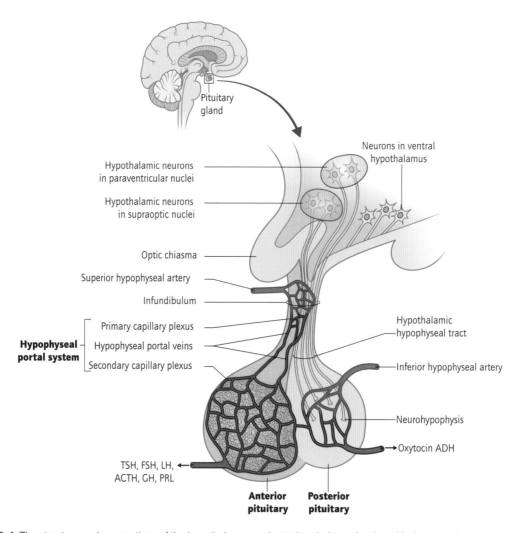

**Figure 12.4** The structure and connections of the hypothalamus and anterior pituitary gland, and its hormonal secretions.

- *ADH release:* reduction in plasma volume, stress, exercise, emotional factors, trauma, morphine and nicotine
- *Oxytocin:* smooth muscle contraction, in myoepithelial cells of mammary glands, causing milk ejection, myometrial contraction

## HYPOTHALAMIC-STIMULATING AND INHIBITORY HORMONES

### Growth hormone-releasing hormone/somatostatin

- Growth hormone-releasing hormone (GHRH) stimulates growth hormone (GH) release from somatotrophs (**Figure 12.5**).
- Somatostatin has the opposite effect.
- *Children:* GH is essential for maintaining a healthy body composition and growth.
- *Adults:* GH aids bone integrity and muscle mass and affects fat distribution.
- Insulin-like growth factor 1 (IGF-1), released from liver in response to GH, exerts negative feedback control on GH secretion.
- GH exhibits pulsatile secretion, particularly at night. Levels during the day are virtually undetectable between pulses.

- GH secretion is *induced* by hypoglycaemia, glucagon and arginine, and *suppressed acutely* by glucose.
- GH mediates retention of substrates for anabolic activity (calcium, phosphorus, nitrogen) and collagen and protein synthesis.
- GH pulse frequency/magnitude is increased during adolescent growth spurts. The circulating peptide Ghrelin displays strong GH releasing activity.

### Gonadotropin-releasing hormone

- Gonadotropin-releasing hormone (GnRH) stimulates LH and FSH synthesis/secretion from gonadotrophs, regulating normal ovarian function (**Figure 12.6**) and testicular function (**Figure 12.7**).
- LH/FSH secretion is pulsatile and is inhibited by oestrogen, testosterone, progesterone and inhibins.
- LH/FSH secretion in women is mediated by a complex feedback mechanism involving oestradiol and progesterone.
- *Women:* FSH stimulates follicle development in the ovary; LH stimulates ovulation (**Figure 12.8**). LH maintains the corpus luteum following ovulation.
- *Men:* FSH stimulates spermatogenesis; LH stimulates testosterone secretion from Leydig cells.

### Thyrotrophin-releasing hormone

- Thyrotrophin-releasing hormone (TRH) releases pituitary TSH, stimulating synthesis and release of thyroid hormones $T_4$ and $T_3$, regulating metabolism, energy growth and development.
- TSH is subject to negative feedback inhibition by $T_4$/$T_3$ (**Figure 12.9**).

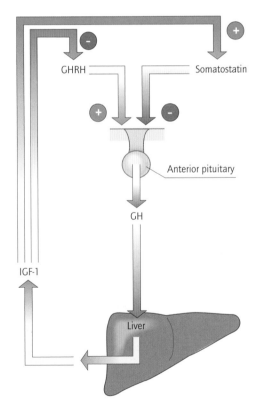

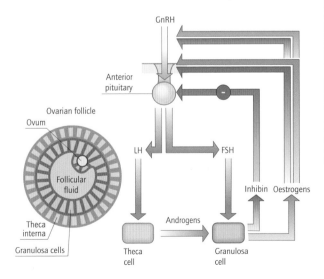

**Figure 12.5** Regulation of GH secretion. GHRH stimulates release and somatostatin suppresses secretion of GH. Liver-derived IGF-1 exerts negative feedback, inhibiting GHRH and stimulating somatostatin secretion. GH secretion is pulsatile, with about seven pulses per day. Circulating GH in health is undetectable for 70% of the day.

**Figure 12.6** The H-P ovarian axis. Pulsatile hypothalamic GnRH secretion induces pulsatile secretion of LH and FSH. LH acts on thecal cells to induce androgen synthesis, whereas FSH induces aromatase activity which converts androgens into oestradiol. FSH also stimulated inhibin A secretion which is involved in the negative feedback regulation of FSH.

475

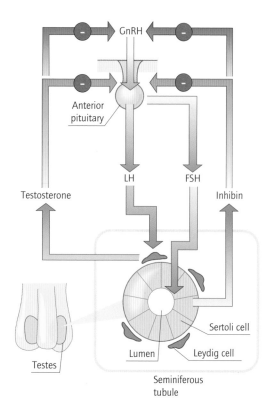

**Figure 12.7** H-P testicular axis. Pulsative GnRH induces pulsatile secretion of LH and FSH. LH acts on Leydic cells to synthesize and release testosterone, whereas FSH acts on Sertoli cells to enable formation of spermatozoa from spermatogonia and also the release of inhibin B, which is involved in negative feedback regulation of FSH. Testosterone is aromatized into oestradiol in the hypothalamus, and the latter mediates the negative feedback regulation of LH.

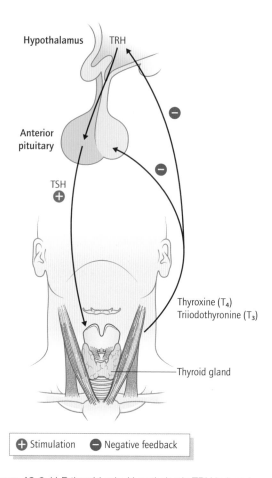

| Stimulation | Negative feedback |

**Figure 12.9** H-P thyroid axis. Hypothalamic TRH induced release of TSH which in turn acts on the thyroid follicular TSH receptor to induce $T_4$ and $T_3$ synthesis and release. Free $T_4$ and free $T_3$ mediate negative feedback at both hypothalamic and pituitary levels.

## Corticotrophin-releasing hormone

- Corticotrophin-releasing hormone (CRH) stimulates adrenocorticotrophic hormone (ACTH) secretion, inducing cortisol synthesis and secretion from the adrenocortical zona fasciculata.

- 90% of cortisol is bound to cortisol-binding globulin in plasma. It is a major regulator of metabolism/immune response.
- ACTH is generated by enzymatic cleavage of pro-opiomelanocortin (POMC; **Figures 12.10** and **12.11**) and inhibited through direct negative feedback control by cortisol.

## Dopamine

- Dopamine inhibits prolactin secretion from the anterior pituitary.
- Prolactin shares considerable structural homology with GH.
- Prolactin secretion is highest at night. It regulates lactation and the development of the mammary duct system (**Figure 12.12**). Secretion increases slowly during pregnancy, in response to postpartum breast/nipple stimulation, stress, physical exercise or hypoglycaemia.

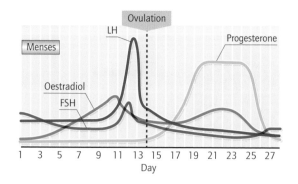

**Figure 12.8** Hormonal regulation of the menstrual cycle. The average 28-day cycle is divided into the pre-ovulatory follicular phase, and a post-ovulatory luteal phase during which progesterone is produced. The rapid rise in oestradiol in the late follicular phase is responsible for the ovulatory LH surge (positive feedback effect of oestradiol).

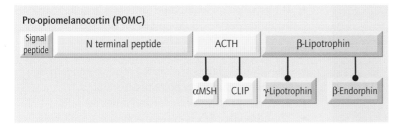

**Figure 12.10** ACTH is derived from the larger pro-opiomelanocortin protein by proteolytic cleavage. The 39 amino-acid ACTH acts on the zona fasciculata of the adrenal cortex to stimulate synthesis and release of cortisol.

## PITUITARY ANATOMICAL RELATIONS

- Located in the sella turcica, connected to the brain by a stalk
- Optic chiasm, above and in front of pituitary
- Cavernous sinuses, containing the carotid artery and cranial nerves 3, 4 and 6

## TARGET ORGANS OF PITUITARY HORMONES

### Thyroid gland

- Weighs about 20 g in health
- Contains 2 months' stores of thyroxine

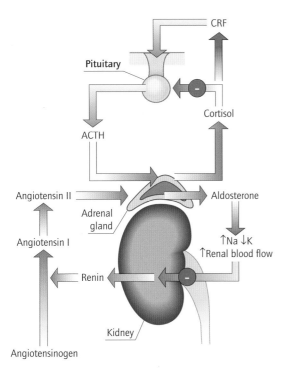

**Figure 12.11** Regulation of GC and MC secretion from the zona fasciculata and glomerulosa layers of the adrenal cortex respectively. ACTH stimulates cortisol secretion. Cortisol circulates in a circadian rhythm; 90% is bound to CBG and 10% free. The free cortisol is responsible for negative feedback regulation of CRF and ACTH. Aldosterone secretion is dependent on the activity of the renin–angiotensinogen–angiotensin II system. It stimulates Na$^+$ reabsorption and K$^+$/H$^+$ elimination in the distal convoluted tubule. Increased body Na$^+$ absorption negatively regulates renin secretion.

- Lateral lobes extend from the thyroid to the cricothyroid cartilages, joined by isthmus (**Figure 12.13**)
- Posteriorly, recurrent laryngeal nerves lie between the trachea and oesophagus

### Thyroid hormones

- $T_4$ and $T_3$ are released from the proteolytic degradation of thyroglobulin, located in protein-rich colloid of thyroid follicles.
- Iodide is avidly taken up via the sodium iodide symporter, oxidized by thyroperoxidase (TPO) and bound covalently to tyrosine residues within thyroglobulin (**Figure 12.14**).
- TPO is inhibited by antithyroid drugs.
- $T_4$ is the major hormone secreted (80%), but $T_3$ (20%) is more active.
- In the liver, heart, kidney and anterior pituitary, $T_4$ is converted to $T_3$ by deiodinase, accounting for approximately two-thirds of $T_3$ production.
- In chronic ill-health and starvation, $T_4$ is converted to inactive reverse $T_3$ by deiodinase 3.
- <1% $T_4$/$T_3$ is free in plasma, as it is bound to thyroid-binding globulin (TBG), transthyretin and albumin.
- Both TRH and TSH are subject to negative feedback inhibition by f$T_4$/f$T_3$ (see **Figure 12.9**).

**12**

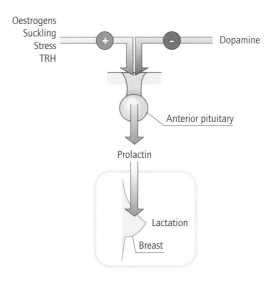

**Figure 12.12** Prolactin secretion is under negative regulation by hypothalamic dopamine. Prolactin secretion is essential for lactation.

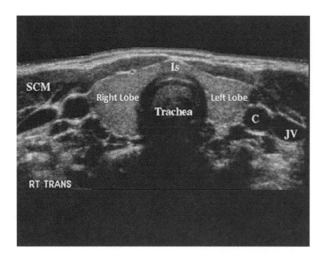

**Figure 12.13** Anatomical relations of the thyroid gland. Two lobes are connected by the midline isthmus. The thyroid strap muscles lie anteriorly, and the sternocleidomastoid anterolaterally. The carotid sheath (c) and, lateral to this, the internal jugular veins (JV) are lateral. A small nubbin of oesophagus protrudes behind the left lobe of the thyroid.

### Action of thyroid hormones

- Essential for normal growth and development
- Affect carbohydrate, protein and fat metabolism
- Stimulate cellular oxygen consumption, controlling basal metabolic rate
- $fT_3/fT_4$ enter cells via the MCT8 transporter, binding to nuclear receptors
- 90% receptor-bound hormone is $T_3$, inducing formation of mRNA encoding various proteins including adrenergic receptors

- Direct effect on membrane functions including amino acid transport, calcium uptake and cAMP formation

### Adrenal glands

- The adrenal glands are located retroperitoneally and attached to the upper poles of the kidneys.
- They comprise outer cortex and inner medulla.
- The adrenal cortex is derived embryologically from mesoderm, comprising 90% of adrenal gland.
- The gland comprises an outer MC-secreting zona glomerulosa, middle cortisol-secreting zone fasciculata, and inner androgen-secreting zone reticularis.
- The androgen dehydroepiandrosterone (DHEA) and its sulphate are weak androgens, have low affinity for androgen receptor and are converted peripherally to more active testosterone.
- In males, the amount released from the adrenals and converted to testosterone is insignificant compared to the amount secreted by the testes.

### Cortisol

Cortisol is the principal GC, which binds to cytoplasmic receptors in the cytoplasm of target cells (see **Figure 12.11**). Ligand–receptor complex is transported to specific GC-binding elements within the cell nucleus, leading to mRNA transcription and protein synthesis.

- It circulates in circadian rhythm, with highest levels between 7 a.m. and 9 a.m., and it is undetectable around midnight.
- This rhythm is disrupted by fever, severe illness, anaesthesia, surgery and hypoglycaemia.

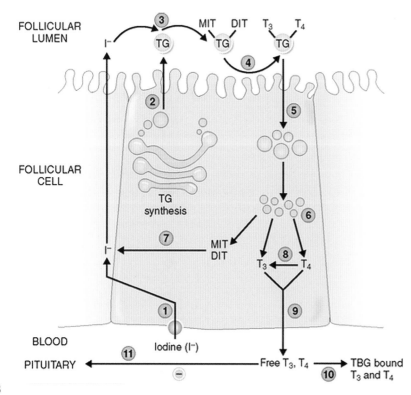

**Figure 12.14** Biosynthesis of thyroid hormones. (1) Iodide trapping. (2) Oxidation of iodide to iodine. (3/4) Organification of tyrosine residues of thyroglobulin (Tg). (5) Pinocytosis of $T_4/T_3$-containing Tg. (6,8) Proteolytic degradation of Tg to release $T_4$ and $T_3$. (7) Dehalogenation of mono-iodotyrosine (MIT) and di-iodotyrosine (DIT) to release iodide for recycling. (9) Release of $T_4$ and $T_3$ into the circulation. (10) Binding to thyroid binding globulin (TBG). (11) Negative feedback of $fT_4$ and $fT_3$ on the pituitary.

### Mineralocorticoids

- Aldosterone is the principal MC produced by zone glomerulosa.
- MCs act on the distal renal tubule, promoting sodium reabsorption and potassium/hydrogen ion excretion (see **Figure 12.11**).

### Renin angiotensin system

- Aldosterone secretion is controlled mainly by the renin angiotensin system (RAS).
- Juxtaglomerular apparatus cells, located close to afferent arterioles, secrete renin in response to intravascular volume depletion, cardiac failure, hypoalbuminaemia and sodium depletion.
- Renin, a proteolytic enzyme, acts on liver-derived angiotensinogen, generating the decapeptide angiotensin I, which is converted to angiotensin II by angiotensin-converting enzyme (ACE), mainly in the lung (see **Figure 12.11**).
- Angiotensin II stimulates aldosterone production and exerts a direct potent vasoconstrictor action.
- Potassium is a potent aldosterone secretagogue.

### Adrenal medulla

- Medullary cells receive preganglionic sympathetic nerve innervation and represent postganglionic sympathetic neurones producing both NE and E.
- Methylation of NE to E requires the cortisol-inducible enzyme phenylethanolamine-N-methyltransferase.
- Secretion of catecholamines occurs in response to exercise, emotion, surgical trauma, pain, hypoglycaemia and fear. Their action is mediated through $\alpha$ and $\beta$ adrenoceptors.
- E binds to both $\alpha$ and $\beta$ receptors; NE is predominantly an $\alpha$ adrenoceptor agonist.
- Catecholamine-O-methyltransferase (COMT), found in liver and kidney, catabolizes circulating catecholamines to normetanephrines and metanephrine. These can be converted by monoamine oxidase (MAO) into vanillyl-mandelic acid (VMA), a major breakdown product of catecholamines in urine.

### Testes

- An adult testis is 15–25 mL in volume.
- Seminiferous tubules, comprising Sertoli and germ cells lying on a basement membrane, make up 80% of the volume.
- Each testis has approximately 200 m of tubules, each converging on the tubuli recti, which empty into the rete testis, which then empties into the ductuli efferentes that lead to the ductus epididymis.
- Germ cells mature into spermatocytes, and spermatids and spermatozoa pass through Sertoli cells towards the tubular lumen.

- Spermatogenesis takes between 60 and 74 days.
- In response to FSH, Sertoli cells manufacture inhibin B (see **Figure 12.7**) which regulates FSH secretion by negative feedback.
- Leydig cells are located between the seminiferous tubules and produce testosterone under the influence of LH. Testosterone exerts paracrine action on Sertoli cells, essential for spermatogenesis.
- In the scrotum, penis and prostate, testosterone is converted to DHT, which is 10 times more potent than testosterone.

### Ovaries

- The volume of a normal ovary is 3–7 mL.
- Cortex encloses follicles of varying FSH-dependent maturity.
- Each follicle comprises an ovum surrounded by granulosa cells, which secretes follicular fluid and aromatizes androgens of theca origin into oestradiol (see **Figure 12.6**).
- The mature follicle measures at least 16 mm and ruptures under the influence of a mid-cycle LH surge, releasing the ovum into the pelvic cavity, later forming a corpus luteum, the source of luteal phase progesterone (see **Figure 12.8**).
- The ovarian medullary stroma synthesizes testosterone/androstenedione under LH influence.
- Androgens are also converted to oestradiol by peripheral aromatization.
- Some androgens reach the circulation unchanged.
- The normal menstrual cycle is 25–34 days.
- *Oligomenorrhoea* is a cycle >34 days.
- *Amenorrhoea* means no menstrual cycle for 6 months.

## APPROACH TO THE PATIENT

### HISTORY

---

**HISTORY 12.1**

#### Questions to be addressed in suspected endocrine diseases

What endocrine disorder is suggested by the initial symptoms?
Are there other associated endocrine disorders that should be sought?
Are there other features suggesting an endocrine syndrome?
What was the earliest onset of symptoms?
What is the differential diagnosis?
What biochemical investigations are required?
Should the gland be imaged?
If there is an overactive gland, does the patient understand the medical and surgical options?
If there is an underactive gland, does the patient understand the timescale of endocrine replacement therapy?

**12**

**General**

When were you last completely well?

How are the following: your sleeping pattern, heat tolerance, weight, appetite, skin and hair?

How have your symptoms developed from when you first noticed them until now? (most endocrine disorders are gradually progressive rather than relaxing)

**Cardiovascular**

Do you get palpitations? (thyrotoxicosis, pheochromocytoma)

Do you get short of breath? (symptom of heart failure which may be a feature of both hypothyroidism and hyperthyroidism)

**Gastrointestinal**

Do you get constipated? (hypothyroidism, hypercalcaemia)

Do your bowels seem overactive? (thyrotoxicosis, neuroendocrine tumour)

**Neurological**

Do your hands shake? (fine tremor is a feature of thyrotoxicosis)

Do you get double vision or any problem with your vision? (Graves' disease and pituitary tumour)

**Musculoskeletal**

Do your muscles feel weak? (thyrotoxicosis, Cushing's syndrome, osteomalacia, hypokalaemia)

**Female reproductive symptoms**

How old were you when you started your periods (menarche)?

How old were you when you had your menopause?

What is the interval between periods?

How many periods do you have a year?

Do you have hot flashes? (sign of oestrogen deficiency)

Do you find intercourse painful? (dyspareunia, a symptom of oestrogen deficiency)

Have you noticed any discharge from your nipples? (galactorrhoea, a feature of hyperprolactinaemi)

If so, is it spontaneous or only on expression?

Do you suffer from excessive unwanted hair? (hirsutism secondary to hyperandrogenism)

**Male reproductive symptoms**

Have you noticed any change in your libido? (low libido may indicate testosterone deficiency)

Do you have early morning erections? (typically reduced in hypogonadism and hyperprolactinaemia)

Do you have difficulty maintaining erections? (may indicate hypogonadism, diabetic vascular damage, venous leaks)

How often do you shave? (frequency typically reduced in hypogonadism)

Do you have problems with fertility? (may indicate gonadal failure, absent vasa)

**Drug history**

What medicines and tonics either prescribed by a doctor or obtained from elsewhere do you take?

Do you take an oral contraceptive? If so, which one?

**Past medical history**

Have you had any thyroid or pituitary surgery?

**Family history**

Does anyone in your family have any thyroid disorder or diabetes?

Has anyone in your family had a similar illness?

Do any illnesses run in your family?

# REPRODUCTIVE PROBLEMS WITH AN ENDOCRINE BASIS

## Women

Menstrual disturbance is common in female gonadal disorders. Such disorders can be divided into:

- Low oestrogen states (e.g. primary and secondary hypogonadism)
- Normal oestrogen states (e.g. polycystic ovary syndrome)

Symptoms of oestrogen deficiency include hot flashes, depression, loss of libido and vaginal dryness. Features of hyperandrogenism include hirsutism, acne, alopecia, seborrhoea and clitoromegaly. Endocrine disorders cause infertility as a result of anovulation and luteal phase insufficiency.

## Men

Impotence is a common symptom. Endocrinopathy is suggested by accompanying features of androgen deficiency (loss of secondary sexual hair, gynaecomastia, loss of libido and erectile dysfunction, and anaemia)

# DRUG HISTORY

Be aware of factitious hypothyroidism in those with access to thyroxine. Lithium reduces thyroxine release, causing hypothyroidism, and amiodarone frequently disturbs thyroid function.

# FAMILY HISTORY

Autoimmune endocrinopathies and multiple endocrine neoplasia (MEN) may be evident in family history.

# PAST MEDICAL HISTORY

## Men and women

- Head injury: hypopituitarism
- Pituitary failure: previous irradiation

## Women

The onset of hypogonadism is usually relatively precise as there will be a history of primary or secondary amenorrhoea or infertility.

## Men

Is there a history of testicular infection, trauma, maldescent, previous chemotherapy in adult hypogonadal men?

# GENERAL INSPECTION

Note:

- Changes in skin, hair quality and fat distribution or features of Cushing's syndrome (CS) and hypothyroidism

- Skin pigmentation and postural hypotension – Addison's disease (AD)
- Bradycardia, signs of heart failure and slow relaxing reflexes – hypothyroidism
- Tachycardia or atrial fibrillation with tremor and pretibial myxoedema – Graves' disease (GD)
- Vitiligo – a marker of autoimmune disease
- Coarsened features, macroglossia, enlarged hands and feet – acromegaly

Perform visual field examination in suspected pituitary tumour (bitemporal hemianopia).

## EXAMINATION OF THE THYROID GLAND

- Look for signs of hyper- or hypothyroidism and thyroid eye disease.
- *Inspect from the front*: The thyroid moves upwards on swallowing (gland enclosed within pretracheal fascia).
- Gently palpate by standing behind the sitting patient, head slightly flexed.
- Document size and consistency (soft, firm or hard).
- Is thyroid uniformly enlarged or nodular, hard or soft, tender or non-tender?
- Ask the patient to swallow water during palpation, facilitating delineation of the lower border of the gland and retrosternal extension.
- A goitre can compress the trachea and/or oesophagus causing breathing difficulty/dysphagia.
- Thyroid carcinoma may invade neighbouring structures.
- Erosion into the trachea/oesophagus may occur. Recurrent laryngeal nerve or cervical sympathetic chain involvement produces hoarseness (Horner's syndrome).
- Metastases may be found in adjacent lymph nodes in papillary carcinoma.
- On thyroid auscultation, bruit is caused by increased vascularity typical of GD.

## EXAMINATION OF THE REPRODUCTIVE SYSTEM

- Sexual development: use Tanner staging for genital development, breast size and pubic hair density (**Figure 12.15**).
- Body-hair distribution/density should be noted although differentiation from normal variation is often difficult.
- Hyperandrogenism in women causes acne, seborrhoea, male pattern baldness and clitoromegaly.
- Testis volume can be measured using Prader orchidometry.
- Scrotal contents should be examined for varicocoeles and testicular neoplasm, with the patient standing.
- Ovaries are best assessed ultrasonically.
- Progesterone causes a mid-cycle rise in body temperature of about 0.5 °C, used to time ovulation.

## INVESTIGATION

### BIOCHEMISTRY

#### Urea and electrolytes

- Hyponatraemia or low PO reflects water retention in the syndrome of inappropriate antidiuresis (SIAD).
- Raised sodium/PO with a low urinary osmolality consistent with water loss is seen in cranial and nephrogenic diabetes insipidus (NDI).
- Hyperkalaemia, hyponatraemia and low bicarbonate are characteristic of MC deficiency in AD.
- Hypernatraemia with hypokalaemia occurs in the MC excess of Conn's syndrome.
- Hypokalaemia is also a feature of CS, due to ectopic ACTH production.

#### Basal pituitary function tests

These comprise GH and IGF-1, LH/FSH, testosterone/oestradiol, TSH/fT$_4$, 9 a.m. cortisol, prolactin and PO/urine osmolality (UO) estimations.

#### Serum growth hormone

- Test serial GH levels to confirm a diagnosis of acromegaly.
- Undetectable GH levels excludes acromegaly but, given the pulsatile nature of GH secretion, a detectable value is non-diagnostic.
- Failure of 75 glucose load to suppress GH to <0.4 µg/L in males and 0.6 µg/L in females, or a paradoxical GH rise following glucose, occurs in acromegaly (**Figure 12.16**).
- Raised IGF-1 levels constitute appropriate cost-effective initial screening test for acromegaly.

#### Plasma prolactin

- Clinical suspicion of prolactinoma is supported by a high plasma prolactin level (usually >3000 mU/L).
- Prolactin is moderately raised in other pituitary tumours causing stalk compression and impairing dopaminergic inhibition of prolactin secretion.

#### Thyroid-stimulating hormone, fT$_4$

See **Table 12.1**.

#### Plasma ACTH/cortisol

See **Table 12.2**.

#### Plasma and urine osmolality

Test PO and UO (**Table 12.3**).

**12**

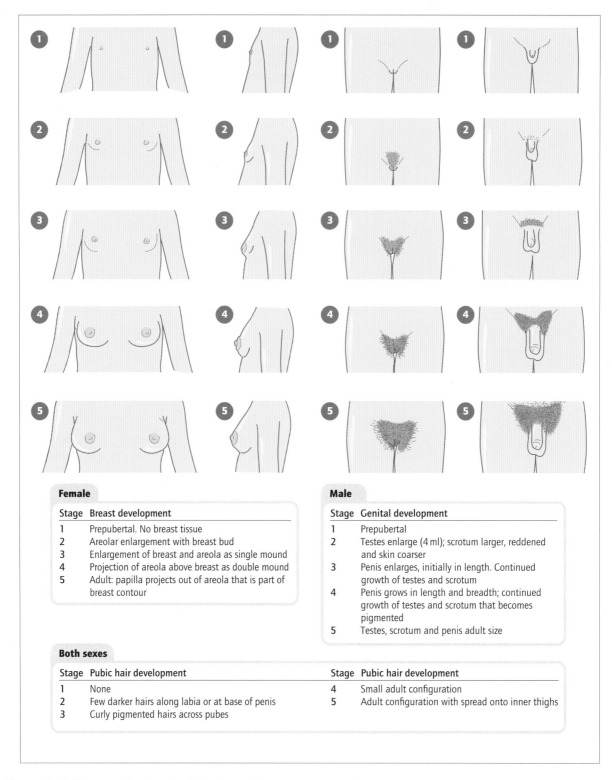

**Female**

| Stage | Breast development |
|---|---|
| 1 | Prepubertal. No breast tissue |
| 2 | Areolar enlargement with breast bud |
| 3 | Enlargement of breast and areola as single mound |
| 4 | Projection of areola above breast as double mound |
| 5 | Adult: papilla projects out of areola that is part of breast contour |

**Male**

| Stage | Genital development |
|---|---|
| 1 | Prepubertal |
| 2 | Testes enlarge (4 ml); scrotum larger, reddened and skin coarser |
| 3 | Penis enlarges, initially in length. Continued growth of testes and scrotum |
| 4 | Penis grows in length and breadth; continued growth of testes and scrotum that becomes pigmented |
| 5 | Testes, scrotum and penis adult size |

**Both sexes**

| Stage | Pubic hair development | Stage | Pubic hair development |
|---|---|---|---|
| 1 | None | 4 | Small adult configuration |
| 2 | Few darker hairs along labia or at base of penis | 5 | Adult configuration with spread onto inner thighs |
| 3 | Curly pigmented hairs across pubes | | |

**Figure 12.15** Tanner staging of pubertal development in males and females.

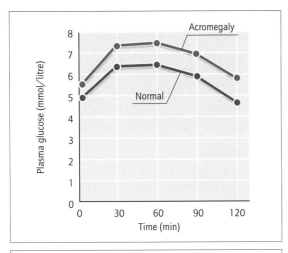

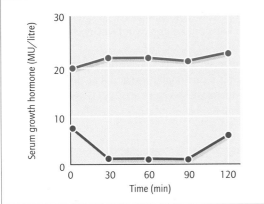

**Figure 12.16** Response of circulating GH to a 75 oral glucose challenge in health and in acromegaly. In the latter, there is incomplete suppression of GH with the OGTT, or level a paradoxical rise in 50% of patients, whereas in health the GH is suppressed.

## Water deprivation test

- The water deprivation test (WDT) helps to exclude borderline diabetes insipidus.
- Fluids are withheld for 8 hours, and PO, UO, urine volume and patient weight are measured at intervals.
- Normally, PO is maintained within the normal range during WDT and UO rises to >600 mOsm/kg at 8 hours.
- In cranial diabetes insipidus (CDI), UO remains inappropriately low and urine output stays high.
- The test should be abandoned if there is excessive urine output and weight reduction >3%.
- Synthetic vasopressin (desmopressin) can be administered and increases UO in CDI but not NDI.

## Insulin tolerance test

- The insulin tolerance test (ITT) is used to diagnose ACTH/GH deficiency.
- Hypoglycaemia stimulates release of counter-regulatory ACTH and GH.
- After IV soluble insulin (0.1–0.15 U/kg), the blood is sampled at intervals for 2 hours for glucose, cortisol and GH estimation.
- Blood glucose should fall to <2.2 mmol/L and the patient should be symptomatic (sweating, palpitations).
- The test is contraindicated in ischaemic heart disease (IHD) or epilepsy.
- It must be conducted on carefully selected patients by experienced staff.
- If ITT is contraindicated, a glucagon or combined arginine/GHRH test may be used.

**Table 12.1** Investigation of TSH and $fT_4$

| Condition | fT$_4$ (12–22 pmol/L) | fT$_3$ (3.7–5.8 pmol/L) | TSH (0.5–4.2 mU/L) |
|---|---|---|---|
| Thyrotoxicosis | Raised | Raised | Suppressed |
| T$_3$ toxicosis | Normal | Raised | Suppressed |
| Primary hypothyroidism | Low | Low | Raised |
| Secondary hypothyroidism | Low | Low | Normal or low |
| Thyroid hormone resistance / TSHoma | Raised | Raised | Normal or raised |

**Table 12.2** Investigation of plasma ACTH/cortisol

| Condition | ACTH | Plasma/urinary free cortisol |
|---|---|---|
| Cushing's syndrome (ACTH-dependent) | Raised in pituitary-dependent Cushing's disease<br>Grossly raised in ectopic Cushing's syndrome (**Figure 12.17**) | Raised with loss of plasma cortisol circadian rhythm |
| Cushing's syndrome (ACTH-independent), due to adrenal adenoma/carcinoma | Low/undetectable | Raised |

**Table 12.3** Investigation of PO and UO

| Condition | Plasma sodium | Plasma osmolality | Urine osmolality | Plasma ADH |
|---|---|---|---|---|
| CDI | Raised | Raised | Inappropriately low | Inappropriately low |
| NDI | Raised | Raised | Inappropriately low | Raised |

**Table 12.4** Investigation of gonadal function

| Condition | LH | FSH | Oestradiol/testosterone |
|---|---|---|---|
| Primary gonadal failure (Klinefelter syndrome, menopause, testicular damage) | Raised | Raised | Low |
| Secondary gonadal failure | Low | Low | Low |

## Gonadal function

See **Table 12.4**.

### Sex hormone-binding globulin

Sex hormone-binding globulin (SHBG) binds circulating oestrogen, testosterone and dihydrotestosterone. Its level is low in obesity and in hyperandrogenic females.

### Progesterone measurement

A detectable progesterone in the luteal phase confirms ovulation (see **Figure 12.8**).

## IMMUNOLOGY

Antibody and autoantibody testing can help differentiate endocrine disorders (**Table 12.5**).

## DIAGNOSTIC IMAGING

### Lateral skull radiography

This will show an expanded pituitary fossa in a large pituitary tumour.

### Magnetic resonance imaging

- Magnetic resonance imaging (MRI) is the optimal way of assessing pituitary tumour extent.
- In women, a prolactinoma, often small (microadenoma <1 cm), may be seen confined to the sella turcica at presentation (**Figure 12.18**); in the case of a macroadenoma, MRI shows the extent of a suprasellar extension (**Figure 12.19**).

- Gadolinium enhancement may enable localization of ACTH-producing adenomas in up to 80% of cases.

### Adrenal imaging

- Adrenal size is assessed by computed tomography (CT).
- Bilateral adrenal hyperplasia is a feature of ACTH-driven CS.
- CT is used for visualization of cortisol, aldosterone-secreting adenomas and pheochromocytoma (**Figure 12.20**).
- In AD the adrenal glands are atrophic in autoimmune adrenalitis but enlarged and calcified in tuberculous disease.
- Unsuspected masses may be discovered during adrenal imaging. Functional tests should be performed; if no evidence of secretory activity is evident, surgical removal of masses >4 cm is recommended.

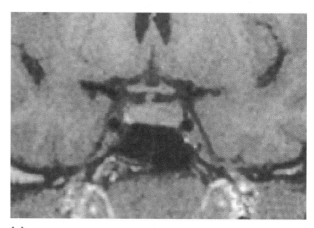

(a)

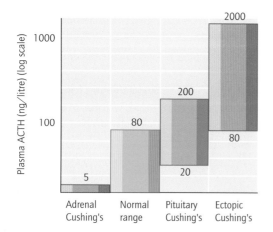

**Figure 12.17** Circulating ACTH levels in pituitary dependent Cushing's disease, ectopic ACTH secretion in adrenal tumours causing Cushing's syndrome. There is an overlap in ACTH levels between CD and ectopic ACTH secretion.

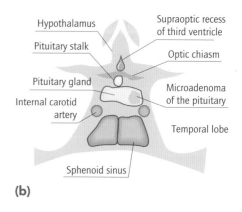

(b)

**Figure 12.18** T1-weighted MRI scan **(a)** and explanatory line diagram **(b)** of the pituitary showing a small defect on the left side of the pituitary fossa, compatible with a microadenoma, in this case, prolactin-secreting. Important anatomical relationships of the pituitary are shown in this coronal scan.

**Table 12.5** Antibodies and autoantibodies in endocrine disorders

| Condition | TPO/Tg antibodies | TSH receptor Ab | 21-hydroxylase Ab | Ovarian autoantibodies | Parathyroid antibodies |
|---|---|---|---|---|---|
| Hashimoto's thyroiditis, primary myxoedema | ++ | Negative | – | – | – |
| GD | + | Positive | – | – | – |
| Autoimmune Addison's disease | – | – | Positive | – | – |
| Hypoparathyroidism | – | – | – | – | Positive |
| Premature ovarian failure | – | – | – | Positive | – |

## Thyroid radioisotope imaging

- Technetium ($^{99m}$Tc) pertechnetate scanning is used because of its short radioactive half-life.
- There is no uptake in thyroiditis and factitious thyrotoxicosis (inappropriate self-administration of thyroxine).

- Distribution of uptake within the thyroid will identify 'hot nodule(s)' (e.g. toxic adenoma and toxic multinodular goitre).
- A thyroid cyst or a thyroid carcinoma will be apparent as a 'cold nodule' with low isotope uptake.
- Tracer uptake is diffusely increased in GD (**Figure 12.21**).

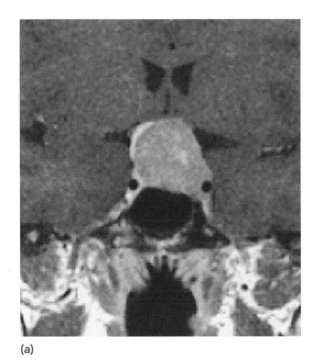

**(a)**

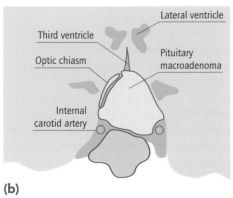

**(b)**

**Figure 12.19** Coronal contrast-enhanced T1-weighted MRI scan **(a)** and explanatory line diagram **(b)** of macroadenoma of the pituitary. The optic chiasm is displaced and compressed.

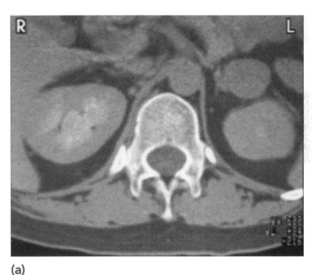

**Figure 12.20** Axial CT scan **(a)** and explanatory line diagram **(b)** of the abdomen showing a left adrenal adenoma.

**12**

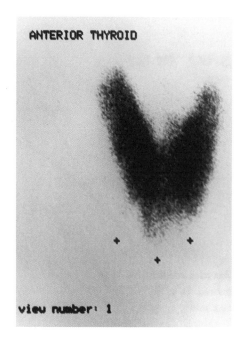

**Figure 12.21** ⁹⁹ᵐTc pertechnetate scan of the thyroid showing increased diffuse uptake typical of GD.

### Thyroid ultrasound imaging

- The cystic or solid nature of a thyroid nodule can be ascertained by thyroid ultrasound (US) examination.
- Papillary carcinoma has specific ultrasonic characteristics (**Figure 12.22**).

### Gonadal ultrasound imaging

- This identifies otherwise improbable testicular tumours or undescended testes in the inguinal canal.
- In females, transabdominal (through full bladder) or preferably transvaginal scans identify ovarian/uterine masses, measure endometrial thickness and assess follicular development (cycle tracking).

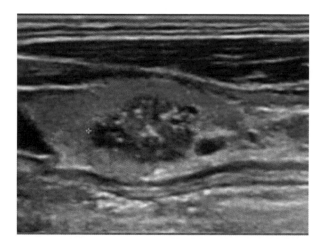

**Figure 12.22** Irregular hypoechoic thyroid nodule showing intralesional microcalcification typical of papillary carcinoma of thyroid.

## HISTOPATHOLOGY

Fine-needle aspiration (FNA) of thyroid masses discriminates between benign and malignant lesions.

## KARYOTYPE

Karyotype analysis may reveal Turner syndrome (TS) (female: XO) and Klinefelter syndrome (male: XXY).

# DISEASES AND THEIR MANAGEMENT

## DISEASES OF THE PITUITARY GLAND

### PITUITARY TUMOURS

- Approximately 10% of intracranial neoplasms
- Functioning/non-functioning
- Functioning tumours usually benign: excessive autonomous production/secretion of GH, ACTH, prolactin, LH, FSH or TSH
- Prolactinoma commonest, then non-secreting pituitary tumours
- GH-/ACTH-secreting tumours moderately rare
- FSH-/LH- and TSH-secreting tumours very rare
- Prolactinomas/Cushing's disease (CD) commoner in females

#### Clinical features

- These depend on tumour size and secretory status.
- Tumours present with local effects or hypopituitarism because of pituitary damage (**Figure 12.23**).

*Local effects*
- Lateral tumour extension: III, IV, VI nerve palsies
- Postnasal space extension
- Cerebral spinal fluid (CSF) rhinorrhoea (CSF leaking into the nose)
- Suprasellar extension, with optic chiasmatic compression and visual field loss (bitemporal upper quadrantinopia initially, then hemianopia; **Figure 12.24**)
- Headaches, signs and symptoms of raised intracranial pressure, occasionally temporal lobe epilepsy
- Hypothalamic pressure causing hyperphagia, disordered thirst/temperature control

*Hypopituitarism*
- This is characterized by decreased or absent pituitary hormone secretion directly or via stalk compression.
- Other causes of hypopituitarism are given in **Table 12.6**. GH secretion is characteristically first to be affected, then LH/FSH, TSH, ACTH. Prolactin secretion is reduced in postpartum pituitary necrosis (Sheehan's syndrome) caused by severe postpartum haemorrhage.

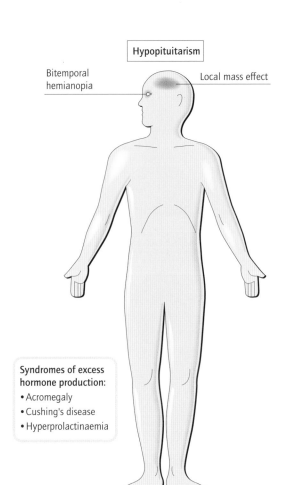

**Figure 12.23** Effects of a sellar mass. Non-functioning tumours may be responsible for hypopituitarism and mass effects such as the neurophthalmic complications of bitemporal hemianopia. Local mass effects can also cause temporal lobe compression and occasionally temporal lobe epilepsy, hydrocephalus. Tumours can also be secretory and cause endocrine syndromes.

- *GH deficiency:* This causes growth failure and features of adult-onset GH deficiency.
- *Gonadotrophin (LH, FSH) deficiency:* This causes hypogonadism.
    - *Women:* Symptoms include decreased libido, amenorrhoea, genital atrophy, reduced body hair and decreased breast size.
    - *Men:* Symptoms include decreased libido, impotence, decreased size/softening of the testes, azoospermia and loss of body hair.
    - *Both sexes:* Features include fine-textured skin with increased fine creasing, particularly around the eyes and mouth.
- *ACTH deficiency:* Symptoms are similar to primary adrenal failure, without pigmentation or the electrolyte changes caused by MC deficiency.
- *TSH deficiency:* This causes hypothyroidism.
- *Vasopressin deficiency:* This is found in CDI (polydipsia, plasma hypertonicity, dilute urine and polyuria). Cortisol deficiency may mask the clinical features of CDI. Symptoms become evident when corticosteroid

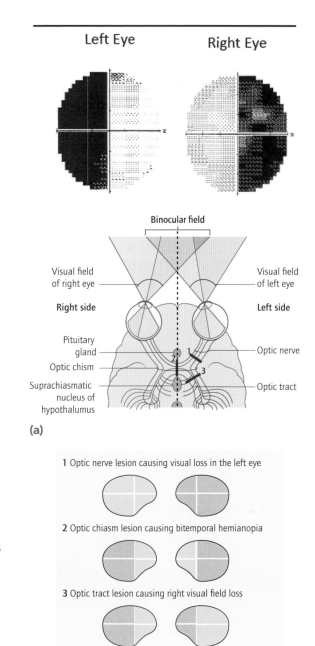

**Figure 12.24 (a)** Bitemporal hemianopia caused by suprasellar extension of pituitary tumour causing optic chiasmatic compression. **(b)** Neuro-ophthalmic abnormalities caused by a suprasellar lesion impacting on the optic nerve (1), the chiasm (2) and the optic tract (3).

replacement is initiated. Other mechanisms causing polyuria are listed in **Table 12.7**.

- Diabetes insipidus can also result from renal tubular resistance to ADH, so-called NDI secondary to interstitial renal disease, hypokalaemia, hypercalcaemia, lithium toxicity (**Figure 12.25**), and also by mutations of V2R. Diabetes insipidus may result from hypothalamus injury (e.g. from pituitary surgery) and may then be transient and recover spontaneously.

**12**

**Table 12.6** Causes of hypopituitarism

**Developmental, congenital**
Defects particularly of midline structures
Kallmann syndrome

**Infiltrations**
Sarcoidosis
Haemochromatosis

**Immunological**
Autoimmune hypophysitis

**Vascular**
Sheehan's syndrome
Pituitary apoplexy

**Tumours**
Pituitary tumours, secondary

**Miscellaneous**
Injury
Radiation
Surgery
Trauma
Infection
Meningitis
Tuberculosis

**Functional**
Anorexia, starvation
Stress
Exercise
Depression

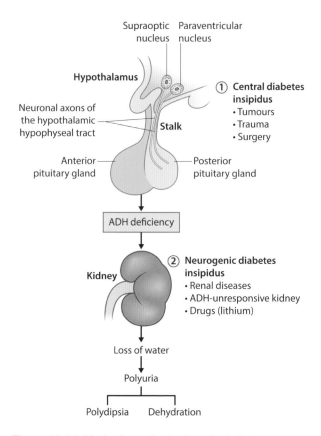

**Figure 12.25** Mechanisms of polyuric and polydipsic states caused by ADH deficiency (1 CDI) and (2) resistance to ADH action (NDI).

### Excessive hormone production

*Prolactinoma* See **Table 12.8**.

Other causes of hyperprolactinaemia have to be excluded (**Table 12.9**).

### Acromegaly

- Excessive GH secretion in post-pubertal adults leads to acromegaly (see ACROMEGALY: CLINICAL FEATURES AND DIAGNOSIS AT A GLANCE). Before epiphyseal fusion, gigantism ensues.
- Clinical progression of acromegaly is shown in **Figure 12.26**.
- Presentation includes the local effects of the tumour itself and the effects of excessive GH production.
- Changes in the face, hands and feet are insidious; diagnosis is often made when the disease has been present for many years (**Figure 12.27**; **Figure 12.28**).

**Table 12.7** Causes of polyuria

Diabetes mellitus
Diabetes insipidus (cranial or nephrogenic)
Psychogenic polydipsia
Diuretic therapy
Hypokalaemia
Hypercalcaemia
Chronic renal failure

- Diagnosis is made on failure of GH to suppress following an oral glucose tolerance test (OGTT) (see **Figure 12.16**).

### Management

- Successful management involves surgery, radiotherapy and/or drugs.
- Treatment is important for the local effects of tumour growth and the regression of clinical features.

#### Drugs

- Dopamine agonists may be used (e.g. bromocriptine, cabergoline). Somatostatin analogues (e.g. octreotide IM, lanreotide sc) are more effective with significant GH/IGF-1 reduction in 40%. Tumour shrinkage is occasionally dramatic (**Figure 12.29**).
- They may cause gallstones.
- Subcutaneous pegvisomant, a GH antagonist, normalizes IGF-1 in 90% of patients. Data are awaited regarding the effect on tumour size and long-term risks.

#### Surgery

- *Transsphenoidal surgery* (TSS) aims to preserve normal tissue if possible. GH levels may normalize after TSS with microadenomas; surgical cure of macroadenomas is not possible.

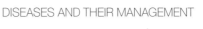

**Table 12.8** Clinical features, investigation and management of prolactinoma

|  | Clinical features in females | Clinical features in males |
|---|---|---|
| **Reproductive phenotype** | Oligomenorrhoea, amenorrhoea, luteal insufficiency, infertility | Often late presentation with larger tumours (macroadenoma), loss of libido, impotence, galactorrhoea, infertility |
| **MRI** | Usually microadenoma/mesoadenoma | Often macroadenoma, with visual field defect |
| **Musculoskeletal phenotype** | Osteopenia/osteoporosis, if associated with long-standing hypogonadism | Osteopenia if associated with long-standing hypogonadism |
| **Biochemical features** | Prolactin elevated sometimes >10 000 mU/L | Prolactin frequently greatly elevated at >100 000 mU/L |
| **Medical management** | Usually medical: cabergoline 0.25 mg twice weekly, dose titrated upwards to get prolactin <360 mU/L<br>Bromocriptine/quinagolide are alternatives | Cabergoline 0.25–2 mg twice weekly; bromocriptine/quinagolide are alternatives<br>Frequent improvement in visual fields, and restoration of pituitary function sometimes seen<br>Treatment usually long-term |
| **Surgical management** | Rarely indicated, except if patient resistant to dopamine agonist, or experiences adverse effect (e.g. development of psychiatric side effects) | Occasionally needed if tumour is unresponsive to dopamine agonists, or with side effects (psychiatric: e.g. gambling addiction) |
| **Radiotherapy** | Rarely indicated | Occasionally indicated if long-term high-dose dopamine agonist therapy needed |
| **Effect of pregnancy** | Treatment usually discontinued with pregnancy<br>Frequent visual field testing needed during pregnancy to guard against oestrogen-mediated tumour enlargement | |

- Expectations should be realistic: the relief of optic chiasmatic compression and tumour debulking.
- Radiotherapy is given adjunctively if GH remains high.

### TSH-secreting tumour
- Very rare
- $fT_4/fT_3$ levels elevated with normal/increased TSH levels
- Tumours often aggressive

*Non-secreting pituitary tumour* TSS surgery is often combined with conventional radiotherapy if complete surgical removal is unachievable

**Table 12.9** Causes of hyperprolactinaemia

**Cranial disease**
- Hypothalamic disease
- Pituitary tumour with stalking disconnection
- Prolactin-secreting tumour (prolactinoma, acromegaly)

**Drugs**
- Neuroleptic drugs
- Metoclopramide, domperidone
- Oestrogens

**Endocrine**
- Hypothyroidism

**Stress**
- Surgical
- Illness
- Venipuncture

*Complications of transsphenoidal surgery*
- CSF leak
- Hyposmia
- Meningitis
- Hypopituitarism
- Haemorrhage and stroke
- Optic nerve or chiasmatic damage with visual impairment
- Transient/permanent CDI
- CDI: treated with long-acting vasopressin analogue dDAVP
- Syndrome of inappropriate antidiuretic hormone secretion (SIADH)

## SYNDROME OF INAPPROPRIATE DIURESIS

- Syndrome of inappropriate antidiuretic hormone secretion (SIADH) has multifactorial causes (**Table 12.10**)

**Table 12.10** Causes of SIADH

| |
|---|
| Lung disease |
| Bronchial carcinoma |
| Tuberculosis |
| Pneumonia |
| Abscess |
| Bronchiectasis |
| Cranial disease (especially tumour or haemorrhage) |
| Drugs |
| Psychotropic agents |

**12**

489

## ACROMEGALY: CLINICAL FEATURES AND DIAGNOSIS AT A GLANCE

**Acromegalic facies**
• Protruding supraorbital ridges
• Enlarged nose
• Coarse facial features
• Prognathia

Headaches
Thickened calvaria

Cardiomegaly

Hypertension

Hepatomegaly

Insulin resistance (diabetes)

Large hands

Impotence and loss of libido
(amenorrhea in women)

Thickened skin

Hyperostosis

Degenerative joint disease

Peripheral neuropathy
(nerve compression)

Large feet and heel pad

**LAB**
↑GH
↑ IGF-I
↑Insulin
↑Ca$^{2+}$, P-
↑Glucose
ACTH (↑ or ↓)

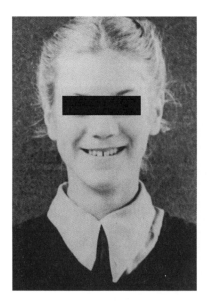
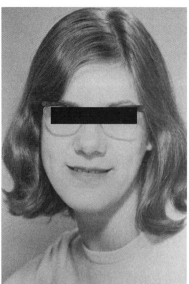
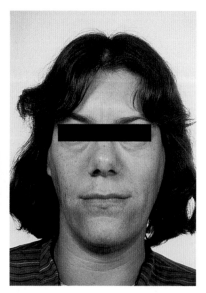

**Figure 12.26 (a–c)** Clinical progression of acromegaly over a 20-year period. Clinical features may be very insidious in onset and time to diagnosis is often >10 years.

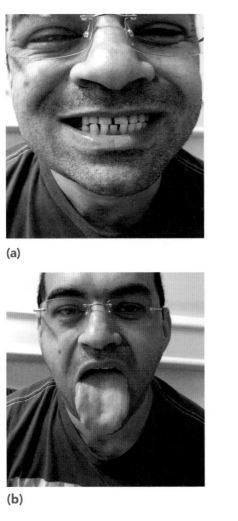

(a)

(b)

**Figure 12.27** Clinical acromegalic features. **(a)** Interdental separation due to maxillary enlargement and malocclusion of the teeth because of prognathism. **(b)** Macroglossia, often the cause of heavy snoring and obstructive sleep apnoea.

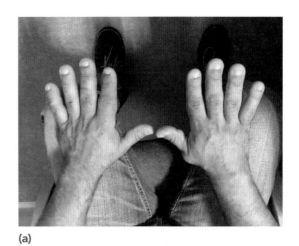

(a)

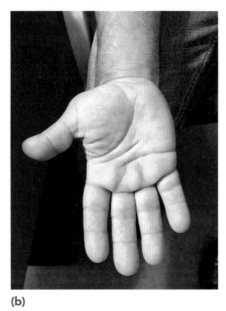

(b)

**Figure 12.28 (a)** The spade-like hands of the acromegalic patient and **(b)** soft tissue overgrowth in the palm of the hand.

**12**

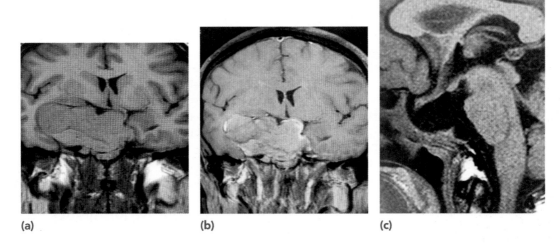

(a)

(b)

(c)

**Figure 12.29 (a,b)** T1-weighted pre- and post-gadolinium contrast-enhanced MRI scan showing massive GH-/prolactin-secreting tumour which responded to combined medical treatment with high-dose cabergoline and a somatostatin analogue over a 2-year period. **(c)** A virtually empty sella turcica with only a rim of pituitary tissue lining it.

**Table 12.11** Investigation of SIADH

| |
|---|
| Low serum sodium |
| Low plasma osmolality |
| UO >100 mOsm/kg |
| Urine sodium excretion >30 mmol/L |
| Normal cortisol and thyroid function tests |

- Pathogenesis often unclear
- Secondary to ectopic ADH production or failure of normal suppression of ADH secretion
- May be caused by drugs (e.g. vincristine, cyclophosphamide) or increased renal ADH sensitivity (e.g. chlorpropamide, carbamazepine)
- Often temporary following TSS
- Water content of all compartments increased (**Table 12.11**)
- Follows excessive dDAVP administration for CDI
- Common cause of hyponatraemia
- Patients not hypotensive or hypovolaemic
- Most are asymptomatic, often identified with U&E measurement
- Rapid-onset sodium <120 mmol/L, confusion, irritability and nausea may develop; as Na+ falls further, fits and coma may occur
- More chronic hyponatraemia leads to cerebral adaptation, fewer symptoms

**Management and prognosis**

- Fluid restriction: 1 L/24 hours
- Treat underlying cause
- Hyponatraemic encephalopathy: hypertonic 3% saline infusion necessary in short term
- Occasionally, demeclocycline (impairs renal tubular response to ADH) used
- Tolvaptan, a V2R antagonist, may also be used
- Prognosis depends on underlying cause
- Avoid over-rapid correction of low sodium to avoid osmotic demyelination (central pontine myelinolysis)

## THYROID DISEASES

## HYPOTHYROIDISM

- Hypothyroidism results from decreased production and secretion of thyroid hormones ($T_4$ and $T_3$).
- It is usually caused by primary thyroid disease, less frequently failure of TSH production.
- Worldwide, the commonest cause is iodine deficiency.
- The autoimmune disease (Hashimoto's thyroiditis) is found in developed countries.
- The next most common cause is previous [131]I treatment for hyperthyroidism (50% of patients develop hypothyroidism within 10 years, especially in the first year after therapy).

- Following partial thyroidectomy, about 30% develop hypothyroidism at 10 years.
- Overall, destructive therapy for hyperthyroidism accounts for one-third of cases of adult hypothyroidism.

**Clinical features and investigation**

- *ECG:* sinus bradycardia, low voltage complexes and ischaemic changes
- *Chest X-ray:* may show pericardial and pleural effusions
- *Histology:* parenchymal infiltration by lymphocytes and lymphoid follicles

See HYPOTHYROIDISM: CLINICAL FEATURES, INVESTIGATION AND TREATMENT AT A GLANCE.

**Management**

- L-thyroxine: initially 50 µg daily, dose titration to 100–200 µg per day
- In the elderly or those at risk of IHD, starting dose lower, with gradual increments to replacement levels
- Optimum replacement L-thyroxine dosage: clinical well-being targeting 1–2 mU/L TSH level
- Secondary hypothyroidism: concomitant ACTH deficiency treated before thyroxine replacement to avoid Addisonian crisis
- Clinical features reverse after 3–4 months of treatment (**Figure 12.30**)

Life expectancy normal except for possible accelerated IHD

## MYXOEDEMA COMA

- Severe presentation of hypothyroidism
- *Precipitating factors:* cold exposure, intercurrent infections, treatment with phenothiazines or barbiturates
- Hyponatraemia and hypoglycaemia
- Most common in the elderly (90% women), especially in poor socioeconomic groups and cold climates
- Clinically, hypothermia, coma and clinical hypothyroidism

**Management and prognosis**

- Hypothermia: gradual rewarming
- IV thyroxine 2–300 µg IV bolus or $T_3$ (5 µg) every 8 hours
- Correct electrolyte disturbances and hypoglycaemia
- Hydrocortisone 100 mg IV, as cortisol secretion impaired with profound hypothyroidism
- Poor prognosis in the elderly

**Investigation**

See **Table 12.12**.

## CONGENITAL HYPOTHYROIDISM

- Complete absence of thyroid gland (athyreosis) or ectopic thyroid and also various genetic defects in $T_4$ biosynthesis

## HYPOTHYROIDISM: CLINICAL FEATURES, INVESTIGATION AND TREATMENT AT A GLANCE

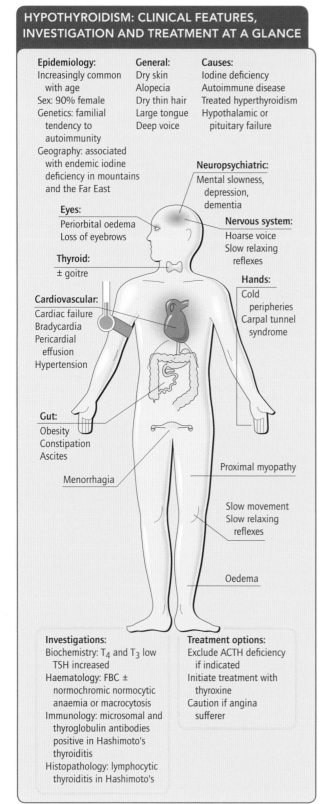

**Epidemiology:**
Increasingly common with age
Sex: 90% female
Genetics: familial tendency to autoimmunity
Geography: associated with endemic iodine deficiency in mountains and the Far East

**Eyes:**
Periorbital oedema
Loss of eyebrows

**Thyroid:**
± goitre

**Cardiovascular:**
Cardiac failure
Bradycardia
Pericardial effusion
Hypertension

**Gut:**
Obesity
Constipation
Ascites

Menorrhagia

**General:**
Dry skin
Alopecia
Dry thin hair
Large tongue
Deep voice

**Causes:**
Iodine deficiency
Autoimmune disease
Treated hyperthyroidism
Hypothalamic or pituitary failure

**Neuropsychiatric:**
Mental slowness, depression, dementia

**Nervous system:**
Hoarse voice
Slow relaxing reflexes

**Hands:**
Cold peripheries
Carpal tunnel syndrome

Proximal myopathy

Slow movement
Slow relaxing reflexes

Oedema

**Investigations:**
Biochemistry: $T_4$ and $T_3$ low TSH increased
Haematology: FBC ± normochromic normocytic anaemia or macrocytosis
Immunology: microsomal and thyroglobulin antibodies positive in Hashimoto's thyroiditis
Histopathology: lymphocytic thyroiditis in Hashimoto's

**Treatment options:**
Exclude ACTH deficiency if indicated
Initiate treatment with thyroxine
Caution if angina sufferer

- In non-iodine deficient areas, incidence 1 in 4000–5000 births
- Frequent in iodine-deficient areas
- Endemic cretinism: mental deficiency, deaf mutism, spastic diplegia, growth-stunting hypothyroidism, goitre

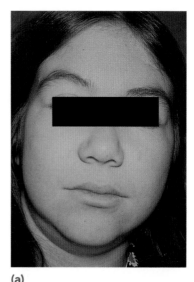

(a)

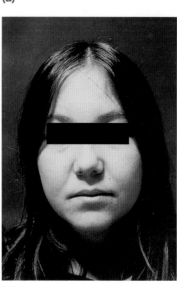

(b)

**Figure 12.30** Facial features of severe myxoedema **(a)** before and **(b)** after 6 months of treatment with L-thyroxine 100 mgg taken 30 min before breakfast on an empty stomach.

- Delayed diagnosis/treatment: permanent mental retardation
- Childhood hypothyroidism: retarded growth and sexual development; skeletal development severely affected; long bones and facial bones fail to develop with epiphyseal dysgenesis or delayed epiphyseal closure

**Table 12.12** Investigation of myxoedema coma

U&E and creatinine
TSH, $fT_4$
Cortisol to exclude Addison's disease
Blood glucose, amylase, chest X-ray
ECG

12

- Puberty delayed; rarely precocious puberty
- TSH routinely assayed in neonates after 5 days to identify neonatal hypothyroidism – does not identify secondary hypothyroidism

### Management and prognosis

- Levothyroxine ($LT_4$) + appropriate dose adjustment
- Neurological deficits irreversible

## HYPERTHYROIDISM

Hyperthyroidism (thyrotoxicosis) is characterized by excessive $T_4/T_3$ secretion. The commonest cause is GD. Other important causes are toxic nodular goitre and toxic adenoma (**Table 12.13**).

See HYPERTHYROIDISM: CLINICAL FEATURES, INVESTIGATION AND TREATMENT AT A GLANCE.

### Clinical features

See **Figure 12.31**.

#### Symptoms and signs of Graves' disease

- Weight loss
- Increased appetite
- Anxiety and irritability
- Goitre
- Fine tremor of the hands or fingers
- Heat intolerance, increased sweating
- Moist skin
- Lighter menstrual flow
- Erectile dysfunction
- Frequent bowel movements
- Fatigue, weakness
- Palpitations, irregular heartbeat, atrial fibrillation
- Sleep disturbance
- Proximal myopathy
- Orbitopathy
- Pretibial myxoedema
- Thyroid acropathy

#### Eye involvement in thyrotoxicosis

- *Lid lag* is present in any form of hyperthyroidism. The levator palpebrae superioris (LPS), partly sympathetically innervated, is affected by increased catecholamine sensitivity. Spasm of the LPS causes upper eyelid retraction and a typical 'stare'. Blinking is frequent with eye grittiness. The sclera is visible above

**Table 12.13** Causes of hyperthyroidism

| |
|---|
| GD |
| Toxic multinodular goitre |
| Toxic adenoma |
| Iodine-induced |
| TSH secreting tumour |
| Drugs |
| Thyroiditis |

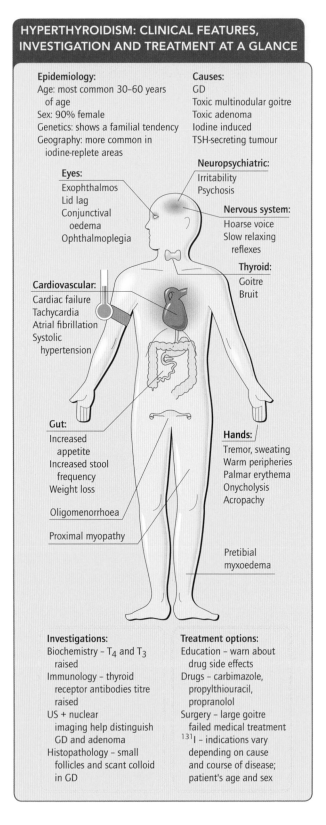

**HYPERTHYROIDISM: CLINICAL FEATURES, INVESTIGATION AND TREATMENT AT A GLANCE**

**Epidemiology:**
Age: most common 30–60 years of age
Sex: 90% female
Genetics: shows a familial tendency
Geography: more common in iodine-replete areas

**Causes:**
GD
Toxic multinodular goitre
Toxic adenoma
Iodine induced
TSH-secreting tumour

**Eyes:**
Exophthalmos
Lid lag
Conjunctival oedema
Ophthalmoplegia

**Neuropsychiatric:**
Irritability
Psychosis

**Nervous system:**
Hoarse voice
Slow relaxing reflexes

**Thyroid:**
Goitre
Bruit

**Cardiovascular:**
Cardiac failure
Tachycardia
Atrial fibrillation
Systolic hypertension

**Gut:**
Increased appetite
Increased stool frequency
Weight loss

Oligomenorrhoea

Proximal myopathy

**Hands:**
Tremor, sweating
Warm peripheries
Palmar erythema
Onycholysis
Acropachy

Pretibial myxoedema

**Investigations:**
Biochemistry – $T_4$ and $T_3$ raised
Immunology – thyroid receptor antibodies titre raised
US + nuclear imaging help distinguish GD and adenoma
Histopathology – small follicles and scant colloid in GD

**Treatment options:**
Education – warn about drug side effects
Drugs – carbimazole, propylthiouracil, propranolol
Surgery – large goitre failed medical treatment
[131]I – indications vary depending on cause and course of disease; patient's age and sex

the cornea. Less severe lid retraction is elicited by demonstrating lid lag.
- *In GD*, there are additional eye symptoms and signs secondary to autoimmune orbitopathy. There is inflammatory infiltrate of the eye muscles,

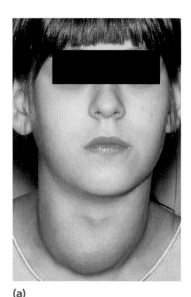

**(a)**

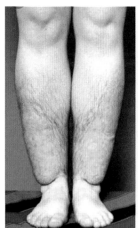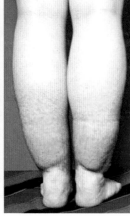

**(c)**

**Figure 12.31** Clinical features of GD. **(a)** A patient showing a smooth diffuse enlargement of a very vascular thyroid. **(b)** Severe ophthalmic GD with exophthalmos, severe lid retraction chemosis, conjunctival injection and periorbital lymphoedema. The caruncular are injected and oedematous. **(c)** Pretibial myxoedema in a patient with active GD. These itchy lesions and the swelling responded well to topical betnovate ointment under occlusion.

orbital fat, and fibrosis. Features can occur without hyperthyroidism (ophthalmic GD). There is forward eyeball protrusion, revealed by white sclera between cornea and lower eyelid in neutral gaze position

(proptosis). Proptosis (exophthalmos) is assessed by exophthalmometry. This may be asymmetrical. Keratitis results from incomplete eye closure. If severe, there is raised intraocular pressure and papilloedema. Weakness or tethering caused by extraocular muscle inflammation causes ophthalmoplegia; the inferior recti are first affected leading to a failure of upward and outward gaze and diplopia. Other muscles may be involved.

### Investigation

- *FBC:* Check FBC before starting treatment as there is a risk of drug-induced agranulocytosis. $fT_3/fT_4$ are raised, TSH suppressed. Thyrotropin receptor (TSHR) and thyroid-stimulating antibodies (TsAB) are raised in GD.
- *Ultrasound/technetium scanning:* This differentiates GD from adenoma.

### Management

- Treatment options: anti-thyroid drugs (ATD), radioactive iodine (RAI), surgery
- ATD: first-line therapy for hyperthyroidism

### *Carbimazole*

- Inhibits TPO and thyroid hormone synthesis; reduces antibody titres
- 40–60 mg daily for 4–6 weeks, maintenance 5–15 mg per day ('titration method')
- 'Block and replace': high-dose together (CBX) with $LT_4$ 100 µg/day.
- Carbimazole: 12–18 months' treatment; 50% patients relapse on stopping drug, especially with large vascular goitres, high TsAB titres, HLA-DR3 haplotype.
- Patients advised about relapses and to report recurrent hyperthyroid symptoms
- Relapse: carbimazole then definitive treatment (RAI/ surgery or continued on carbimazole)
- *Side effects:* skin rash, agranulocytosis (very rare), arthralgia
- *If side effects:* stop drug, seek medical advice with skin rash/sore throat, mouth ulceration (agranulocytosis)
- *Propylthiouracil (150 mg IDS initially):* used with carbimazole intolerance; preferred in pregnancy because less teratogenic, blocks $T_4$ to $T_3$ conversion
- *Propranolol (40–80 mg TDS):* used in early stages of treatment, controlling palpitations/tremor, directly reducing peripheral $T_4$ to $T_3$ conversion

### *Thyroidectomy*

- *This can be partial or total thyroidectomy depending on the severity/size of goitre.*
- Thyroidectomy is appropriate in cases where large goitres, drug intolerance, multiple relapses after drug therapy discontinuation.

**12**

- Ensure euthyroidism before surgery: potassium iodide for 10 days before surgery reduces thyroid vascularity.
- *Surgical complications:*
  - Laryngeal oedema: an early complication that can be life-threatening if not identified early – requires immediate opening of the wound site to allow decompression
  - Left recurrent laryngeal nerve palsy
  - Hypoparathyroidism
  - Transient hypocalcaemia (10%): usually recovers spontaneously; in total thyroidectomy, 0.5 PTH glands are autotransplanted to maintain calcium homeostasis long term
- Calcium levels must be monitored closely postoperatively and supplemented accordingly.
- Depletion occurs if parathyroid glands are damaged during surgery or with calcium influx into bones that have experienced calcium loss during hyperthyroidism.
- Hypothyroidism or recurrent hyperthyroidism may develop later.

### Radioactive iodine therapy

- Radioiodine therapy (RAI) conventionally offered to patients >40 years of age
- Used if disorder difficult to control with drugs, or following recurrence after surgery
- May be offered to younger patients
- Patient rendered medically euthyroid before RAI
- Antithyroid drugs stopped 5–10 days before RAI, to allow gland to retain $^{131}$I
- Treatment may exacerbate GD orbitopathy
- Repeated RAI occasionally needed to control hyperthyroidism; the main complication is hypothyroidism
- Patients informed of hypothyroid symptoms, particularly weight gain: TFTs at intervals following RAI

## THYROID STORM

- Life-threatening
- Precipitated in severely hyperthyroid patients by major stress, injury, infection, surgery
- Exceedingly rare with early, effective hyperthyroidism treatment
- Marked anxiety, agitation, hyperthermia, occasionally frank psychosis + marked tachycardia, tremor, fever, dehydration, cardiac failure
- *Treatment urgent:* see EMERGENCY PRESENTATION 12.1
- Prognosis poor: successful outcome depends on prompt recognition and treatment

## THYROID SWELLINGS

### Endemic goitre

- Endemic goitre is associated with dietary iodine deficiency, and other factors in endemic areas.

---

### EMERGENCY PRESENTATION 12.1

#### Thyroid storm

1 Propylthiouracil 250 mg 6-hourly *or* carbimazole 60–80 mg in divided doses, followed by potassium iodide 15 mg 4–6 hourly)
2 Propranolol 1–5 mg IV 6-hourly, to control cardiac and neuromuscular complications
3 Dexamethasone, parenteral fluids, reducing hyperpyrexia (fans/tepid sponge)

---

- *Pregnancy* places a substantial drain on maternal iodine, and mild enzyme deficiencies involving production of thyroid hormones probably contribute to large goitres seen in iodine-deficient areas.
- Endemic goitre is associated with normal thyroid function; when iodine deficiency is severe, hypothyroidism may develop.
- Babies born to mothers with severe iodine deficiency may develop cretinism. Iodine deficiency is a major cause of goitre worldwide (mountainous regions, Far East).
- *Cretinism* is a severe neurological deficit, with hypothyroidism, goitre and growth stunting.
- Dietary iodine supplements (e.g. iodized table salt) eliminate endemic goitre in developed countries. The introduction of supplements to goitrous areas may unmask GD and precipitate hyperthyroidism. Most patients do not need treatment.

### Simple diffuse goitre

- Goitre not associated with inflammatory or neoplastic processes is common.
- The pathogenesis is poorly understood. It often develops at puberty, suggesting that oestrogens may be involved. It is common, occurring at 10–50 years of age, particularly in women.
- It is often familial.
- The patient is euthyroid.
- No treatment is necessary, except if the gland is large, when size reduction is inducible by thyroxine, suggesting goitre dependency on TSH stimulation.
- Rarely gradual enlargement necessitates surgery.

### Multinodular goitre

- Goitrogens in diet (e.g. excess dietary iodine related to eating seaweed, cassava root) may contribute to multinodular goitre development. Individual nodules may become autonomous, with clinical hyperthyroidism. Toxic adenoma refers to an autonomous hyperfunctioning thyroid nodule with raised $fT_4/fT_3$ and suppressed TSH. The appearance of a multinodular goitre is shown in **Figure 12.32**.
- *Common:* 5% of women >50 years of age. Increasing prevalence with age; high incidence in iodine deficiency areas.

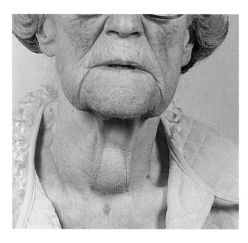

**Figure 12.32** Appearance of a long-standing multinodular goitre in an elderly patient. These lesions may lead to compressive symptomatology with dysphagia and dysphonia.

- *Symptoms:* These include the mass effect, and occasionally hyperthyroidism or hypothyroidism.
- Thoracic inlet X-ray shows tracheal compression.
- Surgery is required for obstructive symptoms (e.g. stridor) and significant retrosternal extension.
- Occasionally, haemorrhage into the nodule can cause rapidly developing obstructive symptoms.
- The dominant nodule within a multinodular goitre requires FNA to exclude malignancy. The overall risk of malignancy is small.

## THYROID MALIGNANCIES

- Thyroid malignancies are classified as well-differentiated papillary (85%: **Figure 12.33**) and follicular (10%), medullary, anaplastic carcinomas or primary thyroid lymphoma (**Table 12.14**).
- They arise in otherwise normal glands. Approximately 10% of medullary carcinomas of thyroid (MCT) are calcitonin-secreting.

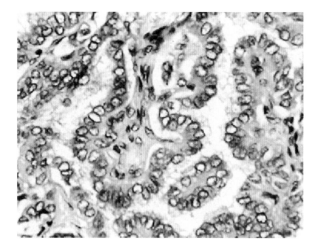

**Figure 12.33** Typical histological appearance of papillary carcinoma of the thyroid, showing the Orphan Annie cells and papillary fronds.

- Head and neck irradiation is the predisposing factor for papillary carcinomas.
- In MEN 2, MCT commonly occurs in association with parathyroid adenomas and pheochromocytoma and *RET* oncogene mutations.
- Primary malignancies of thyroid are rare, accounting for <1% of all cancer deaths and 1–2% of localized thyroid swellings.
- Papillary carcinomas occur at any age, with a median age of 40 years.
- Follicular carcinomas occur in people >40 years.
- Tumours are commoner in women. Occasionally, papillary carcinomas are familial.
- 15% of MCT are familial, autosomal dominant as part of MEN 2.
- Follicular carcinomas are commoner in iodine-deficient areas. Papillary carcinomas are generally seen in areas with high iodine intake.

### Clinical features

- This is a solitary hard nodule in one lobe or in the thyroid isthmus.
- It is difficult to distinguish carcinoma from benign adenoma and colloid nodule.
- Rapidly enlarging glands, dysphonia, dysphagia and/or breathing difficulties suggest malignancy.
- Local secondary lymph nodes deposits occur in papillary carcinoma.
- Any solitary nodule should arouse clinical suspicion of malignancy, particularly in men.
- Calcitonin is produced by MCT, a tumour marker.
- Plasma thyroglobulin is a tumour marker in well-differentiated thyroid carcinoma when TSH is suppressed fully.
- Radioisotope scanning shows a cold nodule; US scan reveals if solid or cystic.
- A solid cold nodule is not necessarily a carcinoma. FNA with cytology is diagnostic.
- A sensible thyroid nodule route of investigation is shown in **Figure 12.34**.

### Management

- Surgery
- Extent of resection determined by physician/thyroid surgeon
- Lobectomy and isthmectomy if disease unilobular
- ROI ($^{131}$I) used if tumour is ROI avid, and useful treatment for residual local or metastatic disease
- Radiotherapy for anaplastic tumours
- Progression variable, depending on age at presentation: growth slower in younger age groups (<40 years of age) and more rapid and invasive in older age groups
- Lifelong follow-up recommended

**12**

**Table 12.14** Classification of thyroid carcinoma

| | Papillary | Follicular | Anaplastic | Medullary | Lymphoma |
|---|---|---|---|---|---|
| **Frequency (%)** | 70–80 | 15 | 5 | 5–10 | 5–10 |
| **Environmental factors** | Exposure to ionizing radiation at young age | Incidence reduced by iodine supplementation | | | Risk increased in patients with autoimmune thyroiditis |
| **Genetic factors** | Associated with rearrangement of *RET* and *NTRK1*, and formation of chimeric genes<br>*BRAF* mutations | Activating point mutations of *RAS* gene<br>*PPARG–PAX8* rearrangements | Associated with mutations in the MAP kinase and PI3K pathways | Typically occurs in MEN 2A and B, but 70% sporadic<br>*Familial:* germline mutations in the *RET* gene<br>Patients with MEN 2B have a more aggressive clinical course than those with MEN 2A<br>Tumour with *RET* / m918T mutation has been associated with poor clinical outcome | |
| **Incidence** | Commoner in younger women (30–50 years) | Peak incidence 40–60 years of age | Occurs in older patients 60–80 years<br>Incidence decreasing | | Very rare<br>2.5% extranodal lymphoma |
| **Histology** | Often multifocal. 15–20% show local extrathyroidal invasion<br>Tumour typically unencapsulated, consisting of 1–2 layers of tumour cells surrounding a fibrovascular core<br>Cells and nuclei large with ground-glass cytoplasm<br>Nuclei have clefts/grooves and holes due to cytoplasmic inclusions (Orphan Annie eyes)<br>50% have calcified psammoma bodies | Follicular differentiation with capsular or vascular invasion | Anaplastic histology<br>Sarcomatoid appearance characterized by spindle cells and giant cells<br>*Thyroglobulin:*0%<br>*Vimentin:*100% (in spindle cells)<br>*EMA:*30–50% (in squamoid cells) | Originates from the parafollicular cells (C cells), which produce the hormone calcitonin and CEA. | Usually arises on top of Hashimoto's thyroiditis.<br>Most are diffuse large B-cell or marginal zone B-cell/MALT lymphoma |
| **Behaviour** | Typically locoregional lymph node metastases | | Spread is haematogenous, distant metastases found in 15–50% at initial presentation<br>Local invasion common<br>Median survival 3–5 months | Typically produces calcitonin<br>*5-year survival:* 65–90%<br>*10-year survival:* 45–85%<br>Up to 75% of patients have nodal metastasis, mostly involving central compartment, ipsilateral and contralateral jugulocarotid chains<br>Serum calcitonin correlates with tumour burden | 80% 5-year survival; marginal zone lymphoma has the best prognosis.<br>Often curable by irradiation or chemotherapy (particularly MALT) |

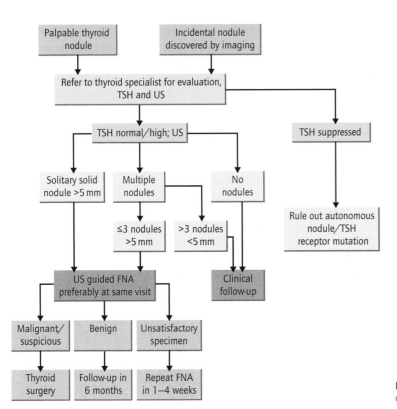

**Figure 12.34** Suggested algorithm for the clinical management of a thyroid nodule.

## PHEOCHROMOCYTOMA

### Epidemiology

- Rare (0.1–0.3% of hypertensive population)
- Commonly 25–55 years of age
- 5% inherited either alone or in combination with other traits

### Disease mechanisms

- Pheochromocytoma produce large amounts of catecholamines, hypertension and pharmacological catecholamine effects.
- They can occur as part of multiple endocrine neoplasia (MEN 2), a familial autosomal dominant syndrome. Mucosal neuromas of the tongue, buccal mucosa and lips suggest MEN 2b.
- Approximately 5% patients with pheochromocytoma have neurofibromatosis, Sturge–Weber and Von Hippel–Lindau syndrome.
- Pheochromocytoma arise anywhere in the sympathetic chain (paragangliomas), 90% develop in the adrenal medulla and 10% are malignant. Paragangliomas secrete predominantly NE, adrenal lesions secrete E and NE. Malignant tumours secrete dopamine.

### Clinical features

- Clinical features secondary to raised circulating catecholamines

- Paroxysmal, precipitated by emotional disturbance, postural change, physical exercise
- Paroxysms last a few minutes to several hours: severe headache, palpitations, tremor and sweating, nausea, vomiting, chest/abdominal pain, hyperglycaemia

### Investigation

- Raised haematocrit, elevated 24-hour urinary E, NE or metabolites normetanephrine, metanephrine, methoxytyramine
- Diagnosis difficult when tumour small or release of catecholamines paroxysmal
- Timed urine collection following a symptomatic episode useful
- Plasma EP/NE measured after 30 min recumbancy
- Tumour localization: CT combined with contrast MRI
- *MIBG/octreoscan imaging:* metaiodobenzylguanidine (MIBG)/octreotide taken up by chromaffin tissue, useful in isotopic imaging of pheochromocytoma and paraganglioma

### Management

- Phenoxybenzamine is an α-adrenergic receptor blocker and is prescribed before invasive imaging such as administration of IV contrast during CT scanning, to avoid hypertensive crises.
- Only administer β-blocking drugs after α blockers, to avoid exacerbating hypertension.
- α/β-adrenergic receptor-blocking drugs control hypertension and restore plasma volume by decreasing vascular resistance.

**12**

- Pre-treatment prevents profound hypotension that follows surgical tumour resection.
- Surgery is usually curative, normalizing hypertension. If unsuccessful, hypertension is controlled by α/β-adrenergic receptor blockade.
- Radiotherapy (external beam or using mIBG) is used for residual malignant tumours although the effect is generally disappointing.

### Prognosis

- 5-year survival >95% for non-malignant tumours
- Recurrence after surgery <10% and surgical cure of hypertension 75%

## DISEASES OF THE ADRENAL CORTEX

### CUSHING'S SYNDROME

The symptoms and signs of CD are caused by chronic inappropriate elevation of free circulating cortisol.
- The commonest cause of CS is iatrogenic.
- CD is commoner in females; ectopic CS is commoner in males.
- ACTH-dependent or ACTH-independent (adrenal tumours).
- CD is caused by an ACTH-secreting pituitary adenoma.
- Ectopic ACTH production is a feature of several carcinomas, especially small-cell lung carcinomas.

    See CUSHING'S SYNDROME: CLINICAL FEATURES, INVESTIGATION AND TREATMENT AT A GLANCE.

### Clinical features

Clinical features are summarized in **Figure 12.35**.

### Differential diagnosis

- Chronic alcoholism (alcoholic pseudo CS) must be ruled out. A careful alcohol intake history is mandatory; blood alcohol level is useful.
- A drug history can establish previous GC treatment.

### Investigation

#### Biochemical investigation of Cushing's syndrome

A screening test for CS is summarized in **Table 12.15**. When screening tests are positive, the patient undergoes more detailed endocrine investigation.

*Urinary cortisol* 24-hour urinary cortisol concentration, measured by radioimmunoassay, is raised in CS:
- *Men:* >259 nmol/24 hour
- *Women:* >409 nmol/24 hour
- False negative rate: 5–10%

*Overnight dexamethasone suppression test*
- Dexamethasone (1 mg) is given orally at bedtime and at 9 a.m. Plasma cortisol is sampled next morning.

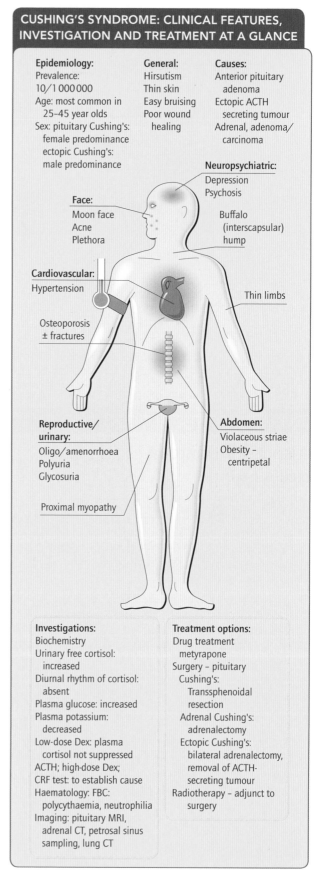

**CUSHING'S SYNDROME: CLINICAL FEATURES, INVESTIGATION AND TREATMENT AT A GLANCE**

**Epidemiology:**
Prevalence:
10/1 000 000
Age: most common in 25–45 year olds
Sex: pituitary Cushing's: female predominance ectopic Cushing's: male predominance

**General:**
Hirsutism
Thin skin
Easy bruising
Poor wound healing

**Causes:**
Anterior pituitary adenoma
Ectopic ACTH secreting tumour
Adrenal, adenoma/ carcinoma

**Neuropsychiatric:**
Depression
Psychosis

**Face:**
Moon face
Acne
Plethora

Buffalo (interscapular) hump

**Cardiovascular:**
Hypertension

Thin limbs

Osteoporosis ± fractures

**Reproductive/ urinary:**
Oligo/amenorrhoea
Polyuria
Glycosuria

Proximal myopathy

**Abdomen:**
Violaceous striae
Obesity – centripetal

**Investigations:**
Biochemistry
Urinary free cortisol: increased
Diurnal rhythm of cortisol: absent
Plasma glucose: increased
Plasma potassium: decreased
Low-dose Dex: plasma cortisol not suppressed
ACTH; high-dose Dex; CRF test: to establish cause
Haematology: FBC: polycythaemia, neutrophilia
Imaging: pituitary MRI, adrenal CT, petrosal sinus sampling, lung CT

**Treatment options:**
Drug treatment metyrapone
Surgery – pituitary Cushing's: Transsphenoidal resection
Adrenal Cushing's: adrenalectomy
Ectopic Cushing's: bilateral adrenalectomy, removal of ACTH-secreting tumour
Radiotherapy – adjunct to surgery

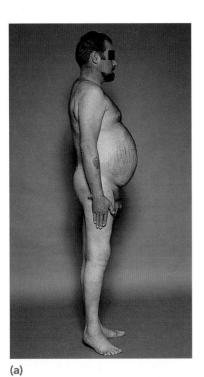

**(a)**

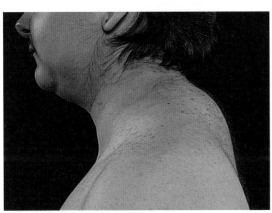

**(b)**

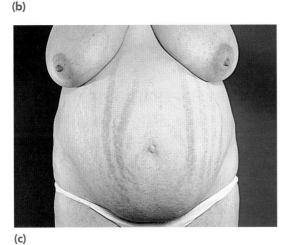

**(c)**

**Figure 12.35** **(a)** Profile of a patient with advanced Cushing's syndrome showing the centripetal fat distribution and the relatively thin arms and legs caused by myopathy. **(b)** Typical dorsocervical hump ('buffalo') in a patient with Cushing's disease. **(c)** Typical violaceous striae in a patient with Cushing's syndrome.

**Table 12.15** Screening test for Cushing's syndrome

1. 24-hour urinary free cortisol (UFC)
2. Overnight 1 mg dexamethasone suppression test (ONDST)

- Normally, plasma cortisol is suppressed (<50 nmol/L) but not in CS.
- False positives are possible in obesity/depression.
- CS is unlikely if both UFC and ONDST are normal.

*Low-dose dexamethasone suppression test (LDDST)*
- This is used to confirm the diagnosis.
- Dexamethasone 0.5 mg is given orally 6-hourly for 48 hours. If the plasma cortisol level is not suppressed to <50 nmol/L = CS.

*Plasma cortisol rhythmicity*
- In CS, there is a loss of normal cortisol rhythmicity. This test should not be performed immediately after hospital admission (affects cortisol rhythm).
- Plasma cortisol measured at 9 a.m./12 midnight with the patient asleep and pre-cannulated.

**Differential diagnosis**

What is the underlying cause?
- *Plasma ACTH:* This discriminates between ACTH-dependent and ACTH-independent aetiologies. Hypokalaemia <3.2 mmol/L occurs in almost 100% of patients with ectopic ACTH secretion but in <10% of patients with CD.
- *High-dose dexamethasone suppression test (HDDST):* This test differentiates CD from other causes of CS. Dexamethasone administered 2 mg 6-hourly for 48 hours suppresses plasma cortisol and urine metabolites by 50% in 90% of patients with CD.
- *IV corticotropin-releasing factor (CRF) (100 mcg):* In CD, CRF provokes exaggerated ACTH release – particularly helpful in equivocal cases of CD when combined with selective venous catheterization.
- *Selective bilateral inferior petrosal sinus ACTH sampling following IV CRF:* This confirms the central origin of ACTH, particularly when a lesion is not demonstrable by MRI.
- *Polycythaemia, neutrophilia and low eosinophil count:* These are all features of hypercortisolism. Glucose intolerance is common and diabetes mellitus results from insulin resistance secondary to glucocorticoid excess. Hypokalaemia results from the MC effect of GC.

**Management**

*Cushing's disease*
- *TSS with selective microadenomectomy* is the treatment of choice. Adjunctive pituitary radiotherapy may be given if surgery is unsuccessful. It may take years to be effective if used without surgery.

**12**

501

- *Bilateral adrenalectomy* is used when other treatments fail. It cures hypercortisolism at the expense of lifelong adrenal replacement therapy. Adrenal surgery has significant morbidity/mortality, reduced by preoperative metyrapone or ketoconazole treatment to reduce plasma cortisol levels enabling correction of metabolic and other features of CS.
- If CD is treated with bilateral adrenalectomy alone, there is a risk of Nelson's syndrome (increasing plasma ACTH levels, pigmentation, enlarging aggressive pituitary tumour growth secondary to loss of negative feedback inhibition from high plasma cortisol). Pituitary irradiation is given after bilateral adrenalectomy for CD, to prevent Nelson's syndrome.
- Metyrapone and ketoconazole are useful oral therapeutic options, especially with uncertainty whether CS results from CD or ectopic ACTH production. Drug dosage is titrated against plasma and urinary cortisol concentrations.

### Ectopic ACTH production

- Ectopic ACTH production caused by rapidly growing bronchial carcinoma may precipitate catabolic state, with pigmention and accelerated weight loss.
- Treatment is often palliative. Hypercortisolaemia is controlled with metyrapone/ketoconazole.
- Resection of benign tumours, though curative, may result in prolonged secondary hypoadrenalism.

### Adrenal adenoma and carcinoma

- Operative removal follows appropriate pre-treatment with metyrapone/ketoconazole. If carcinoma is suspected, pre-treatment is restricted to no longer than 2 weeks.
- Radiotherapy is given postoperatively for malignant tumours. Disseminated adrenal carcinoma is generally unresponsive to cytotoxic therapy, but may respond to adrenolytic drug o'p'-DDD (mitotane).

### Iatrogenic Cushing's syndrome

Where possible, steroid dosage should be reduced and steroid-sparing agents substituted.

### Prognosis

- *Untreated CS:* 5-year 50% mortality, often from cardiovascular disease, thromboembolism or bacterial infection
- *CD:* associated with increased morbidity and mortality; normal pituitary function often sacrificed to secure cure

## PRIMARY HYPERALDOSTERONISM (CONN'S SYNDROME)

- Solitary adrenal adenoma (85%) and bilateral hyperplasia of adrenal glomerulosa cells (15%)
- Hyperaldosteronism causes hypertension, sodium/water retention, potassium loss, alkalosis

- Peak incidence 30–50 years, commoner in females
- Rare glucocorticoid-responsive hyperaldosteronism autosomal dominantly inherited
- Hypokalaemia causes muscle weakness, metabolic alkalosis, tetany, polyuria/polydipsia (NDI); malignant hypertension rare
- Similar electrolyte abnormalities caused by thiazide diuretics
- Plasma aldosterone raised; renin suppressed
- Aldosterone unsuppressed by 4-hour 300 mmol saline infusion, indicating autonomous aldosterone production
- Adenoma and hyperplasia distinguished by different circadian patterns of aldosterone concentrations:
  - Adenoma: aldosterone falls throughout the morning, parallelling cortisol circadian rhythm
  - Hyperplasia: no aldosterone rhythmicity
- High-resolution CT scanning with 2–3 mm cuts shows adenomas as small as 0.5 cm, though lesions sometimes too small to detect; most adenomas <2 cm in diameter
- Selective adrenal venous blood sampling distinguishes unilateral from bilateral disease; simultaneous measurement of cortisol and aldosterone are undertaken to confirm adrenal venous cannulation.

### Management

- Laparoscopic surgery recommended for adenoma and usually cures hypertension; potassium stores replaced before surgery by pre-treatment with specific aldosterone antagonists (spironolactone or eplerinone ± potassium supplementation)
- Bilateral adrenal hyperplasia treated medically with spironolactone, amiloride, triamterene or eplerenone:
  - Spironolactone: decreased libido, gynaecomastia in men
  - Other antihypertensive agents added to control hypertension
- Long-term BP cure rates following surgery 75%

## SECONDARY HYPERALDOSTERONISM

- Activation of RAS results in high aldosterone levels.
- Causes are renal artery stenosis, decompensated liver disease, accelerated hypertension, cardiac failure and nephrotic syndrome.

## ADRENOCORTICAL FAILURE

- In AD there is failure of the adrenal cortex to produce glucocorticoid/MC hormones.
- *Primary adrenocortical failure:* Adrenal gland pathology or rare congenital conditions result from enzyme deficiencies involved in biosynthetic pathway (e.g. congenital adrenal hyperplasia [CAH]).

- *Secondary adrenocortical failure:* Reduced ACTH production may be secondary to hypothalamo-pituitary disease or chronic corticosteroid therapy withdrawal.

## PRIMARY ADRENAL FAILURE

- Autoimmune adrenocortical destruction accounts for 75% in Western countries.
- Tuberculosis accounts for 20% of cases and rare destructive processes (fungal, lymphoma, infarction) for 5%.
- Untreated HIV can cause opportunistic adrenal infection.
- 70% of patients with autoimmune AD have 21-hydroxylase antibodies.
- *Waterhouse–Friderichsen syndrome* is caused by haemorrhagic adrenal destruction associated with meningococcal infection.
- MC deficiency causes sodium loss, hyperkalaemia or acidosis, and extracellular volume loss.
- The disease is commoner in women.
- There is frequently a family history of AD or other autoimmune disorder.

### Clinical features

- Presentation may be precipitated by infection, trauma or surgery, leading to acute hypoadrenalism (Addisonian crisis), which is a medical emergency.
- Clinical features include nausea, vomiting, pigmentation (**Figure 12.36**), apathy, confusion, profound weakness, hypotension/hypovolaemic shock. AD may be a component of polyendocrine syndrome Type 1 (mutations of the *AIRE* gene).

### Biochemical investigation of adrenal insufficiency

- Serum 9 a.m. cortisol often within reference range, inappropriate for degree of stress
- Simultaneous ACTH, renin elevated

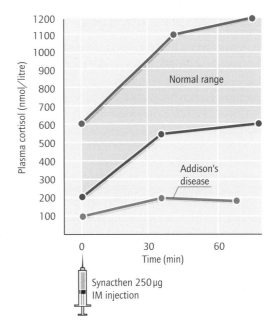

**Figure 12.37** Cortisol response to IM synacthen in health and in a patient with primary adrenal insufficiency.

- Normochromic normocytic anaemia, lymphocytosis and eosinophilia
- Hyperkalaemia, hyponatraemia, low bicarbonate, secondary to MC deficiency, raised urea, creatinine, hypoglycaemia
- Aldosterone low; plasma renin raised
- 21-hydroxylase antibody demonstrable in autoimmune adrenalitis
- *Short synacthen test:*
  - 250 µg synthetic ACTH (1–24: synacthen) injected IM, with plasma cortisol measured at 0, 30 and 60 min following injection
  - Normally, plasma cortisol rises >550 nmol/L (**Figure 12.37**)
- A long (1 mg) depot synacthen test performed if impaired cortisol response in the short test
- In AD, no additional cortisol rise; a poor initial cortisol response followed by progressive rise suggests secondary adrenal failure
- Blood culture and occasionally adrenal biopsy can provide evidence of infection (TB, or fungal infection such as histoplasmosis)
- Adrenal CT useful if non-autoimmune destructive process considered (tuberculous adrenalitis, histoplasmosis, adrenal infarction/haemorrhage)

### Management

#### Addisonian crisis

The acutely ill patient with Addisonian crisis needs immediate treatment (see EMERGENCY PRESENTATION 12.2).

#### Less severe Addison's disease

- Treated with hydrocortisone 10 mg on waking, 5 mg midday, and 5 mg late in the afternoon

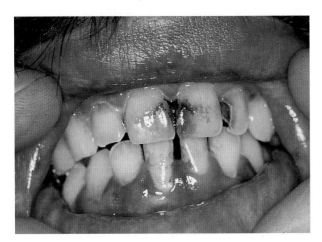

**Figure 12.36** Lip and gingival pigmentation in patient with untreated AD.

**12**

**Addisonian crisis and its management**

Blood is taken to measure plasma cortisol U&E.

Hydrocortisone 100 mg IV is given 6-hourly for 24–48 hours.

Normal saline is given 2–6 litres IV in 12–24 hours.

When stable, convert to maintenance hydrocortisone and fludrocortisone orally.

Seek evidence of precipitating cause and treat accordingly.

Lifelong replacement therapy is required.

- 9-alpha fludrocortisone (MC) 100–200 mcg
- Adrenal insufficiency following withdrawal of chronic corticosteroid treatment avoidable by gradually tapering steroid dosage over weeks
- AD requires lifelong replacement therapy; never stopped; patient given adequate supply of treatment at all times, advised to increase replacement dose during intercurrent stress, mimicking the body's normal response to stress
- Steroid card carried, giving details of medication or medical attendant, and patient encouraged to wear medical identification Medic Alert bracelet/necklace
- *For minor procedures performed under local anaesthetic:* 100 mg of IM hydrocortisone suffices
- *For operative procedures involving general anaesthesia:* 100 mg of hydrocortisone given IM or IV with pre-medication and repeated 6-hourly as required until oral medication resumed

## DISORDERS OF FEMALE REPRODUCTIVE ENDOCRINOLOGY

The endocrine disorders that involve the ovary (**Table 12.16**) are:

- Hypogonadism
- Hyperandrogenism
- Disorders of sexual differentiation

**Table 12.16** Causes of female disorders of reproductive endocrinology

**Hypogonadotrophic hypogonadism**
Hypothalamic and pituitary diseases
Hyperprolactinaemia
Low body weight
Idiopathic

**Hypogonadism with increased gonadotrophins**
Gonadal dysgenesis including TS
POF (autoimmune, idiopathic, iatrogenic)

**Hyperandrogenism**
Polycystic ovary syndrome
CAH
Adrenal and ovarian tumours
Syndromes of extreme insulin resistance

Any of these disorders may present with menstrual disturbance or anovulation.

## FEMALE HYPOGONADOTROPHIC HYPOGONADISM

- Hypothalamic and pituitary diseases (*vide supra*) include hyperprolactinaemia.
- *Weight-related (hypothalamic) amenorrhoea:* Low body weight is frequently not as severe as in anorexia nervosa. The menstrual cycle may not restart for several months after regaining premorbid weight.
- *Stress and exercise-related amenorrhoea:* This is frequently mediated through weight loss. Swimmers commonly maintain fat for buoyancy and thus menstruate, whereas runners have low body fat and are more prone to amenorrhoea.
- *Hypothalamic amenorrhoea:* Sometimes this has no obvious cause.
- Findings include FSH>LH, low serum oestradiol, and absence of gonadotrophin pulsatility.
- Imaging excludes structural lesions.

### Treatment

- Sex steroid replacement
- Treatment for infertility
- With an intact uterus: oestrogen with serial progestagen – avoids endometrial hyperplasia and risk of uterine carcinoma
- Low oestradiol: osteoporosis
- Anovulation responsive to oral anti-oestrogen clomiphene, parenteral therapy with gonadotrophins or pulsatile SC GnRH administered by syringe pump
- Ovulation induction monitored by pelvic US, reducing hyperstimulation and the risk of multiple pregnancies

## FEMALE HYPOGONADISM WITH INCREASED GONADOTROPHINS

### Gonadal dysgenesis

- Mosaicism in TS: A proportion of cells have normal 46,XX karyotype, leading to variable expression of the Turner phenotype.
- 46,XO cell lines result from early mitotic non-dysfunction, causing 'streaks' ovaries. The clinical picture is of premature ovarian failure (POF).
- Germ cell numbers in the second trimester of gestation are initially normal. By birth, oocyte depletion has occurred, resulting in primary gonadal failure and primary (and rarely, secondary) amenorrhoea.
- This occurs in 1 : 2000 live births.
- Features include female phenotype, short stature, sexual infantilism, webbed neck, fish-like mouth,

epicanthic folds, cubitus valgus, aortic coarctation, horseshoe kidney and neonatal lymphoedema.
- LH/FSH levels are raised; oestradiol is low.
- *Treatment:* Hormone replacement therapy (HRT) is started with low-dose ethinyloestradiol (10 µg/day) to minimize side effects and ensure adequate breast development. GH treatment for short stature in TS adds 5–10 cm to the patient's final height.

### Premature ovarian failure

- POF is early ovarian function failure resulting from oocyte depletion.
- Ovarian antibodies are occasionally detectable. POF may coexist with endocrine autoimmunity (e.g. AD, hypothyroidism, pernicious anaemia).
- Patients previously treated for leukaemia and lymphoma develop POF secondary to chemotherapy and radiotherapy.
- POF affects 1% of females, defined as menopause occurring <40 years of age. Familial forms are rare.
- Patients present with primary or (more commonly) secondary amenorrhoea and oestrogen deficiency (flushing, dyspareunia).
- Oestradiol is low; LH/FSH levels are elevated.
- US reveals small ovaries.
- *Treatment:*
  - *Hormone treatment:* simple, but patients may require several consultations before understanding the full implications for fertility
  - *Ovum donation:* donor egg + partner's sperm
- Remission is rarely reported.

## FEMALE HYPERANDROGENISM

### Polycystic ovary syndrome

- Ovarian > adrenal hyperandrogenism
- Unknown aetiology, with several pathological mechanisms, often obesity-related
- Post-pubertal onset, 20–30 years of age, occasionally familial
- Clinical features: hirsuties, seborrhoea, acne (**Figure 12.38**), androgenetic alopecia, obesity, oligomenorrhoea, anovulatory infertility (see Rotterdam criteria below)
- Elevated LH/testosterone in 40%
- US reveals high prevalence of polycystic ovary in women with idiopathic hirsuties; such women considered to have mild polycystic ovary syndrome (PCOS)
- Typical ultrasonic findings: see **Figure 12.39**
- Differentiate from CAH, ovarian and adrenal tumours
- Testosterone >4 nmol/L indicates severe hirsutism; short history suggests underlying androgen-secreting tumour

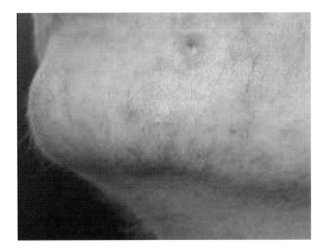

**Figure 12.38** Patient with PCOS with acne, seborrhoea and hirsutism secondary to hyperandrogenism.

### Diagnosis

*Rotterdam criteria* for diagnosis of PCOS (based on two of three criteria):

1. Hyperandrogenism - either clinically by skin manifestations of androgen excess *or* hyperandrogenism (raised testosterone in a blood test)
2. Ovulatory dysfunction (i.e. oligo/anovulation)
3. Polycystic ovaries on US

*and* exclusion of phenotypically similar androgen-excess disorders such as:
- CAH
- Androgen secreting tumours
- CS
- Thyroid dysfunction
- Hyperprolactinaemia

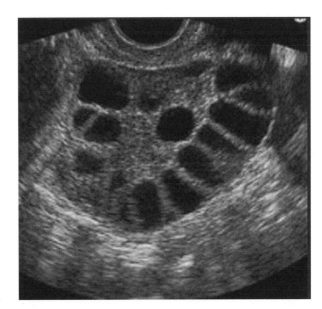

**Figure 12.39** Typical transvaginal appearance of a polycystic ovary, showing multiple immature follicles 5–8 mm in diameter in the periphery of the ovary. The ovarian stroma is relatively dense.

**12**

## Management

- Hirsutism: OCP and antiandrogen (cyproterone acetate or spironolactone) therapy
- Menstrual disturbance: combined OCP
- Anovulation: oral clomiphene citrate/parenteral gonadotrophin treatment
- Metformin/thiazolidinediones induce normal ovulatory cycles and amelioration of clinical picture; metformin reduces insulin/testosterone levels improving fertility prospects in obese PCOS
- Dietary modification and/or regular exercise programme
- Symptomatology varies throughout life, but rarely remits
- 80% of patients with anovulatory infertility respond to ovulation induction

### Congenital adrenal hyperplasia

- CAH is most commonly caused by 21-hydroxylase deficiency (converts 17-α hydroxyprogesterone (17αOHP) to 11-deoxycortisol) in cortisol biosynthesis (see **Figure 12.3**).
- Low cortisol increases ACTH stimulation of the adrenals.
- Build-up of 17-α hydroxy precursors proximal to enzyme block are diverted to androgen production.
- 10% suffer from 11-β hydroxylase or 3-β hydroxysteroid dehydrogenase deficiency.
- Prevalence is 1 in 1000 live births, and presentation is neonatal.
- Inheritance is autosomal recessive.
- Eskimos and Ashkenazi Jews have increased prevalence.

## Clinical features

- Neonatally: ambiguous genitalia/salt-losing crisis
- Females: normal internal genitalia; external virilization variable, depending on severity of enzyme block, varying from penile urethra to, more usually, clitoromegaly
- Late-onset variant results in hirsutism diagnosed as late as fifth decade

## Investigation and management

- 17-αOHP measurements before and 30 min after IV 250 μg synacthen
- 17-αOHP levels: >20 nmol/L in mild forms; >100 nmol/L in severe forms
- Adrenal replacement therapy as in AD

### Adrenal and ovarian tumours

- Adrenal adenomas/carcinomas produce variable quantities of androgens and other steroids.
    - Oestrogen (granulosa – theca cell tumours)
    - Androgens (dysgerminomas, lipoid cell tumours, gonadoblastoma)

- *Clinical features:* depend on relative amounts of androgen, glucocorticoids and MCs secreted
- *Investigation:* sex steroid measurements, CT adrenals and pelvic US required
- *Treatment:* surgery treatment of choice after lesion localization
- *Prognosis:* depends on pathology

### Androgen insensitivity syndrome

- *Androgen insensitivity syndrome (AIS):* 46,XY karyotype: external female phenotype, variable virilization caused by androgen resistance, resulting from mutated androgen receptor
- X- linked recessive
- Prevalence 1 in 50 000 males, usually with neonatal presentation
- *Complete AIS:*
    - 'Testicular feminization' (female phenotype, primary amenorrhoea and absence of secondary sexual hair)
    - Antimüllerian hormone function normal, inguinal testes, absent uterus and Fallopian tubes
- *Partial forms of AIS:* spectrum ranging from phenotypic females to poor virilization with oligospermia (Reifenstein's syndrome)
- Testosterone, LH raised
- Orchidectomy: increased neoplasia risk
- Oestrogen replacement therapy required

## DISORDERS OF MALE REPRODUCTIVE ENDOCRINOLOGY

The male reproductive system may be affected by disease in any part of the H-P testicular axis (**Table 12.17**).

**Table 12.17** Causes of male hypogonadism

**Hypogonadotrophic hypogonadism**
- Hypothalamic and pituitary disease
- IGD
- Kallmann syndrome
- Hyperprolactinaemia
- Haemochromatosis

**Hypogonadism with increased gonadotrophin secretion (testicular failure)**
- Congenital causes
- Testicular agenesis
- Cryptorchidism
- Klinefelter syndrome
- Androgen resistance
- 5α-reductase deficiency

**Acquired causes**
- Testicular trauma or torsion
- Orchitis (mumps, coxsackie viruses)
- Iatrogenic (cytotoxicity irradiation)

# MALE HYPOGONADOTROPHIC HYPOGONADISM

- Hypogonadism is secondary to hypothalamic (GnRH deficiency) or pituitary disease.
- Isolated gonadotrophin deficiency (IGD) is commoner in males and often genetic.
- Kallmann syndrome = IGD + anosmia (**Figure 12.40**).
- Haemochromatosis (autosomal recessive) damages gonadotrophs, affecting both sexes equally.
- Clinical manifestations of hypogonadism occur earlier in men, who lack the protective beneficial effect of menstruation on iron stores.
- Clinical features depend on age of onset of androgen deficiency.
- Hypospadias, microphallus and cryptorchidism occur *in utero*.
- In adults, there is scant body and facial hair, decreased libido and impaired sexual function.
- Prepubertal androgen deficiency leads to late epiphyseal closure of epiphyses, eunuchoidism (arm span > height; heel to pubis length > pubes to crown).
- Full pituitary function tests are required to test other endocrine axes.
- Serum testosterone and LH/FSH are low.

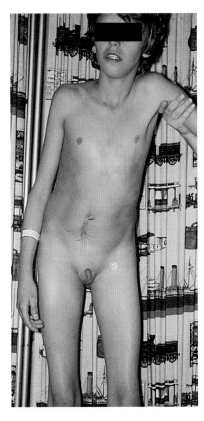

**Figure 12.40** 14-year-old male with hypogonadotrophic hypogonadism, showing infantile genital proportions.

## Management

- Testosterone replacement therapy (TRT) prevents osteoporosis and maintains secondary sexual characteristics.
- Parenteral gonadotrophins (hCG 2000 U twice weekly + FSH 150 U thrice weekly SC) are given for spermatogenesis induction. Pulsative GnRH is an alternative.
- TRT parenterally: 3-weekly (sustanon 250 mg IM) or 3 monthly (nebido 1 gm IM) or transdermal route (e.g. 'Tostran' 2% 50 mg daily).

# HYPOGONADISM WITH INCREASED GONADOTROPHINS (TESTICULAR FAILURE)

## Testicular agenesis

- Impaired testicular function: spectrum ranging from female phenotype if failure occurs before 8 weeks' gestation (46,XY gonadal agenesis), to male phenotype with absent testes if regression occurs after critical phase of male differentiation (13–14 weeks' gestation)
- Prepubertal presentation with a variable phenotype
- *Investigation:* karyotype, pelvic US
- *Management:* TRT

## Cryptorchidism

- Incomplete or maldescent of testes
- Cause unknown
- Testosterone production often reduced; spermatogenesis defective
- Incidence 3% at birth and <1% at 6 months thereafter
- Presents neonatally or prepubertally
- With testicular damage, testosterone low, LH/FSH elevated
- TRT may be indicated
- Orchidopexy performed before aged 2 but does not remove increased malignancy risk
- 10% testicular tumours associated with undescended testes

## Klinefelter syndrome

- 47,XXY karyotype caused by aberrant meiosis in either parent
- Sporadic incidence, associated with advanced maternal age
- 1 in 500–600 males, post-pubertal presentation
- Seminiferous tubule dysgenesis: small testes or azoospermia
- Testosterone deficiency: small phallus, reduced body hair, gynaecomastia, eunuchoidism, osteopenia
- Milder phenotypes recognized (usually mosaic forms XY/XXY); testicular sperm extraction sometimes possible
- Serum testosterone low, LH/FSH raised
- TRT indicated for hypogonadism

**12**

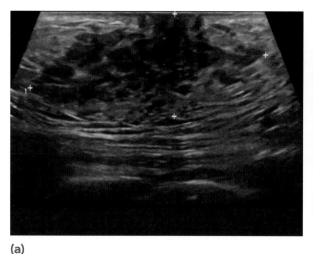

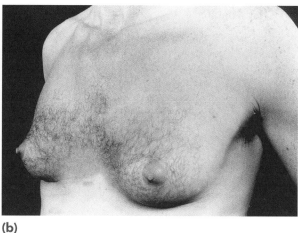

**(a)** **(b)**

**Figure 12.41** **(a)** Gynaecomastia, with typical ultrasonic appearance of glandular tissue **(b)** in a male.

### Acquired testicular diseases

- Causes: infections (mumps, coxsackie, echovirus), radiation, drugs (e.g. cyclophosphamide), renal failure
- Testosterone low, LH/FSH elevated
- TRT indicated

### Gynaecomastia

- Enlargement of male breast tissue (**Figure 12.41**)
- Causes are summarized in **Table 12.18**
- Physiological (newborn, puberty, elderly), or secondary to excess oestrogen or deficiency of androgens, or drugs
- Rarely caused by male breast cancer
- Common condition, occurring 15–70 years of age
- Asymmetry common

**Table 12.18** Causes of gynaecomastia

**Oestrogen excess**
Testicular (Leydig cell) tumour
Increased peripheral production:
- Adrenal tumour
- CAH
- Liver disease
- Starvation
- Hyperthyroidism

**Testosterone deficiency**
Anorchia
Klinefelter syndrome
Androgen resistance
Acquired testicular failure

**Drugs**
Oestrogen derivatives
Digoxin
Spironolactone
Cimetidine
Cannabis

- Testicular examination mandatory to locate a possible source of oestrogen, such as tumour or presence of testicular atrophy
- Gonadotrophins, testosterone, oestradiol, thyroid function tests measured. Testicular US, for occult testicular tumours
- Primary cause identifiable in 50%
- Idiopathic gynaecomastia: tamoxifen, an anti-oestrogen, has variable effects
- Anti-oestrogen therapy ineffective if breast enlargement >2 years (organization of breast tissue or mastectomy needed)

## DISEASE OF MULTIPLE ENDOCRINE ORGANS

## MULTIPLE ENDOCRINE NEOPLASIA SYNDROMES

- Multiple endocrine neoplasia syndromes (MEN): autosomal dominant conditions
- Predisposition to simultaneous/metachronous cancers in two or more endocrine organs
- Two principal forms MEN 1 and MEN 2 (**Figure 12.42**).

### MEN 1

- Caused by *MENIN 1* mutation (chromosome 11)
- Manifestations differ between family members
- Prevalence 2–3 in 100 000; onset variable; sexes equally affected
- Benign parathyroid/pituitary tumours, but pancreatic tumours may undergo malignant change at later age
- Hypercalcaemia (hyperparathyroidism invariant) hypoglycaemia (insulinoma), peptic ulceration (gastrinoma), pituitary tumours (GH/prolactin)
- Genotyping (+ family members): early detection reduces morbidity/mortality

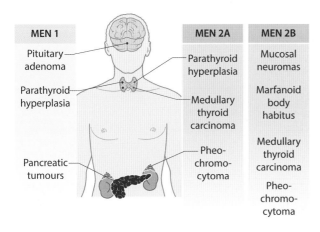

**MEN 1**

Pituitary adenoma

Parathyroid hyperplasia

Pancreatic tumours

**MEN 2A**

Parathyroid hyperplasia

Medullary thyroid carcinoma

Pheo-chromo-cytoma

**MEN 2B**

Mucosal neuromas

Marfanoid body habitus

Medullary thyroid carcinoma

Pheo-chromo-cytoma

**Figure 12.42** The MEN syndromes.

- Screening tests: serum calcium/PTH levels, fasting gut hormones, prolactin, pituitary MRI, pancreatic CT
- Surgery: parathyroid and pancreatic tumours
- Medical treatment: gastrinoma (PPI; somatostatin analogues) and prolactinoma (dopamine agonist)

**MEN 2**

- *RET* proto-oncogene mutation
- Prevalence 2.5 in 10 000
- Variable age of onset

- MCT commonest MEN 2 tumour, occurring in almost all cases >40 years, followed by pheochromocytoma/parathyroid hyperplasia
- Thyroid parafollicular C cells produce calcitonin, acting as tumour marker; serum calcium levels normal
- MEN 2 subdivided into MEN 2A and MEN 2B
- In MEN 2B, mucosal ganglioneuromas, Marfanoid features, visible corneal nerves (slit lamp)
- Familial MCT: MCT sole abnormality
- Early genetic screening of family members for *RET* gene mutations detects carriers before symptom onset
- Biochemical screening: serum calcitonin, calcium, PTH, urinary metanephrines
- Prophylactic thyroidectomy: in carriers, ideally <6 years, eliminating MCT risk
- Adrenalectomy: pheochromocytoma

## AUTOIMMUNE POLYGLANDULAR SYNDROMES

- Autoimmune polyglandular syndromes (APS): defects in cellular or antibody-mediated immunity
- Antibodies against normal cell components are markers of underlying immunological disorder
- Characteristic lymphocytic infiltrate followed by fibrosis of affected organs
- Around 20% of cases familial; disease associations with HLA-B8, HLA-DR3, and HLA-DR4 genotypes
- Features of key syndromes listed in **Table 12.19**

**Table 12.19** Features of APSs

| | Percentage affected (%) | Antibody | Treatment |
|---|---|---|---|
| **Autoimmune polyglandular syndrome 1 (APS1)** | | | |
| Hypoparathyroidism | 90 | Parathyroid | Calcium and 1 alfacalcidol |
| Candidiasis | 70 | | Antifungal agents (e.g. fluconazole) |
| Addison's disease | 60 | 21-hydroxylase | Hydrocortisone + fludrocortisone |
| Ovarian/testicular | 40 | Steroid cell antibodies | HRT |
| Thyroid | 10 | TPO/thyroglobulin | Thyroxine |
| Pituitary | 1 | | |
| Pancreatic islet cells | | GADA, IA-2A, IAA, ZnT8, ICA | Insulin |
| Coeliac disease | | Endomysial, tissue transglutaminase | Gluten-free diet |
| Alopecia | | Tyrosine hydroxylase | – |
| Gastric parietal cells | | Gastric parietal cell | Parenteral vitamin $B_{12}$ |
| Liver | | LKM | Glucocorticoids ± azathioprine |
| Melanocytes | | Complement fixing melanocyte antibodies | |
| **Autoimmune polyglandular syndrome 2 (APS2)** | | | |
| Addison's disease | 95 | 21-hydroxylase | Hydrocortisone and fludrocortisone |
| Hypothyroidism | 70 | Thyroglobulin, TPO | L-thyroxine |
| Type 1 diabetes | 50 | GADA | Insulin |
| Gonadal failure | 20 | Steroid cell | HRT |
| Gastric parietal cells | | Gastric parietal cell, intrinsic factor | Parenteral vitamin $B_{12}$ |
| Myasthenia gravis | | Acetyl choline receptor | Cholinesterase inhibitors |
| Rheumatoid arthritis | | Anti-CCP | |
| Vitiligo | | Melanocyte | |

- Prevalence 5–10 in 10 000
- APS 1 autosomal recessive

- Age of onset and chronology variable
- More common in females

## MUST-KNOW CHECKLIST

- How to manage patients on steroid replacement therapy
- How to diagnose steroid deficiency and interpret short synacthen tests
- How to diagnose and manage an Addisonian crisis
- How to diagnose and manage a hyperthyroid crisis
- How to diagnose and manage myxoedema coma
- Endocrine causes of hypertension
- Endocrine causes of impaired glucose tolerance
- Diagnosis of diabetes insipidus
- Diagnosis of SIADH

**Questions and answers** to test your understanding of Chapter 12 can be found by clicking 'Support Material' at the following link:
https://www.routledge.com/Medicine-for-Finals-and-Beyond/Axford-OCallaghan/p/book/9780367150594

# 13

# Neurological Disease

## MALCOLM MACLEOD

## INTRODUCTION

### NEUROLOGICAL PROBLEMS

About 5 million people will have a stroke in the coming year. Other common neurological disorders such as headache, functional neurological disorders and epilepsy affect many tens of millions of patients throughout the world. About 20% of emergency hospital admissions are primarily neurological, and so all doctors need basic competence in neurological diagnosis.

The impact of neurological disease can leave patients and their doctors desperate for a cure; with the advent of treatments which may alter the course of disease, neurologists also need to have skills in robust critical appraisal of claims of therapeutic effect. Even when cure is not possible, symptomatic treatments can make a significant impact. Active focused neurological rehabilitation can achieve a great deal to restore a patient's dignity, independence and quality of life.

### UNDERSTANDING THE CAUSES

Advances in imaging, neurophysiology, genetics, molecular biology and pharmacology are rapidly increasing our understanding of the causes and pathophysiology of many neurological problems. It is hoped that this will lead to faster and more accurate diagnosis and to rational drug design.

### SOCIAL AND ECONOMIC FACTORS AND NEUROLOGICAL DISEASE

Many neurological conditions, including migraine and epilepsy, impact on economic status, with profound impact on affected individuals and their families. Equally, social factors such as unemployment and poverty impact not only on the incidence of neurological conditions such as epilepsy and stroke but also on its severity and on access to health care.

### DIAGNOSIS OF NEUROLOGICAL DISORDERS

The nervous system is the most functionally complex of all the organ systems. While neurological disorders can therefore produce a wide range of symptoms and signs, the basic clinical skills of careful history-taking and logical thought, coupled with a little knowledge of anatomy and pathology, are all that is required.

DOI: 10.1201/9781003193616-13

## HISTORY AND EXAMINATION

The history is the bedrock of diagnosis in neurology. Meaningful examination and effective investigation is only possible with a well-executed history (see HISTORY & EXAMINATION 13.1). For most problems, the examination contributes little to diagnosis; if the patient cannot give a history – because of language problems or cognitive difficulties or because they were unconscious at the time of an important event – obtain a history from someone who can tell you what has happened.

The patient should be encouraged to tell their own story without too many interruptions. Direct questioning may interrupt the patient's train of thought and may draw them away from the central problem (see HISTORY 13.2). Difficulties in conducting in-person assessments during the COVID-19 pandemic led to a substantial increase in the effective use of teleneurology for diagnosis and management, and many patients may prefer this approach in the future.

### HISTORY & EXAMINATION 13.1

**Purpose of clinical assessment**

To identify the symptoms and their impact
To identify the site(s) of the lesion(s)
To establish the likely pathology of the lesion(s)
To plan appropriate investigations
To initiate appropriate treatment(s)
To avoid unnecessary investigations and treatments
To gauge the patient's understanding of his or her symptoms
To understand the patient's expectations

**The four basic questions to answer**

1  Are the symptoms coming from the nervous system?
2  If so, which part(s) of the nervous system is/are affected?
3  Is the problem localized to one part of the nervous system or is it generalized?
4  Is there one lesion or are there multiple lesions?

### HISTORY 13.2

**Diagnosis in neurology**

Record the history in the patient's own words. The history is their account of their symptoms, not your interpretation of it. Give them time to use their own words, their own descriptions. Often, they will find it difficult to put into words what their symptoms feel like, so try to establish what they mean by the words they use.

Ask about how the symptoms started and how they have developed.

Ask whether there have been any previous episodes and their nature.

Find out what the impact of the illness on the patient has been – e.g. on their independence in activities of daily living.

Where there is any question that the patient's consciousness has been impaired, obtain a first-hand eyewitness account. Where no such witness is available, a telephone call to a relative or to the family doctor can provide high-quality diagnostic information.

## ABOUT THE PATIENT

The patient's age and sex can help decide which diagnoses are likely.

- *Cerebrovascular disease:* This is rare in those under 40 years old.
- *Symptoms of multiple sclerosis (MS):* These usually start between the ages of 20 and 35 years. MS is extremely rare in childhood, and development of MS in those over 60 is unusual. It is twice as common in women as in men, and is rare in non-White populations.
- *Genetic diseases:* Some (e.g. Duchenne muscular dystrophy) are sex-linked and may only affect or be much more severe in males.

## NEUROLOGICAL SYMPTOMS

### Blackouts: fits or faints or 'funny turns'?

The distinction between epilepsy and syncope can usually be made from the history, provided that a first-hand eyewitness account is also available.

- *Was the patient standing, sitting or lying* when the blackout occurred? Simple syncope is unusual in the sitting or lying position.
- *Tongue biting* (specifically the side of the tongue) suggests epilepsy rather than syncope.
- *Speed of recovery:* Rapid recovery suggest syncope rather than epilepsy.

### Headaches

Duration of symptoms is important; headache that has lasted for years rarely have a serious underlying cause; those of shorter duration, particularly when progressive and when associated with other symptoms, are more worrying. The character, location and associated symptoms may suggest the diagnosis, although most headaches have a benign cause. Meningeal irritation (neck stiffness, photophobia and vomiting) can occur with migraine, subarachnoid haemorrhage (SAH) or meningitis; raised intracranial pressure may cause a headache worse in the mornings and while lying flat, which is exacerbated by coughing or sneezing. Scalp tenderness raises a suspicion of temporal arteritis.

### Problems with memory and concentration

Loss of concentration and poor memory are common and usually of no significance. However, association with personality change suggests a frontal tumour, while association with disturbed sleep, anhedonia and low mood suggests depression.

### Difficulty with language, speech and swallowing

Difficulty in articulating words (*dysarthria*) is distinct from difficulties in language processing (*dysphasia*), which may affect the generation of language (*expressive dysphasia*), the understanding of spoken words (*receptive dysphasia*), or both.

Difficulty in swallowing (*dysphagia*) or dysarthria that increase with prolonged effort may be caused by myasthenia gravis. Dysphagia with nasal regurgitation of fluids may be caused by motor neurone disease (MND).

## Blindness, blurred and double vision

Transient monocular visual loss (*amaurosis fugax*) is usually caused by micro emboli in the retinal circulation, and persistent central retinal artery occlusion may cause permanent monocular visual loss. Similar symptoms can be caused by temporal arteritis, where complete and irreversible loss of vision can occur if steroid treatment is not started urgently. Ocular causes of transient visual loss include acute glaucoma and retinal detachment.

When unilateral visual loss is gradual and no cause is immediately apparent, optic nerve compression (e.g. tumour, ophthalmic artery aneurysm) must be assumed until proven otherwise. Other causes of gradual onset monocular blindness include optic neuritis and granulomatous diseases (e.g. sarcoidosis).

Simultaneous complete bilateral visual loss is uncommon, and when it occurs is usually due to reduced cerebral perfusion. Patients may find it difficult to distinguish homonymous hemianopia from monocular blindness, so it is worth taking time to explore what they mean.

Double vision (*diplopia*) may result from lesions of the IIIrd, IVth or VIth cranial nerves, the midbrain or the pons. Alternatively, local pathology in the orbit may interfere with the function of the extraocular muscles. Diplopia is generally abolished by covering one eye; when it persists with one eye closed (monocular diplopia), this may be a result of abnormalities of the cornea, iris, lens or retina. Diplopia may also be caused by myaesthenia gravis, when it is often worse at the end of the day.

## Difficulty with hearing/tinnitus

Hearing loss is part of normal ageing, but progressive unilateral hearing loss suggests a lesion of the vestibulocochlear (VIIIth) cranial nerve such as an acoustic neuroma; and hearing loss with facial weakness and double vision suggest a space-occupying lesion in the cerebellopontine angle, with involvement of the Vth, VIIth and VIIIth cranial nerves.

Ringing in the ear (*tinnitus*), deafness and paroxysms of disabling vertigo suggests Meniere's disease.

## Dizziness and vertigo

Dizziness is one of the most commonly reported neurological symptoms and may refer to the hallucination of movement (vertigo), to light-headedness or to unsteadiness. *Vertigo* is usually caused by disease of the inner ear or brainstem and may be associated with nausea or vomiting. Other dizziness may be due to postural hypotension, functional neurological unsteadiness, anaemia, anxiety, depression or hyperventilation. Patients may report 'poor balance' or 'walking as if drunk' or 'dizziness' because of disease of the inner ear, the vestibulocochlear (VIIIth) nerve, the brainstem, the cerebellum and its connections or of proprioception.

## Difficulties moving the arms or legs

### Weakness

Weakness can be caused by a problem anywhere from the cerebral cortex to the affected muscle. A weak hand may result from a focal lesion of the contralateral cerebral hemisphere, nerve root entrapment in the spine, a lesion in the median nerve or a problem in the muscle itself. A careful history and examination will usually indicate the correct diagnosis.

If just one leg is weak, the problem may be at the level of the peripheral nerve, nerve roots, spinal cord or contralateral cerebral hemisphere. Weakness of both legs can result from a lesion in the spinal cord, a peripheral neuropathy or a parafalcine meningioma.

Weakness of proximal muscles is usually caused by a problem in the muscle itself (a myopathy). Patients have difficulty raising their arms (cannot brush their hair) or legs (difficulty with stairs or getting out of low chairs), or problems with truncal muscles (cannot sit up or turn over in bed). Weakness which gets worse after exertion or at the end of the day may be due to myasthenia gravis.

### Difficulty walking

People with dizziness, poor balance, visual disturbance, leg weakness, cerebrovascular disease, muscle disease or extrapyramidal disease may all present with 'difficulty walking'. The pattern of these associated neurological symptoms should help determine the cause of the difficulty. A host of other non-neurological problems (e.g. arthritis) can cause difficulty with walking.

## Sensory problems

### Sensory loss (numbness)

In general, sensory symptoms are less helpful in guiding diagnosis. Transient positive sensory symptoms (tingling) are common and may be due to local pressure on a peripheral nerve. Migrating positive sensory symptoms are most caused by migraine, although occasionally focal seizures can be responsible. Rarely, demyelination can present with persisting positive sensory symptoms.

## Sphincter and sexual problems

Sphincter and sexual problems are understandably distressing and may not be volunteered by the patient. There may be complete loss of bladder and/or bowel control (incontinence), or a sudden inability to pass urine (retention) or faeces (constipation). Either may be due to problems in the spinal cord. Urinary or faecal incontinence may occur during a generalized seizure.

Erectile failure may occur in multisystem atrophy, but many neurological conditions impact on patients' physical and psychological capacity to enjoy sex. Most sphincter and sexual problems do not, however, have a primary neurological cause; many are associated with drug side effects.

## PATTERN OF DISEASE

### Time course

The pace of the illness provides important diagnostic information. The most important questions are 'What happened?' and 'What happened next?'

- *Abrupt onset of symptoms* suggests a vascular cause (stroke or SAH).
- *A relapsing–remitting pattern* strongly suggests an inflammatory disease such as MS.
- *Gradual onset with a relentless progression* suggests a degenerative process.

### Associated symptoms

Non-neurological symptoms may be relevant in formulating a diagnosis.

- When dealing with dizziness or blackouts, ask about cardiovascular symptoms; arrhythmias and reduced cardiac output can cause neurological symptoms.
- Recent skin rash, joint pain or gastrointestinal disorders may suggest the cause of neurological symptoms (e.g. a facial rash in systemic lupus erythematosus [SLE]).
- Poor general health and weight loss may be caused by covert malignant disease or by other systemic disorders.

## DISEASE IMPACT

Neurological diseases are important because of the impact they have on the activities of daily living. Understanding what capabilities are most important to the individual is central to establishing shared treatment goals.

## DRUG HISTORY

Neurological problems may be side effects of common drugs, sometimes taken for minor ailments. Phenothiazines may cause a movement disorder, anticoagulants may cause a spontaneous intracerebral haemorrhage (ICH), stroke may be caused by 'recreational' drugs such as cocaine and a range of drugs may lead to deterioration in myasthenia gravis.

## PAST MEDICAL HISTORY

Some diseases follow a relapsing–remitting course, and with the benefit of hindsight it may be possible to identify a previously unexplained episode of neurological dysfunction as having diagnostic significance. Equally, established diseases in other organ systems may develop neurological features, so the past medical history may be important.

## FAMILY HISTORY

Some patients with single gene autosomal dominant conditions will give a clear family history. Many other conditions have polygenic inheritance, but this is rarely helpful diagnostically. Importantly, a family history of, for instance, aneurysmal SAH or Huntington's disease (HD) may be a major source of worry, even if the clinical features would not support such a diagnosis.

## NEUROLOGICAL EXAMINATION

The purpose of neurological examination is to test specific hypotheses generated from the history. In many patients, examination is not required; in most others, only selected parts of the neurological examination are needed. But you need to know how to do it all. Patients should be comfortable, and appropriately dressed – it is not possible to see fasciculation through trousers or test sensation through woolly tights.

## CONSCIOUS LEVEL, ALERTNESS AND COGNITIVE FUNCTION

The level of consciousness is assessed using the Glasgow Coma Scale and higher cerebral function may be assessed with the Addenbrooke's Cognitive Examination. Isolated aphasia indicates a focal lesion of the dominant hemisphere, visuospatial dysfunction indicates a lesion of the non-dominant parietal lobe, and amnesia may be caused by temporal lobe lesions

## CRANIAL NERVES

### Visual field defects

See **Figure 13.1**.

- *Homonymous hemianopia or quadrantanopia:* This indicates a lesion of the optic tract, the optic radiation or the occipital cortex. Lesions of the optic radiation in the temporal lobe cause an upper quadrantanopia while lesions in the parietal lobe cause a lower quadrantanopia.
- *Bitemporal hemianopia:* This indicates a lesion at the optic chiasm, typically a large pituitary tumour.
- *Cortical blindness:* This results from bilateral occipital lesions; pathways to the superior colliculi are spared so the pupillary reactions to light are normal.

## PUPILLARY AND EYE MOVEMENT DISORDERS

### Oculomotor (IIIrd) nerve palsy

Painful IIIrd nerve palsy must be investigated urgently because posterior communicating artery aneurysms need immediate treatment. A drowsy patient with a IIIrd nerve palsy may have critically raised intracranial pressure and be on the point of developing fatal herniation of the medial edge of the temporal lobe through the tentorial hiatus.

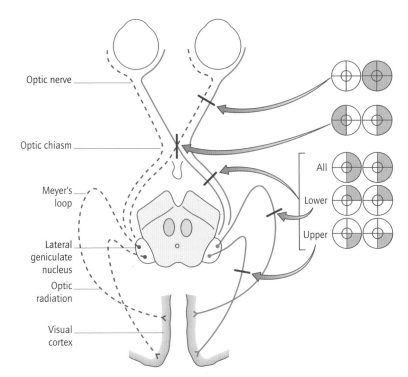

Optic nerve

Optic chiasm

Meyer's loop

Lateral geniculate nucleus

Optic radiation

Visual cortex

All

Lower

Upper

**Figure 13.1** Sites of lesions causing different visual field defects.

## Complete ophthalmoplegia

If all eye movements in one eye are lost, consider lesions in the orbit or cavernous sinus (aneurysm, tumour, cavernous sinus thrombosis, granulomatous disease). Myasthenia gravis and endocrine disease (e.g. dysthyroid eye disease) should be excluded; pupil reactions remain normal in both conditions.

## Internuclear ophthalmoplegia

Internuclear ophthalmoplegia (INO) is demonstrated on lateral gaze; in a left INO, there is a failure of adduction in the left eye and nystagmus in the abducting right eye when looking to the left; gaze to the right is normal (**Figure 13.2**). INOs are caused by a lesion in ipsilateral median longitudinal fasciculus, the tract connecting the IIIrd and VIth nerve nuclei. It may be bilateral. Causes include MS and Wernicke's encephalopathy.

## Horner's syndrome

Interruption of the sympathetic fibres to the pupil causes Horner's syndrome (ptosis, a small pupil [miosis]; ipsilateral loss of forehead sweating and apparent retraction of the eye [enophthalmos]) (**Figure 13.3**).

## THE FACE

### Facial sensation

If loss is confined to one division of the trigeminal nerve, consider demyelination, a structural lesion or, rarely, SLE. An acoustic neuroma may expand and involve the Vth

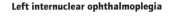

**Left internuclear ophthalmoplegia**

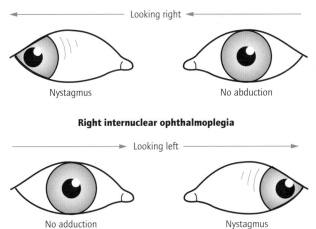

Looking right

Nystagmus

No abduction

**Right internuclear ophthalmoplegia**

Looking left

No adduction

Nystagmus

**Figure 13.2** Findings in INO.

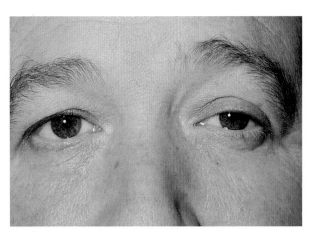

**Figure 13.3** Horner's syndrome.

nerve, resulting in a combination of deafness, ataxia, ipsilateral facial weakness and loss of the ipsilateral corneal reflex.

### Muscles of mastication

Bilateral weakness of jaw opening is not specific to lesions of the motor division of the trigeminal nerve and can occur in MND, myasthenia gravis and myopathies.

### Muscles of facial expression

The upper facial musculature receives input from both cerebral hemispheres; the lower musculature from the contralateral hemisphere only. Therefore, the upper part of the face may be spared in upper motor neurone (UMN) lesions.

## MOTOR SYSTEM

The arms and then the legs are examined, with comparison of each part with its opposite. Power is assessed on the Medical Research Council (MRC) scale.

### Spasticity

This hallmark of UMN lesions is caused by interruption of corticospinal inhibitory pathways, most marked in flexor muscles in the arms and the extensors of the legs, not constant throughout the full range of passive movement, and may be elicited by rapid pronation of the arms, flexion of the legs or dorsiflexion at the ankle.

### Clonus

Clonus is a series of repeated involuntary contractions of the stretched muscle and is a consequence of spasticity and hyper-reflexia. Ankle clonus is demonstrated by flexing the knee slightly then rapidly dorsiflexing the foot.

### Rigidity

This is a general increase in muscle tone. Extrapyramidal ('lead pipe') rigidity is present throughout the whole range of passive movement and may be associated with 'cogwheeling' (like moving the joint over a ratchet). It affects both flexors and extensors and may be exaggerated by simultaneous movements of the contralateral limb.

## SENSORY SYSTEM

The sensory examination is more subjective and contributes less to diagnosis. Comparison of sensation side with side or distal limb with trunk may help establish what is normal. Light touch, pin prick, vibration, joint position sense and temperature should be examined. Where an area of sensory loss exists, its boundaries should be mapped by moving the stimulus outwards from numb to normal.

- *Altered sensation:* This may result from damage to a peripheral nerve, to the spinal cord or to the cerebral hemispheres.
- *Sensory inattention:* With simultaneous symmetrical stimuli, the patient only experiences one, but there is

no abnormality when each side is tested in isolation. This is due to a contralateral parietal lobe lesion.
- *Loss of vibration and/or joint position sense:* This occurs with lesions of the dorsal column in the spinal cord, in a dorsal root ganglionopathy and with peripheral neuropathy.
- *Dissociated sensory loss:* This is loss of pain and temperature sensation with preservation of light touch) and is usually caused by a central cord lesion (e.g. syringomyelia).

## COORDINATION, GAIT AND WALKING SPEED

Coordination is assessed using the finger–nose and heel–shin tests. Lesions in the cerebellar hemispheres produce ipsilateral disturbance of arm and leg coordination. In cerebellar disease, tremor is typically worse when a target is approached (intention tremor). Rhythmic repetitive movements (e.g. rapid tapping with the fingers of one hand on the dorsum of the other) and rapid alternating movements (dysdiadochokinesis) are impaired.

Lesions of the midline cerebellum result in loss of balance when sitting and walking. It is said that Romberg's test is positive when there is loss of postural reflexes or joint position sense in the legs and negative in cerebellar disease, when patients are usually equally unsteady with eyes open or closed.

Gait can be assessed as the patient arrives. Observe walking over 10 metres and turning, looking for a broad-based gait, loss of arm swing or a series of short steps after turning, these last two being features of Parkinson's disease (PD). Ask the patient to walk with the heel of the next foot placed at the toe of the other (tandem walking) to reveal mild ataxia.

## INVESTIGATION

As with examination, the purpose of neurological investigation is not to document every nuance of the human condition but rather to test specific hypotheses regarding the origin of symptoms. There is no such thing as routine neurological investigations; appropriate investigations for different clinical presentations are discussed under those sections.

Imaging of the brain (computed tomography [CT] or magnetic resonance imaging [MRI]), spinal cord (MRI) or vasculature (angiography) can be very helpful diagnostically. Generally, MRI is preferable to CT because of its greater sensitivity and specificity, but in urgent situations CT is preferable because scanning time is shorter and there are fewer contraindications. MRI also carries a risk of identifying incidental findings not relevant to the current presentation, and so, as with all investigations, it should not be used as a screening tool or where there is a very low chance of a positive finding (e.g. chronic headache with normal examination). Imaging of the spine to identify radicular disease is of limited utility if the patient would not be a candidate for surgical intervention.

Lumbar puncture (LP) is a basic clinical technique important in the investigation and management of suspected SAH, acute meningitis or encephalitis, chronic meningeal infiltration or inflammation (e.g. malignant meningitis, sarcoidosis), transverse myelitis, chronic central nervous system (CNS) inflammation or infection (e.g. suspected MS, suspected chronic infection such as neurosyphilis, Borrelia infection, human immunodeficiency virus [HIV] infection and acquired immune deficiency syndrome [AIDS]), demyelinating peripheral neuropathy (e.g. Guillain–Barré syndrome [GBS], chronic inflammatory demyelinating neuropathy), or disorders of cerebrospinal fluid (CSF) dynamics (e.g. idiopathic intracranial hypertension, normal-pressure hydrocephalus). Unless a CT has shown that LP is safe (no mass lesions; open basal cisterns), LP should not be performed if there is papilloedema, focal epileptic seizures, dysphasia, hemianopia, hemiparesis, unequal pupils or oculomotor palsy.

An electroencephalogram (EEG) may be helpful in the categorization of epilepsy and in the investigation of altered consciousness and cognitive decline

## MANAGEMENT

### SPECIALIST NURSES

Specialist nurses working alongside consultant neurology colleagues can make a major contribution to patient well-being, their understanding of their disease and the organization of their care. As well as disease-specific specialist nurses (e.g. MS or epilepsy), generic neurology specialist nurses can have a pivotal role covering the breadth of neurological conditions.

### REHABILITATION

Many neurological conditions cause fixed or progressive impairments resistant to pharmacological or surgical intervention. Rehabilitation aims to help patients maximize their quality of life in those circumstances. Starting with a formal assessment of function, the patient and the rehab team set realistic, achievable and measurable targets. Progress is tracked by repeated formal measurement. Even if impairments are completely physical, it is common for secondary psychological factors such as low mood to become important.

Failure to progress during rehabilitation may be because of unrecognized mood problems (e.g. depression or anxiety) or unrecognized neuropsychological deficits (e.g. visual inattention or neglect). Failure to progress should therefore lead to a reassessment of the patient's mental state and cognitive function.

### Information and communication

Patients and their families need to understand the diagnosis, prognosis and management plan. To the extent that is possible, they should oversee decisions about management. During rehabilitation, regular 'updates' on progress made and goals achieved are important. Patients should be told about the many organizations which provide information and support and offer practical help to patients with specific neurological disorders.

## DISEASES AND THEIR MANAGEMENT

### VASCULAR DISEASE

## STROKE AND TRANSIENT ISCHAEMIC ATTACK

Stroke and transient ischaemic attack (TIA) are common and can result from a variety of pathological lesions affecting blood vessels (see STROKE: CLASSIFICATION AT A GLANCE). They can be mimicked by a variety of non-vascular problems such as migraine, focal epilepsy and cerebral tumour.

### Epidemiology

- Prevalence of stroke-related disability is 800 in 100 000. Annual incidence is 280 in 100 000. Annual incidence of TIA is 35 in 100 000.
- Incidence of stroke and TIA rises exponentially with age, and half of all new patients are older than 70 years.
- Stroke and TIA are slightly more common in females.
- Some rare causes of stroke (cerebral autosomal dominant arteriopathy with subcortical infarcts and leukoencephalopathy [CADASIL]) are caused by single gene defects (*notch*), but increased risk of stroke is also inherited as a polygenic trait.

### Disease mechanisms

The causes of stroke and TIA are listed in **Table 13.1**. Risk factors for both ischaemic and haemorrhagic stroke include:
- Hypertension
- Smoking
- Family history
- Diabetes mellitus (ischaemic stroke only)

Most TIAs and ischaemic strokes are caused by emboli. Composed of fibrin and platelets, the majority form on atheromatous plaques at the origins of the internal carotid and vertebral arteries and are carried by the circulation to the brain. In 10%, the emboli arise from the heart.

Around one in five ischaemic strokes (and a smaller proportion of TIAs) result from *in situ* formation of atheroma in the small deep perforating arteries that supply the internal capsule and the pons; these are lacunar strokes or TIAs.

## STROKE: CLASSIFICATION AT A GLANCE

### Ischaemic stroke (85% of all strokes)

*Large middle cerebral artery territory infarct* (**Figure A**)
*Cause:* Occlusion of main stem of middle cerebral artery

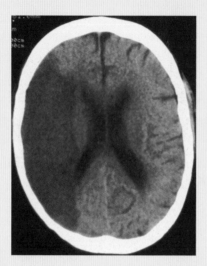

**Figure A** Large middle cerebral artery tertiary infarct (CT).

*Neurological signs:* Hemiplegia, hemianopia, aphasia (if left hemisphere involved), visuospatial disorder (if right hemisphere involved)
*Prognosis:* 40% die within 30 days of onset; 95% probability of death or disability at 6 months

*Cortical infarct* (**Figure B**)
*Cause:* Occlusion of small cortical vessel

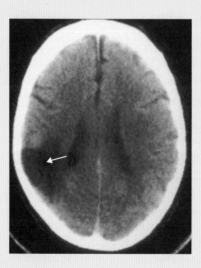

**Figure B** Cortical infarct (CT).

*Neurological signs:* Isolated deficit of cortical function (aphasia or hemianopia, or visuospatial disorder or weakness of hand and/or arm alone)
*Prognosis:* 6% die within 30 days of onset; 45% probability of death or disability at 6 months

*Brainstem infarct* (**Figure C**)
*Cause:* Small vessel disease or embolus

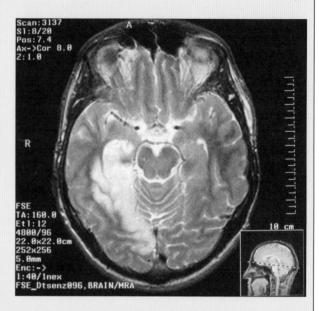

**Figure C** Posterior circulation infarct (MRI).

*Neurological signs:* One or more of double vision, unsteadiness, dysphagia, cranial nerve palsies, Horner's syndrome, quadriparesis, hemiparesis, reduced consciousness
*Prognosis:* 6% die within 30 days; 30% probability of death or disability at 6 months

*Lacunar infarct* (**Figure D**)

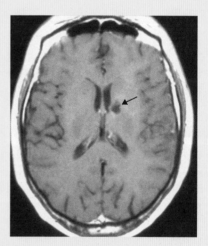

**Figure D** Lacunar infarct (MRI).

*Cause:* Occlusion of single small deep penetrating artery
*Neurological signs:* Hemiparesis or hemisensory loss or unilateral ataxia without disorder of language, memory or visuospatial function

*Continued...*

**13**

*...Continued*

*Prognosis:* 3% die within 30 days; 35% probability of death or disability at 6 months

**Intracranial haemorrhage (15% of all strokes)**

*Primary ICH* (**Figure E**)

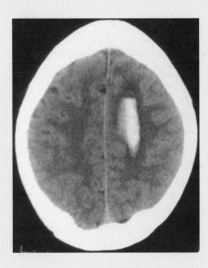

**Figure E** Primary ICH.

*Cause:* Rupture of artery

*Neurological signs:* If severe – coma; if mild – focal neurological deficit, usually indistinguishable from cerebral infarction

*Prognosis:* 30–50% die within 30 days

*SAH* (**Figure F**)

*Cause:* Rupture of cerebral aneurysm or arteriovenous malformation

*Neurological signs:* Sudden headache, neck stiffness, loss of consciousness, some focal signs if the blood spreads into the brain substance

*Prognosis:* 50% die within 30 days. High risk of rebleeding within first few weeks

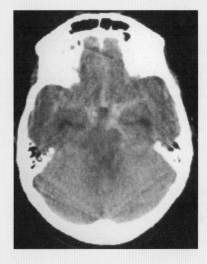

**Figure F** Subarachnoid haemorrhage.

**Table 13.1** Common causes of stroke

**Ischaemic stroke and transient ischaemic attack**

*Thromboembolic infarcts* (about 60%)

- Atheroma of carotid and vertebral arteries

*Lacunar infarcts* (20%)

- Disease of small vessels within the substance of the brain

*Embolism from the heart* (10–20%)

- Left atrial thrombus associated with atrial fibrillation
- Left atrial myxoma (rare)
- Mitral valve endocarditis (bacterial, rheumatic, marantic)
- Mitral valve prosthesis
- Left ventricular mural thrombus complicating myocardial infarction or left ventricular aneurysm
- Cardiomyopathy
- Aortic valve endocarditis (bacterial, rheumatic, marantic)
- Aortic valve sclerosis
- Aortic valve prosthesis
- Congenital cardiac disorders
- Paradoxical embolism from the venous system through a patent foramen ovale
- Atheroma of the aortic arch
- Lupus anticoagulant
- Polycythaemia

*Infection*

- HIV, syphilis

*Multiple mechanisms*

- Drug abuse (e.g. cocaine, amphetamine)

**Primary ICH**

*Ruptured microaneurysm*

- Hypertension

*Small vessel disease*

- Amyloid angiopathy

*Arteriovenous malformation*

*Haemostatic disorders*

- Anticoagulant overdose
- Thrombocytopenia
- Hereditary bleeding disorder

*Multiple mechanisms*

- Drug abuse (e.g. cocaine, ecstasy, amphetamine)

**Subarachnoid haemorrhage**

*Rupture of abnormality*

- Cerebral aneurysm
- Arteriovenous malformation

Primary ICH is usually caused by rupture of a deep penetrating artery within the brain substance and is related to hypertension. Occasionally, rupture of a cerebral aneurysm or an arteriovenous malformation (AVM) may cause haemorrhagic stroke. Superficial lobar haemorrhages may be a result of other causes such as amyloid angiopathy.

### Clinical features

The hallmark of a vascular lesion is the sudden onset of focal symptoms and signs. Ischaemic and haemorrhagic strokes cannot be distinguished on clinical grounds: CT scanning will differentiate between the two. Arterial distributions for some stroke symptoms are given in **Table 13.2**.

The duration of symptoms establishes an arbitrary distinction between stroke (>24 hours) and TIA (<24 hours). However, the differential diagnosis for transient symptoms is broad and includes migraine aura, focal seizures, hypoglycaemia and symptoms of unknown cause. The differential diagnosis for stroke includes functional neurological disorders, cerebral tumour, subdural haematoma and cerebral abscess.

### Investigation

Immediate investigations are important. Brain imaging with CT or MRI should be performed on admission, along with angiography sequences if the patient may be a candidate for thrombectomy. Blood should be taken for glucose, full blood count (FBC), urea and electrolytes (U&Es) and international normalized ratio (INR) and an electrocardiogram (ECG) should be done.

Later investigations include cholesterol, C-reactive protein (CRP), chest X-ray, carotid dopplers (for stroke or TIA in the anterior circulation where the patient is a potential candidate for carotid endarterectomy) and 24-hour

**Table 13.2** Arterial distributions of focal symptoms occurring with TIA or stroke

| Symptom | Arterial distribution |
| --- | --- |
| Dysphasia | Carotid |
| Loss of vision in one eye only | Carotid |
| Weakness of the face/arm/leg* | Carotid or vertebrobasilar, but more often carotid |
| Dysarthria or slurred speech | Carotid or vertebrobasilar |
| Unsteadiness | Carotid or vertebrobasilar |
| Sensory loss of the face/arm/leg* | Carotid or vertebrobasilar |
| Visuospatial disorder | Carotid or vertebrobasilar |
| Quadriparesis | Vertebrobasilar |
| Hemianopia alone | Vertebrobasilar |
| Transient bilateral blindness | Vertebrobasilar |
| Double vision | Vertebrobasilar |

* Symptoms in the face, arm and leg without aphasia, cortical problems or hemianopia are usually caused by ischaemia in the internal capsule or pons. Symptoms restricted to a limb or to the face are usually caused by cortical lesions.

ECG monitoring (to detect paroxysmal atrial fibrillation). Patients without a clear cause for their stroke might also have coagulopathy studies: including proteins C and S and antithrombin III; and autoantibodies: including antinuclear factor (ANF), rheumatoid factor, antineutrophil cytoplasmic antibody (ANCA) and anticardiolipin antibodies; and echocardiography.

### Management

#### Immediate management: ischaemic stroke
Definitive treatment involves immediate removal of the occluding thrombus. If there is an identified large vessel occlusion, this can be achieved through mechanical thrombectomy, which is effective up to 6 hours after symptom onset. In patients without identified large vessel occlusion or where thrombectomy is not possible, intravenous thrombolysis with tissue plasminogen activator (tPA) is effective up to 4.5 hours after stroke onset. Both treatments may be effective up to 24 hours if there is evidence on imaging of potentially salvageable brain tissue.

For all patients, aspirin improves outcome, although the effects are smaller, and it should be avoided in the 24 hours following tPA.

#### Immediate management: intracerebral haemorrhage
Patients should have any anticoagulation stopped and urgently reversed (unless there is intracranial venous thrombosis; and if within 6 hours of ICH onset and sBP >150 mmHg, this should be reduced to <140 mmHg for at least 7 days.

#### Supportive treatment
Otherwise, management of all strokes is based on general supportive treatment including management of complications and identification and management of reversible risk factors. Management in a dedicated stroke unit improves outcome, perhaps because of better attention to the basics of care. A formal swallowing assessment will determine if the patient can safely eat and drink, intermittent pneumatic compression prevents deep venous thrombosis, and good nursing care, with attention to support for a paralysed arm and regular turning to prevent pressure sores, are all important.

#### Secondary prevention
All patients should be encouraged to stop smoking and to adopt a healthy diet. Despite several large trials, the best management of blood pressure in acute ischaemic stroke is not clear. Treatment should probably be withheld until patients are neurologically stable; in the long term, a reduction in diastolic blood pressure of 5–7 mmHg with antihypertensive drugs is associated with a 30–40% reduction in the risk of stroke over the next few years.

*Ischaemic stroke and TIA patients*
- *Antiplatelet drug therapy*: The risk of recurrence is highest early; in patients at low risk of bleeding,

combination aspirin plus clopidogrel can be reduced to clopidogrel alone after 4 weeks.

- *Cholesterol-lowering treatment:* This reduces recurrent vascular events even in those without hypercholesterolaemia.
- *Anticoagulation:* This markedly reduces the risk of recurrent stroke in those with rheumatic mitral valve disease and atrial fibrillation. Depending on risk (which may be estimated using the CHADs-VASC score), it may be indicated in other patients with atrial fibrillation. The best time to start anticoagulation after stroke or TIA is not known but, in practice, it is delayed in larger strokes where there is a greater risk of haemorrhagic transformation.
- *Carotid endarterectomy:* Where carotid dopplers suggest a stenosis of greater than 70% on the relevant side, timely carotid endarterectomy results in a reduced risk of recurrent stroke; the benefit declines with delay to treatment so referral should be immediate.

*Primary intracerebral haemorrhage* If the position of the haematoma is not typical of a hypertensive bleed (if it is central rather than peripheral), and if there is no good explanation for the bleed (haemostatic deficit, cocaine use), cerebral angiography should be performed to detect any underlying aneurysm or AVM.

### Prognosis

The risk of death within 30 days is up to 50% after ischaemic stroke (depending on severity) and less than 1% for TIA. The annual risk of stroke is 5–10% in the first year and 5% thereafter.

## SUBARACHNOID HAEMORRHAGE

### Epidemiology

- SAH accounts for about 5% of all strokes, with an annual incidence of 10 in 100 000.
- It is most common in people over 60 years, and slightly more common in females.

### Disease mechanisms

The causes of SAH are ruptured cerebral aneurysm (90%), ruptured AVM (5%) and, more rarely, mycotic aneurysm associated with, for instance, subacute bacterial endocarditis.

### Clinical features

SAH causes sudden-onset severe headache, which reaches a peak within a few minutes. It is associated with nausea, vomiting and photophobia and the patient may lose consciousness. There may be a focal neurological deficit.

### Investigation

- *CT:* This shows blood in the subarachnoid space in 99% of cases if performed within 6 hours and may suggest which vessel has bled. Patients with a positive CT should undergo immediate CT angiography, to guide management. Later CT may detect complications such as hydrocephalus, haematoma and infarction.
- *Lumbar puncture:* If a negative CT was delayed beyond 6 hours or the suspicion of SAH is high, an LP may show uniform blood staining of the CSF and xanthochromia. LP is most useful at least 8 hours after headache onset.

### Management

Patients should receive nimodipine, analgesia, and have adequate fluid intake. Early definitive endovascular treatment of the aneurysm may be initiated based on the CT angiography alone; but if the architecture is not clear or neurosurgery is being planned, catheter angiography may be required. Deteriorating neurological status may be a result of rebleeding, cerebral ischaemia, hydrocephalus or systemic disturbances such as hypoxia or hypotension. Hyponatraemia, cardiac arrhythmias or neurogenic pulmonary oedema may develop.

Patients should therefore be monitored intensively, and deterioration should prompt consideration of systemic causes (hypoxia; hypotension) and repeat CT.

### Prognosis

About 5–10% of patients die before they get to hospital and 30–50% die within the first month; 50% of the survivors remain dependent.

## CORTICAL VENOUS AND DURAL SINUS THROMBOSIS

These rare conditions are more common in females, and risk factors include oral contraception, pregnancy, dehydration, hypercoagulable states and middle-ear infections.

### Clinical features

Occlusion of cortical veins causes focal neurological signs and seizures, and occlusion of the dural sinuses causes raised intracranial pressure. The diagnosis should be considered in patients with sudden or evolving headache, declining conscious level, seizures, focal neurological deficit or papilloedema.

### Investigation

- *CT scan:* is often normal but may show wedge-shaped infarcts or haemorrhage
- *CT or MR venography:* will confirm the diagnosis

### Management

Those severely affected should receive intravenous heparin, and all should have oral anticoagulation for at least 6 months, and management of risk factors.

## EPISODIC DISORDERS

### BLACKOUTS AND DIZZY TURNS

Transient neurological symptoms such as 'blackouts' and 'dizzy turns' are very common, particularly in the elderly, and do not usually have a serious underlying cause. Cerebral function is diminished if metabolism is impaired (reductions in cerebral perfusion or blood oxygenation or glucose) or neural activity is increased (e.g. in epilepsy). Our perception of ourselves and our environment is an internal neural representation which can be modulated by our expectations and other psychological factors and is not under conscious control.

### Clinical features

Blackouts are transient attacks of loss of consciousness during attacks. Dizziness can mean light-headedness, or vertigo, or a general feeling of unsteadiness.

- *Labyrinthine disorders* cause only vertigo, nausea and nystagmus.
- *Brainstem lesions* cause diplopia, dysarthria, dysphagia, blurred vision, quadriparesis or cranial nerve palsies in addition to vertigo.
- *Cerebellar lesions* may cause unsteadiness, imbalance or 'walking as if drunk', but not vertigo.
- Presyncope comprises light-headedness, faintness, sweating and pallor, which may be relieved by lying flat.
- *Complex partial seizures* may be accompanied by déjà vu, altered smell and/or taste, and vivid memories. Stereotyped movements (e.g. lip smacking), automatisms and an open-eyed trance-like state last a few minutes.
- *Absence seizures* may be accompanied by fluttering of the eyelids.

### Investigation

Investigations are usually unhelpful. If the diagnosis is clear, no tests are required. Very rarely, video EEG monitoring (if attacks are frequent) may be helpful in identifying unusual forms of epilepsy.

### Management

The management of specific conditions is described elsewhere. For syncopal attacks, patients should be advised to avoid precipitants where possible and to lie down if they feel an attack coming on.

## EPILEPSY

Up to 5% of people have one epileptic seizure, but less than half of these have recurrent seizures. There are many different types of seizures.

### Epidemiology

- Active epilepsy occurs in 400–1000 in 100 000 with 200 in 100 000 having more than one seizure per month.

- Peak ages of onset are 0–10 years and over 60 years.
- Some rare forms of epilepsy are inherited as single gene disorders.

### Disease mechanisms

Epilepsy may be secondary to systemic disturbances, drugs or CNS disorders but in 60% no cause is found. Attacks may be provoked by fatigue, hunger, hypoglycaemia or alcohol. Seizures arise from an uncontrolled and recursive recruitment of neighbouring neurones which may remain localized (causing a partial seizure) or spread to the entire cortex (causing a generalized seizure). Seizure thresholds vary but most people, given a sufficient stimulus, have the capacity to have a seizure.

### Clinical features

A narrative account from a first-hand eyewitness describing what happened is often more important than the patient's own description.

### Diagnosis

Even with a good eyewitness account, distinguishing epilepsy from other causes of altered consciousness can be very difficult. Establishing whether attacks are due to epileptic seizures is more important than establishing quite what kind of epilepsy the patient has, although this can be helpful in prognosis and guiding management (**Table 13.3**). Epilepsy is diagnosed when more than one epileptic seizure has occurred.

### Investigation

- *Blood:* Establish whether there is an electrolyte disturbance.
- *ECG* (**Figure 13.4**): This should be performed to seek evidence of a cardiac conduction abnormality (which can sometimes mimic seizures).
- *MRI brain* (**Figure 13.5**): An MRI scan should be done in preference to CT, as it provides more useful information.
- *EEG:* This may be helpful in determining the type of epilepsy, but between attacks is usually normal. Prolonged EEG recording, often with video, can be very helpful if there is diagnostic uncertainty.

### Management

Management aims to identify the cause of the seizures where one exists, to minimize complications and to reduce seizure frequency to the lowest possible level (**Table 13.4**). Attention to the psychological and social aspects of epilepsy is important, and epilepsy nurse practitioners make a valuable contribution. Remember to give advice about driving and pregnancy.

#### Who to treat

In patients where there is no indication of their being at high risk of recurrence (previous brain injury; abnormal EEG or brain imaging; nocturnal seizure), antiepilepsy drugs are not usually started. Some attacks may be so mild or so infrequent that patients would rather not take medication.

**Table 13.3** Common epilepsy syndromes in adults

**GENERALIZED SEIZURES**

**Tonic–clonic epilepsy**

*Clinical features*

- Falls to ground if standing
- Sudden stiffness and loss of consciousness
- Followed by rhythmic jerking of all four limbs
- May be incontinence and biting of the side of the tongue
- Postictal drowsiness and confusion

**PARTIAL SEIZURES**

Partial seizures are:

- *Simple partial* if consciousness is normal
- *Complex partial* if consciousness is impaired

**Temporal lobe seizures**

*Clinical features*

- Onset difficult to describe but may be instantly recognized by the patient, and may have visceral sensory element
- Odd unpleasant smell or taste at onset

- Intense familiarity déjà vu or vivid stereotyped memory
- Speech arrest
- Lip smacking
- Staring into space, uncommunicative for a few minutes
- Amnesic during attack
- Odd semi-purposeful limb movements
- May perform complex stereotyped tasks during complex partial seizure

**Partial motor seizures**

*Clinical features*

- Turning of head and eyes to one side
- Twitching of one hand or arm, or side of face, which may spread from hand to face or from face to hand
- Postictal hemiparesis (Todd's paralysis) sometimes occurs

**Partial sensory seizures**

*Clinical features*

- Tingling or pins and needles ('positive' sensory phenomena), which may spread over one side of the body (leg to arm, or face to hand to leg) over a few minutes

*Choice of antiepilepsy drug*

- Sodium valproate, lamotrigine, topiramate or levetiracetam are reasonable first-choice drugs for patients with generalized seizures, and in partial seizures carbamazepine may also be used. Valproate should not be used in women of childbearing potential, and other antiepilepsy drugs used only after a full discussion of the risks to foetal health.
- Absence seizures and myoclonic epilepsy respond best to sodium valproate or lamotrigine.
- Clonazepam and clobazam are benzodiazepines that can be used as add-on therapy in patients with generalized seizures (tonic–clonic, absence or myoclonic).

*Monitoring therapy*

*Blood levels* These have no role in the routine monitoring of antiepilepsy drug treatment.

- If the patient is still having seizures, the dose is too low.
- If they are getting side effects (impaired concentration, drowsiness, unsteadiness, incoordination and nystagmus), the dose is too high.

- If they are still getting seizures and they are getting side effects, they may need a different antiepilepsy drug.

*Record seizure frequency* The patient's recollection of the frequency and severity of their seizures can be patchy; a seizure diary allows accurate correlation of seizure frequency with factors such as antiepilepsy drug dosage.

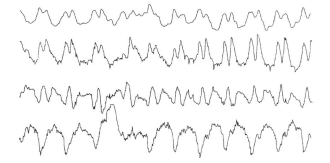

**Figure 13.4** Generalized spike-and-wave EEG.

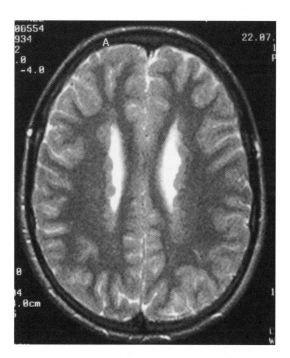

**Figure 13.5** MRI showing grey heterotopia on ventricular surface in a patient with treatment-resistant epilepsy.

**Table 13.4** Management of seizures and of epilepsy

| Supportive treatment | Specific treatment |
|---|---|
| *Advice about driving and other activities* | *Drugs* |
| In the UK, patients who hold a driving licence are required to inform the DVLA that they have had a seizure. After a single seizure, if there are no indications of a high risk of recurrence, the patient will likely be able to return to driving after 6 months. | Use one drug, and increase the dose until seizures are controlled or side effects prohibit further dosage increase. |
| Patients who only ever have seizures arising from sleep may be permitted to drive if this pattern has been established for 3 years. | If one drug does not work, try another 'first-line' drug as monotherapy. |
| Even a single seizure leads to a 10-year suspension on class II (heavy goods vehicles and public service vehicle) licences. | If three first-line drugs have each proved ineffective, move to combination therapy. |
| For other activities (work, swimming, cycling, climbing ladders), patients should be encouraged to make decisions about risk for themselves, based on the likelihood of having a seizure, and the consequences if they do have a seizure in that context. | Consider gradual withdrawal of antiepilepsy drugs after 2 years seizure-free on treatment – but patients who wish to drive generally opt to stay on treatment. |
| | *Surgery* |
| | Where epilepsy is resistant to treatment and disabling, identification of an epileptogenic focus and its surgical resection can in some cases have dramatic benefits. |

*Changing antiepilepsy drug* If seizures are not controlled on the first antiepilepsy drug, change to another first-line agent, withdrawing the first drug after an overlap period of 3–4 weeks. Avoid using more than one antiepilepsy drug until at least three first-line treatments have been tried in adequate dosage.

*Management of epilepsy during pregnancy* Antiepilepsy drugs may cause teratogenicity, neural tube defects and neurodevelopmental delay. However, epilepsy may worsen during pregnancy and the puerperium, in part due to increased volume of distribution and metabolism of antiepilepsy drugs. Teratogenicity occurs early in pregnancy, so women of childbearing age should be on the lowest dose of the safest drug which works for them. Women trying to become pregnant who have been free of seizures for 2 years or more may wish to try coming off medication (recognizing that they should not drive during this period) and should receive folate supplementation. Breastfeeding is generally safe in patients on anticonvulsant drugs, and the sleep deprivation and stress which can accompany parenthood may make seizures worse.

*When to stop antiepileptic drugs* After some years free of seizures, patients may want to find out if their epilepsy has gone away, and if they still need treatment. Actuarial risk of recurrence can be estimated using online algorithms (e.g. http://www.dcn.ed.ac.uk/model/epilepsy.asp). Drugs should be withdrawn one at a time, and gradually. Do not stop sodium valproate therapy in patients with juvenile monoclonic epilepsy as relapse is universal. Patients should be advised not to drive for 6 months after a reduction in their antiepilepsy drug dosage.

Drug-resistant epilepsy is unusual in patients whose nervous system is otherwise normal – so remember that non-epileptic seizures (pseudoseizures) are commonly mistaken for epilepsy.

### Sudden unexplained death
Patients with epilepsy are at risk of sudden unexplained death (SUDEP). This occurs in about 1 in 1000 epilepsy person years and is more common in:
- Males
- Patients who have experienced generalized tonic–clonic seizures in the last year, particularly if they were nocturnal
- Patients who live alone
- Patients with a previous diagnosis of substance abuse or alcohol dependence

Patients should be informed of the risks of SUDEP but encouraged that the risks to them as an individual are low.

### Surgery
Surgical resection of an identified isolated epileptogenic focus can lead to complete remission of seizures, but the number of patients who are likely to derive benefit from surgery is small.

---

**EMERGENCY PRESENTATION 13.1**

## Management of prolonged seizures and status epilepticus

### Definition
A prolonged seizure has a convulsive phase lasting over 5 minutes, and status epilepticus has a convulsive phase lasting more than 30 min, or a sequence of seizures lasting more than 30 min without full recovery between.

### Treatment
- Resuscitate – ensure Airway; Breathing; Circulation
- Exclude hypoglycaemia by checking blood sugar level in capillary (pinprick) blood
- *First-line (5–20 minutes):* intramuscular midazolam or intravenous lorazepam or diazepam
- *Second-line (20–40 minutes):* intravenous fosphenytoin or valproate or levetiracetam
- *Third-line (>40 minutes):* alternative second-line agent, or phenobarbitone or thiopental or propofol

## Prognosis

- Following a first seizure, 50–80% of patients will have a further seizure within 2–3 years.
- Two-thirds of patients with epilepsy go into antiepilepsy drug-free remission within 10 years.

## TRANSIENT GLOBAL AMNESIA

Transient global amnesia (TGA) is a rare condition in the middle-aged and elderly of unknown cause. It is characterized by the sudden onset of an inability to form new memories, and usually also of retrograde amnesia, and lasts for a few hours. During an attack, the patient is fully conscious and alert but is bewildered. They will repeatedly ask the same questions, to the eventual irritation of those around them. Complex actions, including driving a car, can be performed apparently normally. After the attack, amnesia for the attack itself persists.

TGA may occur once or twice but, if attacks are more frequent, they may represent transient epileptic amnesia, which should provoke an MRI of the brain, and which usually responds to antiepilepsy drugs such as carbamazepine.

## SLEEP DISORDERS

In narcolepsy, patients experience the sudden irresistible intrusion of sleep. Some patients also experience cataplexy (a sudden loss of muscle tone and collapse in response to emotional stimuli), vivid dreams, hypnagogic hallucinations and sleep paralysis. There is often a positive family history. It may respond to stimulant drugs such as modafinil, and cataplexy may respond to clomipramine.

## HEADACHE AND FACIAL PAIN

Recurrent or persistent headache is very common and is only very rarely due to brain tumour.

### Epidemiology

About 15% of the population report that they have had a headache of some kind in the last 2 weeks; most of these have no discernible cause but around 2% of the population have severe migraine.

### Disease mechanisms

The mechanism of 'tension' headache is not known, and it is likely to be multifactorial. The mechanism of migraine is also unclear, although increased incidence in women and in those with a family history makes an underlying neurobiological cause likely. Headache may also occur due to changes in intracranial pressure, meningeal irritation, distension, traction or dilatation of the intracranial or extracranial arteries; traction, displacement or occlusion of large intracranial veins or their dural envelopes; or compression, traction or inflammation of the sensory cranial and spinal nerves.

### Clinical features

#### Primary headache

Diagnosis is based on the type, character and pattern of the headache. Typical migraine is a unilateral throbbing headache that may be associated with nausea, vomiting, photo- and phonophobia and is often preceded by visual or sensory auras; the pattern of the attacks is often stereotyped. Migraine can occur with (classical migraine) or without (common migraine) aura; and migraine aura can occur without headache (also known as 'acephalgic' or 'silent' migraine). Clinical examination is usually normal. When no headache is reported, the differential diagnosis, especially in the elderly, includes TIA. The presence of positive visual and somatosensory symptoms (tingling), of malaise, nausea and fatigue, and of a prior history of common or classical migraine all suggest migraine rather than TIA, even in the elderly.

#### Sudden severe headache

Sudden severe headache is much less common than chronic headache, and the differential diagnosis includes SAH, meningitis and cortical venous thrombosis. Sudden severe headache warrants referral to hospital for clinical assessment and a CT scan. Where CT is done within 6 hours and is normal, the risk of 'CT-negative SAH' is very low, and LP is not usually required. Patients over 50 should have an erythrocyte sedimentation rate (ESR) to rule out temporal arteritis (see Chapter 4, Rheumatic disease). CT may show other causes of headache such as subdural haematoma or brain tumour, but MRI may be required to show descent of the cerebellar tonsils through the foramen magnum; in idiopathic intracranial hypotension, imaging may be normal but LP shows a low opening pressure. Extracranial causes of headache include sinusitis, dental abscess and glaucoma.

### Management

In 'tension' headache, non-pharmacological strategies such as ensuring sufficient rest, exercise and hydration and attention to stressors is often more effective than simple analgesia. Codeine-containing preparations may cause medication overuse headache and should be avoided. For migraine, acute treatments such as paracetamol, ibuprofen or naproxen, or triptans may be effective. When migraine is frequent and interferes with usual activities, consider prophylaxis with, for instance, propranolol or amitriptyline.

## FUNCTIONAL NEUROLOGICAL DISORDERS

These disorders are the second commonest reason for referral to a neurologist (around one in six referrals), and functional disorders across the spectrum are involved to some extent in around one-third of secondary care consultations; medically unexplained symptoms are discussed further in

Chapter 14, Psychological medicine. About 40% of patients seen in neurology clinics have symptoms which are either not at all, or only partially, explained by a recognized disease process. Diverse manifestations include non-epileptic attacks, drop attacks, tremor, painful or distressing sensory symptoms, limb weakness, poor balance and unsteadiness, lack of energy and overwhelming fatigue. Often, the symptoms worsen with effort; the patient can sustain more normal function for perhaps a day, but disability is increased in the following days. As with better characterized neurological diseases, stressful life events can be involved with the aetiology in a proportion of patients. Such symptoms appear to be related to and occur with disorders in other organ systems including, for instance, irritable bowel syndrome and fibromyalgia.

Characteristic features on examination include distractibility, where muscle power is weak when examined directly but normal when integral to examination of a different movement. Hip flexion requires bracing (extension) of the contralateral leg. Hoover's sign describes weakness of hip extension on direct examination with preservation of full power when examining contralateral hip flexion. A functional tremor may show entrainment, where the phase of the tremor matches the phase of voluntary movements of the contralateral side. Characteristics of functional alterations in consciousness include long duration, eye closure, recollection of limb shaking, and patients who fall suddenly and lie still with closed eyes. There may be changing patterns of impairment over time and between examinations.

These conditions can be very disabling, yet patients are often unfairly thought to be malingering, or to be in some way weak in the face of their symptoms. Such symptoms can be exceptionally troubling for patients, the more so because the lack of an identifiable cause may lead to a despair that 'if you don't know what's causing this, how can you fix it?' This perception can extend to judgements made by social security (welfare) systems, where, for any given level of disability, patients with functional neurological disorders appear, in the UK at least, to be much less likely to be in receipt of disability benefits. This is particularly unfair, because the nature of their condition renders them among the least able successfully to navigate the complex appeals processes.

Management of functional neurological disorders requires an organized, person-centred, goal-directed approach to rehabilitation. Physiotherapy may be particularly helpful for patients with functional neurological disorders, psychotherapy for patients with non-epileptic seizures, and vestibular rehabilitation exercises (Cooksey-Cawthorne) for patients with unsteadiness. Psychiatric evaluation may be helpful in selected patients where there may be causal stressors, but functional neurological disorders are not primarily psychiatric diseases; patients are not delusional about their symptoms and, while some have symptoms of depression, this is the case for many patients with chronic neurological disability.

Medications for symptom control can be helpful in selected circumstances. However, since neurorehabilitation is based in part on learning or re-learning in the nervous system, and since drugs such as amitriptyline or opiates may inhibit key central signalling pathways required for learning, such drugs should be used at the lowest dose required for the shortest time necessary.

## DISORDERS OF CONSCIOUSNESS AND COGNITIVE FUNCTION

### COMA AND BRAINSTEM DEATH

In general, focal lesions cause coma by compressing the midbrain and brainstem, while coma requiring medical intervention results from a more diffuse pathological process such as hypoglycaemia, meningitis or encephalitis. Acute hydrocephalus can present with a rapid onset of impaired consciousness. Immediate assessment should determine the cause of coma and the need for urgent medical or neurosurgical attention.

The level of consciousness is assessed using the Glasgow Coma Scale. Where coma was preceded by focal neurological symptoms (e.g. focal seizures, hemiparesis), there is usually a focal cause (e.g. subdural haematoma), but hypoglycaemia can cause focal disturbances which resolve when the blood glucose is normalized. A focal cause is also more likely where there are asymmetrical pupils or conjugate deviation of the eyes, or asymmetry of the oculocephalic reflex, the caloric responses, the limb response to pain or the plantar response. Common 'medical' causes of coma include drugs and alcohol intoxication and diabetic hypoglycaemia.

### BRAINSTEM DEATH

There are established criteria which allow the diagnosis of brainstem death. In some patients, extensive damage to the pons causes quadriplegia and loss of speech while the midbrain and cerebral hemispheres function normally. They are therefore awake, able to hear and think, and have a normal EEG, but are unable to communicate except by vertical movements of their eyes. Some such patients recover fully functional independence.

### RAISED INTRACRANIAL PRESSURE

This is an emergency, requiring specialist management.
- Features include a headache which is aggravated by lying flat, coughing, bending or straining, transient visual obscurations, vomiting, papilloedema, false localizing signs (IIIrd or VIth palsy), drowsiness and coma.
- Investigations include urgent blood glucose, U&Es and CT brain. Blood cultures and antigen tests are

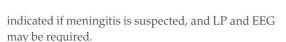

indicated if meningitis is suspected, and LP and EEG may be required.

• The management and prognosis depend on the cause. Dementia and delirium are covered in Chapter 14, Psychological medicine.

## MULTIPLE SCLEROSIS

This inflammatory condition affects first the myelin sheath of central but not peripheral neurones and later causes axon loss. It may present as benign disease, follow a relapsing and remitting course or show inexorable progression from the outset.

### Epidemiology

The prevalence is related to latitude and is highest in the UK and northern Europe. Onset is usually between 20 and 40 years and two-thirds of UK patients are female. There is a genetic contribution to MS, with 15% of MS patients in the UK having an affected first-degree relative.

### Disease mechanisms

The cause of MS is not known. There is increased immunological activity in the CNS (CSF lymphocytosis, intrathecal antibody production). Clinical features arise from slowing of axonal conduction because of loss of the myelin sheath during relapses; following repair, remyelination may be incomplete, resulting in continuing symptomatology and secondary axonal loss.

### Clinical features

MS can affect any parts of the CNS but predominantly involves periventricular deep white matter, optic nerve (causing optic neuritis), brainstem (causing unsteady gait, unilateral facial weakness, or INO) or spinal cord (causing weakness, sensory disturbance, urinary frequency and urgency).

• *Lhermitte's phenomenon* is an electric shock-like sensation shooting down the neck and back and into the arms and legs following flexion of the neck and caused by a lesion in the cervical spinal cord.

• *Uhthoff's phenomenon* is the loss of function in part of the nervous system associated with a rise in body temperature.

After an initial episode of CNS inflammation the patient may make a full recovery, and this is a clinically isolated syndrome. If there is then recurrence, with recovery to baseline, the patient is said to have relapsing–remitting MS. If there then develops progression of neurological impairment between relapses, this is secondary progressive disease. Finally, a small proportion of patients present with the insidious onset of a relentlessly progressive disease, without relapses, and this is primary progressive MS.

### Diagnosis

The diagnostic criteria for MS are established by a committee of experts and are subject to change. Diagnosis is based on history of typical demyelinating events, objective clinical evidence of impairment, and MRI and CSF findings. Confusingly, they come with the caveat that they are not intended to discriminate between MS and other conditions, but rather to stratify patients into those at high or low risk of recurrence, once other diagnoses have been considered unlikely.

In practical terms, the first step is to establish whether a given neurological impairment is likely due to inflammation within the nervous system of the kind seen in MS. The history is usually of onset over a few days to a few weeks, with associated abnormalities on examination and characteristic lesions on brain or spinal cord MRI. CSF may show modest elevation of white cells, along with oligoclonal bands. With no history of previous events, this is a so-called clinically isolated syndrome. If, however, there is dissemination of inflammation in space (affecting different parts of the nervous system, either clinically or by MRI) and time (either from the history, or seeing lesions of different ages at MRI), or if there is a clinically isolated syndrome with dissemination in space (two of periventricular, cortical/juxtacortical, infratentorial brain or spinal cord) and CSF oligoclonal bands, then a diagnosis of MS can be made.

Primary progressive MS does not manifest a relapsing–remitting pattern, and other diagnostic criteria are used.

### Investigation

In a first episode, the primary concern is to exclude a structural lesion as the cause of the symptoms through MRI of the affected CNS region and of *brain* (**Figure 13.6**). Around 90% of patients with clinically definite disease will show areas of high signal with a periventricular distribution. Similar changes may be seen in vasculitis, sarcoidosis and Behçet's disease, but those of MS may be sufficiently typical to allow a diagnosis to be made. If not, other investigations include CSF analysis and visual evoked responses.

### Management

The diagnosis of MS usually has a profound impact on how patients think of themselves, and often the uncertainty about what the future might hold is as disabling as the direct effects of MS. The diagnosis of MS should not, however, be withheld; where there is reasonable suspicion that it is the cause of a patient's symptoms, this should be discussed openly and frankly in an appropriately unhurried, supportive and informative way.

In the acute phase, inflammation may be suppressed by oral or intravenous methylprednisolone, which reduces the duration of relapse but not the extent of recovery. In patients with substantial disease activity, relapse frequency and, possibly, the accumulation of disability (at least in the short term) can be reduced by immunosuppressive drugs such as interferon beta, glatirimer acetate, teriflunomide, fingolomod or dimethylfumarate. In patients with highly active disease (relapses despite immunosuppressive treatment), natalizumab or alemtuzumab may be effective. However,

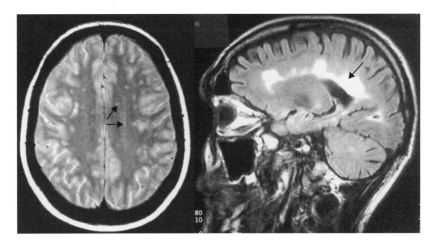

**Figure 13.6** MRI showing periventricular white matter lesions in a patient with MS.

powerful immunosuppression can be associated with development of a serious opportunistic viral brain infection, progressive multifocal leucoencephalopathy, so the benefits of treatment need to be balanced against the risks, and patients receiving such treatments should be under the continuing review of a specialist MS clinic.

Attention should be given to any disability and handicap, and symptomatic relief is available for spasticity, dysaesthetic pain and bladder symptoms. Involvement of an MS nurse practitioner can be invaluable.

### Prognosis

Around 50% of patients with a single episode of demyelination and an abnormal MRI will develop clinically definite MS within 3 years. American World War II veterans with a diagnosis of MS in 1956 had median survival times of 30 and 40 years for males and females, respectively. For patients with established relapsing–remitting disease, more than half are still able to walk 500 metres without assistance 10 years into their illness.

## MOVEMENT DISORDERS

## PARKINSON'S DISEASE AND EXTRAPYRAMIDAL DISORDERS

PD is a neurodegenerative disease affecting dopaminergic neurones of the extrapyramidal system (**Figure 13.8**) and is characterized by disturbance of the control of movement and of posture, abnormalities of cognition and mood, and autonomic disturbance. The extrapyramidal system may also be affected by small vessel vascular disease, drug side effects, multiple system atrophy, progressive supranuclear palsy and toxins.

### Clinical features

Extrapyramidal disease is characterized by tremor, rigidity and bradykinesia and postural instability. These features may occur in isolation (e.g. in PD), alongside dysfunction of other CNS systems (e.g. in multiple system atrophy) or as features of more generalized conditions (e.g. multi-infarct dementia).

The features of early PD (general slowness, expressionless face, shaking) may be falsely attributed to the effects of age, arthritis, depression, alcohol, stroke or brain tumour, and the correct diagnosis may take some time to establish. PD is often asymmetrical at onset.

### Diagnosis

A clinical diagnosis of PD can be made if:
- There is tremor, cogwheel rigidity and bradykinesia
- Abnormalities are restricted to the extrapyramidal system
- There is no other obvious cause
- There is a good response to L-DOPA (**Figure 13.7**)

Other features include postural instability, loss of facial expression, soft monotonous voice, stooped posture, festinating gait, loss of arm swing, cognitive deficits, mood disturbance and abnormalities of autonomic function.

If there is an obvious underlying cause (such as drugs or toxins), or there are features of disease outside the extrapyramidal system, the patient does not have PD and it is better to diagnose an 'extrapyramidal disorder' than 'parkinsonism' in such patients.

### Investigation

Uncomplicated patients who meet the criteria above do not require investigation. Liver function tests, calcium levels, copper, caeruloplasmin and urinary copper will exclude treatable metabolic causes, and a DATSCAN may demonstrate the characteristic loss of presynaptic dopamine terminals.

### Management

There are no treatments which halt the degeneration of dopaminergic neurones, but the consequences can be mitigated by:
- Increasing dopamine production (L-DOPA, with a peripheral DOPA decarboxylase inhibitor)

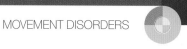

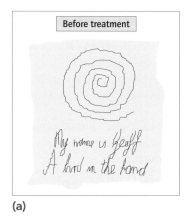
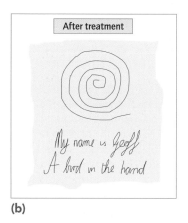

(a)          (b)

**Figure 13.7** Writing and spiral drawn by a patient with PD **(a)** before and **(b)** after treatment.

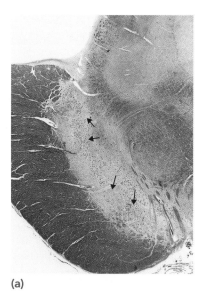

(a)

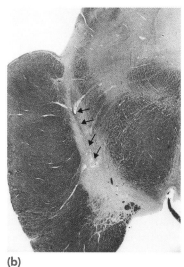

(b)

**Figure 13.8 (a)** Substantia nigra, showing a normal population of large pigmented cells. Klüver–Barrera stain. **(b)** Same area as in **(a)** but here with PD. There is severe depletion of pigmented cells, and the whole area is shrunken. Reproduced from Esiri M (1996) *Oppenheimer's Diagnostic Neuropathology*, 2nd edn (Wiley-Blackwell, Oxford), with the permission of the author.

- Direct dopamine agonists
- Drugs which inhibit dopamine breakdown (COMT inhibitors)

Symptoms of constipation, depression or musculoskeletal pain should be treated, and involvement of a PD nurse practitioner can be invaluable.

Those who initially respond to L-DOPA may find that, over time, the benefit of each tablet is shorter, with rapid transitions to an unmedicated state; this is the 'on–off' effect. In the first instance, smaller, more frequent dosing may help; in the longer run, subcutaneous apomorphine infusion may be required.

### Prognosis

This is a disease of the elderly, and many patients die with their PD rather than dying of PD.

## ESSENTIAL TREMOR

Essential tremor is common (2/1000), and 60% of patients have an affected first-degree relative. Tremor affects the arms (94%), head (titubation, 33%) and voice (16%). The tremor is worse when drinking from a cup of water and when anxious and improves following small amounts of alcohol in 70%. Coordination and gait are otherwise normal.

With a typical history and examination, no investigation is required; if treatment is required, propranolol, primidone or topiramate may be effective.

## OTHER MOVEMENT DISORDERS

### Clinical features and disease mechanisms

#### Chorea

Chorea describes continuous irregular random movements that appear semi-purposeful and fidgety. All parts of the body appear to be involved at random and the gait has a jerky dance-like quality.

*Huntington's disease (HD)* This is an autosomal dominant condition resulting from an expanded trinucleotide repeat in the Huntingtin gene. Accumulation of the Huntingtin gene product in intracellular inclusions disrupts cellular metabolism and leads to cell death, most marked in the striatum and the cortex. It causes chorea, fidgetiness, impaired judgement and impaired cognitive function.

*Wilson's disease* This is a rare autosomal recessive disorder of copper metabolism due to mutations in the gene encoding ATP7B, a copper transporting-P-type ATPase. Patients may present with liver disease in childhood or with the neurological syndrome in adolescence. Neurological symptoms include impaired concentration, declining intellect, behavioural problems, involuntary movements and generalized dystonia, ataxia or an akinetic–rigid syndrome. Patients have a typical smiling facial appearance with drooling and often have slurred speech. There may be copper deposition in Descemet's membrane of the cornea, giving a greenish brown pigmentary (Kayser–Fleischer) ring, which may only be visible at slit-lamp examination.

*Serum copper and caeruloplasmin* are low, *urinary copper excretion is* increased and *liver biopsy* shows increased copper content. Management involves the use of chelating agents such as penicillamine, and if treatment is begun promptly, the prognosis is good.

Chorea may also be caused by drugs, SLE, thyroxicosis or rare neurodegenerative diseases.

### Hemiballismus

This is characterized by sudden and unpredictable throwing movements of one limb and is usually caused by infarction of the contralateral subthalamic nucleus.

### Myoclonic jerks

These are brief jerks of a muscle and are usually caused by a metabolic disturbance. Unlike chorea, the movements are infrequent and discontinuous. Early morning myoclonus suggests juvenile myoclonic epilepsy, and myoclonus in the context of a rapidly evolving dementia suggests CJD.

### Dystonia

This is a slow sustained irregular twisting posture of a limb or the trunk. Some dystonias are focal (affect one limb only), whereas others are generalized.

### Management

Management consists of supportive treatment; genetic counselling where appropriate; correcting any underlying disorder; drug treatment with, for instance, haloperidol (for chorea), tetrabenazine (chorea, generalized dystonia), benzhexol (generalized dystonia) or botulimium toxin (focal dystonia), although the response to drug treatment is often disappointing.

## CEREBELLAR DISORDERS

These typically present with slurred speech (dysarthria), unsteady walking (ataxia), incoordination of hand and arm movements and nystagmus. Patients complain of unsteadiness 'as if drunk'. They may stumble when trying to change direction and the gait is broad-based. Finger–nose testing may show a tremor that increases in amplitude as the finger nears the target (intention tremor) or misses the target altogether (past-pointing).

Cerebellar disorders are most commonly due to stroke, MS, the effects of drugs or alcohol or a space-occupying lesion. Less frequent causes include the Miller Fischer variant of GBS, paraneoplastic cerebellar degeneration or inherited disorders such as Friedreich's or spinocerebellar ataxia.

Investigation begins with *MRI*. If no cause is found:

- *CSF:* seeking evidence of MS, or lymphocytes or malignant cells suggesting an underlying inflammatory or malignant disorder
- *Chest CT:* to exclude a bronchial neoplasm
- *Pelvic ultrasound* in females: to exclude an ovarian tumour

## STRUCTURAL LESIONS OF THE BRAIN

### Epidemiology and disease mechanisms

#### Cerebral tumours

Annual incidence:

- Malignant brain tumour 5–15 in 100 000
- Metastatic brain tumour 3–15 in 100 000
- Benign brain tumour 10 in 100 000

#### Cerebral abscess

- The annual incidence of cerebral abscess is 1 in 100 000.
- The clinical manifestations include headache, fever and malaise in a tachycardic, drowsy and confused patient. However, abscesses may occur in the absence of fever or other signs of systemic infection.

#### Extradural and subdural haematoma

- *Extradural haematoma* is usually an early consequence of head trauma, where a damaged middle meningeal artery bleeds into the extradural space. Blood accumulates rapidly, causing mass effect and dysfunction of underlying brain, often with significant midline shift. Without treatment, it is often fatal.
- *Subdural haematoma* usually presents some weeks after head injury. It is caused by bleeding into the subdural space from small veins crossing between the brain surface and the dura. There is an insidious onset of headache, confusion, dementia or evolving focal deficit.

#### Subdural empyema

Infection in the frontal sinuses or middle ear may extend to the subdural space, causing local pain and tenderness, fever, headache and impaired conscious level. There are often focal signs including hemiplegia, hemisensory disturbance, a unilateral extensor plantar or paralysis of lateral gaze.

### Clinical features

Space-occupying lesions may cause hemiparesis, headache, papilloedema, vomiting, epilepsy, dysphasia, cognitive defect or personality change.

## Investigation

- *CT scanning*: This will determine whether a space-occupying lesion is present. Patients with subdural empyema may have a 'normal' scan initially, with changes only becoming apparent on repeated scanning 24–48 hours later.
- *MRI*: This may provide additional information in differentiating tumour from abscess, in the posterior fossa, and in surgical planning.
- Where a mass lesion is identified, CT chest abdo pelvis may be indicated, along with ultrasound of testicles or breast.
- For tumours and abscesses, a histological or microbiological diagnosis should be made on tissue obtained at biopsy.

## Management

Extradural and subdural haematomas are usually drained surgically, and cerebral abscesses should be drained and treated with appropriate antibiotics. The management of a cerebral tumour depends on its type, site and size and on the general condition of the patient. Cerebral oedema is managed with dexamethasone, and obstructive hydrocephalus may be managed with ventricular drainage. Meningiomas and pituitary tumours may be managed by surgical excision, sometimes followed by radiotherapy; or, if they are low-risk, may simply undergo surveillance. Lesions with features characteristic of low-grade glioma may also be managed conservatively. Following tissue diagnosis, malignant gliomas may be managed by surgical excision, radiotherapy and chemotherapy, alone or in combination.

## Prognosis

The prognosis for promptly treated extradural and subdural haematoma, subdural empyema and cerebral abscess is good, but delays in treatment can be fatal. Epilepsy is a frequent complication of cerebral abscess, subdural empyema and brain tumour. The prognosis for glioblastoma is poor, but patients with a solitary cerebral metastasis may do well following successful excision.

## STRUCTURAL LESIONS OF THE SPINE

## SPINAL CORD LESIONS

Prompt recognition and treatment of compressive lesions of the spinal cord can prevent the development of severe neurological disability. Rapidly progressive symptoms are a neurological and potentially a neurosurgical emergency, especially if faecal or urinary continence is impaired. It is important to determine when the patient was last able to walk, stand unaided, pass urine and open their bowels (EMERGENCY PRESENTATION 13.2).

---

### EMERGENCY PRESENTATION 13.2

**Management of suspected spinal cord compression**

**Diagnosis**

Consider the diagnosis in any patient with:
- Spinal pain
- Weakness in legs

Other signs include:
- Sphincter disturbance
- Sensory level
- Loss of reflexes

Look for evidence in the history and examination of malignant disease, which may have metastasized to the cord.

**Investigation**
- Urgent MRI imaging of cord
- Plain radiography
- Chest X-ray
- Biopsy of extradural compressive lesions

**Treatment**
- Dexamethasone may reduce cord oedema
- Urgent referral to neurosurgeon and/or radiation oncologist as appropriate

---

### Epidemiology

- Spinal cord lesions are uncommon.
- In the developed world, spinal cord compression occurs in older people because of cervical spondylosis or metastatic disease. In Africa and South America, tuberculous abscess of the spine is common.
- Non-compressive spinal cord syndromes include MS in the developed world, human T-cell lymphotropic virus (HTLV-1) infections in the tropics (tropical spastic paraplegia), and AIDS myelopathy where HIV infection is endemic.

### Disease mechanisms

- Acute spinal cord dysfunction is commonly due to spinal metastases, cord infarction, demyelination or trauma.
- Other causes of cord compression include spondylitic myelopathy, tumours (e.g. lymphoma, meningioma); syringomyelia or intrinsic cord tumours; paraspinal abscess, central disc prolapse and atlantoaxial subluxation in rheumatoid arthritis.
- Other non-compressive causes include transverse myelitis, vitamin $B_{12}$ deficiency, neurosyphilis and genetic causes.

### Clinical features

- *General clinical features of spinal cord lesions* (**Figure 13.9**):
  - Weak or absent voluntary movement below the lesion

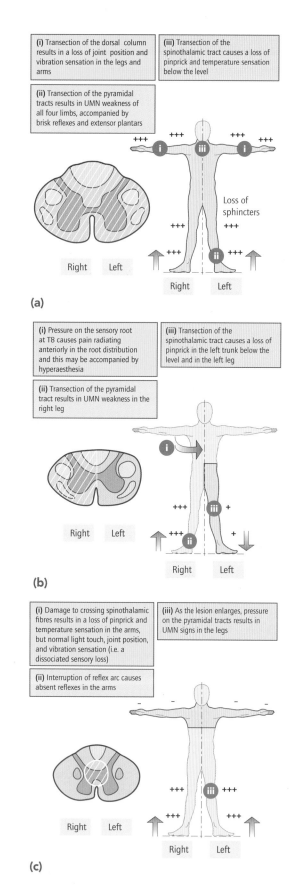

**(i)** Transection of the dorsal column results in a loss of joint position and vibration sensation in the legs and arms

**(iii)** Transection of the spinothalamic tract causes a loss of pinprick and temperature sensation below the level

**(ii)** Transection of the pyramidal tracts results in UMN weakness of all four limbs, accompanied by brisk reflexes and extensor plantars

Loss of sphincters

Right    Left

Right    Left

**(a)**

**(i)** Pressure on the sensory root at T8 causes pain radiating anteriorly in the root distribution and this may be accompanied by hyperaesthesia

**(iii)** Transection of the spinothalamic tract causes a loss of pinprick in the left trunk below the level and in the left leg

**(ii)** Transection of the pyramidal tract results in UMN weakness in the right leg

Right    Left

Right    Left

**(b)**

**(i)** Damage to crossing spinothalamic fibres results in a loss of pinprick and temperature sensation in the arms, but normal light touch, joint position, and vibration sensation (i.e. a dissociated sensory loss)

**(iii)** As the lesion enlarges, pressure on the pyramidal tracts results in UMN signs in the legs

**(ii)** Interruption of reflex arc causes absent reflexes in the arms

Right    Left

Right    Left

**(c)**

**Figure 13.9** Common patterns of cord lesion. **(a)** Cord transection; **(b)** cord hemisection (Brown-Séquard syndrome) at T8; **(c)** cervical central cord syndrome.

○ Reduced or absent sensation below the affected level
○ Brisk reflexes below the level of the lesion and loss of bladder and bowel function

- *Metastatic disease:* There is usually back pain, tenderness on percussing the spine, or radicular (nerve root compression) pain.
- *Infection:* Tuberculous infection can cause severe kyphosis because of destruction of the vertebral body; acute bacterial abscesses cause acute severe back pain and tenderness.
- *MS:* There may be a history of a relapsing–remitting neurological disorder with onset over days and weeks.
- *Acute transverse myelitis:* The onset of symptoms is over minutes or hours and there may be a history of recent infection.
- *Vitamin $B_{12}$ deficiency:* This causes degeneration of both the pyramidal (corticospinal) and dorsal column (posterior spinothalamic) tracts, causing UMN signs in the legs and loss of vibration sensation and proprioception in the feet. An axonal peripheral neuropathy may also occur, giving absent ankle jerks.
- *Acute spinal cord infarction:* This is usually caused by anterior spinal artery occlusion and gives sudden-onset loss of power and spinothalamic (pain and temperature) sensation below the lesion, with preservation of dorsal column sensation (proprioception, vibration and light touch).

### Is the lesion really in the spinal cord?

Patients with brainstem lesions or with bilateral hemisphere lesions may mimic a cord lesion, with UMN and sensory signs in all limbs, but the presence of dysphasia or confusion or cranial nerve palsies places the lesion *above* the spinal cord. UMN signs restricted to one limb are usually caused by intracranial rather than spinal cord pathology.

## SPINAL NERVE ROOT LESIONS

Root lesions are rarely associated with serious underlying disease. They are commonly caused by compression due either to spondylitic disease or to prolapsed intervertebral disc (PLID). Other causes include herpes, meningitis and metastatic disease. Root lesions are a major cause of distress and work absences.

Root lesions cause pain, weakness and loss of sensation and tendon reflexes in the cutaneous distribution (dermatome) and muscles (myotome) supplied by that root. The pain often radiates down the limb and may be exacerbated by traction on the root (e.g. neck turning, coughing). An aching pain that does not radiate below the knees is often due to facet joint disease.

Specific manifestations include:

- *Cauda equina syndrome,* giving sensory loss over the genitalia, perineum and buttocks, with urinary retention and faecal incontinence and usually due to a central disc prolapse

- *An isolated T1 root lesion* causing weakness and wasting of the small muscles of the hand, numbness over the medial aspect of the forearm and an ipsilateral Horner's syndrome due to a cervical rib or an apical chest tumour (Pancoast's syndrome)

### Investigation of cord and root lesions

MRI is the investigation of choice. If the MRI is normal, CSF analysis and various blood tests (protein electrophoresis, angiotensin-converting enzyme, vitamin $B_{12}$ levels) may be helpful.

### Management of spinal cord and root lesions

- Seek immediate specialist neurological or neurosurgical advice where there is a rapidly progressive weakness, especially with sphincter involvement: emergency discectomy is indicated for acute central disc prolapse, and malignant cord compression may respond to emergency radiotherapy with reversal of the neurological deficit. Dexamethasone may reduce cord oedema.
- For acute disc prolapse without cord involvement, most cases will improve spontaneously over 4–6 months without surgical intervention.
- For other presentations, the management is largely that of the underlying cause, alongside supportive treatments to prevent the complications of tetraparesis or paraparesis.

## SYRINGOMYELIA

In this rare condition, a central fluid-filled cavity develops in the spinal cord (syringomyelia) or brainstem (syringo-bulbia). It may be associated with congenital abnormalities at the foramen magnum or occur secondary to a tumour of the cord or to trauma. The expanding cavity compresses sensory fibres crossing the midline on their way to join the lateral spinothalamic tract; later, it may also compress the corticospinal tracts. There is loss of pain and temperature (but not light touch, proprioception or vibration) sensation at the segmental levels of the syrinx along with reflex loss at that level. As symptoms progress UMN signs may develop in the legs.

The syrinx and any associated pathologies are seen at MRI. Placement of a syringoperitoneal shunt may relieve pain and arrest progression of the neurological deficit.

## DISORDERS OF CEREBROSPINAL FLUID DYNAMICS

## HYDROCEPHALUS

Hydrocephalus is an increased ventricular volume, usually associated with increased CSF pressure. If it is developed before closure of the skull sutures (about 2 years of age), the

**Table 13.5** Management of disorders of CSF dynamics

**Obstructive hydrocephalus**
- Temporary (ventricular access device with external ventricular drainage) or permanent (ventriculoperitoneal or ventriculoatrial shunting) may be required

**Idiopathic intracranial hypertension**
- Exclude cerebral sinus thrombosis with CTV or MRV
- Identify and discontinue drugs associated with IIH (OCP, vitamin A, tetracyclines)
- Measure and monitor visual fields
- In the longer term, usually responds to weight loss and diuretics (e.g. acetazolamide)
- Progressive visual loss indicates need for permanent CSF drainage procedure such as lumboperitoneal shunting or optic nerve sheath fenestration

CTV, CT venogram; IIH, idiopathic intracranial hypertension; MRV, MR venogram; OCP, oral contraceptive pill.

skull will be enlarged. While long-standing hydrocephalus can be asymptomatic, acute dilatation of the ventricular system or rises in CSF pressure are almost always symptomatic.

Obstructive hydrocephalus may occur at the third ventricle (Colloid cyst), cerebral aqueduct or in the posterior fossa. Non-obstructive (communicating) hydrocephalus may be due to impaired CSF reabsorption (SAH, meningitis) or excessive CSF production (choroid plexus papilloma) or may simply be a reflection of reduced brain volume.

- *Manifestations:* These include impaired consciousness, gait abnormalities, seizures, pituitary dysfunction and bilateral UMN signs.
- *Investigation:* This includes brain imaging and, where there is a communicating hydrocephalus of unknown cause, CSF examination may be helpful.
- *Management:* Long-standing compensated hydrocephalus is managed conservatively. Patients with symptomatic hydrocephalus may require surgical drainage (with a ventriculoperitoneal shunt) (**Table 13.5**).
- *Prognosis:* If appropriately treated, the prognosis is that of the underlying cause.

## IDIOPATHIC INTRACRANIAL HYPERTENSION

### Epidemiology

- Rare
- Occurs in young and middle-aged women
- 75% of patients female

### Disease mechanisms

This condition of unknown aetiology usually occurs in obese females; it may be drug-related (e.g. tetracyclines, oral contraceptives, vitamin A overdosage) or related to endocrine dysfunction (e.g. Addison's disease), and in some patients it may be associated with cortical venous thrombosis.

### Clinical features

Patients present with headaches typical of raised intra-cranial pressure with papilloedema but without focal neurological signs. There may be episodes of transient visual loss caused by waves of increased intracranial pressure reducing retinal perfusion. Visual fields should be charted every 6 months to ensure there is no progressive field defect.

### Investigation

- *Urgent CT scan:* This is required to exclude a mass lesion or obstructive hydrocephalus.
- *Lumbar puncture:* CSF should be obtained by LP if the CT scan is normal; the diagnosis is confirmed if the pressure is elevated, the CSF is acellular and its protein level is normal.
- *CT or MR venography:* This is required to exclude thrombosis of the cerebral sinuses

### Management

- Where present, venous thrombosis should be treated.
- Most patients respond to weight loss and carbonic anhydrase inhibitors such as acetazolamide.
- Those whose symptoms progress may require neurosurgical treatment in the form of optic nerve fenestration or thecoperitoneal shunting.

### Prognosis

With appropriate treatment only a few patients develop persistent visual loss. In some, the headache symptoms evolve into chronic migraine.

## DISEASES OF CRANIAL NERVES

Cranial nerves dysfunction may be a component of other problems discussed elsewhere. Here we focus on those problems with a primary effect on the cranial nerves.

## COMPRESSION

Brain swelling may lead to herniation of the uncus downwards through the tentorium cerebri and compression of the oculomotor (IIIrd) nerve as it passes over the free edge of the tentorium. This is the cause of a fixed dilated pupil and indicates severe brain swelling requiring immediate treatment. The abducens (VIth) nerve has a long intracranial course and may be compressed or stretched by raised intracranial pressure. Conversely, patients may experience a transient VIth nerve palsy following LP.

More distally, the oculomotor nerve runs near the posterior communicating artery and expanding aneurysms of the posterior cerebral artery (PCA) may cause a IIIrd nerve palsy (ptosis; fixed eye; dilated unreactive pupil) with pain around the eye on that side. Similarly, the optic nerve may be compressed by aneurysms of the carotid, anterior communicating or ophthalmic arteries causing a visual field defect or a monocular visual loss.

Neuromas of the auditory (VIIIth) nerve may emerge from the internal auditory meatus and grow in the space between the anterolateral aspect of the cerebellum and the posterolateral aspect of the pons (the cerebellopontine angle). As well as causing deafness because of involvement of the auditory nerve, there may also be compression and dysfunction of the facial (VIIth) and the trigeminal (Vth) nerve.

Intermittent or pulsatile compression from aberrant loops of blood vessel is thought to be the cause of some cases of trigeminal neuralgia (trigeminal [Vth] nerve) and hemifacial spasm (facial [VIIth] nerve); surgical decompression may give dramatic relief of symptoms in those patients unresponsive to medical treatment (gabapentin; carbamazepine; amitriptyline).

## IMPAIRED VASCULAR SUPPLY

Each nerve carries with it its own blood vessels or vasa nervorum, and occlusion of the arterial supply to a nerve causes it to cease to function. In most cases, function returns, usually over 4–8 weeks. The oculomotor (IIIrd) and abducens (VIth) nerves are most often affected, and causes include diabetes, hypertension, arteriosclerosis and, less commonly, vasculitides including temporal arteritis. Such 'medical' causes of IIIrd nerve palsies may be painful, but the pupillary response to light is almost always normal. However, this clinical distinction is often difficult to make with certainty, and so it is reasonable to exclude a posterior communicating artery aneurysm in all patients presenting with a IIIrd nerve palsy.

## INFLAMMATION

An inflammatory demyelinating neuropathy can affect cranial nerves, either in isolation or as part of a more generalized neuropathy.

*Bell's palsy* is a benign, self-limiting, lower motor neurone facial weakness of unknown cause and is the most common lesion of a single cranial nerve. All facial muscles on that side are affected. It needs to be differentiated from more serious causes of a peripheral lesion, and from facial weakness resulting from a central lesion (e.g. hemisphere or brainstem), by the absence of other symptoms or signs.

Bilateral lower motor neurone facial weakness can be difficult to spot and sometimes the only clue is that the patient is unable to smile.

Other causes of VIIth cranial nerve lesions include GBS, HIV infection, Lyme disease, lymphoma and sarcoidosis.

## DISEASES OF PERIPHERAL NERVES AND THE NEUROMUSCULAR JUNCTION

## MOTOR NEURONE DISEASE

### Epidemiology

- MND is rare before the age of 50. The incidence rises with age.
- Prevalence is around 8 in 100 000.
- Around 10% of cases have an affected first-degree relative, and some of these kindreds have mutations in genes for superoxide dismutase, C9ORF and others.

### Clinical features

MND commonly starts with progressive weakness, wasting and fasciculation of initially one but later all four limbs. Reflexes are brisk, with increased tone, clonus and extensor plantars. This combination of upper and lower motor neurone features in the absence of sensory changes is strongly suggestive of MND. There may be slurred speech, difficulty swallowing, choking, and nasal regurgitation of food and fluid due to bulbar involvement, with increased jaw jerk, and a slow, stiff, waster fasciculating tongue. Involvement of the intercostal muscles and the diaphragm may lead to type II respiratory failure. There may be wasting and fasciculation of the intercostal muscles.

### Investigation

- *Electromyography* (EMG): shows widespread denervation and reinnervation
- *MRI of the cervical and lumbar spine:* may be needed to rule out cervical spondylosis

### Management and prognosis

Patients should be managed in a specialist multidisciplinary MND clinic. There is no disease-modifying treatment, but riluzole may slow disease progression. Chronic respiratory failure may be managed with non-invasive nocturnal ventilation, and enteral feeding (percutaneous endoscopic gastrostomy [PEG] or radiologically inserted gastrostomy [RIG]) may be required for dysphagia.

Median survival is 3 years from symptom onset, and shorter if bulbar signs are present.

## PERIPHERAL NEUROPATHY

Peripheral neuropathy is a dysfunction of lower motor neurones or sensory neurones or both. Hereditary motor and sensory neuropathy (HMSN) has at least 76 recognized genetic causes, which may be autosomal dominant or recessive, or X-linked. Some are due to genes integral to normal nerve function while others may be secondary to metabolic disturbance.

Acquired peripheral neuropathy may occur:
- In systemic disorders such as diabetes or chronic renal failure
- Due to toxins such as alcohol or lead
- Due to deficiency of, for instance, vitamin $B_{12}$
- In endocrine disorders such as hypothyroidism
- In inflammatory conditions such as SLE or vasculitis

### Disease mechanisms

The three main mechanisms underlying generalized neuropathies are:
- *Demyelinating:* loss of the myelin sheath, often the result of immune-mediated damage
- *Axonal:* loss of nerve cells, often related to metabolic or toxic processes (e.g. alcohol)
- *Vasculitic*

### Clinical features

Motor neuropathies cause distal weakness and wasting in the hands and feet (**Figure 13.10**) and sensory neuropathies cause sensory loss in the hands and feet ('glove and stocking'). Autonomic neuropathies cause features of autonomic failure including postural hypotension, loss of sinus arrhythmia, reduced sweating, diarrhoea, impotence and, if severe, retention of urine or constipation. Hereditary neuropathies may manifest pes cavus, slowly progressive distal leg weakness, atrophy and sensory loss, marked hypertrophy of peripheral nerves, tremor, or ataxia.

### Investigation and management

Often no cause can be identified. Investigation aims to demonstrate pathology in the peripheral nerves, and then to attempt to identify the cause. Extensive tests are required to screen for infective and metabolic causes and to rule out other illnesses that may give rise to neuropathy as a secondary phenomenon. Nerve conduction studies confirm that a

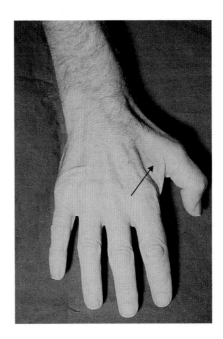

**Figure 13.10** Wasting of first dorsal interosseous in ulnar neuropathy.

neuropathy is present and may help to distinguish between demyelinating and axonal neuropathies. Nerve biopsy may be helpful, especially if infection (e.g. leprosy), vasculitis or demyelinating neuropathy is suspected.

Treatment comprises physiotherapy and occupational therapy, and treatment of any underlying cause.

## GUILLAIN–BARRÉ SYNDROME

GBS is the most common acute neuropathy (annual incidence 1.5 in 100 000); early recognition and appropriate management are essential because death can result from respiratory failure or autonomic dysregulation. Antibodies raised in response to infection cross-react with particular sugars (gangliosides) found on Schwann cell membranes, resulting an autoimmune inflammatory demyelinating polyradiculopathy.

GBS begins a few days after an acute infection, with distal tingling and then weakness; there may be back pain. The weakness is accompanied by areflexia and may progress rapidly to a complete flaccid quadriparesis with respiratory paralysis, and 25% of patients require ventilation. Autonomic involvement can lead to cardiac arrhythmias and labile blood pressure.

### Investigation

- *Lumbar puncture:* shows elevated CSF protein but the white cell count is usually normal; if the white cell count is elevated, consider alternative diagnoses
- *Nerve conduction studies:* usually show marked slowing of nerve conduction velocities, and antiganglioside antibodies may be detected in serum; however, in acutely ill patients these tests may not be available in time to influence management
- *Respiratory function:* should be monitored by measuring vital capacity, with arrangements for respiratory support if vital capacity falls below 1 litre

### Management and prognosis

Treatment with either plasma exchange or intravenous immunoglobulin speeds recovery. Patients may have a prolonged period of paralysis requiring ventilation; they will require considerable psychological support and should receive daily physiotherapy to prevent flexion contractures, heparin as deep-vein thrombosis prophylaxis, and analgesia if required.

Two-thirds of patients will eventually recover completely, but there is significant mortality (8%), principally from respiratory failure or pulmonary embolism.

## CHRONIC INFLAMMATORY DEMYELINATING POLYNEUROPATHY

This rare condition is, like GBS, caused by immune-mediated demyelination; however, it is distinguished from GBS in that, by definition, it continues to worsen for at least 2 months from onset; preceding infection is less commonly identified, and the natural history is of a chronic progressive course.

### Clinical features

These are similar to those of GBS, but respiratory muscle, cranial nerve and autonomic involvement is less common in chronic inflammatory demyelinating polyneuropathy and reflex loss is often asymmetrical.

### Investigation

- *CSF:* shows elevation of CSF protein, perhaps also a CSF pleocytosis, unlike GBS
- *Nerve conduction studies:* show slowed conduction

### Management and prognosis

Management includes intravenous immunoglobulin or plasma exchange, and long-term low-dose corticosteroids, perhaps with a steroid sparing agent such as azathioprine.

Some patients accumulate mild persistent disability with recurrent episodes.

## MONONEUROPATHIES

Mononeuropathy (dysfunction of a single peripheral nerve) is usually caused by local compression or trauma, but there may be increased vulnerability to such lesions because of an otherwise subclinical generalized neuropathy. Most commonly involved sites are the median nerve at the wrist (carpal tunnel syndrome); the ulnar nerve at the elbow; the common peroneal nerve at the fibular head; and the lateral cutaneous nerve of the thigh (meralgia paraesthetica). Carpal tunnel syndrome is common, and causes pain in the hand, especially at night, which may be relieved by rubbing or shaking the hand. There can be sensory loss in the lateral side of the hand and weakness and wasting of the thenar eminence muscles (abductor pollicis brevis, opponens pollicis, flexor pollicis brevis). Carpal tunnel syndrome is more common in pregnancy, hypothyroidism, rheumatoid arthritis and acromegaly.

Nerve conduction studies are not required with a typical presentation if surgery is not being considered.

Most patients improve spontaneously. Carpal tunnel syndrome may respond to surgical decompression and weight loss may cure meralgia paraesthetica.

## OTHER PERIPHERAL NERVE PROBLEMS

### Mononeuritis multiplex

This may be caused by diabetes mellitus, polyarteritis nodosa, SLE and rheumatoid arthritis. Rarer causes include sarcoidosis, paraproteinaemia, carcinomas, leprosy, AIDS and intravenous drug abuse.

More than one nerve is affected at the same time, and enough nerves may be affected for the features to be indistinguishable from those of a peripheral neuropathy. Nerve conduction studies and nerve biopsy may be required.

### Brachial plexus lesions

Lesions can be caused by trauma, malignant infiltration, radiation fibrosis or inflammation. Complete lesions give a wasted, weak, numb and areflexic arm; partial lesions may also cause pain in the arm.

### Brachial neuritis (neuralgic amyotrophy)

This is characterized by severe pain in the shoulder for 1–3 days followed by the development of weakness and wasting of the shoulder and upper arm muscles as the pain resolves; reflexes may be absent. While the cause is unknown, it is thought to be caused by inflammation of the plexus.

## MYASTHENIA GRAVIS

Patients complain of weakness, double vision, drooping eyelids, impaired voice and difficulty swallowing that worsen as the day progresses. At examination, there may be fatiguable weakness of ocular, bulbar, respiratory or limb muscles. The pupils remain normal, reflexes are preserved and there is no sensory loss. Problems may be restricted to the ocular muscles.

Antibodies to the nicotinic acetylcholine receptor cause competitive inhibition of transmission at the neuromuscular junction. Some drugs, including penicillamine, may cause myasthenia gravis and others, including gentamicin and tetracycline, may worsen pre-existing disease. There may be an associated thymoma, particularly in patients over 40 years of age.

Anti-acetylcholine receptor antibodies are positive in 85% of patients, and EMG shows decrementing responses to repetitive stimulation. CT thorax is required to exclude a thymoma.

In acute disease, check that the patient's swallowing is safe, and give heparin for prophylaxis of deep-vein thrombosis. Monitor forced vital capacity, and respiratory support may be required. Anticholinesterase drugs may provide immediate relief of symptoms: these prolong the action of acetylcholine by inhibiting the anticholinesterase enzyme. Side effects include bradycardia, increased sweating and salivary secretion, and a depolarizing block (cholinergic crisis) in excessive dosage. Muscarinic side effects can be managed with antagonists such as probantheline. Immunomodulatory treatment with steroids, intravenous immunoglobulin, plasma exchange or azathioprine may be required. Thymectomy is indicated for patients under 40 years whose symptoms are not controlled by anticholinesterase drugs or where CT has suggested the presence of a thymoma.

## LAMBERT–EATON MYASTHENIC SYNDROME

Lambert–Eaton myasthenic syndrome is caused by circulating antibodies to presynaptic voltage-gated calcium channels, leading to impaired recruitment of synaptic vesicles following depolarization. About half of cases are a paraneoplastic phenomenon, usually associated with small cell carcinoma of the bronchus. The main feature is fatiguable limb weakness. Other features include absent reflexes and autonomic features such as dry mouth or impotence. Absent reflexes may return if the relevant muscle groups are exercised (post-tetanic accentuation). Bulbar and ocular features are rare.

EMG shows increased response to repeated stimulation, and patients may respond to pyridostigmine, 3,4-diaminopyridine, and immunomodulation with prednisolone, azathioprine, intravenous immunoglobulin or plasma exchange.

## MUSCLE DISEASE

Causes of muscle disorders are listed in **Table 13.6**.

## PRIMARY MUSCLE DISORDERS

Most muscle disorders have greatest impact on proximal limb and truncal musculature. The characteristic symptoms are of difficulty raising the arms above the head, getting up from low chairs, climbing stairs and sitting up in bed.

## POLYMYOSITIS AND DERMATOMYOSITIS

See Chapter 4, Rheumatic disease.

## DUCHENNE AND BECKER MUSCULAR DYSTROPHIES

### Epidemiology

- Rare
- Occur in childhood (Duchenne) or adult (Becker)
- Males only
- X-linked recessive because of mutations in *dystrophin*

### Disease mechanisms

Dystrophin, a protein needed for the proper functioning of muscles, is subject to many mutations; those in one region are associated with the more common and more aggressive Duchenne muscular dystrophy, while those of another are associated with the less severe Becker dystrophy.

### Clinical features

Symptoms typically begin after the affected boy has learned to walk (**Figure 13.11**); they may develop strategies to overcome their proximal weakness, such as 'climbing' their arms up their legs to rise from the floor (Gower's manoeuvre).

### Management

There is no treatment. Genetic counselling in affected families gives parents the option of, for instance, *in vitro* fertilization (IVF) with pre-implantation genetic testing.

**Table 13.6** Causes of muscle disorders

**Anterior horn cell disease** (spinal muscular atrophy)
- Infantile (Werdnig–Hoffman type)
- Juvenile (Kugelberg–Welander type)
- Adult spinal muscular atrophy

**Mitochondrial disease**
- Mitochondrial myopathy with ophthalmoplegia
- Mitochondrial encephalopathy with lactic acidosis and stroke-like episodes
- Mitochondrial myopathy with myoclonus, epilepsy and typical 'ragged-red fibres' on muscle biopsy

**Inflammatory muscle disease**
- Polymyositis
- Dermatomyositis
- Inclusion body myositis

**Genetically determined muscle disease**
- Duchenne and Becker muscular dystrophies
- Emery–Dreifuss muscular dystrophy
- Limb girdle muscular dystrophy
- Carnitine palmitoyl-transferase deficiency
- Myophosphorylase deficiency
- Phosphofructokinase deficiency
- Acid maltase deficiency
- Dystrophia myotonica
- Glycogen storage diseases

**Periodic paralysis**
- Hypokalaemic periodic paralysis
- Hyperkalaemic periodic paralysis

**Non-metastatic effect of malignancy**
- Paraneoplastic myopathy

**Electrolyte imbalance**
- Hypokalaemia
- Hypocalcaemia

**Endocrine disease**
- Hypo- or hyperthyroidism
- Hypo- or hyperparathyroidism
- Addison's disease
- Cushing's syndrome
- Acromegaly

**Drugs and toxins**
- Alcohol
- Corticosteroids
- Clofibrate
- Zidovudine
- HMG-CoA reductase inhibitors (e.g. simvastatin)

## Prognosis

In Duchenne muscular dystrophy, most patients use wheelchairs by their teens and die in their twenties. Becker muscular dystrophy is much less severe, and most patients die with their disease rather than because of it.

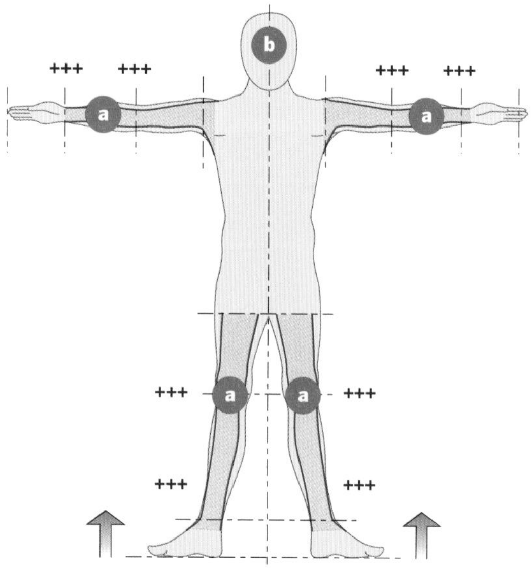

**Figure 13.11** Symptoms and signs of neuromuscular disease.

# DYSTROPHIA MYOTONICA (MYOTONIC DYSTROPHY)

## Epidemiology

- Affects 5 in 100 000 (Type 1) and 9 in 100 000 (Type 2)
- Autosomal dominant trinucleotide (DM1) and tetranucleotide (DM2) repeat disorder affecting the genes for *myotonic dystrophy protein kinase* (DM1) or CCHC-type zinc finger nucleic acid-binding protein (DM2)

## Clinical features

These include distal muscle weakness and wasting, frontal balding, cataracts, ptosis, type 1 diabetes and a typical facial appearance (**Figure 13.12**). Patients have difficulty relaxing muscles after use, which may reveal itself as an inability to let go after shaking hands.

## Investigation

- *EMG:* findings are typical
- *DNA testing*

## Management

Annual review is needed to detect the development of complications. Procainamide or phenytoin may be used for the weakness, and some patients require a cardiac pacemaker. Genetic counselling in affected families gives parents the

**13**

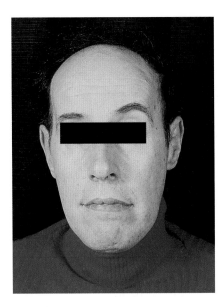

**Figure 13.12** Typical facies of myotonic dystrophy.

option of, for instance, IVF with pre-implantation genetic testing.

**Prognosis**

The condition is slowly progressive.

## SYSTEMIC DISORDERS AND THE NERVOUS SYSTEM

Changes in the periphery such as pregnancy, systemic diseases, drugs and toxins can all impact on the functioning of the nervous system; further, services must adapt to meet the hitherto unmet neurological needs of the elderly patients who primarily have neurological disorders and often have impairments in other organ systems. Close integration between neurology and other medical teams is therefore very important.

## EVIDENCE-BASED NEUROLOGY

The practice of neurology should, where possible, be based on firm evidence that a treatment is likely to be effective. As new evidence becomes available, so treatments should also change. The pace at which new information becomes available means that treatment decisions should be based not on what is written in books but on more up-to-date systematic reviews, meta-analyses, or formal evidence-based management guidelines.

### MUST-KNOW CHECKLIST

- What is the most important source of information in reaching a diagnosis in neurology?
- Describe the characteristic lesions causing the immediate, slow and very slow development of neurological symptoms.
- Describe the difference between upper and lower motor neurone weakness.
- What is the role of drug monitoring in treatment for epilepsy?
- From whom does one obtain a history of cognitive impairment or altered consciousness?
- Describe the modes of action available for the treatment of PD.
- Differentiate between clinical and biological significance in the interpretation of drug treatment trials.
- Is CT scanning sufficient to make the diagnosis of brain tumour?
- Describe treatment options in patients with stroke.
- What sources of information, help and advice are there for patients newly diagnosed with a neurological condition?

**Questions and answers** to test your understanding of Chapter 13 can be found by clicking 'Support Material' at the following link: https://www.routledge.com/Medicine-for-Finals-and-Beyond/Axford-OCallaghan/p/book/9780367150594

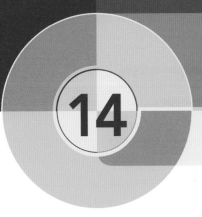

# Psychological Medicine

## 14

### HARRISON HOWARTH, JIM BOLTON & GARY BELL

## INTRODUCTION

There is an artificial division between the mind and body in our thinking, demonstrated in the way psychiatric services are often delivered separately to general medical services. Illnesses of all kinds have biological, psychological and social components, and it may be counterproductive to separate them on the basis of affliction of mind or body.

Advances in understanding the causes, course and management of a number of physical disorders highlight the relevance of psychological and social factors and demonstrate the need for an integrated approach to patient care.

## APPROACH TO THE PATIENT

The aims of the psychiatric assessment are to:
- Take a detailed history and mental state examination
- Make a diagnosis
- Perform a risk assessment
- Formulate a management plan

Establishing a good working relationship with the patient is essential for obtaining a full and accurate history.

## HISTORY AND EXAMINATION

### HISTORY TAKING

#### Demographics

Document the patient's age, sex, marital status, racial and cultural background, and present occupation.

#### Current symptoms

Ask about the nature of the symptoms, their duration and the extent to which they impair the patient's daily function. Ask if the patient receives any support.

#### Past medical and psychiatric history

Record details of:
- Previous illnesses
- Hospital admissions
- Treatments prescribed

#### Family history

Ask the patient if anyone in their family has a history of physical or psychiatric illness, including drug or alcohol misuse. It is also important to ask about a family history of suicide. Relationships with family members should also be discussed.

#### Personal history

A full personal history should include:
- Birth and developmental milestones
- Early family life
- Educational attainments
- Occupational history
- Psychosexual development (sexual abuse, sexual orientation, number of partners)
- Interpersonal relationships

#### Social history

The personal history leads into an up-to-date account of the current social situation, including home, family and work.

DOI: 10.1201/9781003193616-14

## Forensic history

Note any past criminal offences and periods in prison or on probation.

## Current medication

Many drugs prescribed for physical illnesses can affect mood. Drugs prescribed for psychological illnesses can have physical side effects.

## Tobacco, alcohol and substance misuse

Ask about the substance used, frequency and context of use. The CAGE questionnaire is a useful screening instrument for excessive alcohol use (see 'Alcohol misuse and dependence' below).

## Premorbid personality

Attempting to make an assessment of a person's personality before the onset of their illness is often one of the most challenging, but revealing, aspects of eliciting the history. Consider their coping style, relationships, interests and activities prior to becoming unwell. Personality trait models may help you to determine changes in personality that have occurred with illness (e.g. Costa's Big Five personality traits: openness to experience, conscientiousness, extroversion, agreeableness and neuroticism). Premorbid personality may need to be obtained through a collateral history.

# PHYSICAL EXAMINATION

Examine for potential causes of a presentation (e.g. hyperthyroidism in a presentation of mania) and possible complications (e.g. self-harm in a patient with personality disorder). General systems examination is also recommended.

# MENTAL STATE EXAMINATION

The mental state examination is described in detail in HISTORY & EXAMINATION 14.1.

## DIFFERENTIAL DIAGNOSIS

## CLASSIFICATION OF MENTAL DISORDERS

In physical medicine, a diagnosis usually depends on identifying the cause of a condition; in psychological medicine, it more often relies on identification of syndromes. We then group symptoms together and classify them, for example as mood disorders or psychotic disorders.

## DIAGNOSTIC HIERARCHY

When considering the differential diagnosis of mental illness, it is helpful to use a diagnostic hierarchy where a diagnosis in one group of conditions takes precedence over those in the groups below (**Table 14.1**).

---

## HISTORY & EXAMINATION 14.1

### Mental state examination

#### Appearance and general behaviour
Consider rapport, eye-contact and look for:
- Signs of self-neglect
- Abnormalities in movement/posture
- Defence mechanisms (hostility/denial)
- Visible self-harm

#### Affect and mood
Record the patient's emotional state, both observed and reported, and note inconsistencies between the two. All patients should be asked about suicidal ideation. There is no evidence that asking a patient about suicidal ideation increases the risk that they will harm themselves.

#### Flow of thought and speech
Comment on the rate, volume and tone of speech. Listen for:
- Pressure of speech (i.e. fast and difficult to interrupt)
- Retardation of speech (i.e. slow and often inaudible)

#### Content of thought and speech
Document *what* the patient says. Look out for evidence of obsessions or delusions.
- *Obsession:* A thought, image or idea that repeatedly intrudes upon consciousness. It is recognized by the patient as a product of his or her own mind.
- *Delusion:* A firmly held false belief which is inconsistent with the patient's social, cultural and religious background. Note whether a delusion is consistent with a patient's emotional state.

#### Form of thought and speech
Listen to how ideas are linked together. Record examples. Listen for:
- Flight of ideas (a rapid shift from one idea to the next)
- Loosening of associations (i.e. the logical connections between ideas breaks down)
- Neologisms (i.e. new words, e.g. 'blattered')

#### Abnormal perceptions and experiences
Note any abnormal behaviour during the interview that suggests that the patient is experiencing hallucinations or illusions. Observe for and ask about passivity experiences.
- A *hallucination* is an abnormal perception occurring in the absence of an external stimulus.
- An *illusion* is a misinterpretation of an external stimulus.
- *Passivity* is the experience that one's body actions, thoughts, feelings and impulses are being controlled by someone or something.
- *Depersonalization and derealization* are the feelings that one is unreal or that everything around one is unreal.

#### Cognitive state
Assess:
- Level of consciousness
- Orientation in time, place and person
- Attention and concentration
- Registration, or immediate recall
- Short-term memory, i.e. learning new material
- Long-term memory, both for general knowledge and autobiographical information

#### Insight
Ask the patient to explain their understanding of their symptoms, and whether they see themselves as ill and in need of treatment.

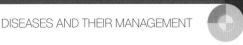

**Table 14.1** Diagnostic hierarchy of psychiatric disorders

A diagnosis in one group takes precedence over those in the groups below.
1. Organic mental disorders and conditions secondary to alcohol and substance misuse
2. Psychotic disorders, including schizophrenia
3. Mood disorders, including depressive disorder and bipolar affective disorder
4. Neurotic disorders, including anxiety-related disorders

## INVESTIGATION

A list of general investigations that might be considered in a case of mental disorder is given in **Table 14.2**. Investigations should not be routine; the choice should be guided by the clinical presentation.

## PRINCIPLES OF MANAGEMENT

The management of any psychiatric disorder must be comprehensive and requires a team approach to physical, psychological and social treatments. Possible causative factors should be considered, divided chronologically into those factors which predispose to an illness, precipitate its manifestation and perpetuate the symptoms.

**Table 14.2** General investigations

**Corroborative information**
Observations of medical staff
Collateral history from relatives, friends and other health professionals
Previous medical, psychiatric or primary care records

**Laboratory investigations**
*Haematology*
Full blood count: to detect anaemia, infection, and a raised mean corpuscular volume (MCV) in alcohol misuse
*Biochemistry*
U&Es: to reveal electrolyte disturbances, and dehydration
CRP: to detect inflammation and infection
Calcium: hyper- and hypocalcaemia can cause depression and anxiety respectively
Thyroid function tests: hyper- and hypothyroidism can cause mania/anxiety and depression respectively
Liver function tests: to detect liver dysfunction in alcohol misuse
Urinary drug screen: to detect illicit drug use
*Microbiology*
MSU, blood cultures, virology, lumbar puncture: to detect infection

**Diagnostic imaging**
*Chest radiography:* to reveal chest infection and malignancy
*CT or MRI head scan:* to detect intracranial pathology
*EEG:* to investigate possible epileptic seizures

## DISEASES AND THEIR MANAGEMENT

There are a number of ways in which physical and psychiatric disorders can interact. Medical patients may have coincidental psychiatric disorders; hence a working knowledge of the range of common psychiatric disorders is required.

## PSYCHIATRIC COMPLICATIONS OF PHYSICAL ILLNESS

Psychiatric complications of physical illness include disease- and/or treatment-induced organic mental disorders, as well as psychological reactions to physical illnesses and their treatments.

### ORGANIC MENTAL DISORDERS

Organic mental disorders are those where the symptoms are attributable to an independently diagnosable cerebral or systemic disease (**Figure 14.1**; **Table 14.3**).

#### Delirium

Delirium is a common and serious acute neuropsychiatric syndrome with core features of inattention and cognitive impairment, and associated features including changes in arousal, altered sleep–wake cycle, and other changes in mental status. It should be considered in any medical patient with a sudden deterioration in mental state.

*Epidemiology*
- Delirium most commonly occurs in the elderly.
- It affects an estimated 14–56% of hospitalized elderly patients, but only 25% of cases are identified.

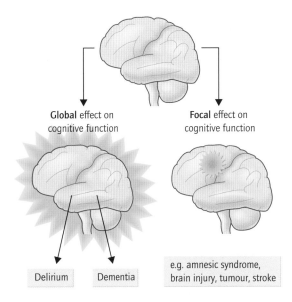

**Figure 14.1** Organic mental disorders.

**Table 14.3** Organic mental disorders

**Dementia (chronic)**
- Alzheimer's disease
- Vascular dementia
- Frontotemporal dementia
- Dementia with Lewy bodies

**Delirium (acute)**
- Primary cerebral pathology
- Systemic disease
- Drug-induced
- Drug withdrawal

**Organic amnesic syndrome**
- Korsakov syndrome

**Other organic disorders**
- Traumatic brain injury
- Personality disorders due to brain disease and dysfunction or physical illness

### Causes

Delirium has many possible causes; both intra- and extracerebral. Causes include:
- Infections (particularly chest and urine)
- Brain tumours or haemorrhages
- Medication-induced (analgesia, hypnotics, psychotropics)
- Drug-induced (alcohol, stimulants, opioids)
- Drug withdrawal

### Clinical features

Delirium usually develops suddenly and often lasts no more than a few days, following a fluctuating course. Cognitive function tends to be globally impaired. The level of consciousness (and therefore confusion) varies, often being worse at night.

Clinically it presents as hyperactive, hypoactive or mixed states. The hyperactive presentation is associated with restlessness, agitation, hallucinations and delusions. Hypoactive delirium presents with lethargy and drowsiness.

Hallucinations and illusions are common and are usually visual.

### Investigation

Investigations should be carried out to identify the underlying cause of the delirium, including blood tests, urine analysis, and imaging scans if appropriate (chest X-ray, CT head).

### Management

The most important aspect of management is to identify and treat the underlying cause.

Symptomatic relief is also important. Consider discontinuing contributing medications. Provide well-lit, quiet surroundings. Correct any sensory deficits (e.g. missing hearing aids or glasses) and encourage relatives to visit.

Keep a fluid balance chart to avoid dehydration and prescribe adequate pain relief. Sedative medication should be avoided if possible and only prescribed when other measures are ineffective and the patient's behaviour poses a significant risk to themselves or others.

### Prognosis

Delirium is a medical emergency and is associated with a high mortality both during hospital admission and in the following months.

## Dementia

Dementia is a syndrome of acquired chronic global impairment of higher mental functions (i.e. personality, intellect and memory), *without* impairment of consciousness. Certain clinical features help to differentiate dementia from delirium (**Table 14.4**).

### Epidemiology
- Approximately 20% of those aged 80 years and over are affected
- Primarily the elderly
- Overall prevalence is similar between sexes, but Alzheimer's disease more common in women
- Sporadic Alzheimer's disease is three times more prevalent in heterozygotes for the apolipoprotein ε4 allele and 15 times in homozygotes

### Causes and disease mechanisms

The two most common types of dementia in the elderly are Alzheimer's disease (50%) and vascular dementia (25%). The cause of Alzheimer's disease is unknown, but genetic factors appear to be involved. Vascular dementia results from cerebral ischaemic changes due to hypertension, generalized atherosclerosis or stroke. Other less common

**Table 14.4** Differential diagnosis of delirium and dementia

| Feature | Delirium | Dementia |
|---|---|---|
| Onset | Acute | Usually insidious |
| Duration | Transient | Persistent |
| Course | Fluctuating over hours, worse at night, lucid intervals | Stable over days |
| Conscious level | Reduced | Normal |
| Sleep–wake cycle stages | Disrupted | Often normal in early |
| Perception misidentifications | Impaired (illusions, hallucinations) | Uncommon in early illness |
| Autonomic changes | Common | Uncommon |
| Psychomotor changes | Common | Uncommon |

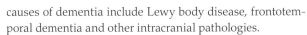
causes of dementia include Lewy body disease, frontotemporal dementia and other intracranial pathologies.

In Alzheimer's disease, there is progressive atrophy that predominantly affects the medial temporal and parietal cortex.

Larger-vessel vascular dementia is caused by discrete large strategic infarcts, and small-vessel vascular dementia by widespread subcortical micro-infarcts and incomplete infarction and ischaemia.

### Clinical features
Dementia usually develops gradually, and the most common symptom is poor memory. Presentation is, however, highly variable and often characterized by changes in many higher functions, including personality, behaviour, mood and intellect.

- *Alzheimer's disease* is characterized by a slow and progressive course in which there is an early loss of memory and a global deterioration of higher functions.
- *Large-vessel vascular dementia* causes a stepwise deterioration of mental and physical function with focal neurological lesions associated with successive vascular events.
- *Small-vessel vascular dementia* develops slowly and progressively. Symptoms include motor and cognitive slowing, forgetfulness, mood changes, urinary symptoms and short-stepped gait.

### Investigation
Treatable causes of dementia are rare but should be screened for on initial investigations. These include vitamin $B_{12}$ and folate deficiencies, hypothyroidism and anaemia.

### Management
*Psychological and social support* Treatment is largely symptomatic and supportive. In moderate to severe dementia, evaluation of daily living skills by an occupational therapist and of appropriate community-based supports by a social worker are essential.

*Drug treatments*
- *Acetylcholinesterase inhibitors* (donepezil, rivastigmine and galantamine) are recommended in mild to moderate Alzheimer's to improve cognitive function. The N-methyl-D-aspartic acid (NMDA) receptor antagonist memantine is recommended in moderate Alzheimer's intolerant to acetylcholinesterase inhibitors and in severe Alzheimer's. They have a modest effect and should only be started by an experienced specialist.
- *Antipsychotic medication* (e.g. risperidone) *or hypnotics* (short-acting benzodiazepines such as temazepam) in small doses are helpful for agitated and disturbed behaviour or poor sleep, but care is needed as medication can increase confusion and stroke risk.

### Prognosis
Death generally occurs several years after diagnosis, but effective treatment can result in a good quality of life.

## FOCAL ORGANIC DISORDERS

Focal organic disorders occur as the result of discrete brain injuries. Causes include trauma, tumours and strokes. How such disorders are managed often depends on the nature of the symptoms.

### Organic amnesic syndrome

The *amnesic syndrome* results predominantly in memory impairment, while other cognitive functions remain relatively intact.

### Cause
The most common cause is alcohol-related thiamine deficiency, also known as Korsakov's syndrome. A variety of other causes, both thiamine- and non-thiamine-related, have also been described.

### Disease mechanisms
The amnesic syndrome results from degenerative changes in areas of the brain which are involved in forming and retrieving memories, specifically the mammillary bodies, the hippocampus and the medial aspect of the thalami.

### Clinical features
Memory impairment occurs in clear consciousness. There is mixed anterograde and retrograde amnesia.

### Investigation
MRI head may be used to look for atrophy of the mammillary bodies or other areas of the limbic system.

### Management
Profound memory deficit may preclude independent living. Neurorehabilitation may maximize a patient's abilities. Treatment with thiamine (vitamin $B_1$) occasionally results in improvement.

### Prognosis
Prognosis depends on the cause of the underlying lesion; however, with degenerative changes, substantial improvement is unlikely.

## ACUTE BEHAVIOURAL DISTURBANCE

Organic mental disorders may be associated with acute disturbed or violent behaviour, the management of which is discussed in EMERGENCY PRESENTATION 14.1.

## PSYCHOLOGICAL REACTIONS TO PHYSICAL ILLNESS

Physical illness can have profound effects on the mental state of a patient. While some degree of mood disturbance is considered normal, more pronounced reactions include:
- Anxiety-related disorders (see page 554)
- Depressive disorder (see page 552)
- Adjustment disorder

## Adjustment disorder

Adjustment disorder is a state of distress arising in the period of adaptation to a significant life event, such as the diagnosis of a severe physical illness. It occurs in around one-quarter of medical patients.

General management of adjustment disorder is supportive with the aim of facilitating adjustment to a new situation. Patients should be given a clear explanation of their illness, the treatment, and prognosis. They should be allowed to express their feelings and encouraged to explore coping resources.

For further discussion of common emotional reactions to life-threatening illness, see Chapter 16, Palliative medicine.

## Abnormal illness behaviour

Abnormal illness behaviour describes a range of behaviours which occur in response to a physical illness. These include excessive concern about physical health, seeking different medical opinions, and disability out of proportion to the physical disease.

## SOMATIC PRESENTATION OF A PSYCHIATRIC DISORDER

### MEDICALLY UNEXPLAINED SYMPTOMS

A large number of patients throughout health services have physical symptoms which cannot be wholly accounted for by organic disease. Physicians and psychiatrists tend to use different terms when diagnosing medically unexplained symptoms.

- Physicians tend to describe syndromes that commonly present to their specialty, such as 'irritable bowel syndrome' in gastroenterology and 'fibromyalgia' in rheumatology – though these syndromes often arrive in specialty services pre-labelled from general practice (see Chapter 13, Neurological disease).
- Psychiatrists describe syndromes which are often based on causative hypotheses, such as 'somatization disorder' or 'dissociative disorder' (see below).

### Epidemiology

More than one-quarter of new medical outpatients experience bodily symptoms that cannot be explained by organic disease.

### Cause and disease mechanisms

Some medically unexplained symptoms are the somatic (bodily) symptoms of anxiety or depression (see 'Depressive disorder' and 'Anxiety-related disorders' below), although the precise cause of symptoms is often unknown. We all experience bodily sensations, but only a small proportion of these are interpreted as symptoms of disease.

### Clinical features

A number of psychiatric syndromes that include medically unexplained symptoms are described.

- *Somatization disorder:* multiple chronic physical symptoms for which no adequate physical explanation can be found
- *Hypochondriacal disorder:* persistent preoccupation with the possibility of a serious disease
- *Dissociative (conversion) disorder:* patients have symptoms of a neurological disorder (e.g. amnesia, paralysis, convulsions) but no evidence for a primary illness to account for the symptoms

### Investigation

Appropriate investigations for the patient's presenting problem should be carried out. A balance needs to be struck between missing disease and the potential of excessive investigations to perpetuate the disorder.

### Management

Recent stresses and chronic worries should be identified. Provide a coherent explanation of the symptoms, relating mind and body. More severe cases may require specialist cognitive behavioural therapy (CBT).

### Prognosis

For most patients, the symptoms are transient and usually respond to simple reassurance and explanation.

## SIMULATED DISORDERS

Simulated disorders involve the intentional production or feigning of physical or psychological symptoms.

### Clinical features

#### Factitious disorders

Factitious disorders, of which a severe form is often known as Munchausen's syndrome, are characterized by the conscious feigning of physical or psychological symptoms to simulate disease. The motivation for this behaviour is usually obscure, with patients having a psychological need to assume the sick role.

#### Malingering

This is characterized by intentional production of physical or psychological symptoms, motivated by identifiable external incentives (e.g. evading the police or criminal proceedings, financial compensation or obtaining drugs).

### Management

Patients should be confronted about their behaviour but also offered support. A joint medical and psychiatric approach is ideal.

## PHYSICAL COMPLICATIONS OF PSYCHIATRIC DISORDER

## SELF-HARM

Self-harm is most commonly by self-poisoning or self-cutting. People who self-poison are more likely to seek medical attention; 80% of cases presenting to an emergency department are as a result of overdose with prescription or over-the-counter medication.

The signs and symptoms of self-harm are summarized in **Table 14.5**.

### Epidemiology

- Estimated lifetime prevalence is 5–6% in the UK
- Most common in adolescence and young adulthood
- More common in females than males

### Causes

In many cases, self-harm is an impulsive act, precipitated by a recent life stress against a background of chronic social and interpersonal difficulties. In a minority of cases, self-harm is carried out with high suicidal intent.

**Table 14.5** Signs and symptoms of self-harm

| |
| --- |
| **Characteristics more often associated with non-fatal self-harm** |
| Female |
| Younger |
| Marital status: single, divorced, young wife |
| Unemployed |
| Urban environment |
| Lower socioeconomic class |
| **Characteristics more often associated with suicide** |
| Male |
| Older – especially over 45 years |
| Unemployed or retired |
| Socially isolated |
| Poor physical health – especially chronic or painful illnesses |
| Poor mental health – especially schizophrenia, bipolar affective disorder, depressive disorder, alcohol or substance misuse |
| **Features indicating high suicidal intent** |
| Evidence of planning |
| Preparation for a final event, e.g. leaving a note, making a will |
| Act performed alone |
| Act unlikely to be discovered |
| Precautions taken to avoid discovery |
| No effort to get help |
| All available drugs taken |
| Expectation of a fatal outcome |

### Management

- *Assessment of suicide risk:* Initial assessment should include suicidal intent at the time of the act, and ongoing suicide risk.
- *Associated mental disorders:* Of patients who harm themselves, one-third will have had previous contact with psychiatric services and one-third will receive a psychiatric diagnosis following self-harm.
- *Psychosocial assessment:* Anyone presenting to health services following self-harm should receive a psychosocial assessment.

### Prognosis

Following self-harm, risk of further self-injury and suicide is high. Around 15% will self-harm again within 1 year.

## ALCOHOL MISUSE AND DEPENDENCE

Alcohol misuse causes a wide range of physical, psychological and social problems, and places a significant burden on the NHS. In the UK, there are more than one million hospital admissions per year related to alcohol. For more information on the specific physical complications of alcohol

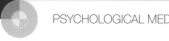

misuse, see Chapter 9, Liver, biliary tract and pancreatic disease.

- *Sensible drinking limits:* Men and women are advised not to consume more than 14 units per week.
- *Hazardous drinking:* This is where an individual's drinking pattern poses a health risk.
- *Harmful (or problem) drinking:* Alcohol at this level contributes to physical, psychological or social harm.
- *Alcohol dependence syndrome:* This represents a severe form of harmful drinking. It consists of a combination of physical and psychological factors.

### Epidemiology

- Around 4% of those aged 16–65 are dependent on alcohol.
- Older people drink more frequently, whereas young people drink more on a single occasion.
- About 75% of patients are male.

### Causes

The cause of alcohol misuse and dependence is a complex interaction of biological, psychological and social factors.

- *Physical*: About 20% of people with chronic alcohol dependence may inherit some genetic predisposition; the evidence is stronger for men than women.
- *Psychological*: The pleasurable effects of intoxication can reinforce drinking behaviour.
- *Sociological*: There may be reinforcement from the social situation where drinking takes place; people who lack other sources of pleasure may be especially susceptible to this.

### Clinical features

#### Screening

A simple screening questionnaire is the CAGE (**Table 14.6**). Two or more questions answered positively should trigger a more detailed assessment.

#### Complications of alcohol misuse

The complications of alcohol misuse include neurological, psychiatric and social disorders.

#### Withdrawal symptoms

Features range from mild discomfort to life-threatening.

- *Early withdrawal:* In the first 12 hours, symptoms include nausea, sweating, anxiety and insomnia.
- *Moderate withdrawal:* Signs are more marked. Transient auditory hallucinations may occur.

**Table 14.6** History taking in alcohol and substance misuse: the CAGE screening questionnaire for alcohol dependence

| |
|---|
| Have you ever felt you ought to **c**ut down on your drinking? |
| Have people **a**nnoyed you by criticizing your drinking? |
| Have you ever felt bad or **g**uilty about your drinking? |
| Have you ever had a drink first thing in the morning (an '**e**ye-opener') to get rid of a hangover? |

- *Withdrawal seizures:* These can occur 12–48 hours after the last drink.
- *Delirium tremens:* This usually occurs 72 hours after the last drink. Clinical features include tremor, confusion, agitation, illusions, hallucinations and pyrexia.

#### Wernicke's encephalopathy

This is the presence of neurological symptoms resulting from central nervous system (CNS) lesions caused by exhaustion of thiamine and other B-vitamin stores. It is most commonly seen in malnourished people with alcohol misuse. The classic triad of symptoms – confusion, ataxia, and eye signs (nystagmus and ophthalmoplegia) – occurs in only 10% of patients. Wernicke's encephalopathy carries a high risk of irreversible brain damage and may lead onto Korsakov's syndrome (see 'Organic amnesic syndrome' above).

### Investigation

Common laboratory findings are a raised mean corpuscular volume (MCV) and gamma-glutamyl transferase (GGT).

### Management

- Patients who experience withdrawal symptoms will need to be detoxified.
- Benzodiazepines such as chlordiazepoxide are used in a reducing regimen to prevent seizures and reduce symptoms of withdrawal.
- Incipient Wernicke's encephalopathy is treated with IV vitamin B+C (Pabrinex).
- Low-risk patients are given thiamine and vitamin B compound strong tablets as prophylaxis.
- Subsequent management is best coordinated by a specialist alcohol team.

### Prognosis

At follow-up, 30–40% of problem drinkers either have successfully abstained from alcohol or practise controlled drinking.

## SUBSTANCE MISUSE AND DEPENDENCE

Substance misuse occurs when a drug is used in a way which is socially unacceptable, illegal or harmful. Misused drugs include the following:

- *Stimulants:* amphetamines, cocaine
- *Hallucinogens:* cannabis, LSD, solvents
- *Opioids:* heroin, morphine, pethidine, codeine, methadone, oxycodone
- *Hypnotics:* benzodiazepines, barbiturates

### Epidemiology

- Around one-third of adults in England and Wales have used illicit drugs at some point in their lives.
- Prevalence of substance misuse is commoner in younger age groups.
- Substance misuse is commoner among men.

## Causes

As for alcohol misuse, the cause of substance misuse in an individual is a complex interaction of biological, psychological and social factors.

## Clinical features

Clinical features will depend on the drug used.

- Opioid misusers often present to general medical services with a disease for which they have increased susceptibility (e.g. infective endocarditis or HIV), or with complications of repeated intravenous injection, such as an abscess. The symptoms of opioid withdrawal are unpleasant but rarely life-threatening (see OPIOID WITHDRAWAL: CLINICAL FEATURES AT A GLANCE). They include:
  - o *Psychological:* anxiety, agitation, fatigue, irritability and insomnia
  - o *Physical:* runny nose, teary eyes, hot and cold sweats, shivers, yawning, muscle aches and pains, abdominal cramps, nausea, diarrhoea and vomiting

In overdose, opioids lead to reduced consciousness, pinpoint pupils and reduced respiratory rate.

- Acute intoxication with stimulant drugs is characterized by agitation, dilated pupils, tremor, pyrexia and cardiac arrhythmia.
- Cocaine induces increased energy associated with an increase in blood pressure and heart rate. There have been reports of abnormalities of cardiac conduction.

## Investigation

- *Biochemistry:* urinary drug screen
- *Microbiology:* hepatitis and HIV serology

## Management

For many substance misusers, medical admission or attendance at the emergency department may be their only contact with health services. This provides an important opportunity to detect substance misuse, assess and treat immediate medical problems, and to facilitate referral to specialist services.

### Opioid overdose

Opioid overdose is a medical emergency. Intravenous naloxone can be life-saving and is often diagnostic as the level of consciousness will improve immediately.

### Medical inpatients

Medical inpatients with opioid misuse should be discussed with specialist services for advice on the management of drug dependency.

### Withdrawal symptoms

Patients may report withdrawal symptoms and request prescriptions for drugs. It is not necessary, or ideal, to prescribe controlled drugs in the majority of cases.

### Psychiatric complications

Many substances of misuse, both in intoxication and withdrawal, can give rise to acute psychiatric complications. Management is aimed at treating specific symptoms (e.g. with benzodiazepines) rather than being drug-specific.

## Prognosis

The prognosis depends primarily on the individual's motivation. One study found 57% of patients with opioid dependence were on methadone maintenance therapy, while 23% were abstinent 2–3 years after inpatient treatment. Naltrexone, an opioid antagonist, is now the preferred treatment for opioid abstinence.

## EATING DISORDERS

There is no obvious discontinuity between normal and disordered eating. Around 90% of women have been on weight loss diets and 10% have used vomiting or laxatives in an attempt to lose weight. Hence, as well as the recognized disorders of anorexia and bulimia nervosa, there are also

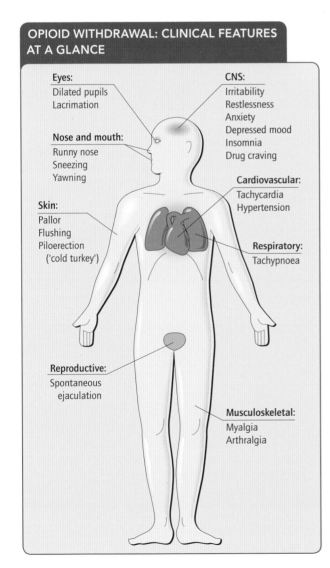

**OPIOID WITHDRAWAL: CLINICAL FEATURES AT A GLANCE**

**Eyes:**
Dilated pupils
Lacrimation

**Nose and mouth:**
Runny nose
Sneezing
Yawning

**Skin:**
Pallor
Flushing
Piloerection
('cold turkey')

**Reproductive:**
Spontaneous ejaculation

**CNS:**
Irritability
Restlessness
Anxiety
Depressed mood
Insomnia
Drug craving

**Cardiovascular:**
Tachycardia
Hypertension

**Respiratory:**
Tachypnoea

**Musculoskeletal:**
Myalgia
Arthralgia

sub-threshold disorders, and disorders with a mixture of anorectic and bulimic symptoms.

### Anorexia nervosa

#### Epidemiology

- Lifetime risk for females is 2–4% and for males 0.3%
- Peaks at age 15–19 years

#### Causes

The causes of anorexia nervosa are multifactorial, involving physical, psychological and social factors.

- *Physical:* Family and twin studies indicate a genetic susceptibility to anorexia nervosa.
- *Psychological:* There are no definite personality types associated with the eating disorders, although certain traits, such as low self-esteem and perfectionism, are more common.
- *Social:* Social and cultural pressures on women influence attitudes to weight and shape.

#### Clinical features

There are three components to the diagnosis of anorexia nervosa:

- *Core psychopathology*: Patients experience a tremendous drive to lose weight and find being at normal weight abhorrent. Weight is below a minimally normal weight for age and height (often defined as BMI ≤17.5).
- *Abnormal eating behaviour resulting in weight loss*: Patients severely restrict their intake of food beyond normal dieting. Other weight-reducing behaviours may include self-induced vomiting, excessive exercise and abuse of laxatives.
- *Endocrine disturbance and physical features*: Amenorrhoea occurs in the majority of women. The physical consequences of anorexia nervosa are shown in ANOREXIA NERVOSA: CLINICAL FEATURES AT A GLANCE.

Presentation to general medical or gynaecological outpatient departments with weight-related amenorrhoea is common. Focus history taking at initial presentation on eating habits and beliefs, and the meaning of thinness.

#### Investigation

The investigations carried out will depend on the situation and severity of the illness. Other causes of weight loss, both physical and psychiatric (e.g. schizophrenia, depressive disorder and obsessive–compulsive disorder [OCD]), must be excluded.

- *Haematology:* full blood count (FBC ), Erythrocyte sedimentation rate (ESR)
- *Biochemistry:* U&Es, liver function tests, calcium and phosphate, thyroid function tests; reproductive hormone assay
- *Electrocardiogram (ECG)*
- *Bone densitometry*
- *Pelvic ultrasound: maturity of reproductive organs*

#### Management

- *Medical outpatients*: Patients with an identified eating disorder should be referred to psychiatric services.

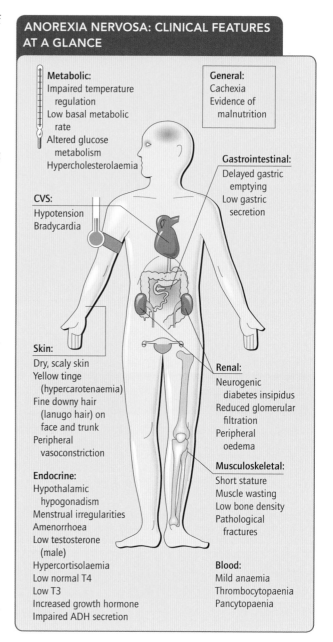

**ANOREXIA NERVOSA: CLINICAL FEATURES AT A GLANCE**

**Metabolic:**
Impaired temperature regulation
Low basal metabolic rate
Altered glucose metabolism
Hypercholesterolaemia

**General:**
Cachexia
Evidence of malnutrition

**Gastrointestinal:**
Delayed gastric emptying
Low gastric secretion

**CVS:**
Hypotension
Bradycardia

**Skin:**
Dry, scaly skin
Yellow tinge (hypercarotenaemia)
Fine downy hair (lanugo hair) on face and trunk
Peripheral vasoconstriction

**Renal:**
Neurogenic diabetes insipidus
Reduced glomerular filtration
Peripheral oedema

**Endocrine:**
Hypothalamic hypogonadism
Menstrual irregularities
Amenorrhoea
Low testosterone (male)
Hypercortisolaemia
Low normal T4
Low T3
Increased growth hormone
Impaired ADH secretion

**Musculoskeletal:**
Short stature
Muscle wasting
Low bone density
Pathological fractures

**Blood:**
Mild anaemia
Thrombocytopaenia
Pancytopaenia

- *Medical inpatients*: Inpatient treatment is necessary for patients at an extremely low weight (less than 70% of expected weight for height) and severe physical complications. Refeeding and gradual weight gain are the main focus of treatment.
- *Specialist treatment*: Treatment must address both the behavioural and psychological aspects of the disorder. The goals are weight gain to a normal healthy weight, resumption of normal eating behaviour and addressing individual and family conflicts.

#### Prognosis

Approximately 50% of patients make a complete recovery, 33% make a partial recovery and 20% run a chronic course. The mortality rate is 4%.

## Bulimia nervosa

### Epidemiology

- Peak onset is later than anorexia nervosa (age 15–25)
- Estimated prevalence of 1–2%

### Cause

Factors are similar to anorexia nervosa. Overall, heritability of bulimia nervosa appears to be less than for anorexia nervosa. Depression is common and may precede the onset of the illness.

### Clinical features

- *Core psychopathology*: Individuals judge themselves in terms of their weight and shape, rather than feeling they have intrinsic value.
- *Abnormal eating behaviour*: The primary feature is binge-eating, where an individual consumes a larger than normal quantity of food in a discrete period of time. Patients compensate for binge-eating by engaging in behaviours to prevent weight gain, such as self-induced vomiting, laxative abuse, exercise and dietary restriction.
- *Physical symptoms:* Weight is often normal or slightly under- or overweight. Bulimia nervosa is associated with menstrual irregularities and infertility. Signs of repeated self-induced vomiting include enlarged salivary glands, dental erosion and calluses on the dorsum of the hands.

### Investigation

- *Biochemistry:* U&Es, calcium and phosphate
- *ECG*
- *Pelvic ultrasound*

### Management

- *Medical:* Bulimia nervosa should be considered in patients with unexplained abdominal and gynaecological symptoms. Repeated vomiting or laxative use is a cause of hypokalaemia.
- *Specialist*: The majority of patients can be treated as outpatients. The principles of treatment are education, behavioural methods to regain normal eating habits and addressing the underlying emotional causative factors.

### Prognosis

Up to 80% recover fully.

## PSYCHIATRIC DISORDER AND PHYSICAL ILLNESS COEXISTING INDEPENDENTLY

Psychiatric disorder and physical illness are both common, so comorbidity is inevitable, but each is over-represented in the other. Physical illness, particularly if it requires hospitalization, can be particularly stressful for those with a psychiatric disorder. It is therefore essential that all past and present psychiatric disorders and treatments are adequately documented on admission and that any current psychotropic medication is continued.

## PSYCHOTIC DISORDERS

### Schizophrenia

Schizophrenia is the most common of the psychotic disorders. It is a major cause of distress, both to individual sufferers and their families, and carries a high mortality.

### Epidemiology

- Lifetime prevalence is around 1%.
- Onset is typically in early adulthood.
- Sex distribution is equal.
- Adoption studies consistently demonstrate a 10–20% incidence if one parent has schizophrenia and a 49% incidence if both parents have the disorder.

### Causes and disease mechanisms

The syndrome of schizophrenia may represent the end point of a number of different causal pathways. Genetic studies have shown evidence for inherited causative factors. Those with a lower inherited predisposition to schizophrenia may require additional environmental triggers for the onset of the disorder, whereas those with a higher genetic load may develop the illness with minimal additional environmental factors.

### Clinical features

Schizophrenia is a syndrome characterized by disturbances of thinking, perception and mood, occurring in clear consciousness. Symptoms of schizophrenia fall into two groups:

- *Positive symptoms:* These can be considered as an *addition* to normal psychological function. They include delusions, hallucinations and thought disorder.
- *Negative symptoms:* These can be considered as *diminished* psychological functioning. Individuals may have a flattening and lack of reactivity in their mood and problems with attention, appear apathetic and have a reduced output and content of speech.

The pattern of illness varies between individuals but is most commonly one of acute relapses against a background of persistent chronic symptoms.

### Investigation

Investigations should be considered to rule out drug-induced or organic psychotic conditions, especially in patients presenting with their first episode of illness.

### Management

Management of schizophrenia incorporates medical, psychological and social approaches, which are usually coordinated by a community mental health team. Antipsychotic medication is particularly useful for treating

**14**

positive symptomatology but is of little benefit for negative symptoms.

Psychological and social support, of both the patient and the family, are essential given the chronic course of the illness and the associated social deterioration.

### Prognosis
Factors associated with a poor prognosis include:
- Early or insidious onset
- Lack of affective component
- Low IQ
- Lower social class
- Predominance of negative symptoms
- Poor response to antipsychotics

### Schizoaffective disorder

Schizoaffective disorder is a term usually reserved to describe the illness of a small group of patients in whom the clinical picture is equally dominated by symptoms of both schizophrenia and a mood disorder (mania or depressive disorder).

### Delusional disorder

Delusional disorder is characterized by a well-organized set of delusions in an individual whose occupational and social functioning is otherwise normal.

## MOOD (AFFECTIVE) DISORDERS

The fundamental disturbance in these disorders is a change in mood to either depression or elation. The disorders tend to be recurrent, and the onset of individual episodes is often related to stressful events.

### Depressive disorder

The distinction between normal sadness and depressive disorder depends upon the severity and chronicity of symptoms, and the effect on an individual's level of psychological and social functioning. Depressive episodes may be single or recurrent. A depressive episode can be graded as mild, moderate or severe.

### Epidemiology
- Around 5% of people will have an episode of depression each year.
- The average age of onset is mid-twenties.
- It is twice as common in women.
- 20% of first-degree relatives of a person with depressive disorder have a mood disorder.

### Causes and disease mechanisms
Depressive disorder covers a heterogeneous range of disorders with different causes. For some, there is an inherited vulnerability. Depressed mood is accompanied by neurochemical changes, including serotonin, noradrenaline and dopamine. Predisposing factors include separations from caregivers in childhood and parental violence. In at least

**Table 14.7** Physical illness and depressive disorder

Depressive disorders are particularly common in the following groups:
- Illnesses affecting the brain (e.g. stroke, head injury)
- Acute, painful or life-threatening illnesses (e.g. myocardial infarction)
- Chronic, painful, disabling and disfiguring illnesses (e.g. rheumatoid arthritis)
- Major and unpleasant treatments (e.g. surgery, chemotherapy)
- Elderly people

**Physical disease**
Certain illnesses have been specifically linked to depression, with the assumption that there is a physical effect related to the disease or treatment. These include:
- Tumours (primary and secondary)
- Infections and post-infection states
- Hypothyroidism
- Hyperparathyroidism
- Cushing's syndrome
- Vitamin deficiencies (especially $B_1$, $B_6$, $B_{12}$)
- Neurological disorders (especially multiple sclerosis and Parkinson's disease)
- Autoimmune rheumatic diseases

**Drug-related**
Drug-induced depressive disorder is common and may relate to direct or indirect CNS toxicity. Iatrogenic causes include:
- Endocrine agents (e.g. corticosteroids, oral contraceptive pill)
- Antihypertensives (e.g. propranolol, nifedipine)
- Antiarrhythmics (e.g. lidocaine, procainamide)
- Antibiotics (e.g. penicillins, tetracycline)
- Antiparkinsonian drugs (e.g. levodopa, amantadine)
- Anticonvulsants (e.g. carbamazepine, vigabatrin)
- Antineoplastic drugs (e.g. interferon, vincristine)
- Antihistamines (e.g. cimetidine)

70% of cases there is an identifiable stressful trigger to an episode of depressive disorder.

The relationships between depressive disorder and physical illness are described in **Table 14.7**.

### Clinical features
Symptoms of a depressive episode include:
- Depressed mood
- Loss of interest and enjoyment (anhedonia)
- Reduced energy and fatigue
- Poor concentration and attention
- Reduced self-esteem and self-confidence
- Ideas of guilt
- A pessimistic view of the future
- Disturbed sleep
- Reduced appetite and weight loss

A severe depressive episode may be accompanied by psychotic symptoms (delusions and hallucinations) which are congruent with the low mood (e.g. delusional guilt, illness or poverty).

## Investigation

For many cases of depressive disorder, physical investigations are not required unless physical disease is suspected. Thyroid disease should be ruled out in females.

## Management

Mild to moderate episodes of depression may respond to either antidepressant medication (usually a selective serotonin reuptake inhibitor first-line, e.g. sertraline) or psychotherapeutic approaches (**Table 14.8**), or a combination of the two. Severe depression requires antidepressant medication, and antipsychotic medication if psychotic symptoms are present.

When a patient is prescribed an antidepressant, they should be told that it usually takes 2–3 weeks before the antidepressant effect becomes apparent. A course of antidepressants should be continued for at least 6 months to 1 year after recovery, to minimize the risk of relapse on discontinuation.

**Table 14.8** Psychotherapy

### Definition
The treatment of emotional, behavioural or personality problems by psychological means

### Classification
Different forms of psychotherapy can be classified according to their rationale. Commonly used psychotherapies with medical patients are described below.

*Counselling*
- Supportive and non-judgemental listening, to help the patient find solutions to personal difficulties
- Less stressful than other kinds of psychotherapy
- Used to help patients to adjust to a life crisis, such as bereavement, or coping with physical illness

*Cognitive behavioural therapy*
- Combines cognitive and behavioural psychotherapies
- Focuses on changing unhelpful thoughts, feelings and behaviours
- Commonly used in the treatment of anxiety and depression

*Dialetic behavioural therapy*
- A specific type of CBT used in the treatment of personality disorders

*Psychodynamic psychotherapy*
- Concerned with the way that a person's mental representation of themselves and the world may lead to problems in current personal relationships
- Used in depressive disorder, eating disorders and personality disorders

*Systemic therapy (family therapy)*
- Considers problems in the social context in which they arise
- May be used where an individual's illness impacts significantly on the family

For severe episodes of depressive disorder, particularly where the patient is unresponsive to antidepressants, or where a faster response is required, a course of electroconvulsive therapy (ECT) may be appropriate.

## Prognosis

Individual episodes of depressive disorder typically last between 3 and 12 months. Following a first depressive illness, 50% of people will experience a recurrence.

## Bipolar affective disorder

Bipolar affective disorder (manic-depressive disorder) is characterized by repeated episodes of mood disorder, with at least one episode of elation (mania).

### Epidemiology
- Lifetime prevalence of around 2%
- Peak age of onset 15–19 years old
- Sex ratio of 1 : 1
- 20–25% of first-degree relatives of a person with bipolar disorder have a mood disorder

### Causes
Bipolar affective disorder has a relatively high genetic contribution, with a heritability of 0.8. Episodes of illness are often precipitated by stressful life events.

### Clinical features
Patients have repeated episodes of mood disturbance, although individual patients will have different patterns of illness. Characteristically recovery is complete between episodes. Symptoms of a depressive episode are described above. Symptoms of a manic episode include:
- Persistent elevation of mood, out of keeping with circumstances
- Irritability and suspiciousness
- Increased energy and over activity
- Speech is fast and difficult to interrupt (pressure of speech)
- Decreased need for sleep
- Loss of normal social inhibitions
- Poor attention and concentration with marked distractibility
- Inflated self-esteem
- Grandiose or overoptimistic ideas

### Investigation
Investigations should be carried out where indicated to exclude a potential physical cause for the first presentation of the disorder, particularly thyroid disease in female patients (see 'Depressive disorder' above).

### Management
The main prophylactic for bipolar affective disorder is a mood-stabilizing drug. NICE guidance recommends using lithium first-line. Antipsychotic drugs may also be used, either in the treatment of an acute relapse of the illness where there are psychotic symptoms or as a prophylactic medication in

patients who are intolerant of lithium. Antidepressant drugs should be used with caution as there is a risk that they might precipitate a manic episode. ECT may be used in the treatment of manic or depressive episodes, particularly when the patient is suicidal, psychotic, stuporous or not responding to medication.

### Prognosis

There is wide variation in the long-term outcome of the disorder, with a trend towards shorter remissions and longer depressive episodes after middle age.

## ANXIETY-RELATED DISORDERS

Anxiety-related disorders are common. All of the disorders described below have anxiety as either the primary symptom or a major component of the illness. Anxiety becomes pathological when the optimal level of anxiety is exceeded, when it becomes pervasive, or when it occurs in inappropriate situations.

### Epidemiology

- Generalized anxiety disorder and panic disorder have a lifetime prevalence of 5% and 3% respectively. Anxiety-related disorders are twice as common in medical patients as in the general population.
- Peak age of onset is around 30 years of age.
- Two-thirds of patients with generalized anxiety disorder, panic disorder or phobic anxiety disorder are female; there is an equal sex distribution for OCD and women are more likely to develop post-traumatic stress disorder (PTSD) than men.
- Genetic factors are thought to be important in the anxiety-related disorders.

### Causes and disease mechanisms

Individuals may be predisposed to excessive anxious arousal due to inherited factors or the effect of environmental factors on the developing brain. Physical factors implicated include abnormal regulation of the central adrenergic system in panic disorder. Vulnerability may also be acquired later in life through traumatic experience.

### Clinical features

The symptoms of anxiety fall into three main groups (see ANXIETY: CLINICAL FEATURES AT A GLANCE).

### Generalized anxiety disorder

Patients describe primary symptoms of anxiety for most days for several weeks at a time.

### Panic disorder

Anxiety occurs in discrete, unpredictable episodes, or 'panic attacks'.

### Phobic anxiety disorder

Anxiety is provoked in certain well-defined situations which are not objectively dangerous. The fear experienced

**ANXIETY: CLINICAL FEATURES AT A GLANCE**

Cognitive symptoms:
Apprehension
Worry about the future
Feeling 'on edge'
Difficulty concentrating

Symptoms due to autonomic overactivity:
Dizziness, light-headed
Dry mouth
Tachycardia
Tachypnoea
Abdominal discomfort
Sweating

Symptoms due to motor tension:
Tremor
Fidgeting
Tension headache

is recognized as irrational by the individual, but it cannot be reasoned away and leads to an avoidance of such situations.

- *Simple phobias* are circumscribed fears of specific objects, situations or activities.
- *Social phobia* is a fear of humiliation or embarrassment in front of others.
- *Agoraphobia* is a fear of situations from which there is no easy escape (usually to home).

### Obsessive–compulsive disorder

OCD is characterized by obsessional thoughts and compulsive rituals (repetitive and purposeless behaviours performed in response to obsessional thoughts), which are not secondary to another disorder and are of sufficient severity to interfere with normal social and occupational functioning. Patients see them as abnormal, and attempts to suppress them result in increasing anxiety, which can only be relieved by the compulsive act.

### Post-traumatic stress disorder

PTSD arises as a response to an exceptionally catastrophic or threatening event, which is re-experienced in recurrent and intrusive distressing recollections, dreams and flashbacks. This often occurs against a background of a sense of numbness. There is usually a state of autonomic hyperarousal and hypervigilance.

### Investigation

Investigations may be required when an underlying physical disorder is suspected as a cause for anxiety-related symptoms.

### Management

In mild to moderate cases, behavioural and cognitive psychotherapies are the most common treatment (see **Table 14.8**). Pharmacological strategies can be very effective, however, and include selective serotonin reuptake inhibitors (SSRI) antidepressants, venlafaxine, trazodone and pregabalin.

### Prognosis

Overall response to treatment is good but very variable, depending on the severity of the illness and the presence of complicating factors (e.g. personality, alcohol and substance misuse).

## PERSONALITY DISORDERS

Personality disorder occurs when an individual's enduring behaviour causes long-standing difficulties for themselves or those around them. They can be seen as the extreme end of a spectrum of personality. Classification systems describe a number of personality disorders. The most common type encountered in clinical practice is usually emotionally unstable personality disorder, also known as borderline personality disorder.

### Epidemiology

- Estimates of general population rates depend on the definitions used, with up to 1% having a severe personality disorder, and 10% having a mild disorder or problematic personality traits. This rate increases to 20% of GP attenders, with a similar rate likely in medical patients.
- Personality disorders develop in adolescence and persist into adult life.
- Emotionally unstable personality disorder is more common in women.

### Causes

A common problem in personality disorder is the appropriate control of emotional responses, which may be related to adverse childhood experiences.

### Clinical features

Emotionally unstable personality disorder is characterized by a difficulty in controlling emotions, which may become overwhelming. Individuals may have outbursts of anger or use maladaptive behaviours to reduce tension (e.g. self-harm or alcohol misuse).

### Management

The treatment of choice for most people with a personality disorder is long-term psychotherapy. Dialectic behavioural therapy is particularly helpful for self-harm (see **Table 14.8**).

### Prognosis

Personality disorder tends to persist through adult life. Benefiting from treatment depends on the patient's ability to sustain a therapeutic relationship and continue with long-term treatment.

---

**MUST-KNOW CHECKLIST**

- Carry out a psychiatric assessment in a patient with physical illness, including history, mental state examination and appropriate physical examination
- Suggest and justify a differential diagnosis, supported by a discussion of possible contributory factors
- Suggest a management plan, including physical, psychological and social investigations and treatments
- Describe the presentation and possible causes of delirium
- Describe the presentation and pathophysiology of dementia
- Describe the range of psychological reactions to physical illness
- Discuss the presentation and management of medically unexplained symptoms
- Describe the assessment and management of a patient following deliberate self-harm
- Describe the presentation and management of alcohol and substance misuse in medical patients
- Describe the physical complications of eating disorders
- Briefly describe the common psychiatric disorders that may coexist with physical illness

---

**Questions and answers** to test your understanding of Chapter 14 can be found by clicking 'Support Material' at the following link: https://www.routledge.com/Medicine-for-Finals-and-Beyond/Axford-OCallaghan/p/book/9780367150594

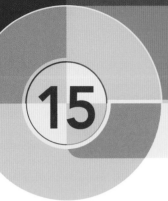

# 15

# Haematological Disease

THOMAS A. FOX AND EMMA C. MORRIS

## INTRODUCTION

Haematology is the study of blood and the diseases that affect it. It covers a broad spectrum of conditions from inherited disorders such as the haemoglobinopathy to aggressive malignancies such as acute leukaemia. Haematologists are heavily involved in the diagnostic process and in many countries have dual qualifications in clinical medicine and pathological sciences. With the advent of the 'genomic era', haematology has made huge strides forward in our understanding of disease processes and new therapeutic approaches. Haematology can seem impossibly complicated initially, but a basic understanding of how blood and its different components (cells and molecules) function and interact will give any inquisitive student the keys to a fascinating, varied specialty that is at the cutting edge of modern medicine and advanced therapeutics including gene therapy.

## STRUCTURE AND FUNCTION OF THE BLOOD

### HAEMATOPOIESIS (BLOOD FORMATION)

*Definitive haematopoiesis* occurs in the foetal liver and spleen between 2 and 7 months, and finally the bone marrow between 5 and 9 months post-conception. In adult life, active haematopoiesis retreats to the axial skeleton. Huge numbers of blood cells ($250 \times 10^9$ red cells plus $63 \times 10^9$ white cells in an adult male) must be replaced every day. These numbers escalate during infection, bleeding or other stresses.

DOI: 10.1201/9781003193616-15

## COMPONENTS OF BLOOD

Blood consists of *red cells* (*erythrocytes*), *white cells* (*leucocytes*) and *platelets* (*thrombocytes*) suspended in *plasma* (**Figure 15.1**). Depending on the test needing to be performed, clotted or unclotted blood can be collected from patients by using different collection tubes which contain varying reagents. Clotting can be prevented by adding a calcium chelator (ethylenediaminetetra-acetic acid [EDTA] or citrate). Blood collected in EDTA is used to determine the full blood count (FBC).

When blood clots in a tube, the resulting supernatant is called *serum*. This facilitates the study of other plasma proteins, particularly antibodies – hence the study of antibody reactions in human blood is called *serology*. Clotted blood is used for many biochemical tests including the determination of electrolyte concentrations.

## RED CELLS (ERYTHROCYTES)

The function of red blood cells (RBCs) is to transport oxygen from the lungs to the tissues. Importantly, RBCs do *not* contain a nucleus and are therefore unable to synthesize

new proteins or proliferate and they have a fixed lifespan in the circulation.

After maturation in the bone marrow, young red cells (*reticulocytes*) pass into the bloodstream. The *reticulocyte count* (normally approximately 1% of the total red cells) represents new red cell production and is a useful measure of how effective the bone marrow is at producing new cells (for the normal range, see **Table 15.1**). In disease states such as haemolytic anaemia, a very high reticulocyte count would be expected as the bone marrow tries to compensate for the cells being lost. After about 120 days in the circulation, the cell is recycled by macrophages in the spleen. Premature destruction of red cells is called *haemolysis*.

Tissue oxygen concentration governs the rate of erythropoiesis via erythropoietin (Epo), which drives proliferation of red cells. Epo is mainly secreted in the *kidney* by tubular and interstitial cells that sense tissue *hypoxia* (low oxygen tension). In chronic renal failure, anaemia results from suppressed erythropoiesis because of failure of this mechanism.

### Red cell antigens

The red cell membrane carries many immunogenic protein or carbohydrate molecules on its surface, known as *blood*

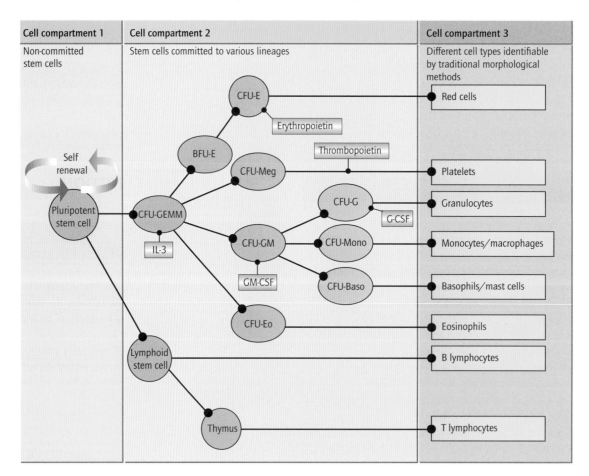

**Figure 15.1** Bone marrow pluripotent stem cell development. Diagram to show how non-committed stem cells develop into stem cells committed to the various lineages and lead to the formation of different cell types identifiable by traditional morphological methods. Baso, basophil; BFU-E, burst forming unit-erythroid; CFU, colony forming unit; CFU-E, colony forming unit-erythroid; Eos, eosinophil; G, granulocyte; GEMM, granulocyte, erythroid, monocyte, megakaryocyte; Meg, megakaryocyte; Mono, monocyte.

**Table 15.1** Normal haematological values

| Haematological parameter | | Value |
|---|---|---|
| Haemoglobin | Men | 130–170 g/L |
| | Women | 120–160 g/L |
| Red blood cell count (RBC) | Men | $4.5$–$6.0 \times 10^{12}$/L |
| | Women | $3.8$–$5.2 \times 10^{12}$/L |
| Mean cell volume (MCV) | | 78–95 fL |
| Packed cell volume (PCV) | Men | 40–52% |
| | Women | 37–47% |
| Reticulocyte count | | 0.2–2.0% |
| White blood cell count (WBC) | | $4$–$11 \times 10^9$/L |
| Platelets | | $150$–$400 \times 10^9$/L |

*group antigens.* These antigens are grouped into *blood group systems* of which the two most important are the ABO and Rhesus (Rh) systems. Blood groups are important because an individual who lacks an RBC antigen (antigen-negative) can produce antibodies to it, if transfused with antigen-positive red cells. RBC antibodies can lead to *transfusion reactions*. The consequent rapid destruction of large numbers of red cells in the circulation can cause severe systemic symptoms including hypotensive shock, acute renal failure and disseminated intravascular coagulation (DIC) (**EMERGENCY PRESENTATION 15.1**). Expert advice from the on-call transfusion medicine or haematology consultant should always be sought.

Another way that RBC immunization occurs is across the placenta if the foetus inherits a paternal red cell antigen that the mother lacks. Small numbers of foetal red cells can pass into the maternal circulation and immunize her against it. Transfer of maternal IgG back across the placenta results in destruction of the antigen-positive foetal RBCs, causing haemolytic disease of the newborn.

### ABO (or ABH) blood group system

This is coded by three allelic genes: A, B and O (**Table 15.2**). ABO antigens are oligosaccharides widely expressed on bacteria. Universal exposure (in early postnatal life) to gut bacteria causes the key property of ABO antigens: *no red cell exposure is needed* to immunize us against them thus severe reactions occur immediately on transfusion of ABO incompatible blood. From early infancy we all possess naturally occurring IgM ABO antibodies. *ABO-mismatched* transfusions cause the most dangerous (complement-mediated intravascular) reactions, accordingly, named *major haemolytic transfusion reactions.*

---

**EMERGENCY PRESENTATION 15.1**

### Incompatible blood transfusion (wrong blood)

#### Prevention

- Identify the patient (blood recipient) correctly – name, date of birth, hospital number.
- Label the sample tube fully and accurately *in writing* with the recipient's details *at the patient's bedside.*
- Blood for transfusion should be collected from the blood bank only by trained staff.
- Two trained staff members should check that the details on the blood label match those of the recipient *at the bedside.*

#### Symptoms of incompatible blood transfusion (blood transfusion reaction)

- Hypotension (shock)
- Chest, back or abdominal pain
- Fever
- Dark urine (intravascular haemolysis)
- Rigors
- Rash

If there are symptoms of a blood transfusion reaction:

- *Stop the transfusion immediately* and detach the giving set from the patient.
- Attach a new giving set, keeping the line open to infuse saline.
- Check the identity of the patient against the details on the blood bag label.
- Monitor the patient closely to support vital functions, airway, etc.
- Take new blood samples (FBC, coagulation screen, urea and electrolytes, direct antiglobulin test [DAT], re-crossmatch) and send these to laboratory with the blood unit and giving set associated with the reaction.

---

### Rh blood group system

This complex system of protein antigens is encoded by allelic genes (Cc, D, Ee) at three closely linked loci inherited as haplotypes (e.g. *CDe/cde*). Confusingly, there is no little 'd' antigen but individuals who lack 'D' are denoted as being 'd'. Individuals are termed Rh-positive (85% of the UK population) if their red cells carry the *D* antigen, or Rh-negative (15% of the UK population) if they lack the *D* antigen (and are thus denoted as 'd'). Rh (D)-positive individuals may

**Table 15.2** ABO blood group system

| Blood group (phenotype) | Genotype | Red cell antigen | Antibodies | Frequency in UK (%) | Blood suitable for transfusion |
|---|---|---|---|---|---|
| O | OO | H | Anti-A, anti-B | 46 | O |
| A | AA or AO | A | Anti-B | 42 | A or O |
| B | BB or BO | B | Anti-A | 9 | B or O |
| AB | AB | A and B | None | 3 | AB or O |

therefore inherit a single (*Dd*) or double (*DD*) dose of the D antigen.

Rh IgG antibodies result from antigen exposure during transfusion or pregnancy. It is therefore important to avoid transfusing a Rh-negative recipient (*d*) with the strongly immunogenic *D* antigen (with Rh-positive blood). Thus, in most countries, children and women of childbearing age are typically given D-negative blood if their D status is unknown. Because Rh antibodies are IgG, they do not cause the violent intravascular haemolysis seen in ABO-mismatched transfusions.

## HAEMOGLOBIN: THE 'MOLECULAR LUNG'

All human haemoglobin molecules consist of four globin chains: two α- and two β-chains. The major haemoglobins produced during definitive haematopoiesis are composed of two α chains plus two γ chains in the fetus ($\alpha_2\gamma_2$ = foetal haemoglobin [HbF]), and two α plus two β chains in the adult ($\alpha_2\beta_2$ = adult haemoglobin [HbA]).

### Why do foetuses need different haemoglobin?

HbF binds poorly to 2,3-diphosphoglycerate and foetal blood pH is low, so the amount of oxygen carried at any partial pressure is greater than in adult blood. This *increased oxygen affinity* ensures that HbF can 'steal' $O_2$ from maternal HbA across the placental interface, thus maintaining an adequate oxygen supply to foetal tissues (**Figure 15.2**).

### Haemoglobin synthesis

Haemoglobin production in humans is characterized by three major switches in haemoglobin composition (**Figure 15.3**). From 9 months post conception, HbF is progressively replaced

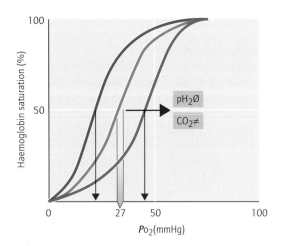

**Figure 15.2** Haemoglobin oxygen dissociation curve. The $P_{50}$ is the partial pressure of oxygen at which haemoglobin is 50% saturated and is normally 27 mmHg (red curve). $P_{50}$ values increase (reflecting decreased oxygen affinity) as the pH decreases (the Bohr effect) and as carbon dioxide concentration increases (green curve). $P_{50}$ values decrease when oxygen affinity increases (e.g. high-affinity haemoglobins).

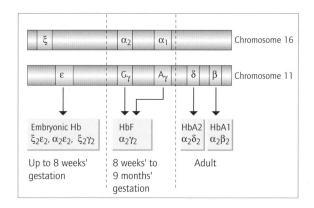

**Figure 15.3** Organization of the human globin gene cluster. The genes expressed and haemoglobins synthesized during embryonic, fetal and adult life are illustrated.

by HbA. At 1 year, the HbA pattern is fully established. HbA ($\alpha_2\beta_2$) comprises more than 95%, while the minor haemoglobin HbA$_2$ ($\alpha_2\delta_2$) accounts for approximately 2.5%.

## HAEMOGLOBIN CONCENTRATION IN THE BLOOD

### Anaemia

The haemoglobin concentration in blood (Hb) is expressed as grams per litre (g/L) or grams per decilitre (g/dL).

The haemoglobin concentration in an individual depends on:

- Age
- Sex
- Pregnancy
- Diet
- Altitude at which the individual lives
- Presence of diseases that reduce/suppress production (e.g. infection, lack of red cell production), increase losses through bleeding (e.g. colonic carcinoma) or other mechanisms (e.g. malaria)

*Anaemia* is the term for an abnormally low Hb concentration. Consensus 'diagnostic' *normal ranges* for Hb concentration at sea level are:

- *Males:* 130–180 g/L; therefore anaemia = Hb <130 g/L
- *Non-pregnant females:* 120–170 g/L; therefore anaemia = Hb <120 g/L
- *Pregnant females:* 110–160 g/L; therefore anaemia = Hb <110 g/L

## WHITE CELLS (LEUCOCYTES)

The primary function of white cells is defence against pathogens. The normal adult differential white cell count is shown in **Table 15.3**.

### Polymorphonuclear neutrophils

Polymorphonuclear neutrophils (PMNs) phagocytose and kill micro-organisms. PMNs have a unique 'polymorphic' nucleus with two to five lobes. A grossly elevated PMN count

**Table 15.3** Normal adult differential white cell count

| White cell | Absolute number (×10⁹/L) | Relative number (%) |
|---|---|---|
| Neutrophils | 2.0–7.5 | 40–75 |
| Lymphocytes | 1.5–4.0 | 20–45 |
| Monocytes | 0.1–0.8 | 2–10 |
| Eosinophils | 0.04–0.45 | 1–6 |
| Basophils | <0.1 | 1 |

in the absence of infection or inflammation should raise the suspicion of a haematological malignancy such as chronic myeloid leukaemia (CML) or chronic neutrophilic leukaemia.

## Eosinophils

The function of eosinophils is defence against multicellular parasites (e.g. helminths) and participation in IgE-mediated immune responses.

- *Normal eosinophil count:* $0.05–0.35 \times 10^9$/L
- *Increased eosinophil count:* $>0.35 \times 10^9$/L = eosinophilia
- *Reduced eosinophil count:* $<0.05 \times 10^9$/L = eosinopenia

Eosinophils have bilobed nuclei and large, orange-stained cytoplasmic granules. Eosinophilia is seen in allergic reactions, in response to endo- or ectoparasitic infections and secondary to a range of other diseases including inflammatory lung and gastrointestinal disorders and certain malignant diseases including Hodgkin's lymphoma (HL). Occasionally, a primary hypereosinophilia occurs due to a clonal myeloproliferative disorder.

## Basophils

- *Normal basophil count:* $0.00–0.09 \times 10^9$/L
- *Increased basophil count:* $>0.1 \times 10^9$/L = basophilia

While their exact function remains unknown, basophils contain high levels of histamine and heparin and are involved in allergic (IgE-mediated) responses: sustained basophilia in the absence of other causes is usually a sign of CML.

## Monocytes

Mononuclear phagocytes = monocytes in the blood, macrophages in the tissues.

The function of monocytes is to phagocytose invading microbes and other foreign material, process resulting peptides, and present them bound to surface MHC-2 complexes for recognition and response by T and B lymphocytes.

- *Normal monocyte count:* $0.4–1.1 \times 10^9$/L
- *Increased monocyte count:* $>1.1 \times 10^9$/L = monocytosis
- *Decreased monocyte count:* $<0.4 \times 10^9$/L = monocytopenia

## Lymphocytes

The function of lymphocytes is to recognize non-self antigens and to generate the adaptive cellular (T lymphocyte) and humoral (B lymphocyte) immune responses to them.

- *Normal lymphocyte count:* $1.0–4.0 \times 10^9$/L

- *Increased lymphocyte count:* $>4.0 \times 10^9$/L = lymphocytosis
- *Decreased lymphocyte count:* $<1.0 \times 10^9$/L = lymphopenia

Lymphocytes leave the bone marrow and migrate to the secondary lymphoid organs (thymus for T cells, lymph node follicles for B cells) where they further differentiate into mature antigen-specific T and B cells. Blood lymphocytes are 80% T cells and 20% B cells. Lymphocytes and the immune system are discussed in detail in Chapter 2, The scientific basis of medicine.

## Platelets

The function of blood platelets is to prevent haemorrhage by forming platelet plugs at sites of blood vessel damage.

- *Normal platelet count:* $150–400 \times 10^9$/L
- *Increased platelet count:* $>400 \times 10^9$/L = thrombocytosis
- *Decreased platelet count:* $<150 \times 10^9$/L = thrombocytopenia

Platelets are produced in the bone marrow by cytoplasmic budding from *megakaryocytes*, in turn derived from the pluripotent HSCs via committed megakaryocyte precursors (CFU-Meg). Proliferation, maturation and platelet budding are all governed by the platelet growth factor thrombopoietin (THPO). Platelets are important in haemostasis, with the formation of a platelet plug at the site of injury being one of the first steps in bringing about the cessation of bleeding (see below).

## HAEMOSTASIS

Haemostasis is the process of stopping bleeding. There is tight control of the process as thrombosis formation when it is not warranted results in thromboembolic disease and failure of clot formation results in bleeding disorders.

## PRIMARY HAEMOSTASIS

Vessel wall trauma results in damaged vascular endothelial cells and exposes the underlying subendothelium. Platelets adhere to the site, due to interactions with *von Willebrand factor (vWF)* and *collagen* (**Figure 15.4**). Platelets then aggregate, blocking the defect in the vessel wall.

## SECONDARY HAEMOSTASIS

The primary platelet plug disintegrates unless strengthened by a fibrin net generated by a complex interaction of clotting factors (the *coagulation pathway;* **Figure 15.5**).

### Clot initiation

*Tissue factor (TF)* on endothelial cells activates *factor VII.* TF–factor VIIa complexes bind and activate factor X. Acting like a starter motor, this cleaves a small amount of thrombin (from prothrombin), which activates factors VIII and V, and then enzymatic factor IX. If this activation is sufficient, coagulation proceeds to the next stage.

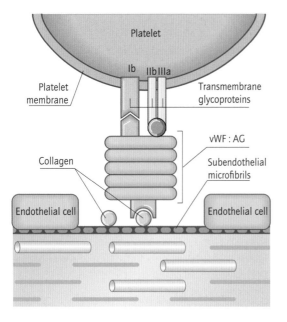

**Figure 15.4** Platelet adhesion to damaged endothelium. The adhesion of platelets to damaged vascular endothelium is mediated by multimeric von Willebrand factor (vWF: Ag). It binds to glycoprotein Ib on the platelet membrane as well as to subendothelial collagen. Deficiencies of glycoprotein Ib (Bernard–Soulier syndrome), IIb/IIIa (Glanzmann's thrombaesthenia), and vWF: Ag (von Willebrand's disease) all result in haemorrhagic disorders.

### Clot amplification and propagation

Factors VIIIa and IXa form a membrane complex that increases factor Xa generation tenfold. Factor Xa forms *prothrombinase* complexes with *factor Va* on platelet surfaces,

speeding *thrombin* generation from *prothrombin*. Thrombin cleaves fibrinogen to form a durable fibrin clot.

### *Where has the 'intrinsic pathway' gone?*

*In vivo* there are no separate intrinsic and extrinsic clotting pathways involved in clot formation. In the circulating blood, all clotting factors act together and are simultaneously available. Because the laboratory 'coagulation screen' tests occur in test tubes (*in vitro*), different clot-initiation pathways can be tested separately (**Figure 15.6**). Knowledge of the intrinsic and extrinsic clotting pathways is still useful in order to understand which clotting factors are being assessed by different laboratory tests.

## CLOT REGULATION AND REMOVAL

### Clot regulation: the protein C system and antithrombin

Thrombin generation is modulated by the naturally occurring anticoagulant proteins (protein C, protein S and antithrombin). There are genetic conditions which cause deficiencies of protein C and S which result in a marked increase in risk of pathological thrombosis formation. Affected patients often suffer a venothromboembolism at a young age and need to be managed with anticoagulation.

### Fibrinolysis

Clots contain the seeds of their own destruction, *plasminogen*. This is cleaved by *tissue plasminogen activator (tPA)* or *urokinase* to the fibrinolytic enzyme *plasmin*. Plasmin cleaves fibrin into D-dimer fragments. This dissolves the clot, while plasmin also activates repair of the original vessel damage (angiogenesis).

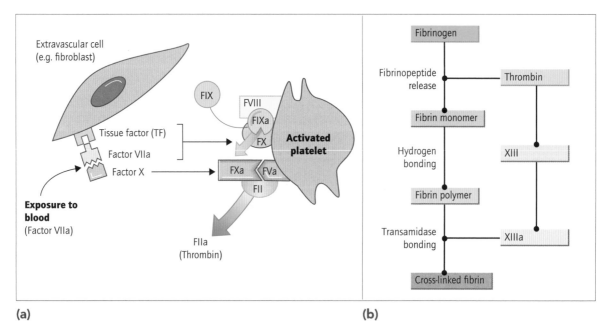

**(a)**

**(b)**

**Figure 15.5 (a)** The cell-based pathways for the formation of thrombin. **(b)** Conversion of soluble fibrinogen into a cross-linked fibrin clot. Thrombin specifically cleaves small peptides from α and β chains of fibrinogen. The resultant fibrin is stabilized by activated factor XIII (XIIIa).

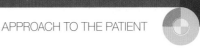

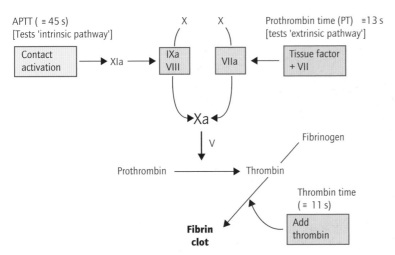

APTT ( ≡ 45 s)
[Tests 'intrinsic pathway']

Prothrombin time (PT) ≡13 s
[tests 'extrinsic pathway']

Thrombin time
( ≡ 11 s)

**Figure 15.6** Extrinsic and intrinsic coagulation pathways. APTT: activated partial thromboplastin time.

## APPROACH TO THE PATIENT

### PRESENTING SYMPTOMS OF HAEMATOLOGICAL DISEASE

Haematological disease causes aberrant function of one or more components of the blood. The symptoms of blood diseases are directly caused by this loss or gain of function (**Figure 15.7**).

#### Anaemia (reduced red blood cell function)

Symptoms of anaemia:
- Reduced exercise tolerance
- Sleepiness
- Breathlessness on minimal effort or at rest
- Headache
- Palpitations
- Chest pain
- Pallor

#### Infection

Loss of white blood cell number or function increases the risk of infection. Because of the short lifespan of neutrophils in the circulation, *neutropenia* can develop acutely, so the symptoms may be of short duration. Neutrophils defend against bacterial pathogens, while lymphocytes are important for controlling viral and opportunistic pathogens. Increased risk of infection can also be due to reduced immunoglobulin production (hypogammaglobulinaemia) in some diseases.

#### Bleeding (reduced platelet or coagulation function)

Symptoms of thrombocytopenia or coagulation factor deficiency:
- Skin rash (purpura)
- Bruises
- Nosebleeds (epistaxis)

15

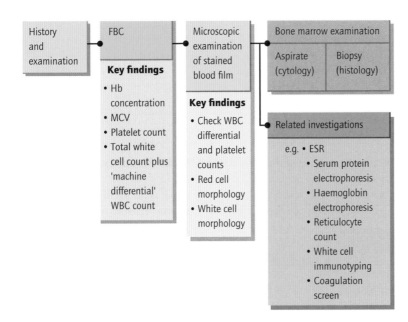

**Figure 15.7** Sequence of steps in haematological investigation.

- Oral bleeding or 'blood blisters'
- Heavy periods (menorrhagia)
- Prolonged bleeding after surgery or dental extraction

### Lumps and swellings

- *Enlarged glands:* may be caused by lymphoma (commonly) or leukaemia (rarely) but may signal infection or other malignancies
- *Abdominal swelling and/or fullness:* may be caused by splenomegaly in lymphoma and related diseases (e.g. non-Hodgkin's lymphoma [NHL], chronic lymphocytic leukaemia [CLL]) or myeloproliferative disorders (e.g. CML, myelofibrosis [MF])
- *Abdominal pain:* may be caused by splenic infarction in splenomegaly

### Pain

Back pain may signify myeloma bone disease. Acute episodes of excruciating pain involving back, limbs, chest or the whole body are typical of sickle cell disease (SCD). Bone pain combined with symptoms of pancytopenia suggests acute leukaemia. Pain in the calf or thigh may be caused by deep-vein thrombosis (DVT) and, if accompanied by pleuritic chest pain, may signify pulmonary embolism (PE).

### Weight loss and fever

Significant weight loss (more than 10% body weight) may occur in lymphoma and chronic leukaemias. Fever may be caused by the blood disease itself or infection as a result of leucopaenia. When weight loss, fever and drenching night sweats are present (without infection), they are termed 'B' symptoms.

### Drug history

Notable drugs which result in haematological abnormalities include aspirin (bleeding disorders), antiepileptic drugs (folate deficiency), oestrogen-containing drugs (increased risk of thrombosis), antidepressants, antipsychotics and antirheumatic drugs (neutropenia).

### Past medical history

Previous medical disorders may provide clues to the aetiology of the current haematological disorder (e.g. a history of gastrectomy in a patient with macrocytic anaemia caused by vitamin $B_{12}$ deficiency).

### Family history

A positive family history suggests an inherited disorder. In bleeding disorders, a sex-linked inheritance pattern may be evident, increasing the likelihood of a diagnosis of *haemophilia.*

## EXAMINATION

Details of how to approach clinical examination can be found in the earlier part of this book. Examination findings in haematological patients can be dramatic

**Table 15.4** Causes of splenomegaly

| Aetiology | Example |
|---|---|
| Infection | |
| Acute bacterial | Septicaemia |
| | Infective endocarditis |
| | Typhoid |
| Acute viral | Infectious mononucleosis, viral hepatitis |
| Chronic bacterial | Brucellosis, tuberculosis |
| Parasitic | Malaria, schistosomiasis, kala-azar |
| Inflammation | Rheumatoid arthritis, systemic *lupus* erythematosus, sarcoidosis |
| Haematological | Leukaemia, lymphoma, myeloproliferative disorders, haemoglobinopathies, chronic haemolytic anaemia |
| Venous congestion | Portal hypertension (liver disease), hepatic and portal vein thrombosis |
| Other mechanisms | Metabolic storage diseases, amyloidosis |

Causes of massive splenomegaly include chronic malaria and kala-azar (endemic areas). In the UK, CML and MF are more common. Rarely, Gaucher's disease.

(haemophilic arthopathy in haemophilia, severe pulmonary hypertension in SCD, massive splenomegaly in MF) or subtle (pallor in a patient with acute leukaemia). Particular attention should be paid to the spleen and lymph nodes (**Table 15.4**).

## INVESTIGATION

### HAEMATOLOGY

#### Full blood count

When an automated analyser processes an FBC sample, it measures:

- Haemoglobin concentration (Hb conc, g/L)
- MCV, femtolitres (fL)
- WBC
- Neutrophil count
- Lymphocyte count
- Platelet count

#### *Simple diagnosis using the full blood count*

1 *Is the patient anaemic?*
2 *If the patient is anaemic, what is the MCV?*
   o If the MCV is <78 fL, the anaemia is microcytic (iron deficiency or thalassaemia trait).
   o If the MCV is >100 fL, the anaemia is macrocytic (megaloblastic anaemias, thyroid disease).
   o If the MCV is normal (80–100 fL), the anaemia is normocytic (anaemia of chronic disease, bone marrow failure).

Answering questions 1 and 2 therefore gets us halfway towards the cause of anaemia – by reading two numbers!

3 *Is the WBC increased or decreased?If the WBC is increased, which cell type is responsible?* Compare the absolute neutrophil, lymphocyte, monocyte and eosinophil counts with the normal ranges (see **Table 15.3**).

4 *If the WBC is decreased, which cell type is lacking?* As for question 3.

5 *Is the platelet count low (thrombocytopenia) or high (thrombocytosis)?* Compare the platelet count with the normal range (see **Table 15.1**).

Answering questions 3–5 allows an initial classification into neutrophilia/neutropenia, lymphocytosis/lymphopenia, etc.

## *Reticulocyte count*

Reticulocytes normally comprise approximately 1% of circulating red cells. They increase in number if there is increased red cell production. Any reticulocyte count over 7% (more than $300 \times 10^9$/L) in the presence of other markers of haemolysis (e.g. raised bilirubin and anaemia) is suggestive of a haemolytic anaemia.

## Blood film microscopy

Microscopy of a stained peripheral blood film is necessary in the workup of any potential haematological disorder. Key observations are intended to:

- Confirm the automated FBC findings
- Identify any *abnormal white cells* (e.g. leukaemic blasts)
- Recognize *red cell abnormalities* (e.g. sickled cells, oval macrocytes, red cell fragments)
- Detect intracellular *parasites* (e.g. malaria)

## Bone marrow aspirate, trephine biopsy and phenotyping

### *Bone marrow aspirate*

In bone marrow aspiration, a sample of fluid is drawn by syringe through a hollow needle inserted into the posterior iliac crest (under local anaesthetic). This is then stained and microscopically examined. The marrow cells can also be subjected to cytogenetic analysis, cell culture and molecular studies. Microscopy of stained films obtained by bone marrow aspirate is a key diagnostic test in the presence of:

- Unexplained anaemia (? myelodysplasia, haematological malignancy or infection)
- Unexplained cytopenias
- Significant paraproteinaemia (? myeloma)

### *Bone marrow trephine biopsy*

This biopsy, in which a small core of bone marrow is removed from the posterior iliac crest using a trephine (cutting) needle, is often performed immediately following aspiration. The trephine gives a more accurate measure of total marrow cellularity and architecture than the aspirate.

### *Immunophenotyping, flow cytometry and molecular genetics*

These investigations are now routinely used in the diagnosis of haematological malignancies. They can be performed on peripheral blood or cells taken from the bone marrow aspirate (which contains precursor cells, not normally found in the peripheral blood).

## Haemoglobin electrophoresis

This separates all the haemoglobin species present in a blood sample by their differing mobility in an electric field.

## Direct antiglobulin test

The DAT indicates that there are anti-red cell antibodies bound to the surface of circulating red cells. It is used in two situations:

- If there is evidence of a haemolytic anaemia (when a positive DAT indicates autoimmune haemolytic anaemia [AIHA])
- If there is suspicion of an antibody-mediated blood transfusion reaction

## Coagulation screening tests

These tests should be performed *if there is any evidence of a bleeding disorder.* Their use in patients without a bleeding history to 'screen' for disease is controversial and can lead to misleading results.

### *Prothrombin time*

Prothrombin time (PT) tests the TF-driven 'extrinsic' clotting pathway (factor VII) and final common pathway (II, V, X). It is usually expressed as a ratio, the international normalized ratio (INR). An INR of more than 1.2 indicates a deficiency of *any or all* of *coagulation factors VII, X, V, II and fibrinogen.*

### *Activated partial thromboplastin time*

Activated partial thromboplastin time (APTT) tests the contact activated 'intrinsic' clotting pathway (factors VIII, IX, XI and XII) and final common pathway. It is usually expressed as a ratio, the *APTTr*. Prolongation indicates a deficiency of *any or all* of coagulation factors *XII, XI, IX, VIII, X, V, II and fibrinogen.* Note that deficiency of factor XII does not result in bleeding.

### *Thrombin clotting time*

Thrombin clotting time (TCT) tests fibrinogen and prolongation-indicated fibrinogen deficiency.

### *Simple diagnosis using the coagulation screen*

See **Figure 15.6**.

The three tests make diagnostic sense when their results are viewed together. Five main patterns occur:

1 *PT ↑, others normal:* factor VII deficiency or early warfarin therapy (note this would result in a raised INR as this is derived from the PT).

2 *APTTr ↑, others normal:* factor (XII), XI, IX or VIII deficiency; pattern is seen in haemophilia A (factor VIII

**Table 15.5** Normal serum haematinic levels

| Haematinic | Level |
|---|---|
| Serum iron | 18–48 µmol/L (men) |
| | 120–30 µmol/L (women) |
| Serum total iron-binding capacity (TIBC) | 45–72 µmol/L |
| Serum ferritin | 20–250 µg/L (men) |
| | 15–150 µg/L (women) |
| Serum folate | 3–15 ng/mL |
| Red cell folate | 150–500 mg/mL |
| Serum vitamin $B_{12}$ | 160–1000 pg/mL |

deficiency) and haemophilia B (factor IX deficiency), both severe inherited bleeding disorders

3 *INR ↑ and APTTr ↑, TCT normal:* vitamin K deficiency or established oral anticoagulant therapy (deficiency of factors II, VII, IX and X)

4 *TCT ↑, others normal:* indicates hypofibrinogenaemia or inteference with fibrin formation (e.g. paraprotein); TCT is more sensitive to fibrinogen abnormalities that the INR or APTTr

5 *All abnormal (usually with ↓ platelet count):* hepatic failure or DIC

### Fibrin D-dimer assay

This detects a plasmin-mediated breakdown product of fully formed fibrin (clot). It is increased in venothromboembolic disease (DVT and PE) and in DIC.

## BIOCHEMISTRY

### Haematinic assays

These include iron, folate and cobalamin (vitamin $B_{12}$) assays (**Tables 15.5** and **15.6**).

### Other biochemical changes

- *Hypercalcaemia:* common in myeloma
- *Renal failure* (creatinine ↑, urea ↑, K ↑): commonly occurs in myeloma and can be marked at presentation
- *Hyperuricaemia:* occurs in tumour lysis syndrome after chemotherapy of high-grade malignancies

## DIAGNOSTIC IMAGING

### Radiology

#### Chest radiography

This could be chest X-ray or high-resolution computed tomography scan (HRCT).

- Lung infiltrates in opportunistic pneumonia and sickle cell acute chest syndrome
- Abscess formation in fungal infection
- Wedge shadows in PE
- Hilar and mediastinal lymphadenopathy

#### Skeletal radiography

- Lytic bone disease
- Aseptic necrosis of the hip in SCD
- Joint damage and cartilage loss in haemophilia

#### Ultrasound

- Confirmation of spleen and liver size
- DVT (Doppler compression technique)
- Ultrasound-guided biopsy

#### Nuclear medicine

- Lung (V/Q) scans for pulmonary emboli
- Positron emission tomography (PET)/CT, and PET/MRI scanning using radiolabelled glucose (FDG) (widely used in the diagnosis and staging of lymphoma)

#### Computerized tomography and magnetic resonance imaging

- Detection of lymphadenopathy/tumour masses in inaccessible sites (abdominal, pelvic, retroperitoneal, CNS)
- Cord compression in myeloma
- CT and MRI are used in preference to skeletal survey (where available) in the diagnosis of patients with mutliple myeloma.
- Joints in SCD and haemophilia (magnetic resonance imaging [MRI])
- CT-guided biopsy

## HISTOPATHOLOGY

Histopathological examination of bone marrow specimens and lymph node biopsies are essential in the diagnosis of haematological disorders. Core biopsy of lymph nodes is now used in preference to fine-needle aspiration.

**Table 15.6** Serum iron, TIBC and ferritin in different diseases

| Disease | Serum iron | TIBC | Percentage transferrin saturation | Ferritin |
|---|---|---|---|---|
| Iron deficiency | ↓ | ↑ | ↓↓ | ↓ |
| Chronic disease | ↓ | → or ↓ | ↓ | → or ↑ |
| Sideroblastic anaemia | ↑ | → | ↑ | ↑↑ |
| Haemochromatosis | ↑ | → | ↑ | ↑↑ |
| Ineffective erythropoiesis | ↑ | → | ↑ | ↑↑ |
| Hypoproteinaemia | ↓ | ↓ | → | → |

↓, Decreased; ↑, increased; →, normal.

## TRANSFUSION: BLOOD COMPONENT SUPPORT

Transfusion support is a cornerstone of the management of haematology patients. It permits high-dose chemotherapy and is used to support patients with conditions such as haemoglobinopathies. Transfusion should be avoided in haematinic deficiency and the deficient factor should be replaced instead (e.g. iron infusion). The reason for any transfusion must always be written in the case notes and patients should, if able, give their informed consent.

### Red cells

Transfusion is usually justifiable when Hb concentration falls below 70–80 g/L. Each unit of red cells raises Hb concentration by 7–10 g/L.

### Platelets

The purpose of platelet transfusion is to increase the platelet count from a level causing bleeding or increased bleeding risk to one that does not. Surgery requires different platelet thresholds depending on the site and bleeding risk. Abdominal surgery including caesarean section can safely be performed with platelet counts >50 × 10$^9$/L while neurosurgery and ophthalmic surgery require the platelet count to be 100 × 10$^9$/L or greater.

### Fresh frozen plasma

The purpose of infusing (thawed) plasma is to correct deficiencies of several clotting factors in acute situations (e.g. hepatic failure, massive blood transfusion). In cases of major haemorrhage, red cells and fresh frozen plasma (FFP) should be transfused at a ratio of at least 2 : 1.

### Clotting factors

These are used to correct a deficiency of a single factor (e.g. factor VIII in haemophilia A). Plasma-derived concentrates are being replaced by synthetic recombinant clotting factors as the treatment of choice. Recombinant factors do not carry a risk of blood-borne infections and should be used in preference to plasma-derived products where available.

## RISKS OF TRANSFUSION

### Acute haemolytic transfusion reaction

This is the most serious adverse event of transfusion and is usually due to the transfusion of ABO-incompatible blood. In ABO-incompatible reactions, transfused red cells are destroyed by the recipient's preformed anti-A or anti-B antibodies resulting in intravascular haemolysis and sudden and dramatic clinical deterioration (see EMERGENCY PRESENTATION 15.1). Incompatible blood transfusion should be

considered a 'never event'. Life-threatening consequences can occur after transfusion of less than 10 mL incompatible blood.

- *Usual cause:* transfusing red cells intended for a different person (*wrong blood*), when the risk of ABO mismatch is 1 in 3
- *Symptoms:* fear; flushing; pain at drip site; back and/or abdominal pain
- *Signs:* fever; hypotension; bleeding; red urine (resulting from haemoglobin – microscopy shows no red cells)
- *Management: stop the transfusion immediately;* keep the drip open; resuscitate and support the circulation (see EMERGENCY PRESENTATION 15.1).

### Transfusion-associated circulatory overload

Transfusing too much blood, or too fast, leads to acute cardiac decompensation and acute pulmonary oedema. Transfusion-associated circulatory overload (TACO) is now one of the commonest serious adverse transfusion events reported in the UK's annual SHOT (Serious Hazards of Transfusion) report. Particular care should be taken in adults with a low body mass index or history of congestive cardiac failure. All patients requiring transfusion should be assessed for their risk of developing TACO and, if necessary, measures should be taken to reduce the risk (e.g. using diuretics with transfusion and only transfusing one unit).

- *Symptoms:* breathlessness; cough
- *Signs:* basal crepitations; jugular venous pressure (JVP) ↑; tachycardia
- *Management:* oxygen, diuretic therapy

### Transfusion-associated acute lung injury

Transfusion-associated acute lung injury (TRALI) is caused by passive transfer of human leukocyte antibodies (HLA) or human neutrophil antibodies (HNA) in the donor sample. This results in a clinical picture that resembles acute respiratory distress syndrome (ARDS) and in the acute setting can be difficult to distinguish from TACO. Any suspected cases should be reported to the blood service so that they can be investigated and, if the donor is found to have HLA/HNA antibodies, any other products made from their donation are withdrawn and they are retired as a donor.

- *Symptoms:* dyspnoea, hypoxia without evidence of circulatory overload; occurs within 6 hours of transfusion
- *Signs:* bilateral pulmonary infiltrates on chest X-ray; bilateral coarse crackles
- *Management:* supportive; may require ICU admission for respiratory support

### Delayed haemolytic transfusion reaction

Immune IgG anti-red cell antibodies react with incompatible transfused cells to cause phagocytosis in the reticuloendothelial system and antibody-dependent cellular cytotoxicity (ADCC). The result is rapid extravascular destruction of

**15**

the cells (over 24–48 hours). It can occur with any of the blood groups and antibodies against a particular antigen are usually detectable in the patient's plasma after the event. Further transfusion should be avoided (if possible) until the causative antigen has been identified.

- *Symptoms:* fever, chills, malaise
- *Signs:* jaundice, Hb rapidly falls to pretransfusion level
- *Management:* symptomatic

### Transfusion-transmitted infection

In order of magnitude, current UK risk estimates of acquiring infection from a single blood component unit are:

- *Hepatitis B:* 1 in 1.6 million units transfused
- *Hepatitis C:* 1 in 40.5 million units transfused
- *HIV:* 1 in 5.7 million units transfused
- *New variant Creutzfeldt–Jakob disease (vCJD) prion:* has been known to be transmitted by blood transfusion and, while the risk is thought to be small, extensive measures have been taken to reduce the risk of contaminated blood from entering the blood supply

### Iron overload (transfusion haemosiderosis)

Patients on chronic long-term transfusion regimens (e.g. thalassaemia major) will develop endocrine and cardiac failure due to iron toxicity unless regular chelation therapy is administered.

## DISEASES AND THEIR MANAGEMENT

### ANAEMIA

Broadly speaking, the causes of anaemia (**Table 15.7**) are:

- Decreased red cell production
- Increased red cell destruction
- Red cell loss through haemorrhage

### MICROCYTIC ANAEMIAS

Microcytic anaemia is defined as anaemia associated with a low MCV (less than 78 fL) and is due to the shortage of one of the building blocks of haemoglobin: iron deficiency,

globin chain deficiency (thalassaemia, inherited, common) or haem deficiency (lead poisoning,).

## IRON-DEFICIENCY ANAEMIA

### Epidemiology

This affects all ages but is commoner in women (10–15% of women of reproductive age).

### Disease mechanisms

The underlying cause of iron deficiency must be found.

- *In a woman of reproductive age,* iron deficiency is nearly always caused by imbalance between dietary intake and iron losses (menstrual and pregnancy related blood loss).
- *In all males and postmenopausal women,* the development of iron deficiency must be *assumed to be caused by a gastrointestinal malignancy* until proven otherwise by full gastrointestinal investigation, including endoscopy.

#### Control of iron absorption and turnover

In humans, the amount of iron in the body is controlled through increased or decreased uptake from the gut. There are no mechanisms that can increase iron excretion if iron is in excess. Viamin C favours iron absorption by converting ferric ions to ferrous ions.

*Hepcidin* is the master iron regulator and plays a crucial role in iron homeostasis by reducing iron absorption in the gut. Iron deficiency results in decreased hepcidin production and thus increased iron absorption in the gut. Similarly, hepcidin production is decreased in genetic haemochromatosis (and thus causes increased iron uptake). In iron overload states, hepcidin production is increased thus reducing gut absorption of iron.

### Investigation

Diagnosis is based on the presence of a microcytic anaemia accompanied by a low serum ferritin (a marker of iron stores, but also an acute phase protein), and confirmed by a response to iron therapy.

- *FBC:* anaemia with MCV less than 78 fL; increased platelet count (thrombocytosis) often seen, particularly in the case of chronic blood loss

**Table 15.7** Diagnostic approach to anaemia

| Anaemia | MCV (fL) | Platelets | White cell count | Diagnosis |
|---|---|---|---|---|
| Microcytic | <80 | | | Iron deficiency |
| | | | | Thalassaemia |
| Normocytic | 80–96 | Normal | Normal | Anaemia of chronic disorder, rheumatoid arthritis |
| | | Low/normal | Abnormal | Marrow invasion by cancer (leucoerythroblastic anaemia) |
| | | | | Haematological malignancy |
| | | Normal | Increased | Chronic haematological malignancy |
| Macrocytic | >96 | Normal | Normal | Vitamin B$_{12}$ or folate deficiency, liver disease, haemolysis |
| | | Low | Normal/low | Vitamin B$_{12}$ or folate deficiency, acute haematological malignancy |
| | | Normal/low | Abnormal | Myelodysplastic syndromes (MPS) |

- *Blood film:* pale hypochromic red cells and 'pencil' cells
- *Serum iron measurements:* iron ↓; TIBC ↑; transferrin saturation ↓; ferritin ↓. (*Ferritin* is a water-soluble protein present in minute amounts in the serum, where its concentration correlates with total body iron)

## Management

Treatment is with oral iron therapy. In patients with severe iron deficiency anaemia who require relatively urgent treatment or in patients who are not responding or tolerating oral therapy, intravenous (IV) iron preparations can be given.

## IRON-DEFICIENCY ANAEMIA AT A GLANCE

### Epidemiology

*Prevalence*
500–600 million people worldwide

*Age, sex and ethnicity*
Common in children, women of reproductive age and vegans

*Genetics*
N/A

*Geography*
Less economically developed countries with malnutrition and hookworm infestation

*Incidence*
Most common in women of reproductive age (menstruation plus multiple pregnancies)

### Findings on investigation

*Haematology*
FBC: Hb less than 13 g/dL (males), less than 12 g/dL (females): MCV less than 78 fL
Blood film: hypochromic RBCs: 'pencil cells' (**Figure A**)

*Biochemistry*
Ferritin ↑, serum iron ↓, TIBC ↑, transferrin saturation ↓

*Diagnostic imaging*
Iron deficiency should be investigated by endoscopy for gastro-intestinal cancer in:
All men
All postmenopausal women
Anyone with gastrointestinal symptoms

*Histopathology*
Bone marrow cytology is needed in people with other potential causes of anaemia: in iron deficiency, there is absent iron staining (Perls' stain), erythroid hyperplasia and poorly haemoglobinized RBC precursors

### Clinical features

*Symptoms associated with reduced oxygen transport*
Tiredness and sleepiness
Loss of interest in usual pursuits
Breathlessness on effort
Palpitations

*Mucocutaneous*
Mucosal pallor
Angular stomatitis
Koilonychia (very rare)
Brittle hair and nails

**15**

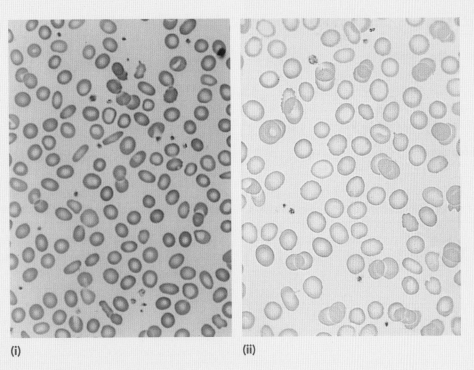

(i)   (ii)

**Figure A** Iron-deficiency anaemia. Peripheral blood films showing hypochromic, cells with poikilocytosis: **(i)** pencil cells; **(ii)** hypochromasia.

*Continued...*

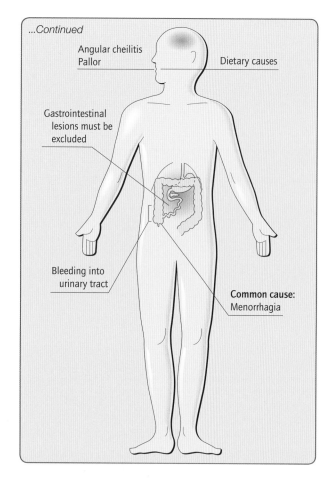

...*Continued*

Angular cheilitis
Pallor

Dietary causes

Gastrointestinal
lesions must be
excluded

Bleeding into
urinary tract

Common cause:
Menorrhagia

## NORMOCYTIC ANAEMIA: ANAEMIA OF CHRONIC DISEASE

### Epidemiology

- About 10–15% of all hospitalized patients
- Commonly seen in acute infections and chronic inflammatory states
- More common in those over 65 years

### Disease mechanisms

Anaemia of chronic disease is normocytic. It is associated with impaired iron mobilization from iron stores, aimed at depriving microorganisms of iron. Chronic infections (e.g. tuberculosis), carcinoma, chronic kidney disease and connective tissue disorders (e.g. rheumatoid arthritis) are typical causes (see **Table 15.7**).

### Clinical features

The clinical picture is non-specific and largely that of the underlying chronic disorder.

### Diagnosis

This is anaemia (usually in the range 80–100 g/L) in the presence of any chronic or subacute inflammatory disorder. The anaemia is often refractory to therapy. It is often a diagnosis of exclusion.

### Investigation

- *FBC:* This shows normochromic or mildly hypochromic anaemia.
- *Iron status:* Iron stores, as reflected in serum ferritin, are normal or increased, but serum iron is low. TIBC is normal or mildly reduced, so that the percentage iron saturation is not as markedly reduced as in iron deficiency (see **Table 15.7**).

### Management

Management includes successful treatment of the underlying chronic disorder. In severe cases where there is haemodynamic compromise, blood transfusion may be required.

## MACROCYTIC ANAEMIAS

## MEGALOBLASTIC ANAEMIA

Megaloblastic anaemia is characterized by distinctive morphological features. Deficiencies of vitamin $B_{12}$ and/or folate are the most common causes (**Table 15.8**).

### Vitamin $B_{12}$ deficiency and pernicious anaemia

$B_{12}$ deficiency may result from insufficient dietary intake or due to autoimmune destruction of gastric parietal cells which secrete the intrinsic factor necessary for absorption of $B_{12}$ in the terminal ileum.

### *Epidemiology*

- 25 cases/100 000 people over 40 years of age per year
- More common in women
- Dietary deficiency commoner in vegans and ethnic groups which adhere to strict vegetarian diets

**Table 15.8** Causes of vitamin $B_{12}$ and folate deficiency

| Cause | Example |
|---|---|
| **Vitamin $B_{12}$ deficiency** | |
| Nutritional deficiency | Vegan diet |
| Gastric malabsorption | PA, gastrectomy |
| Intestinal malabsorption | Ileal resection, Crohn's disease, stagnant loop syndrome caused by an anatomical blind loop, intestinal stricture, or jejunal diverticulosis, tropical sprue |
| **Folate deficiency** | |
| Nutritional deficiency | Alcoholism, old age, psychiatric disturbance |
| Malabsorption | Coeliac disease, Crohn's disease |
| Excessive use | Haemolytic anaemia |
| Increased requirements | Myeloproliferative disorders, pregnancy |
| Folate-antagonist drugs | Methotrexate, trimethoprim, anticonvulsants |

## Pathogenesis

Classic pernicious anaemia (PA) results from an 'auto-immune' gastritis leading to atrophy of parietal cells (which secrete intrinsic factor needed for $B_{12}$ absorption). Autoantibodies against intrinsic factor are found in 55% of patients. Rare patients have poor vitamin $B_{12}$ absorption because of past gastrectomy or damage to the terminal ileum (e.g. by Crohn's disease).

## Clinical features

Awareness of the disease and the sensitivity of automated MCV measurement in the routine FBC has led to earlier diagnosis, often at the asymptomatic (macrocytic but not yet anaemic) stage of the disorder. Gastrointestinal features of weight loss, diarrhoea and constipation are common. An important subgroup of patients presents with neurological effects of vitamin $B_{12}$ deficiency, without any macrocytosis or megaloblastic change. Neurological manifestations include peripheral neuropathy, optic atrophy, subacute combined degeneration of the cord (posterior column and pyramidal tract involvement) and mental abnormalities such as irritability, somnolence and dementia.

## Diagnosis

The findings of megaloblastic anaemia with a low total serum cobalamin level and the presence of anti-intrinsic factor antibodies have a high predictive value (95%) for a diagnosis of PA. Gastric parietal cell antibodies have a low specificity for the diagnosis of PA. The previously well-known Schilling test is no longer widely available and is rarely used.

## Investigation

- *FBC:* macrocytic anaemia (red cell MCV more than 100 fL); if severe, with accompanying leucopenia and thrombocytopenia
- *Blood film:* shows oval macrocytes, marked variation in red cell size (anisocytosis, with RBC fragments) shape (poikilocytosis), and hypersegmented (more than four lobes per cell nucleus) neutrophils
- *Bone marrow aspirate:* not needed unless there is diagnostic uncertainty
- *Serum cobalamin:* <200 ng/L
- Positive anti-intrinsic factor antibodies in combination with low serum cobalamin produce a high predictive value for diagnosis of PA

## Management

Malabsorption of vitamin $B_{12}$, irrespective of aetiology, is treated with *1 mg hydroxocobalamin* administered by intramuscular injection every 3 months for life. Initially 5–6 doses are given over 3 weeks. Daily oral $B_{12}$ supplement in the form of cyanocobalamin 50 μg tablets can be used in dietary deficiency.

## Folate deficiency

### Epidemiology

Folate deficiency occurs worldwide in all age groups.

## Pathogenesis

It occurs in six main settings:

- Decreased dietary intake (often associated with iron deficiency)
- Malabsorption (e.g. coeliac disease)
- Acute starvation
- Increased folate requirement of pregnancy
- Increased folate requirement because of rapid red cell turnover in haemolytic anaemias (e.g. sickle cell anaemia [SCA])
- Chronic therapy with antiepileptic agents (e.g. phenytoin)

## Diagnosis

- Macrocytic anaemia with oval macrocytes and/or hypersegmented neutrophils
- Low serum folate (<2.5 μg/L)

## Investigation

- *FBC:* macrocytic anaemia
- *Biochemistry:* low serum folate

## Management

Oral folic acid tablets (5 mg) are given once daily in established folate deficiency anaemia. In malabsorption, daily doses of up to 15 mg may be required. Before prescribing folate, vitamin $B_{12}$ deficiency must be excluded because folate replacement can provoke neuropathy if vitamin $B_{12}$ deficiency is also present. For prophylaxis during pregnancy, a daily dose of 400 μg is given, unless there is a high risk of neural tube defects, when at least 800 μg/day is indicated.

### Other causes of macrocytic anaemia

The other most frequent cause of a macrocytic anaemia is *chronic excess alcohol ingestion. Non-alcoholic liver disease* and *hypothyroidism* can also be causes. If macrocytosis is unexplained, bone marrow examination may be required to exclude an MDS.

## HAEMOLYTIC ANAEMIAS

### Disease mechanisms

Haemolysis can be primary or secondary to another cause (e.g. haemolytic transfusion reaction), drug-induced haemolysis or due to abnormal red cells (e.g. SCA) or enzyme deficiencies such as glucose-6-phosphate dehydrogenase (G6PD) deficiency.

### Intravascular haemolysis

This refers to red cell destruction within the blood vessels. Free Hb appears in the blood (*haemoglobinaemia*) and is lost in the glomerular filtrate (*haemoglobinuria*), causing dark-coloured urine which can be mistaken for haematuria. If intravascular haemolysis is part of an explosive (IgM-mediated) immune reaction, such as in ABO-incompatible red cell transfusion, it provokes life-threatening systemic upset with acute renal failure and DIC.

15

### Extravascular haemolysis

Binding of IgG to the red cell membrane leads to recognition and clearance by macrophages of the reticuloendothelial system in the spleen, liver and bone marrow. In haemolytic anaemias caused by red cell membrane defects (including SCD), the red cell destruction occurs mainly extravascularly.

### Increased red cell breakdown products

In all forms of haemolytic anaemia, the turnover of haem increases, reflected in the levels of unconjugated and conjugated bilirubin processed by the liver. In long-term chronic haemolytic states, oversaturation of bile may result in gallstone formation.

### Investigation

- *FBC:* normocytic or mildly macrocytic anaemia
- *Reticulocyte count:* increased
- *Blood film microscopy:*
  - Polychromasia caused by the presence of young red cells
  - Diagnostic abnormalities of red cell shape (e.g. sickle cells, elliptocytes, spherocytes)
  - Red cell fragments (schistocytes) indicate a *microangiopathic* haemolytic process
- *Haemoglobin electrophoresis:* may show abnormal haemoglobin (e.g. HbS)
- *Red cell enzyme assay:* may reveal G6PD deficiency
- *Haemoglobinuria:* in intravascular haemolysis
- *Lactic dehydrogenase (LDH):* increased
- *Serum bilirubin:* increased
- *DAT:* postive in immune mediate haemolysis
- *Serum haptoglobin:* reduced

## AUTOIMMUNE HAEMOLYTIC ANAEMIA

### Epidemiology

- Incidence is 1 in 100 000
- Affects people of any age, including children

### Disease mechanisms

AIHA is caused by an autoantibody to the patient's own red cells. The antibodies are active either at body temperature (37 °C – 'warm antibody' = IgG) or at room temperature (15 °C – 'cold antibody' = IgM; **Table 15.9**). Cold antibody AIHA often causes red cell autoagglutination on blood films and is therefore sometimes called cold agglutinin disease. Haemolysis is usually extravascular, resulting from phagocytosis of antibody and/or complement-coated red cells within the spleen and liver.

### Clinical features

Mild jaundice and moderate splenomegaly are typical of chronic warm AIHA. Worsening of haemolysis on exposure

**Table 15.9** Causes of warm-reacting antibody (often IgG) and cold-reacting antibody (often IgM)

| Cause | Example |
|---|---|
| **Warm-reacting antibody** | |
| IgG (± complement fixation) directed | Idiopathic |
| against very 'public' antigen | Lymphoproliferative disorders (or common) erythrocyte (e.g. CLL, NHL) |
| | Autoimmune rheumatic diseases (e.g. systemic lupus erythematosus) |
| Haptens | Drugs (e.g. quinine) sulphonamides, chlorpromazine, penicillin |
| Immune complexes | |
| Autoantibodies | |
| **Cold-reacting antibody** | |
| Lymphoproliferative disease producing monoclonal IgM that reacts with the red cells at low temperatures | Cold haemagglutinin disease |
| Autoantibody with anti-I and anti-I specificity | Mycoplasma infection, infectious mononucleosis |
| IgG directed against P blood group system | Paroxysmal cold haemoglobinuria |

to cold (or even normal ambient) temperatures is typical of cold antibody (IgM) AIHA.

- *Primary AIHA:* occurs without evidence of an underlying disease
- *Secondary AIHA:* occurs in the context of an existing autoimmune disorder (rheumatoid arthritis, SLE) or lymphoma or chronic leukaemia (NHL or CLL)
- *Mycoplasma-associated (acute) cold agglutinin AIHA:* associated with atypical pneumonia and cold agglutinins (anti-I antibodies)
- *Drug-induced AIHA:* e.g. methyldopa, cephalosporin antibiotics, others

### Investigation and diagnosis

- *FBC:* shows anaemia, mild macrocytosis; WBC and platelets usually normal
- *Reticulocyte count:* increased (more than $100 \times 10^9$/L)
- *Blood film:* shows polychromasia; *red cell agglutination* may be seen in cold antibody AIHA
- *DAT:* a positive test detects immunoglobulin and/or complement on the red cell membrane
- *Cold agglutinins* (IgM antibodies directed against the red cell I antigen): detected in warm separated serum in cold AIHA

## Management

- Warm (IgG-mediated) AIHA usually responds to corticosteroids (e.g. prednisone 1 mg/kg body weight). Other immunosuppressive agents, such as the anti-CD20 monoclonal antibody rituximab, may be needed in steroid refractory cases. Splenectomy is reserved for severe refractory cases. In possible drug-induced AIHA, the suspected drug is stopped.
- Treatment of cold haemagglutinin disease includes control of the underlying disorder (e.g. with anti-*Mycoplasma* antibiotics) and warming the patient. Rituximab may be useful in some cases.

## HAEMOGLOBINOPATHIES

Genetic disorders of haemoglobin are caused by abnormalities of globin genes. A single abnormal allele, inherited from one parent, results in an asymptomatic *heterozygous* carrier state (a trait). If a person inherits abnormal alleles from both parents, they are affected (*homozygous*) and usually suffer from severe anaemia, together with other features arising from abnormal red cell structure and function.

Haemoglobinopathies can be divided into two broad groups:
- *Reduced synthesis of globin chains (the thalassaemias):* These disorders are caused by a wide range of genetic mutations affecting both α-globin and β-globin genes.
- *Structural haemoglobin variants:* These are caused by genetic mutations encoding single nucleotide/amino acid substitutions (haemoglobin S, haemoglobin C, haemoglobin E and more than 200 other variants), many of which have no clinical effect. Clinically important structural variants *all affect β-globin chains*.

## THALASSAEMIAS

Thalassaemia is caused by inherited globin gene abnormalities that result in underproduction or absence of either the β-globin or the α-globin chain. The resulting reduction in haemoglobin level causes variable degrees of anaemia (the most severe forms being incompatible with life), haemolysis, cell death in the bone marrow and consequent massive bone marrow hypertrophy and iron overload.

### α-thalassaemia

#### Epidemiology
- Carried by many millions worldwide, depending on ethnicity
- Worldwide: highest in Africa (mostly α+) and South East Asia (China, Thailand, Vietnam: mostly α0); also found in Middle Eastern and Mediterranean populations

### Clinical syndromes
The clinical subtypes are determined by the number of expressed α genes:
- *Deletion of all four α genes:* There is no α chain production so neither HbF nor HbA is synthesized (**Figure 15.8**). Hb Bart's (γ4) self-assembles but cannot transport oxygen. The foetus develops severe congestive heart failure (Bart's hydrops fetalis) and dies *in utero* or at term.
- *Deletion of three α-globin genes:* This results in HbH disease, in which excess α chains are synthesized and precipitate within the red cell as HbH. Clinically, HbH disease is classified as a thalassaemia intermedia.
- *Deletion of one or two α genes:* This causes α-thalassaemia trait, which is asymptomatic.

### Investigation
- *HbH disease:* Clinically, this is a thalassaemia intermedia: moderate anaemia (haemoglobin 80–100 g/L), marked microcytosis, anisocytosis and poikilocytosis.
- *Deletion of two α genes:* Typical findings are a normal haemoglobin level, a low red cell MCH (<25 pg) and MCV, and a high red cell count.

### Management and prognosis
HbH disease requires prophylactic folic acid and occasional transfusion in times of stress. α-thalassaemia trait does not require any treatment, but genetic counselling of carriers of reproductive age is important.

### β-thalassaemia

#### Epidemiology
β-thalassaemia is found worldwide, but highest rates (5–15%) occur in the Mediterranean region (Cyprus,

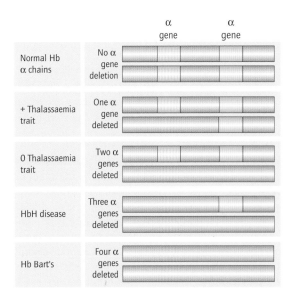

**Figure 15.8** Genetic basis of α-thalassaemia. The clinical subtypes of α-thalassaemia are determined by the number of α genes expressed.

southern Italy and Greece), African, Middle Eastern and South East Asian ethnic groups.

### Genetics and pathogenesis

In β-thalassaemia, β-globin chain synthesis is reduced (β$^{++}$-thalassaemia) or absent (β$^0$-thalassaemia). Inheritance of various pairs of defects causes variation in clinical severity (see below). β-thalassaemia and α-globin chain abnormalities can coexist in the same individual.

### β-thalassaemia syndromes

There are three major clinical phenotypes:
- *Thalassaemia major:* severe, transfusion-dependent anaemia
- *Thalassaemia intermedia:* lifelong anaemia but infrequent transfusion needs
- *Thalassaemia minor:* the asymptomatic carrier 'trait'

There are several genotypes that can result in each clinical phenotype.

### β-thalassaemia major

*Clinical features*
- Affected individuals present in the first year of life (as haemoglobin production changes from HbF to HbA1) with failure to thrive because of severe anaemia.
- If not enlisted in an effective transfusion and iron chelation regimen, patients will develop:
  o Hepatosplenomegaly
  o Bone marrow expansion with disfiguring bone deformity (e.g. facial bones)
  o Pigment gallstones
  o Cardiac damage and endocrinopathies resulting from iron overload

*Investigation*
- *FBC:* anaemia (Hb may be as low as 20–30 g/L)
- *Blood film:* target cells, hypochromia, microcytosis, red cell fragments, nucleated red cells
- *Haemoglobin electrophoresis:* HbA1 is absent, HbF is greatly increased (from less than 1% to 80–100% of Hb)
- *Radiography:* bone X-rays show medullary expansion because of marrow hypertrophy (e.g. 'hair-on-end' appearance of skull X-ray)

*Management* Regular (4–6-weekly) red cell transfusion is needed, aiming to keep Hb more than 100 g/L to suppress marrow hypertrophy and iron absorption from the gut (hypertransfusion regimen). Continuous iron chelation with oral agents is now preferred by the majority of patients to continuous subcutaneous desferrioxamine infusions. Allogeneic bone marrow transplantation in young patients with appropriately matched allogeneic stem cell donors is the only curative treatment option but carries a risk of morbidity and mortality. Gene therapy approaches have recently shown promise in clinical trials.

*Prognosis* Increasingly, with effective transfusion programmes and iron chelation, many patients survive to adulthood, which was previously rare. Allogeneic stem cell transplantation can offer a cure.

### β-thalassaemia intermedia

*Clinical features* Symptoms are similar to β-thalassaemia major, but less severe. Bone deformity and hepatosplenomegaly may occur. Patients usually maintain their haemoglobin at 6–9 g/dL without transfusion. The blood film appearances are similar to those of thalassaemia major. Iron overload may occur because of increased iron absorption.

*Management and prognosis* Intermittent transfusion may be indicated in some patients. Patients have near-normal life expectancy.

### β-thalassaemia minor (β-thalassaemia trait)

This describes the heterozygous state (one normal β-globin gene plus either a β$^0$ or a β$^+$ gene). Affected individuals are asymptomatic and are often diagnosed incidentally but should always be provided with access to antenatal diagnosis. Haemoglobin levels are 11–12 g/dL. MCV is <78 fL. The condition mimics iron deficiency but with normal iron levels.

## SICKLE CELL HAEMOGLOBINOPATHIES

- *SCA:* refers to the homozygous (disease) state HbSS
- *SCD:* refers to all patients with compound heterozygote states involving HbS (HbSS, HbSC, HbS/β$^0$ Thal, HbSO$^{Arab}$, etc.)
- *Sickle cell trait:* refers to the asymptomatic healthy HbAS heterozygote

### Epidemiology

- 25% of individuals in sub-Saharan Africa are heterozygous for HbAS.
- In the UK, 20% of West African and 10% of Afro-Caribbean ethnicity carry a single copy of the sickle cell gene.
- There are at least 5000 patients in the UK.

### Sickle cell anaemia

The disorder results from a single point mutation in the β-globin gene. Deoxygenated HbS forms self-organizing polymers, leading to red cell distortion, shortened red cell survival (haemolytic anaemia) and blockage of the microcirculation causing infarction and tissue death. SCA is characterized by anaemia, asplenism and acute and chronic organ damage resulting from vaso-occlusion (vascular obstruction by sickle cells) and consequent infarction.

### Clinical features

There is wide clinical variability in SCA.
There are several types of sickle crisis:
- *Painful crisis:* Severe localized or generalized pain is a result of sickling in tissues and consequent tissue hypoxia. Opiate analgesia is usually required. Painful

crises can be triggered by acute insults such as infection and these should be actively looked for.

- *Splenic sequestration:* This occurs in younger patients and results in an extremely rapid fall in Hb (often to 2–3 g/dL) with rapid spleen enlargement.
- *Acute chest syndrome:* This is a medical emergency. It is usually provoked by infection or other insults but can also occur in isolation. Sickle vaso-occlusion in the lung circulation causes rapidly spreading infarction and consolidation with a vicious cycle of profound hypoxia and further sickling. Treated with oxygen, positive airway pressure and blood transfusion (often exchange transfusion) to reduce circulating HbS.
- *Cerebral infarction:* Stroke is a major complication of SCA in childhood.
- *Priapism:* This is painful persisting penile erection. Severe cases can result in permanent loss of erectile function. Treatment options include needle aspiration or surgery.

### Investigation

- *FBC:* There is usually an anaemia with a haemoglobin level of 60–80 g/L and an elevated reticulocyte count. Symptoms of anaemia may be less than expected because HbS is a low-affinity Hb that releases oxygen readily in the tissues.
- *Blood film:* This shows sickle cells and target cells.
- *Haemoglobin electrophoresis*: The trace is characterized by the migration of a single band between HbA2 and HbA.
- *Sickle solubility test:* This detects the presence of HbS (is positive in sickle trait) and can be used as a screening test to exclude the presence of a sickling disorder.

### Management

SCA is managed by preventing infections that may precipitate haemolytic and aplastic crises with lifelong penicillin and folic acid. Sickle cell patients have functional hyposplenism and are poor at dealing with encapsulated bacteria. Long-term oral hydroxyurea (HU) therapy has been shown to increase haemoglobin levels and reduce the number of crises in severely affected individuals by increasing HbF levels. HU should be offered to all patients from infancy to reduce risk of complications. Patients with recurrent chest crises or stroke should be offered a regular exchange transfusion programme. Iron chelation therapy is crucial to ameliorate the toxic effects of iron. There was previously only one effective chelator (desferrioxamine), which had to be given by prolonged subcutaneous infusion. New oral iron chelators (e.g. deferiprone and desferasirox) are much more convenient for patients and are better tolerated.

Surgery is hazardous if carried out without appropriate precautions in patients with SCA. Strict attention to adequate hydration and oxygenation before and during anaesthesia is essential. Preoperative exchange transfusion is widely recommended before major surgical procedures. Similar precautions are required during pregnancy in women with SCA.

### Other sickle cell disorders

- *HbSC disease:* This results from inheritance of a HbS gene from one parent and a HbC gene from the other. The clinical features are similar to (although usually milder than) those of homozygous SCA (HbSS).
- *HbS/β⁰ thalassaemia:* The clinical phenotype is indistinguishable from SCA.

### Antenatal screening with specialist counselling

Antenatal screening with specialist counselling of prospective parents is extremely important for all sickle cell disorders, including asymptomatic heterozygous carriers (HbAS).

## RED CELL ENZYMOPATHIES

### Epidemiology

- G6PD is the commonest enzymopathy; others are rare or very rare
- G6PD deficiency more common in males (X-linked)
- May be seen in any ethnic group, but G6PD deficiency most frequent in individuals of African, Mediterranean and South East Asian descent

### Disease mechanisms

#### Glucose-6-phosphate dehydrogenase deficiency
The enzyme G6PD performs a rate-limiting step in the pentose phosphate pathway, which generates NADPH, the red cell antioxidant. G6PD deficiency renders the red cell vulnerable to the oxidant stress of:
- Infection and fever
- Oxidant drugs (primaquine, sulphonamides)

Haemolysis can be brisk and result in severe life-threatening anaemia.

#### Glycolytic pathway enzyme deficiencies
These deficiencies (e.g. pyruvate kinase deficiency) reduce the ATP energy supply to the red cell and thereby limit its survival in the circulation.

### Clinical features

The general features are those of haemolytic anaemia, with an evident provoking cause in G6PD deficiency.

### Investigation

- *FBC:* anaemia (usually normocytic)
- *Blood film:* polychromasia; red cells may show 'bitemarks' (G6PD deficiency) or 'sputnik' projections (pyruvate kinase deficiency); reticulocytosis
- *RBC enzyme assay:* demonstrates the enzyme deficiency

## SICKLE CELL ANAEMIA AT A GLANCE

### Epidemiology

*Prevalence*

- In the UK, 25% of African descent and 10% of Afro-Caribbean descent have sickle cell trait (heterozygous AS).
- In tropical Africa, about 1 in 100 births results in a child with SCD.
- There are at least 5000 people with SCA in the UK.

*Sex*

- Equal sex distribution

*Genetics*

- Homozygous for haemoglobin S gene (HbSS)

*Geography*

- Gene originated in malarious zones (tropical Africa, Mediterranean, India) and followed diaspora to Caribbean, Europe, USA, Brazil

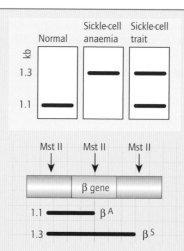

**Figure C** Prenatal diagnosis. Trophoblast DNA, obtained by sampling at 6–9 weeks of gestation, is used to detect the base substitution. Different fragment lengths are produced depending on the presence of a normal (HbA) or sickle (HbS) gene. Restriction enzyme analysis of fetal DNA reveals a single 1.3 kb band in homozygotes, a 1.3 kb band in heterozygotes, and a single 1.1 kb band corresponding to the normal β gene in normal individuals. Using the polymerase chain reaction this test can be performed in less than 6 hours, with as little as 0.25 µg of DNA.

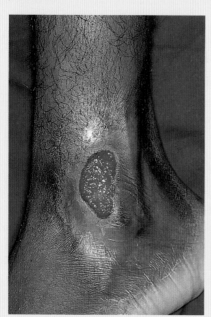

**Figure A** Typical sickle ulcer, lateral malleolus.

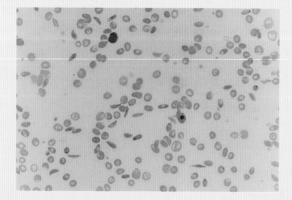

**Figure B** Peripheral blood film showing sickle-shaped cells, polychromasia and target cells. Many of the red cells appear irregular and elongated – sickle cells. Target cells are present, together with a nucleated red cell: these indicate functional hyposplenism present in SCD.

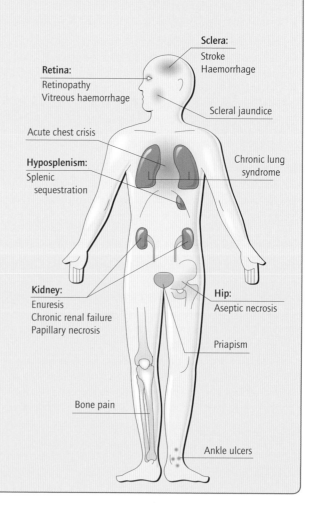

**Sclera:**
Stroke
Haemorrhage

**Retina:**
Retinopathy
Vitreous haemorrhage

Scleral jaundice

Acute chest crisis

**Hyposplenism:**
Splenic
sequestration

Chronic lung syndrome

**Kidney:**
Enuresis
Chronic renal failure
Papillary necrosis

**Hip:**
Aseptic necrosis

Priapism

Bone pain

Ankle ulcers

## Management

- Withdraw provoking drug and treat underlying infection
- Folate supplementation
- Red cell transfusion only if anaemia severe

# MICROANGIOPATHIC HAEMOLYTIC ANAEMIAS

These are a subgroup of haemolytic anaemias in which haemolysis occurs in the microvasculature due to a variety of factors. The microangiopathic haemolytic anaemia (MAHAs) are rare but are important to recognize as they can be *rapidly fatal*; if identified, they can be treated effectively. Any suspicion of MAHA should prompt immediate discussion with a haematologist.

## Epidemiology

- Rare (5 in 1 000 000/year)
- Can occur at any age in all ethnic groups

## Disease mechanisms

Haemolysis occurs in small blood vessels due to a variety of causes.

- *Haemolytic–uraemic syndrome (HUS):* Platelet and endothelial damage is related to toxigenic *Escherichia coli* infection.
- *Thrombotic thrombocytopenic purpura (TTP):* Damage is related to inherited or acquired deficiency of a protease (ADAMTS13) that normally cleaves very large forms of vWF.

## Clinical features

There is acute severe intravascular haemolytic anaemia:
- With thrombocytopenia and CNS symptoms (encephalitis and coma) in *TTP*
- With diarrhoea and renal failure in *HUS*
- In the context of pregnancy in *eclampsia* and haemolysis, elevated liver enzymes and low platelet count (*HELLP*) syndrome
- With uncontrolled severe (malignant) hypertension

## Investigation

- *FBC:* anaemia, thrombocytopenia
- *Blood film:* red cell fragments (schistocytes), polychromasia
- *LDH elevation:* often a sensitive marker of response to therapy
- *Urea and creatinine:* markers of renal failure
- Stool culture for verotoxin-secreting *E. coli* 0.157

## Management

- MAHA is a medical emergency and plasma exchange (PEX) should be initiated as soon as possible as this is life saving in TTP – this diagnosis is indistinguishable from other causes of MAHA at presentation. If PEX is delayed pending transfer to an appropriate centre, FFP (which contains the missing protease ADAMTS13) can be given.
- PEX is effective in most cases of TTP.
- Renal replacement therapy is indicated in many cases of HUS.
- Delivery of the infant is indicated in eclampsia and HELLP.

## Prognosis

- *TTP:* This is rapidly fatal if left untreated. PEX has transformed outcomes, but mortality remains high. Recurrence can occur.
- *HUS:* The majority of patients recover with supportive therapy, but permanent renal impairment can result.
- *Eclampsia, HELLP, malignant hypertension:* The outcome is good with rapid recognition and treatment.

# WHITE BLOOD CELL DISORDERS (HAEMATO-ONCOLOGY)

## GENERAL PRINCIPLES OF TREATMENT AND MANAGEMENT IN HAEMATO-ONCOLOGY

### Aim of treatment

Before discussing different haematological malignancies and their therapeutic agents it is important to consider what a particular treatment is trying to achieve.

### Curative intent

Many malignant blood diseases are curable. Acute lymphoblastic leukaemias (ALL) in children and HL in young adults are both highly curable with long-term remissions in over 90% of patients in these groups. Remission rates are dependent on patient factors (e.g. comorbidities and ability to tolerate intensive therapy) and disease biology (e.g. cytogenetic risk group, stage). Furthermore, many haematological malignancies are curable with allogeneic haematopoietic stem cell (HSC) transplantation, but in the over 60s this mode of treatment is high risk, carrying a transplant-related-mortality risk of up to 30% or more.

### Disease-modification

Many malignant blood diseases are indolent and not yet curable. They are often chronic disorders with a sluggish tumour growth rate. Myeloma, CLL and low-grade NHLs fall into this group. In these diseases, therapy is given with the aim of disease modification – it is accepted that the disease cannot be cured but long remissions of up to several years at a time would be expected.

### Palliative intent

Not all malignant blood disorders respond to therapy and recognizing patients for whom palliative care is the most appropriate option is an important skill. Palliative care includes analgesia, transfusion support, steroids or low-dose chemotherapy that aims to reduce symptoms such as night sweats.

## Drugs

### Cytotoxic chemotherapy
The purpose of cytotoxic therapy is to kill abnormal cells, thereby reducing the size of the malignant clone. If this reduction is enough, the patient enters remission. Complete remission (CR, defined as a complete lack of detectable malignant cells) is a vital endpoint in therapy because cure is largely not possible without it. Recent research has highlighted the importance of controlling the proliferation of malignant or leukaemic stem cells in the long-term control of haematological malignancies. Cytotoxic drug classes useful in haematological malignancies are as follows.

*Alkylating agents*
- *Typical drugs:* chlorambucil and cyclophosphamide; work by inducing DNA damage
- *Side effects:*
  o Early: pancytopenia, mucositis, hair loss, cystitis
  o Late: infertility, secondary leukaemia

*Antimetabolites*
- *Typical drugs:* methotrexate, cytosine arabinoside; work by inhibiting DNA synthesis
- *Side effects:*
  o Early: pancytopenia, hair loss, mucositis
  o Late: few

*Anthracyclines*
- *Typical drugs:* daunorubicin, doxorubicin; inhibit DNA and RNA synthesis
- *Side effects:*
  o Early: mucositis, pancytopenia, hair loss, nausea
  o Late: cardiotoxicity

*Vinca alkaloids*
- *Typical drug:* vincristine binds tubulin, arresting metaphase
- *Side effects:*
  o Early: abdominal pain, neuropathy
  o Late: neuropathy

### Combination chemotherapy
The therapeutic effects of cytotoxic agents are summative while the toxicities, although similar, show just enough difference to be able to combine agents *without* lethal summation of toxicity. Lasting remissions were first obtained (in HL) by exploiting this fact with a drug combination. Typically, *cycles* of combination chemotherapy are given with gaps for recovery, allowing targeting of multiple malignant cells as they pass through the cell cycle. Chemotherapeutic agents are increasingly used in combination with immunotherapy (e.g. monoclonal antibodies such as rituximab) or gene-engineered T cells (e.g. CAR-T cells).

### Immunotherapeutic agents
Harnessing the power of the immune system is increasingly important in the fight against haematological malignancies. Monoclonal antibody drugs conjugates are able to target specific proteins on a cell's surface thus selectively killing cancer cells. Rituximab is an example of such a drug, which binds to the protein CD20 which is expressed on the surface of many B-cell malignancies.

In addition to monoclonal antibody therapies, the last 2 years has seen the introduction of cellular immunotherapy for ALL and B-cell lymphomas. These approaches have utilized gene-engineered T cells, modified to express new cell surface recognition receptors (CAR or TCR), which can bind to target antigens on the surface of the malignant cell and trigger the T cell to kill the target cell.

### Biological agents and small molecules
Imatinib, a tyrosine kinase inhibitor (TKI), was hailed as a 'magic bullet' when it was introduced in 2001 for CML. This previously fatal condition was transformed into a chronic disorder. Imatinib targets the disease-causing genetic mutation by blocking the effect of a protein tyrosine kinase continuously activated as the result of the mutation. These drugs have had a dramatic response in most patients. Since then, many other 'next generation' TKIs have been developed. Other examples of using drugs for molecular targets include Ruxolitib targeting the JAK2 mutation in polycythaemia vera and MF and new agents targeting different molecular abnormalities in acute myeloid leukaemia (AML).

### Haematopoietic stem cell transplantation
This high-risk therapy offers the only chance of a long-term cure for the most aggressive haematological malignancies. HSCs can be harvested from the patient themselves (*autologous stem cells*) or a relative or an unrelated donor who has the same tissue type as the patient (*allogeneic stem cells*). The patient then undergoes chemo- and/or radiotherapy to obliterate their own bone marrow cells, including any residual malignant cells, before being infused with the stem cells from the donor.

*Autologous HSC infusion (autograft, also referred to as 'stem cell rescue')* This is performed in patients in certain haematological malignancies (e.g. myeloma and lymphoma) as part of a course of treatment, if their disease is considered to be sensitive to *high-dose chemotherapy*. The patient's own HSCs are harvested and stored. The patient can then be treated with a dose of chemotherapy that would otherwise cause dangerous marrow suppression. The stored HSCs are infused to 'rescue' the patient and normal blood counts return in 11–14 days.

*Allogeneic HSC transplantation* This is where HSCs harvested from a *donor* are infused and repopulate the marrow of a *recipient* with a bone marrow disease. The reason for doing allogeneic HSC transplantation is twofold.
- The donor marrow cells are healthy and not contaminated with malignant cells.

- A new immune system develops in the recipient after the transplant where the circulating immune cells arise from the donor haematopoietic stem cells and these immune cells are able to recognize and kill any residual malignant cells in the patients (referred to as the graft versus leukaemia/lymphoma effect [GVL]).

However, because the bone marrow is the source of immune effector cells, there is a risk that the transplanted immune system will attack its new host causing *graft-versus-host disease* (*GVHD*), which may cause severe morbidity or mortality. Also, as the transferred stem cells are non-self, if the recipient is not sufficiently immunosuppressed, graft rejection may occur resulting in failure of blood counts to recover after the transplant. In order to minimize the risk of these severe complications, the donor and recipient must be closely matched at the molecular level for their *human leucocyte antigen* (*HLA*) molecules (also referred to as tissue typing). In addition, the pre-existing stem cells must be eliminated by an appropriate *conditioning regimen*, which typically contains a combination of chemotherapy and radiotherapy. Finally, *immunosuppression* with ciclosporin A (or other immunosuppressive agents) must be given to prevent GVHD in the first few weeks and months after the transplant. Allogeneic HSC transplantation treats aggressive malignancies through the GVL effect. In bone marrow failure syndromes or immunodeficiencies, donor HSCs replace the patient's defective HSCs and give rise to healthy immune and blood cells.

Allogeneic HSC transplantation is a challenging therapy used in carefully selected and counselled patients with the following disorders:

- Haematological malignancies, particularly AML, ALL in adults and relapsed lymphomas
- Aplastic anaemia
- Thalassaemia major
- SCA
- Severe immunodeficiency

### Emergency treatment

A neutropenic patient with a fever must be treated as an emergency (EMERGENCY PRESENTATION 15.2).

## HAEMATOLOGICAL MALIGNANCIES

## ACUTE LEUKAEMIA

### Disease mechanisms

Leukaemia results from mutations or translocations involving oncogenes or transcription factors that affect cell replication and apoptosis in haematopoietic cells. A multi-step chain of several such events culminates in the development of a clone of cells with a growth advantage over their normal counterparts. Proliferating leukaemia cells replace normal haemopoiesis causing bone marrow failure with pancytopenia.

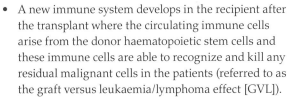

**EMERGENCY PRESENTATION 15.2**

**Fever in a neutropenic patient**

**Problem**

Fever (more than 37 °C for 2 hours or longer, or one reading of greater than 38 °C) may be the only sign of life-threatening infection in a patient with neutropenia (polymorph count less than $1.0 \times 10^9$/L).

The most common causative organisms are Gram-positive bacteria.

The most dangerous causative organisms are Gram-negative bacteria.

**Action**

Take blood and urine cultures.

Immediately start therapy with a combination of IV broad-spectrum antibiotics that cover both Gram-negative and Gram-positive pathogens (e.g. gentamicin plus tazocin): do not wait for culture results.

If the patient is already on antibiotics, a new second-line combination is commenced.

If the patient has been neutropenic for many days and febrile for 72 hours or longer, consider antifungal therapy.

G-CSF therapy may improve neutrophil counts in this situation.

If patients are also lymphopenic, consider other opportunistic pathogens.

### Classification of acute leukaemia

There are two types of acute leukaemia, defined by the lineage to which the blast cells belong:

- ALL
- AML

### Clinical features

Both types of acute leukaemia present as bone marrow failure, with symptoms and signs of anaemia, infection and bleeding. General malaise and bone pain are frequent. Time from first symptoms to diagnosis is usually short.

### Diagnosis

Diagnosis usually requires the presence of >20% blast cells in the bone marrow (in normal bone marrow the blast percentage is <5%) and the presence of any blasts in the peripheral blood (peripheral blood should not contain any blasts). Increasingly, molecular techniques (e.g. identification of a particular chromosomal abnormality or genetic mutation) can be used to diagnose acute leukaemia irrespective of the blast percentage or morphological appearances of the peripheral blood smear and/or bone marrow.

Distinguishing AML and ALL is vital because therapy is different. Using the incorrect drugs will fail to kill the leukaemic cells. In addition, it is always important to recognize the acute promyelocytic subtype of AML (APML) as this

**15**

has a different treatment and requires urgent management of any associated coagulopathy.

- *Blast cell morphology (appearance):* blood and bone marrow smears
- *Blast cell immunophenotyping:* using a panel of lineage-specific monoclonal antibody 'markers'
- *Cytogenetic study of blast cells in marrow/blood* (by karyotyping): demonstrates leukaemia-specific chromosome abnormalities
- *Molecular diagnosis:* by fluorescence *in situ* hybridization (FISH), PCR or other DNA technique demonstrates leukaemia-specific DNA sequences; more recently, targeted genome sequencing and/or microarrays have also been used

### Investigation

- *FBC:* may show a pronounced leukocytosis or the WBC may be in the normal range or even low; often there is reduction of normal cell types (pancytopenia)
- *Blood film:* leukaemic *blast* cells are usually seen
- *Bone marrow examination:* must be performed to make the diagnosis
- *Coagulation screen:* may show INR ↑, TT ↑ (see **Figure 15.6**) and fibrinogen ↓, resulting from DIC
- *Hypercalcaemia and hyperuricaemia:* may be present
- *Urea and creatinine:* may be high, indicating renal impairment

## ACUTE MYELOID LEUKAEMIA

### Epidemiology

AML incidence increases with age.

### Management

Aims of therapy:
1 Prevention of death from bone marrow failure by *supportive therapy* is the primary aim.
2 Aim for induction of *complete remission*, defined as non-detectability of leukaemic blasts plus return of normal cell counts. Increasingly, clinicians are able to detect minimal residual disease (MRD) by molecular or immunological methods. Patients who are MRD-negative after induction chemotherapy have a much better prognosis than those who are MRD-positive.
3 *Consolidation* of cytotoxic therapy, which may include further cycles of chemotherapy or, in high-risk patients, allogeneic stem cell transplantation, offers the best chance of cure.

APML is sensitive to the vitamin A derivative all-*trans*-retinoic acid (ATRA) and this drug in combination with chemotherapy or arsenic results in very high (>95%) cure rates for this subtype of AML. It is important to identify this subtype urgently at diagnosis as the treatment is very different

and at presentation many patients develop DIC, which can be managed with blood product support but can be rapidly fatal if unrecognized.

### Prognosis

Survival rates for all patients are in the region of 50% at 5 years, but there is huge variability in this group depending on patient characteristics. Older age, high-risk cytogenetics, comorbidities, MRD positivity and failure to enter remission after induction chemotherapy all confer a worse prognosis. Patients with the APML variant have an over 90% chance of a cure with appropriate treatment.

## ACUTE LYMPHOBLASTIC LEUKAEMIA

### Epidemiology

Peak incidence of ALL is at 1–5 years. It then occurs infrequently in all age groups until the rate rises again over 60 years.

### Management

Aims of therapy are the same as in AML, but *CNS-directed therapy* is also needed because ALL often infiltrates the meninges of the brain and spinal cord. ALL therapy includes an extra sequence of intrathecal chemotherapy (injected directly into the spinal canal via lumbar puncture). In children and some adult patients, *maintenance therapy* with oral drugs is needed for 2 years.

There are several new exciting therapies in B-ALL. New immunotherapeutic agents such as blinatumumab and engineered T-cell therapies (CAR-T cells) have shown dramatic results in treatment-resistant B-ALL. They are now used to manage patients with chemorefractory disease and in patients who have relapsed after bone marrow transplant.

### Prognosis

More than 90% of children between the ages of 2 and 10 are cured with chemotherapy. Prognosis is poorer and more variable in infants, teenagers and adults and is dependent on MRD status, cytogenetic risk group and response to chemotherapy. In adults, the presence of particular cytogenetic abnormalities can confer a dismal prognosis.

## MYELODYSPLASTIC SYNDROMES

MDS are a heterogeneous group of disorders characterized by dysplasia in multiple blood cell lineages. The natural disease course is progression to AML. MDS is much commoner in older patient. It presents insidiously with subtle abnormalities and progressive cytopenias.

### Diagnosis

Diagnosis is made on FBC (cytopenias or macrocytosis), bone marrow examination (dysplastic changes) and cytogenetic findings.

## Investigation

- *FBC:* cytopenias
- *Blood film:* characteristic appearance of neutrophils, with hypogranulation (empty appearance) of cytoplasm, marked monocytosis in chronic myelomonocytic leukaemia (CMML)
- *Bone marrow aspirate and trephine:* dysplastic changes and other changes specific to MDS subtype (e.g. presence of 10% or more blasts in the highest-risk subtype)

## Management

- Supportive care (e.g. blood and platelet transfusion, Epoetin Alpha [EPO] injections)
- Low-dose chemotherapy agents (e.g. azacitadine)
- Intensive anti-AML chemotherapy and bone marrow transplantation in patients with high-risk disease able to tolerate these regimes

## Prognosis

This is dependent on subtype. Those patients able to tolerate intensive chemotherapy have similar prognoses to patients with AML (dependent on cytogenetic risk group, etc.).

# CHRONIC MYELOID LEUKAEMIA

### Epidemiology

- Incidence is 1 in 100 000/year
- Slightly more common in males

### Disease pathogenesis

In CML, normal haematopoiesis is replaced by a clone of cells containing an abnormal chromosomal translocation t(9;22), the Philadelphia (Ph) chromosome. Translocation of the *abl* oncogene from chromosome 9 results in the creation of a fusion gene (*bcr-abl*) on chromosome 22. Transcription and translation of this hybrid gene result in a hybrid abnormal signalling kinase, which is continuously activated and drives the production of myeloid cells.

### Clinical features

Splenomegaly is prominent, often larger than 10 cm at diagnosis, and may cause discomfort. Other features include hepatomegaly, anaemia because of bone marrow suppression (secondary to infiltration of abnormal cells), hyperviscosity, hyperuricaemia and gout.

The clinical course follows a sequence of phases:

1 *Chronic phase* lasting 3–5 years
2 *Accelerated phase* with increasing white cell counts and splenomegaly
3 *Blast crisis* (median duration 2–4 months) with rapidly progressive and poorly treatable AML or ALL

## Investigation

- *FBC:* anaemia; WBC is increased, often massively (e.g. $250 \times 10^9$/L)
- *Blood film:* dominant feature is neutrophilia, with numerous myelocytes and basophils

## Management

- *TKIs* (e.g. imatinib) have radically changed the treamtent of CML. These oral agents have transformed a previously incurable disease into a chronic condition. Patients are monitored several times a year to ensure their disease continues to respond. There is new evidence that patients who have a 'deep molecular response' for several years may be able to stop their treatment completely and remain in remission.
- *Allogeneic bone marrow transplant* is now reserved only for patients who fail to respond or develop resistance to TKIs.

## Prognosis

CML is now thought of as a chronic disease and TKIs can result in long-term disease control. Blast crisis still carries a poor prognosis but fortunately this is now an increasingly rare event.

# CHRONIC LYMPHOCYTIC LEUKAEMIA

CLL is a chronic leukaemia caused by a clonal expansion of mature, differentiated lymphocytes, involving the blood, bone marrow and lymphoid tissues.

### Epidemiology

- Age-dependent; prevalence increases with age
- Two-thirds are male
- CLL is the most common haematological malignancy

### Disease mechanisms

CLL is a clonal proliferation of normal-looking but functionally useless B lymphocytes. In progressive CLL, they slowly accumulate in the blood, marrow and lymphoid tissues, compromising normal marrow and immune function.

### Clinical features

Many patients are diagnosed after a routine FBC and the disorder progresses slowly or not at all. Others present with a high lymphocyte count, lymphadenopathy and heavy bone marrow infiltration, with symptoms of general malaise, B symptoms, bone marrow failure and recurrent infections. Secondary AIHA (in 5–10% of patients) or autoimmune thrombocytopenia sometimes develops.

### Diagnosis

Diagnosis depends on the demonstration of a peripheral blood lymphocytosis ($>7 \times 10^9$/L) composed of B cells with a unique immunophenotype.

**15**

## Investigation

- *FBC:* lymphocytosis (>5 × 10⁹/L); cytopenias may be present
- *Blood film:* typical small lymphocytes and abundent 'smear' cells
- *Marrow and trephine:* CLL infiltrate varies from patchy to diffuse and massive
- *Molecular analysis:* presence of p53 mutations and deletions of chromosome 11 (del(11q)) confer a poor prognosis

## Management

Many patients are asymptomatic when diagnosed on routine blood counts and require no active therapy apart from monitoring. If the CLL progresses (e.g. with cytopenias, lymphadenopathy or B symptoms), treatment is indicated. Treatment depends on the patient's functional status and can vary from chemoimmunotherapy (with fludarabine- and rituximab-containing regimes) to low-dose single-agent chemotherapy. The Bruton's TKI ibrutinib and the pro-apoptotic agent venetoclax are promising and are increasingly used in difficult-to-treat cases.

## Prognosis

Many patients with non-progressive CLL will die of other age-related diseases. In the progressive form, careful therapy may help the patient to achieve a good quality of life for several years or so, however the disease is incurable. Infectious complications can result in significant mortality in advanced CLL.

---

### CHRONIC LYMPHOCYTIC LEUKAEMIA AT A GLANCE

**Epidemiology**

*Incidence*
- 200/million people over 60 years

*Age*
- Rarely seen in people under 40 years old

*Sex*
- Male : female 2 : 1

**Findings on investigation**

*Haematology*
- *FBC:* normochromic or haemolytic anaemia common. ↑ WBC because of lymphocytosis (more than 10 × 10⁹/L). ↓ Platelet count because of bone marrow infiltration or autoimmune thrombocytopenic purpura (AITP)
- *Blood film:* excess small lymphocytes and 'smear' cells
- *Bone marrow aspirate and trephine:* varying degrees of marrow infiltration with small B lymphocytes

- *Cell markers:* essential test to show clonality and typical CD5⁺ B-cell phenotype
- *Genetics:* p53 mutations, etc.

*Immunology*
- Immunoglobulin quantitation reveals hypogammaglobulinaemia in 60%

*Diagnostic imaging*
- *Chest X-ray:* to detect opportunistic pneumonia secondary to hypoimmunoglobulinaemia
- *CT:* of chest and abdomen to detect the extent of lymphadenopathy and splenomegaly

**Clinical features**
- Lymphadenopathy may be absent, localized or massive
- Splenomegaly often found, may be massive
- Systemic symptoms: anorexia, weight loss (more than 10% body weight), fever and night sweats; in late stages, cachexia may develop
- Bone marrow involvement: anaemia, neutropenia, thrombocytopenia
- Immune suppression with opportunistic infection
- CLL is often diagnosed coincidentally on routine FBC in an asymptomatic elderly patient

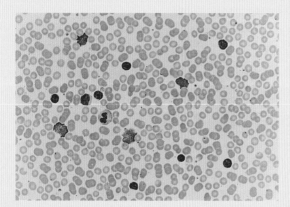

**Figure A** Chronic lymphatic leukaemia (CLL). Blood film showing immature B lymphocytes and smear cells. In this low-power field most of the cells are typical CLL lymphocytes. These are small cells with a high nuclear cytoplasmic ratio in which the nuclei contain very heavily clumped chromatin. One rather larger lymphocyte is present and some lymphoid heterogeneity is often present in CLL. At least four damaged lymphocytes are present – smear cells.

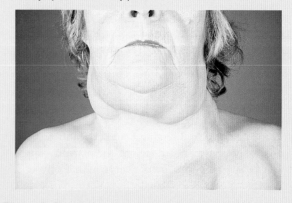

**Figure B** CLL: bilateral cervical lymphadenopathy in a 67-year-old woman. Haemoglobin 12.5/dL; white blood count 150 × 19⁹/L (lymphocytes 146 × 10⁹/L); platelets 120 × 19⁹/L. Reproduced from Hoffbrand AV & Pettit JE (1993) *Essential Haematology*, 3rd edn (Wiley-Blackwell, Oxford), with the permission of the authors.

*Continued...*

...Continued

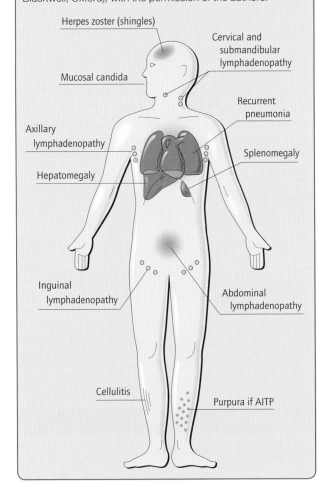

**Figure C** Chronic lymphatic leukaemia: herpes zoster infection in a 68-year-old female. Reproduced from Hoffbrand AV & Pettit JE (1993) *Essential Haematology*, 3rd edn (Wiley-Blackwell, Oxford), with the permission of the authors.

*(Body diagram labels:)* Herpes zoster (shingles); Cervical and submandibular lymphadenopathy; Mucosal candida; Recurrent pneumonia; Axillary lymphadenopathy; Splenomegaly; Hepatomegaly; Inguinal lymphadenopathy; Abdominal lymphadenopathy; Cellulitis; Purpura if AITP

## MYELOPROLIFERATIVE DISORDERS

Myeloproliferative disorders (MPD) are chronic low-grade malignant disorders resulting from the clonal proliferation of myeloid cells with or without bone marrow fibrosis as a result of pro-fibrotic cytokine production (**Figure 15.9**).

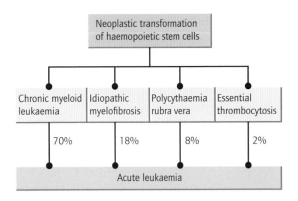

**Figure 15.9** Interrelationships between myeloproliferative disorders. Intermediate myeloproliferative disorders having features of more than one type of myeloproliferative disease may occur.

MPD are divided into three main types depending on the most prominent finding:

- *Overproduction of red cells:* polycythaemia rubra vera (PRV)
- *Overproduction of platelets:* essential thrombocythaemia (ET)
- *Overproduction of bone marrow matrix (stromal) elements:* idiopathic MF

There is significant overlap between these conditions and PRV and ET can progress to MF. All MPDs can transform to AML and, in young patients, aggressive treatment is indicated to prevent this.

## POLYCYTHAEMIA RUBRA VERA

Causes of polycythaemia are listed in **Table 15.10**.

### Epidemiology

- Older age groups: average age at diagnosis 60 years
- Incidence is 1 in 100 000/year

**Table 15.10** Causes of polycythaemia

| Pathogenesis | Disorder |
|---|---|
| **True polycythaemia** | |
| Primary | Polycythaemia rubra vera |
| Secondary | |
| Appropriate erythropoietin increase | High altitude, congenital cyanotic heart disease, pulmonary disease, hypoventilation (including obesity), high-affinity haemoglobins, heavy smoking |
| Inappropriate erythropoietin increase | Renal disease (hypernephroma, cysts), hepatoma, cerebellar haemangiomas, uterine fibromas (large) |
| **Relative polycythaemia** | |
| Unknown | Stress or pseudopolycythaemia |
| Dehydration | Vomiting, diarrhoea, diuretics |

### Clinical features

Many patients are diagnosed after a routine FBC. Nearly 50% of patients present with arterial or venous thrombosis. Pruritus affects 15% of patients at presentation and is especially noticeable after a warm bath or shower.

### Investigation

- Hb >165 g/L (men), Hb >160 g/L (women) or haematocrit >49% (men) or 48% (women)
- Presence of the JAK2 V617F or Jak 2 exon 12 mutation
- Bone marrow examination (if performed) shows increased cellularity

### Management

- *Venesection* (removal of venous blood every 1–2 weeks): initially used to reduce the haemoglobin concentration to normal, but may aggravate thrombocytosis
- *Aspirin:* to reduce risk of thrombosis
- *Myelosuppressive therapy with hydroxyurea or interferon:* often required to achieve long-term normalization of blood counts

### Prognosis

Many patients live for more than 10 years with few symptoms and well-controlled disease. PRV may transform to MF and AML, with a poor prognosis.

## ESSENTIAL THROMBOCYTHAEMIA

In ET, there is chronic elevation of the platelet count above $450 \times 10^9$/L, associated with megakaryocytic hypertrophy in the bone marrow.

### Epidemiology

Incidence is 1 in 100 000/year.

### Disease mechanisms

In this variant of MPD, it is the platelet number increasing progressively which leads to increased risk of both bleeding and thrombosis.

### Investigation

- *FBC:* normal Hb; normal WBC; platelet count *persistently* >$450 \times 10^9$/L
- *Bone marrow and trephine:* aspirate shows increased megakaryocytes and is needed to exclude fibrosis (MF can present in a similar way)
- Identification of a clonal marker (JAK2, CALR or MPL mutation) using various molecular techniques

### Management

The aim of management is to reduce the risk of thrombosis by normalizing the platelet count. As in PRV, aspirin is given while HU, anagrelide and interferon are used to reduce the platelet count.

## IDIOPATHIC MYELOFIBROSIS

This is chronic progressive haemopoietic failure caused by infiltration of the marrow space by fibrosis. Progressive cytopenias develop and can be severe. Extramedullary spread of haematopoiesis to the spleen produces dramatic and uncomfortable splenomegaly. Transformation to AML is commoner than with other MPNs.

### Epidemiology.

- Incidence 1 in 1 000 000/year
- Older age groups: average age at diagnosis 60 years

### Disease mechanisms

Marrow fibrosis results from uncontrolled release of growth factors (e.g. platelet-derived growth factor [PDGF]) from clonal myeloid cells.

### Investigation

- *FBC:* progressive cytopenias
- *Peripheral blood film:* a leucoerythroblastic film, with typical 'teardrop' poikilocytes
- *Bone marrow and trephine:*
  o Aspiration frequently unsuccessful – a 'dry tap' – because of the fibrosis
  o Trephine biopsy vital and reveals the extensive fibrosis (**Figure 15.10**)
- Clonal marker (e.g. JAK2, CALR or MPL mutations) often detected

### Management

- Care is supportive with blood and platelet transfusions.
- JAK2 inhibitors such as ruxolitinib are now used to improve symptoms such as splenomegaly and B symptoms.
- High-risk patients are referred for allogeneic bone marrow transplantation.

### Prognosis

Although JAK2 inhibitors have improved survival rates, MF still carries the worse prognosis of any MPD. Allogenic bone marrow transplantation offers a cure for younger patients.

## LYMPHOMA

## HODGKIN'S LYMPHOMA

HL consists of a clonal B-cell tumour mixed with a large population of 'reactive' non-malignant cells. Often the majority of the tumour mass/bulk is made up of these reactive cells, rather than the malignant cells.

### Epidemiology

- Peak incidence 18–28 years
- A second small peak after 60 years involves the diffuse subtype

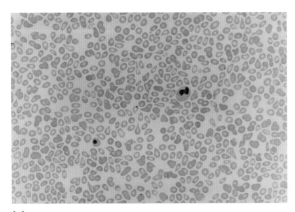

**(a)**

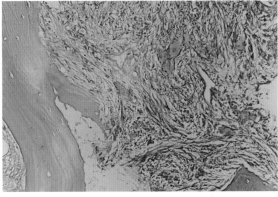

**(b)**

**Figure 15.10** Idiopathic MF. **(a)** Typical peripheral blood appearances in MF. Many of the red cells have the elongated teardrop appearance (teardrop poikilocytes). A nucleated red cell is present and is part of the leukoerythroblastic picture typical of MF. **(b)** Bone marrow trephine stained with reticulin showing complete replacement of the intertrabecular space by dense connective tissue. The dense fibres represent reticulin and are grossly increased. Megakaryocytes are abundant and are responsible for stimulating the fibrosis.

## Diagnosis

Diagnosis requires the detection of classic binucleate Reed–Sternberg cells in lymph node biopsy tissue. These cells have a typical immunohistochemical staining pattern.

## Clinical features

Typically there is painless, sometimes massive, rubbery lymphadenopathy, commonly affecting cervical and supra-clavicular lymph nodes. B symptoms are present in a third of patients at diagnosis and their presence worsens the prognosis and may warrant higher intensity therapy.

## Investigation

### Haematology

- *FBC:* usually normal; cytopenias only present if there is bone marrow involvement
- *ESR and/or CRP:* raised
- *LDH:* raised
- *CT or CT/PET of thorax, abdomen and pelvis:* identifed sites of disease and nodes which are accessible for biopsy

### Histopathology

Fine-needle aspiration often fails to yield a diagnosis, so core or excision lymph node biopsy is used.

## Management

The treatment selected for HL depends on the stage of the disease and is individualized for each patient.

- *Early stage HL* (Stages IA and IIA): This can be cured by targeted radiotherapy and a short course of combination chemotherapy.
- *Late stage HL:* This requires six or more courses of chemotherapy with or without radiotherapy. Patients are typically scanned halfway through their treatment and their chemotherapy reduced or intensified depending on how well they are responding.
- Patients with relapsed or refractory disease may be treated with newer agents such as brentuximab (for CD30+ disease) and/or allogeneic HSCT.

## Prognosis

HL is an eminently treatable disease with over 90% of patients achieving long-term remissions. Patients can suffer long-term and late effects from treatment which is why it is important to risk-stratify patients and to give as little chemotherapy as is needed to treat their stage of disease.

## NON-HODGKIN'S LYMPHOMAS

NHLs are malignant tumours of B or T lymphocytes affecting lymph nodes and/or other organs of the lymphoreticular system (spleen/liver). B-cell lymphomas are more common and generally have a better prognosis than T-cell lymphomas. Extranodal disease can occur.

## Epidemiology

- All types of NHL combined are a common form of cancer (1 in 1000/year).
- There are many subtypes, the most common of which are follicular lymphoma (a B-cell neoplasm) and diffuse large B-cell lymphoma (DLBCL).
- T-cell lymphomas are rare and aggressive.
- Incidence increases with age.

## Disease mechanisms

NHLs are heterogeneous and may arise anywhere in the body (including the gut and brain) but most commonly in the main lymph node groups. They are a clonal proliferation of B or T cells.

## Clinical features

Most NHLs present with *lymphadenopathy*. B symptoms are often a presenting feature. Lymphomas follow one of two clinical patterns: they grow rapidly (*high-grade lymphomas*, e.g. Burkitt's lymphoma and DLBCL) or slowly (*low-grade*

**15**

*lymphomas*, e.g. follicular lymphoma). The rapid growth rate seen in high-grade NHL makes these tumours more sensitive to chemotherapy and therefore potentially *curable*. Low-grade lymphomas progress much more slowly but are generally *incurable* although multiple courses of chemotherapy can be given which can keep the disease under control for many years, and allogeneic HSCT can be curative for carefully selected patients.

### Diagnosis

Diagnosis requires the demonstration of infiltration of enlarged lymph nodes and/or other tissues by clonal B or T cells.

### Investigation

- *FBC:* may be normal; cytopenias seen if there is marrow involvement
- *Blood film:* may be normal or lymphoma cells may be seen
- *Bone marrow and trephine:* infiltration by lymphoma cells may be evident
- *Liver function tests:* elevated alkaline phosphatase and/or alanine aminotransferase suggest liver infiltration
- *Lactate dehydrogenase (LDH):* usually raised
- *CT scanning and ultrasound-guided biopsy:* useful for staging
- *Histopathology:* core or excision biopsy of involved lymph nodes demonstrate a clonal lymphoid population
- *Molecular*: a number of NHL are associated with characteristic chromosomal translocations, e.g. mantle cell lymphoma t(11:14)

### Management

#### High-grade non-Hodgkin's lymphoma

Rapid growth rate makes high-grade NHL sensitive to chemotherapy and therefore potentially curable. Intensive chemoimmunotherapy (e.g. rituximab, cyclophosphamide, doxorubicin, vincristine and prednisolone; R-CHOP) is given as a series of cycles. Relapsed cases may sometimes be salvaged by high-dose therapy and autologous or allogeneic stem cell transplant.

#### Low-grade non-Hodgkin's lymphoma

As with CLL (see above), a watchful waiting technique saves the patient from unnecessary therapy and toxicity in early asymptomatic stages. Progressive disease requires treatment with chemoimmunotherapy, which can induce remissions that can last years. Autologous and allogeneic stem cell transplant is used in younger patients in some low-grade subtypes.

### Prognosis

Prognosis for individual patients is variable and depends on precise histology, stage and tumour sensitivity.

## MULTIPLE MYELOMA AND OTHER PARAPROTEINAEMIAS

A *paraprotein* is an abnormal monoclonal immunoglobulin produced by a malignant clone of antibody-producing B cells (usually plasma cells). *Multiple myeloma* is a malignant tumour of plasma cells, terminal cells of the B-cell lineage, which secrete immunoglobulins (antibodies), thus myeloma is typically associated with the presence of a paraprotein. Other clonal disorders of B cells can also be associated with a paraprotein: these are also classified (with myeloma) as *paraproteinaemias*. Very high paraproteins can be associated with the hyperviscosity syndrome.

### MULTIPLE MYELOMA

#### Epidemiology

- Commonest haematological malignancy
- Incidence increases with age

#### Diagnosis

Diagnosis requires 10% or more clonal plasma cells to be present in the bone marrow and the presence of the *CRAB* criteria:
- Hypercalcaemia
- Renal impairment
- Anaemia
- Bone lesions (seen on skeletal survey or increasingly on CT or MRI)

In the absence of CRAB features, >60% plasma cells are needed in the bone marrow before a diagnosis of active myeloma can be made. Patients with <60% plasma cells and no CRAB features are said to have 'smouldering' (asymptomatic) myeloma.

#### Clinical features

- *Pathological bone fractures:* common presentation; tumours of the spine can cause *spinal cord compression*
- *Hypercalcaemia:* occurs because of rapid bone resorption; can require emergency treatment
- *Anaemia and pancytopenia:* due to bone marrow infiltration
- *Renal failure:* immunoglobin light chains obstruct renal tubules

#### Investigation

- *FBC:* frequently cytopenias at diagnosis
- *Blood film:* often normal; plasma cells in the peripheral blood indicate very aggressive disease (and/or the rare plasma cell leukaemia)
- *Bone marrow and trephine:* >10% malignant plasma cells
- *Protein electrophoresis:* demonstrates a paraprotein
- *Urinalysis:* will detect free clonal light chains (Bence Jones proteinuria) in nearly all cases

## LYMPHOMA AT A GLANCE

### Clinical features

- Lymphadenopathy is the key feature, with painless enlargement of single or multiple lymph nodes
- Symptoms and signs of a space-occupying tumour in any body compartment (e.g. brain, abdomen), because lymphoma can involve any organ
- Systemic symptoms: anorexia, weight loss (more than 10% body weight), fever and night sweats
- Bone marrow involvement: anaemia, neutropenia (susceptible to infections), thrombocytopenia (easy bruising)
- Immune suppression with opportunistic infection (e.g. shingles)

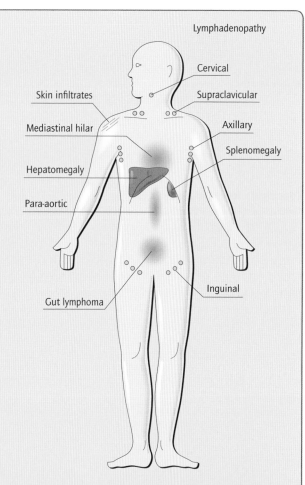

Lymphadenopathy

Skin infiltrates

Cervical

Supraclavicular

Mediastinal hilar

Axillary

Splenomegaly

Hepatomegaly

Para-aortic

Gut lymphoma

Inguinal

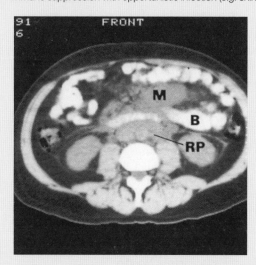

**Figure A** CT scan of the abdomen showing enlarged mesenteric (M) and retroperitoneal (RP; para-aortic) lymph nodes. B, bowel.

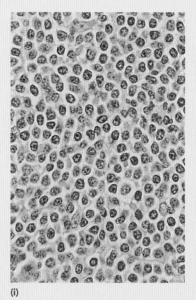

(i)

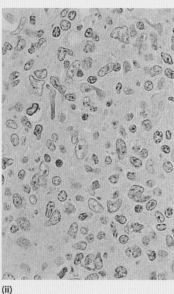

(ii)

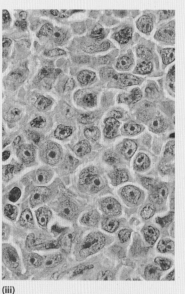

(iii)

**Figure B** Non-Hodgkin's lymphoma: high-pose view of lymph node biopsies showing: **(i)** lymphocytic lymphoma showing predominantly small lymphocytes with round nuclei containing densely clumped heterochromatin; **(ii)** centrocyte lymphoma showing medium-sized cells with nuclear pleomorphism but characteristically having a cleaved nucleus and pale indistinct cytoplasm. The nuclei have a light chromatin pattern and may contain nucleoli; **(iii)** immunoblastic lymphoma showing large neoplastic cells with a single prominent nucleolus and abundant darkly staining cytoplasm. All figures reproduced from Hoffbrand AV & Pettit JE (1993) *Essential Haematology*, 3rd edn (Wiley-Blackwell, Oxford), with the permission of the authors.

15

- $\beta_2$-*microglobulin:* a useful marker of the activity of the disease (high = active = bad)
- *Diagnostic imaging:* needs to be performed at diagnosis to diagnose lytic lesions; plain radiography used to be the gold standard but increasingly MRI and CT used

### Management

*Urgent initial supportive treatment* may include:
- Immediate rehydration for renal failure
- Bisphosphonate drugs for hypercalcaemia
- Urgent radiotherapy or surgery to decompress the spinal cord

#### Specific antimyeloma treatment

Combination chemotherapy is given, tailored to the patient's comorbid condition. Younger, fitter patients typically receive high-dose chemotherapy with autologous stem cell 'rescue' (autologous stem cell transplant). The idea is to reduce the burden of disease, and remissions lasting several years can be seen. Patients typically undergo multiple courses of different chemotherapy drugs which usually include a drug of the proteasome inhibitor class. New immunotherapeutic drugs targeting proteins on the surface of malignant plasma cells (e.g. daratumumab) are increasingly used. Patients typically receive many lines of different treatment.

#### Supportive care

This is of the utmost importance in myeloma in order to preserve quality of life. Patients should receive regular bisphosphonates and many require opioid analgesia for bone pain.

### Prognosis

Prognosis is dependent on cytogenetics, comorbid state and response to treatment. Myeloma is an incurable disease but new drugs have prolonged overall survival to >10 years from diagnosis for many patients.

## OTHER PARAPROTEINAEMIAS

### Monoclonal gammopathy of undetermined significance

The elegant term monoclonal gammopathy of undetermined significance (MGUS) is applied to the finding of a low-level paraprotein *alone* (e.g. IgG paraprotein <20 g/L), without increased plasma cells in the marrow or any symptoms, signs or investigational findings suggesting myeloma activity. It is a very common finding in patients over 65 years and might be found in up to 1% of individuals over 80 years. Patients have a small annual risk of progressing to multiple myeloma and require annual follow-up.

### Waldenström's macroglobulinaemia

This rare chronic lymphoproliferative disease is defined by the presence of an IgM paraprotein in the serum. IgM paraproteins can make the blood very viscous and patients can present with symptoms of *hyperviscosity* (blurred vision, headaches, transient ischaemic attacks [TIAs] and confusion). It is a low-grade disorder that is managed with watchful waiting and cycles of chemoimmunotherapy.

## BONE MARROW FAILURE

In bone marrow failure states, haematopoiesis fails as a result of stem cell damage. The most common acquired bone marrow failure syndrome is aplastic anaemia while inherited diseases which present in childhood include Diamond–Backfan anaemia, Fanconi anaemia and dyskeratosis congentia (DKC). They all present with significant cytopenias, and allogeneic stem cell transplantation is the cornerstone of treatment for many.

## APLASTIC ANAEMIA

### Epidemiology

- Incidence is 1–2 in 1 000 000/year
- Occurs in all age groups

### Disease mechanisms

*Causes* can be immune, exposure to drugs/chemicals/radiation or unknown. The result is damaged stem cells which cannot generate mature blood cells.

### Clinical features

Severe aplastic anaemia with marked neutropenia and thrombocytopenia resembles acute leukaemia clinically, and life-threatening infections (see EMERGENCY PRESENTATION 15.2) and bleeding episodes are common.

### Diagnosis

Aplastic or hypoplastic anaemia is diagnosed on the basis of a pancytopenia in the absence of other abnormalities with an 'empty marrow' seen on bone marrow trephine biopsy sections.

### Investigation

- *FBC:* pancytopenia, and reduced or absent reticulocytes
- *Bone marrow and trephine:* aspiration reveals hypocellular particles; trephine reveals hypoplasia or aplasia showing reduced cellularity and increased fat spaces

### Management

Supportive treatment includes blood and platelet transfusions, and management of infection. Severe aplastic anaemia is treated with rabbit or horse antithymocyte globulin (ATG) and ciclosporin. Bone marrow transplantation is the first-line treatment in severely affected younger patients.

## MYELOMA AT A GLANCE

### Clinical features

*Musculoskeletal*
- Bone pain
- Pathological fractures
- Vertebral collapse
- Kyphosis and loss of height

*Neurology*
- Spinal cord compression

*Haematology*
- Anaemia
- Thrombocytopenia

*Immunology*
- Infections of the respiratory tract as a result of hypogammaglobulinaemia

*Renal*
- Protein (light chain) cast disease (myeloma kidney)
- Renal tubular atrophy and degeneration
- Pyelonephritis

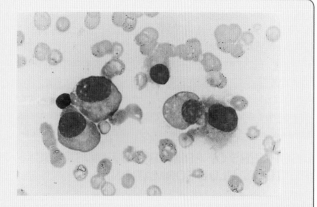

**Figure C** Bone marrow aspirate in myeloma. This high-power field shows five plasma cells, together with a small lymphocyte. Note the very basophilic cytoplasm with a paler area corresponding to the Golgi apparatus. The nucleus has a typically eccentric location.

*Metabolic*
- Hypercalcaemia
- Amyloid
- Cryoglobulinaemia

*Vascular*
- Hyperviscosity syndrome

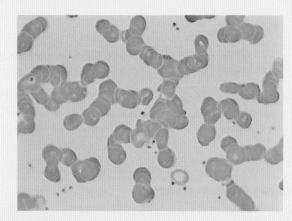

**Figure A** Blood film showing rouleaux formation, which is a common finding in multiple myeloma.

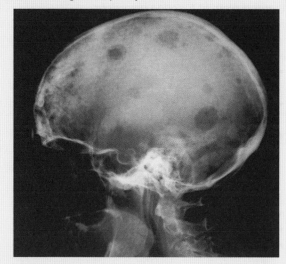

**Figure B** Radiograph showing multiple small 'punched-out' osteolytic lesions (rounded lucent areas) of multiple myeloma in the skull.

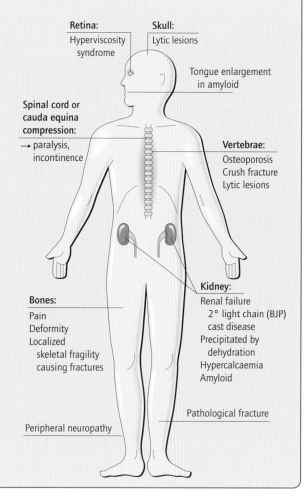

### Prognosis

Allogeneic stem cell transplantation is curative but it carries a significant risk of morbidity and mortality. Prognosis in older patients depends on what treatment can safely be given. Thrombopoietin agonists have been shown to improve all cytopenias and immunosuppression can be effective.

## HAEMOSTATIC DISORDERS

## DISORDERS OF PRIMARY HAEMOSTASIS (PLATELET PLUG FORMATION)

If formation of the platelet plug is delayed, abnormal bleeding tends to be immediately obvious from cuts, surgical incisions or mucous membranes (e.g. epistaxis). Careful history-taking is needed to exclude a drug effect mimicking a platelet function disorder (e.g. aspirin use).

## PLATELET DISORDERS

## THROMBOCYTOPENIA (PLATELETS ↓)

A reduced platelet count is a common finding in many disorders, because the lifespan of circulating platelets is reduced in:
- All types of infection
- Any disorder causing widespread activation of the haemostatic system (e.g. major trauma)
- Complications of pregnancy (e.g. pre-eclampsia)

Beware of two common laboratory artefacts that can mimic thrombocytopenia:
- *A small clot in the blood sample*
- *Platelet clumping caused by a reaction with the anticoagulant EDTA – repeat FBC in a tube containing citrate*

### Immune thrombocytopenic purpura
#### Epidemiology
- Estimated incidence is 1 in 1000/year
- Can occur at any age
- More common in females

#### Disease mechanisms
There are acute (self-limiting) and chronic forms of immune thrombocytopenic purpura (ITP). Acute ITP is the usual form in children and often follows viral infection, remitting spontaneously as the infection is cleared. Chronic ITP mostly affects adults.

#### Clinical features
The typical symptom is *purpura* and other bleeding symptoms (e.g. epistaxis, gum bleeding or menorrhagia). Severe bleeding (e.g. intracranial, retinal or abdominal haemorrhage) is relatively uncommon, even with very low platelet counts.

#### Diagnosis
ITP is a diagnosis of exclusion; patients should be screened for viral infections and a blood film examined. If other cytopenias are present or there are other concerning features, a bone marrow aspiration will need to be performed.

#### Investigation
- *FBC:* normal Hb (unless major bleeding); normal WBC; low platelet count
- *Blood film:* red and white cells normal; platelets reduced and may be bigger than normal

#### Management
Treatment is rarely needed for ITP in children: bleeding (see below) is rare, and the condition usually spontaneously remits in 1–4 weeks. Chronic ITP may require treatment.

Treatment options in ITP include:
- Corticosteroids
- IV immunoglobulin (IVIG) if a rapid response is needed
- Thrombopoietin receptor agonists and/or rituximab increasingly used in steroid-refractory cases
- Splenectomy now rarely used and should only be considered when all ither treatment options have been exhausted

#### Prognosis
Acute ITP commonly has a self-limited course with spontaneous remission occurring within days to weeks. In chronic ITP, symptoms usually stabilize, and the platelet count slowly improves with time.

### Platelet function disorders

Primary haemostasis may fail if the platelet count is normal but platelet function is reduced.

#### Inherited platelet function disorders
These are extremely rare. Affected individuals have a lifelong bleeding tendency, which can pose difficulties in surgery and childbirth.
- *Glanzmann's thrombocythaemia:* autosomal recessive inherited deficiency of platelet fibrinogen receptors
- *Bernard–Soulier disease:* autosomal recessive inherited deficiency of platelet vWF receptors
- *Platelet storage pool deficiency and transduction disorders:* a larger group of inherited mild bleeding disorders in which platelet activation mechanisms are disturbed

#### Investigation
- *FBC:* platelet count often normal
- *Blood film:* may show abnormal platelet granulation or size
- *Platelet aggregometry:* a specialized test performed in tertiary centres that can identify platelet disorders based on their response to different agonists

### Management and prognosis

Hereditary platelet disorders require registration with a haemophilia centre for advice and therapy in case of bleeding or surgery. Minor bleeds can be arrested by firm pressure or use of tranexamic acid (which helps stop clot breakdown). Major bleeds require urgent treatment (EMERGENCY PRESENTATION 15.3) and may require platelet transfusion.

### Von Willebrand's disease

The most common inherited bleeding disorder caused by deficiency (Type 1 von Willebrand's disease [vWD]) or abnormality (Type 2 vWD) of the large adhesive plasma protein vWF. Type 3 is rare and results in almost complete deficiency of vWF.

### Epidemiology

- Most common inherited bleeding disorder
- Around 1 in 1000 people affected
- Autosomal dominant inheritance in Type 1 and most of Type 2; some rare Type 2 variants and the rare Type 3 disease display autosomal recessive inheritance patterns

---

**EMERGENCY PRESENTATION 15.3**

**Major haemorrhage**

**Definition**

Sudden, unexpected and ongoing blood loss resulting in haemodynamic compromise

**Problems**

Loss of circulating volume (hypovolaemia) is an immediate threat and also leads to further bleeding via activation of DIC.
A dilutional coagulopathy can develop rapidly if adequate blood product replacement is not given.

**Actions**

Ensure good vascular access: maintain blood volume with saline or plasma expanders.
Notify the blood bank of the situation (hospitals should have a major haemorrhage protocol).
If red cells must be given prior to compatible blood issue by the blood bank, give ABO group-compatible uncross-matched blood. If the blood group of the patient is not known, universal donor O negative (or O positive blood for males) can be given in an emergency.
Samples should be sent to the blood bank as soon as possible so the group can be identified but this should not delay giving emergency group O blood if needed.
FFP should be given at least after every second unit of red cells.
Cryoprecipitate should be given to treat/prevent hyper-fibrinogenaemia.
Tranexamic acid is a useful adjunct in many situations and particularly in trauma.

---

### Disease mechanisms

Reduced or dysfunctional vWF results in abnormalities of primary haemostasis.

### Clinical features

- Easy bruising
- Epistaxes (nosebleeds that run like a tap)
- Menorrhagia
- Early excess bleeding during dentistry or surgery
- Peripartum bleeding (Type 2)
- Joint, muscle and CNS bleeds are very rare

### Diagnosis

Note the coagulation screen (PT, APTT, etc.) is often normal. The bleeding history should prompt investigation with assays that measure the amount of vWF (antigen assay) and vWF function.

### Investigation

- *Coagulation screen:* may show APTTr ↑, but *often normal*
- *Platelet aggregometry:* abnormal response to ristocetin
- *vWF assay:* amount of vWF can be assessed by detection of antigens on the surface of the protein; its function can be assessed by the protein's ability to bind collagen or its response to the agonist ristocetin

### Management

This depends on the subtype and the patient's bleeding phenotype. It may not require any specific management apart from after trauma or before surgery, etc. The vWF content of plasma is increased (often to normal) by injection of the synthetic vasopressin analogue desmopressin and this can be used to temporarily normalize vWF levels (e.g. for an operation). Infusion of vWF concentrate is only required for major bleeding challenges (e.g. major surgery or patients with very severe phenotypes). Type 3 disease is a severe bleeding disorder which requires lifelong replacement of vWF similarly to haemophilia.

### Prognosis

The vast majority live normal lives. Some Type 2 vWD patients and all Type 3 patients have a severe bleeding disorder which requires extensive lifelong specialist care.

## DISORDERS OF SECONDARY HAEMOSTASIS

A durable clot depends on the coordinated action of the plasma coagulation factors in thrombin generation. Deficiency of any of the key coagulation factors will impact clot formation.

## INHERITED DISEASE: HAEMOPHILIA

Haemophilia is one of the severe inherited bleeding disorders. Haemophilia A is due to deficiency of factor VIII and

**15**

is more common than haemophilia B (deficiency of factor IX). Both disorders are inherited in an X-linked manner and result in a similar clinical phenotype (see **Figure 15.5**).

### Haemophilia A (factor VIII deficiency)

#### Epidemiology

- Incidence 1 in 10 000 male births
- Inherited in an X-linked recessive manner

#### Disease mechanisms

Haemophilia A results from deficiency of factor VIII, arising from a number of different factor VIII gene lesions. Nearly half occur *sporadically*, in families with no history of haemophilia.

#### Clinical features

There is recurrent haemorrhage into joints (haemarthrosis) and muscles (intramuscular haematoma), beginning when the child starts to walk. Typically, a sequence of bleeds affects a single joint (target joint). Spontaneous haemorrhage may occur and intracranial haemorrhage is the most feared complication.

Until the development of recombinant factors VIII and IX, plasma-derived factor concentrate was used, which exposed many recipients to blood-borne viruses. Successive epidemics of hepatitis B and C and HIV therefore occurred in the haemophilia community. The risks of blood-borne infection are now minimized with recombinant clotting factors.

#### Investigation

- *Coagulation screen:* APTTr is raised with normal INR and TCT. As the factors deficient in haemophilia form part of the *in vitro* intrinsic coagulation pathway, it is important to remember this when thinking about which tests will be abnormal.
- *50 : 50 mixing studies (APTT after mixing patient plasma with the same volume of normal plasma):* In haemophilia A and B, the APTT should correct on addition of normal plasma (the plasma provides a source of functional factor VIII or IX).
- *Factor VIII assay:* Less than 1% (severe); 1–5% (moderate); >5% (mild).

#### Management

*Mild haemophilia* Desmopressin (DDAVP) injection (see vWD above) also boosts factor VIII level in mild haemophilia because vWF is the carrier protein for factor VIII. This can be used 'on demand' (e.g. to cover the patient for a dental extraction). Mild haemophilia still has a significant effect on the lives of those affected despite the nomenclature.

*Severe and moderate haemophilia* This requires a comprehensive care approach, in which every aspect (bleeding, joint and muscle rehabilitation, surgery, genetics, treatment of associated infections, dentistry, surgery, social care, etc.) is delivered by a specialized clinical team.

Central to care is prompt treatment of bleeds with effective doses of factor VIII concentrate, often injected by the patient or a family member. It is sometimes begun in infancy after inserting a permanent vascular access device (e.g. portacath). The concentrate used should be recombinant (non-plasma-derived) factor VIII if available. New prolonged half-life factor concentrates have reduced the frequency of injections. A cure is on the horizon following exciting developments in gene therapy.

## HAEMOPHILIA B (FACTOR IX DEFICIENCY, CHRISTMAS DISEASE)

### Epidemiology

- Incidence is 2 in 100 000 male births
- Presents at birth or early childhood
- X-linked recessive inheritance pattern

### Disease mechanisms

Haemophilia B results from deficiency of factor IX, arising from a number of factor IX gene lesions. Most cases occur in families with a history of haemophilia.

### Investigation and management

As for haemophilia A, the APTT is typically prolonged but it is factor IX that is deficient whereas factor VIII levels are normal. Management is the same as for haemophilia A, but therapy is IV *factor IX concentrate*. Gene therapy has also recently proven highly effective in haemophilia B.

### Prognosis of haemophilia A and B

Before effective factor replacement began in the early 1960s, the median age of death for boys with severe haemophilia was around 16 years. Life expectancy for both types normalized by the early 1980s, but then fell back again because of the HIV epidemic of the later 1980s. Today, with good care, patients have a normal life expectancy. Early clinical trials of gene therapy have demonstrated very promising results, and this may transform the treatment landscape in the not-too-distant future.

## ACQUIRED BLEEDING DISORDERS

### Vitamin K deficiency

#### Epidemiology

- Haemorrhagic disease of the newborn (HDN) occurs in 1 in 10 000 births if vitamin K prophylaxis is not given
- Haemolytic disease in the newborn; older patients are vulnerable to vitamin K starvation.

#### Disease mechanisms

Vitamin K is:

- Required as a cofactor for the synthesis of the functional forms of coagulation factors II (prothrombin), VII, IX and X – these are termed the vitamin-K-dependent coagulation factors
- Present at very low levels in human breast milk
- Antagonized by the commonly used vitamin K antagonist drugs (e.g. warfarin)

## HAEMOPHILIA AT A GLANCE

### Epidemiology

*Incidence*

- 1 in 10 000 males (haemophilia A); 1 in 50 000 males (haemophilia B)

*Genetics*

- X-linked recessive inheritance

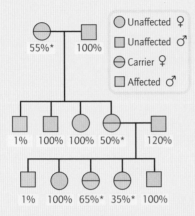

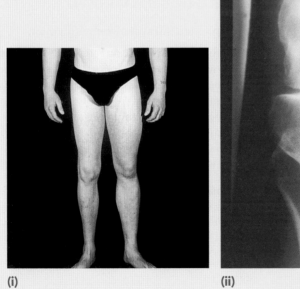

**Figure B** Abnormal bruising in severe haemophilia A.

**Figure A** A typical family tree in a family with haemophilia. Note the variable levels of factor VIII activity in carriers (*) due to random inactivation of X chromosome (lyonization). The percentages show the degree of factor VIII activity as a percentage of normal. Reproduced from Hoffbrand AV & Pettit JE (1993) *Essential Haematology*, 3rd edn (Wiley-Blackwell, Oxford), with the permission of the authors.

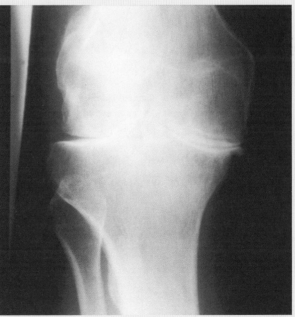

(i)                    (ii)

**Figure C (i)** Haemophilia: target joint in otherwise fit patient. In this patient the right knee is a target joint damaged by repeated haemarthroses. As a result the muscles of the thigh are wasted. The patient has been promptly treated with on-demand factor VIII over the years. **(ii)** Chronic haemophilia arthropathy. Radiograph of the right knee joint showing marked narrowing of the joint space, subchondral cyst formation and osteoarthritic changes. Progressive damage despite on-demand therapy is the rationale for prophylaxis.

*Continued...*

15

...Continued

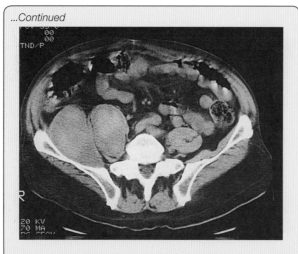

**Figure D** CT scan of the pelvis showing iliopsoas (retroperitoneal) haematoma.

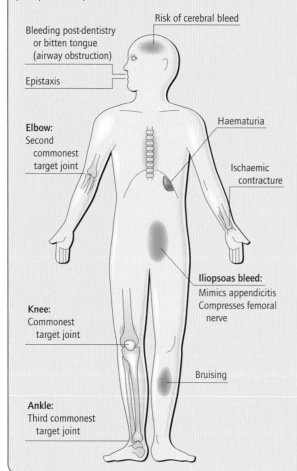

Risk of cerebral bleed

Bleeding post-dentistry or bitten tongue (airway obstruction)

Epistaxis

Elbow:
Second commonest target joint

Haematuria

Ischaemic contracture

Iliopsoas bleed:
Mimics appendicitis
Compresses femoral nerve

Knee:
Commonest target joint

Bruising

Ankle:
Third commonest target joint

### Diagnosis
Awareness of the possibility of vitamin K deficiency is crucial. The INR is very sensitive to the factor VII level, and to vitamin K deficiency.

### Clinical features
Babies with HDN also have heavy bruising, and sometimes present with gastrointestinal, pleural, pericardial or CNS bleeding.

### Investigation
*Coagulation screen* shows INR ↑ (>1.5), usually APTTr ↑, and normal TCT.

### Management
*HDN* is prevented by:
- Intramuscular injection of 1 mg vitamin K (phytomenadione) at birth
- Two doses of oral vitamin K in the first postnatal week, plus a third at 1 month in exclusively breastfed babies

## Acquired haemophilia
### Disease mechanisms
Acquired haemophilia is a rare autoimmune condition in which autoantibodies are produced against factor VIII or more rarely factor IX.

### Clinical features
It commonly presents in the elderly with widespread subcutaneous bruising which can be dramatic.

### Investigation
*Coagulation screen* shows APTT ↑ that does *not* correct on 50 : 50 mixing.

### Management
Acquired haemophilia can be rapidly fatal if untreated. Prompt treatment with immunosuppression (steroids, cyclophosphamide and rituximab) suppresses antibody formation while haemostatic bypass agents (such as recombinant factor VII) are used to stop bleeding. Treatment is challenging as patients are often elderly and frail. Of those successfully treated, 50% will relapse.

## Disseminated intravascular coagulation

DIC is caused by systemic activation of haemostasis resulting in widespread activation of thrombotic mechanisms and consumption of coagulation factors. Patients can have a 'thrombotic', 'bleeding' phenotype or a mixed picture. Thrombosis in the microvasculature can rapidly result in multi-organ failure. DIC is *always* due to an underlying disorder and prompt management of the underlying cause is needed to resolve the haematological disorder.

### Diagnosis
*Risk assessment* Does the patient have an underlying disorder known to be associated with overt DIC? If yes, proceed to scoring system.

*Order global coagulation tests* PT, APTT, platelet count, fibrinogen

*Score the test results*
- Platelet count (>100 × 10⁹/L = 1; <100 × 10⁹/L = 1; <50 = 2 × 10⁹/L = 2)
- Elevated fibrin marker (e.g. D-dimer, fibrin degradation products) (no increase = 0; moderate increase = 2; strong increase =3)

- Prolonged PT ($<3$ s = 0; $>3$ but $<6$ s = 1; $>6$ s = 2)
- Fibrinogen level ($>1$ g/L = 0; $<1$ g/L = 1)

*Calculate score*

- $>5$ compatible with overt DIC; repeat score daily
- $<5$ suggestive for non-overt DIC; repeat in 1–2 days unless clinical deterioration

There is a strong correlation between increasing score and mortality. The diagnosis of DIC should encompass both clinical and laboratory information. It is important to repeat the tests to monitor this dynamic scenario.

## Clinical features

Clinical features of the underlying cause:

- Trauma, massive blood transfusion (especially if blood not warmed)
- Pregnancy, labour, postpartum
- Sepsis – fever, hypothermia, shock
- Metastatic carcinoma

Clinical features of thrombi in the microvasculature:

- Acute renal failure
- ARDS
- Delirium, altered conscious level, coma
- Digital gangrene, progressing to limb ischaemia and gangrene
- Haemorrhagic infarction of the adrenals

Clinical features of consumption coagulopathy:

- Widespread bruising and purpura
- Fresh bleeding from old wounds and skin puncture sites

## Investigation

- *FBC:* thrombocytopenia
- *Blood film:* red cell fragments may be present
- *Coagulation screen:* usually (but not always) INR ↑, APTTr ↑, TCT ↑
- *Fibrinogen assay:* usually reduced ($<1.5$ g/L)
- *Fibrin degradation products (FDP or D-dimers):* increased

## Management

Treatment of the underlying cause is paramount (e.g. broad-spectrum antibiotics in sepsis). Aggressive management of the coagulopathy with blood products may be needed if the patient develops bleeding complications but expert advice should be sought.

## THROMBOSIS AND THROMBOPHILIA

### Epidemiology

- The vast majority of venous thromboembolisms (VTEs) are sporadic or due to some transient risk factor (e.g. surgery, pregnancy).
- A minority of patients who develop a VTE have an inherited thrombophilia, antithrombin deficiency, protein C or S deficiency.

## Disease mechanisms

Clot regulation depends on controlling thrombin via two mechanisms: direct inhibition by antithrombin, and negative feedback regulation by the protein C pathway. Inherited thrombophilias change proteins with roles in thrombin control, in directions that increase thrombin activity.

### Inherited thrombophilia

- Factor V Leiden
- Prothrombin gene mutation
- Protein C deficiency
- Protein S deficiency
- Antithrombin deficiency

### Acquired thrombophilia

Acquired thrombophilia usually involves interference with thrombin control arising from underlying disease processes or autoantibodies. The most important is antiphospholipid syndrome.

### Risk factors for VTE

- Pregnancy and puerperium
- Surgery, particularly lower limb orthopaedic procedures
- Trauma and immobility, particularly spinal injury
- Oestrogen therapy

The likelihood that an individual will sustain a thrombotic event is therefore a multifactorial risk. When deciding how (or whether) to protect someone against VTE, or in performing diagnostic imaging for DVT, all the factors listed above are combined in a clinical risk score.

### Diagnosis

The vast majority of VTE is sporadic and screening for an inherited thrombophilia is not indicated in unselected patients with VTE. Thrombophilia testing should be considered in young patients with unprovoked VTE with a family history of thromboses.

### Clinical features

VTE disease usually presents as:

- DVT of the leg, either distal (calf veins only) or proximal (popliteal vein or above)
- PE caused by embolization of clot from proximal DVT

In addition, thrombophilia may present as:

- Atypical venous thrombosis in axillary, mesenteric or cerebral veins
- Recurrent mid-trimester foetal loss (secondary to placental thrombosis)
- Recurrent DVT
- Sagittal sinus thrombosis (rare)

**15**

## Investigation

The key investigation is objective confirmation of the presence of a DVT. This is because clinical diagnosis (by symptoms and signs) is incorrect in approximately 70% of cases.

- *Coagulation screen:* may show ↑ APTTr that does not correct on addition of normal plasma; evidence of an antiphospholipid antibody (lupus inhibitor)
- *D-dimer assay:* can be used to risk-stratify patients to guide further investigations (e.g. to rule out VTE in patients with a low probability of disease)

### Diagnostic imaging

- *Compression duplex ultrasound:* commonly used to diagnose DVT
- *CT pulmonary angiogram:* is the gold standard imaging modality for the diagnosis of PE

## Management

For treatment of proven acute DVT or PE, see Chapter 6, Respiratory disease.

### Acute therapy: heparin

Heparin is the drug of choice in the initial treatment, but the original standard therapy (IV unfractionated heparin) has largely been replaced by low-molecular-weight heparin (LMWH) therapy administered subcutaneously once or twice a day. LMWH is the main therapeutic agent used in pregnancy for women who have suffered a VTE or are thought to be at high risk of VTE during pregnancy.

### Continued therapy: vitamin K antagonists (warfarin)

This used to be the standard of care for continued therapy of VTE, aiming to prevent recurrence. Six months' therapy is usual after a first VTE and long-term therapy is sometimes required for recurrent VTE or in the presence of thrombophilia. Regular monitoring with the INR test ensures safe and protective intensity of anticoagulation.

### Continued therapy: direct oral anticoagulants (DOACs)

Direct oral anticoagulants (DOACs) are oral, once or twice daily, and work by directly inhibiting either thrombin (dabigatran) or factor Xa (rivaroxaban, apixaban). They are well tolerated and do not require regular monitoring like warfarin. In uncomplicated VTE, these are often used as first-line therapy. They cannot be used in pregnancy and their anticoagulant effect is unpredictable in patients at extremes of weight or in those with poor renal function.

### Prevention of deep-vein thrombosis and pulmonary embolism

Patients who have already sustained more than one proven DVT or PE benefit from lifelong anticoagulation. VTE risk assessment should be performed on all patients on admission to hospital and thromboprophylaxis prescribed (usually with LMWH) if the risk score indicates.

---

**MUST-KNOW CHECKLIST**

- The normal limits of haemoglobin concentration, neutrophil, lymphocyte and platelet counts
- Identify abnormalities of the FBC, suggest likely causes and appropriate investigations
- The human ABO and Rhesus blood group systems and what they mean in blood transfusion
- The hazards of blood transfusion
- The different clinical impacts of:
  - Acute versus chronic leukaemia
  - Low-grade versus high-grade lymphoma
- How to examine a patient for:
  - Lymphadenopathy
  - Hepatomegaly and splenomegaly
  - Signs of anaemia
  - Signs of abnormal bleeding
- How to use the coagulation screen to locate the underlying cause of abnormal bleeding

**Questions and answers** to test your understanding of Chapter 15 can be found by clicking 'Support Material' at the following link: https://www.routledge.com/Medicine-for-Finals-and-Beyond/Axford-OCallaghan/p/book/9780367150594

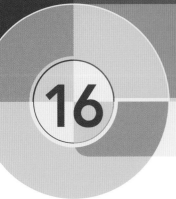

# Palliative Medicine

## 16

ADRIAN TOOKMAN & FAYE GISHEN

## AIMS OF PALLIATIVE MEDICINE

A key aim of palliative medicine is symptom control for people with advanced, progressive, life-limiting illness. These people may have complex symptoms and palliative care focuses on the whole patient rather than simply taking a disease-orientated approach by:

- Addressing psychological, social, spiritual and financial needs as well as physical symptoms
- Offering control, independence and choice, to allow participation in their care, including negotiating the most appropriate place to die (home, hospice or hospital)
- Supporting 'the family' (all those who are important to the patient) alongside the patient
- Providing bereavement counselling after death
- Providing support and expert advice to other professionals involved in the care

A team approach is essential. Close liaison between the hospital, community and hospice is key. The multidisciplinary palliative care team might include palliative medicine physicians, clinical nurse specialists and allied healthcare professionals. In the home, the GP and district nurse are often key workers. The palliative care team generally coordinates care and local resources to maximize the quality of care.

## COMMUNICATION IS KEY

A substantial proportion of medical students qualify without having had significant experience in the management of dying patients. Death may be perceived as a failure in medicine and can generate feelings of inadequacy, fear and despair in doctors. These fears can lead to avoiding difficult conversations. The principles of good communication are to address the patient's concerns openly and honestly, to assess needs holistically before giving advice or attempting to formulate solutions, to watch for non-verbal as well as verbal clues, and to clarify and summarize what the patient reports. It is not just a question of 'What should the patient know?', but an assessment of 'What does the patient want to know?'

## HISTORY AND EXAMINATION

Take a full history from the patient and examine them (HISTORY & EXAMINATION 16.1).

## SET A TREATMENT AND MANAGEMENT PLAN

### Explain symptoms to the patient and discuss the treatment options

Patients should be given adequate and accurate information about the treatment options so that they can make informed choices.

It is important to consider that prescribed medications are:

- *Rational* (e.g. use laxatives and not analgesics for the pain of constipation)
- *Regular* (e.g. laxatives, antiemetics and analgesics must be given regularly for persistent symptoms)
- *The right dose*
- *Given at the right interval*
- *Given by the correct route* (e.g. rectally, transdermally, subcutaneously or intramuscularly)

DOI: 10.1201/9781003193616-16

Keep the regimen simple, and explain it to the patient, in writing if appropriate. Supervise and review it regularly.

## Anticipate

Symptoms can change rapidly in the context of advanced illness, and distress may be avoided if such changes are anticipated. A deterioration that makes it impossible to continue with oral medication should be anticipated to ensure that injectable preparations are available. This can avert an unnecessary crisis.

Discuss patients' future preferences and wishes where appropriate (advance care planning).

## COMMON SYMPTOMS IN PATIENTS WITH ADVANCED DISEASE

A number of symptoms are common in patients with advanced disease.

## PAIN

Pain is sometimes feared by cancer patients and can also be a significant issue in people with non-malignant disease. It can normally be modified or alleviated. Thorough pain assessment is likelier to result in effective management.

### Diagnose the cause of the pain

Patients may experience pain at multiple sites; therefore, each site of pain should be evaluated individually. To establish the cause of any pain, it is essential to take a careful history, particularly noting:

- Site of pain and any radiation
- Type and severity of pain
- Exacerbating and relieving factors
- Previous history, including analgesic use

Physical examination may confirm a diagnosis. It may be appropriate to image a patient, or perform other investigations, if management will be altered by the results. Always assess how significant the pain is for a patient and how it impacts on function and quality of life.

### Common causes of pain

Common cause of pain are given in **Table 16.1**.

### Set realistic objectives and treat appropriately

Realistic objectives should be set. For most patients, pain can be significantly modified, and complete pain relief may be achieved in many. For some patients, however, pain can prove intractable and refractory to treatment. These patients provide the greatest challenge and multiple avenues of pain control should be considered. Treatment normally depends on cause. Not all pain requires analgesia; for example, the pain of urinary retention is best treated by catheterization. When analgesics are indicated, however, they must be prescribed appropriately.

### Analgesic treatment of pain

The authors advocate the following simple three-step regimen (based on the WHO analgesic ladder) shown in **Figure 16.1**. Simpler regimens are usually best and will lead to better concordance.

### Principles of prescribing opioids

Opioids are commonly used to control background pain. This usually requires regular prescribing. Doses should be adequate and titrated upwards until pain is controlled. Medication should be prescribed 'as required' for any additional breakthrough pain.

#### Choice of opioid

The gold standard strong opioid in the UK is morphine (**Table 16.2**).

Alternative opioids can also be used (**Table 16.3**).

**Table 16.1** Common causes of pain

| Type of pain | Common causes |
| --- | --- |
| Bone pain | Common in patients with cancer and can be caused by metastatic disease or by local infiltration by tumour |
| | Characteristically worse on movement, with bones sometimes tender to palpation |
| Visceral pain | Commonly caused by tumour in internal organs of the thorax, abdomen or pelvis |
| | Often a deep-seated pain resulting from stretching of a capsule (e.g. stretching of the liver capsule causes right hypochondrial pain and tender hepatomegaly) |
| | Can result from distension of a hollow organ (e.g. small and large intestines, bladder, ureters) causing spasmodic colicky pain |
| Neuropathic (or nerve) pain | Nerves may be infiltrated or compressed |
| | Pain may be described as 'burning', associated with abnormal sensations (e.g. hyperaesthesia) |
| | Destruction of nerve plexi, nerve roots or peripheral nerves may result in deafferentation pain (sensory changes in the painful area) |
| | Pain arising centrally (from the brain or spinal cord) may manifest as unilateral spontaneous pain and hypersensitivity, associated with dysaesthesiae (abnormal sensation) |
| Myofascial pain | Common in patients with cancer and other conditions (e.g. multiple sclerosis, motor neurone disease) |
| | May radiate in a non-dermatomal pattern with localized hypersensitive areas of muscle as tender 'trigger' points |
| Superficial pain | Bed sores may be unavoidable in debilitated patients |
| | Scars may also be painful (for example, post-surgery) |

### Routes of administration

The oral route is preferred if the patient can swallow, but it may be necessary to administer parenterally or transdermally (**Table 16.4**). If regular injections are required, consider a continuous subcutaneous infusion (CSCI), also known as a syringe pump or driver. If converting between opioids, always use conversion charts and seek specialist advice from the palliative care team.

### Opioid-resistant pain

Some pains are either partially sensitive or insensitive to opioids and may be managed with additional or alternative drug or other techniques (e.g. radiotherapy, nerve block).

**Step 1 Non-opioids**

Mild pain
Simple analgesia e.g. Paracetamol/NSAIDs
If pain is not relieved, move to

**Step 2 Weak opioid**

Mild/moderate pain
Weak opioids can be used alone or in combination with simple analgesia
If pain is not relieved, move to

**Step 3 Strong opioid**

Moderate/severe pain
Morphine (or equivalent strong opiod) can be used alone or in combination with simple analgesia
At any step, adjuvant analgesic agents (such as anti-epileptics, antidepressants, bisphosphonates or steroids) can be added in.

**Figure 16.1** Three-step regimen for treating pain.

**Table 16.2** Strong opioids: prescribing oral morphine

**Normally start with Immediate-release morphine preparations**

- Available as tablets or liquids
- Prescribed 4-hourly; NB prescribed less frequently e.g. in hepatic impairment
- Use when patient first starts on strong opioids, and then 'as required' for breakthrough or episodic pain

**Then convert to sustained-release morphine preparations**

- Available as tablets
- 12-hourly sustained release preparations available
- Use when patient's pain is stable on the immediate-release preparation

**Getting the dose right**

- Dose of immediate-release morphine is reviewed, and the regular prescription adjusted every 24 hours (or sooner if pain severe)
- Regular dose is titrated upwards in line with the total 'breakthrough' doses given in the preceding 24 hours

16

**Table 16.3** Strong opioids: alternative opioids

| Alternative strong opioid | Comments |
| --- | --- |
| Fentanyl | Applied topically as a patch, and changed every 3 days |
| | Useful in patients unable to swallow or absorb oral opioids or in whom compliance is problematic |
| | Safer in renal impairment |
| Oxycodone | Comes as immediate and long-acting preparations |
| | Safer in renal impairment |
| Diamorphine | Highly soluble therefore may be used when large doses of opioids required |
| Alfentanil | Used in renal impairment |
| Methadone | Long-acting with range of receptor activation, e.g. NMDA, 5-HT receptors indicate possible role in pain that is relatively insensitive to morphine |
| | Long action due to lipophilicity results in accumulation, for specialist use only |

### Bone pain

- Although usually partially sensitive to opioids, bone pain may need additional treatment with a non-steroidal anti-inflammatory drug (NSAID).
- If the pain is localized, radiotherapy may be indicated
- Surgical fixation may be indicated if there is a pathological fracture or a high risk of this.

### Neuropathic pain

- Nerve pain may be relatively insensitive to opioids.
- Corticosteroids may be useful where there is nerve compression.
- Nerve infiltration, irritation and destruction may respond to drugs that alter neurotransmission. Options include:
  - Low-dose tricyclic antidepressants (e.g. amitriptyline)
  - Anticonvulsants (e.g. gabapentin)
- Consider radiotherapy and nerve block injections.

### Liver capsule pain

- This may be partially opioid-sensitive.
- Corticosteroids should be considered as they may reduce hepatic distension and relieve capsular stretching and NSAIDs (e.g. ibuprofen) may be effective.

### Colic

- Treat colic caused by constipation with laxatives.
- If colic is caused by tumour obstruction, antispasmodics (e.g. buscopan) may be indicated.

### Muscle spasm

- Muscle spasm may be treated with benzodiazepines or baclofen.

**Table 16.4** Indications for parenteral opioids

| |
| --- |
| The last few hours/days of life when the patient is unconscious or unable to swallow |
| Dysphagia |
| Nausea and vomiting |
| Bowel obstruction or malabsorption |
| Inability to tolerate tablet burden |
| Best used when pain is stable |

### Prescribing opioids: fears and side effects

Opioids are safe and effective for the treatment of patients in pain. **Table 16.5** considers some of the fears and myths surrounding their use. Some predictable side effects are summarized in **Table 16.6**.

### Psychological factors in pain

Pain may be exacerbated by psychological factors as well as physical ones. Management directed only at physical factors may fail to control pain adequately in some patients. Coexistent depression or anxiety should be addressed and, if appropriate, talking therapies (such as counselling) should be offered.

### Use of complementary therapies

Although sometimes lacking a rigorous evidence base, certain complementary therapies (e.g. massage) seem to benefit some groups of patients. If patients perceive these therapies as adding to their overall well-being, carers and healthcare professionals should support them, provided the treatment does not harm or interfere with their conventional management. Patients report that hypnotherapy, acupuncture, aromatherapy and relaxation therapy may be useful.

### Injection techniques for cancer pain

Nerve blocks can have a place in palliative care and are highly effective when used judiciously in a select group of patients. Various injection techniques can be used. Some of these techniques need expertise and specialized equipment and can be considered with:

- Localized pain
- Pain resulting from involvement of nerve roots
- Abdominal pain arising from neural (e.g. coeliac) plexus
- Rib pain

## FATIGUE AND WEAKNESS

These can be common and distressing symptoms in patients with advanced illness, who can lose muscle mass and become deconditioned. When caused by general debility, they are difficult to treat. Reversible causes, such as cord

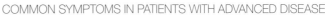

**Table 16.5** Fears and myths around prescribing opioids

**Addiction**

*'Patients will become dependent on opioids.'*

Studies in this population have shown that 'psychological' addiction is rare. Chemical dependence does occur (as with many drugs) and this must be considered when morphine is reduced. In these instances, morphine should be reduced gradually and not stopped abruptly.

**Tolerance**

*'I must not start morphine too early in case the patient becomes used to it and the dose will need increasing.'*

Tolerance has been shown to occur when opioids are taken over a long period. If a dose increase is clinically indicated, this should be done.

**Respiratory depression**

*'I cannot use morphine in frail patients or those with respiratory problems because it precipitates respiratory depression.'*

This does not occur with careful attention to dosage. Opioids are used in the palliative care setting for dyspnoea because they reduce the sensation of breathlessness.

**Hastening death**

*'I can't prescribe morphine until the patient is very close to death. I like to reserve morphine until the very end.'*

Opioids do not hasten death. Indeed, relieving pain may actually prolong life and improve quality of life.

**Indicating death is imminent**

*'Morphine signals imminent death.'*

A prescription of morphine is often perceived by the patient as an unspoken sign that death is imminent. The physician should always be aware of this, explaining that, when an opioid is prescribed, the intention is to treat pain and that opioids are not reserved only for the terminal phase of illness.

**Table 16.6** Side effects of opioids

| Side effect | Frequency (%) | Suitable action |
| --- | --- | --- |
| Constipation | >95 | Regular laxative prescription should be considered prophylactically as well as to treat established constipation. |
| Nausea and vomiting | 30 | *Prescribe antiemetic.* A prophylactic antiemetic (e.g. cyclizine or haloperidol) can be prescribed when starting an opioid. |
| | | Opioid-induced nausea usually subsides within a few days so a regular antiemetic can be withdrawn (unless there is also nausea from another cause). |
| Drowsiness | 20 | This *normally subsides in* about 5 days on a stable dose. |
| Other side effects | | A dry mouth is very common and should be treated with simple local measures such as artificial saliva sprays. |
| | | Confusion and hallucinations are rare (<1% of patients) and other causes should be excluded. |

**16**

compression and cerebral metastases, in patients with cancer should be excluded (see ONCOLOGICAL EMERGENCIES IN PALLIATIVE MEDICINE AT A GLANCE).

## Management

It is important to acknowledge the issue and explain to the patient that the weakness is often multifactorial (underlying illness, medication, cachexia etc.). This allows for realistic goals to be set, which can reduce the patient's distress. Corticosteroids can be useful for some patients, but their effect (increase in energy and sense of well-being) is temporary; lasting only a few weeks. They should not therefore be introduced without careful consideration and their short-term benefit must be weighed against possible side effects such as proximal myopathy and peptic ulceration (hence,

they are normally prescribed with gastric protection such as a proton pump inhibitor).

## DYSPNOEA

Dyspnoea is a subjective difficulty in breathing. It may be experienced by cancer patients, especially those with lung cancer or lung pathology, but it occurs in non-malignant disease too (**Table 16.7**).

## Management

Coexistent medical problems such as infection and congestive cardiac failure should be treated. Management of dyspnoea caused by tumour is outlined below. Explanation should always precede prescription and can itself lead to

**Table 16.7** Causes of dyspnoea in palliative care patients

**Cancer**
Primary tumour
Secondary or metastatic cancer, including *lymphangitis carcinomatosis*
Malignant pleural effusion
Massive ascites splinting the diaphragm

**Other causes**
Infection
Anaemia
Post-radiotherapy or post-chemotherapy fibrosis
Congestive cardiac failure
Chronic obstructive airways disease
Dysfunction of respiratory muscles due to progressive neurological disease
Anxiety

improvement. Severe dyspnoea resulting from large airway compression may cause stridor, is extremely distressing and requires prompt action (see ONCOLOGICAL EMERGENCIES IN PALLIATIVE MEDICINE AT A GLANCE).

Drug treatment of dyspnoea in terminal illness includes:

- Corticosteroids for lymphangitis, bronchospasm, large bulk tumour and superior vena cava obstruction
- Bronchodilators for bronchospasm
- Low-dose morphine to reduce the sensation of dyspnoea
- Anticholinergics to reduce respiratory secretions
- Anxiolytics for anxiety

Non-drug treatments include:

- Attention to the environment (e.g. upright position, fan, calm surroundings)
- Radiotherapy
- Blood transfusion for anaemia
- Aspiration of fluid from the chest or abdomen (thoracocentesis)
- Counselling and reassurance
- Alternative methods (e.g. hypnotherapy, relaxation techniques)

# DYSPHAGIA

Dysphagia (difficulty in swallowing) may occur with progressive neurological disease. It is important to explain the cause of the dysphagia and advise the patient about diet (soft or liquid diet) (**Table 16.8**). A speech and language therapist or dietician may be important to involve in the care. Any concurrent pain should be treated. If the patient is not in the terminal phase (commonly patients with progressive non-malignant neurological disease) and all other avenues have been exhausted, consideration should be given to gastrostomy (e.g. percutaneous endoscopic [PEG]; or radiologically inserted [RIG]) feeding. It is better to discuss this option sooner rather than later to allow the patient to make a considered and informed decision.

# ANOREXIA (DECREASED APPETITE) AND CACHEXIA (WASTING)

Causes of anorexia are:

- Disease itself, with high metabolic rate
- Fear of vomiting
- Presentation of food (too much, unappetizing)
- Constipation
- Oral problems (e.g. oral candidiasis, mouth ulcers, dry mouth)
- Oral tumour
- Biochemical abnormality (e.g. hypercalcaemia, uraemia, hyponatraemia)
- Medications, radiotherapy
- Depression or anxiety

If the above factors have been addressed and it is still felt to be a problem for the patient, corticosteroids or mirtazapine (an antidepressant with appetite-stimulating effects) may be considered.

# NAUSEA AND VOMITING

Nausea and vomiting are relatively common in the palliative care population. Rational treatment is based on the

**Table 16.8** Causes and management of dysphagia

| Type of dysphagia | Implication | Cause | Management |
| --- | --- | --- | --- |
| Solids then liquids | Obstruction | Tumour mass, external compression (e.g. lymphadenopathy) | Corticosteroids, radiotherapy, laser dilatation, stent |
| Solid and liquids simultaneously | Neuromuscular | Terminal neuromuscular dysfunction in very weak patients | |
| | | Progressive neurological disease | Dry secretions, anticholinergics ± PEG feeding |
| | | Perineural tumour infiltration with head and neck tumours that damage cranial nerves (V, IX, X) | Corticosteroids ± PEG feeding |
| Painful | Mucosal causes | *Candida* (not always clinically obvious) | Antifungals |
| | | Postradiotherapy | Analgesia |
| Psychogenic | | | Counselling, anxiolytics |

**Table 16.9** Common causes of nausea and vomiting in patients with advanced disease

| Cause of emesis | Management |
| --- | --- |
| Anticancer treatments such as chemotherapy or radiotherapy | Prescribe antiemetics as per oncology protocol (not HT3 antagonists as this is quite prescriptive). |
| Drugs (e.g. opioids) | Stop offending drug, if possible, and consider alternative |
| Vestibular causes (associated vertigo) | Labyrinthine sedatives (e.g. antihistamines) |
| Psychosocial, anxiety, fear | Counselling, anxiolytics |
| Anticancer treatments such as chemotherapy or radiotherapy | Prescribe antiemetics as per oncology protocol |
| Bowel obstruction | |
| Constipation | Laxatives |
| Gastric stasis secondary to drugs or compressed stomach (hepatomegaly or ascites) | Prokinetic antiemetic ± antacid Consider ascitic drainage |
| Biochemical uraemia, hypercalcaemia, hyponatraemia, abnormal liver function | Treat cause if reversible Use centrally acting antiemetic |
| Cerebral tumour (primary or metastatic, meningeal metastases ± cerebral oedema | Antiemetic acting on vomiting centre (NB neuroleptics lower seizure threshold therefore should be avoided) Steroids ± radiotherapy |
| Gastric irritation due to drugs or blood | Stop offending drug, if possible, give proton pump inhibitor or H2 receptor antagonist |

assessment of the most likely underlying cause (**Table 16.9**). Antiemetics are often indicated. Most antiemetics act at one of the three sites shown in **Table 16.10**.

Sometimes more than one antiemetic will be necessary to control symptoms. If so, it is logical to combine drugs that act by different mechanisms or on different neurotransmitters.

## CONSTIPATION

Constipation is common in debilitated patients and can be exacerbated by the use of opioids. The need to treat constipation is often a consequence of failing to concomitantly prescribe prophylactic laxatives. Most patients on opioids should be prescribed a regular laxative. A rectal examination is indicated to assess for faecal loading or impaction. Laxatives can have softening, stimulant or osmotic actions and again should be tailored to the cause of constipation, where known.

## ANXIETY

Anxiety can be a normal response to serious illness. The most common emotional reaction to a life-threatening

**Table 16.10** Sites of action of antiemetic drugs

| Site of action | Class of drug | Example |
| --- | --- | --- |
| Centrally acting Chemoreceptor trigger zone | Neuroleptic | Haloperidol |
| Vomiting centre | Antihistamine | Cyclizine |
| Peripherally acting | Prokinetic | Domperidone |
| Broad spectrum | Phenothiazine | Levomepromazine |

illness is fear and uncertainty, and many anxieties are based on fears that may be addressed and resolved.

Common fears are concerned with:
- Unrelieved symptoms, especially pain
- Death and the process of dying
- Uncompleted tasks (e.g. a will has not been made)
- Loss and separation from family, job, income
- Loss of dignity and autonomy
- Altered body image

It is therefore important to recognize and accept normal levels of anxiety but monitor for features of anxiety: feelings of tenseness, restlessness and insomnia, panic attacks and autonomic hyperactivity (e.g. palpitations, sensation of choking). Anxiolytics may be helpful, as may counselling.

## DEPRESSION

Despair may also be a normal response to a life-threatening illness and should be recognized and acknowledged. However, it is important to consider treating this.
- Common somatic symptoms of depression (e.g. weight loss, anorexia, lethargy) may be less reliable symptoms here as they may also be a manifestation of advanced physical disease
- Presence of a low mood depressed mood most of the time
- Patient's awareness that their mood is different from normal sadness
- Lowering of interest and enjoyment of social activities (anhedonia)
- Crying, irritability, poor concentration, poor sleep
- Suicidal ideation

Such patients may be treated with antidepressants and psychosocial support.

**16**

## ONCOLOGICAL EMERGENCIES IN PALLIATIVE MEDICINE AT A GLANCE

Listed are some of the reversible problems which are commonly underdiagnosed.

### Superior vena cava obstruction

*Symptoms*
- Dyspnoea, oedema of face, neck and arms, headache

*Cause*
- Tumour mass compressing superior vena cava

*Management*
- Immediate high-dose steroids
- Urgent radio- or chemotherapy ± venous stent and anticoagulation

### Stridor

*Symptoms*
- Severe dyspnoea

*Cause*
- Tumour mass obstructing upper airways

*Management*
- Steroids, radiotherapy/chemotherapy ± stenting of airway

### Malignant spinal cord compression

*Symptoms*
- Back pain, progressive or acute
- Weakness in legs, sensory loss and/or urinary retention/incontinence

*Cause*
- Extradural compression by tumour mass arising in vertebral body, or spinal/paraspinal tumour mass

*Management*
- Time is of the essence: if left untreated, cord compression tends to become irreversible
- Immediate high-dose steroids and urgent investigation with MRI of spine
- Radiotherapy and sometimes neurosurgical intervention may be considered

### Hypercalcaemia

*Symptoms*
- Malaise, anorexia, nausea, vomiting, constipation, thirst, polyuria, drowsiness, confusion

*Cause*
- Tumour-related humoral factors
- Often but not always associated with bone metastases

*Management*
- Fluids and bisphosphonates, together with treatment of underlying malignancy if possible (e.g. chemotherapy)
- Steroids or calcitonin may be considered

### Bowel obstruction

*Symptoms*
- Abdominal distension, pain, absolute constipation, vomiting

*Management*
Depends on site, whether proximal (obstruction of the stomach or small bowel) or distal (large bowel). Surgical intervention should be considered but is rarely indicated in obstruction caused by advanced malignancy. Intravenous fluids and nasogastric tube may be indicated. The aim is symptom control with drugs to reduce nausea and vomiting using antiemetics, avoiding gastrokinetic antiemetics such as metoclopramide or domperidone as they may exacerbate symptoms. Cyclizine and levomepromazine are usually effective. Steroids, analgesia and antisecretories are also used.

### Acute renal failure

*Symptoms*
- Oliguria, anuria, or symptoms of uraemia, e.g. confusion, twitching

*Cause*
- Ureteric obstruction due to pelvic/para-aortic tumour mass
- Drugs, especially NSAIDs

*Management*
- Renal imaging (e.g. ultrasound)
- Steroids, radiotherapy/chemotherapy and/or ureteric stents
- Discontinue any contributing drugs where possible

### Fracture

*Symptoms*
- Severe pain, immobility
- Usually pathological fracture through a bone metastasis

*Cause*
- Bone metastasis or local bony invasion

*Management*
- If prognosis warrants, consider surgical fixation

### Urinary retention
- Quite common and often missed

*Symptoms*
- Difficulty passing urine, abdominal pain, but sometimes, in patients who are unable to communicate, only manifestation may be agitation

*Cause*
- Drugs, cord compression, local obstruction, general debility

*Management*
- Catheterization

## CARE OF THE DYING PATIENT

When a patient with advanced illness enters the dying phase (normally a day or so before death), all medication should be reviewed; *all* drugs should be stopped apart from those indicated for symptom control. The route of administration may need to be reviewed. Communication is vital; anticipate problems and changes in the patient's condition and explain them to the patient and their carers. Reassure them that the patient will be kept comfortable. Often it is appropriate to use a syringe pump to administer medications (**Figure 16.2**; **Table 16.11**).

### ANALGESIA

Analgesia should be continued even if a patient becomes unconscious, as the patient may still experience pain. Abrupt withdrawal of opioids can result in unpleasant reactions. If a patient is on regular opioids, they normally need to be continued at an equivalent dosage subcutaneously, often via a syringe pump. It is rare to remove an analgesic transdermal patch at this stage.

### AGITATION

Agitation can be a problem and reversible causes should be sought and treated appropriately (e.g. retention of urine requires catheterization). It is not uncommon for patients to become agitated and confused shortly before death. If sedation is indicated, use subcutaneous midazolam or levomepromazine, either as single doses or as a subcutaneous infusion using a syringe pump or administered as required.

**Table 16.11** Drugs suitable for use in the syringe pump in the terminal phase of illness

| Indication | Drug |
|---|---|
| Analgesic | Diamorphine, morphine, oxycodone, alfentanil |
| Antiemetic | Haloperidol, levomepromazine, cyclizine |
| Terminal secretions | Hyoscine hydrobromide, glycopyrronium, hyoscine butylbromide |
| Terminal agitation | Midazolam, levomepromazine |

### TERMINAL SECRETIONS ('DEATH RATTLE')

Terminal secretions can be controlled using subcutaneous hyoscine or glycopyrronium as required. Either can be added into the syringe pump or administered as required.

### CRISES

Occasionally it may be appropriate to prophylactically prescribe drugs for a crisis situation or emergency, such as a major bleed (haemoptysis or haematemesis) (e.g. midazolam). Such crises can greatly distress the patient and their family and need to be handled with speed and sensitivity.

### RELIGIOUS AND SPIRITUAL CONSIDERATIONS

People of different spiritual beliefs and faiths have different needs at the time of death. The professionals involved at this time need some understanding of the different religions and beliefs and associated practices so that they can provide support or call in expert colleagues.

## BEREAVEMENT

Support offered to the family both during a patient's illness and at the time of their death may help the family to cope better afterwards. Factors associated with an increased risk of difficult bereavement include:

- A close, dependent or ambivalent relationship
- Concurrent stress at the time of bereavement
- Memories of a 'bad' death (e.g. uncontrolled symptoms)
- Perception of a low level of support (perception may be more important than the actual support in determining outcome)
- Strong feelings of guilt and reproach
- Lack of opportunity to say goodbye and things left unsaid (e.g. as a result of a sudden or traumatic death or absence at the time of death)

**16**

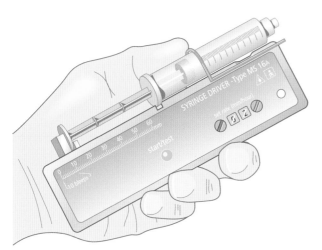

**Figure 16.2** Subcutaneous infusion pump. A subcutaneous infusion pump is a small battery-driven device that will inject the contents of a syringe over a 24-hour period. It can be used in the home and in the inpatient setting.

## CONCLUSIONS

The assessment and treatment of patients with palliative care needs can be challenging. There is a clear imperative to assess patients accurately and speedily attend to their physical symptoms. This requires specialist skills in managing patients with complex illness. The picture is made more difficult when one takes into account the considerable emotional and social problems that patients and families face when trying to cope with life-threatening illness. All physicians will treat patients who have palliative care needs and so they should be familiar with the palliative approach to patient care and be able to respond to the diverse needs of such patients.

### MUST KNOW CHECKLIST

- Understand the principles of palliative medicine and be aware that they are applicable to people with a wide variety of life-threatening illnesses
- Have an understanding of palliative care delivery including the concept of the multidisciplinary approach
- Be able to assess patients' physical, emotional, social and spiritual needs and be aware of the wider dimension of the family
- Understand the importance of hope and that this may have other goals than cure
- Understand the importance of diagnosing and treating the cause of each symptom
- Be aware of the common symptoms in patients with advanced progressive illness and their management
- Have a working knowledge of analgesics and their indications and side effects
- Be able to weigh up the benefits and burdens of treatment
- Be familiar with the major problems encountered by patients and families during the dying process
- Be aware of the risk factors for abnormal bereavement reactions

**Questions and answers** to test your understanding of Chapter 16 can be found by clicking 'Support Material' at the following link: https://www.routledge.com/Medicine-for-Finals-and-Beyond/Axford-OCallaghan/p/book/9780367150594

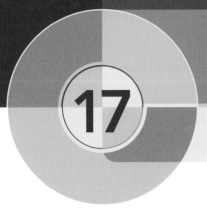

# Poisoning

## 17

PAUL DARGAN

## INTRODUCTION

Poisoning is a common reason for emergency department presentation, and early recognition of clinical features of toxicity is essential to ensure appropriate targeted management.

Over-the-counter and prescribed medications are common causes of both intentional and unintentional poisonings. Recreational drug use can result in significant intoxication, with alcohol and opioid poisonings in particular being responsible for many deaths across the world. It is important to bear in mind that drugs may have been administered to someone, perhaps in 'spiked' drinks, without their knowledge and this includes sedating drugs, such as benzodiazepines. Less commonly, patients may be accidentally exposed either at home or in the workplace to toxins such as carbon monoxide, heavy metals and organophosphates.

## APPROACH TO THE PATIENT

Although some poisoned patients may be drowsy, confused or unconscious, the majority are able to provide a history of events leading up to their presentation and a detailed history is an important component of the risk assessment of the poisoned patient. Clinical examination should assess the cardiovascular, respiratory and neurological function of the patient, followed by identifying features of specific toxins. Resuscitation of patients who present with significant features of toxicity should follow the standard approach to the resuscitation of any patient.

## HISTORY

This should specifically focus on:
- The agent(s) the patient was exposed to
  - Patients often take more than one medication, chemical or recreational drug and may have additionally ingested alcohol.
  - Herbal remedies and other alternative remedies, and over-the-counter medications must be included when taking a drug history
- The quantity of the toxin that the patient has been exposed to
- The timing of the poisoning.
  - Was this a single exposure and, if so, what time did it occur?
  - Or was it a staggered overdose? For a staggered overdose, record information on the time the ingestion started/finished and the quantities taken.
- The route of exposure – oral ingestion, topical, inhalation, or injection
- Symptoms experienced since exposure
- Whether the poisoning occurred due to deliberate self-harm, in which case ongoing risk of self-harm or suicidal ideation should be assessed

Find out about the patient's past medical and psychiatric history.

DOI: 10.1201/9781003193616-17

## EXAMINATION

As with any unwell patient, the initial approach should focus on assessing the patient's airway, breathing and circulation. Further examination should focus on:

- *General inspection:*
  - Does the patient appear diaphoretic?
  - Is there evidence of toxins or drug-related paraphernalia on or around the patient?
  - Does the patient have skin lesions, such as burns, blisters or rashes? Look specifically for needle track-marks (injection sites) or cuts/scars from deliberate self-harm.
  - Measure the temperature.
- *Cardiovascular system:*
  - Monitor the heart rate and blood pressure.
- *Respiratory system:*
  - Observe for tachypnoea or respiratory depression; in patients with a low respiratory rate assess respiratory depth.
  - Auscultate to assess for wheeze or crepitations.
- *Gastrointestinal system:*
  - Look for evidence of corrosive burns within the oral cavity (the absence of these does not exclude corrosive ingestion).
  - Inspect for jaundice or other stigmata of liver disease.
  - Examine the abdomen to assess for localized tenderness (specifically examine for a palpable bladder).
- *Central nervous system:*
  - Assess the Glasgow Coma Score.
  - Assess pupil size and reaction to light
  - Examine the eye movements, looking for nystagmus.
  - Assess for the presence of increased tone (including clonus) and hyper-reflexia.
  - Assess for the presence of cerebellar signs.
- *Mental health assessment:*
  - Is the patient agitated, withdrawn or confused?
  - Assess whether the patient's exposure to the toxin(s) was accidental or intentional. All patients with deliberate self-poisoning should have a formal psychiatric assessment.

## GENERAL MANAGEMENT

- In patients with significant clinical features, obtain intravenous (IV) access.
- All patients with deliberate self-poisoning should have a blood sample taken for a plasma paracetamol concentration.
- In patients with significant clinical features, a blood gas sample should also be taken to assess the patient's acid–base status, as well as lactate, carboxyhaemoglobin and methaemoglobin levels.

- All drowsy patients or those with a seizure should have a capillary glucose.
- An electrocardiogram (ECG) trace will identify abnormalities in the PR, QRS or QT interval durations, which can predict the risk of brady- or tachyarrhythmias.
- Access online guidance from TOXBASE® (https://www.toxbase.org) – the information portal of the National Poisons Information Service – and, where necessary, consult toxicology experts at the National Poisons Information Service.

## GUT DECONTAMINATION AND ELIMINATION OF POISONS

Activated charcoal can be given orally or via a nasogastric tube to those who present within an hour of a potentially toxic ingestion. The large surface area and high adsorptive capacity of activated charcoal enable it to bind to and reduce gastrointestinal absorption of most toxins. Due to the risk of serious complications, gastric lavage is no longer routinely recommended. Whole bowel irrigation is given for slow-release preparations and for body packers; its use should be guided by a clinical toxicologist.

Haemodialysis or other extracorporeal techniques may be indicated to increase elimination of drugs (e.g. lithium, salicylates) or toxins (e.g. toxic alcohols) in patients with significant ingestions; the use of these techniques should always be discussed with a clinical toxicologist.

# MANAGEMENT OF SPECIFIC POISONS

## PARACETAMOL

### Background

Paracetamol-induced liver failure is the leading cause of acute liver failure in the United Kingdom (UK) and the United States (US) and there are around 150 deaths each year in the UK related to paracetamol toxicity.

### Pharmacology

When therapeutic quantities of paracetamol are used, the majority of the drug is metabolized by glucuronide and sulphate conjugation; 5–10% of paracetamol is metabolized by cytochrome P450 isoenzymes to an intermediate metabolite, NAPQI, which subsequently is detoxified by conjugation with glutathione. In paracetamol overdose, glutathione stores become depleted and therefore NAPQI accumulates leading to hepatocyte damage and renal tubular necrosis.

### Clinical features

Patients may develop nausea, vomiting and abdominal pain in the first few hours of paracetamol overdose and following this there can be a period in which the patient is asymptomatic. Clinical signs of liver injury, such as jaundice and right upper quadrant tenderness, typically develop 24–48 hours post-overdose.

### Management

In patients with a single ingestion, bloods should be taken to assess the patient's liver, renal and coagulation function. Plasma paracetamol concentrations should be measured at presentation (or 4 hours post-ingestion if the patient presents earlier) and then plotted on the paracetamol overdose treatment nomogram to determine whether the patient needs treatment with the antidote acetylcysteine; nomograms may vary depending on national guidance; in the UK, current guidance is that patients with a paracetamol concentration above 100 mg/L at 4 hours post-ingestion require treatment (this is often known as the '100-line'). If the level is near or above the line, or if there is any doubt about the timing of the overdose, treatment with acetylcysteine should be commenced. Up to 25% of those treated develop an anaphylactoid reaction, typically involving pruritis, flushing and nausea, which should be managed by stopping the infusion; some patients may also require 10 mg IV chlorpheniramine.

Patients with signs of progressive liver injury, a coagulopathy, metabolic acidosis or kidney injury should be discussed with a liver unit as liver transplantation may be required in cases of severe organ failure.

## TRICYCLIC ANTIDEPRESSANTS

### Background

An estimated 4–5% of the global population suffer from a depressive disorder and, in the UK, 1 in 3 people are prescribed an antidepressant. The two main classes of antidepressants are tricyclic agents (e.g. amitriptyline and dosulepin) and selective serotonin reuptake inhibitors (e.g. fluoxetine and sertraline).

### Pharmacology

Tricyclic antidepressants (TCAs) act primarily by inhibiting serotonin and norepinephrine transporters; additionally, they antagonize muscarinic anticholinesterase receptors and block sodium channels. TCAs have a narrow therapeutic index and overdoses are associated with high mortality rates.

### Clinical features

- Anticholinergic signs (xerostomia, mydriasis, tachycardia, fever, urinary retention)
- Neurological signs (nystagmus, hyperreflexia, clonus, seizures, reduced consciousness or coma)
- Cardiovascular signs (tachycardia, transient hypertension followed by profound hypotension, ventricular arrhythmias)
- Metabolic acidosis

### Management

Bloods should be taken to assess electrolytes, in addition to a blood gas to evaluate acid–base status. TCAs are weak bases and thus, when an acidaemia is present, there is a greater proportion of ionized drug (which increases bioavailability of the TCA). An ECG should be obtained in all patients. ECG features of a TCA overdose include a prolonged corrected QT interval and QRS prolongation. QRS prolongation is an important prognostic marker – patients with a QRS greater than 110 ms and particularly greater than 160 ms are at increased risk of ventricular arrhythmias and seizures. Patients with TCA toxicity should be on a cardiac monitor because of the risk of arrhythmias and may require supportive care in a critical care setting. Hypertonic (8.4%) sodium bicarbonate should be given to patients with QRS prolongation, hypotension, seizures or arrhythmias. Recurrent doses may be required aiming for a pH of 7.45–7.50.

## OPIOIDS

### Background

Opioids are prescribed for their analgesic properties although this drug class is frequently used recreationally. Fatal overdoses of both prescription and non-prescription opioids are increasing throughout the world, particularly in the US. Commonly used opioids include morphine, heroin, codeine, tramadol, oxycodone and fentanyl.

### Pharmacology

Opioids primarily act on three classes of receptor – μ (mu), κ (kappa), and δ (delta) – located throughout the central and peripheral nervous systems.

### Clinical features

In addition to their analgesic properties, opioids have numerous adverse effects, including nausea and vomiting, pruritis, miosis and constipation. At higher doses, patients may develop reduced consciousness and respiratory depression that can progress to respiratory arrest. Physical dependence is common in those who use opioids regularly.

### Management

Patients with significant opioid toxicity typically present with pinpoint pupils, respiratory depression and unconsciousness. The opioid antagonist naloxone should be administered in titrated boluses in those with significant respiratory depression – ideally intravenously, although the intramuscular route can be used if venous access cannot be achieved. Naloxone has a rapid onset of action and patients often respond within seconds. Naloxone has a short half-life, however, and thus further boluses or an infusion may be required to maintain consciousness and adequate ventilation.

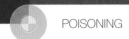 

## MUST-KNOW CHECKLIST

- Poisoning is a common reason for attending the emergency department.
- The initial approach should focus on assessing the patient's airway, breathing and circulation.
- Activated charcoal can adsorb some toxins successfully if given within 1 hour of the overdose.
- In patients who have taken a paracetamol overdose, acetylcysteine can reduce the risk of developing an acute liver injury.
- TCAs have a narrow therapeutic index, and patients who have taken an overdose can present with anticholinergic symptoms, as well as cardiovascular and neurological compromise.
- Patients with significant opioid toxicity typically present with pinpoint pupils, respiratory depression and unconsciousness. The opioid antagonist naloxone should be administered in those with significant respiratory depression.

**Questions and answers** to test your understanding of Chapter 17 can be found by clicking 'Support Material' at the following link: https://www.routledge.com/Medicine-for-Finals-and-Beyond/Axford-OCallaghan/p/book/9780367150594

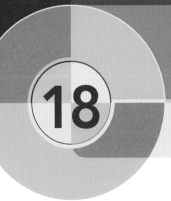

# Skin Disease

## 18

CHRISTOPHER BUNKER & RICHARD WATCHORN

## INTRODUCTION

The skin is a large complex organ, with multiple roles (**Table 18.1**).

## APPROACH TO THE PATIENT

### HISTORY

Dermatology is a visual subject, but an accurate history is essential (HISTORY & EXAMINATION 18.1):

- It is possible to recognize patterns of disease from the history alone.
- It is vital to assess the impact of the disease on the patient. Details of occupation, personal and family medical history are frequently of diagnostic importance. Sexual history should be sensitively elicited.

### SKIN SYMPTOMS

Skin symptoms include itch, rash, lump, ulceration, cracking, blistering, redness, scaling, flushing, pain, body-image issues, hair loss and nail changes. Temporal and spatial characteristics of the presenting symptoms should be established (HISTORY & EXAMINATION 18.1).

**Table 18.1** Functions of the skin

| Function | Examples |
|---|---|
| Barrier function | Prevention of fluid/electrolyte loss |
| | Protection from microorganisms, toxic materials and ultraviolet (UV) radiation |
| Immune defence | Innate and adaptive immunity |
| Sensation | Touch, pain |
| Thermoregulation | Core temperature; water loss |
| Metabolic | Vitamin D, hormones |
| Psychosexual | Individual recognition, sexual attraction |

### DISEASE IMPACT

The impact of skin disease can be profound. Itch may interfere with sleep. Real or perceived cosmetic disfiguration can cause psychosocial and sexual dysfunction. Activities of daily living or ability to walk can be impaired. Determination of disease impact can influence treatment decisions.

### DRUG HISTORY

Drugs rashes are common; all medications taken must be identified. Some may not be volunteered, such as over-the-counter treatments, herbal agents or illicit drugs.

DOI: 10.1201/9781003193616-18

### Important questions to ask a patient with a skin disorder

#### About the patient

What is your occupation?

How much time have you spent in the sun? Do you tan or burn?

Do you have any specific concerns or ideas regarding this skin problem?

#### Symptoms

Itch, pain, etc.

#### Pattern of disease

*Onset and progression*

When did the symptoms start?

Where on your skin did it develop first?

How have they changed with time?

#### Associated features

Are your symptoms associated with your lifestyle, work, or home?

Have you noticed any changes affecting your hair, eyes, mouth, nails, genitals, joints?

Have you noticed any other symptoms?

Does anybody else at home have similar symptoms?

#### Disease impact

How do your symptoms affect you at work and at home (mobility, social activities, sexual life, personal hygiene or sleep)?

#### Drug history

Which treatments have been attempted? Have they helped?

#### Travel history

Where have you travelled recently?

#### Family history

Atopy (e.g. asthma, eczema or hay fever), psoriasis, skin cancer, etc.

#### Past medical history

Have you had any skin disorder previously (e.g. eczema, psoriasis, skin cancer)?

Have you had any other disorder such as asthma, hay fever, diabetes?

## EXAMINATION

A general skin examination must:

- Be performed in adequate light
- Include scalp, nails and mucosae
- Establish distribution pattern, site and morphology of lesions using appropriate terminology (CLINICAL EXAMINATION AT A GLANCE)

Skin type (**Table 18.2**) may influence clinical findings (e.g. erythema may be less evident in darker skin types).

## INVESTIGATION

- *Dermoscopy:* visualization of microscopic structures not visible with naked eye

**Table 18.2** Classification of skin sensitivity to the sun

| Type I | Always burns |
|---|---|
| Type II | Usually burns, sometimes tans |
| Type III | Sometimes burns, usually tans |
| Type IV | Always tans Asian / Middle Eastern |
| Type V | Asian > Afro-Caribbean |
| Type VI | Afro-Caribbean > Asian |

- *Histology* (**Figure 18.1**): direct microscopy of tissue to establish cell populations, morphology, presence of invasion in neoplasia, pattern of inflammation in inflammatory disorders, immunohistochemistry to identify cell lineage in neoplasia
- *Immunofluorescence* (**Figure 18.2**): detection of skin antibodies in suspected autoimmune disease
- *Microbiology:* swabs or tissue for microscopy, culture and antibiotic sensitivities and/or viral PCR; skin (biopsy specimens), skin scrapings, nail clippings or hair may be examined for fungal microscopy, culture and PCR

## GENERAL PRINCIPLES OF MANAGEMENT

### SUPPORTIVE TREATMENT

In general, supportive treatment includes:

- Emollients and soap avoidance (an irritant)
- Sun protection
- Psychological support

### SPECIFIC TREATMENT

Modalities include withdrawal of drugs, or prescription of drugs, phototherapy or surgery.

#### Drugs

Topical dermatological medications are summarized in **Table 18.3** and **Table 18.4**.

#### Phototherapy

- This is therapeutic controlled exposure to UV light.
- Ultraviolet B (UVB) phototherapy is safer than psoralens plus ultraviolet A photochemotherapy (PUVA); psoralen may be applied topically (e.g. bath PUVA) or taken orally.
- It is effective in psoriasis, eczema, pruritus, mycosis fungoides and other dermatoses.
- Mechanisms of action include T-cell apoptosis.
- Risks include phototoxicity (sunburn), skin cancer, exacerbation of underlying condition or reactivation of cold sores.

#### Surgery

Surgery may be diagnostic (biopsy) or curative (for skin tumours).

**CLINICAL EXAMINATION AT A GLANCE**

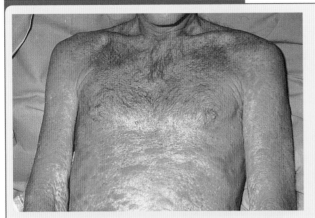

**Figure A** Confluent (contiguous) erythema and erythematous nodules (drug eruption and histoplasmosis – AIDS).

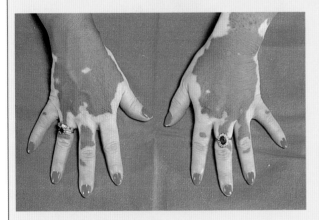

**Figure B** Flat lesions: macules (small) and patches (large area) of hypopigmentation (vitiligo).

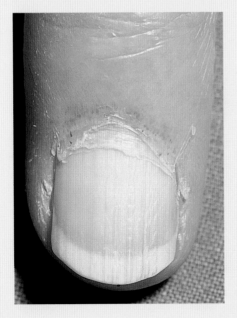

**Figure C** Nailfold telangiectasia (systemic sclerosis).

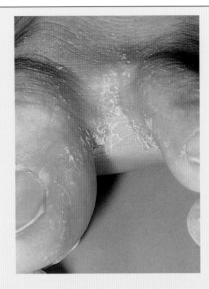

**Figure D** Interdigital scale (Norwegian scabies).

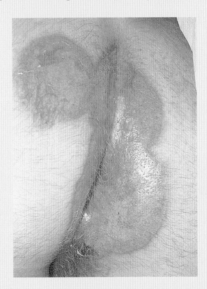

**Figure E** Perianal erosion (partial focal epidermal loss) (herpes simplex – AIDS).

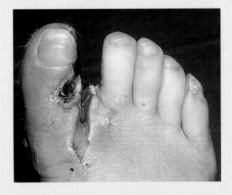

**Figure F** Interdigital ulcer (focal full-thickness epidermal loss) (diabetes mellitus).

*Continued...*

18

...*Continued*

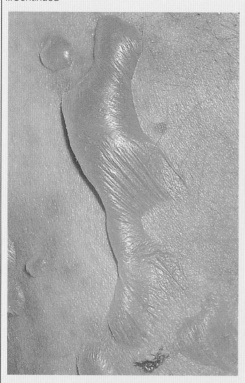

**Figure G** Fluid-filled lesions: vesicles (<5 mm) and bulla (>5 mm) (bullous pemphigoid).

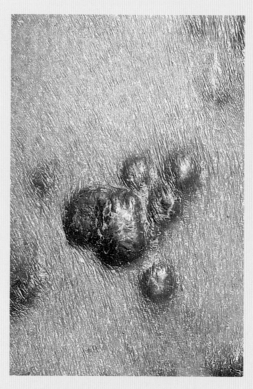

**Figure I** Raised solid lesions: papules (nodules are papules with deep component) (Kaposi's sarcoma – AIDS).

**Figure H** Café au lait macule (McCune–Albright syndrome).

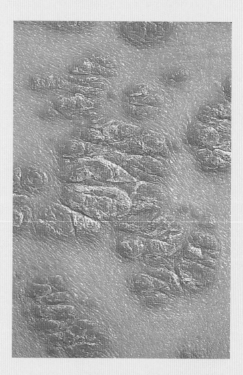

**Figure J** Hyperkeratotic (scaly), erythematous plaques (psoriasis).

*Continued...*

*...Continued*

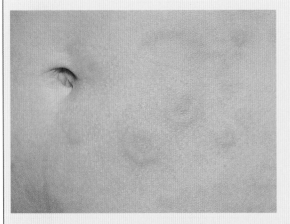

**Figure K** Weals (oedematous plaques) (acute urticaria).

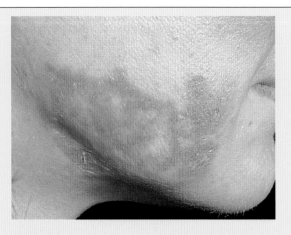

**Figure N** Erythema, atrophy, scarring (discoid lupus erythematosus [DLE]).

**18**

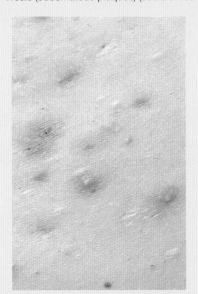

**Figure L** Comedones (hair follicles filled with keratin), pustules (pus-filled lesions) and scars (acne vulgaris).

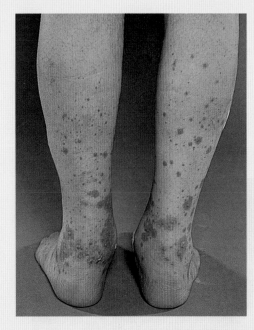

**Figure O** Palpable purpuric papules (allergic vasculitis of the leg).

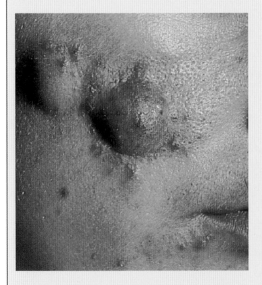

**Figure M** Cysts (fluid-filled sac) (pyoderma faciale).

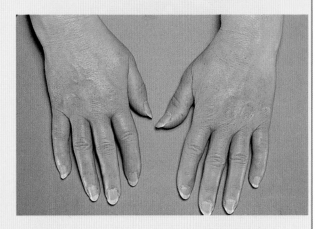

**Figure P** Sclerosis (sclerodactyly—systemic sclerosis).

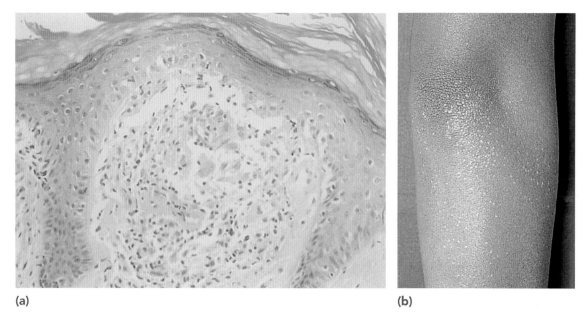

**(a)**                                                           **(b)**

**Figure 18.1 (a)** Photomicrograph of skin showing: histology (haematoxylin and eosin) papillary dermal inflammatory cell infiltrate of lichen nitidus; **(b)** clinical photograph of lichen nitidus (micropapular variant of lichen planus).

# DISEASES AND THEIR MANAGEMENT

## INFLAMMATORY DERMATOSES

### URTICARIA AND ANGIOEDEMA

Urticaria (hives) describes a clinical finding: an eruption of weals.

#### Disease mechanisms

- Mast cell degranulation occurs with release of histamine and vasoactive mediators.
- Acute urticaria is triggered by various substances including allergens, infections and food or drugs (by allergic and non-allergic mechanisms). Type I hypersensitivity mediates acute urticarias, but not chronic (>6 weeks) urticarias, which are probably autoimmune or multifactorial in aetiology.

#### Clinical features

- Weals (CLINICAL EXAMINATION AT A GLANCE, **Figure K**) are pruritic pink or pale dermal swellings (**Table 18.5**).
- Individual weals resolve in less than 24 hours.
- Deeper dermal swelling causes angioedema (without erythema).
- Purpura or weals persisting beyond this timeframe can signify urticarial vasculitis.
- Angioedema without weals requires exclusion of angiotensin-converting enzyme (ACE) inhibitor-induced angioedema or C1-esterase inhibitor deficiency (hereditary or acquired).
- 'Spontaneous urticaria' indicates absence of an identifiable trigger.

**Figure 18.2** Direct immunofluorescence of lupus erythematosus showing speckled basement membrane zone (BMZ) deposition of IgM. Courtesy of BS Bhogal, Institute of Dermatology. Reproduced from Champion RH *et al.* (eds) (1992) *Textbook of Dermatology*, 5th edn (Wiley-Blackwell, Oxford), with the permission of the authors.

**Table 18.3** Topical treatments

| | Action | Indications | Side effects |
|---|---|---|---|
| **Emollients and soap substitutes** | | | |
| Paraffin, emulsifying ointment, aqueous cream | Hydrate skin | Dry scaly dermatoses, pruritus | May contain preservatives and other ingredients that irritate or sensitize Highly flammable |
| **Topical steroids (corticosteroids)** | | | |
| Hydrocortisone (mildly potent), clobetasone (moderately potent), betamethasone (potent), clobetasol (superpotent – note similarity in name to clobetasone, a moderately potent topical steroid) | Anti-inflammatory | Inflammatory dermatoses Use as a lotion, cream or ointment, foam or with an antibacterial (e.g. fusidic acid) or antifungal (e.g. hydrocortisone, clotrimazole) A 'finger-tip unit' should suffice to cover an area equal to two hands laid flat | Striae, infection, atrophy, tinea incognito, systemic absorption, allergic contact sensitivity, tachyphylaxis (loss of response with prolonged use) |
| **Topical antibiotics** | | | |
| Fucidic acid, mupirocin, neomycin, clindamycin, erythromycin, metronidazole | | Superficial infections (e.g. impetigo, pitted keratolysis) or acne, rosacea | Irritant |
| **Topical antifungals** | | | |
| Clotrimazole, ketoconazole, nystatin | | Tinea, seborrheic dermatitis | Irritant |
| **Topical keratolytics** | | | |
| Benzoyl peroxide, salicylic acid | | Acne, warts, hyperkeratosis | Irritant |
| **Topical retinoids** | | | |
| Adapelene, isotretinoin | Downregulate collagenase and elastase; sebostatic | Photodamage, acne | Irritant, photosensitivity |
| **Topical cytotoxics** | | | |
| 5-fluorouracil | Cytotoxic | Actinic keratoses, Bowen's disease | Toxic reaction and irritation (essential for mode of action) |

- 'Inducible' urticaria indicates an identifiable trigger, and includes the solar, aquagenic, cholinergic (exercise), contact and cold forms of urticaria.
- *Differential diagnosis:* Other conditions may manifest with urticarial-like lesions or angioedema (**Table 18.6**).

### Investigation

- Full blood count (FBC), eosinophil count and erythrocyte sedimentation rate (ESR)
- Thyroid function tests
- Antinuclear antibody (ANA), complement (C4) levels and viral (human immunodeficiency virus [HIV]/hepatitis)
- *Microbiological investigations:*

**Table 18.4** Immunosuppressants

| |
|---|
| Azathioprine, prednisolone, methotrexate, ciclosporin, mycophenolate mofetil |
| *Indications:* connective tissue disease; bullous disease; eczema; psoriasis |

- o Throat swabs
- o Stool sample for *Helicobacter pylori* antigen, and ova, cysts and parasites
- If urticaria other than common urticaria is suspected, specialist assessment is indicated.

### Management

- Avoidance of the offending agent
- Antihistamines ($H_1$-antagonists) up to four times daily

**Table 18.5** Types of urticaria

| Type | Features |
|---|---|
| Spontaneous urticaria Acute (<6 weeks) Intermittent Chronic (>6 weeks) Angioedema | No identifiable trigger |
| Inducible urticaria | Including cholinergic, aquagenic, cold, heat, solar, contact (allergic), dermographism |

**Table 18.6** Differential diagnosis of urticaria

| Type | Features |
|---|---|
| Urticarial vasculitis | Lesions lasting > 24 hours, ecchymosis |
| Insect bites (papular urticaria) | |
| C1 esterase inhibitor deficiency | Angioedema without weals – due to acquired or hereditary C1 esterase inhibitor deficiency |
| ACE inhibitor-induced angioedema | Angioedema without weals |
| Autoinflammatory syndromes | Systemic symptoms and internal organ involvement (e.g. cryopyrin-associated periodic syndromes, Schnitzler's syndrome) |

- Omalizumab (IgE-antagonist) for resistant cases; other options include montelukast, ciclosporin, propanolol
- Systemic steroids if required as rescue therapy

## LICHEN PLANUS

### Disease mechanisms

The disease mechanism is unknown; viruses and autoimmunity are proposed aetiological factors.

### Clinical features

- Pruritic violaceous papules with white lines (Wickham's striae, **Figure 18.3**)

- Oral involvement common (sometimes present in absence of skin involvement); nail dystrophy may be observed
- Lichen planopilaris: subtype that causes scarring alopecia

### Investigation

Skin biopsy is needed.

### Management

- Potent topical steroids; sometimes phototherapy or oral therapy (prednisolone or tetracyclines)
- Oral, genital, hair or nail disease usually requires expert input

## PITYRIASIS ROSEA

### Disease mechanisms

This is a reactive rash associated with human herpes virus (HHV)-6, HHV-7 and HHV-8.

### Clinical features

- Itchy oval erythematous patches with a 'collarette' of scale (**Figure 18.4**)
- A larger lesion (herald patch) precedes the generalized eruption
- Common in young adults
- Spontaneously resolves

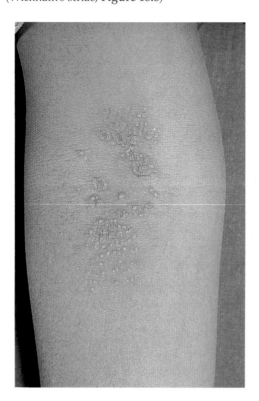

**Figure 18.3** Lichen planus. Polygonal papules with superficial shiny scale (Wickham's striae).

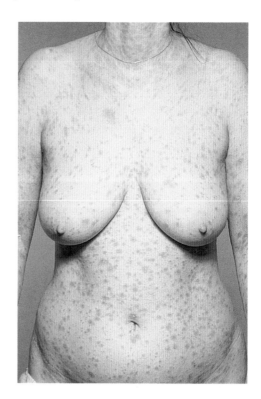

**Figure 18.4** Pityriasis rosea. Oval scaly patches. Herald patch centre right chest.

## Investigation

Serology will exclude secondary syphilis (a clinical mimicker).

## Management

- Emollients
- Reassurance

## KERATOSIS PILARIS

- Hyperkeratosis of hair follicles, manifesting as spiky follicular lesions, often on the upper limbs
- A *normal variant*, rather than a true skin condition
- *Treatment:* not usually required; urea-based moisturizers may ameliorate itching

## ECZEMA (DERMATITIS)

Eczema can be subdivided aetiologically or clinically (**Table 18.7**). The physical signs are listed in **Table 18.8**.

## ATOPIC ECZEMA

This is a relapsing inflammatory condition usually beginning in infancy (see ECZEMA AT A GLANCE).

### Disease mechanisms

- The pathogenesis is complex and involves immune dysregulation and epidermal barrier dysfunction.
- A personal or first-degree family history of eczema, asthma or hay fever increases the risk.

### Clinical features

Ill-defined erythematous scaly patches occur with flexural predilection (extensor in infancy) (ECZEMA AT A GLANCE, **Figure A**).

- Scratching and rubbing lead to skin thickening (lichenification).
- *Eczema herpeticum* occurs when herpes simplex virus (HSV) supervenes and is an emergency that requires treatment with systemic aciclovir.
- Vesicles are immediately destroyed by scratching, leaving characteristic monomorphic 'punched-out' erosions (ECZEMA AT A GLANCE, **Figure B**).

**Table 18.7** Classification of eczema

| Endogenous eczema | Exogenous eczema |
|---|---|
| Atopic eczema | Irritant contact dermatitis |
| Autosensitization | Allergic contact dermatitis |
| Seborrhoeic eczema | Chronic actinic dermatitis |
| (Venous) stasis eczema | |
| Asteatotic eczema | |
| Pompholyx | |
| Discoid eczema | |
| Eczematous drug reactions | |

**Table 18.8** Physical signs of acute and chronic eczema

| Acute | Chronic |
|---|---|
| Erythema | Lichenification |
| Oedema | Scaling |
| Vesicles | |
| Serum exudation/crusts | |
| Excoriations | |

## Investigation

- Diagnosis is clinical; in atypical or recalcitrant cases, biopsy is required to exclude mycosis fungoides, and patch testing may be required to exclude contact allergy.
- Recalcitrant nipple eczema requires biopsy to exclude Paget's disease.
- Microbiological testing is used if infection is suspected (e.g. eczema herpeticum).

## Management

- Topical emollients to support barrier function and topical corticosteroids to control inflammation are the cornerstones.
- Soaps desiccate the skin; they should be replaced with emollient soap substitutes.
- Scratching can perpetuate the 'itch–scratch cycle'.
- Counselling may be needed regarding eczema herpeticum and how to recognize it.
- For recalcitrant cases:
  o UVB phototherapy
  o Hand PUVA (for hand dermatitis)
  o Systemic treatment with methotrexate, mycophenolate mofetil, azathioprine, or ciclosporin
  o Dupilumab (an IL-4Rα antagonist)

## OTHER TYPES OF ENDOGENOUS ECZEMA

### Stasis eczema (varicose eczema)

This affects the lower legs (see 'Lower limb oedema'; ECZEMA AT A GLANCE, **Figure D**).

### Discoid eczema

- Itchy, coin-shaped plaques
- Requires potent or superpotent topical steroids

### Pompholyx

This is vesicular eczema of the palms and soles.

### Seborrhoeic dermatitis

- A scaly, erythematous form of eczema with a predilection for the scalp (dandruff), face (ECZEMA AT A GLANCE, **Figure C**), chest, axillae and groins; often asymptomatic
- Can be severe and extensive in HIV

**ECZEMA AT A GLANCE**

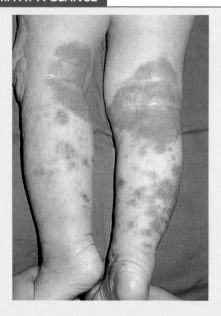

**Figure A** Atopic-like dermatitis (Wiskott–Aldrich syndrome).

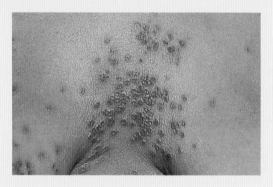

**Figure B** Eczema herpeticum. Erosions and crusts.

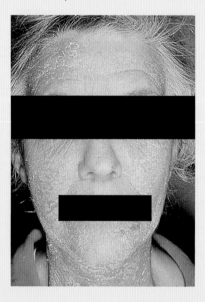

**Figure C** Severe seborrhoeic dermatitis. Reproduced from Champion RH *et al.* (eds) (1992) *Textbook of Dermatology*, 5th edn (Wiley-Blackwell, Oxford), with the permission of the authors.

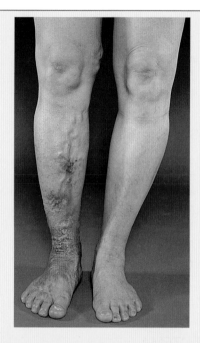

**Figure D** Varicose eczema (stasis dermatitis).

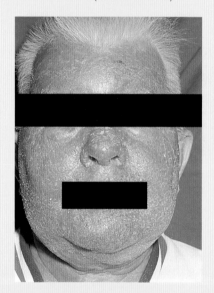

**Figure E** Acute contact dermatitis.

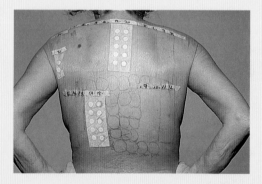

**Figure F** Contact dermatitis under evaluation by patch testing.

- Represents a reaction to commensal *Malassezia* spp.
- Responds to topical steroids and antifungals (e.g. ketoconazole)

## CONTACT DERMATITIS

### Disease mechanisms

Contact dermatitis (ECZEMA AT A GLANCE, **Figure E**) is irritant in 80% of cases and allergic (type IV, cell-mediated) in 20%.

### Investigation

*Patch testing* is used. Potential allergens are determined with a thorough history, including occupational exposures, applied in patches to a non-inflamed back (ECZEMA AT A GLANCE, **Figure F**), removed at 48 hours and the reactions read. Examination for late responses is undertaken at 72 hours.

### Management

Allergen avoidance is recommended but this may prove challenging (e.g. in airborne allergic contact dermatitis).

### Prevention

- Atopic, irritant and allergic factors may coexist (e.g. with hand eczema). For wet work, cotton gloves inside rubber gloves are recommended.
- Barrier creams are important in industrial and domestic prophylaxis.

## PSORIASIS

This is a chronic inflammatory disorder, with variable distribution and morphologic subtypes.

### Disease mechanisms

- Complex pathogenesis: T-cells (particularly Th17 cells) activation and cytokine secretion (TNF-alpha, IL-17 and IL-23) cause inflammation and keratinocyte proliferation (see PSORIASIS AT A GLANCE).
- Flares are precipitated by infections (e.g. with *Streptococcus* spp.), stress, trauma (Koebner phenomenon) and drugs.

### Clinical features

- Plaque psoriasis (most common subtype): red, silver-scaled plaques
- Predominant scalp and extensor distribution
- Guttate psoriasis: 'teardrop' plaques
- Flexural: lacks scale
- Nail involvement (PSORIASIS AT A GLANCE, **Figure E**): pitting, onycholysis, dystrophy and subungual hyperkeratosis); signifies higher risk of joint involvement (psoriatic arthritis; PSORIASIS AT A GLANCE, **Figure F**)

- Pustulosis has distinct IL-36-mediated pathogenesis: frequently affects palms and soles (PSORIASIS AT A GLANCE, **Figure D**)
- Erythroderma

### Management

- Tailored to extent, comorbidities and impact on quality of life
- Psychological support
- Assessment for psoriatic arthritis
- Emollients and soap substitutes
- Avoidance of aggravating factors (smoking, alcohol, obesity)
- Topical agents (localized disease): vitamin D analogues (calcipotriol), corticosteroids, calcineurin inhibitors (tacrolimus or pimecrolimus)
- Phototherapy
- Systemic therapies if unresponsive:
  o Methotrexate
  o Acitretin
  o Ciclosporin
  o Advanced therapies for severe resistant disease: apremilast (phosphodiesterase-4 inhibitor), biologic therapies that antagonise cytokines such as TNF-α (adalimumab) interleukin-17 (secukinumab, ixekizumab) and interleukin-23 (guselkumab, risankizumab)

## ACNE VULGARIS

This is a chronic inflammatory disorder of the pilosebaceous unit.

### Disease mechanisms

Hyperseborrhoea and inflammation are triggered by *Cutibacterium acnes*.

### Clinical features

Acne causes comedones, papules, pustules, nodules, cysts and scars (**Figure 18.5**) on face, back or chest.

### Investigation

Endocrine assessment is needed if there is evidence of polycystic ovarian syndrome (PCOS) or Cushing's syndrome.

### Management

Early treatment is advised to minimize the risk of scarring.
- *Mild (predominantly comedonal):* topical therapy (benzoyl peroxide, topical retinoids, azaleic acid)
- *Moderate–severe:* oral tetracyclines (in conjunction with topical agents above); for females, androgen antagonists (cyproterone acetate or spironolactone) may be considered
- *Severe (recalcitrant, nodulocystic, scarring or severe psychosocial impact):* isotretinoin (teratogenic)

## PSORIASIS AT A GLANCE

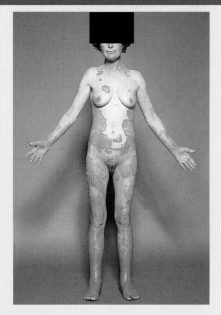

**Figure A** Pre-erythrodermic psoriasis.

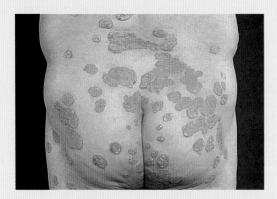

**Figure B** Chronic plaque psoriasis.

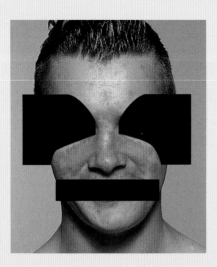

**Figure C** Sebopsoriasis (clinical overlap with seborrhoeic dermatitis; compare with ECZEMA AT A GLANCE, **Figure C**).

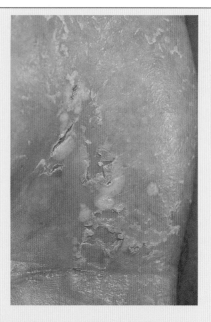

**Figure D** Palmoplantar psoriasis (pustular hypothenar eminence).

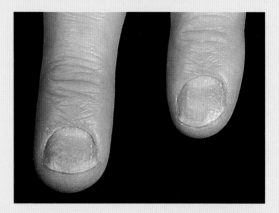

**Figure E** Nail psoriasis. Note dystrophy, pits and onycholysis.

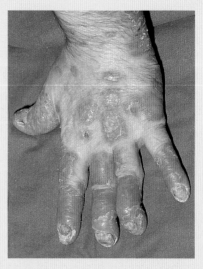

**Figure F** Psoriatic arthropathy (arthritis mutilans); severe nail dystrophy.

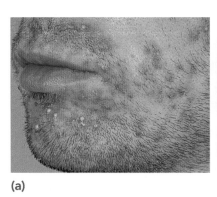
(a)

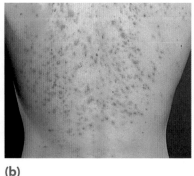
(b)

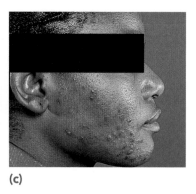
(c)

**Figure 18.5 (a–c)** Acne vulgaris (seborrhoea, comedones, papules, pustules, nodules, scars and postinflammatory hyperpigmentation).

**18**

# ROSACEA

This is a chronic dermatosis predominantly affecting fair-skinned, middle-aged individuals. UV light, innate immunity and demodex mites are proposed aetiological factors.

## Clinical features

Nomenclature of subtypes reflects clinical features: erythematotelangiectatic, papulopustular (**Figure 18.6**), phymatous (thickened skin, with distortion of features if severe) and ocular.

## Management

- *Erythematotelangiectatic subtype:* sun protection, topical vasoconstrictors (e.g. brimonidine) or vascular laser

- *Papulopustular subtype:* topical (azeleic acid, metronidazole or ivermectin), or oral agents (tetracycline or isotretinoin)
- *Phymatous rosacea:* electrocautery or laser ablation
- *Ocular rosacea:* oily lubricating gels and lid hygiene, careful lid massage and antibiotics

# HIDRADENITIS SUPPURATIVA

This chronic relapsing inflammatory disorder is characterized by painful lesions in apocrine-rich skin (axillae, inframammary areas and groin).

## Disease mechanisms

- Unknown; associations with obesity and smoking
- Genetic predisposition in a subset of patients

## Clinical features

- Comedones, nodules or abscesses in axillae, groins, breasts or behind ears
- Sinus tract formation and scarring

## Investigation

- Swabs
- Tissue cultures and histopathology in atypical disease
- Imaging to determine involvement of underlying structures (e.g. gastrointestinal tract in perianal disease)

## Management

- Multidisciplinary: dermatologists, surgeons and microbiologists
- Complications include superinfection, lymphoedema and psychosocial impairment
- Analgesia, psychological support, weight loss
- First line: long-term oral tetracyclines
- If unresponsive: dapsone, acitretin, clindamycin and rifampicin (dual regimen) or intravenous ertapenem
- TNF-α antagonists (adalimumab) for moderate-to-severe disease
- Surgery: incision and drainage, abscess 'de-roofing', excision of affected areas

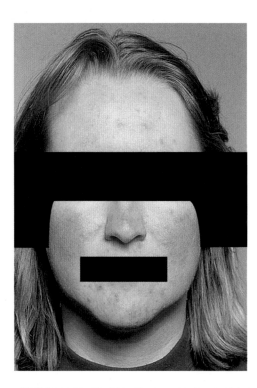

**Figure 18.6** Rosacea. Facial erythema, papules, pustules and telangiectasia.

## MORPHOEA (LOCALIZED SCLERODERMA)

### Disease mechanisms

The disease mechanisms are unknown.

### Clinical features

- There are circumscribed (**Figure 18.7**), linear or facial (en coup de sabre) fibrotic (thickened and hardened) plaques.
- Disease overlying joints causes contractures and requires aggressive immunosuppression (prednisolone and methotrexate or mycophenolate mofetil).

## DISCOID LUPUS ERYTHEMATOSUS

### Disease mechanisms

DLE is an autoimmune disorder.

### Clinical features

- Red scaly patches (**Figure 18.8**) on face, scalp and sun-exposed areas, with scarring and follicular plugging (CLINICAL EXAMINATION AT A GLANCE, **Figure N**)
- ˜5% eventually develop systemic lupus erythematosus (SLE)

### Investigation

Biopsy for histology and immunofluorescence.

### Management

- Sun protection
- Potent topical steroids
- Hydroxychloroquine

## DERMATOMYOSITIS

Cutaneous features include:

- Oedematous maculopapular erythematous plaques on the interphalangeal and metacarpophalangeal joints (Gottron's papules)

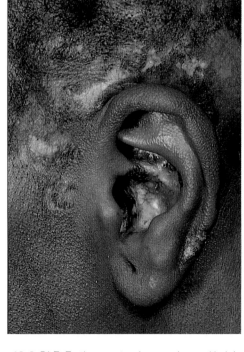

**Figure 18.8** DLE. Erythema, atrophy, scarring and hair loss.

- Erythema of sun-exposed areas
- Heliotrope sign of eyelids: oedema and lilac colour (**Figure 18.9**)
- Subcutaneous calcification and ulceration
- Facial erythema
- Photodistributed poikiloderma (hyper and hypopigmentation)
- 'Flagellate' erythema (linear streaks)
- Abnormal periungual capillary loops and ragged cuticles
- Digital ulceration (anti-MDA5 dermatomyositis)

For more information on dermatomyositis, see Chapter 4, Rheumatic disease.

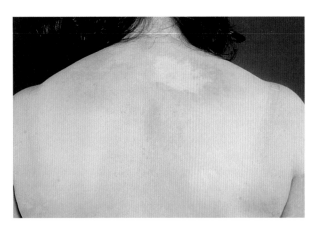

**Figure 18.7** Localized scleroderma (morphoea). Plaques on back.

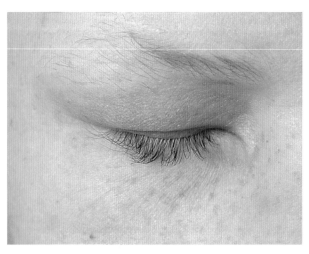

**Figure 18.9** Dermatomyositis. Lilac heliotropic rash on eyelids.

# LICHEN SCLEROSIS

This is a chronic inflammatory scarring dermatosis with genital predilection.

## Disease mechanisms

Proposed mechanisms include chronic occlusive exposure to urine, autoimmunity or dysbiosis.

## Clinical features

- Whitened, atrophic skin, fissures, adhesions, anatomical distortion (partial or complete resorption of labia minora, burying of clitoris in women [**Figure 18.10**], effacement of frenulum and/or loss of coronal sulcus in men)
- May be asymptomatic, or may cause itch, redness or pain, including dyspareunia
- May present as inability to retract foreskin ('phimosis') in men
- May manifest as non-specific inflammation (vulvitis or balanoposthitis), leading to misdiagnosis as 'thrush'
- Anatomical distribution varies by gender:
  o In men: urethral extension may occur, disrupting urinary stream
  o In women: perineal and perianal extension may occur ('figure of eight' pattern)
- Risk of malignant transformation, manifesting as persistent, erythematous patches, ulcers or papules
- Extragenital lichen sclerosis appears as atrophic ivory patches (**Figure 18.11**)

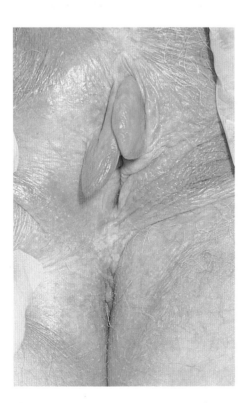

**Figure 18.10** Vulval lichen sclerosus. Note loss of vulval architecture. Courtesy of Dr RCD Staughton.

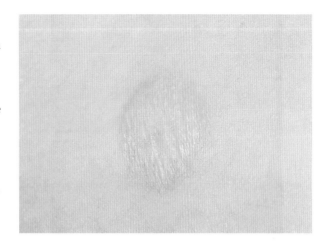

**Figure 18.11** Lichen sclerosus.

## Investigation

The diagnosis is clinical; the role of biopsy is mainly to exclude malignant transformation.

## Management

- Superpotent topical corticosteroids (e.g. clobetasol) and barrier emollient
- Recalcitrant cases in men require circumcision (usually curative)
- Self-monitoring for malignant transformation

# SARCOIDOSIS

- Cutaneous manifestations are highly variable; known as the 'great mimicker'
- Typical manifestations include:
  o Erythema nodosum (**Figure 18.12**)
  o Lupus pernio (**Figure 18.13**)
  o Papules, nodules and plaques
- *Skin-specific investigations:* biopsy for histology and microbiology (culture/mycobacterial PCR)
- *Treatment:* options include intralesional triamcinolone and systemic agents (see Chapter 6, Respiratory disease)

For more information on sarcoidosis, see Chapter 6, Respiratory disease.

# IMMUNOBULLOUS DISORDERS

- May be subepidermal or intraepidermal
- Investigated with biopsy of involved skin for histology and perilesional skin for immunofluorescence (**Figure 18.14**; **Figure 18.15**)

## Bullous pemphigoid

This is the most common autoimmune blistering disorder.

### Disease mechanisms

It is caused by autoimmunity against basement membrane components (subepidermal).

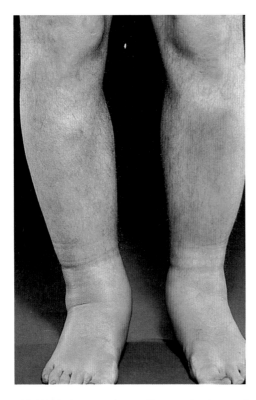

**Figure 18.12** Erythema nodosum. Causes: streptococcal infection, sarcoid, tuberculosis.

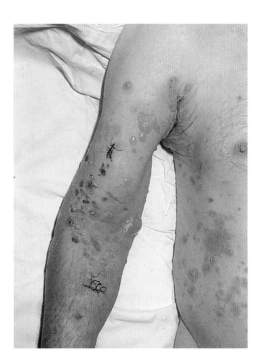

**Figure 18.14** Bullous pemphigoid. Tense blisters (bullae) on an erythematosus and urticated base.

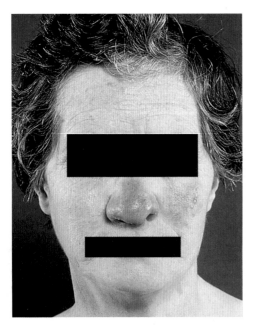

**Figure 18.13** Sarcoidosis (lupus pernio of the nose and cheek). Infiltrated plaques and nodules.

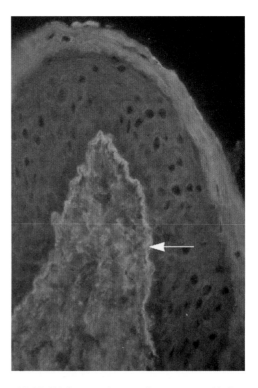

**Figure 18.15** Bright green immunofluorescence of IgG at the BMZ (indicated by arrow) in a patient with pemphigoid. Reproduced from Champion RH *et al.* (eds) (1992) *Textbook of Dermatology*, 5th edn (Wiley-Blackwell, Oxford), with the permission of the authors.

**18**

### Clinical features

- Initial manifestations are pruritus with urticated erythematous and eczematous areas (see **Figure 18.14**; CLINICAL EXAMINATION AT A GLANCE, **Figure G**).
- Tense (subepidermal) blisters develop later.
- The oral mucosa may be involved.

### Management

- Superpotent topical corticosteroids
- Systemic therapy (prednisolone and/or doxycycline) in extensive involvement
- Steroid-sparing agents: methotrexate, azathioprine or mycophenolate mofetil, IV-Ig or rituximab

## Mucous membrane pemphigoid

- Subepidermal blistering disorder with *scarring*
- May present as asymptomatic gingivitis, or erosions or ulcers of oral mucosa or conjunctivae, which may be asymptomatic or painful
- May involve skin, nasal cavity, genitalia, pharynx, rarely larynx or oesophagus
- May cause blindness; ophthalmological involvement is essential
- *Treatment:* multidisciplinary and includes topical steroids with steroid-sparing agents (dapsone, sulfasalazine, mycophenolate mofetil, azathioprine, cyclophosphamide, IV-Ig or rituximab)

## Pemphigus vulgaris

Intraepidermal blistering is caused by antibodies targeting the cell desmosomal structure.

### Clinical features and investigation

- Blistering may initially solely affect the oral mucosa.
- The blisters are intraepithelial and rupture easily, leaving erosions (**Figure 18.16**).
- *Direct immunofluorescence* demonstrates intercellular IgG and C3 (**Figure 18.17**).

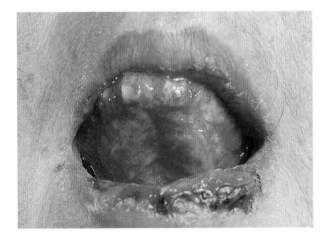

**Figure 18.16** Pemphigus vulgaris. Severe mucocutaneous erosions.

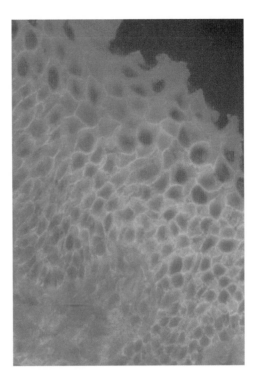

**Figure 18.17** Bright green immunofluorescence of IgG in the intercellular space in a patient with pemphigus vulgaris. Reproduced from Champion RH *et al.* (eds) (1992) *Textbook of Dermatology*, 5th edn (Wiley-Blackwell, Oxford), with the permission of the authors.

### Management

Use high-dose prednisolone, with adjuvant steroid-sparing agents (azathioprine or mycophenolate mofetil); cyclophosphamide, rituximab and IVIG are alternatives.

## Dermatitis herpetiformis

### Disease mechanisms

- Subepidermal blistering due to antibodies targeting skin antigens with substantial homology with tissue transglutaminase
- Requires duodenal biopsy due to associated coeliac disease

### Clinical features

- Intensely itchy grouped vesicles form on extensor surfaces or the face.
- Due to itching, blisters rarely remain intact and often only excoriations remain evident (**Figure 18.18**).

### Management

- Dapsone
- Gluten avoidance

## DISORDERS OF PIGMENTATION

- Hypo- and hyperpigmentation can complicate inflammatory dermatoses.
- Both are more evident in more pigmented skin types.

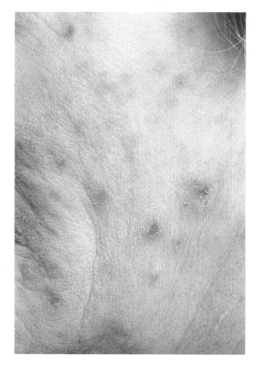

**Figure 18.18** Dermatitis herpetiformis. Excoriations and erosions.

# HYPERPIGMENTATION

Hyperpigmentation may be observed in genetic conditions, sometimes appearing as café au lait patches (CLINICAL EXAMINATION AT A GLANCE, **Figure H**). Other causes are listed in **Table 18.9**.

# HYPOPIGMENTATION

Hypopigmentation may be genetic:

- Albinism
- Hypopigmented ash leaf patches may be found in tuberous sclerosis

## Vitiligo

The depigmentation of vitiligo is due to melanocyte destruction.

### Disease mechanisms

It is an autoimmune disorder.

### Clinical features

- Depigmented macules (CLINICAL EXAMINATION AT A GLANCE, **Figure B**)
- May by induced by trauma (Koebner phenomenon)
- Wood's light: stark white lesions
- *Differential diagnoses:* post-inflammatory hypopigmentation, pityriasis versicolor and idiopathic guttate hypomelanosis (**Figure 18.19**)

**Table 18.9** Causes of hyperpigmentation

| Type | Condition | Affected area(s)/Feature |
|---|---|---|
| Melasma | | Facial predominance |
| Endocrine disorders | Addison's disease | Diffuse with accentuation in photodistribution |
| | | Sites of trauma |
| | | Palmar creases |
| | | Mucous membranes |
| | | Nails |
| | | Axillae, perineum, areolae |
| | Acromegaly | |
| | Nelson's syndrome | |
| | Insulin resistance | Velvety hyperpigmentation of flexural areas |
| | Hyperthyroidism | Localized or generalized hyperpigmentation |
| Cirrhosis | | Jaundice |
| Haemolysis | | |
| Renal failure | | |
| Haemochromatosis | | Bronzing of skin |
| Genetic conditions | Peutz–Jeghers syndrome | Melanotic macules on mucosal surfaces |
| | Neurofibromatosis | Café au lait macules, axillary freckling (type 1) |
| | McCune–Albright syndrome | Café au lait macules |
| Primary cutaneous amyloidosis | | Confluent or rippled macules or papules |
| Pellagra | | Photodistributed hyperpigmentation |
| Drugs | Antimalarials | Blue–grey |
| | Amiodarone | Grey |
| | Bleomycin | Flagellate |

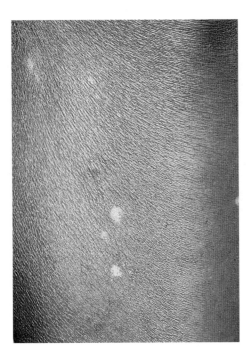

Figure 18.19 Idiopathic guttate hypomelanosis. Macular hyperpigmented lesions.

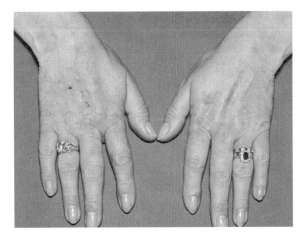

Figure 18.20 Porphyria cutanea tarda. Blisters, erosions and scars on dorsal aspect of hands.

*Management*
- Topical steroids or calcineurin inhibitors (pimecrolimus or tacrolimus)
- Phototherapy
- Sun protection and cosmetic camouflage
- Poorly responsive to treatment; Janus kinase inhibitors show promise as future strategy

## PHOTODERMATOLOGY

- Sun-exposed areas affected: face, anterior chest 'V' and hands
- Periorbital, retroauricular and submental skin usually spared
- Classification:
  o *Phototoxic* (no immune reaction): porphyria, sunburn, drug-induced, phytophotodermatitis
  o *Photoallergic* (hypersensitivity): polymorphic light eruption (PLE), chronic actinic dermatitis and drug-induced (NB may also be phototoxic), photo-allergic contact dermatitis, solar urticaria
  o *Photoexacerbated:* SLE, dermatomyositis, atopic dermatitis (minority), psoriasis (minority)
  o *Metabolic:* porphyrias

## POLYMORPHIC LIGHT ERUPTION

- PLE is most common photoallergic dermatosis
- Variable (polymorphic): erythema, papules, urticarial weals
- Eruption within hours of sun exposure

- Onset in spring or early summer; characteristically improves within days due to a 'hardening' phenomenon
- Sun avoidance and sunscreens essential
- Treatment options include topical or oral steroids or phototherapy (to induce 'hardening')

## PORPHYRIAS

### Porphyria cutanea tarda

- May be familial or sporadic
- Associated with impaired or deficient uroporphyrinogen decarboxylase
- Associated with liver disease
- Skin fragility, photosensitive blistering with milia, scarring and hypertrichosis occur on exposed sites (e.g. the hands) (**Figure 18.20**)
- *Treatment:* includes avoidance of alcohol, oestrogen and sunlight, venesection and low-dose hydroxychloroquine

### Erythropoietic protoporphyria

- Burning pain on sunlight exposure
- Scarring but no blistering

### Congenital erythropoietic porphyria

- Photosensitivity, scarring, hypertrichosis
- Red fluorescence of urine and teeth

### Variegate porphyria

- Drug-provoked, photosensitive blistering
- Neuropsychiatric attacks

## DISORDERS OF HAIR AND NAILS

### DIFFUSE NON-SCARRING ALOPECIA

The differential diagnosis is given in **Table 18.10**.

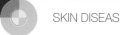

**Table 18.10** Causes of diffuse non-scarring alopecia

Androgenetic alopecia
Telogen effluvium

**Endocrine disorders**
Hypothyroidism
Hypopituitarism
Virilizing syndromes (e.g. adrenal or ovarian tumours,
  congenital adrenal hyperplasia, PCOS)

**Other causes**
Skin diseases
SLE
Psoriasis
Alopecia areata

**Metabolic/other**
Nutritional
Iron deficiency
Chronic illness
HIV infection
Renal disease
Liver disease
Malignant disease
Drugs (multiple, including lithium, cytotoxics)

### Androgenetic ('pattern') alopecia

- This affects men and women.
- Young women require screening for endocrine disorders.

### Alopecia areata

- This is a form of non-scarring alopecia that typically manifests in discrete patches (**Figure 18.21**).

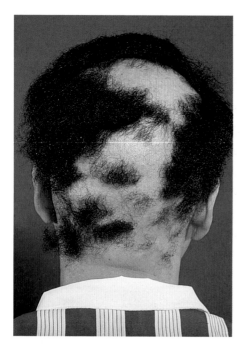

**Figure 18.21** Alopecia areata.

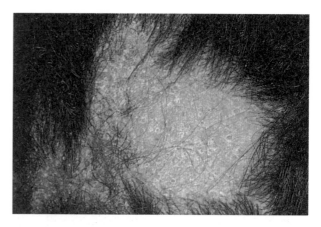

**Figure 18.22** Tinea capitis. Erythema, scale, scarring alopecia. An inflammatory mass is called a kerion.

- It may involve the entire scalp (alopecia totalis) or body (alopecia universalis) or cause generalized thinning (diffuse alopecia areata).
- The prognosis is variable.
- Janus kinase inhibitors are an emerging therapeutic strategy.
- Patchy alopecia with erythema and scale may indicate tinea capitis (**Figure 18.22**).

## SCARRING ALOPECIA

In scarring alopecia, hair follicles are destroyed. Treatment aims to prevent further hair loss (**Table 18.11**; **Figure 18.8**; **Figure 18.22**; **Figure 18.23**). Tetracyclines are indicated in folliculitis decalvans and lichen planopilaris. Hydroxychloroquine is used in DLE.

## NAIL DISORDERS

Nail changes may indicate underlying illness (**Figure 18.24**; **Figure 18.25**). Causes are given in **Table 18.12**.

### Finger clubbing

There is increased curvature of the nail, with an increase in the base angle with the nailfold to >180° (**Figure 18.27** Causes are listed in **Table 18.13**.

**Table 18.11** Causes of scarring alopecia

Tinea capitis (**Figure 18.22**) and kerion
Folliculitis decalvans
Syphilis
Central centrifugal cicatrizing alopecia
Lichen planopilaris (**Figure 18.23**)
Sarcoid
Lupus erythematosus (especially DLE; see **Figure 18.8**)
Scleroderma
Metastatic carcinoma

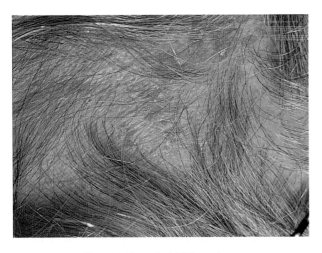

**Figure 18.23** Cicatricial (scarring). Lichen planus.

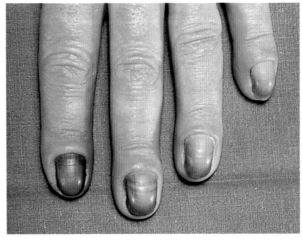

**Figure 18.25** Yellow nail syndrome.

**18**

## VASCULAR DISORDERS

### LOWER LIMB OEDEMA

#### Disease mechanism

- *Primary:* congenital lymphatic anomalies
- *Secondary:* cardiac failure, venous defects (e.g. thrombosis, incompetence), hypoalbuminemia, pelvic mass, infections (recurrent cellulitis, lymphatic filariasis)

#### Clinical features

- Causes lipodermatosclerosis, stasis (varicose) eczema, haemosiderin pigmentation and risk of ulceration
- Capillaritis (manifesting as red dots) often evident

#### Investigation

- *Lymphoscintigraphy:* map lymphatic abnormalities
- *Echocardiogram:* systolic/diastolic dysfunction
- *Pelvic imaging:* pelvic masses

#### Management

- Compression therapy
- Withdrawal of exacerbatory drugs (e.g. amlodipine) where possible

- Treatment of superimposed eczema
- Vascular assessment to identify surgically correctable defects
- Other treatment for underlying cause

### LEG ULCERS

- *Most common causes:* venous insufficiency, arterial disease and diabetes mellitus
- *Other causes:* listed in **Table 18.14** (see also LEG ULCERATION AT A GLANCE)

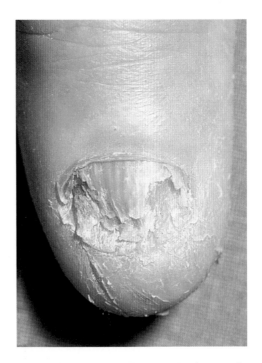

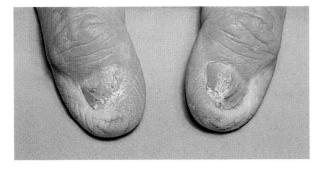

**Figure 18.24** Scarring nail dystrophy. Lichen planus.

**Figure 18.26** Onychomyosis. Tinea unguium/gross nail dystrophy. Linear burrows in web space.

**Table 18.12** Causes of nail changes

| Nail change | Cause |
| --- | --- |
| Pits | Psoriasis (PSORIASIS AT A GLANCE, **Figure E**) |
| | Alopecia areata |
| Ridges | Psoriasis (PSORIASIS AT A GLANCE) |
| Nicks | Darier's disease |
| Dystrophy | Psoriasis (PSORIASIS AT A GLANCE, **Figures E and F**) |
| | Raynaud's phenomenon |
| | Arterial disease |
| | Lichen planus (**Figure 18.23; Figure 18.25**) |
| | Onychomycosis (**Figure 18.26**) |
| White spots | Trauma |
| Red bands | Darier's disease |
| Longitudinal black bands (melanonychia) | Physiological: skin types III–VI |
| | Lichen planus |
| | Melanoma |
| | Addison's disease |
| | Malnutrition |
| Black spots | Trauma (haemorrhage) |
| | Naevi |
| | Melanoma |
| Red spot | Glomus tumour |
| Onycholysis | Psoriasis, trauma (PSORIASIS AT A GLANCE, **Figure E; Figure F**) |
| | Drugs |
| Paronychia | Nailfold infection |
| Beau's (transverse) lines | Acute illness, drugs or trauma |
| | Psoriasis (PSORIASIS AT A GLANCE, **Figure E**) |
| White bands | Arsenic poisoning |
| | Hypoalbuminaemia |
| Leuconychia | Cirrhosis |
| | Diabetes mellitus |
| | Cardiac failure |
| | Anaemia |
| Yellow nail syndrome (curved nail, reduced growth, **Figure 18.25**) | Bronchiectasis, lymphoedema |
| | Bronchogenic carcinoma |
| Blue lunulae | Wilson's disease |
| Koilonychia (spoon-shaped nails) | Iron deficiency |
| Splinter haemorrhages | Trauma |
| | Autoimmune rheumatic disease |
| | Endocarditis |
| Ragged cuticles | Autoimmune rheumatic disease (CLINICAL EXAMINATION AT A GLANCE, **Figure C**) |
| Nailfold telangiectasia | Autoimmune rheumatic disease (CLINICAL EXAMINATION AT A GLANCE, **Figure C**) |

## Clinical features

These may suggest the underlying cause:
- *Livedo* (**Figure 18.28**): vasculitis or calciphylaxis
- *Purpura* (**Figure 18.29**): vasculitis or embolic phenomena
- *Oedema* (**Figure 18.30**): venous stasis ulceration (LEG ULCERATION AT A GLANCE, **Figure A**).
- *Undermined edge:* pyoderma gangrenosum, an idiopathic extending ulcer (LEG ULCERATION AT A GLANCE, **Figure E**; **Figure 18.31**). Associations include ulcerative colitis, Crohn's disease and rheumatoid arthritis.

## Investigation

- *Skin biopsy:* to determine cause (e.g. carcinoma, vasculitis, embolic phenomena)
- *Doppler studies:* to exclude arterial insufficiency

## Management

- *Multidisciplinary:* dermatologists, tissue viability nurses, vascular surgeons and podiatrists
- *Specific treatments:* prednisolone, ciclosporin or infliximab for pyoderma gangrenosum; compression therapy for venous ulceration

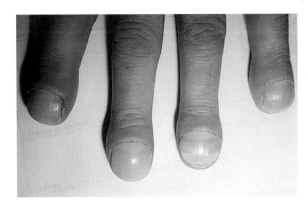

**Figure 18.27** Finger clubbing associated with bronchial carcinoma (see other causes **Table 18.13**). Reproduced from Champion RH *et al.* (eds) (1992) *Textbook of Dermatology*, 5th edn (Wiley-Blackwell, Oxford), with the permission of the authors.

**Table 18.13** Causes of clubbing

| |
|---|
| **Lung diseases** |
| Bronchiectasis |
| Cystic fibrosis |
| Tuberculosis |
| Lung carcinoma |
| Mesothelioma |
| Pulmonary fibrosis |
| **Cardiac diseases** |
| Congenital heart disease (cyanotic) |
| Bacterial endocarditis |
| Atrial myxoma |
| **Gut diseases** |
| Crohn's disease |
| Tropical sprue |
| Cirrhosis |
| **Idiopathic/familial** |
| Vascular disorders |
| Axillary artery aneurysm |
| Hyperthyroidism |
| Acropachy |

**Table 18.14** Causes of leg ulcers

| |
|---|
| Trauma |
| Pressure |
| Venous insufficiency |
| Arterial disease |
| Calciphylaxis |
| Cholesterol emboli |
| Neuropathy (e.g. diabetes mellitus, multiple sclerosis) |
| Pyoderma gangrenosum |
| Haemoglobinopathy and haemolysis |
| Infection (tropical ulcer, tuberculosis, Leishmaniasis) |
| Vasculitis |
| Gout |
| Thrombophilia |
| Immunobullous diseases |
| Skin cancer (SQUAMOUS CELL CARCINOMA AT A GLANCE, **Figure E**) |
| Necrobiosis lipoidica |

18

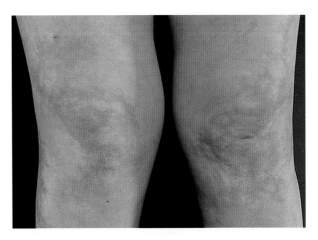

**Figure 18.28** Livedo reticularis. Network of cyanotic vascularity in the knees. Causes: lupus erythematosus, polyarteritis nodosa, drugs.

## RAYNAUD'S PHENOMENON

This phenomenon causes episodic digital ischaemia in response to cold temperatures.

### Disease mechanisms

Causes are listed in **Table 18.15**.

### Clinical features

There is an episodic painful digital cold-induced response with characteristic sequential colour changes of white, blue and red (**Figure 18.32**).

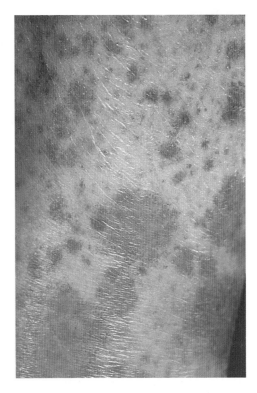

**Figure 18.29** Purpura (cryoglobulinaemia).

## LEG ULCERATION AT A GLANCE

**Complications**

- Contact dermatitis
- Infection
- Squamous cell carcinoma (Marjolin's ulcer)

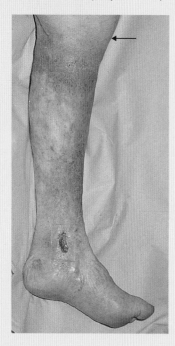

**Figure A** Venous ulceration. Note the margin of allergic contact dermatitis due to rubber in the compression bandaging (arrow).

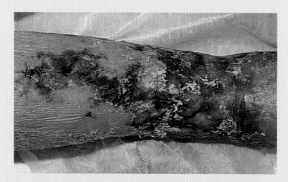

**Figure B** Cholesterol emboli. Necrotic ulcers.

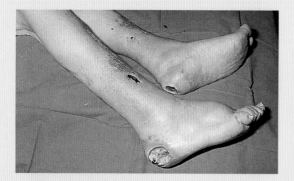

**Figure C** Calciphylaxis causing leg ulceration (chronic renal failure and replacement therapy).

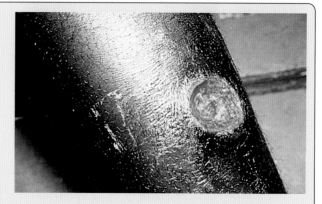

**Figure D** Tropical ulcer. Aetiology uncertain: malnutrition and infection incriminated. Courtesy of Institute of Dermatology, London. Reproduced from Champion RH *et al.* (eds) (1992) *Textbook of Dermatology*, 5th edn (Wiley-Blackwell, Oxford), with the permission of the authors.

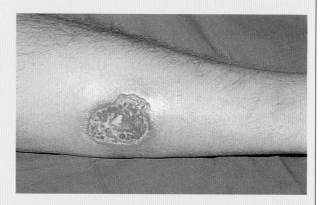

**Figure E** Pyoderma gangrenosum (rheumatoid arthritis). Ulcer with indurated edge.

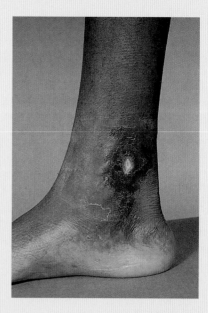

**Figure F** Haemolysis (sickle cell anaemia). Chronic ulcer.

*Continued...*

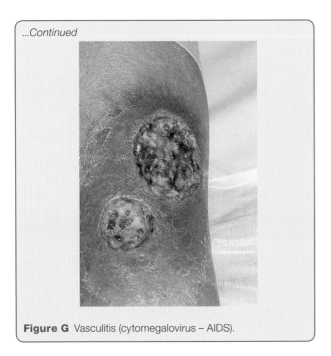

**Figure G** Vasculitis (cytomegalovirus – AIDS).

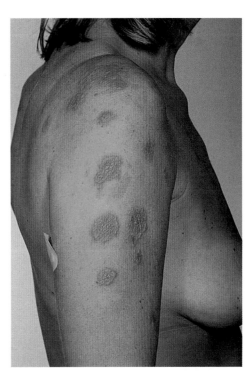

**Figure 18.31** Pyoderma gangrenosum. Vesicobulbous and nodular lesions. Causes: rheumatoid arthritis, inflammatory bowel disease (IBD), myeloma.

## Management

- Protection from cold temperatures
- Phamacologic: nifedipine, sildenafil, losartan

## PERNIOSIS (CHILBLAINS)

- Sore or itchy tender dusky red papules resulting from vasospastic reactions to low temperatures
- *Treatment:* may be supportive or may include nifedipine

**Table 18.15** Causes of Raynaud's phenomenon

| |
| --- |
| Idiopathic |
| Cervical rib |
| Vibrating tools |
| Autoimmune rheumatic disease |
| Arteritis (e.g. giant cell arteritis) |
| Drugs (e.g. beta-blockers and ergot alkaloids) |
| Hyperviscosity |

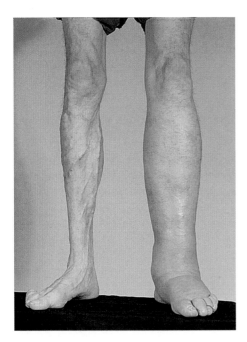

**Figure 18.30** Lymphoedema of the lower limb. Swelling and deep crevices. Reproduced from Champion RH *et al.* (eds) (1992) *Textbook of Dermatology*, 5th edn (Wiley-Blackwell, Oxford), with the permission of the authors.

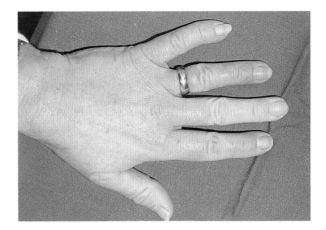

**Figure 18.32** Raynaud's phenomenon. Digital pallor of left middle finger. Causes: idiopathic, cervical rib, vibrating tools, autoimmune rheumatic disease, arteritis, drugs (beta blockers, ergot alkaloids), hyperviscosity syndromes.

**Table 18.16** Causes of livedo reticularis

| |
|---|
| Physiological (cutis marmorata in young girls) |
| Vasculitis (as in autoimmune rheumatic disease) |
| Cholesterol emboli |
| Thrombocythaemia |
| Cryoglobulinaemia |
| Paralysis |
| Heart failure |
| Hyperviscosity |
| Drugs (e.g. amantadine) |
| Idiopathic |

## LIVEDO

- Mottled net-like discoloration
- *Livedo reticularis:* a network of cutaneous cyanosis (see **Figure 18.28**); causes are listed in **Table 18.16**
- *Erythema ab igne:* develops with chronic heat exposure (e.g. an electric fire in the elderly)

## VASCULITIS

- May be exclusively cutaneous or systemic (with or without cutaneous involvement)
- Cutaneous manifestations depend on size of vessel involved:
  - *Medium vessels:* livedo reticularis, retiform (net-like) purpura, ulcers, subcutaneous nodules, digital necrosis
  - *Small vessels:* palpable purpura, urticarial papules

See Chapter 4, Rheumatic disease, for detailed information on vasculitis syndromes.

## CUTANEOUS SMALL VESSEL VASCULITIS

Cutaneous small vessel vasculitis (CSVV) is common.

### Disease mechanisms

- Often idiopathic
- Minority due to underlying infections (e.g. pneumonia).
- Less commonly, drug-induced or autoimmune (e.g. Henoch–Schönlein purpura or IgA vasculitis)
- Thorough history required to detect systemic involvement

### Clinical features

- Variable: palpable purpura, urticarial papules or petechiae
- Urticarial vasculitis may be indistinguishable from urticaria; clues include ecchymosis or persistence of lesions for >24 hours
- Predominantly affects lower limbs

### Investigation

- If review of systems is negative, only FBC, renal profile and urinalysis required
- Complement (C3/C4) in urticarial vasculitis

- Persistent cases: viral hepatitis serology, HIV, Antistreptolysin O titer (ASOT), rheumatoid factor and chest X-ray, cryoglobulins, ANCA (latter may both involve cutaneous small vessels)
- Biopsy to exclude clinical mimickers (e.g. emboli)

### Management

- Often spontaneously resolves within weeks
- Persistent, recurrent or symptomatic cases require oral prednisolone or anti-inflammatories (e.g. tetracycline) and compression stockings

## SKIN INFECTIONS

Most skin infections are caused by Gram-positive cocci and are listed in **Table 18.17**.

## BACTERIAL INFECTIONS

### Folliculitis

- Inflammation of hair follicles
- Follicular erythema; sometimes pustular
- May be infectious or non-infectious
- Eosinophilic (non-infectious) folliculitis is associated with HIV
- Recurrent cases may arise from nasal carriage of *Staphylococcus aureus*, particularly strains expressing Panton–Valentine leukocidin (PVL)
- Deep follicular infection causes furuncles; involvement with adjacent connected follicles results in a carbuncle
- *Treatment:*
  - Antibiotics (usually flucloxacillin or erythromycin)
  - Incision and drainage required for furunculosis
  - Decolonization regimens of nasal mupirocin and chlorhexidine body wash required if swabs indicate nasal carriage of *Staphylococcus aureus* or if PVL-positive

**Table 18.17** Gram-positive cocci and the skin infections they cause

| Examples of staphylococcal skin infections | Examples of streptococcal skin infections |
|---|---|
| Folliculitis | Ecthyma |
| Sycosis barbae | Erysipelas |
| Furunculosis | Cellulitis |
| Ecthyma | Impetigo |
| Impetigo | Scarlet fever |
| Cellulitis | Necrotizing fasciitis |
| Staphylococcal scalded skin syndrome (SSSS) | Erythema nodosum |
| Vasculitis | Superinfects other dermatoses (e.g. leg ulcers) |
| Superinfects other dermatoses (e.g. atopic eczema, HSV, leg ulcers) | |

**Figure 18.33** Impetigo. Vesicopustules with golden crust.

## Impetigo

- Superficial skin infection with yellow crust, caused by streptococci (non-bullous) or staphylococci (vesiculobullous; **Figure 18.33**)
- Often affects face (perioral, ears, nares)
- Swabs to establish the culprit microcrobe and determine antimicrobial sensitivity
- *Treatment:* topical ± systemic antibiotics

## Cellulitis

- Infection of subcutaneous connective tissue
- Tender swelling with ill-defined erythema or oedema (**Figure 18.34**)

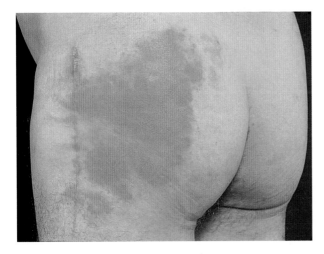

**Figure 18.34** Cellulitis complicating hip replacement operation site.

- Oedema is a predisposing factor and recurrent episodes may be caused by destruction of local lymphatics
- *Treatment:* systemic antibiotics

### Staphylococcal scalded skin syndrome

- Generalized erythema and exfoliation in a child or immunocompromised adult due to a toxin-producing staphylococcus
- Organism cannot be cultured from denuded skin
- Clinically resembles Stevens–Johnson syndrome (SJS)/ toxic epidermal necrolysis (TEN)
- *Management:*
  o Hospitalization to support skin function (emollients to support barrier function, fluid, electrolyte and nutritional monitoring)
  o Systemic antibiotics

### Ecthyma

- Pyogenic ulceration with adherent crusts
- Streptococci and staphylococci implicated
- Systemic antibiotics required

### Erysipelas

- Infection of deep dermis and subcutis (**Figure 18.35**)
- Painful, sharply defined erythema, often on the face or limb (**Figure 18.36**); there may be desquamation
- Sometimes a red streak of lymphangitis and local lymphadenopathy
- A portal of entry should be sought (e.g. tinea pedis)
- Systemic symptoms (fever, malaise)
- *Treatment:* intravenous antibiotics

### Scarlet fever

This is caused by upper respiratory tract infection with erythrogenic toxin-producing streptococci.

### Necrotizing fasciitis

- Initial dusky induration (usually of a limb), followed by rapid painful necrosis of skin, connective tissue and muscle
- Potentially fatal

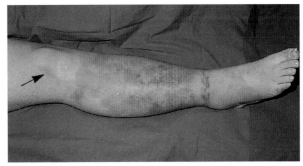

**Figure 18.35** Erysipelas. Note superior linear track of lymphangitis indicated by arrow.

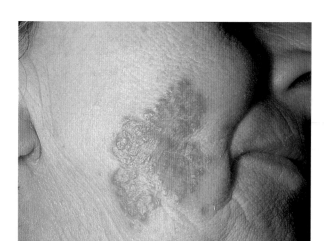

**Figure 18.36** Lupus vulgaris of the cheek. Erythematous indurated granulomatous plaque. Courtesy of Professor JAA Hunter, Edinburgh Royal Infirmary. Reproduced from Champion RH *et al.* (eds) (1992) *Textbook of Dermatology*, 5th edn (Wiley-Blackwell, Oxford), with the permission of the authors.

- Usually synergistic, involving streptococci, staphylococci, enterobacteriaceae and anaerobes
- Prompt diagnosis essential (requires high index of suspicion), followed by broad-spectrum parenteral antibiotics and surgical debridement
- MRI can aid diagnosis
- Blood and tissue cultures can determine organisms and sensitivities
- High mortality
- Can affect the scrotum (Fournier's gangrene)

**Cutaneous tuberculosis**

This may develop from distant internal disease (miliary), direct inoculation (lupus vulgaris, chancres, gummas), or extension from underlying focus (scrofuloderma).

**Atypical mycobacterial infection**

- Important cause of infection in immunosuppressed states
- *Mycobacterium marinum:* causes indolent granulomatous ulcers (fish-tank granuloma) in healthy people
- *Mycobacterium ulcerans:* an important cause of limb ulceration in Africa (Buruli ulcer) and Australia (Searle's ulcer)

**Borreliosis (Lyme disease)**

Lyme disease is discussed in Chapter 3, Infectious disease.

**Erythrasma**

- Well-defined wrinkled red-brown patch in intertriginous areas (**Figure 18.37**)
- *Corynebacterium minutissimum*
- *Treatment:* topical or systemic erythromycin

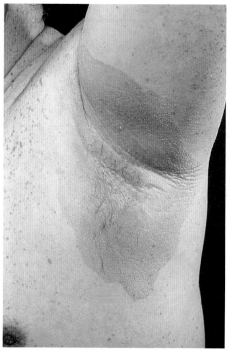

**(a)**

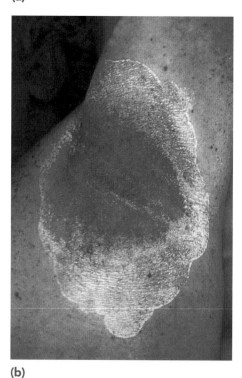

**(b)**

**Figure 18.37** Erythrasma: **(a)** normal light; **(b)** coral pink axillary fluorescence, resulting from proporphyria III elaborated by *Corynebacterium minutissimum* in erythrasma, under Wood's light.

**Pitted keratolysis**

- Pitted erosions of soles caused by *Corynebacteria* infection
- *Treatment:* topical clindamycin

**18**

### Erysipeloid

- Erythema and oedema of the hand that extends slowly over weeks
- Caused by *Erysipelothrix rhusiopathiae* after handling contaminated raw fish or meat

### Anthrax

- Painless necrotic ulcer with surrounding oedema and regional lymphadenopathy at the site of contact with hides, bone meal or wool infected with *Bacillus anthracis*
- Painful systemic symptoms with regional lymphadenopathy
- *Treatment:* doxycycline or ciprofloxacin
- *Pseudomonas* infection

*Pseudomonas* infection can cause otitis externa, folliculitis with systemic symptoms (after immersion in hot tub) and necrotic ulcers (ecthyma gangrenosum) in immunocompromised individuals.

## VIRAL INFECTIONS

### Herpes simplex virus infection

- Any skin or mucosal site may be infected by HSV
- Genital infections more often caused by HSV-2
- Prodromal tingling/burning
- Painful vesicles, erosions and crusts on an erythematous base (**Figure 18.38**)
- Viral PCR for diagnostic confirmation, but treatment must be initiated immediately
- *Management:*
  - Oral aciclovir (IV if extensive or in immunosuppressed individuals)
  - Recurrent infection may require long-term low-dose oral aciclovir

### Varicella zoster virus

Varicella zoster virus (VZV) is discussed in Chapter 3, Infectious disease (**Figure 18.39**; **Figure 18.40**).

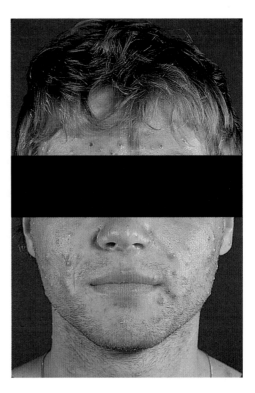

**Figure 18.39** Chickenpox. Crops of vesicles and pustules.

### Hand, foot and mouth disease

- An acute self-limiting coxsackievirus infection
- Vesicular lesions in the mouth and on the palms and soles

### Orf

- Zoonotic parapoxvirus from sheep
- Large tender solitary nodule on hand or face

### Warts

- Caused by human papillomavirus (HPV) (**Figure 18.41**)
- Often eventually self-resolve; active treatment options include salicylic acid or cryotherapy

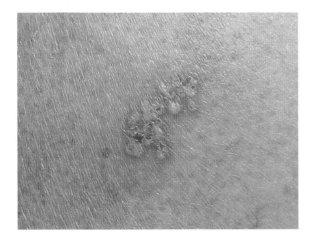

**Figure 18.38** Herpes simplex. Erythema and vesicles.

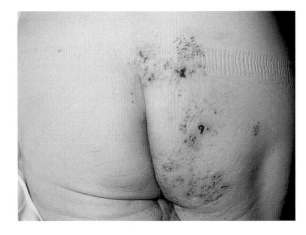

**Figure 18.40** Shingles. Healing with pain, crusts and scars.

SKIN DISEASE

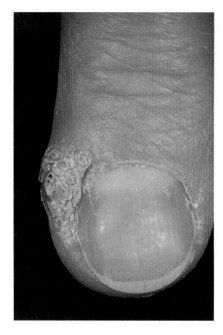

Figure 18.41 Periungual viral wart. Papillomatosis, hyperkeratosis and loss of dermatoglyphics.

## Molluscum contagiosum

- Poxvirus infection
- Umbilicated dome-shaped papules (**Figure 18.42**)
- Common in children
- Usually resolves spontaneously
- Cryptococcosis must be considered as differential diagnosis in immunosuppressed

## FUNGAL INFECTIONS

### Candidosis

- Usually an intertriginous infection (affecting the axillae, submammary folds [**Figure 18.43**], crurae and digital clefts) or of oral mucosa

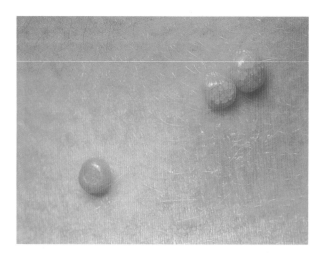

Figure 18.42 Molluscum contagiosum. Dome-shaped papules with central umbilication.

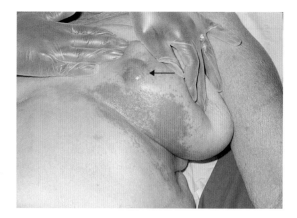

Figure 18.43 Candidosis. Erythematous, almost eroded intertrigo. Note satellite lesions and nodular breast carcinoma (arrow).

- A common cause of vulvovaginitis
- May affect the mucosae
- *Treatment:* topical nystatin, imidazole or clioquinol

### Pityriasis versicolor

- Superficial *Malassezia* infection, manifesting as hyperpigmented or hypopigmented patches with fine scale (**Figure 18.44**)
- *Treatment:* topical imidazole or selenium sulphide shampoo

### Dermatophytosis

- Infection by fungal genera *Trichophyton*, *Microsporum* and *Epidermophyton*

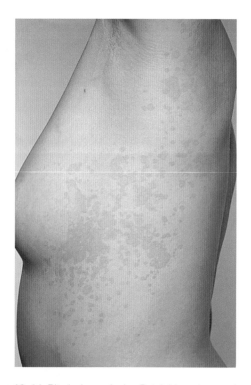

Figure 18.44 Pityriasis versicolor. Petaloid, scaly macules.

640

**18**

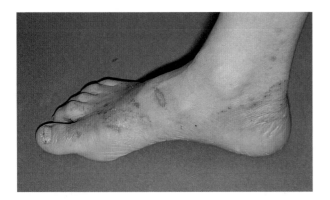

**Figure 18.45** Tinea pedis. Well-marginated erythematous scaly eruption (moccasin pattern).

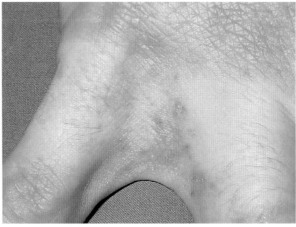

**Figure 18.46** Scabies.

- Red, scaly, sometimes annular ('ringworm') patches or plaques
- Usually itchy
- Frequently affects groins and feet (**Figure 18.45**); flexural involvement manifests with macerated erythema with a scaly edge
- Nails may be involved (onychomycosis; see **Figure 18.26**)
- Kerion, an infected inflammatory plaque, may develop as a boggy purulent lump on the scalp; requires systemic antifungal treatment
- *Treatment:* topical antifungals (e.g. miconazole or terbinafine)
- Widespread dermatophytosis, nail or scalp involvement requires systemic therapy

## SKIN INFESTATIONS

### SCABIES

- It is important always to enter differential diagnosis of pruritus.
- A history of affected contacts is suggestive.
- It typically involves digital clefts (**Figure 18.46**), axillae and genitalia.
- Excoriations are evident; close examination may reveal burrows (**Figure 18.47**).
- Hyperkeratosis and crust are observed in immunosuppression (Norwegian scabies; CLINICAL EXAMINATION AT A GLANCE, **Figure D**).
- *Treatment* is with topical permethrin application over the entire skin overnight, repeated 7–10 days later. Clothing (including bedclothes) is washed concurrently. Oral ivermectin is an alternative.
- Cohabitants also require treatment.

### PEDICULOSIS

Pediculosis is caused by *Pthirus pubis* (crab louse), or head lice.

## SKIN TUMOURS

### BENIGN TUMOURS AND NORMAL VARIANTS

#### Epidermoid cysts

These are smooth subcutaneous nodules with a central punctum.

#### Seborrhoeic keratoses

- Skin-coloured or brown papules that appear 'stuck-on' (**Figure 18.48**)
- Increase in prevalence with age

#### Port-wine stain (naevus flammeus)

- This is a congenital capillary malformation.
- Facial examples may be associated with intracranial vascular anomalies and neurological deficits such as epilepsy (Sturge–Weber syndrome).
- Early treatment with pulsed-dye laser gives optimal cosmesis.

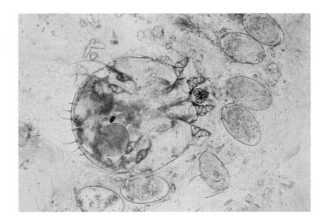

**Figure 18.47** *Sarcoptes scabiei*, the scabies mite. Female with eggs. Reproduced from Champion RH *et al.* (eds) (1992) *Textbook of Dermatology*, 5th edn (Wiley-Blackwell, Oxford), with the permission of the authors.

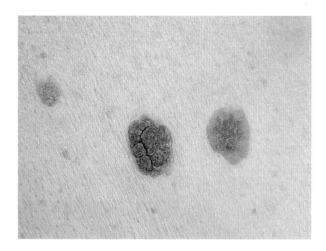

**Figure 18.48** Seborrhoeic keratoses. Tan to black, warty, flat papules and nodules.

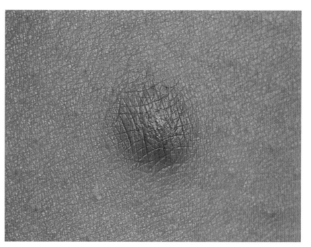

**Figure 18.49** Dermatofibroma/histiocytoma. Firm pigmented papule.

### Infantile haemangioma

- Superficial: bulbous red tumour (strawberry nevus)
- Deep examples: blue or purple
- Appears in the first month
- Complications include infection, ulceration, feeding difficulties, airway compromise, ocular (including proptosis, amylopia, amblyopia)
- Lumbosacral haemangiomas or segmental examples of the head may be associated with congenital anomaly syndromes
- Most involute by 6 years of age; scars, fibrofatty residua or telangectasia may remain
- *Treatment:* active treatment with propanolol if periocular, subglottic (risk of stridor), multifocal, risk of disfigurement

### Campbell de Morgan's spots

These are small (1–2 mm) 'cherry' angiomas.

### Telangiectasia

- Dilated capillaries
- May represent a normal variant, photo-aging or an underlying dermatosis (CLINICAL EXAMINATION AT A GLANCE, **Figure C**)

### Spider naevi

- Arteriolar dilatations that blanch on pressure
- Typically found in area drained by the superior vena cava
- May increase in number in pregnancy and portal hypertension

### Angiokeratomas

- Red papules commonly found on the scrotum (Fordyce's angiokeratoma)
- *Angiokeratoma corporis diffusum* (Fabry's disease): must be considered where multiple smaller and hyperkeratotic examples occur in a bathing trunk distribution

### Dermatofibromas

- Firm round red or brown papules or nodules
- Commonly seen on the legs (**Figure 18.49**)

### Xanthomas

- Yellow tumours representing massive lipid deposition within dermal cells
- May be associated with underlying lipid disorders (**Figures 18.50–18.52**)

### Lipomas

These are soft subcutaneous adipose tumours.

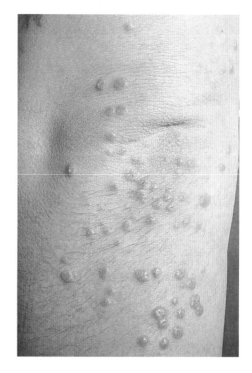

**Figure 18.50** Extensive eruptive xanthomas in a patient with chylomicronaemia syndrome. Yellow infiltrated papules.

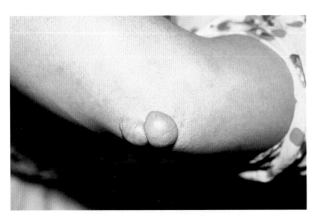

**Figure 18.51** Tuberous xanthoma in a patient with hypercholesterolaemia.

## Lentigines

- Large tan macules
- Associated congenital disorders include *Peutz–Jeghers* and *LEOPARD* syndromes

## EPIDERMAL TUMOURS/PRECANCERS

### Keratoacanthoma

- A benign, dome-shaped papule with a crateriform centre with a keratin plug
- Most frequently observed on sun-exposed areas
- Grows rapidly initially, before undergoing involution
- Usually excised as clinical and histological distinction from squamous cell carcinoma (SCC) is difficult

### Actinic keratoses

- Scaly erythematous macules or plaques (see SQUAMOUS CELL CARCINOMA AT A GLANCE, **Figures A** and **C**)
- Represent sun-induced epidermal dysplasia
- May evolve into SCC
- *Treatment:* options include cryotherapy, photodynamic therapy and topical 5-fluorouracil

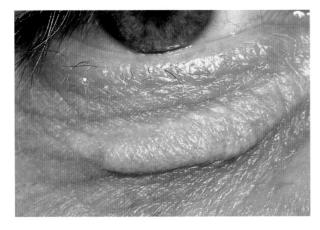

**Figure 18.52** Xanthelasma. Most patients do not have a hyperlipidaemia.

### Bowen's disease (SCC-in situ)

- Bowen's disease (or SSC-in situ) is a red scaly patch or papule (SQUAMOUS CELL CARCINOMA AT A GLANCE, **Figure B**) which can become invasive
- *Treatment:* This is similar to that of actinic keratoses although excision is required if invasion is suspected.

### Basal cell carcinoma

Basal cell carcinoma (BCC) is the most common form of skin cancer. It is more common in older age groups and in paler complexions.

#### Disease mechanisms
It is UV-mediated mutagenesis.

#### Clinical features
- Classically described as pearly papules (BASAL CELL CARCINOMA AT A GLANCE, **Figure A**), but may be pigmented or resemble scars, or simply red patches (BASAL CELL CARCINOMA AT A GLANCE, **Figures C–E**)
- Indolent growth may delay diagnosis
- Locally invasive but virtually never metastasizes

#### Management
- Surgical excision with clear histological margins
- For aggressive subtypes (e.g. infiltrative), recurrence or high-risk sites (e.g. periocular), Mohs' micrographic surgery is indicated; this involves removal of successive layers of tissue with concurrent histological examination prior to closure
- Curettage and cautery or topical therapy (imiquimod, 5-fluorouracil) for superficial subtype
- Radiotherapy if surgery unsuitable
- Vismodegib (Hedgehog pathway inhibitor) for locally advanced or metastatic disease
- Counselling regarding sun protection and skin self-monitoring

### Squamous cell carcinoma

#### Clinical features
- Most common in sun-exposed areas in patients >50 years of age
- May manifest as an enlarging ulcer, a rapidly growing nodule or a verrucous plaque
- Often painful
- May invade local structures and metastasize

#### Treatment
- Surgical excision with clear histological margins
- Radiotherapy if unsuitable for surgery *or* as adjuvant treatment in high-risk tumours
- Radiotherapy or PD-1 inhibitors for metastatic disease
- Counselling regarding sun protection and skin self-monitoring

## BASAL CELL CARCINOMA AT A GLANCE

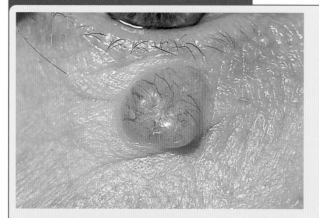

**Figure A** BCC below the right eye. Nodule.

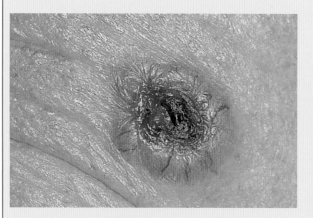

**Figure B** Classical crateriform BCC. Ulcerating nodule.

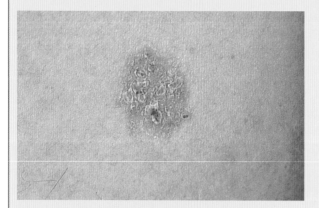

**Figure C** Superficial BCC on posterior shin. Red scaly patch.

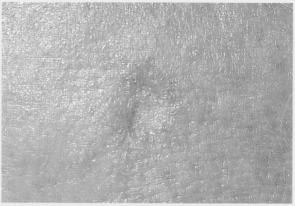

**Figure D** Morphoeic BCC on the face. Irregular plaque.

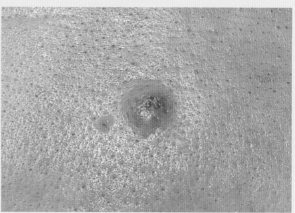

**Figure E** Pigmented BCC. Courtesy of Dr RCD Staughton.

## MELANOCYTIC TUMOURS

Assessment of pigmented lesions (**Table 18.18**) requires experience, skills in dermoscopy and a low threshold for biopsy.

### Melanocytic naevi (moles)

Moles are benign melanocyte tumours (**Figure 18.53**).

### Congenital melanocytic naevi (CMN)

- Congenital melanocytic naevi (CMN) present from birth (**Figure 18.54**)
- Mutations in *NRAS* or *BRAF*
- Smooth to mamillated surface
- May have associated proliferations in leptomeninges or brain parenchyma (neurocutaneous melanosis); risks include seizures, nerve dysfunction,

## SQUAMOUS CELL CARCINOMA AT A GLANCE

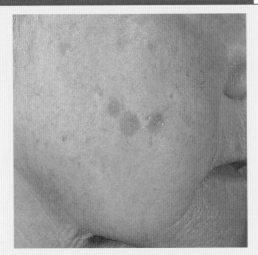

**Figure A** Actinic keratoses on a cheek. Red scaly patches

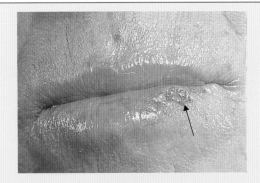

**Figure D** SCC on the lip (early ulcer).

**18**

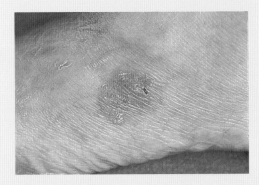

**Figure B** Bowen's disease. A red scaly patch.

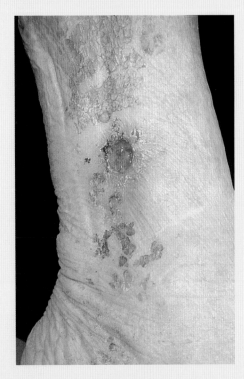

**Figure E** SCC of the leg (Marjolin's ulcer) complicating long-standing venous disease.

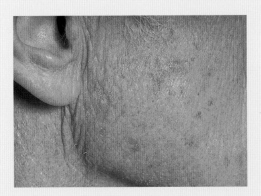

**Figure C** Actinic keratoses. Biopsy showed that the central lesion was an SCC.

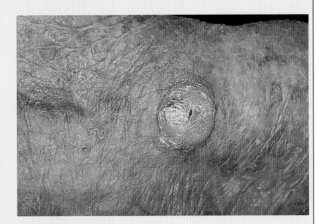

**Figure F** Nodule of SCC.

**Table 18.18** Assessment of pigmented lesions

**History**
Change in size, shape, colour, bulk
Congenital or acquired
Family history of melanoma
Sun exposure/sunbed use
Skin type

**Examination**
Irregular size, shape, pigmentation, surface
Dermoscopic features

**Phenotype**
Numerous naevi
Atypical naevi
Actinic damage

sensorimotor deficits and increased intracranial pressure
- If >1 cm, MRI brain/spine required prior to 6 months of age
- Risk of melanoma if >60 cm, multiple or abnormalities on initial MRI

## Dysplastic (atypical) naevi

These are naevi (**Figure 18.55**) that are <5 mm, irregular in shape, size, surface or colour. They may resemble melanoma and confer increased risk thereof.

## Melanoma

Melanomas are malignant melanocyte tumours (MALIGNANT MELANOMA AT A GLANCE).

### Risk factors
- Family history
- Skin type (I–II)
- UV exposure (severe sunburns or sunbed use)
- Numerous (>100) or atypical naevi

### Clinical features
- The *ABCDE* rule may aid detection:
  - *A* – asymmetry
  - *B* – border irregularity
  - *C* – colour variation
  - *D* – diameter >5 mm
  - *E* – evolving

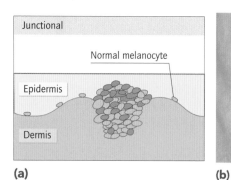

**(a)**

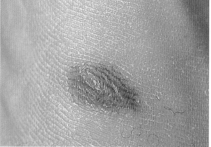

**(b)**

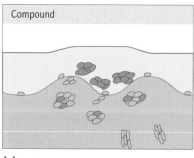

**(c)**

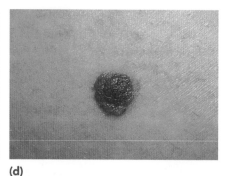

**(d)**

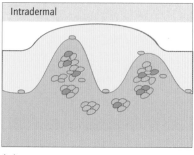

**(e)**

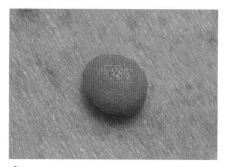

**(f)**

**Figure 18.53** Drawings and clinical pictures of melanocytic naevi. **(a,b)** Junctional melanocytic naevus. **(c,d)** Compound melanocytic naevus. **(e,f)** Intradermal melanocytic naevus.

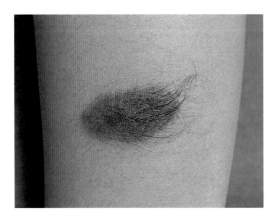

**Figure 18.54** Congenital melanocytic naevus.

- Nodular melanoma does not respect the *ABCDE* rule, with the exception of *E*.
- Lesions may appear clinically *non-specific* or mimic harmless lesions (e.g. haemangiomas)
- A *high index of suspicion* is required for early diagnosis.
- Clinical subtypes are summarized in MALIGNANT MELANOMA AT A GLANCE.

### Investigation

- *Histopathology:* Excision biopsy of the complete lesion is needed (punch or shave biopsy can cause misdiagnosis or underestimate thickness); ulceration and increased Breslow indicate worse prognosis.
- *Genetic analysis: BRAF* mutation is associated with worse prognosis but indicates responsiveness to *BRAF* inhibitors.
- *Imaging:* This is important in the context of suspected metastasis or surveillance of established metastasis.

### Management

- Excision biopsy for confirmation
- Further management determined by a dermatology-led multidisciplinary team of plastic surgeons, oncologists, specialist nurses, radiologists and histopathologists

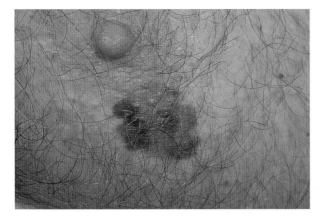

**Figure 18.55** Dysplastic naevus. Large, irregular edge, irregular pigmentation.

- Subsequent wide local excision margins are determined by thickness
- Sentinel node biopsy for prognostication
- *For advanced melanoma:* inhibitors of oncogenic signalling (*BRAF, MEK*) or immunotherapy to promote immune response against melanoma (PD-1/PD-L1, CTLA-4 inhibitors)
- Counselling on self-monitoring and sun protection

### Kaposi's sarcoma

- Associated with HHV8 infection
- May signify AIDS but also endemic in Mediterranean populations
- Purple nodules (solitary or acral), sometimes ulcerated

### Mycosis fungoides

- This is a cutaneous T-cell lymphoma (**Figure 18.56**).
- Diagnostic confirmation often takes years due to non-specific clinical and histological features and resemblance to eczema.

### Clinical features

- Early stage manifests in fixed scaly patches (like eczema or psoriasis) or plaques (favourable prognosis).
- These often remain stable for decades.
- Evolution into nodules or ulcers signifies aggressive behaviour and a poor prognosis.
- *Sézary syndrome* is a variant manifesting with erythroderma, lymphadenopathy and abnormal circulating lymphocytes.

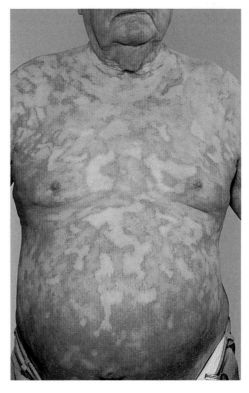

**Figure 18.56** Mycosis fungoides. Advanced plaque stage.

## MALIGNANT MELANOMA AT A GLANCE

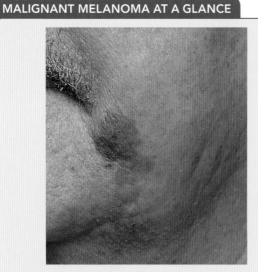

**Figure A** Lentigo maligna (Hutchinson's freckle).

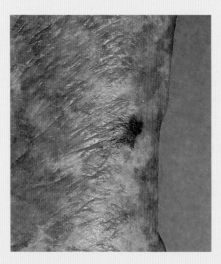

**Figure B** Area of actinic damage (arm) containing superficial spreading melanoma.

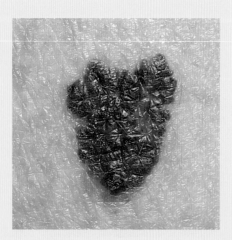

**Figure C** Superficial spreading melanoma (back).

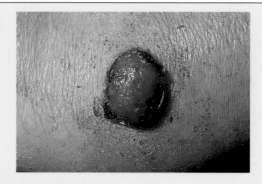

**Figure D** Nodular melanoma (arm).

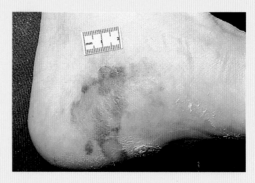

**Figure E** Acral lentiginous melanoma (foot). Reproduced from Champion RH *et al.* (eds) (1992) *Textbook of Dermatology*, 5th edn (Wiley-Blackwell, Oxford), with the permission of the authors.

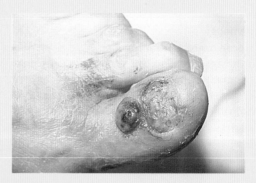

**Figure F** Subungual melanoma causing nail destruction. Note the pigmentation of the nailfold.

*Investigation*
Take biopsy for histology and T-cell receptor gene rearrangement studies.

*Management*
- Clinical monitoring
- Topical steroids, PUVA, and bexarotene for symptomatic relief (do not alter course of condition)
- *Advanced disease:* radiotherapy, extracorporeal photochemotherapy, targeted treatment (e.g. Brentuximab vedotin)

## THE SKIN AND SYSTEMIC DISEASE

## NON-SPECIFIC SKIN MANIFESTATIONS

Hair and nail manifestations, Raynaud's phenomenon, vasculitis and livedo reticularis have been discussed earlier. Facial flushing is discussed below.

### Morbilliform (maculopapular) rash

- Extensive involvement yields confluent appearance.
- Supportive treatments (emollients) and topical steroids give symptomatic relief although the trigger must be sought.
- It is most frequently caused by a drug (type IV allergy) or infection.
- The culprit drug may precede the eruption by weeks and may prove difficult to identify; sequential withdrawal of drugs may be required.
- Viruses are the most common infectious cause (measles, rubella, EBV, CMV, HHV6 and HHV7) but others include syphilis, toxoplasma, disseminated fungal infections, leptospirosis and rickettsia.
- Other causes include arthropod reactions, early guttate psoriasis and early SJS/TEN (clues suggesting the latter include dusky erythema, tenderness, fever or mucosal involvement).
- Facial oedema, eosinophilia, atypical lymphocytosis, or renal, pulmonary or liver impairment or fever may suggest drug reaction with eosinophilia and systemic symptoms (DRESS), a potentially life-threatening hypersensitivity reaction.

### Erythroderma

- Confluent erythema affects ≥90% of the body surface area (BSA). Causes are listed in **Table 18.19**.
- Systemic manifestations reflect impaired skin function: peripheral edema, tachycardia, fluid and protein loss, thermoregulatory compromise, and risk of sepsis.
- Hospitalization may be required to manage the haemodynamic and immunological effects of skin failure. TEN is discussed below.

**Table 18.19** Causes of erythroderma

| |
|---|
| Eczema |
| Psoriasis |
| Drugs |
| Mycosis fungoides (Sézary syndrome) |
| Photosensitivity |
| Toxic erythema |
| Toxic shock syndrome |
| SSSS |
| TEN |
| Infestations (scabies and lice) |
| Congenital disorders |

### Erythema multiforme

*Disease mechanisms*
This is a hypersensitivity reaction with multiple triggers (**Table 18.20**).

*Clinical features*
- A symmetrical eruption of 'targetoid' lesions (**Figure 18.57**), particularly on the hands and feet
- Malaise, fatigue
- Erythema multiforme *major* refers to the presence of fever, blistering and/or mucocutaneous involvement
- May be recurrent

*Management*
- Treatment is supportive with emollients and topical (and sometimes oral) steroids.
- Underlying infections should be treated, although this may not influence the course of the eruption.

### Stevens–Johnson syndrome/toxic epidermal necrolysis

SJS/TEN is a potentially fatal idiosyncratic reaction along a spectrum of severity, caused either by a drug or by intercurrent illness.

**Table 18.20** Causes of erythema multiforme

| |
|---|
| **Idiopathic** |
| *Infection* |
| Herpes simplex (causes), mycoplasma pneumonia, psittacosis, hepatitis B, orf, infectious mononucleosis, histoplasmosis |
| *Autoimmune rheumatic diseases* |
| Lupus erythematosus or SLE (Rowell's syndrome), polyarteritis nodosa |
| **Drugs** |
| Non-steroidal anti-inflammatory drugs (NSAIDs), sulphonamides, antiepileptics, allopurinol |
| **Tumours** |
| Carcinoma, leukaemia |
| **Endocrine** |
| Pregnancy and premenstrual |
| **Sarcoid** |

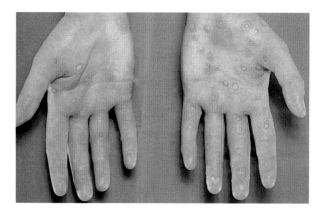

**Figure 18.57** Erythema multiforme. Target lesions. Causes: HSV, mycoplasma, orf, SLE.

### Clinical features
- This may initially manifest as a non-specific maculopapular rash (dusky erythema, tenderness or fever are suggestive of SJS/TEN).
- Mucocutaneous involvement is universal and may extend into the respiratory or gastrointestinal tracts.
- Epidermal necrosis and detachment cause denudation and skin failure, risking shock, high output cardiac failure, infection and thermoregulatory failure.
- Epidermal detachment:
  - <10% BSA is termed 'SJS'
  - >30% BSA is termed 'TEN'
  - 10–30% BSA is termed 'overlap SJS/TEN'
- *Complications:* These include scarring, blindness, renal tubular necrosis, eroded gastrointestinal tract, interstitial pneumonitis and psychological sequelae.

### Management
- Withdrawal of potential culprit drugs
- Admission to specialist unit for:
  - Emollient application
  - Minimal manipulation (to prevent further detachment)
  - Fluid and electrolyte monitoring
  - Temperature management
  - Nutritional support
  - Identification and treatment of infection

### COVID-19
Cutaneous manifestations:
- *Most common:* erythematous, chilblain-like and urticarial lesions
- *Less common:* vesicles, livedo and petechiae

See Chapter 3, Infectious disease, for further information on SARS-CoV-2/COVID-19.

### Erythema nodosum
This is a form of panniculitis (inflammation of subcutaneous fat) manifesting as tender nodules with bruise-like colour changes (see **Figure 18.12**), frequently on the lower limbs. An underlying cause must be sought (**Table 18.21**).

### Generalized pruritus
- Cause must always be sought (**Table 18.22**)
- May prove intractable
- May eventuate in nodular prurigo, an eruption of nodules also seen in eczema

**Table 18.21** Causes of erythema nodosum

| |
|---|
| **Idiopathic** |
| *Infection* |
| Streptococcal infections, tuberculosis, cat-scratch disease, psittacosis, *Yersinia*, kerion, histoplasmosis, blastomycosis, coccidioidomycosis, erythema nodosum leprosum |
| **Sarcoid** |
| *Inflammatory bowel disease* |
| Crohn's disease, ulcerative colitis |
| **Drugs** |
| Oestrogens (e.g. oral contraceptives), sulphonamides, penicillin, iodides, bromides |
| **Neoplasia** |
| Leukaemia, Hodgkin's disease |

**Table 18.22** Causes of generalized pruritus (without diagnostic skin lesions) and recommended investigations

| Pathology | Disorder | Investigation |
|---|---|---|
| Haematological | Iron deficiency | FBC, ferritin, faecal occult blood |
| | Polycythaemia rubra vera | FBC |
| | Lymphoma | FBC, chest X-ray |
| | Leukaemia | FBC |
| | Myeloma | Urea, Ca, serum free light chains / protein electrophoresis |
| Neoplasia | Lung | Examination, tumour markers, imaging |
| | Abdomen | |
| | Central nervous system | |
| Infestation | Scabies, pediculosis, | Eosinophils |
| | Intestinal parasites | Stool ova, cysts and parasites |
| Renal | Chronic kidney disease | Renal profile |
| Hepatic | Cholestasis | Liver function |
| Drugs | Opiates, alcohol, gold | |
| Miscellaneous | Senile pruritus | |
| | Psychogenic | |

**Table 18.23** Causes of facial flushing

**Endocrine**
Carcinoid syndrome
Phaeochromocytoma
Medullary carcinoma of the thyroid
Zollinger–Ellison syndrome
Angioneurotic oedema
Menopause

**Foods**
Alcohol
Glutamate, nitrite, capsicum

**Drugs**
Bromocriptine, nifedipine, tamoxifen

**Skin disease**
Rosacea, urticaria, erythromelalgia

- *Treatment:* includes emollients, soap substitute, menthol creams and removal of trigger; phototherapy may alleviate symptoms

### Facial flushing

This is observed in rosacea but also due to other causes, summarized in **Table 18.23**.

## SPECIFIC SKIN MANIFESTATIONS

### Gastrointestinal disease

#### Inflammatory bowel disease

- IBD is often associated with hidradenitis suppuritiva, psoriasis, pyoderma gangrenosum, Sweet's syndrome, clubbing and erythema nodosum.
- Crohn's disease may be associated with orofacial granulomatosis, oral ulceration, perianal abscesses and fistulae.

#### Dermatitis herpetiformis

This is the cutaneous manifestation of coeliac disease.

#### Gastrointestinal malignancy

- Causative genetic syndromes may also manifest in the skin.
  - *Gardner's syndrome:* a variant of familial adenomatous polyposis caused by autosomal domintant mutations in the APC gene; skin

findings including epidermoid cysts, lipomas, and benign skin tumours (neurofibromas)
- *Peutz–Jeghers syndrome:* caused by autosomal dominant mutations in the *STK11/LKB1* gene, mucocutaneous manifestations include pigmented macules of the lips, oral mucosa, eyes, hands and feet, and anogenital areas
- *Muir–Torre syndrome:* autosomal dominant mutations in the *MSH2/MLH1* genes; cutaneous manifestations include sebaceous gland tumours, SCC
- *Cowden syndrome:* autosomal dominant mutations in the *PTEN* gene; mucocutaneous findings include benign papules on the face, 'cobblestone' oral mucosa, and benign scaly lesions of the hands and feet
- *CDKN2A* mutations are associated with glioblastoma, melanoma and pancreatic cancer.

### Liver disease

Manifestations include jaundice, spider naevi, leuconychia, pruritus, xanthomas and striae.

### Nutritional diseases

Skin signs of nutritional disease are listed in **Table 18.24**.

### Endocrine disease

Skin signs of endocrine diseases are listed in **Table 18.25**.

### Metabolic disease

Gout may present with painful dactylitis or a nodule (classically on the ear). The porphyrias are discussed under photodermatology. Xanthomas (see **Figures 18.50–18.52**) are associated with dyslipidaemia.

### Haematological disease

The skin signs of haematological disorders are listed in **Table 18.26**.

### Graft-versus-host disease (GvHD)

- Affects 10–80% of allogenic haematopoetic stem cell transplant recipients
- Donor T-lymphocytes immunological activity against recipient tissues
- Can develop any time after transplant

**Table 18.24** Skin manifestations of nutritional disease

| Skin sign | Features | Nutrient deficiency |
|---|---|---|
| Scurvy | Purpura, perifollicular corkscrew hairs | Vitamin C |
| Pellagra | Photosensitive dermatitis (Casal's necklace) | Nicotinic acid |
| Acrodermatitis enteropathica | Neonatal perioral, perianal and acral dermatitis | Zinc |
| Glossitis and angular cheilitis | Sore tongue/lips | B complex |
| Hyperkeratosis | Itch, dryness | Essential fatty acids |
| Kwashiorkor/marasmus | Exfoliation | Protein/calorie |

**Table 18.25** Skin manifestations of endocrine disorders

| Disorder | Skin signs |
|---|---|
| Diabetes mellitus | Neuropathic foot ulceration, candidiasis, staphylococcal skin infections, diabetic dermopathy, necrobiosis lipoidica (**Figure 18.58**), granuloma annulare, xanthomas, injection site lipoatrophy and hypertrophy, acanthosis nigricans |
| Hypothyroidism | Cold, dry skin (peaches and cream), fine thin hair, eyebrow loss |
| Hyperthyroidism | Hot, moist skin, diffuse hair loss, thyroid acropachy (clubbing) |
| PCOS | Acne, hirsutism, irregular periods, acanthosis nigricans |
| Autoimmune thyroid disease | Vitiligo, pretibial myxoedema |
| Cushing's syndrome | Striae, moon face, buffalo hump, acne, hirsutes, truncal obesity, acanthosis nigricans |
| Addison's disease and Nelson's syndrome | Hyperpigmented scars, palmar creases, pigmented oral macules |

- Affects skin, liver and gut
- Highly variable cutaneous findings

### Amyloidosis

#### Disease mechanisms

This is caused by deposition of immunoglobulin light-chain material derived from circulating paraprotein.

#### Clinical features

- About 40% of patients with primary myeloma-associated systemic amyloidosis have cutaneous manifestations:
  - Macroglossia
  - Carpal tunnel syndrome
  - Waxy purpuric mucocutaneous lesions
- Secondary amyloidosis usually has no cutaneous manifestations.

- Primary cutaneous amyloidosis is usually localized and nodular (amyloid derives from plasma cells) or macular/papular (macular/lichen amyloidosis: amyloid derives from keratin filaments).

### Rheumatological disease

#### Systemic lupus erythematosus

- Malar butterfly rash
- Photosensitivity
- Oral ulcers
- Non-specific manifestations:
  - Urticaria
  - Non-scarring alopecia
  - Raynaud's phenomenon (see **Figure 18.32**)
  - Cutaneous vasculitis

See Chapter 4, Rheumatic disease, for further information on cutaneous lupus.

#### Systemic sclerosis

- Raynaud's phenomenon (see **Figure 18.32**)
- Sclerodactyly: tight shiny skin or waxy swollen sausage fingers (CLINICAL EXAMINATION AT A

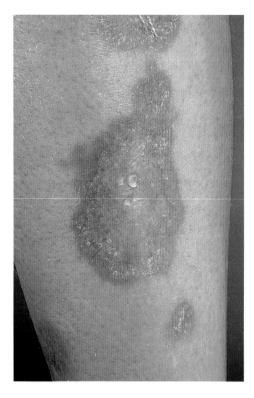

**Figure 18.58** Necrobiosis lipoidica diabeticorum. Atrophic plaques. Causes: diabetes mellitus.

**Table 18.26** Skin manifestations of haematological disorders

| Skin sign | Haematological disorder |
|---|---|
| Purpura | Thrombocytopenia |
| Leuconychia | Anaemia |
| Jaundice (lemon-yellow tinge) | Haemolytic anaemia |
| Leg ulcers | Haemolysis (e.g. thalassaemia and fibrinolytic disorders – proteins C and S) |
| Pyoderma gangrenosum | Monoclonal gammopathy |
| Vasculitis | Monoclonal gammopathy and myeloma |
| Leukaemic infiltration (especially myelomonocytic types) | Leukaemia |
| Granulomatous | Human T-cell lymphotropic virus type I (HTLV-I/ATLL) adult T-cell lymphoma leukaemia papules |
| Urticaria pigmentosa | Mast cell leukaemia |
| Non-melanoma skin cancer | Chronic lymphatic leukaemia |

GLANCE, **Figure P**), dorsal erythematous patches, digital ulceration, calcinosis, flexion deformity, muscle wasting, nail dystrophy, periungual erythema and telangiectasia, and ragged cuticles (CLINICAL EXAMINATION AT A GLANCE, **Figure C**)

• Characteristic facies: perioral radial furrowing, microstomia and telangiectasia

For more information, see Chapter 4, Rheumatic disease.

## MALIGNANT DISEASE AND THE SKIN

Cutaneous metastases have highly variable clinical features. Other signs of internal malignancy are detailed in Table 18.27.

## HUMAN IMMUNODEFICIENCY VIRUS

HIV may cause severe eruptions of common dermatoses; other manifestations are also seen, summarized in Table 18.28.

**Table 18.27** Cutaneous associations of malignant disease

| Feature | Cause |
|---|---|
| Invasion of skin by neoplastic cells | Metastases and infiltration by reticuloses and leukaemic cells |
| | Paget's disease |
| Non-specific skin markers | Infections (e.g. varicella-zoster in lymphoproliferative disease) |
| | Purpura, petechiae and ecchymoses (e.g. leukaemia and dysproteinaemias) |
| | Viscosity syndromes (Raynaud's, acral infarction, erythromelalgia, polycythaemia rubra vera and dysproteinaemias) |
| Accepted skin markers | Acanthosis nigricans |
| | Dermatomyositis |
| | Endocrine (e.g. ectopic ACTH, Nelson's syndrome, acromegaly) |
| | Necrolytic migratory erythema (glucagonoma) |
| | Episodic facial flushing |
| | Pyoderma gangrenosum |
| | Erythema elevatum diutinum |
| | Radiodermatitis |
| | Acquired ichthyosis |
| | Generalized pruritus |
| | Urticaria pigmentosa |
| Genetic syndromes | Palmoplantar keratoderma |
| | Gardner's syndrome |
| | Peutz–Jeghers syndrome |
| | Muir–Torre syndrome |
| | Cowden syndrome |
| | Hereditary leiomyomatosis and renal cell cancer |

**Table 18.28** Cutaneous manifestations of HIV

**Inflammatory dermatoses**
• Seroconversion toxic erythema
• Psoriasis
• Seborrhoeic dermatitis
• Eosinophilic pustular folliculitis
• Generalized granuloma annulare
• Papular eruption of HIV
• Severe drug reactions

**Infections**
• Dermatophytosis
• Candidosis
• Hairy leucoplakia (**Figure 18.59**)
• Papulonodular demodiciosis
• Atypical primary, secondary and late syphilis
• Bacterial folliculitis
• Bacillary haemangiomatosis
• Viral warts
• Molluscum contagiosum
• Cutaneous atypical mycobacterial infection
• Herpes simplex
• Herpes zoster

**Other skin manifestations**
• Porphyria cutanea tarda
• Atypical pityriasis rosea
• Xerosis/eczema
• Acquired ichthyosis and keratoderma
• Aphthous stomatitis

**Neoplasia**
• Kaposi's sarcoma
• Cutaneous lymphoma
• Melanoma and non-melanoma skin cancer

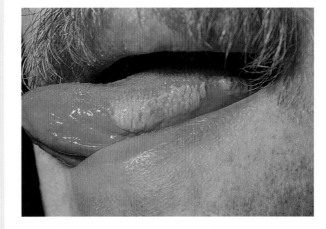

**Figure 18.59** Hairy leucoplakia.

## OROGENITAL DISORDERS

### MOUTH

**Oral ulceration**

Oral ulceration is common. Differential diagnoses are given in **Table 18.29**.

**Behçet's syndrome**

- A multisystemic disease of unknown cause
- Oral ulceration is universal; other cutaneous manifestations and criteria for diagnosis are listed in **Table 18.30**
- Extracutaneous involvement (non-exhaustive)
- Ocular (keratitis, uveitis, optic neuritis) (90%)
- Joint arthritis (50%)
- Bowel haemorrhage, infarction, perforation
- Central nervous system involvement (e.g. vasculitis, meningoencephalitis, thrombophlebitis) (10–20%)
- Cardiopulmonary: arteritis, vulvar disease, myocarditis, arrhythmias
- Glomerulonephritis
- Treatment is challenging

**Table 18.29** Differential diagnosis of oral ulceration

| |
| --- |
| Lichen planus |
| Behçet's syndrome |
| Herpes simplex |
| SJS |
| Aphthous stomatitis |
| Reactive arthritis |
| Pemphigus (erosions) |
| Mucous membrane pemphigoid |
| Lupus erythematosus |
| Syphilis |
| Oral cancer |
| Drugs (nicorandil, hydroxyurea) |

**Table 18.30** International Study Group criteria for diagnosis of Behçet's disease

| | |
| --- | --- |
| Recurrent oral ulceration | Aphthous or herpetiform oral ulceration at least three times in a 12-month period |
| *Plus any 2 of the following:* | |
| Recurrent genital ulceration | |
| Eye lesions | Anterior or posterior uveitis; cells in the vitreous chamber or retinal vasculitis |
| Cutaneous lesions | Erythema nodosum-like lesions, pseudofolliculitis, papulopustular lesions or cuneiform nodules |
| Positive pathergy test | |

## ANOGENITAL PRURITUS

- Causes include dermatoses (psoriasis, lichen planus, contact dermatitis [irritant/allergic], lichen sclerosis), infectious (lice, tinea, threadworms) and colorectal carcinoma.
- Copious barrier emollient and soap avoidance are crucial.
- Patch testing may be required for allergies to preservatives (e.g. methylisothiozoloninone) and fragrances (in creams) or dyes (in clothing).

## PSYCHOGENIC DERMATOSES

### DERMATITIS ARTEFACTA

- Self-inflicted lesions in accessible sites
- Denial of responsibility
- Causes include 'cries for help' or secondary gain (monetary, social)
- *Treatment:* involves identifying stressors, counselling, cognitive behavioural therapy, and may require psychiatric input

### TRICHOTILLOMANIA

This is deliberate pulling of hair.

### DELUSIONAL INFESTATION

- May concern small living creatures (e.g. insects) or inanimate objects (e.g. fibres)
- Examination reveals excoriations, without evidence of infestation
- Patients offer a bag or matchbox containing dust, debris and hair as evidence
- Substantial psychosocial morbidity
- Sometimes dangerous attempts at self-eradication (e.g. pesticides or bleach)
- *Treatment:* antipsychotics

### BODY DYSMORPHIC DISORDER

- A distorted perception of self-image
- More often obsessional than delusional
- *Treatment:* pharmacological (antidepressant) and non-pharmacological (cognitive behavioural therapy)

### VULVODYNIA, PENODYNIA AND SCROTODYNIA

Burning or shooting pain is felt in the absence of overt dermatological disease.

# IATROGENIC SKIN DISEASE

Drugs cause many skin disorders. Types of drug rash and some culprits are listed in **Table 18.31**.

## IMMUNOSUPPRESSION (THERAPEUTIC)

Cutaneous complications include:
- Infections
- Viral warts
- Actinic keratoses, and skin cancer, particularly SCC

## RADIOTHERAPY

- Radiodermatitis (acute/chronic)
- SCC

**Table 18.31** Frequent drug causes of skin disease (non-exhaustive)

| Skin disease | Drug causes |
| --- | --- |
| Morbilliform rash | Penicillins, cephalosporins, thiazides |
| TEN | Penicillins, phenytoin and other antiepileptics, allopurinol, sulphonamides, NSAIDs |
| Erythema multiforme | Sulphonamides, penicillins, phenytoin, NSAIDs |
| Eczema | Thiazides, beta-blockers, aminophylline, sulphonamides |
| Photosensitivity | Tetracyclines, phenothiazides, amiodarone, thiazides, hypoglycaemics |
| Urticaria | Aspirin, opioids, contrast media, penicillins |
| Pigmentation | Tetracyclines (especially minocycline), oral contraceptives, antimalarials, amiodarone, phenytoin |
| Fixed drug eruptions | NSAIDs, paracetamol, codeine |

**Medicine for Finals and Beyond**

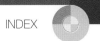

volume receptors 317
vomiting
in advanced illness 602–3
causes and diagnosis 386
drug treatments 394, 395
opioid use 601
von Gierke's disease 465–6
von Hippel–Lindau disease 314, 499
von Willebrand factor (vWF) 562
assay 591
von Willebrand's disease 15, 562, 591
vulva, lichen sclerosus 625
vulvitis, candidiasis 76–7
vulvodynia 654

Waldenström's macroglobulinaemia 588
walking difficulty, neurological disease 513
walking speed 516
warfarin 596
reversal 378
warts 639–40
anogenital 75
periungual 640
water absorption 363
water deprivation test 483
Waterhouse–Friderichsen syndrome 503
weakness 513
advanced illness 600–1
weals 615, 616
Wegener's granulomatosis, *see* granulomatosis with polyangiitis
weight loss 388, 390
approach to diagnosis 390
causes of unexplained 390
diabetes mellitus management 434, 435
haematological disease 564
investigation 390
obesity 453–4
Well's criteria (pulmonary embolism) 196
Wernicke's encephalopathy 515, 548
West Nile virus 54
wheeze 156
Whipple's triad 428, 450

white blood cells (WBCs/leucocytes) 560–1, 565
count in rheumatic disease 86
formation 558
normal adult counts 561
white matter lesions, periventricular 527, 528
Wickham's striae 618
Wilson's disease 340, 344, 530
Wiskott–Aldrich syndrome 620
Wolff–Parkinson–White syndrome 235–6
Wolfram syndrome 431
World Health Organization (WHO), neglected tropical diseases 69, 70
wounds
botulism 56
tetanus 56
wrist disorders 125
tenosynovitis 89
writing, in Parkinson's disease 529

X chromosome 13
X-linked disorders 15
haemophilia 592–3
xanthelasma 365, 459, 643
xanthine stones 312
xanthomas 460, 642–3
eruptive 460, 642
primary biliary cholangitis 343
tendon 459
tuberous 643
Xpert MTB/RIF 35, 55

yaws 70
yellow nail syndrome 631, 632
*Yersinia pestis* 69
Young's syndrome 176

zanamivir 39, 45
zidovudine (AZT) 39
Ziehl–Neelsen staining 35, 36, 55, 168, 170
Zika 66
zoledronate 148, 150
Zollinger–Ellison syndrome 428